Integrated Pharmacology

Page • Curtis • Sutter • Walker • Hoffman

Clive P Page PhD

Professor of Pharmacology
Department of Pharmacology
King's College
London
UK

Michael J Curtis PhD

Reader in Pharmacology
Department of Pharmacology
King's College
London
UK

Morley C Sutter MD PhD

Professor of Pharmacology and
Honorary Associate Professor of
Medicine
Departments of Pharmacology
& Therapeutics and Medicine
University of British Columbia
Vancouver
Canada

Michael JA Walker PhD

Professor of Pharmacology
Department of Pharmacology
& Therapeutics
University of British Columbia
Vancouver
Canada

Brian B Hoffman MD

Professor of Medicine
Stanford University School of Medicine
and Geriatrics, Research, Education and
Clinical Center
Veterans Affairs Health Care System
Palo Alto
USA

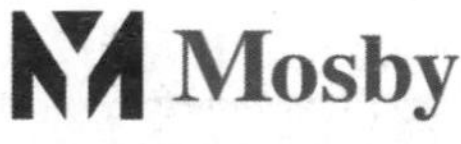

Mosby

London • Chicago • Philadelphia
St Louis • Sydney • Tokyo

Publisher: **Dianne Zack**

Development Editor: **Louise Crowe**

Senior Project Manager: **Linda Horrell**

Project Manager: **Elizabeth Payne**

Production: **Gudrun Hughes**

Design: **Greg Smith**

Layout: **Rob Curran**

Illustration Management: **Danny Pyne**

Illustrators: **Danny Pyne**
Mike Siaz
Sandie Hill
Diane Kinton
Marion Tasker
Jenni Miller
John Cheung

Cover Design: **Greg Smith**

Index: **Janine Ross**

Published by Mosby, an imprint of Mosby International (a division of Times Mirror International Publishers Ltd), Lynton House, 7–12 Tavistock Square, London WC1H 9LB, UK

ISBN 0 7234 2556 6

Originated in Hong Kong by Imago

Printed in Barcelona, Spain by Grafos S.A. Arte sobre papel, 1997

Cataloguing in Publication Data
Catalogue records for this book are available from the British Library and the US Library of Congress.

Foreword

As a teacher of pharmacology for almost thirty years, I have often heard students lament their dissatisfaction with the enormous amount of information that must be memorized during their introductory course in medical pharmacology. I have also heard teachers attempt to encourage their students by telling them that once all the information is memorized it can then be assimilated into lasting understanding. These same teachers express their disappointment (and amazement) when they re-encounter their students two years later on a clinical pharmacology course and find that much, if not most, of the information presented in the second year of medical school has been forgotten.

The authors and editors of *Integrated Pharmacology* have recognized that learning, i.e. understanding of concepts and retention of useful information, requires a framework in which the information can be interrelated. Pharmacology is, by definition, an integration. It is the integration of chemistry, anatomy, physiology, molecular biology, and pathology that enables the student to understand why, when, and how drugs can be used to treat disease. It is therefore only logical that it would be more efficient and longer lasting to learn pharmacology by first reviewing the normal physiology, then the pathophysiology and how it can be perturbed to treat a disease. A fresh understanding of the physiologic mechanisms responsible for normal control of blood pressure and a vivid picture of the end organ damage brought about by hypertension give the student a vivid and memorable mental framework upon which to hang the different actions of antihypertensive drugs.

This textbook is a refreshing change from the past. Unlike many pharmacology texts, it is eminently readable because of the logical flow of information that builds into therapeutic concepts. The outstanding illustrations display complex processes in attractive and easily understood figures. The use throughout the text of a common set of icons to describe the targets of drugs is a welcome innovation that will facilitate learning. I believe many of today's students will find this approach to learning pharmacology less onerous and hopefully more rewarding than their predecessors who have waded into the morass of unrelated pharmacologic facts only to be frustrated.

The practice of medicine relies immensely on the appropriate use of medications to treat diseases. However, all too often physicians are overwhelmed by the seemingly unrelated fragments of information that must be remembered to safely and effectively prescribe and monitor drug therapy. Too often, drugs that interact adversely are co-prescribed, dosages are not reduced appropriately for patients with impairment of the critical route of drug elimination, etc. The presentation of the necessary information in an integrated fashion, building upon an understanding of how diseases alter normal physiology, has the potential to provide lasting understanding and improved therapeutics.

An academic who only presents facts is not a teacher; a teacher is one who nurtures the learning process and thereby modifies behavior and patterns of thinking for a lifetime. I trust that *Integrated Pharmacology* is a teacher's tool that will result in improved therapeutics.

Raymond L Woosley MD PhD
Professor and Chairman, Pharmacology
Georgetown University
President 1996–1998
The Association for Medical School of Pharmacology

Preface

Integrated Pharmacology takes a new approach by presenting drugs and their mechanisms of action in the context of the diseases they are used to treat.

This textbook is written in two sections. The first concerns principles of drug action, and introduces concepts of how drugs exert their actions. It offers insights into how our overall knowledge and use of drugs is influenced by many factors, including history and myths. A system of simple icons to explain the main molecular and cellular actions of drugs is introduced.

Section 2 is concerned with drug treatment of diseases in a framework of the body's systems. The pertinent background biochemistry, physiology, and pathology are provided. The reader is also introduced to increasingly important aspects of pharmacology, such as risk–benefit, pharmacoeconomics, and pharmacovigilance. When using section 2, the reader can delve more deeply into the principles governing the use and actions of drugs by cross-referencing to section 1.

Throughout *Integrated Pharmacology*, illustrations, key facts boxes, tables of adverse actions and drug interactions are used to highlight important issues. At the end of each chapter a set of multiple choice questions, and an extended case study, test the knowledge acquired.

The prescribing of drugs is the endpoint of many contacts between physicians and their patients. Therefore, it is essential that students of medicine acquire a full and detailed understanding of pharmacology integrated with disease in order to make rational prescribing possible.

Integrated Pharmacology is designed with problem-based learning in mind, but is not intended exclusively for medical students. The book will also be useful to biomedical scientists and students interested in pharmacology, as it bridges the gap between fundamental mechanisms and the use of drugs to treat human disease.

Acknowledgements

We would like to acknowledge the sterling efforts of our contributors who have made what seemed like an impossible task come to fruition in record speed. Our thanks also go to our colleagues at Mosby for seeing this textbook through to completion and for keeping the editors on track! In particular, we would like to thank the driving forces of Dianne Zack, Linda Horrell, and Louise Crowe. Many of the illustrations have benefited from the superb imagination of Danny Pyne who undoubtedly now has a greater understanding of pharmacology than most professionals! We would also like to thank Greg Smith for the design of the book.

Picture credits

Figures 7.1, 11.1, 14.1, 14.2, and 14.3 adapted from *Human Histology 2e*, by Dr A Stevens and Professor J Lowe, Mosby International 1997.

Figures 15.1, 15.2, 15.5, 15.6, 15.7 and 15.8 adapted from *Immunology 4e*, by Professor I Roitt, Dr J Brostoff, and Dr D Male, Mosby International 1996.

Chapter 19 image of eye courtesy of Dr P-M Bouloux, Department of Endocrinology, Royal Free Hospital, London, UK.

Contents

Contributors

Shlomo Abraham PhD
Department of Pharmacology
Israel Institute for Biological Research
Ness Ziona, Israel

PG Adaikan PhD
Department of Obstetrics & Gynaecology
National University of Singapore
Singapore

Karl Erik Anderson MD PhD
Department of Clinical Pharmacology
University Lund Hospital
Sweden

Fred Y Aoki MD
Department of Medical Microbiology
University of Manitoba
Winnipeg, Canada

Kathy Banner PhD
Dept of Pharmacology
King's College London
London, UK

Chris J Bowmer PhD
Department of Pharmacology
University of Leeds
Leeds, UK

Graham E Bryce MD
Division of Otorhinolaryngology
University of British Columbia
Vancouver, Canada

Paul Eder MD
Dana-Farber Cancer Institute
Boston, USA

Robin Ferner MSc MD FRCP
City Hospital
Birmingham, UK

Tommy W Gage DDS PhD
Division of Pharmacology
Baylor College of Dentistry
Dallas, USA

Keith Hillier PhD
Clinical Pharmacology Group
University of Southampton
Southampton, UK

Zhuo-Wei Hu MD PhD
Department of Medicine
Stanford University School of Medicine
Stanford, USA

Itsuo Iwamoto MD
Department of Internal Medicine 2,
Chiba University School of Medicine
Chiba, Japan

Akira Kaneko MD
Tokyo Women's Medical College
Dept of International Affairs & Tropical Medicine
Tokyo, Japan

Robert Kerwin MA PhD FRCP
Department of Psychological Medicine
Institute of Psychiatry
London, UK

Richard Z Lin MD
Department of Medicine
Stanford University School of Medicine
Stanford, USA

John Littleton PhD MB BS
Department of Pharmacology
King's College
London, UK

Richard D Mamelok MD
Mamelok Associates
Palo Alto, USA

Ronald D Mann MD FRCP FFPM FCP
Drug Safety Research Unit
Burlesdon Hall
Southampton, UK

Jeffrey W Miller MD
Lilly Laboratory for Clinical Research
Wishard Memorial Hospital
Indianapolis, USA

Philip K Moore PhD
Department of Pharmacology
King's College
London, UK

R Naylor BPharm PhD DSc FRCP
School of Pharmacy
University of Bradford
Bradford, UK

Toshimasa Nishiyama MD
Department of Parasitology
Nara Medical University
Nara, Japan

Ravinder Pabla PhD
Department of Cardiology
University of Utah
Salt Lake City, USA

Michael K Pugsley PhD
Department of Microbiology & Medical Genetics
University of California, Irvine
Irivine, USA

DMJ Quastel MD PhD
Department of Pharmacology & Therapeutics
University of British Columbia
Vancouver, Canada

Sian Rees PhD
University Laboratory of Physiology
Oxford, UK

Craig R Ries MD
Department of Anesthesia
University of British Columbia
Vancouver, Canada

Jon Robbins PhD
Department of Pharmacology
King's College
London, UK

Nerys Roberts MD MRCP BSc
Department of Dermatology
Queen Mary's University Hospital
London, UK

Stephen D Shafran MD
Division of Infectious Diseases
University of Alberta
Edmonto, Canada

O Simons PhD
Department of Pharmacology
University of West Indies
Kingston, Jamaica

Daniel S Sitar BScPharm MSc PhD
Clinical Pharmacology Section
University of Manitoba
Winnipeg, Canada

F Michelle Sutter MD
Department of Surgery
University of British Columbia
Vancouver, Canada

Reza Tabrizchi PhD
Department of Pharmacology & Therapeutics
University of British Columbia
Vancouver, USA

Michael John Travis BSc MB BS MRCPsych
Department of Psychological Medicine
Institute of Psychiatry
London, UK

John P Wade MD
Division of Rheumatology
University of British Columbia
Vancouver, Canada

Katherine Wilson BPharm PhD DSc
Department of Obstetrics & Gynaecology
St. George's Hospital Medical School
London, UK

Dr Mike S Yates PhD
Department of Pharmacology
University of Leeds
Leeds, UK

Principles

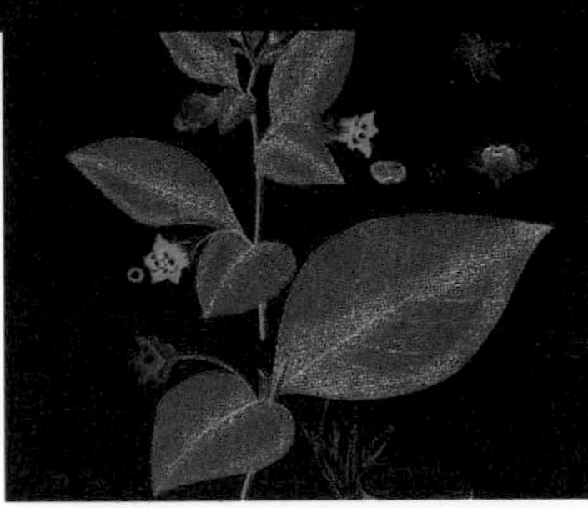

1. Introduction

WHAT IS PHARMACOLOGY?

Pharmacology is the science that deals with the mechanism of action, uses, and adverse effects of drugs

The word 'pharmacology' comes from the Greek word for drug, *pharmakon*, and is the study of what biologically active compounds do in the body, and how the body reacts to them.

The word 'drug' has many meanings, but is most commonly used to describe a substance used as a medicine for the treatment of disease. However, if the word drug is used to refer to any biologically active compound, then it includes:

- Everyday substances such as caffeine, nicotine, and alcohol.
- Drugs of abuse, such as cannabis, heroin, and cocaine.
- Food additives.
- Cosmetics.

Pharmacology does not include pharmacy, which is the preparation and dispensing of drugs.

> **What is pharmacology?**
>
> - Pharmacology is the study of what drugs do and how they do it
> - A drug is a chemical that is usually used to treat disease
> - Drugs are intended to have a selective action, but this ideal is seldom achieved
> - There is always a risk of adverse effects as well as a benefit connected with using any drug
> - A knowledge of pharmacology is essential for using drugs effectively in therapy

Pharmacology is concerned with the effects of drugs on living systems or their closely related components such as cells, membranes, or enzymes. As a result, many levels of organization or system complexity can be studied, ranging from the molecular interaction of drugs to the effect of drugs on populations. Pharmacologists therefore often identify themselves according to the level at which they study drugs.

A knowledge of pharmacology is important in the practice of both human and veterinary medicine, where drugs are used to treat disease. The principles of pharmacology also apply to toxicology, where the effects of the biologically active substances that are studied are harmful rather than therapeutic. Whether a drug is used for therapy or as a poison, a knowledge of its pharmacology is essential if it is to be used so that it does primarily what is wanted of it (i.e. so that its effect is selective).

Ideally, all drugs should have a selective action, but often they do not. A selective action can be achieved if:

- A relatively high concentration of the drug can be obtained at the target cell, tissue, or organ where its action is required.
- The drug is chemically tailored so that it interacts selectively with the discrete cell, tissue, or organ at the location where it is to have its effect.

Research pharmacologists spend much time and effort attempting to achieve such selective action, and understanding its mechanisms and limitations forms the basis of understanding both therapeutics and toxicology.

PHARMACOLOGIC TERMINOLOGY

As with all scientific disciplines, pharmacology has its own vocabulary and language. Such terms include pharmacodynamics, pharmacokinetics, pharmacotherapeutics, selectivity, selective toxicity, risk–benefit ratio, pharmacoepidemiology, pharmacoeconomics, toxicology, toxins, toxinology, poisons, and toxicity (see below).

Pharmacodynamics and pharmacokinetics

Pharmacodynamics describes what a drug does to the recipient of the drug, while pharmacokinetics describes what the recipient of the drug does to the drug. A knowledge of both pharmacodynamics and pharmacokinetics is essential to understand what drugs do and how they do it.

Pharmacodynamics is the detailed study of how drugs act

Quantitative methods and mathematical analyses are often used in pharmacodynamic studies to compare the effects of drugs and to ensure accuracy and completeness in describing these effects. Such studies include the measurement of the effects of the drug at different drug concentrations, and this information is often presented in the form of a graph as a dose–response curve. Dose–response curves can be plotted and analyzed in a variety of ways so that drugs and their effects can be understood and compared (Fig. 1.1).

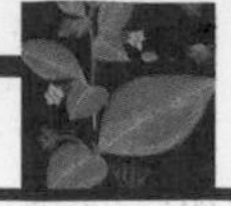

Pharmacologic definitions

- Pharmacodynamics is the study of how drugs act
- Pharmacokinetics is the study of how the body absorbs, distributes, metabolizes, and excretes drugs
- Pharmacotherapeutics is the use of drugs to treat disorders
- Pharmacoepidemiology is the study of the effect of drugs on populations
- Pharmacoeconomics is the study of the cost-effectiveness of drug treatments

Pharmacokinetics is the study of how the body absorbs, distributes, metabolizes, and excretes drugs

Drug exposure may be deliberate, as when prescribing a medicine to treat a disease, or inadvertent, as a result of contaminated food, water or air.

A drug can be taken by several different routes. The most common is by mouth (*per os*). The drug is swallowed and travels to the intestine. There it must disintegrate, if it is a pill or capsule, before dissolving in the gut fluids to diffuse across the intestinal mucosa and be absorbed into the blood stream. The drug is then distributed by the blood to various parts of the body and diffuses out of the blood into the tissues, according to the blood flow to any particular region and other factors. Depending on its nature, the drug may then be metabolized or remain unchanged in the body. Metabolism can render a drug more (or less) active than the original drug. The liver is an important site for drug metabolism (see Chapters 5 and 9). Excretion is primarily via the kidney but may occur by other routes, depending on the drug (see Chapter 5).

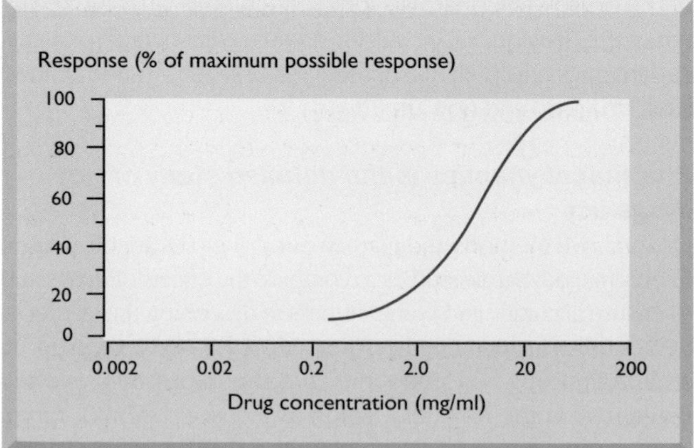

Fig. 1.1 A standard dose–response curve. This shows that the effect of a drug increases with increasing concentrations to reach a maximum.

Pharmacotherapeutics (pharmacotherapy)

Pharmacotherapeutics, pharmacotherapy, or simply therapeutics is the use of drugs to treat disease, for example:

- To alter symptoms or signs, such as pain or fever.
- To replace substances that are not present, or are not present in sufficient quantity, such as insulin in patients with Type 1 diabetes mellitus.
- To kill parasites.

Clearly, a knowledge of pharmacology is essential to use drugs rationally. A knowledge of the disease and its pathology is also required. A clinical pharmacologist is usually trained as both a physician and a pharmacologist and often provides advice on the therapeutic use of drugs.

Selectivity

The aim of all therapy is to use a drug that has only one effect on a particular problem or a set of problems. In pharmacotherapy there is an attempt to alter some physiologic or pathophysiologic process selectively in a way that benefits the recipient of the drug (Fig. 1.2).

However, drugs are only relatively selective in their effects. All drugs are capable of producing adverse effects as well as their beneficial effects, depending on the circumstances of their use. The selectivity of a drug depends on:

- The nature of the drug.
- The dose administered.
- Special features of the recipient, such as genetic make-up, age, and coexisting disease.

Selective toxicity

Selective toxicity is the term applied to the use of drugs as chemotherapeutic (antimicrobial and anticancer) agents or pesticides (insecticides, antiparasitic agents, or herbicides), which are used to kill the parasite or unwanted cells, but leave the host or environment relatively unharmed. The more closely the unwanted cell or parasite resembles the host, the more difficult it is to achieve selective toxicity. Therefore, although drugs can be relatively effective against bacteria, they are relatively nonselective against cancer cells.

Risk–benefit ratio

The phrase 'risk–benefit ratio' is used when considering the risk of the adverse effects produced by a drug in relation to its likely beneficial effects (Fig. 1.3). Whenever drugs are used therapeutically the benefits from their use should be greater than the risks. How much greater depends on the severity of the disease being treated. A greater risk would be accepted in the treatment of an otherwise fatal disease than in the treatment of a less serious one. All aspects of the pharmacology of the drug need to be considered, from basic to economic, to determine what the risk–benefit ratio is for a particular case.

Each activity of everyday life such as driving a car or swimming has an associated risk, and our perception of these risks may be quite erroneous. Accurate information about the risks of a prescribed drug in relation to those of daily life is needed to keep the risks in perspective. This is obtained by studying the effects of the drug on large populations (see Chapter 6).

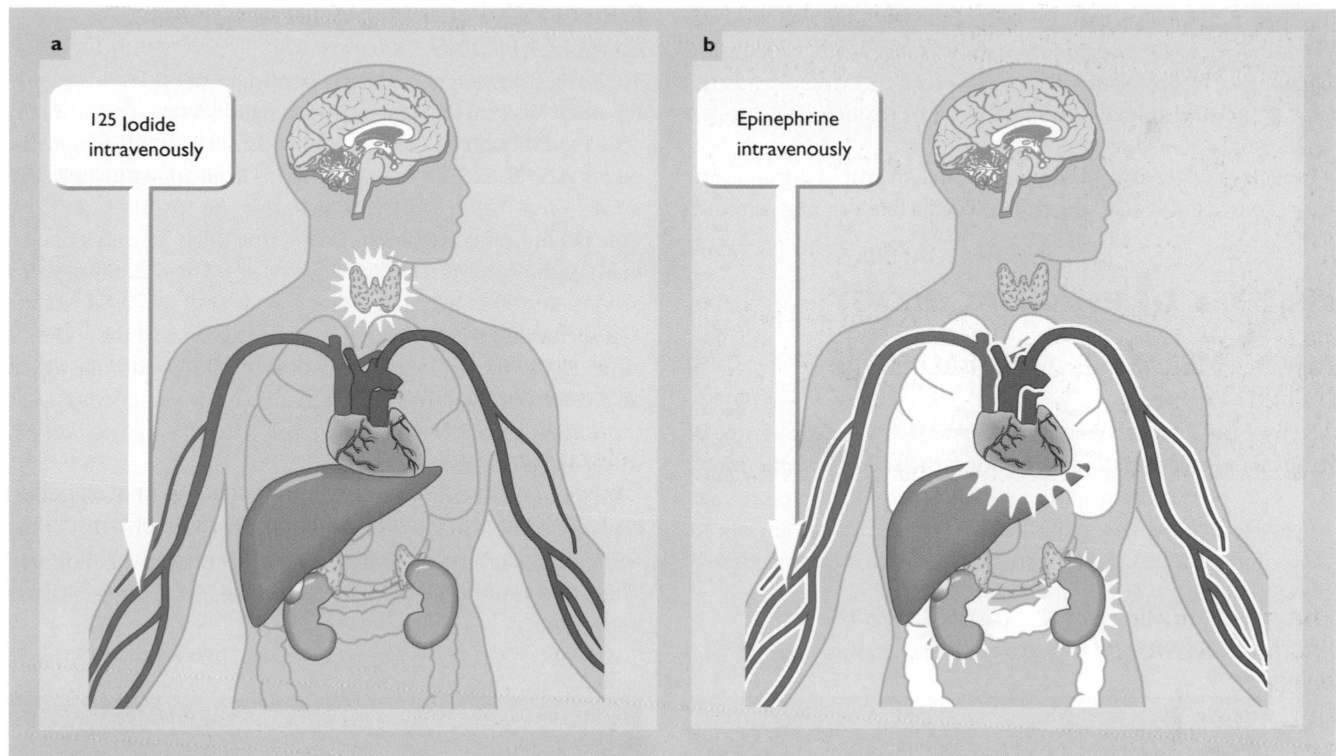

Fig. 1.2 Ideally, all drugs have a selective effect. However, complete selectivity is seldom achieved. (a) ^{125}I (radioactive) is selectively taken up by the iodide uptake system of the thyroid gland. Therefore, radioactivity is high in the thyroid and not elsewhere in the body. (b) Epinephrine will have an effect wherever adrenoceptors occur. For example, such receptors are present in the heart and blood vessels, so blood pressure and heart rate are raised. Adrenoceptors occur throughout the body and therefore the effects of epinephrine are widespread.

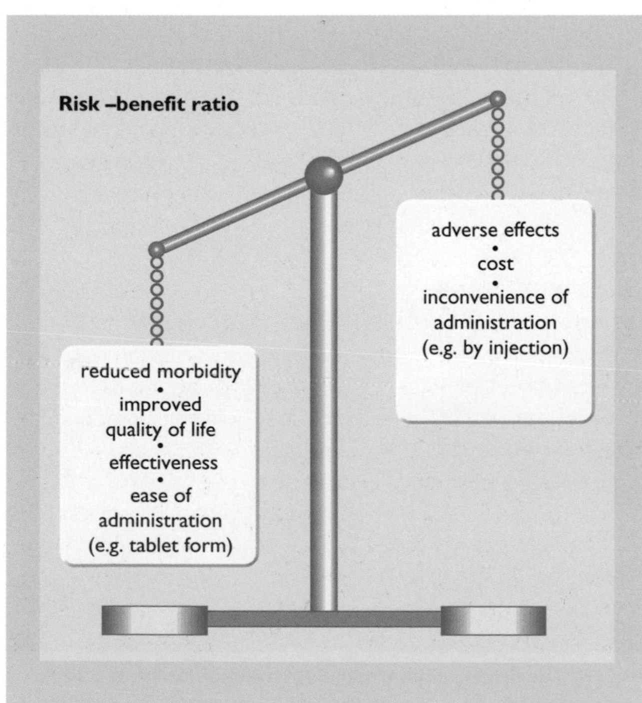

Fig. 1.3 Risk–benefit ratio. The beneficial effects of a drug should outweigh the adverse effects. All drugs are capable of producing bad effects as well as the wanted good effects

Pharmacoepidemiology and pharmacoeconomics

Pharmacoepidemiology is the study of both the beneficial and the adverse effects of a drug on large numbers of people, for example:

- The study of the effect that widespread use of antibiotics in a community has on the type of pneumonia prevalent in that community.
- The effectiveness of drugs in altering disease pathology and mortality.

Similarly, it is also important to know the financial cost of using a drug and therefore the discipline of pharmacoeconomics has evolved. This is the study of the cost of medicines, taking into account:

- The financial cost of the disease involved.
- The total financial cost of developing, manufacturing, and marketing the drug.

Pharmacoepidemiology is often linked to pharmacoeconomics since determining the financial costs of a drug usually involves studying large populations.

Toxicology, toxins, toxinology, poisons, and toxicity

Toxicology is the study of the harmful effects of chemicals on humans, animals, or plants, including chemicals used as medicines or pesticides. The concepts of pharmacodynamics, pharmacokinetics, pharmacoepidemiology, and pharmacoeconomics apply to toxicology just as they do to pharmacotherapeutics.

The only difference is that the endpoints differ: harm is the endpoint in toxicology and benefit that in pharmacotherapeutics.

Toxins are harmful substances produced by living organisms, both plants and animals (see Chapter 29). Toxinology is the scientific study of such compounds.

Poisons are chemicals that kill or inhibit growth of living organisms. These effects may be produced deliberately or inadvertently.

HISTORY OF PHARMACOLOGY

MAGIC, MEDICINE, AND RELIGION INTERTWINED

The roots of pharmacology are entwined with the knowledge of drugs and their uses that were often the secrets of the priest, holy man, or shaman in ancient societies, and the effects of drugs were often viewed as magical. The person who knew about drugs and potions was respected and often feared since intentional poisoning was not unknown.

Ancient and modern pharmacology

- Ancient civilizations used a mixture of magic, religion, and drugs to treat diseases, and drugs were often thought to be magical
- Most drugs in antiquity came from plants and animal parts or fluids
- Knowledge of drugs increased in parallel with knowledge of body function (anatomy, physiology, and biochemistry) and chemistry
- Modern drug development depends on academia and industry working together

Knowledge of drugs has evolved in parallel with an increased understanding of disease

Despite the need to treat disease, knowledge of the mechanisms causing any disease is always limited. If a disease is believed to be caused by gods, spirits, or supernatural forces, the treatment must invoke magic as it is believed that supernatural causes can only be counteracted by supernatural means. Drugs in the past were therefore often believed to be magical and were given magical names such as 'eye of the sun.'

The sources of drugs were plants, minerals and animals. A frieze from Mesopotamia dated to the eighth century BC shows priests carrying a goat, mandrake flowers, and opium poppy heads. This illustrates the important combination of religion, plants, and animals in therapeutics as practiced by ancient peoples, and confirms that opium is an ancient medicinal plant (Fig. 1.4).

DRUG DEVELOPMENT IN ANCIENT CIVILIZATIONS

The earliest written record that specifically mentions drugs is the Egyptian Medical Papyrus of Smith dating from approximately 1600 BC, although it deals primarily with surgery and other treatments. The Ebers Papyrus, which dates from approximately 1550 BC, also lists some 700 remedies, their preparation and use. Concoctions ranged from the occult (the thigh bone of a hanged man) to the familiar (opium or castor oil). These last two preparations are still in use after some 3500 years!

Medicine and the use of drugs was evolving in China and India in parallel to their evolution in Ancient Egypt, but there was little Western contact with Asia at that time. Vaccination was practiced in India in 550 BC, but was only introduced into Western medicine some 2000 years later.

Ancient Greek culture contributed a great deal to the development of pharmacy and drugs. Hippocrates (460–377 BC) wrote on the ethics of medicine as well as the causes of disease. The Greeks attributed disease to an imbalance of humors in the

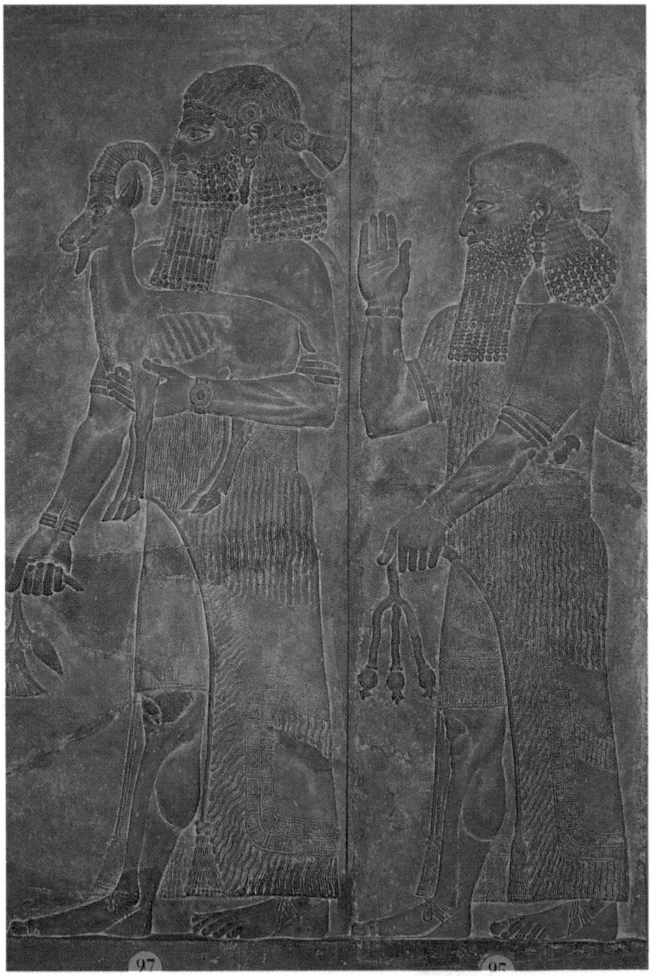

Fig. 1.4 The origins of pharmacology: religion, animals, and plants. Frieze from the palace of King Sargon II, in Kharasabad. Musée du Louvre, Paris, Antiquités Orientales. (Courtesy of Service de Documentation Photographique de la Réunion des Musées Nationaux, Chateau de Versailles.)

body, the humors being blood, phlegm, black bile, and yellow bile. This doctrine was elaborated by Galen (130–201 AD), a Greek physician, who practiced in Alexandria and in Rome. Galen's influence on medicines persisted right through to the 1500s, and can still be seen today in the use of herbal mixtures. The Romans organized and regulated the practice of medicine, including the use of drugs, but contributed little new knowledge to pharmacology. Theophrastus (372–287 BC) listed all that was then known about medicinal plants, and Dioscorides (57 AD), Nero's surgeon, used this list as his basis for a compendium of substances used as medicines—materia medica—which described nearly 500 plants and how to prepare remedies from them.

The Persians sustained Greek views of medicines and transmitted these to the Arabs when Persia was conquered. The traditions of medicine and of pharmacy were maintained and developed by the Arabs from approximately 700 to 1000 AD, who regulated the practice of medicine and pharmacy and established apothecary shops, hospitals, and libraries. They built on the published works of Galen and introduced several new ways of preparing drugs. The English word 'alcohol' is from the Arabic word 'al-kuhl,' meaning 'all things very fine,' and originally referred to ground sulfides of lead and antimony used as eye make-up (Fig. 1.5). The Arabs also introduced alchemy to Europe. Alchemy combined Egyptian ideas, astronomy, astrology, and Greek natural philosophy, with Christian metaphysics in an attempt to discover the origin and meaning of all things. Alchemy was the parent of chemistry and therefore an ancestor of modern pharmacology.

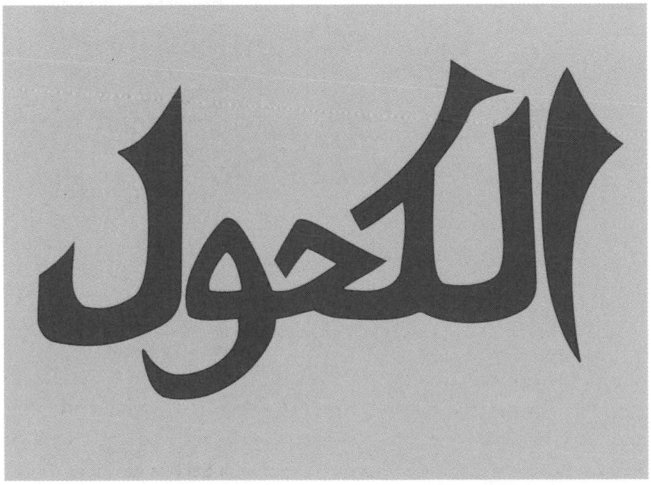

Fig. 1.5 The arabic word al-kuhl or alcohol. It originally referred to one of the first ways of preparing drugs for external use.

DRUG DEVELOPMENT SINCE THE MIDDLE AGES

In the Middle Ages the practice of medicine and use of drugs in Europe was often associated with monasteries. Many of them had herbal gardens which provided their medicines.

The grandfather of pharmacology is generally agreed to be Paracelsus, who was born in 1493 in Switzerland. He was the son of a physician, travelled widely in Europe, and graduated as a doctor of medicine from Ferrara. Many of his writings were prescient. He advised against the complicated mixtures that were common medications at that time and believed that each drug (or plant) should be used alone. He wrote 'It is the task of chemistry to produce medicines for the treatment of disease since the vital functions of life are basically chemical in nature... . All things are poisons, for there is nothing without poisonous qualities. It is only the dose which makes a thing a poison.' These statements are cornerstones of pharmacologic thought. Today it is recognized that drugs are chemicals that alter biologic chemistry and that their selectivity depends on the dose.

Developments in pharmacology depended on the developing sciences of chemistry, pathophysiology, physiology, and botany

The development of pharmacology depended on increasing understanding of human physiology and disease processes (pathophysiology). Understanding in turn depended on the application of scientific method to these problems. In the 1600s

Important figures in the history of pharmacology

- Dioscorides (57 AD), Greek, compiled materia medica of 500 plants and remedies
- Galen (130–201 AD), Greek living in Rome, developed a Theory of Disease, which persisted for hundreds of years
- Paracelsus (1493–1541), itinerant Swiss scholar and alchemist, the 'grandfather of pharmacology'
- Sertürner (1805), German pharmacist, isolated morphine, the first pure drug
- Ehrlich (1909), German pathologist and Nobel prize winner, developed chemotherapy
- Domagk (1935), German pathologist and Nobel prize winner, noticed the antibacterial effect of Prontosil, a prototype of sulfonamides, the first selective antimicrobial agents
- Beyer (1950s), US pharmacologist, instrumental in the development of thiazides, derivatives of sulfonamides, and several other drugs
- Black (1960–today), British pharmacologist and Nobel prize winner, developed propranolol and cimetidine

there were many contributors to the understanding of physiology and diseases. These included William Harvey (1578–1657), who introduced experimentation (demonstration of the circulation of the blood), and Sydenham (1624–1689), who introduced classification into the study of diseases, their causes, and their treatment.

Developments in chemistry

The idea of using chemicals as drugs seems to have been first suggested by van Helmont (1515–1564), who discovered carbonic acid and who also introduced the term gas into chemistry, while the theory that an imbalance of body chemicals could cause disease was first proposed by the Dutch physician, Sylvius (1614–1672). The physicist/chemist Boyle (1627–1691) was the first to demonstrate that drugs had an effect when given intravenously as well as by mouth. The activities and thoughts of chemists and physicians were therefore closely linked.

Developments in botany

In the ancient and recent past, most drugs came from plants and not from known chemicals, for example, the Egyptians used the opium poppy (see above). Plant use continued and, in the 1640s, cinchona bark from South America was introduced into Europe by the Jesuit priests of the Roman Catholic Church to treat malaria. However, one of the problems associated with botanicals as medicines is consistent identification of plants. This was improved by the system of plant classification introduced by the Swedish botanist Linnaeus (1707–1778).

Several Swiss and French botanists such as Schröder (1641) and Lémery (1698) published books on vegetable materia medica, as had the Ancient Egyptians, Babylonians, Indians, and Chinese. Universities of the Middle Ages established botanic gardens to learn more about medicinal plants. The botanic works of Haller (1708–1777), a physician in Berne and Göttingen who combined the study of both physiology and botany, were collected into a publication by Vicat in 1776, which in turn was translated into German by Hahnemann, the founder of homeopathy.

William Withering published his treatise *An Account of the Foxglove and Some of its Medical Uses* in 1785. In this text he described observations made over a ten-year period on the therapeutic use of *Digitalis purpurea*. The principles he laid down then for the use of digitalis to treat dropsy (swelling of the ankles and abdomen) are largely still valid today (Fig. 1.6).

Isolation of pure compounds Progress in understanding plants and the drugs they contain was aided by the Swedish chemist Carl Wilhelm Scheele (1742–1786). He produced pure chemicals by crystallization, among which were glycerin and malic acid. Scheele's work laid the foundation for the isolation of the first pure drug, morphine, by Sertürner (1783–1841) in 1805. Pure substances rather than crude extracts could be isolated and tested for their pharmacologic effect.

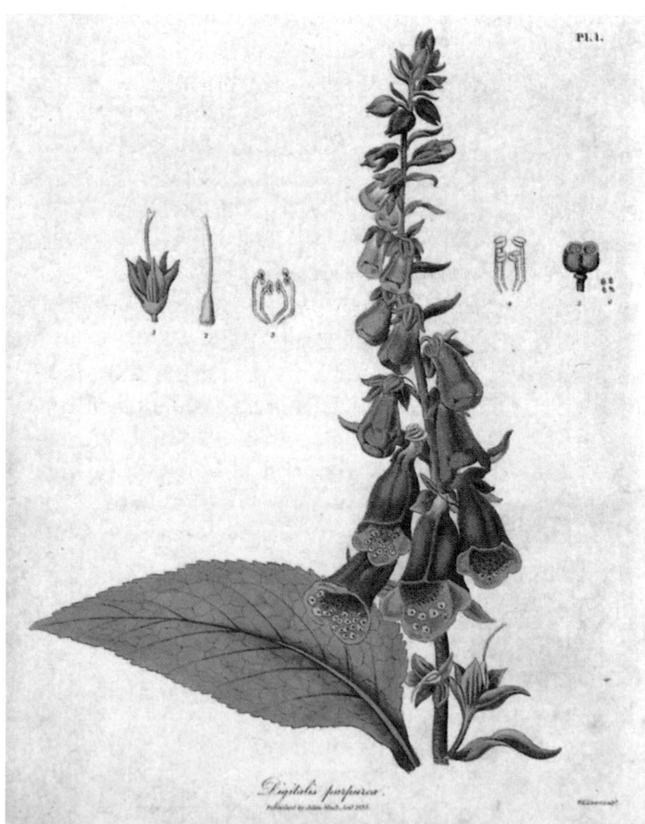

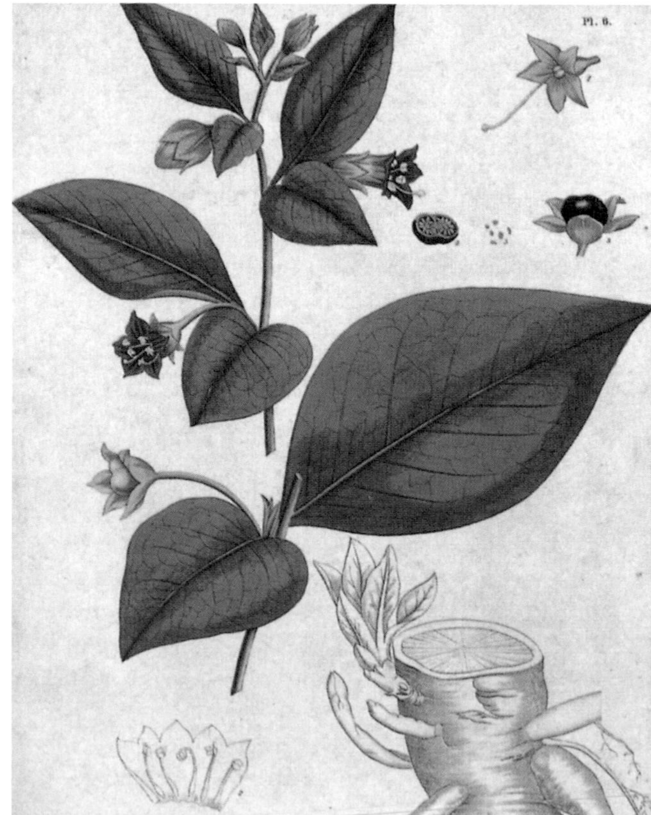

Fig. 1.6 Foxglove and deadly nightshade. These are the plant sources of digoxin and atropine, respectively. (Reproduced with permission from George Graves, *Medicinal Plants*, New York: Crescent Books. Copyright 1990 Bracken Books.)

Developments in physiology

Understanding how and where drugs act requires a detailed knowledge of biologic function (i.e. physiology and biochemistry). Such knowledge and understanding were advanced by the work of French physiologists such as François Magendie (1783–1855) and his pupil Claude Bernard (1813–1878). Their techniques of investigation localized the sites in the body where drugs act. Claude Bernard, for example, had clearly demonstrated by 1856 that curare paralysed skeletal muscle by acting at nerve junctions.

Developments in pharmacologic concepts

Pharmacology uses information derived from physics, chemistry, and the biologic sciences to understand what drugs do and how they do it. A few principles are, however, special to and underlie pharmacology, and include:

- The concept first suggested by Felix Fontana (1720–1878) that in plant or other biologic material there is an active principal responsible for the effect of the original mixture.
- The concept that there is a distinct relationship between the dose of a drug and its effect. This is attributed to Peter John Andrew Daries who wrote of it in his doctoral dissertation of 1776. Paracelsus also made an important contribution to this concept. The dose–response curve is an expression of this phenomenon (see Fig. 1.1). Its quantification is derived from the physicochemical constructs of Langmuir, which were first interpreted into a biologic context by Clarke (1885–1941). The appropriate mathematic analysis of the relationship between dose and response is still evolving (see Chapter 4).
- The concept of structure–activity relationships among drugs. The study of how altering a chemical structure could alter the effect of a drug had its beginnings when James Blake (1815–1841) systematically altered a series of inorganic salts and observed their differing pharmacologic effects. Paul Ehrlich (1854–1915) exploited this technique in searching for compounds that would selectively kill invading organisms—the search for a 'magic bullet.'

MODERN DRUG DEVELOPMENT

Interaction between academic theories and the practices of industry has been highly productive

The development of modern drugs is closely allied to the development of the dye industry in Germany, from which emerged the modern pharmaceutical industry. Many scientists have contributed to the development of drugs while working in industry, but only a few selected drugs and individuals can be mentioned here.

- Salicylic acid was synthesized from phenol in 1860 by Kolbe and Lautemann.
- Acetylsalicylic acid (aspirin) was synthesized in 1899 by Dreser.
- Prontosil, which is transformed in the body to a sulfonamide, was developed by Domagk in 1935.

Other sulfonamides quickly followed Prontosil and gave rise to a series of chemically related drugs developed by the pharmaceutical industry: acetazolamide (a carbonic anhydrase inhibitor), the thiazide diuretics developed by Karl Beyer, and then the sulfonylurea oral hypoglycemics.

Meanwhile, academic pharmacology was making headway in the classification of receptors, work that had been initiated by Barger and Dale in industry and Gaddum in academia. Antihistamines of the H_1 type were developed by Bovet, while β adrenoceptor antagonists such as propranolol were developed by James Black. Later he went on to develop H_2 antagonists, such as cimetidine, which became the biggest-selling drug in the world.

Pharmacology is now using the tools of molecular biology to develop new drugs based on new insights into diseases. These insights are often derived from studying cell function at a molecular level. Proving the effectiveness and safety of such drugs, however, still depends on studies involving individual patients and populations of patients. Pharmacology is so fascinating because it spans the spectrum from molecules to the patient.

CONTINUED EVOLUTION OF THE DRUG DEVELOPMENT PROCESS

Drugs improve the quality of life for millions of people and prevent disease on a global scale. It is estimated that drugs have added 3–5 years to the average life expectancy, and have revolutionalized the treatment of many different diseases. However, today's pharmacologists are faced with the formidable task of finding novel drugs for the treatment of diseases that pose a significant health risk to society such as cystic fibrosis, Alzheimer's disease, stroke and acquired immunodeficiency syndrome (AIDS). Furthermore, although there are effective medications against some infectious organisms, resistant strains are developing all the time; there is, therefore, a continual need to develop even better drugs to treat infection.

It is estimated that it takes an average of 7–10 years to develop a new drug from first identifying a novel chemical entity through to its successful use in patients, at a financial cost of up to US$250 million. As pharmacologists are involved in nearly every stage of this development process, pharmacology is an important branch of modern science.

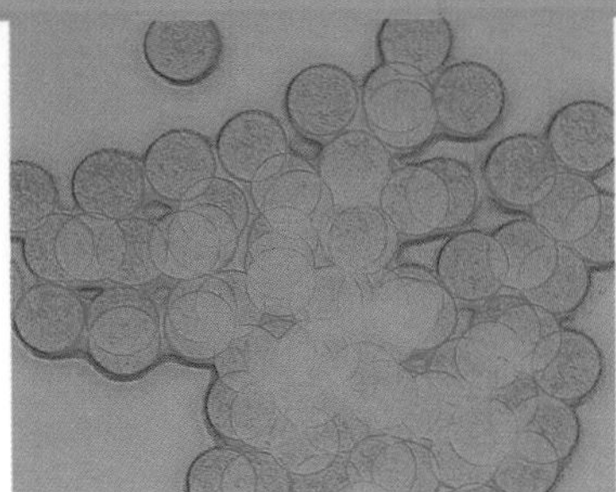

2. Drug Names and Classification Systems

METHODS FOR CLASSIFYING DRUGS

Pharmacology has been a recognized scientific discipline for over 100 years, but pharmacologists cannot agree about what exactly pharmacology is. Confusion and disagreement also exist over the classification and even the naming of drugs. It is tempting to draw an analogy between the present classification systems for drugs and those for pre-Linnean botany.

Current systems of drug classification result in a confusion of systems, procedures, names, and implications. There are many systems for naming and organizing drugs, but no system is universally accepted. The pharmacology student therefore has to become familiar with extensive lists of drugs, which may be contradictory and confusing. The existing drug classification systems are reviewed and discussed in this chapter, which aims to provide some clarity in this confusion.

WHAT IS A DRUG?

There is less confusion about what a drug is:

- Webster defines a drug as 'a substance intended for use in the diagnosis, cure, mitigation, treatment, or prevention of disease.'
- Collins defines a drug as 'any synthetic or natural chemical substance used in the treatment, prevention or diagnosis of disease.'

Regardless of definition, many pure and impure substances are used by humans to produce changes in their pathophysiology, or physiology, or that of animals. Synonyms for the word 'drug' include medicine, agent, compound, and pharmacologic tool:

- 'Medicine' in the past was a plant or animal substance that was used to treat diseases (i.e. materia medica or medical matter).
- 'Agent' is used as a collective noun, as in antitubercular, antihypertensive, anticancer, or anesthetic agent.
- 'Compound' is a chemical used for pharmacologic purposes, but not as a therapeutic agent.
- A pharmacologic tool is a drug used to produce a controlled change in living tissue or tissue components.

DRUG NAMES

A single drug can have a variety of names and belong to various classifications. There is no truly international body in pharmacology to impose standard nomenclature. Different national committees can impose different names on the same drug. Classifications are even less official. This book contains examples of regional and national variations in drug names, but the process for officially naming drugs is becoming more consistent. Generic names are not attractive, but can have common roots and endings providing clues to their use and actions. Sometimes they include part or the whole of a researcher's name. Some generic names contain a root ending indicating the main actions or properties of the drug.

In the commercial world, brand names will never follow a consistent pattern

When a patent on a drug expires it will be manufactured by different pharmaceutical companies, each imposing its own brand name. Copyrighted brand names are chosen to be catchy, pleasing, and easy to remember; their creation is one of the skills of marketing. Marketing departments of pharmaceutical companies go to great lengths to find attractive names and use computers to generate thousands of possibilities.

The naming of drugs is therefore complex and based on source, chemistry, effects, regulation, and marketing. It is, however, necessary to know the names of different drugs and, although brand names are often easier to remember than generic names, generic names should be used wherever possible.

There are several approaches to classifying drugs

The various approaches for classifying drugs are not exclusive because a drug can belong to many classes. For example, atropine can be classified:

- On the basis of its molecular mechanism as a nonselective competitive antagonist at muscarinic receptors (i.e. a muscarinic antagonist, see Chapter 3).
- On the basis of its actions on the autonomic nervous system as a parasympathetic antagonist.
- As the prototypical atropinic because it was the first of this type of drug to be discovered.
- On the basis of its pharmacotherapeutic actions as an antiulcer drug that has been used in the treatment of peptic ulcer.
- As a belladonna alkaloid.

A drug's classification provides information about its chemical nature, pharmacologic actions, and pharmacotherapeutic use. Unfortunately, such information is often not systematic. It is not clear how long it will be before drugs are classified and named in a systematic manner analogous to that used for living organisms. IUPHAR (International Union of Pharmacology) and WHO (World Health Organisation) are attempting to make drug definitions and classifications consistent.

It is useful to classify drugs according to a pattern such as:

- Pharmacotherapeutic class.
- Pharmacologic class.
- Molecular mechanism.
- Chemical nature (but not full chemical name).
- Group or special features.
- Generic name.

Thus, atropine can be classified as:

- An antimuscarinic (spasmolytic).
- Muscarinic antagonist.
- Competitive antagonist at M_1, M_2, and M_3 receptors.
- Solanaceous (belonging to the plant family Solanaceae—potato, tobacco, nightshade) alkaloid.
- Atropinic alkaloid.
- Atropine.

Main factors for classifying drugs

- **Pharmacotherapeutic actions (may be multiple)**
- **Pharmacologic actions (may be multiple)**
- **Molecular actions (both site and mechanism)**
- **Other factors (source and chemistry)**

DRUG CLASSIFICATION SYSTEMS

The systematic approach to classification discussed above relies upon agreed definitions of drug actions, which are selective, exclusive, precise, and definite in both pharmacotherapeutic and pharmacologic terms. These prerequisites are rarely found in either medicine or pharmacology.

Any definition of a disease can be precise if the pathology is understood, but will be imprecise if the pathology is not understood. For example, the definition of tuberculosis is clear and unambiguous: the causative organism is known and well understood, and there is no confusion arising from the many possible clinical presentations. Thus an antitubercular drug is used to treat infections with *Mycobacterium tuberculosis*. On the other hand, hypertension is a syndrome characterized by a blood pressure that is high relative to arbitrary levels for normal blood pressure. Definitions of 'normal' blood pressure can vary, as can the definition of 'high.' To add further complication, some causes of hypertension are known, but the cause(s) of most cases remains unknown. As a result, the term 'primary hypertension' is used. The classification 'antihypertensive drug,' therefore, reveals only that the drug is, or has been, used to lower blood pressure.

FUNCTIONAL CLASSIFICATIONS

In the following text, 'functional' refers to the actions of drugs on disease or physiologic (pharmacologic) functions and on the critical biochemical entities with which drugs interact. Pharmacotherapeutic actions are those intimately concerned with diseases and therapy, whereas pharmacologic actions may not be related to therapy. Although the actions of drugs on biochemical entities are not truly functional responses, they are nevertheless included in this section.

Classification based on pharmacotherapeutic actions

A classification based on pharmacotherapeutic action can cause problems if it is ill-defined or imprecise, and there are widespread and limiting restrictions to the use of such a classification. Such a classification can lead to inappropriate extrapolations about the use of drugs. It is wrong to assume that drugs with a common pharmacotherapeutic classification have common mechanisms or adverse effects. Some pharmacotherapeutic classes of drugs may have much in common and share mechanisms of action, but their effectiveness, toxicity, and adverse effects can be very different. The only certain conclusion that can be drawn from the pharmacotherapeutic classification of a drug is that the drug has been used or is currently in use for the condition indicated.

Pharmacotherapeutic classifications are inconsistent and imprecise

Pharmacotherapeutic classifications can be broad (e.g. antiviral, antibacterial, anticancer) or restrictive (e.g. neuromuscular antagonists, which are used almost exclusively for producing muscle relaxation during surgery).

A major problem with pharmacotherapeutic classifications is imprecision. Consider the classification 'antiarrhythmic.' A cardiac arrhythmia is a disorder of the heart rhythm arising from cardiac nodal tissue, atria, or ventricles. Arrhythmias may be tachyarrhythmias or bradyarrhythmias, and be due to any one of, or a combination of, a variety of underlying conditions. The only common feature is a disorder of heart rhythm. As a result, the term 'antiarrhythmic' only indicates that the drug has been used to treat an arrhythmia either clinically or experimentally.

In considering the above example, it is obvious that the classification can be improved by subclassification. For example, classification of antiviral drugs can be improved if a particular family of viruses or a single virus is included in the classification (e.g. antiherpes antiviral). Subclassification is particularly useful for antibacterial and antiparasitic drugs for which a hierarchy of classification can be achieved. For antiparasitic drugs a subclassification according to the infecting parasite is useful. 'Antimalarial' is therefore a clear classification, as is 'antitubercular' for antibacterial drugs.

It is clear that the pharmacology student has to be careful in drawing conclusions from pharmacotherapeutic classifications. In addition, a knowledge of disease conditions and their classification and subclassification is vital for the accurate use of pharmacotherapeutic classifications.

Classification based upon pharmacologic actions

Pharmacologic actions are useful classifiers, but may be physiologic, as in the use of the term 'sympathomimetic' applied to norepinephrine because of its ability to mimic stimulation of the sympathetic nervous system. Pharmacologic actions are often defined in terms of the receptor with which a drug interacts (see Chapter 3). Norepinephrine is therefore also an α adrenoceptor agonist because it activates α adrenoceptors to produce pharmacologic actions. However, this produces difficulties in differentiating between pharmacologic and molecular actions. A useful hierarchy when considering drug actions comprises:

- The whole body.
- Body systems.
- Body tissues.
- Cellular effects.
- Molecular effects.

This hierarchy is used in subsequent chapters of this book.

Pharmacologic classifications are often imprecise

A lack of precision in describing pharmacologic actions complicates any classification based upon them. Often synonyms exist for the same action, for example with the anesthetics. Anesthetic means 'lack of feeling,' and both local and general anesthetics produce this effect, but at different sites and with different modalities and mechanisms of action. In the case of anesthetics, this ambiguity is overcome by a subclassification into local and general anesthetics. However, subclassifications are not always possible. In addition, pharmacologic terms often have widely different meanings in different contexts.

Pharmacologic classifications can be precise

However, a pharmacologic classification can be precise. For example, a drug that relaxes vascular smooth muscle can be classified as a smooth muscle relaxant, a vasodilator, and a hypotensive. These classifications are interrelated because arteriolar smooth muscle relaxation causes vasodilation. Vasodilation, in the presence of a maintained cardiac output, lowers blood pressure (i.e. produces hypotension). The precision can, however, be further improved because vasodilation describes smooth muscle relaxation in arterioles and arteries, while venodilation refers to dilation of veins. The use of the word 'direct' describes direct relaxant actions on smooth muscle, while the use of the word 'indirect' implies that the vasoconstrictor mechanisms have been antagonized.

Drug actions on the heart can also be precisely defined. An inotropic drug alters the contractility of the heart, a positive inotropic drug increasing contractility and a negative inotropic drug decreasing contractility. Using the words 'direct' and 'indirect' indicates whether or not the drug acts directly on heart cells:

- The cardiac glycoside (chemical classification) digoxin, is a directly acting positive inotropic drug because it acts directly on heart cells to increase contractions.
- A β adrenoceptor antagonist (molecular site and mechanism classification) such as propranolol is an indirectly acting negative inotrope because it antagonizes actions of the sympathetic system on the heart.

Drugs that increase heart rate are tachycardics, while bradycardics slow heart rate. Such actions can be direct or indirect:

- The sympathomimetic (pharmacologic classification) amine (chemical classification) dobutamine, a β adrenoceptor agonist (molecular site and mechanism classification), is a directly acting tachycardic drug.
- Atropine can have indirect tachycardiac actions. As a muscarinic antagonist (molecular site and mechanism classification) it antagonizes the action of bradycardic nerves on the heart and can therefore increase heart rate.

Imprecise pharmacologic classifications are widely used

Inhibitors, antagonists, depressants, excitants, and activators are all examples of widely used pharmacologic classifications. However, although they are relatively familiar words, they lack scientific precision:

- 'Inhibitor' is used to describe drugs that prevent or reduce physiologic, biochemical, or pharmacologic activity. Inhibition can therefore take place at the level of substrates and enzymes; at regulation sites for neuronal, hormonal, and autacoid systems; on receptors; on ion channels; on cellular activity; and even on cell membranes.
- 'Activators' have actions opposite to those of inhibitors.

With this classification almost any drug can be classified as being either an inhibitor or an activator. A great disadvantage of using such terms is that inhibition in one situation may be activation in another. It is therefore possible to produce excitation at one site by inhibiting another site.

Classification based upon actions on molecular targets

This method of classification depends on two factors:

- The nature of the molecular site.
- The nature of a drug's interaction with the site.

As is discussed in more detail in Chapter 3, there are many targets at which drugs can act to produce pharmacotherapeutic and pharmacologic responses. In most cases these targets are proteins and include receptors, ion channels, enzymes, and cell transporter molecules.

Classification of drugs according to their molecular actions can be precise

A classification based on a drug's molecular actions can be precise, but only if the molecule and its interaction sites are well understood. The site on such molecules with which drugs interact is sometimes known with certainty (e.g. the hydrolytic site on acetylcholinesterase and the recognition site on β adrenoceptors).

Many drugs interact with proteins to initiate processes that ultimately result in cellular and tissue responses

An agonist is a drug that produces a response when it interacts with a receptor. An antagonist (also known as an inhibitor or blocker) is a drug that prevents the response produced by an agonist, or inhibits the molecule's normal functions. Such classification terms cannot, however, be considered to be mutually exclusive and are often used too loosely without sufficient thought.

Classification is easy if a drug interacts with well-identified receptors

β Adrenoceptor antagonists are drugs that bind to β adrenoceptors. Since the binding does not produce a response, but instead prevents molecules that normally interact with the receptor from producing their response, such drugs are also known as β blockers. A more precise classification would be competitive, nonselective, β adrenoceptor antagonists. On the other hand, the bronchodilator albuterol used to treat asthma acts upon the β_2 subtype of β adrenoceptors to cause smooth muscle relaxation (bronchodilation) (i.e. it is an agonist). Albuterol is therefore a β_2 adrenoceptor agonist.

There are many different receptors with which drugs interact and by which they can be classified. Such receptors are subdivided into different families on the basis of their molecular structure and the mechanism linking them to cell responses. Others are classified on the basis of the endogenous molecules (e.g. neurotransmitter, hormone, autacoid) with which they interact. There are two subfamilies of adrenoceptors for the neurotransmitter norepinephrine: α and β. These are further subdivided into subtypes (e.g. α_1, α_2, β_1, β_2).

Drugs interact with their protein targets by a limited number of mechanisms

A drug interaction with a protein target almost always involves discrete binding. Binding to the protein will:

- Activate the protein if the drug is an activator.
- Prevent protein activation if the drug is an inhibitor.

However, since such classification terms are of limited use, it is preferable to use descriptive terms. In terms of receptor activation, terms such as agonist, partial agonist, and inverse agonist (see Chapter 3) form a good basis for classification. Similarly, 'antagonist' describes a molecule that denies agonists the opportunity to bind and activate the receptor, sometimes by binding at the identification site for agonists. This type of competitive antagonism can be overcome by increasing the quantity of agonist. Antagonism occurring at the same receptor, but not the same binding site, is noncompetitive antagonism.

Competitive antagonism is usually readily reversible and the drug is easily lost from its binding site on the receptor. However, the competitive antagonism produced by some drugs is irreversible:

- Phenoxybenzamine produces an irreversible antagonism at α adrenoceptors by covalently binding.
- Large polypeptides from snake venoms (such as α-bungarotoxin from kraits) bind irreversibly to the nicotinic receptors at the skeletal neuromuscular junction.

Analogous types of inhibition can occur for drugs acting on enzymes. Comparatively few drugs act on enzymes as the substrate, but many drugs act as enzyme inhibitors. Inhibition can be competitive or noncompetitive, reversible, or irreversible. Classic examples are:

- Reversibly acting drugs such as neostigmine, which acts on the enzyme acetylcholinesterase.
- Irreversible inhibitors such as the organophosphates (e.g. parathion) which act on acetylcholinesterase.

Some drugs act upon ion channels in cell membranes

Some drugs make ion channels (sites of selective ionic permeability) open up, while others prevent them opening. Such drugs can be classified according to channel type. The best-known channels are those for Na^+, K^+, and Ca^{2+}. Various subtypes are recognized on the basis of their molecular structure and properties (e.g. responsiveness to voltage or drugs). There are at least four subtypes of Na^+ channel, four for Ca^{2+}, and many (at least nine) for K^+. A drug that prevents opening of a Na^+ channel may therefore be classified as a Na^+ channel blocker. A selective drug acting on a particular channel subtype may be further classified according to the subtype (e.g. L type).

Ion channels can respond to drugs in one of two ways

A drug acting on an ion channel may either prevent opening or prevent closing. Those that inhibit opening are classified as ion channel blockers. Verapamil is a Ca^{2+} channel blocker. It is also classified as a Ca^{2+} antagonist because at the physiologic level it antagonizes the actions of Ca^{2+}. The latter classification is, however, less acceptable since it confuses the mechanism of action, particularly as it has not been clearly established just how verapamil antagonism occurs in terms of binding to a physiologically specific site. The term 'blocker' is probably more satisfactory, since it encompasses the idea that such drugs may act to block channels physically. It is equally possible that such drugs disturb channel function by binding at a remote site and allosterically disrupting channel function.

Drugs that open channels are known as channel activators or channel agonists. The neurotransmitter γ-aminobutyric acid (GABA) is a true agonist since it binds to a specific receptor on Cl^- channels and makes them open. Exogenous drugs are also capable of opening ion channels (e.g. K^+ channel openers such as cromakalim). These drugs bind to the adenosine triphosphate (ATP)-dependent K^+ channel, which opens in response to the binding, leading to vascular smooth muscle relaxation and blood vessel vasodilation. Because of this vasodilation such drugs can be used as antihypertensives.

SOURCE (PLANT OR ANIMAL) AND CHEMICAL CLASSIFICATIONS OF DRUGS

Although most drugs are totally synthetic in origin and discovered as a result of systematic and rational drug design, some drugs are still obtained from natural sources. The main natural source is the botanic world. When the source of a drug is a particular species of plant or animal it, and related drugs, are classified according to the species, genus, or family of the organism in which it is found. Such substances are usually organic molecules which, if they contain nitrogen, are known as alkaloids. Alternatively, if the molecule contains an amino acid it is often a polypeptide. Nature seems to make rather prolific use of the C17 hydrocarbon ring, the steroid ring, found in cholesterol. This ring forms the chemical base for many naturally occurring drugs and hormones.

Classifications based on the botanic or animal sources of drugs

Both the source and chemistry of drugs of natural origin may be combined in a classification, as with the digitalis glycosides or belladonna alkaloids. Digitalis glycosides are found in plants of the *Digitalis* genus (e.g. *Digitalis purpurea*), are chemically glycosides, and are therefore classified as digitalis glycosides. Similarly, the weak bases found in plants of the *Atropa* genus are called belladonna alkaloids. One of these belladonna alkaloids, atropine, is named after the genus.

Classifications based on the chemical nature of drugs

Some drug classifications rely purely on the drug's chemistry. The chemical identity of most drugs is known and can therefore be described according to the rules of IUPAC (International Union of Pure and Applied Chemistry) in a completely unambiguous manner. For example, atropine is endo($\pm$)-α-(hydroxymethyl)benzeneacetic acid 8-methyl-8-azobicyclo[3.2.1.]oct-3-yl ester and norepinephrine is 4-(2-amino-1-hydroxyethyl)-1,2-benzenediol. Obviously, such complexity cannot be used routinely, and exact chemical names are never used to describe drugs. A variety of shorthand methods have therefore been developed. As a result, there is no consistent method for naming drugs chemically, although the generic name often indicates a component chemical group.

A chemical group name is commonly used to identify groups of drugs with similar basic chemical structures that often have similar pharmacologic profiles (e.g. catecholamines). Catecholamines include the neurotransmitters norepinephrine and dopamine, and the hormone epinephrine. The term 'catechol' is the chemical description of a benzene ring containing two hydroxyl groups in the *meta* and *para* positions. Many catechols occur naturally or have been synthesized, but few have biologic activity. The term 'amine' refers to a nitrogen group. Catecholamines are therefore molecules with a catechol moiety and an amine group. The term 'catecholamine' is purely a chemical description and has no biologic implications, but a pharmacologist uses the term exclusively to describe those molecules that have biologic activity or compounds metabolically related to the pharmacologically active catecholamines.

Many group names are used for classification

Commonly used examples of group names are:

- Steroids. Many drugs contain a steroid group; some are endogenous, while others are exogenous and synthetic. Glucocorticosteroids, mineralocorticsteroids, sex hormones, and anabolic steroids are all steroids.
- Barbiturates (from barbituric acid).
- Benzodiazepines.
- Dihydropyridines.

Such groupings are useful classifiers both for official drugs and for understanding the actions of chemically related drugs.

Classifications based on generic names

All drugs available on prescription and many over-the-counter drugs have a generic name. This is the name which appears in official national pharmacopeias. Pharmacopeias were originally published as source books for medical materials and indicated the animal or plant source of individual drugs, manner of extraction, and assay. They were the original source of the generic names for a drug. Since most of today's drugs are available in a pure form, modern pharmacopeias are concerned principally with pure drugs. As publication of pharmacopeias is a national concern, generic names can vary, for example:

- Norepinephrine or levarterenol in the US is noradrenaline in Europe and the UK.
- Furosemide in the US is frusemide in the UK.
- Cromolyn in the US is cromoglycate in the UK.

However, such disagreement is limited. Often the only international differences between generic names is a minor difference in spelling. Major differences between the generic names used in the USA, Europe, and Japan are indicated in the index at the end of this book.

There are now increasing attempts to harmonize naming between the European Union, Japan, and the US. In recent years there has been success in making common roots and names consistent. As a result, the word ending:

- 'olol' is used for most β adrenoceptor antagonists.
- 'dipine' for Ca^{2+} channel blockers of the dihydropyridine chemical type.
- 'tilide' for antagonists of the delayed rectifier K^+ channel.

It should not be assumed, however, that the rules for such naming are absolute, since for every rule there is an exception.

Classifications based on commercial needs

A synthetically prepared drug developed by a pharmaceutical company starts life as a chemical with a code name, usually letters and a number. The letters are for the pharmaceutical company, the number a simple numbering sequence starting at 1 for the first compound synthesized. In some companies such numbers approach one million. A potential drug is only given a generic name when it is considered to be commercially viable. Before this stage it is known as a compound. The company can suggest generic names, but any suggestion requires approval from the appropriate national committee, which may suggest

Drug names

- The generic name for a drug should be used, if possible
- The existence of multiple brand names is confusing
- Generic names can vary between countries
- The generic name may provide a clue to the pharmacotherapeutic action and/or pharmacotherapeutic classification

another name. Such committees often accept the name given by the country of origin and continue to use common route and group names to identify common pharmacologic actions.

The generic name should be used in biomedical science and by physicians

When writing orders for drug treatment or prescriptions, using the generic name causes less confusion and lessens the chance of error. In many countries it gives the dispensing pharmacist the right to dispense the cheapest form of the drug.

With new patented drugs, which are usually marketed by the one manufacturer who discovered it, there is often only one generic name and one brand name. However, once a patent expires, the generic name remains but the brand names proliferate.

Indicate which is the correct answer for each question.

1. A pharmacopeia is
- a) a reference book for drugs
- b) a β adrenoceptor antagonist
- c) a drug
- d) a plant
- e) a medicine

2. Drugs have been classified on the basis of all of the following, except
- a) pharmacotherapeutic action
- b) source
- c) chemical nature
- d) color
- e) molecular size

3. In scientific and medical usage, drugs should be referred to by their
- a) clinical name
- b) generic name
- c) color
- d) botanic origin
- e) brand name

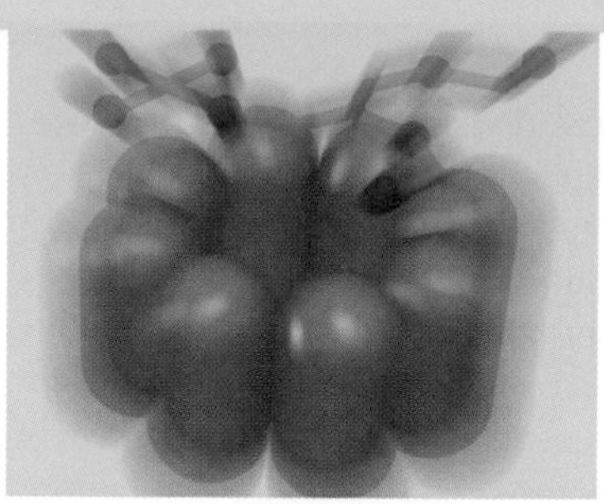

3. General Principles of Drug Action

WHAT DOES A DRUG DO, AND HOW DOES IT DO IT?

The purpose of this chapter is to illustrate the mechanisms by which drugs produce their actions.

MECHANISM OF ACTION OF DRUGS

The mechanism of action of a drug can be considered at the following four different levels:

- Body systems.
- Component tissues.
- Constituent cells.
- Molecules.

The term 'mechanism of action' therefore has different meanings according to this hierarchy of complexity (i.e. system, tissue, cellular, and molecular).

Drug action at the four different levels can be explained using propranolol as an example

Propranolol is a useful drug for treating angina pectoris, a condition resulting from relative ischemia (i.e. insufficient blood flow) in a portion of the heart:

- At a system level, propranolol reduces the heart's normal response to increased sympathetic nervous system activity, namely an increase in heart rate and force of contraction.
- At the tissue level, propranolol is negatively inotropic and chronotropic (reducing cardiac contractile force and heart rate, respectively) as a result of blocking the actions of the neurotransmitters released by the cardiac sympathetic nervous system.
- At a cellular level, propranolol prevents the elevation of intracellular cyclic adenosine monophosphate (cAMP), protein phosphorylation, Ca^{2+} mobilization and oxidative metabolism induced by sympathetic nervous system activity.
- At the molecular level, propranolol acts by competitive, reversible, antagonism of the binding of epinephrine and norepinephrine to β_1 adrenoceptors.

Drug action at the four different levels can be explained using rifampin even though it does not act on human tissue

The mechanism of action of any drug can be dissected in this manner, even if the drug does not act directly on human tissue to be beneficial. For example, rifampin is an effective drug in the treatment of tuberculosis:

- At a system level, rifampin prevents progressive loss of respiratory function.
- At a tissue level, rifampin prevents lung damage arising as a result of infection with the *Mycobacterium tuberculosis*.
- At a cellular level, rifampin inhibits mycobacterial ribonucleic acid (RNA) synthesis leading to death of mycobacteria.
- At the molecular level, rifampin binds to mycobacterial RNA polymerase.

THE FOUR LEVELS OF DRUG ACTION AND DRUG CLASSIFICATION

Looking at the four levels of drug action helps classify a drug according to its mechanism of action. Propranolol is therefore always classified as a β adrenoceptor antagonist, and in the context of the treatment of angina, as an anti-anginal drug. However, such a classification is not exclusive. In the context of the treatment of hypertension, propranolol is still a β adrenoceptor antagonist, but is also referred to as an antihypertensive drug with specific system and tissue level mechanisms of action that are unique to its role in the treatment of hypertension.

In this chapter, the general principles of mechanism of drug action are described at each of the four levels, using examples to illustrate the issues. First, however, it is necessary to define the concept of response.

Response to a drug can also be defined at molecular, cellular, tissue, and system levels

Since the mechanism of action of a drug can be defined at four levels of complexity, the responses to a drug can also be defined in the same way. A drug may therefore elicit molecular, cellular, tissue, and system responses (Fig. 3.1). Generally, drugs that produce a response at each of these levels are defined as agonists. Drugs that simply block the actions of agonists are defined as antagonists. Their molecular response does not directly produce a response at the cellular, tissue and system level although antagonists may cause a cellular, tissue, and system response as a result of the block of the molecular response to an endogenous or exogenous agonist.

Drugs may be classified according to their clinical effects

Medicines have a pharmacotherapeutic mechanism of action defined as treatment, and the response component is the disease process. Poisons have a toxic mechanism of action

The four levels of drug action and drug classification

Mechanism	Definition	Response components
System	An effect on system function	Integrated systems including linked systems (e.g. nervous system, cardiovascular system)
Tissue	An effect on tissue function	Electrogenesis, contraction, secretion, metabolic activity, proliferation
Cellular	Transduction	The biochemicals linked to the drug target (e.g. ion channel, enzyme, G proteins)
Molecular	Interaction with the drug's molecular target	The drug target (e.g. receptor, ion channel, enzyme, carrier molecule)

Fig. 3.1 The four levels of drug action and drug classification.

defined as toxicity, and the response component is health. Pharmacotherapeutic drugs may also have toxic properties.

MOLECULAR TARGETS FOR DRUGS

In order to produce an effect, a drug must first interact with a molecular target. The 'target' for most drugs is a protein, although for some drugs it is a macromolecular lipid or proteolipid component of a cell membrane, and some drugs act directly on nucleic acids. The most common type of proteins with which drugs interact are receptors, ion channels, enzymes, and transport molecules. These will be discussed first.

HORMONE AND NEUROTRANSMITTER RECEPTORS

A drug receptor is a macromolecular protein target with which an endogenous or exogenous agonist drug binds to initiate a cellular response. Thus, a receptor must be connected to cellular response elements such as enzymes, second messengers, or ion channels (see p. 29).

Although most drug targets that have been described as receptors are macromolecular proteins, not all macromolecular proteins that are drug targets are what would traditionally have been called receptors. Such targets include ion channels, enzymes, symporters, antiporters, and pumps. Moreover, there is no fundamental reason why a drug receptor must necessarily be a protein as a matter of definition, it just so happens that this is usually the case. Perhaps the best way of understanding the difference between receptors and other molecular targets for drugs is as follows. Ion channels, enzymes, symporters, antiporters, and pumps respond at the molecular level in a major and substantial way to drugs when they act as molecular targets for drugs.

- Ion channels, symporters, and antiporters open or close.
- Enzymes activate or switch off.
- Pumps are turned on or off.

The effects of this may be dramatic; the molecular response is unsubtle and tangible. Receptors, on the other hand, usually undergo only subtle changes in configuration that usually require a linkage to transduction components for any dramatic effect of the drug to be apparent; the molecular response is therefore usually subtle and barely tangible. Throughout this text, receptors are shown as an icon (Fig. 3.2).

Receptors can be identified from radioligand binding studies. Binding studies can be performed using antagonists labeled with radioactive markers (e.g. tritium, ^3H) to demonstrate the presence of specific binding. Today, the powerful techniques of molecular biology allow determination of the protein and amino acid molecular structure of the receptor as well as its genetic code. From this, the receptor for study can be expressed as a functioning unit in a suitable living cell (e.g. frog oocyte) or in an artificial medium with the appropriate transduction system so that function can be measured at the level of the cellular response.

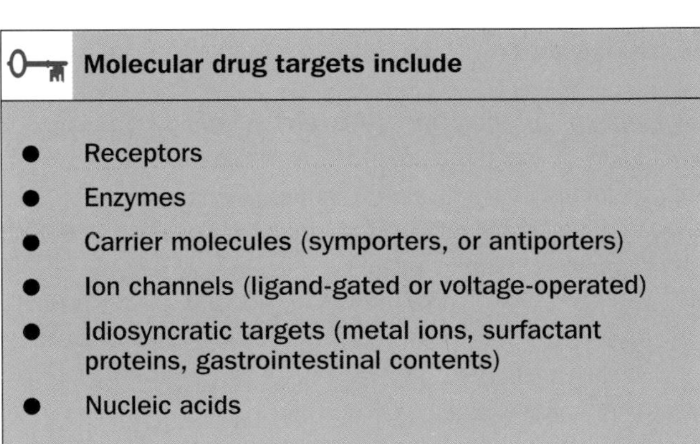

Molecular drug targets include

- Receptors
- Enzymes
- Carrier molecules (symporters, or antiporters)
- Ion channels (ligand-gated or voltage-operated)
- Idiosyncratic targets (metal ions, surfactant proteins, gastrointestinal contents)
- Nucleic acids

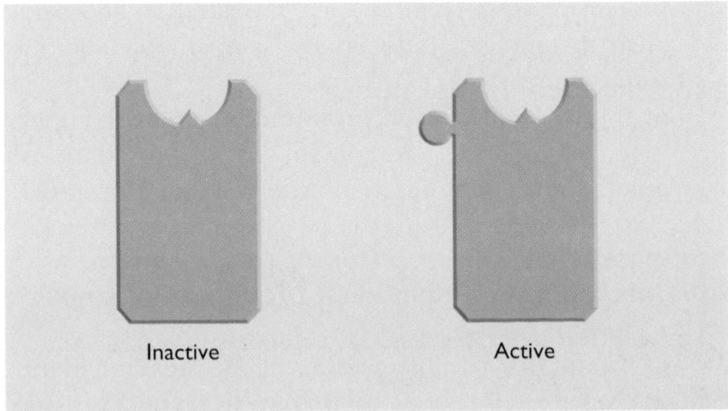

Fig. 3.2 The icon used throughout the text for receptors .

Agonism describes binding of a drug to a receptor so activating the receptor to produce molecular and cellular responses

Agonism is the production of a response by a drug interacting with a receptor. The production of the activated state of the receptor is the molecular response to an agonist. Each interaction between an agonist molecule and a receptor produces a molecular response, which is subsequently amplified at the intracellular level.

In most cells the maximum cellular response to an agonist is achieved with only a small proportion of the maximum number of molecular responses possible for that cell. In other words, the number of receptors is usually much higher than that required for obtaining a maximum cellular response. These excess receptors are usually referred to as 'spare receptors,' and are important because they increase the sensitivity of the cell to small changes in the concentration of agonist (see Chapter 4).

In the past, it has been assumed that, in the absence of an agonist, a receptor is never in an activated state, but this is now known to not be the case for many receptors. On a random basis, and in the absence of an agonist, a receptor may convert to an activated state for a certain period of time and thereby produce a low-level cellular response. Receptors therefore oscillate between inactive and active states, with the active state being heavily favored in the presence of agonist.

The relationship between agonist (A) and response is defined by binding to the receptor (R) with the response being defined as a product of agonist–receptor binding (AR). Therefore $A + R \Leftrightarrow AR \Rightarrow$ (response). The mathematical basis of this relationship will be discussed in more detail in Chapter 4. Throughout the text, agonists will be shown using an icon (Fig. 3.3).

Partial agonism describes binding of a drug to a receptor producing relatively inefficient responses

A drug that interacts or binds with a receptor in a relatively inefficient manner is a partial agonist. Conceptually, a partial agonist is a drug for which each interaction between it and the receptor produces less than a maximal molecular response, or randomly produces either a molecular response or no response (a failed molecular response). In both cases, the maximum cellular response to the partial agonist is less than the maximum cellular response to a full agonist acting on the same receptor, provided that there are no spare receptors.

If there are many spare receptors, it is inherently possible for a partial agonist to elicit a maximum cellular response. Partial agonists are required to interact with a large proportion of the receptor pool to produce a maximum cellular response, leaving only a small reserve of receptors or none at all.

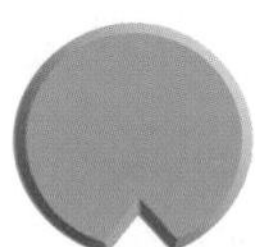

Fig. 3.3 The icon used throughout the text to indicate agonists.

Inverse agonism describes binding of a drug to a spontaneously activated receptor leading to deactivation of the receptor

Certain drugs can bind to a receptor that is in an activated state when not bound to an agonist, thereby inactivating the receptor. This is called inverse agonism. The molecular response to an inverse agonist is therefore either:

- Deactivation of the activated receptor.
- Stabilization of receptors in an inactive conformation.

Production of a deactivated state of receptor is the molecular response to the inverse agonist.

Antagonism describes binding of a drug to a receptor that prevents a response to an agonist occurring

Historically, the existence of receptors was recognized because it was found that specific agonists produced responses in such a way that the concentration dependence of the effects was conserved between different tissues (and indeed between species). A similar conservation of concentration dependence was seen for drugs that blocked responses to agonists. These drugs are defined as antagonists. The explanation for these findings was that the agonist and antagonist were acting on a conserved target, which was thereafter defined as a receptor.

A competitive antagonist is a drug that competes for the same binding site on the receptor as an agonist. The kinetics of these reactions are defined by the affinity constants for the two reactions: K_A for the agonist reaction, and K_B for the antagonist reaction, which are described in more detail in Chapter 4. It is these rate constants, K_A and K_B, that are conserved among different tissues if the drugs A and B act on the same receptor in these different tissues.

Antagonism can result from a variety of molecular mechanisms

Molecular mechanisms producing antagonism include the following:

- Interaction between the antagonist and the same binding site as that for the agonist. This denies the agonist access to its binding site (competitive antagonism).
- Interaction between the antagonist and a site different to the agonist binding site, leading to allosteric distortion of the binding site for the agonist. This prevents either agonist binding or the ability of the agonist, when bound to the receptor, to elicit a molecular response. If the antagonist can bind only when the agonist is not bound, it is called noncompetitive. If the antagonist can bind even when an agonist is bound, it is called uncompetitive.

Since antagonist action can be reversible or irreversible, there are six possible types of antagonism, which are shown in Fig. 3.4. The effect that an antagonist can have on the responses to an agonist is described in mathematical terms in Chapter 4.

Some drugs may act as agonists yet inhibit the cellular response to a second agonist. Although the first and second agonists do not act on the same receptor type, and the receptors are not physically linked, the outcome at the cellular level may be

	Competitive	Noncompetitive	Uncompetitive
Reversible	✓	✓	✓
Irreversible	✓	✓	✓

Fig. 3.4 The six possible types of antagonism.

similar to that of antagonism. This would occur if the first drug's receptor were linked to the same transduction mechanism as the second, but affected it in the opposite direction. This kind of antagonism is conventionally known as physiologic or functional antagonism, although it would be more precise to describe it as cellular level antagonism. It is not antagonism at the receptor level, which is the level at which we have defined antagonism and agonism.

Similarly, two agonists may act on different receptors, have different cellular mechanisms of action, and produce opposite tissue responses. Again, conventionally one of the drugs is said to be a functional or physiologic antagonist of the other, although a more precise term would be tissue level antagonist. A good example is the action of norepinephrine and acetylcholine on arterioles. Norepinephrine causes contraction and acetylcholine causes relaxation. However, it is obviously not helpful to describe norepinephrine as an acetylcholine antagonist. Equally, at the cellular level, drugs may activate transduction pathways that act in opposition to each other and therefore produce tissue level antagonism.

We do not believe that the word antagonism should be used as described in the previous two paragraphs, given its specific meaning in pharmacology. We suggest that the term antagonist is restricted to drugs that inhibit the molecular response to other drugs that act on receptors, and throughout the text antagonists will be shown using an icon (Fig. 3.5).

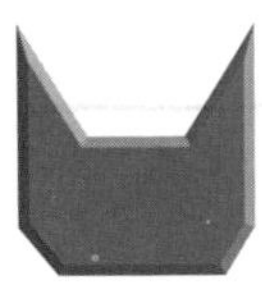

Fig. 3.5 The icon used throughout the text to indicate antagonists.

Definitions

- Affinity is the tendency to bind to receptors
- Efficacy is the relationship between receptor occupancy and the ability to initiate a response at the molecular, cellular, tissue or system level
- Intrinsic activity is the capacity of a single drug–receptor complex to evoke a response

Agonism

- Agonism is the production of a molecular and cellular response to an interaction between a drug (agonist) and a receptor that activates the receptor. The intrinsic activity of a full agonist is defined as equal to 1
- Partial agonism occurs when a drug interacts with a receptor to produce an average of less than 1 unit of molecular response. The average molecular intrinsic activity lies between 0 and 1
- Antagonism occurs when a drug interacts with a receptor to inhibit the action of an agonist. The molecular intrinsic activity is 0
- Inverse agonism occurs when a drug interacts with a receptor to reduce its resting level of molecular activity. The molecular intrinsic activity is –1
- Partial inverse agonism occurs when a drug interacts with a receptor to reduce the resting level of molecular activity. The molecular intrinsic activity lies between 0 and –1

Ligands

Generally, 'ligand' means 'that which binds.' Conventionally, ligand means a molecule (e.g. agonist, antagonist, etc.) that binds with a molecular target. When the term ligand is used, it indicates that binding occurs, but it does not give any indication of the nature of the molecular response (agonism versus antagonism).

First and second messengers

Endogenous ligands and drugs, acting on molecular targets, are sometimes known as first messengers. The reason is that the molecular action is the first message that the ligand elicits. Later, in the section that discusses transduction, we will explain how the molecular response elicits a cellular response. Unsurprisingly, the cellular components that participate in the cellular response are known commonly as second messengers although we have avoided the use of this term in favor of 'transduction component.'

VOLTAGE- AND RECEPTOR-OPERATED ION CHANNELS

Ion channels have an important role as molecular targets for drugs (and, in many cases, as transduction components).

Ion channels are transmembrane spanning proteins that allow the selective passage of specific ions when the channel is opened. The passage of ions occurs when the molecular structure of the channel permits it. The molecular structure of the channel therefore defines the state of the channel. The states of the channel are:

- Rested (i.e. closed, but openable in response to a stimulus).
- Activated (open).
- Inactivated (i.e. closed and not openable in response to a stimulus).

Some drugs have a molecular mechanism of action that involves modulating the transition of the ion channel between states. The state transition of an ion channel is known as gating. If gating is normally controlled by membrane potential, the channel is said to be voltage operated (VOCs). If gating is normally controlled by an endogenous molecule (e.g. a neurotransmitter), the channel is said to be receptor operated; perhaps it ought to be called receptor gated, but this is not the convention.

Voltage-gated ion channels are modulated at the molecular level by membrane potential (voltage)

Ion channels that are normally modulated by membrane potential are known as voltage-operated ion channels. Their molecular response to drugs is a change in their voltage dependence. Throughout the text, voltage-gated ion channels will be shown using an icon (Fig. 3.6).

Voltage-gated ion channels have a similar number of transmembrane domains and extracellular and intracellular components (Fig. 3.7). When responding as a molecular target, a voltage-gated channel can be viewed functionally as possessing a ligand-recognition site and a gating component. The ligand-recognition site interacts with exogenous ligands (e.g. drugs). The gating component provides the molecular response.

Electrophysiologic studies using patch clamping allow electrical visualization of the opening process of an ion channel to the level of a single opening of a single channel. It is therefore possible to record the minute currents that flow through a single ion channel.

The selectivity of channels for different ions is determined by specific protein configurations within the channel pore.

The simplest way of explaining how voltage gating works is to consider the voltage-gated Na^+ channel in cardiac tissue

The voltage-gated Na^+ channel in cardiac tissue possesses two voltage sensors (gates), which open or close according to the membrane potential (voltage).

- One (the fast gate) opens and closes quickly (msec).
- The other (the slow gate) opens and closes slowly (tens of msec).

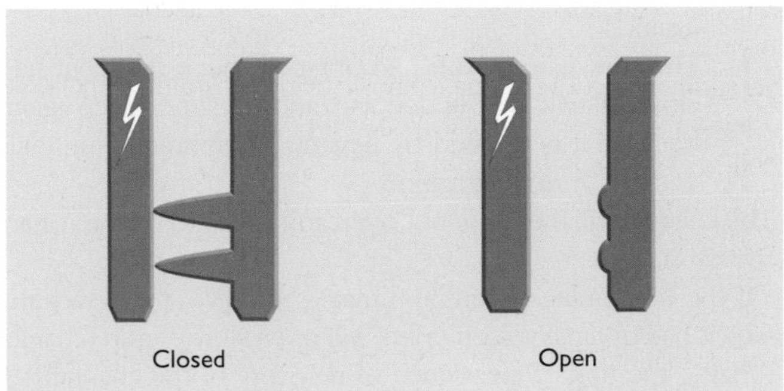

Fig. 3.6 The icon used throughout the text for a voltage-gated ion channel, showing the channel closed and open. The icon is drawn with two gates, although some channels have only one, or three or more gates.

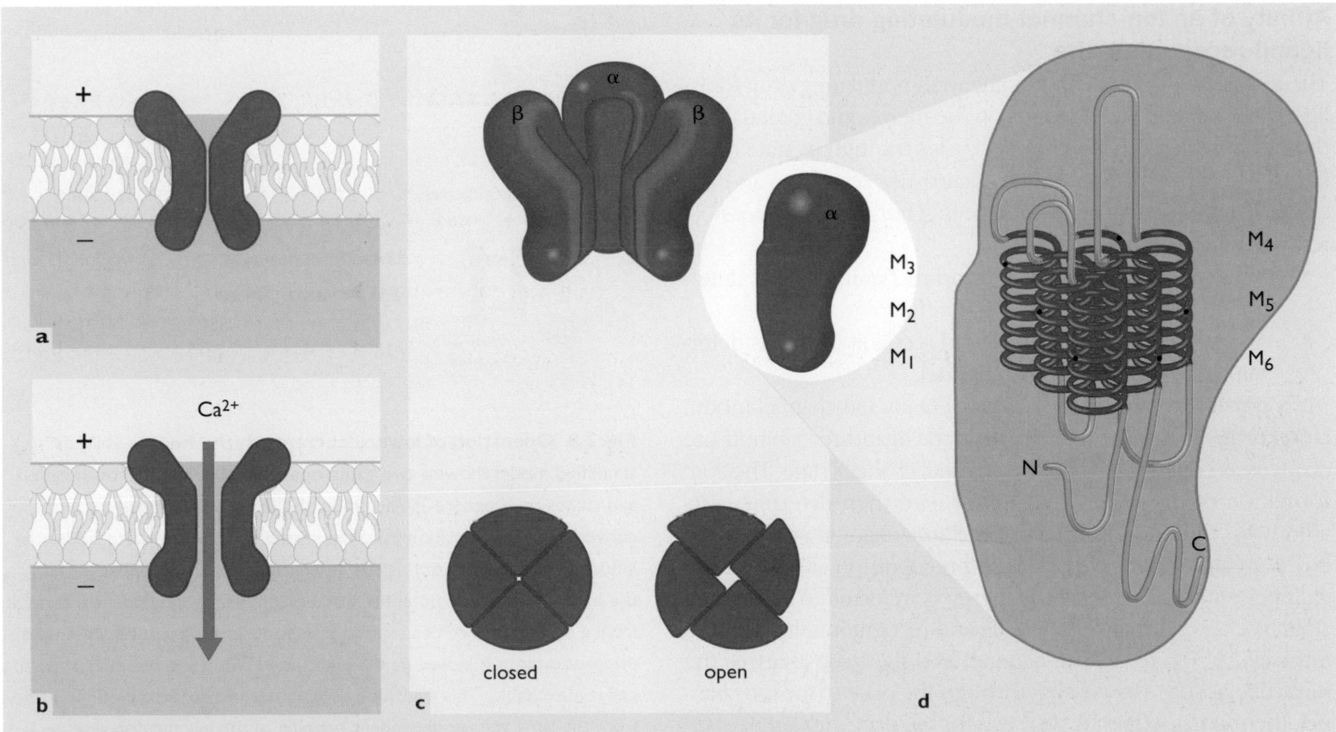

Fig. 3.7 Voltage-gated ion (Ca^{2+}) channel showing structure. (a) The rested channel is closed and ion passage is not possible. (b) When the channel opens, ions move down their concentration and charge gradients. (c) Re-orientation of two α and β subunits is responsible for channel opening. (d) The complete structure of one of the α subunits. M_1–M_6 refer to subunits of the channel.

During diastole, when the membrane potential is negative, the slow gate is open and the fast gate is closed. The net effect is that the channel is closed, and is said to be rested (Fig. 3.8). However, if the membrane potential becomes more positive, the fast gate opens very quickly, so both gates are open and the channel is said to be in the activated state. The slow gate then slowly closes in response to the change in voltage. As a result, if the membrane potential stays positive, the channel will, with time, become closed again. This represents the time dependence of the channel.

If the membrane potential then becomes negative again, the open gate quickly closes. Now both gates, and the channel, are closed. If the membrane is depolarized (made positive) again:

- The fast gate, which had rapidly opened before, will open again.
- The slow gate, which had originally been open but had closed slowly during depolarization, will not open again, because it is opened by negative membrane potentials and not by depolarization.

The channel will therefore not open and is said to be in the inactivated state.

If the membrane potential remains negative, the slow gate, which had originally been open, will open slowly again (characterizing the time dependence of recovery of the channel). A second depolarization will now be able to open the channel again, because the fast gate will open before the slow gate has had time to close again.

Drugs that interact with voltage-dependent ion channels as their molecular mechanism of action bind to a ligand-recognition site, which is part of the channel.

Affinity of an ion-channel-modulating drug for its ligand-recognition site

The apparent affinity of an ion-channel-modulating drug for its ligand-recognition site depends on the membrane potential and the rate at which the ion channel cycles through its state transitions. This gives rise to the characteristics of voltage and frequency dependence of drug action. There are two possible reasons for this behavior:

- Affinity of the drug for its ligand recognition site is determined by the state of the channel.
- Access of the drug to its ligand-recognition site is determined by the state of the channel.

It is possible to model the action of many ion-channel-modulating drugs by conceptualizing that the ligand-recognition site changes its conformation as the channel changes state. The conformation of the ligand-recognition site then determines its affinity for the drug. A drug that reduces channel opening and has a greater affinity for its ligand-recognition site when the channel is in the open state is therefore referred to as an open state blocker. Alternatively, if the ligand-recognition site is on the intracellular surface of the channel and the drug accesses the intracellular space by passing through the pore of the ion channel, then access would be the basis for the drug's apparent open state blockade. An example of such a drug is lidocaine when used as a local anesthetic.

It is difficult to separate all the possible ligand-recognition regions within the channel, and therefore a variety of terms are used to describe the actions of drugs on ion channels. The terms ion-channel blocker, ion-channel plugger, channel agonist and channel antagonist have been used to describe drugs that modulate channel function. The specific terms commonly used by convention often differ (e.g. Na^+-channel blocker and Ca^{2+} antagonists). Such words, however, do not represent the exact mechanism by which the drugs modulate channel function.

Drugs that impair channel opening have certain characteristics if they act through one of the following mechanisms:

- By binding to the ligand-recognition site when the channel is in the inactivated state and keeping the channel in the inactivated state.
- By entering the open channel and binding.
- By binding when the channel is in the rested or activated state and converting it to the inactivated state.

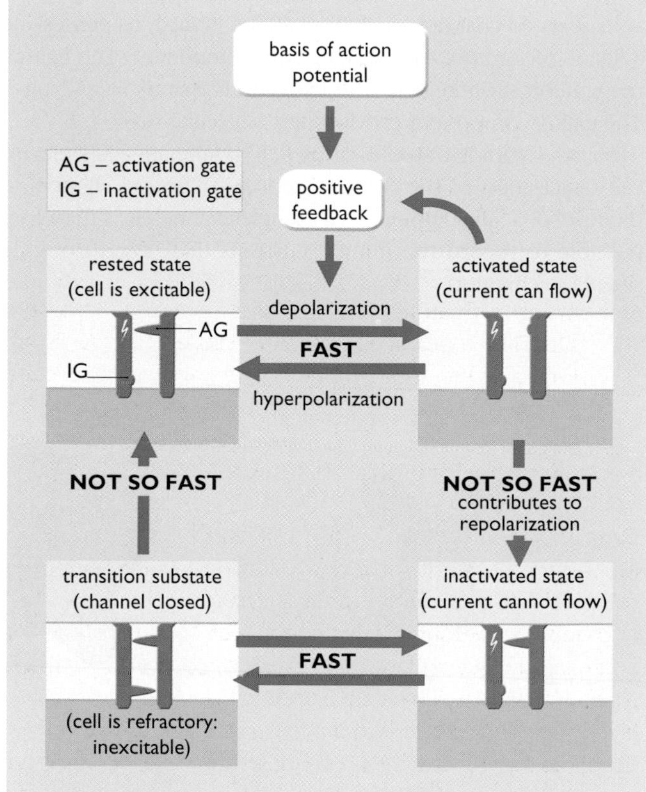

Fig. 3.8 Operation of inward currents in the heart. This is a simplified model showing two gates: one which opens on depolarization and closes on hyper-(re-)polarization, the other which functions in the converse mode. Transition from the rested to activated state, under the influence of depolarization, is fast and elicits a positive feedback. This is the basis of the action potential. Inactivation is time dependent and results from a slower closure of a second gate at positive potentials. When the inactivation gate is closed (in the inactivated and transition substates), the cell is inexcitable. This transition contributes to repolarization. Transition from the slow voltage-dependent opening of the inactivation gate determines the refractory period (the period of inexcitability during the action potential).

Drug interactions with Na^+ channels

Neuronal, cardiac muscle and skeletal muscle Na^+ channels differ slightly in structure and protein composition. Drugs that impair Na^+-channel opening during membrane depolarization are commonly known as Na^+-channel blockers, and discriminate to a certain extent between the different subtypes. For example, tetrodotoxin (a toxin found in puffer fish, some salamanders, and one type of octopus) can block neuronal and skeletal muscle Na^+ channels at concentrations as low as 10 nM, but the concentration needed to block cardiac muscle Na^+ channels is 100 times higher.

Two common types of Na^+-channel blockers are used therapeutically

Local anesthetics and Class I antiarrhythmic drugs block Na^+ channels:

- Local anesthetics such as lidocaine and bupivacaine may have some relative selectivity for the neuronal form of the Na^+ channel, but this selectivity is not marked. Current evidence suggests that most local anesthetics interact with a ligand-recognition site on the intracellular surface of the channel and that the drug has to access the intracellular space to reach its site of action. This mechanism differs from that of tetrodotoxin, which is a highly charged molecule that accesses its ligand-recognition site towards the extracellular surface of the channel.
- Class I antiarrhythmic drugs used to treat certain forms of cardiac arrhythmia are currently believed to interact mainly with an intracellularly-located ligand-recognition site. They appear to fall into three classes (Class Ia, Ib, and Ic), according to how their activity depends on the ion-channel state and on the apparent kinetics of binding and dissociation (called 'unbinding' in this context) with the channel in its three states (see Chapter 8).

Drug interactions with Ca^{2+} channels

At least four types of Ca^{2+} channel in the plasma membrane selectively allow the entry of Ca^{2+} ions into cells. These Ca^{2+} channels can be found in many different types of tissue. The best-characterized and most important clinically is the L (large)-type Ca^{2+} channel, which opens during depolarization and then inactivates (more slowly than the Na^+ channel) by voltage-dependent gating. It is the predominant Ca^{2+} channel in cardiac and smooth muscle and is blocked by a variety of clinically important drugs. The voltage dependence of the channel's state and relative apparent selectivity of drugs for specific states of the channel result in the tissue-selective actions of certain therapeutic drugs. The most important Ca^{2+} channels as molecular targets for drugs are the L-type channels.

There are three common classes of clinically important L-type Ca^{2+} antagonists

These classes are:

- The benzothiazepine derivatives (e.g. diltiazem).
- The phenethylalkylamines (e.g. verapamil).
- The 1,4-dihydropyridines (e.g. nifedipine, amlodipine).

1,4-Dihydropyridines show marked tissue selectivity for vascular smooth muscle cells

As 1,4-dihydropyridines show marked tissue selectivity for vascular smooth muscle cells, they cause selective relaxation of vascular smooth muscle (vasodilation). This is the basis for their use in the treatment of high blood pressure. A likely reason for this selectivity is that vascular smooth muscle cells have a relatively depolarized membrane potential for much of the time. This increases the probability of the L channels being in the activated and the inactivated state rather than in the rested state. Nifedipine has a relative selectivity for the activated and inactivated state of the L channel, and so blocks the vascular smooth muscle L channels at lower concentrations than, for example, the L channels in cardiac tissue, which are more likely to be in the rested state because the membrane potential is negative for a greater proportion of the time.

Although phenethylalkylamine Ca^{2+} antagonists such as verapamil are vascular selective, they have the additional ability to block L-type Ca^{2+} channels in the atrioventricular (AV) node of the heart. The average membrane potential in the AV node lies between that of vascular tissue and other cardiac tissues (i.e. ventricular and atrial muscle) so the AV node is relatively depolarized compared with the other regions of the heart. Unlike nifedipine, verapamil is therefore of value in the treatment of cardiac arrhythmias that involve the AV node (see Chapter 8). This is a good example of how selectivity for tissue action (see p. 37) is determined by subtleties in molecular mechanism of action).

Other types of Ca^{2+} channels Other types of Ca^{2+} channels, namely N, P, and T, may be selectively blocked by a variety of compounds, particularly peptides derived from certain combshell venoms. Novel drugs with a pharmacotherapeutic efficacy in humans may emerge from the selective blockade of these channels.

Drug interactions with K^+ channels

The opening of channels that are selective for K^+ results in the generation of outward-going (hyperpolarizing) currents. There are many types of K^+ channel, and they are a very mixed group in terms of their voltage and time dependency and ligand gating. There are more than ten different types, and their expression varies between tissue types, with some tissues expressing many types.

The nomenclature for some of the K^+ channels and currents is confusing, since certain individual types expressed in different parts of the body are named differently according to the tissue in which they are expressed. For example, the rapid Ca^{2+}-independent transient outward K^+ current in the heart (Ito_1) is identical to the current named IA in neuronal tissue.

Responsiveness to voltage and time varies between different K^+ channels

The varied responsiveness to voltage and time between different K^+ channels is illustrated in the heart (Figs 3.9, 3.10): the rapid delayed rectifying K^+ current (I_{Kr}) is activated by depolarization, whereas the inwardly rectifying K^+ current (I_{K1}) is activated by hyperpolarization. Also, some K^+ channels exhibit inactivation but others do not. In the heart, the mixed properties of the different K^+ channels contribute to the unusual shape of the cardiac action potential.

Other voltage-operated ion channels

Although the majority of the scientific literature on ion channels has focused on cation (Na^+, Ca^{2+}, and K^+) channels, recently it has become more apparent that voltage-gated channels exist for anions, for example, Cl^-. Chloride channels are found both peripherally and in the central nervous system (CNS). There are a variety of other ion channels with peculiar characteristics. Some are not selective for a single ion. For example, the channel responsible for the funny current (I_f) in the heart allows the passage of both Na^+ and Ca^{2+} ions.

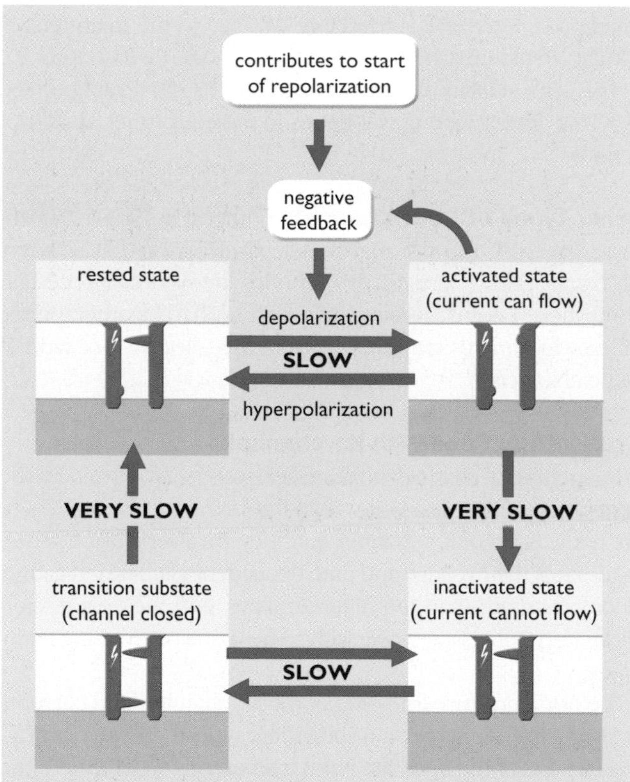

Fig. 3.9 Operation of the rapid delayed rectifier K^+ current (I_{Kr}) found in the heart. The channel possesses two gates, and can thus cycle between four states. Depolarization shifts the channel state from rested to activated, allowing hyperpolarizing outward current to flow. This has a negative feedback influence on depolarization, thus contributing to the initiation of re-(hyper-)polarization. Time dependence occurs because of slow voltage-dependent transition to an inactivated state. This cycles, via a substate, to the basal state (rested). The relative speed of the state transitions (kinetics) is shown.

Drug interactions with receptor-operated ion channels

There are numerous receptor-operated ion channels. All known receptor-operated channels are, physically, channels that possess, as part of their structure, a ligand-recognition site that interacts with an endogenous ligand. Thus, the principal difference between them and voltage-operated channels is that they are not gated by voltage and can be gated by an endogenous ligand. In the case of many receptor-operated channels, 'receptor' is the term used conventionally to describe the entire receptor-operated channel. Thus, the nicotinic cholinoceptor is actually a receptor-operated channel. The nicotinic receptor is a complex transmembrane-spanning molecule. It was the first receptor–ion-channel complex to be isolated, sequenced, and reconstructed in three dimensions, and exists as a tetramer with the acetylcholine ligand-recognition site on its external 'lip.' When two molecules of acetylcholine bind to the two binding sites on the ligand-recognition site, the configuration of the channel changes so that that it opens. The opening of the channel results in a sudden increase in permeability to Na^+ and K^+ ions. The movement down their concentration gradients depolarizes the cell.

Tubocurarine blocks the nicotinic receptor-operated channel in skeletal muscle

A drug that blocks the nicotinic receptor in skeletal muscle is tubocurarine. It was isolated many years ago from plant extracts used to coat the tips of darts used by American Indians in the Amazon basin.

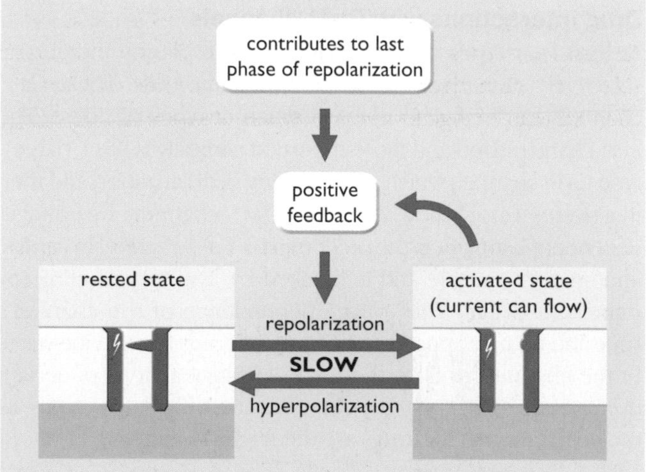

Fig. 3.10 Operation of the inward rectifier K^+ current (I_{K1}) found in the heart. The channel possesses one gate and can thus cycle between two states only. Repolarization shifts the channel to the activated state. The K^+ current that flows causes further repolarization so a positive feedback ensues. There is no inactivation because there is no second gate that closes after repolarization. However, the outward K^+ current is reduced by intracellular Mg^{2+}.

Receptor-operated channels have a hybrid function, being both molecular target and transduction component

Receptor-operated channels are discussed in more detail on p. 28. This is because their operation represents the first stage of the transduction that is caused by ligand binding. Therefore, they represent molecular targets that actually participate in the cellular response to drugs that affect them.

CARRIER MOLECULES

There is a need to regulate a cell's internal content of both small ions and large molecules. Passage of specific ions and molecules is facilitated by carrier molecules. Energy-independent carriers are transporters (which move one type of ion or molecule in one direction), symporters (which move two or more ions or molecules), or antiporters (which exchange one or more ions or molecules for one or more other ions or molecules). Energy-dependent carriers are called pumps. They are oriented enzymes. Enzymes that are not pumps are described later. Carrier molecules can be active or inactive. Some are activated by drugs, and others rendered inactive by drugs.

Energy-dependent carriers (pumps)

Na^+/K^+-dependent adenosine triphosphatase (ATPase) is a classic membrane pump. If left uncorrected, the opening and closing of ion channels that generate electrical activity across the cell membrane would lead to Na^+ accumulation within the cell and a corresponding loss of K^+. However, Na^+/K^+-dependent ATPase activity ensures that this does not occur. As Na^+ begins to accumulate as a result of action potentials, Na^+/K^+-dependent ATPase transfers Na^+ ions across the membrane to the extracellular fluid in exchange for K^+ ions from the extracellular fluid (two Na^+ ions for three K^+ ions). The energy for this is supplied by the hydrolysis of ATP. Throughout the text, pumps will be shown using an icon (Fig. 3.11).

Energy-independent carriers (which are not enzymes) can transport, symport, and exchange. One example of this is the Na^+/Ca^{2+} exchanger, which normally acts to move Ca^{2+} out of the cell in exchange for Na^+ (three Na^+ for one Ca^{2+}).

A variety of carriers are present in the various component membranes of the cell and in addition to ions, may carry important molecules such as sugars, and nucleic and amino acids.

Energy-independent carrier molecules will be represented by an icon throughout the text (Fig. 3.12).

ENZYMES

The cell and body fluids contain a large variety of enzymes, each of which is a potential target for drugs that either mimic the enzyme's substrate or inhibit the enzyme's activity. The icon that is used throughout the book for those enzymes that are not pumps is shown in Fig. 3.13.

Drugs may act upon a variety of ligand-recognition sites on an enzyme. If the site of inhibitory drug action is the substrate-recognition site for the enzyme, the interaction between the drug and the enzyme is competitive.

However, drugs can interfere with enzymes in other ways. If the site of drug action is separate from the substrate-recognition site, inhibition can result from allosteric mechanisms or by

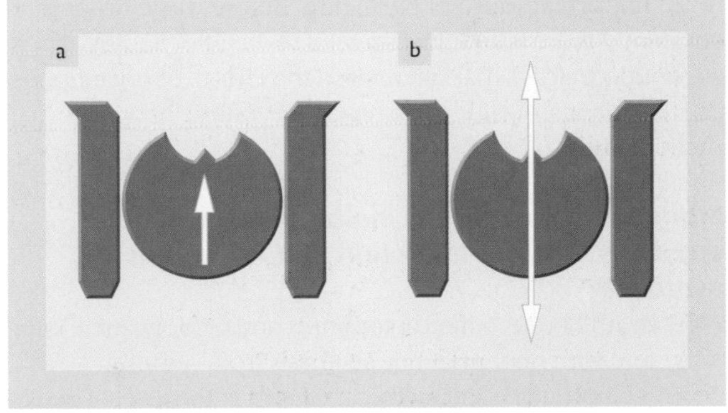

Fig. 3.12 The icon used throughout the text for an energy-independent carrier molecule. (a) An inactive transporter or symporter characterized by unidirectional transport. (b) An active antiporter characterized by two-way transport.

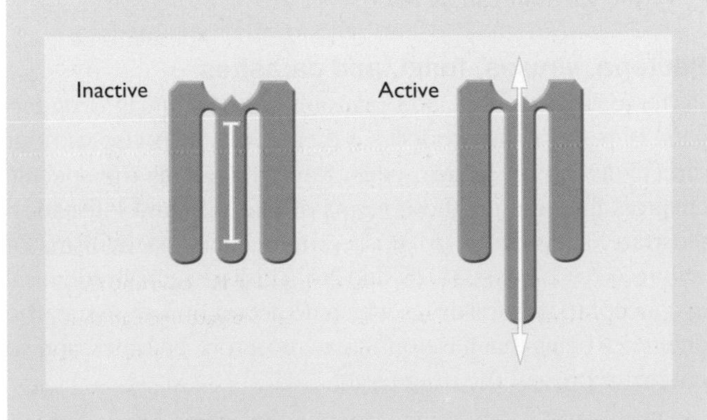

Fig. 3.11 The icon used throughout the text for a pump showing the inactive and active states.

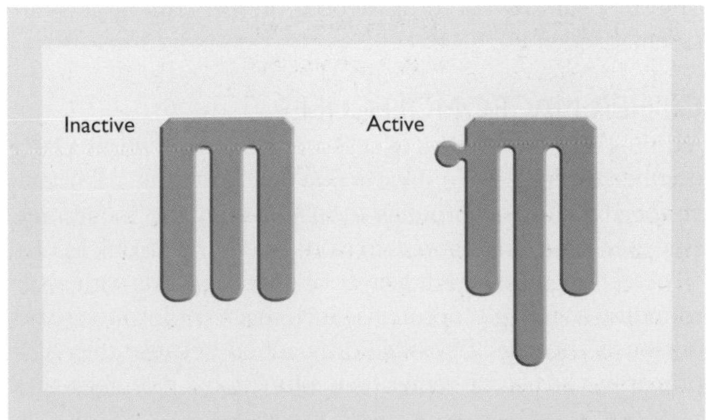

Fig. 3.13 The icon used throughout the text for an enzyme showing the inactive and active states.

disruption of the enzyme's integrity. This is very similar to non- and uncompetitive antagonism by drugs on classical receptors (discussed on p. 19 and in detail in Chapter 4). A typical example of this is inhibition of the enzyme acetylcholinesterase, which is the enzyme responsible for degrading the neurotransmitter acetylcholine. Acetylcholinesterase has a substrate-recognition site with two components, one of which recognizes the esteratic moiety, and the other which recognizes the charged moiety in acetylcholine. The molecule of acetylcholine, located and oriented by the substrate-recognition site, then undergoes hydrolysis (i.e. separation of acetylcholine into its component molecules choline and acetate). Some cholinester analogs of acetylcholine can bind with both components of the substrate-recognition site while other analogs bind with only one. In doing so, they inhibit the hydrolysis of endogenous acetylcholine. The interaction is competitive but can be reversible or irreversible.

There is a group of molecules that bind covalently with the esteratic component of the substrate-recognition site. The most important of these are the organophosphates. The irreversibly inhibited enzyme then degenerates. Such organophosphate compounds have been used as nerve gases in chemical warfare and as insecticides. As insecticides they can be an important cause of poisoning. Before these drugs bind covalently there is an initial stage of reversible binding. There are antidote drugs that can reverse the effects of organophosphate poisons during their reversible phase of action (e.g. pralidoxime).

Many anticancer drugs inhibit the activity of enzymes involved in protein and nucleic acid synthesis

- Azathioprine, 6-mercaptopurine, and 6-thioguanine interfere with ribonucleotide synthesis from purines.
- 5-Fluorouracil and methotrexate act at the level of deoxyribonucleotides by disturbing 2' deoxythymidylate synthesis.
- Cytarabine inhibits DNA polymerase and RNA synthesis.
- Doxorubicin, etoposide, amsacrine, and dactinomycin inhibit DNA replication and RNA transcription.

SUMMARY OF THE MECHANISMS OF DRUG ACTION ON PROTEIN TARGETS

The mechanisms of drug action on protein targets are summarized in Fig. 3.14.

OTHER MACROMOLECULES

Although the membranes of cells are the sites at which a large number of drugs have their action, such actions are usually at specific sites on proteins located within the membrane. However, some drugs appear to work on other macromolecules.

The cell membrane is a bilayer of phospholipids with a surrounding coat of glycoproteins. Such macromolecules are not obviously the site of possible drug action because they have primarily a structural rather than a functional role. Structural molecules have fewer specific ligand-recognition sites with which a drug can interact, and when such a molecule consists of many repeated chemical motifs a huge number of drug molecules would be required to saturate the sites, indicating a need for drug concentrations to be in the millimolar range for effectiveness, whereas most drugs act at submillimolar concentrations down to femtomolar or even lower concentrations.

The plasma membrane is just one of many membranes in the cell, and they are usually composed of a bilayer of lipids. Intracellular membranes include those surrounding cellular organelles such as the nucleus and mitochondria.

In addition, certain drugs (particularly glucocorticosteroids) interact with intracellular receptors that are actually free molecules which participate in cell nuclear modulation (see Fig. 3.15).

DRUG ACTIONS ON NUCLEIC ACIDS

The most prominent drugs that utilize nucleic acids—deoxyribonucleic acid (DNA) and ribonucleic acid (RNA)—as their molecular targets are anticancer drugs. Different anticancer drugs have their mechanism of action at different stages of nucleic acid synthesis, for example:

- The bleomycins damage DNA and prevent its repair.
- Alkylating agents, mitomycin, and cisplatin cross-link DNA.

EXAMPLES OF MOLECULAR TARGETS FOR DRUG ACTION

Examples of molecular targets for drug action are listed in Fig. 3.15.

MOLECULAR TARGETS THAT ARE NOT PART OF HUMAN CELLS

Chemical targets

Some drugs achieve their therapeutic effect without interacting with cells at all, for example:

- Chelating drugs act by binding to ions (such as Fe^{2+}, Fe^{3+} and Al^{3+}).
- Surfactants alter the surface physical properties of biologic fluids.
- Certain drugs used in the treatment of gastrointestinal disorders adsorb substances in the gut and so alter the consistency and transit time of the bowel contents through the gastrointestinal tract.

Bacteria, viruses, fungi, and parasites

Bacteria, viruses, fungi, and parasites are nonhuman drug targets. Here the drug produces a therapeutic response without directly acting on human cells. Nevertheless, as the specific chapters focusing on these forms of infection and infestation illustrate, such drugs do possess molecular mechanisms of actions (see Chapters 24, 25, and 26). This is essentially identical in concept to that for drugs which do act on human tissue; the difference being that it is nonhuman receptors, enzymes, and so on, that represent the drug target.

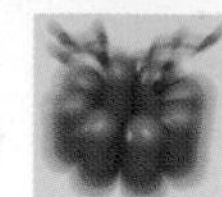

CELLULAR TARGETS FOR DRUGS (TRANSDUCTION)

Molecular targets for drugs such as receptors are linked to a variety of cellular response components (such as enzymes, ion channels, etc.). The operation of this linkage is known as transduction. The most important and varied forms of transduction are those that are associated with a receptor as the molecular target. Because of this, receptors are actually classified in relation to the transduction component with which they are directly linked. A discussion of this linkage and classification system is a good way of introducing the concept of transduction.

Four families of receptors are distinguished by their transduction systems. In terms of receptor structure and the ensuing cellular response following occupation of the receptor, these four families (Fig. 3.16) are referred to as the receptor superfamilies: receptor-operated channels; G protein-linked receptors; receptors that are enzymes; and DNA-linked receptors.

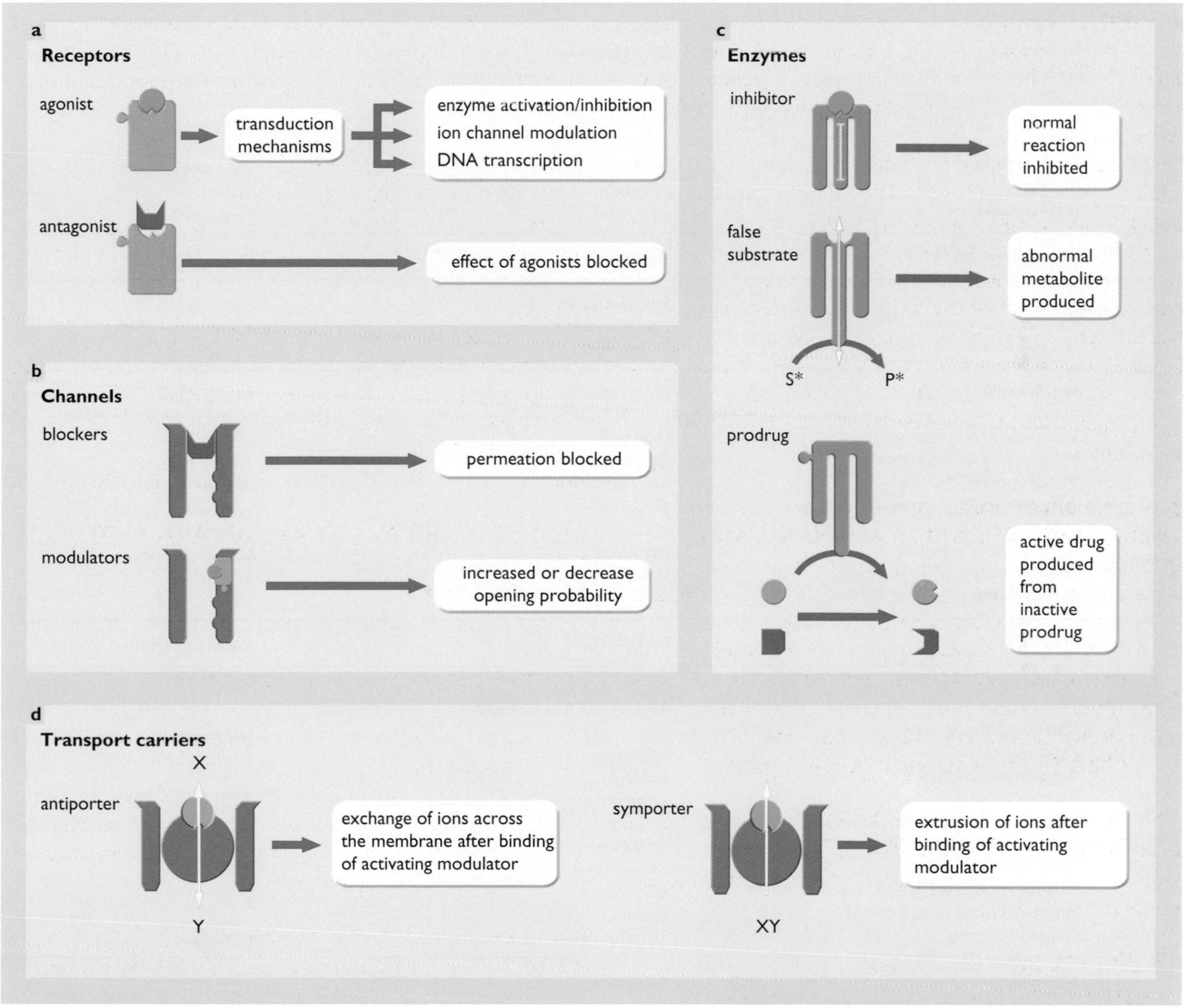

Fig. 3.14 Protein targets for drug action. These can be broadly divided into three classes. (a) Agonists can bind to receptors to initiate changes in transduction mechanisms leading to a variety of cellular effects. Antagonists bind to receptors to block the effect of the agonist. (b) Drugs can block the passage of materials across channels or bind to components of the channel proteins to modulate the opening of ion channels. (c) Drugs can interact directly with the action of enzymes via a variety of mechanisms. S* and P* are false substrate and false product, respectively. (d) Drugs can bind to exchange proteins (antiporters) to move ions across the membrane. The direction of ion movement is shown by the direction of the arrow. Here, transporters are shown being activated by drugs, but note that some transporters are active at rest, and blocked by drugs. X and Y represent ions, which may have a postive or negative charge.

RECEPTOR-OPERATED ION CHANNELS

Receptor-operated ion channels were mentioned on p. 24 in the context of their role as molecular drug targets. Their role in transduction follows ligand binding. In most cases an agonist opens the channel, whereas antagonists prevent this opening. As noted earlier, for reasons that are largely convention (i.e. historical), the ligand-recognition site together with the remainder of the receptor-operated ion channel is commonly called a receptor, although in effect it is a hybrid of a molecular target and a coupled transduction component.

Some examples of molecular targets for drug action

Membrane receptors	**Agonists**	**Antagonists**
α_1 Adrenoceptor	Norepinephrine	Prazosin
α_2 Adrenoceptor	Norepinephrine	Yohimbine
β Adrenoceptor	Isoproterenol	Propranolol
Histamine (H_1 receptor)	Histamine	Terfenadine
Histamine (H_2 receptor)	Impromidine	Cimetidine
Opiate (μ-receptor)	Morphine	Naloxone
5-HT_2 receptor	5-HT	Ketanserin
Thrombin	Thrombin	Hirudin
Insulin receptor	Insulin	Not known
Intracellular receptors	**Agonists**	**Antagonists**
Estrogen receptor	Ethinyl estradiol	Tamoxifen†
Progesterone receptor	Norethinderone	Danazol
Glucocorticosteroid receptor	Budesonide	Mifepristone
Ion channels	**Drugs that block channels**	**Modulators**
Voltage-gated Na^+ channels	Lidocaine	
Voltage-gated Ca^{2+} channels	Dyhydropyridine	Dihydropyridines
Voltage-gated K^+channels	4-aminopyridine	Ibutilide
ATP-sensitive K^+ channels	Glyburide	Lemakalim
		Sulfonylureas
GABA-gated Cl^- channels	Picrotoxin	Benzodiazepines
Glutamate-gated (NMDA) cation channels	Dizocilpine	Glycine
Enzymes	**Inhibitors**	**False substrates**
Acetylcholinesterase	Neostigmine	
	Organophosphate insecticides	
Choline acetyltransferase		Hemicholinium
Cyclooxygenase	Indomethacin	Eicosatetraynoic acid
Angiotensin-converting enzyme	Enalapril	
Carbonic anhydrase	Acetazolamide	
HMG-CoA reductase	Simvastatin	
Dopa decarboxylase	Carbidopa	Methyldopa
DNA polymerase	Cytarabine	Cytarabine
Enzymes involved in DNA synthesis	Azathioprine	
Enzymes of blood clotting cascade	Heparin	
Phosphodiesterase	Theophylline	
Carriers	**Inhibitors**	
Choline carrier (nerve terminal)	Hemicholinium	
Norepinephrine Uptake 1	Tricyclic antidepressants	
	Cocaine	
5-HT uptake	Fluoxitine	
Renal weak acid transfer	Probenecid	
Na^+ pump	Digitalis	
Na^+/H^+ exchanger	Amiloride	

†Can act as a partial agonist in certain tissues.

Fig. 3.15 Examples of molecular targets for drug action. (GABA, γ-aminobutyric acid; 5-HT, 5-hydroxytryptamine; HMG–CoA, 2-hydroxy-3-methylglutaryl coenzyme A; NMDA, *N*-methyl D-aspartate)

This large family of receptors includes receptors for:

- Acetylcholine (nicotinic receptors).
- GABA ($GABA_A$ receptors).
- Glycine.
- 5-hydroxytryptamine ($5\text{-}HT_3$ receptors).
- Purine (P_2x receptors).

The receptor is composed of subunits, each of which has four transmembrane domains. These domains form complexes of varying stoichiometry (Fig. 3.17).

The most completely understood of the receptor-operated ion channels is the nicotinic receptor on skeletal muscle and electric organ membranes from the electric eel (*Torpedo eel*). This receptor was one of the first to be sequenced and its mode of function is understood in great detail. Other receptor-operated ion channels show considerable homology with it. There are different types of nicotinic receptors. This presumably accounts for the fact that although all nicotinic receptors respond to acetylcholine, antagonists and other agonists can have fairly selective actions on

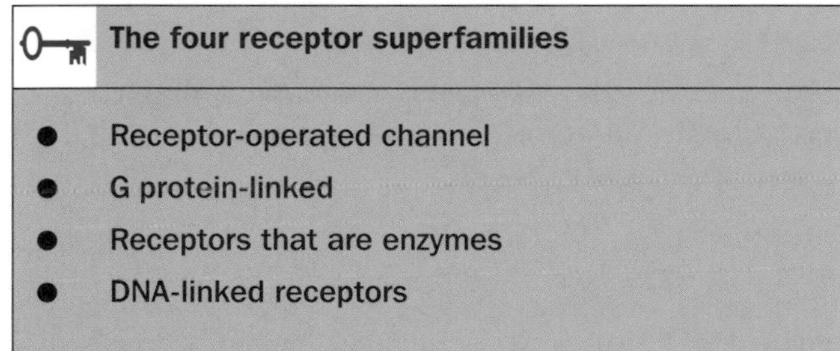

The four receptor superfamilies

- Receptor-operated channel
- G protein-linked
- Receptors that are enzymes
- DNA-linked receptors

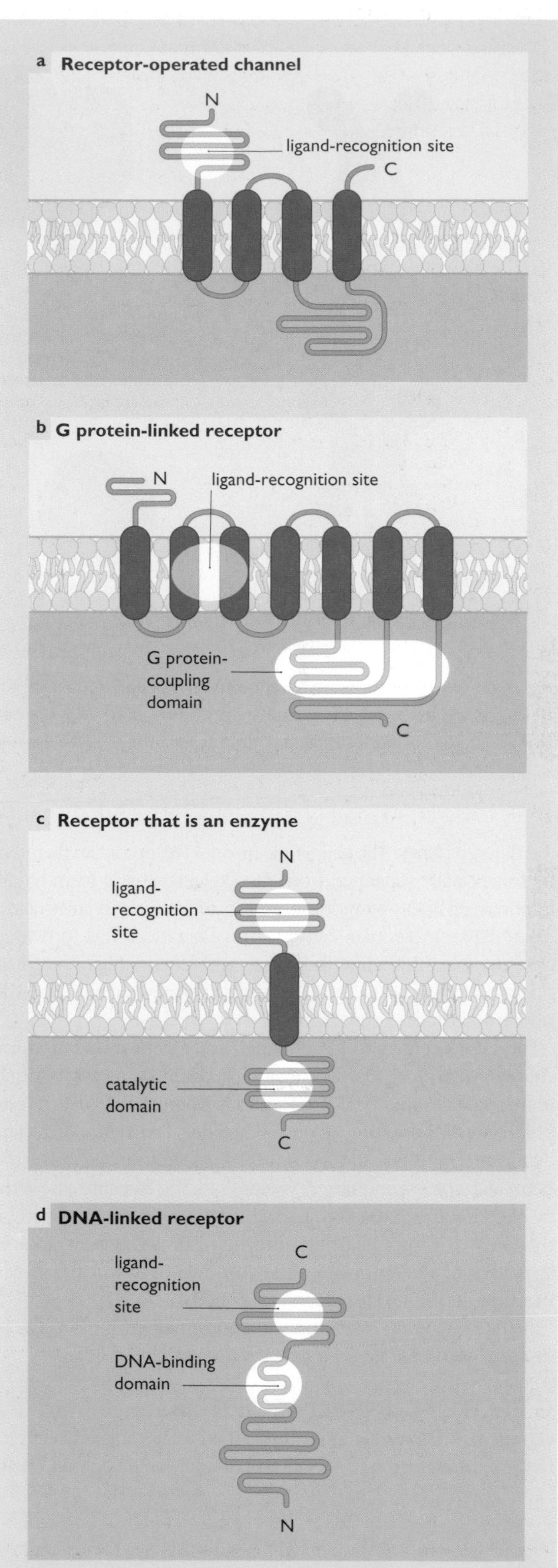

Fig. 3.16 Schematic representation of the general structure of the four receptor superfamilies. (a) An extracellular binding domain is coupled to a hydrophobic α helical region of the protein that forms the membrane-spanning domain. Up to five subunits that have this general structure form a complex surrounding a central ion channel. This is best examplified by the nicotinic acetylcholine (ACh) receptor. Typically, this type of receptor mediates the very fast action of neurotransmitters. (b) The ligand-recognition site is found within the α helices and the membrane-spanning domain is connected to an intracellular domain that couples to G proteins. This is a typical receptor structure for very many hormones and slower-acting neurotransmitter systems that act via G protein-coupled transduction systems (e.g. ACh acting on muscarinic receptors on smooth muscle). (c) The receptors for various growth factors and insulin have an extracellular ligand-recognition site linked directly to an intracellular catalytic domain that has either tyrosine kinase or guanylyl kinase activity when the ligand-recognition site is occupied by an appropriate agonist. These may be defined as receptors that are enzymes. (d) The ligand-recognition site is linked to a DNA-binding domain. It is typified by the receptors for steroid and thyroid hormones. These may be defined as DNA-linked receptors. 'C' is the *C*-terminal, and 'N' the *N*-terminal of the protein. (Adapted with permission from *Pharmacology, 3rd edn*, by Rang, Dale, and Ritter, Churchill Livingstone, 1995.)

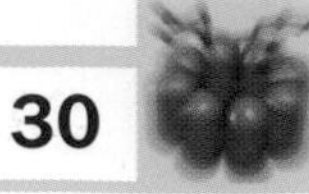

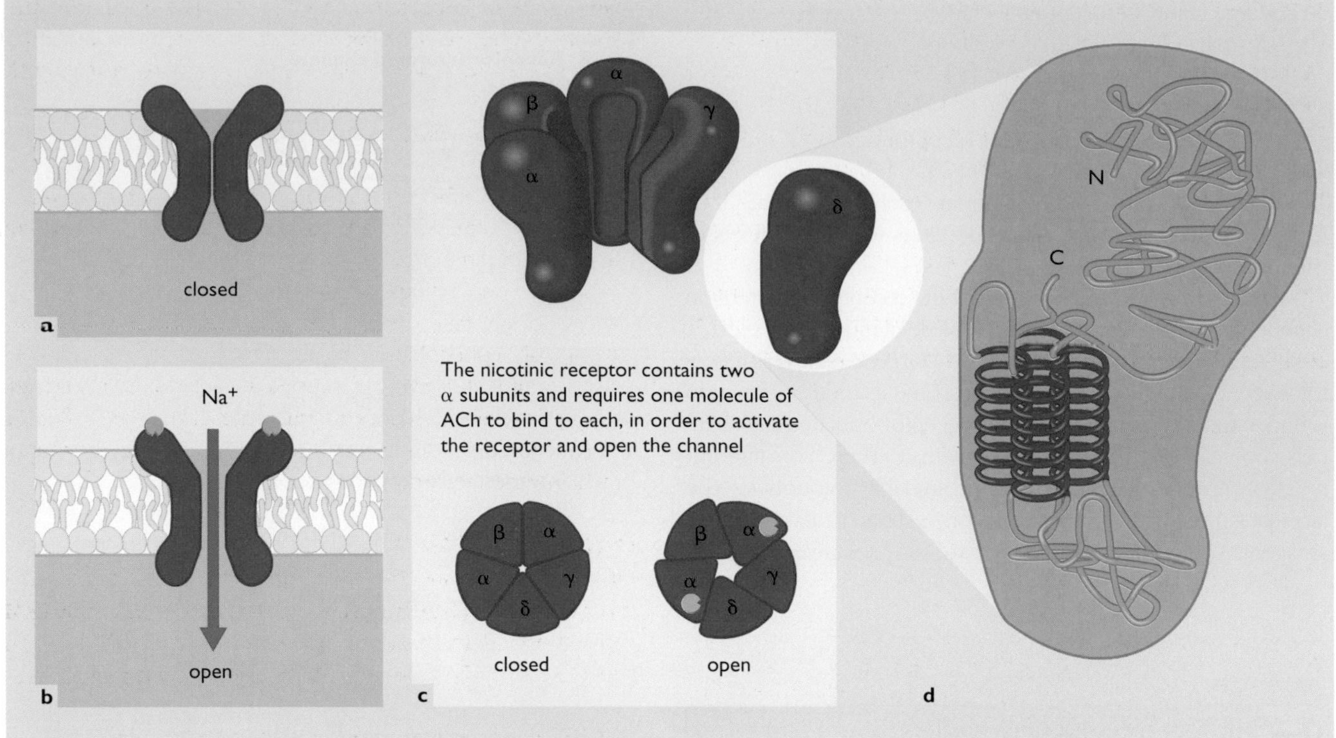

Fig. 3.17 The nicotinic acetylcholine (ACh) receptor. The receptor-operated ion channel consists of five protein subunits (2α, β, γ, and δ) all of which traverse the membrane and surround a central pore. ACh binds to the α subunits and the two ACh molecules must bind in order to open the channel (c). The complete structure of the δ subunit (d). 'C' is the *C*-terminal, and 'N' the *N*-terminal of the protein.

the different types. The ganglionic nicotinic receptor can therefore be functionally separated from the skeletal muscle form by differential sensitivity to agonists, and to antagonists in particular.

Extensive molecular biologic investigation has provided considerable insight into the nature and functioning of receptor-operated channels in terms of their cation selectivity and the phenomenon of desensitization.

The GABA-regulated Cl^- channel is a receptor-operated ion channel with more than one ligand-recognition site and is found in many places in the CNS. Its activation generally causes hyperpolarization, inhibiting neuronal activity. The benzodiazepine ligand-recognition site recognizes exogenous ligands (the benzodiazepine tranquilizers) whose binding facilitates the activity of GABA. In addition, inverse agonists have been identified for the GABA receptor, although they have no known therapeutic application. Receptor-operated ion channels will be shown throughout the text as an icon (Fig. 3.18).

In the remaining cases, transduction involves the linkage of discrete and separate molecules to the coupled receptor.

G PROTEIN-LINKED RECEPTORS

G proteins are transduction components that are linked directly to, but are distinct from, a specific superfamily of receptors. The G protein is linked with secondary transduction components such as ion channels. A classic example of this is the opening of K^+ channels in cardiac muscle following acetylcholine binding to muscarinic receptors.

G protein-linked receptors are composed of seven transmembrane helices (I–VII) (Fig. 3.19).

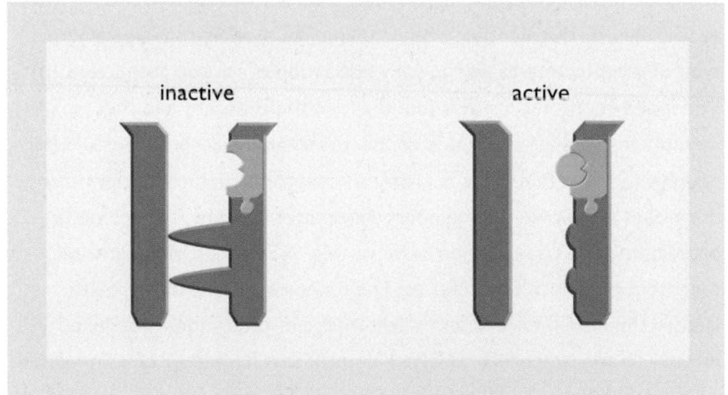

Fig. 3.18 Icon for receptor-operated ion channel. Note that in certain cases the inactive (agonist unbound) state is 'channel open' and the agonist closes the channel.

G proteins consist of three subunits, α, β, and γ (Fig. 3.20) and act as on–off switches for cell signaling

In the cell membrane, specialized G proteins exist as a complex of subunits (α, β, and γ). In the 'off' or resting state for G proteins, the guanine nucleotide diphosphate (GDP) is tightly bound to the α subunit of the G protein. When the G protein-linked receptor is occupied by an agonist molecule, the GDP dissociates from the α subunit. The GDP is then replaced by guanine triphosphate (GTP), which activates the G protein causing dissociation of the α subunit from the $\beta\gamma$ complex, each of which can then influence secondary transduction components inside the cell (the 'on' state, see below). There are many types of G protein in most cells. The α subunit then hydrolyzes GTP to GDP, which in turn inactivates the α subunit, allowing it to reassociate with the $\beta\gamma$ complex, resetting the G protein to the 'off' position.

G proteins are shown throughout the text as an icon (Fig. 3.21).

Stimulation or inhibition of G proteins results in modulation of the enzyme system responsible for producing the following transduction components:

- Cyclic nucleotides.
- Diacylglycerol (DAG).
- Inositol phosphates.

For example following β_1 agonism, a G protein activates adenylyl cyclase, which catalyzes the formation of cAMP. Transduction procedes by cAMP activating enzymes, the identity of which varies according to tissue type.

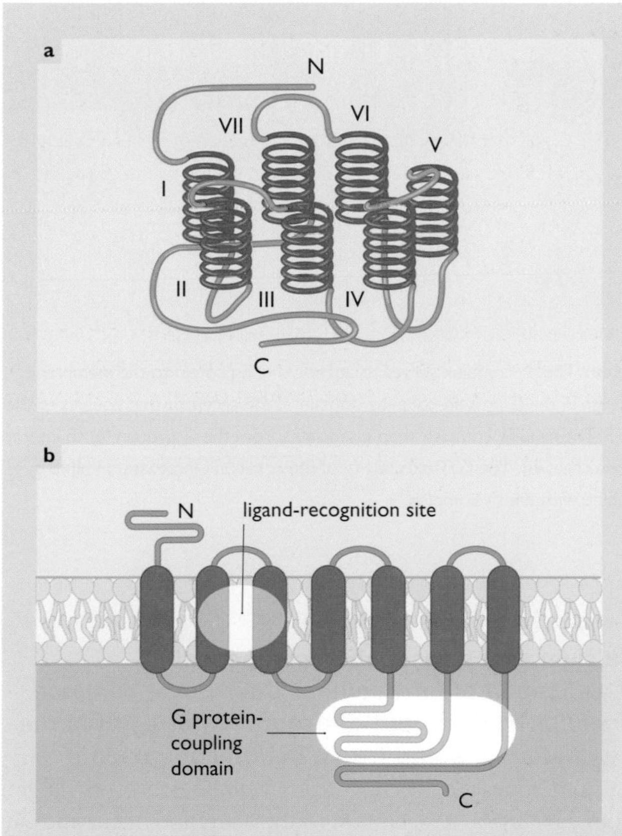

Fig. 3.19 Schematic representation of a G protein-linked receptor. (a) There are seven transmembrane helices (I–VII). (b) The G protein coupling domain is the part of the receptor that interacts with the α subunit of the G protein to facilitate transduction following binding of an agonist to the binding domain. 'C' is the *C*-terminal, and 'N' the *N*-terminal of the protein.

Cyclic nucleotides

Of the three transduction components linked to G proteins, the most widespread is adenylyl cyclase. The cyclic nucleotide cAMP is synthesized from adenosine triphosphate (ATP) by the enzyme adenylyl cyclase. cAMP has diverse biologic actions.

cAMP has an effect on energy metabolism, cell differentiation, ion-channel functioning, and contractile proteins

cAMP phosphorylates intracellular proteins (many are enzymes) through the action of cAMP-dependent protein kinases.

The protein kinases activated by cAMP phosphorylate the amino acid residues serine and threonine, using ATP as a source of phosphate groups (Fig. 3.22). This can lead to:

- Activation of hormone-sensitive lipase.
- Inactivation of glycogen synthase.
- Activation of phosphorylase kinase and therefore conversion of inactive phosphorylase b to active phosphorylase a.

This pattern of changes in enzyme activity results in:

- Increased lipolysis.
- Reduced glycogen synthesis.
- Increased glycogen breakdown.

In addition, the Ca^{2+} channels and sarcoplasmic reticulum in cardiac cells are phosphorylated, so increasing Ca^{2+} currents and Ca^{2+} release.

G proteins activate the diacylglycerol–inositol pathway

One G protein, termed G_q, stimulates phospholipase C. This enzyme in turn leads to the production of DAG and inositol (1,4,5) triphosphate (IP_3) from the hydrolysis of polyphosphotide inositides. An alternative pathway involves activation of membrane phospholipase A_2 by G proteins, leading to the formation of DAG and phosphatidic acid. These transduction components have a diversity of actions.

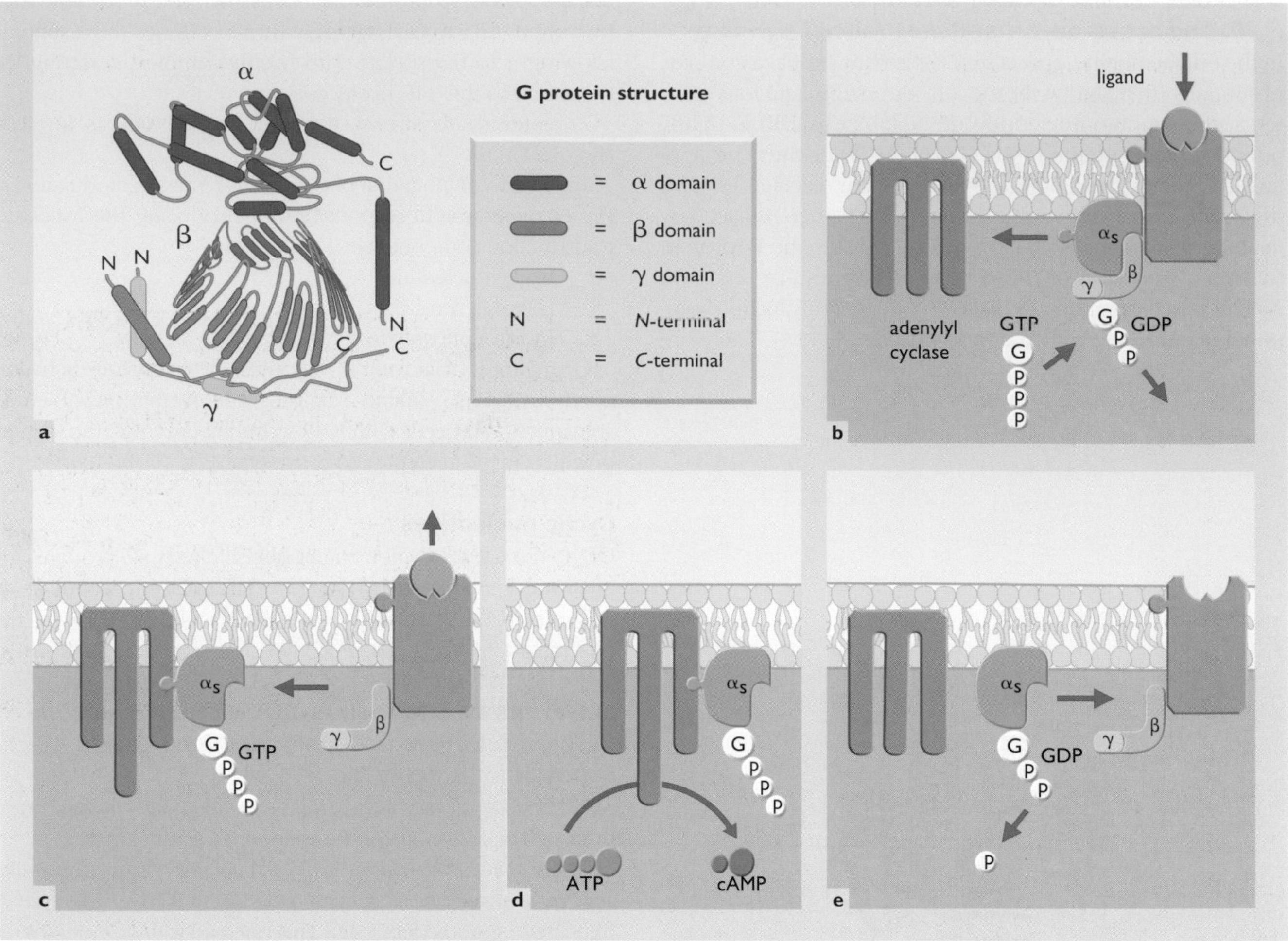

Fig. 3.20 Schematic representation of the α, β, and γ subunits of the G protein. The βγ complex serves to anchor the G protein to the membrane. When an agonist binds to a G protein-linked receptor (b), there is a conformation change in the G protein-coupling domain of the receptor that couples to the α subunit of the G protein, causing the bound GDP to exchange with intracellular GTP. The α–GTP complex then dissociates from the G protein (c) to interact subsequently (d) with a target protein (e.g. an enzyme such as adenylyl cyclase, or an ion channel). The GTPase activity of the α subunit increases on binding, leading to hydrolysis of the bound GTP to GDP, which allows the α subunit to recombine with the βγ complex.

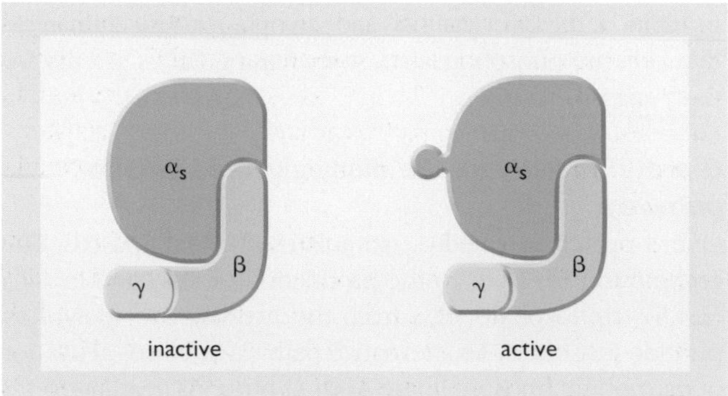

Fig. 3.21 The icon used throughout the text for the G protein in the inactive and active states. Note that the α_s subunit dissociates when the G protein is active (see Fig. 3.20) but, for simplicity, the icon for the active G protein is shown 'intact,' but with an 'appendage' (as for 'active' receptors, see Fig. 3.2).

Calcium as a transduction component

Mobilization of intracellular Ca^{2+} is the common final link in the chain of events resulting from the production of some transduction components

Calcium appears to control many cellular processes ranging from contraction to secretion to the activation of enzymes. Its mobilization is linked to the activity of other transduction components.

Calcium is stored on the membrane of endoplasmic reticulum of smooth muscle and is released when IP_3 acts on a specific intracellular 'IP_3 receptor.' IP_3 is not the only inositol phosphate produced in the cell by phospholipase. There appears to be a bewildering array of such compounds, which may have different functions. The tetraphosphate inositol (1,3,4,5) phosphate appears to facilitate the entry of Ca^{2+} into different cellular compartments (Fig. 3.23).

DAG released by the actions of phospholipase C (and D) directly affects the activity of a membrane-bound protein kinase C, which is the enzyme responsible for phosphorylating serine and threonine and the subsequent change in activation state of various proteins (over 50 types). There are at least six types of protein kinase C, each with its own substrate specificity.

Protein kinase C is involved in transduction in the following processes:

- Modulation of the release of endocrine hormones and neurotransmitters.
- Smooth muscle contraction.
- Inflammation.
- Ion transport.
- Tumor promotion.

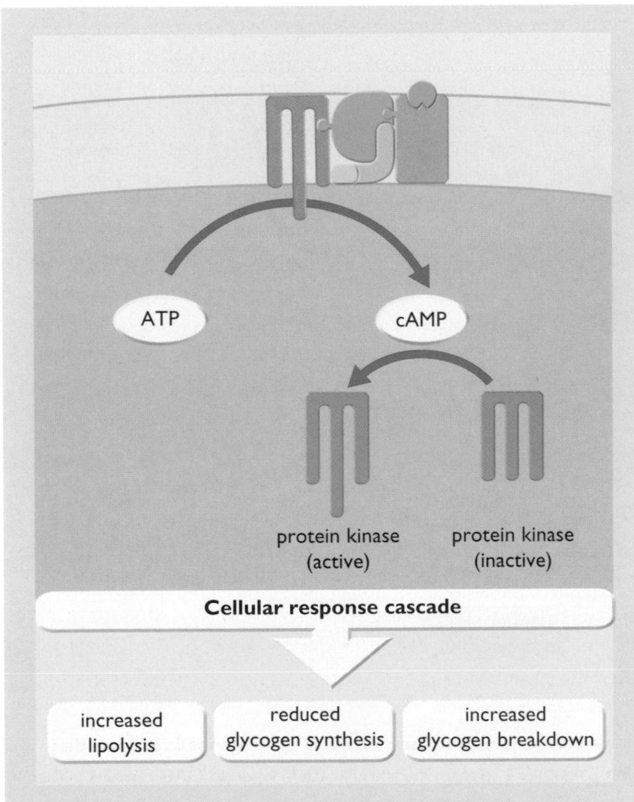

Fig. 3.22 The effect of cAMP as a transduction component. cAMP production increases in response to activation of a G protein linked receptor. Protein kinases, activated by cAMP, are secondary transduction components which participate in a cellular response cascade.

Calcium is involved in transduction in the following processes:

- Smooth muscle contraction.
- Increased rate of contraction and relaxation of cardiac myocytes.
- Secretion of transmitter molecules or glandular secretions.
- Hormone release.
- Cytotoxicity.
- Activation of certain enzymes.

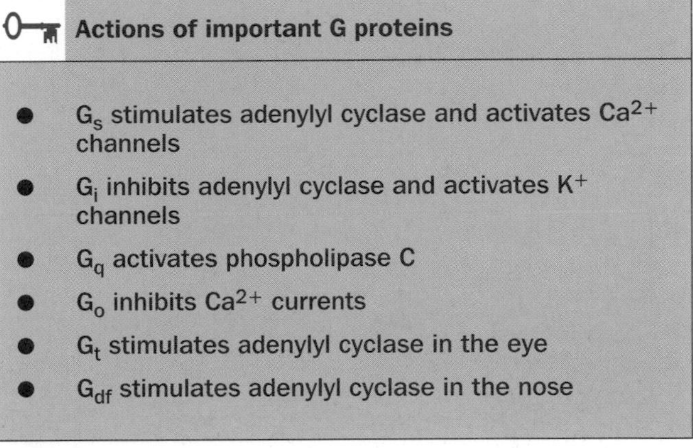

Actions of important G proteins

- G_s stimulates adenylyl cyclase and activates Ca^{2+} channels
- G_i inhibits adenylyl cyclase and activates K^+ channels
- G_q activates phospholipase C
- G_o inhibits Ca^{2+} currents
- G_t stimulates adenylyl cyclase in the eye
- G_{df} stimulates adenylyl cyclase in the nose

RECEPTORS THAT ARE ENZYMES

Tyrosine kinases

Tyrosine kinase receptors (Fig. 3.24) are involved in the regulation of growth, differentiation, and responses to metabolic stimuli. They include the receptors for insulin, epidermal growth factors, and platelet-derived growth factor. These receptors act as intracellular tyrosine kinases and are responsible for the phosphorylation of tyrosine residues. They are structurally quite different from G protein or channel-linked receptors.

The activation of tyrosine kinase receptors allows autophosphorylation of tyrosine residues, which serve as high-affinity sites for a variety of intracellular proteins. The tyrosine-phosphorylated receptor can then act as a platform for other proteins to bind to, leading to the activation of pathways involving multiple protein kinases. Receptor-linked tyrosine kinases couple to multiple signaling pathways, and coordinated activation of many pathways may be required to evoke a full cellular response.

These proteins typically have sequences that provide ligand-recognition sites for other proteins involved in signal transduction. A frequently exposed binding domain is termed SH_2. The binding of SH_2-containing proteins is specific and leads to a highly selective activation of particular enzyme pathways and gene transcription, mediated by classes of protein kinases. After receptor recognition and SH_2 binding, the steps leading to a tissue response can involve activation of phospholipase C, IP_3 production and Ca^{2+} release. Many growth factors act through this mechanism. There is therefore considerable interest in potential drugs that interact with or mimic the SH_2 domain because they could have profound effects on growth and differentiation, and, by implication, cancer, immunologic disease, and other disorders.

Guanylyl cyclase

The membrane-bound form of guanylyl cyclase provides an example of a structurally related receptor system. The binding of atrial natriuretic peptide (ANP) causes part of the ANP receptor to exhibit guanylyl cyclase activity, resulting in the formation of the transduction component cyclic guanosine monophosphate (cGMP). The ANP receptor–guanylyl cyclase molecule is a transmembrane protein. However, the guanylyl cyclase may be cytoplasmic; for example in endothelial cells, bradykinin activates membrane receptors to generate nitric oxide (NO), which then acts as a messenger to activate cytoplasmic guanylyl cyclase.

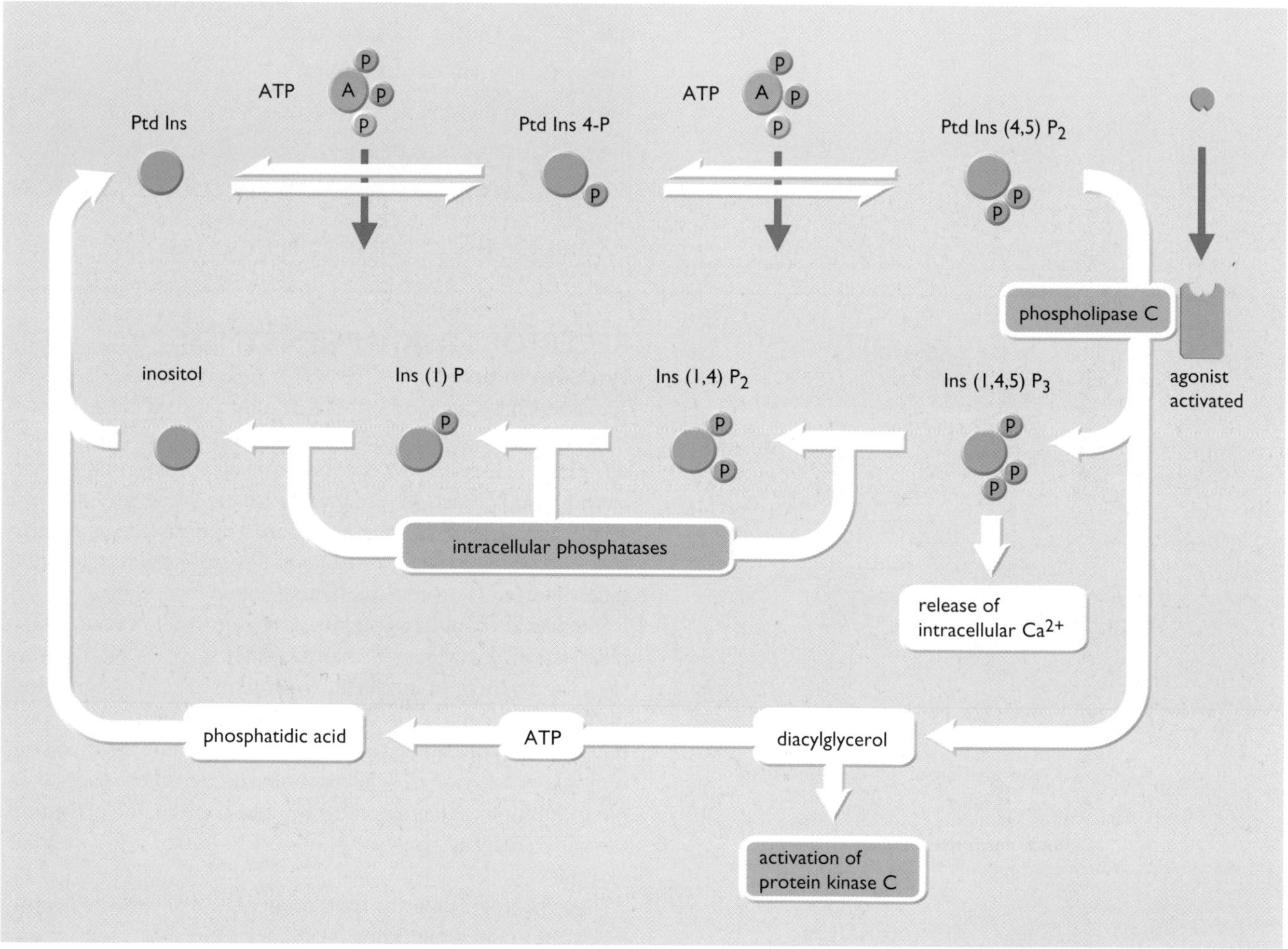

Fig. 3.23 The phosphatidyl inositol cycle as a transduction system. The membrane enzyme phospholipase is activated by an agonist to produce the second messengers Ins (1,4,5) P_3 (inositol triphosphate, IP_3) and diacylglycerol (DAG). Intracellular IP_3 releases intracellular Ca^{2+} whereas DAG remains in the membrane where it activates protein kinase C. Activation of protein kinase C initiates protein phosphorylation, IP_3 undergoes sequential dephosphorylation by intracellular phosphatases to give inositol which can then be incorporated into the membrane to form phosphatidyl inositol, which, via ATP, is phosphorylated in steps to phosphatidyl inositol diphosphate from which IP_3 can be cleaved by phospholipase C. The recycling of IP_3 and DAG into phosphatidyl inositol is blocked by lithium, which depletes inositol lipids in the brain and is used as a drug in the treatment of manic depression (see Chapter 7).

DNA-LINKED RECEPTORS

Intracellular receptors that can interact with DNA exist for some molecules such as retinoic acid, corticosteroids, thyroid hormone, and vitamin D. These receptors are mainly composed of nuclear proteins. As a result, the agonists have to pass through the cell membranes to reach their receptor. For example, a steroid first enters the cell and binds with a cytoplasmic receptor, which often has an inhibitory component bound to it, for example heat shock protein 90 (HSP90). The steroid displaces HSP90 and the resulting steroid–receptor complex then translocates to the nucleus. Once in the nucleus and bound to the receptor, the steroid–receptor complex can recognize specific base sequences and activate specific genes.

Secondary transduction following DNA-linked receptor activation involves a change in the synthesis of specific proteins

Secondary transduction involves an increase or decrease in the synthesis of specific proteins as a result of activating specific genes. This is a slow process compared with that of the millisecond responses that are found in other forms of transduction (Fig. 3.25).

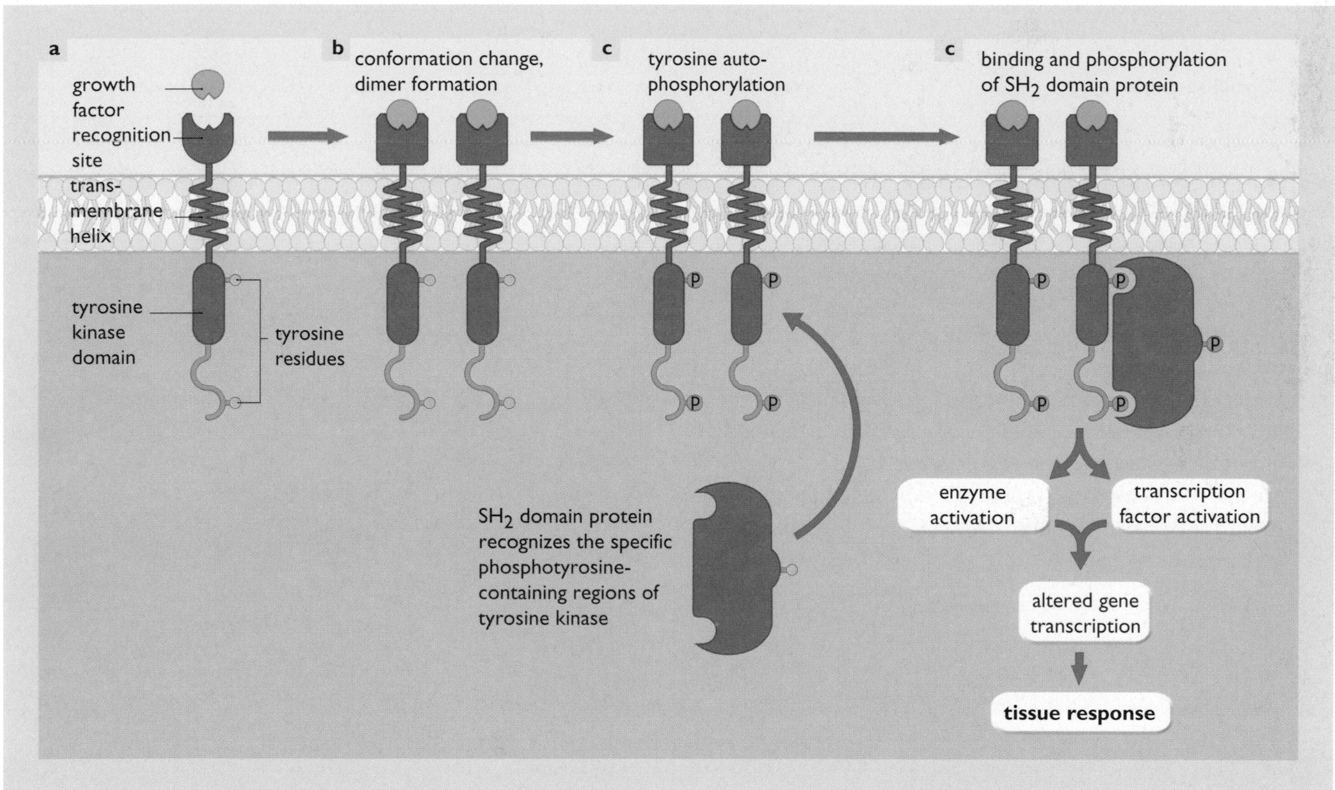

Fig. 3.24 Transduction mechanisms for receptors that act as enzymes. (a) The binding of a growth factor to its receptor domain (b) leads to conformational changes resulting in dimer formation. This results in autophosphorylation of the tyrosine residues in the tyrosine kinase domain of the receptor (c). The specific phosphotyrosine-containing regions of the tyrosine kinase domain then bind the SH_2 domain which results in activation of various intracellular responses leading to the tissue response (d). (Adapted with permission from *Pharmacology, 3rd edn*, by Rang, Dale, and Ritter, Churchill Livingstone, 1995.)

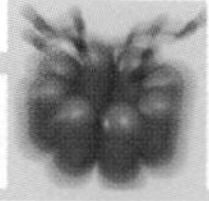

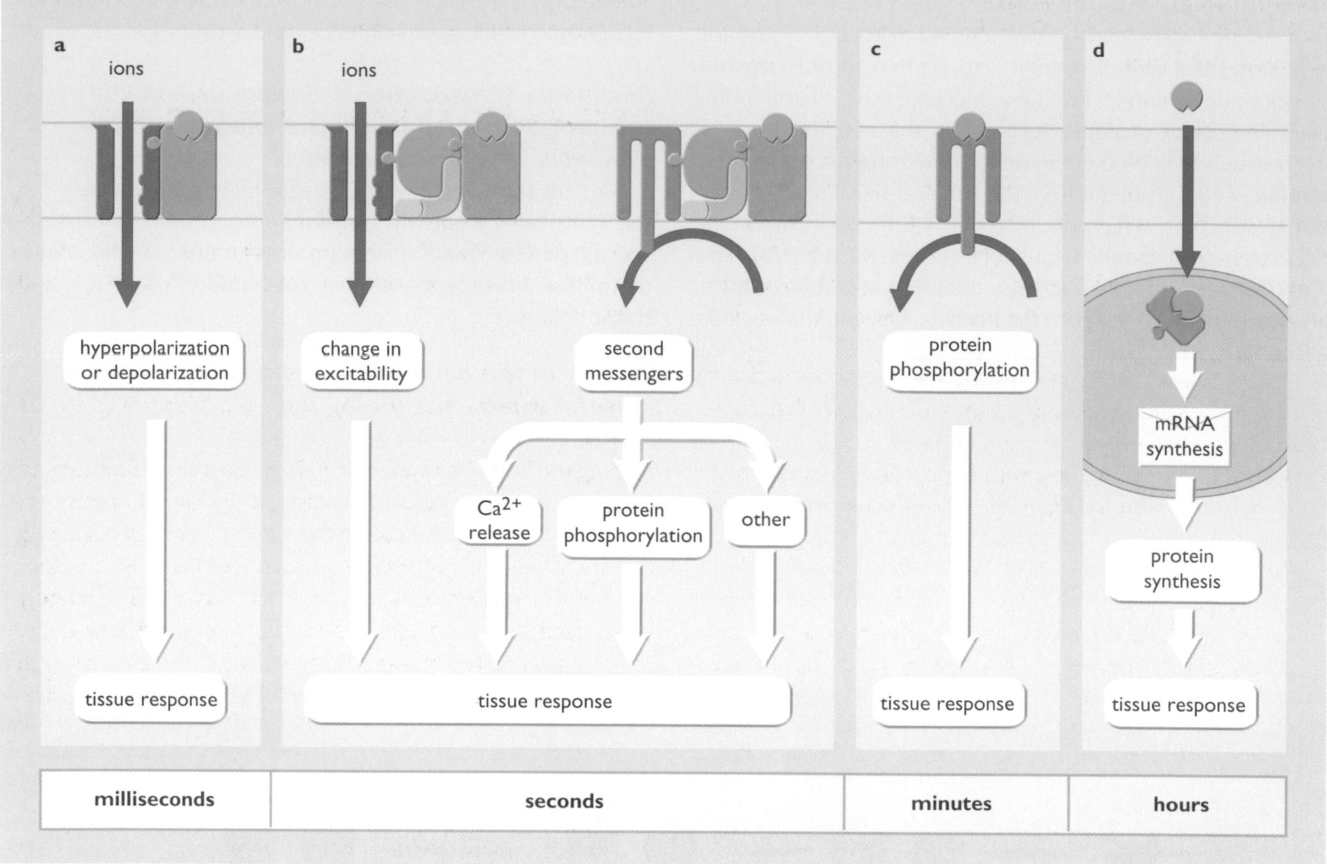

Fig. 3.25 Integration of molecular and cellular mechanisms. (a) Receptor-operated ion channel-linked transduction is very rapid. (b) G protein-linked transduction is rapid. (c) G protein-independent enzyme-initiated transduction is slow. (d) DNA-linked transduction is very slow.

The receptors for steroid hormones provide a good example of how transduction operates:

- Glucocorticosteroids increase the production of lipocortin, which accounts for some of their actions as anti-inflammatory drugs (see Chapter 11).
- Mineralocorticosteroids increase the production of specific renal transport molecules involved in the renal tubular transport of Na^+ and K^+ (Fig. 3.26).

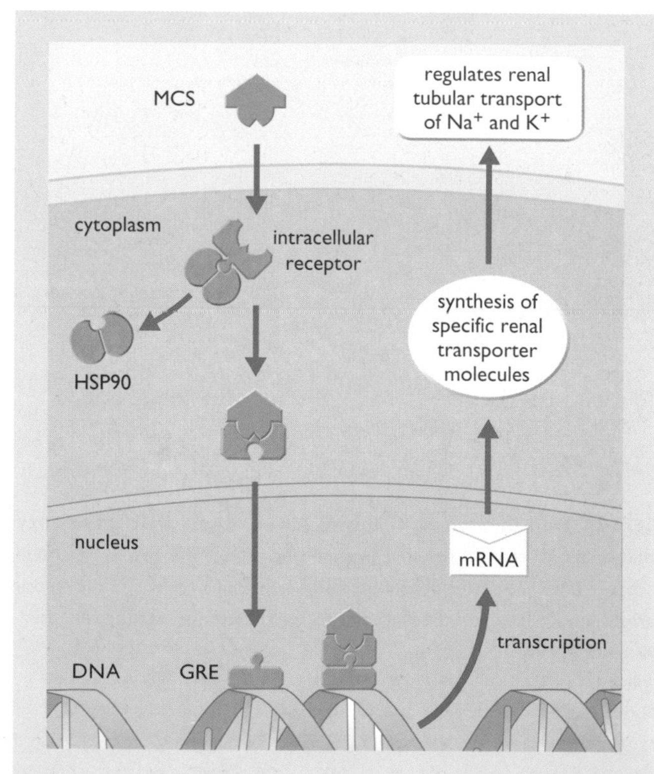

Fig. 3.26 Example of transduction involving DNA-linked receptors. Mineralocorticosteroids (MCS) bind to intracellular receptors (GR) which are normally associated with two molecules of a 90 kDa heat shock protein (HSP90). The MCS–receptor complex translocates to the nucleus and binds to glucocorticosteroid response elements (GRE) in the promoter sequences of target genes. This leads to an increase in transcription of new proteins (such as renal transporter molecules, which enhance Na^+ reabsorption).

EXAMPLES OF INTEGRATION OF MOLECULAR AND CELLULAR MECHANISMS

Receptors and other molecular targets link to the cellular response components in the transduction cascade. Here, some examples of this integration of molecular and cellular mechanisms are described. Characteristically, the speed of transduction, and production of the tissue response, is determined by both molecular and cellular components (see Fig. 3.25). The speed of transduction determines the onset of the tissue response. For example:

- Interaction of an agonist with a receptor-operated ion channel produces rapid (milliseconds) hyperpolarization or depolarization.
- Interaction of an agonist with G protein-linked receptor may lead to one of many responses on a timescale of seconds.
- Interaction of a drug with a G protein-independent enzyme may lead to changes on a timescale of minutes.
- Interaction of a drug with DNA-linked transduction may lead to altered gene expression and the synthesis of a new protein over a period of hours.

Some examples of these types of transduction and their molecular initiation are shown in Figs 3.26–3.31.

TISSUE AND SYSTEM TARGETS FOR DRUGS

It can be relatively simple to determine the mechanisms of action of a drug at a molecular and cellular level, but it is more difficult to determine the mechanisms of action at the tissue and system level.

Division of the body into systems is artificial, but is useful when considering a drug's mechanisms of action

Dividing the body into systems can be subject to preference and prejudice, but most researchers accept that certain body systems can be effectively compartmentalized, while recognizing that the whole body integrates all such systems. It is therefore possible to consider the action of drugs on the CNS separately from their actions on the cardiovascular or endocrine systems.

As an example, the actions of some drugs used to treat high blood pressure can be easily explained solely in terms of their

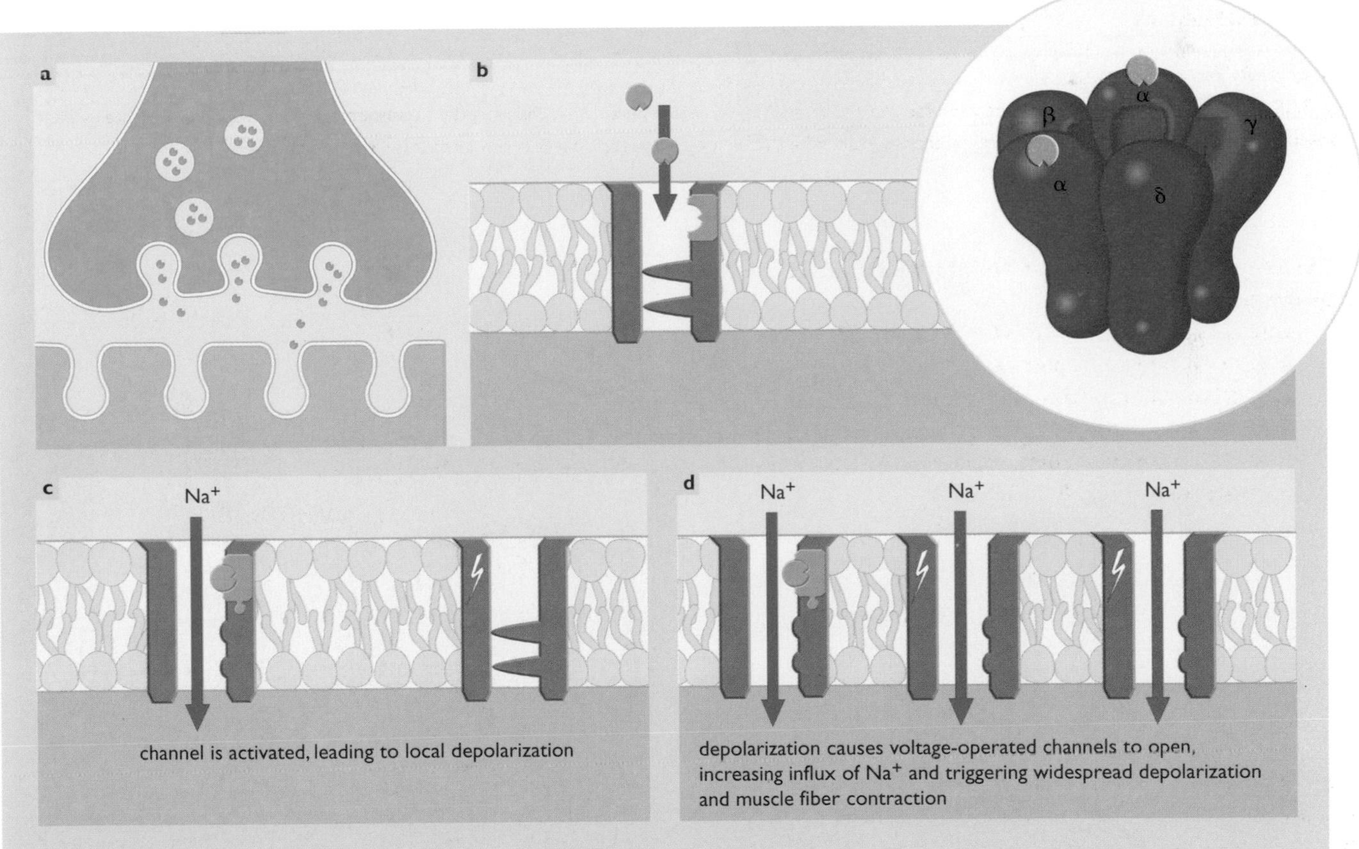

Fig. 3.27 Example of receptor-operated ion channel-linked transduction. (a) In response to an electrical impulse arriving at the nerve ending, vesicles of acetylcholine (ACh) fuse with the membrane of the nerve terminal, resulting in liberation of ACh into the synaptic cleft. (b) ACh binds to ligand-recognition sites within the α subunits of the ion channel (insert) leading to opening of the ion channel, allowing an influx of Na^+, causing local depolarization (c). This depolarization initiates transduction, causing voltage-operated channels to open in the adjacent regions of the membrane, increasing a further influx of Na+ and thus triggering widespread depolarization and muscle fiber contraction (d).

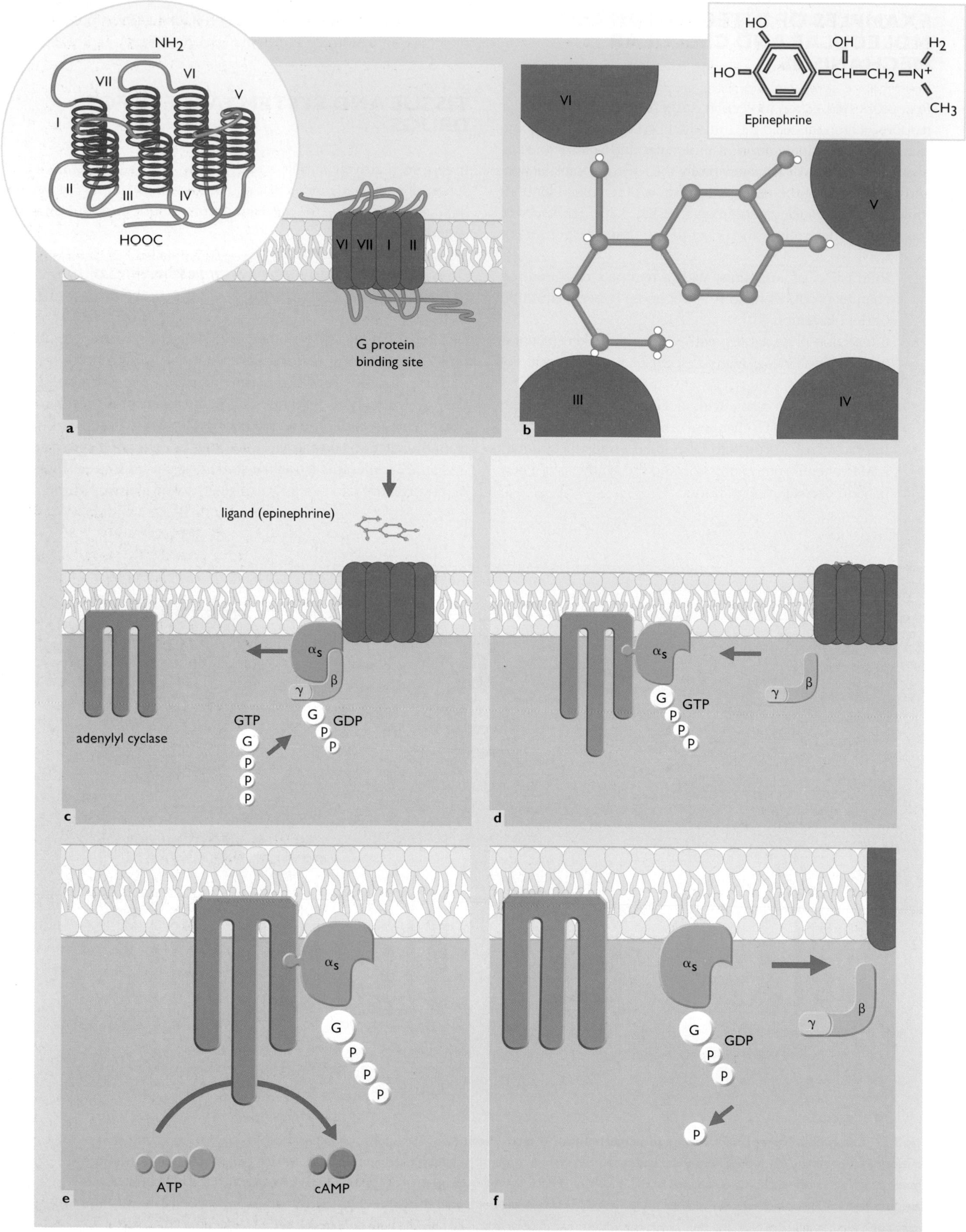

NH2
VII
VI
V
I
II
III
IV
HOOC
VI VII I II
G protein binding site
a

HO
OH
H2
HO
CH
CH2
N+
CH3
Epinephrine
VI
V
III
IV
b

ligand (epinephrine)
αs
β
γ
G
GDP
P
P
GTP
G
P
P
P
adenylyl cyclase
c

αs
G
GTP
P
P
P
γ
β
d

αs
G
P
P
P
ATP
cAMP
e

αs
G
GDP
P
P
P
γ
β
f

Fig. 3.28 Example of G protein-linked transduction. (a) Seven-domain transmembrane-spanning receptor (in this example, the β adrenoceptor). (b) Agonist (e.g. epinephrine). (c) Molecular action of epinephrine (β adrenoceptor agonism) and the first stage of transduction (dissociation of the α subunit from the G protein). (d) Next stage of transduction: activation of effector protein (adenylyl cyclase enzyme) by the α subunit of the G protein. (e) Next stage of transduction: hydrolysis of ATP by activated adenylyl cyclase enzyme. (f) Transduction ceases when the α subunit of the G protein dissociates from the effector protein.

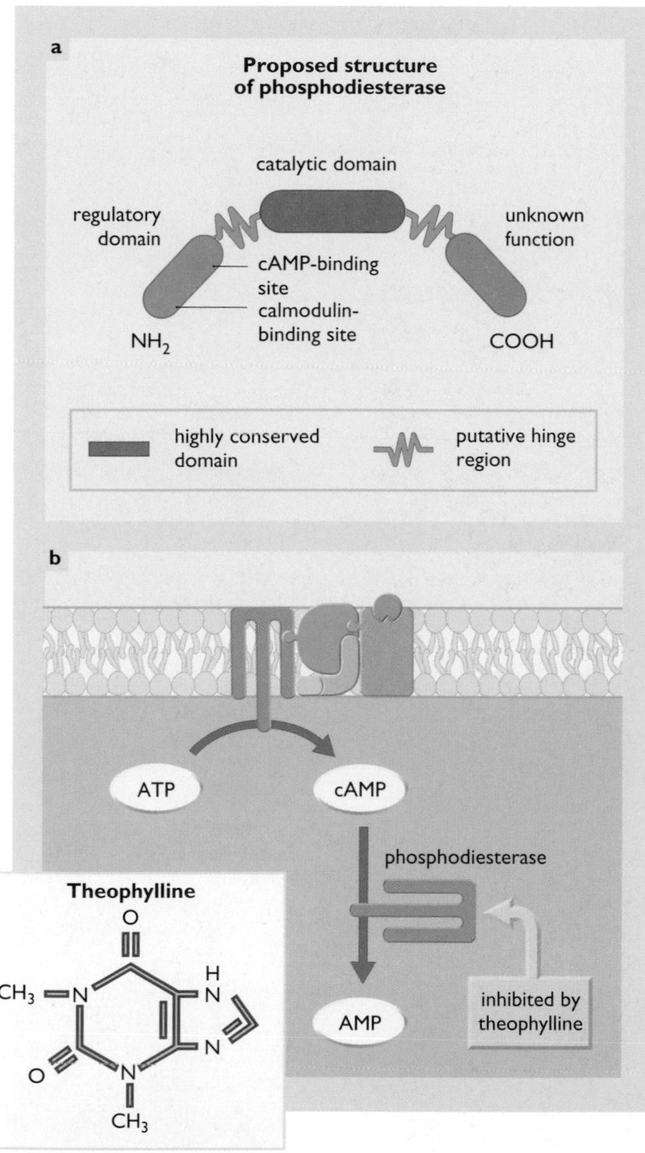

Fig. 3.29 Example of enzyme-initiated transduction. Phosphodiesterase enzymes are involved in the metabolism of the cyclic nucleotides (e.g. cAMP). This family of enzymes is inhibited by theophylline. Inhibition leads to accumulation of cyclic nucleotides within cells. Note that cyclic nucleotides accumulate in response to the action of drugs on G protein-linked nucleotide cyclase enzymes.

actions on the cardiovascular system. Obviously, actions on the cardiovascular system must have implications for the rest of the body. However, when examining mechanisms of drug action it is reasonable for the sake of simplicity sometimes to consider only the target system itself and regard all other actions as a consequence of the effects on the target system.

A limited number of systems are considered in this section. Special emphasis is given to the autonomic nervous system, which has an effect on the activity of other systems and represents one of the most pharmacologically explored of the body systems.

Tissue and system responses are intimately linked. The tissue mechanism of drug action has been considered along with the system mechanisms in this section. The reason is that it is difficult to divorce a tissue response (such as muscle contraction, electrical activity, secretion, or cell division) from the system that the tissue is part of (e.g. heart and cardiovascular system).

The influence of nerves, hormones, and vascular factors varies with different tissues

Most tissues are innervated by one or all of the various subdivisions of the autonomic nervous system, but each tissue has its own individual pattern of innervation. In some tissues autonomic innervation is unimportant in controlling the function of that tissue or its response to drugs, whereas in others it plays a major role. Some tissues are dominated by the adrenergic system and others by the cholinergic system, while in others there is an equal balance between the two systems. Although the classic adrenergic and cholinergic autonomic nervous systems are important, there is a growing realization that the NANC system also has an important role.

Tissues have widely varying mechanisms for controlling their blood flow

Tissues vary widely in the mechanisms they use to control their blood flow, although in most there is a standard arterial and venous vasculature. The only major differences in vascular anatomy is that some tissues may contain only end arteries whereas others have collaterals. The control of flow in such vessels, however, varies markedly, in that each tissue has its own balance of autoregulation of blood flow versus adrenergic or other ubiquitous blood-vessel controlling mechanisms such as endothelin, NO, or angiotensin. Those tissues that exhibit marked autoregulation, such as the brain and heart, do so by autoregulation systems that are relatively specific to that particular tissue.

KIDNEY

The kidneys are the major excretory tissues in the body for many substances. They control the salt and water content of the blood and therefore of the entire body. In addition, they excrete the waste products of metabolism, such as urea, uric acid, and creatinine.

The kidneys filter renal blood flow in the glomerulus and produce an ultrafiltrate, which then can be added to or subtracted from during its passage through the renal tubule. Renal function depends upon the adequacy of blood flow through

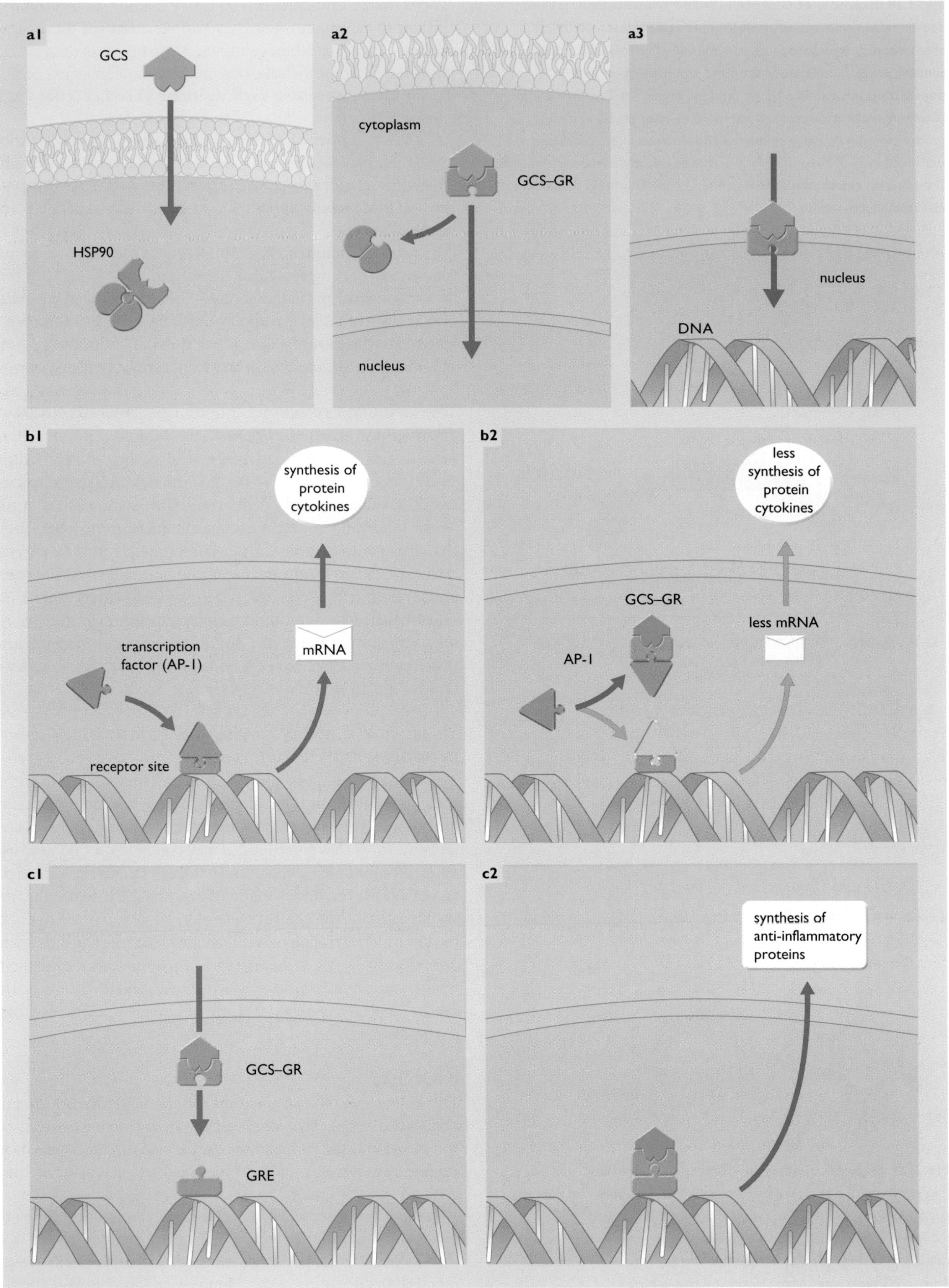

a1
GCS
HSP90

a2
cytoplasm
GCS–GR
nucleus

a3
nucleus
DNA

b1
synthesis of protein cytokines
transcription factor (AP-1)
mRNA
receptor site

b2
less synthesis of protein cytokines
GCS–GR
less mRNA
AP-1

c1
GCS–GR
GRE

c2
synthesis of anti-inflammatory proteins

Fig. 3.30 Example of DNA-linked transduction Glucocorticosteroids are thought to exert anti-inflammatory effects by at least two distinct mechanisms. (a1) Glucocorticosteriods (GCS) cross the cell membrane and bind with receptors located in the cytoplasm (here bound in an inactive form to heat shock protein 90, HSP90). (a2) First stage of transduction: dissociation of the glucocorticosteroid receptor complex (GCS–GR) from HSP90. (a3) Next stage of transduction: translocation of GCS–GR into the cell nucleus. (b1) In some cells, the synthesis of a protein (e.g. pro-inflammatory cytokines) can be initiated by transcription factors acting on their own receptors. (b2) Once in the nucleus, GCS–GR binds to (and 'mops up') the transcription factor (e.g. AP-1), thereby reducing the amount of new protein synthesized. If this protein is a pro-inflammatory mediator (e.g. a cytokine), the net effect is to reduce inflammation. (c1) Alternatively, GCS–GR may bind with a glucocorticosteroid response element (GRE, a receptor on DNA). (c2) Binding of GCS–GR to the GRE inhibits the synthesis of proteins (e.g. anti-inflammatory lipocortins).

the kidney, the renal nerves, and hormones present in the blood. Blood flow through the kidney is autoregulated. There are therefore a number of possible tissue mechanisms by which drugs can exert renal actions. The most important of such drugs are the diuretics (see Chapter 10).

In addition, the kidney secretes renin, which results in the subsequent release of hormones such as aldosterone. The following description of the mechanisms by which drugs can influence the renal system is based upon the structure of the nephron, discussed in detail in Chapter 10.

Drugs acting on the glomerulus

At the level of the glomerulus, blood is filtered by hydrostatic forces to form an ultrafiltrate. This ultrafiltrate contains the small molecular components of the blood, since proteins are unable to pass through the glomerular filtration membrane. However, if the membrane is damaged, protein will pass into the urine.

Drugs acting on the renal tubule

Once the ultrafiltrate leaves the glomerulus it is exposed to the absorptive and secretive processes of the various cells that line the renal tubule. Diuretic drugs can influence both these processes. Different types of diuretics inhibit the reabsorption of Na^+, K^+, and bicarbonate ions.

> **Sites of drug action in the kidney**
>
> - The glomerulus
> - The tubule
> - The loop of Henle
> - The distal tubule and collecting ducts

The tisssue action of diuretics is to increase the flow of urine from the kidneys. It is possible to achieve this by a variety of different mechanisms (see Chapter 10).

Antidiuretic hormone acts on the distal tubule and collecting ducts

The free water content of the ultrafiltrate can also be reduced as the filtrate passes through the distal tubule and down the collecting ducts into the ureters and bladder. The permeability of this part of the kidney is altered by antidiuretic hormone, and high concentrations of this hormone result in the production of a highly concentrated urine.

HEART

The mechanisms of action of drugs on the heart may be direct or indirect

For example, β adrenoceptor agonists directly produce inotropic effects (i.e increase force of contraction). However, drugs that activate sympathetic nerves in the heart indirectly have inotropic effects mediated by the release of norepinephrine. Other drugs, such as α_1 receptor agonists, indirectly modulate cardiac function by changing peripheral vascular resistance or rate of return of blood to the heart.

The types of tissue responses produced in the heart are electrical, mechanical, and secretory. Electrical responses involve changes in propagation of the cardiac action potential relevant to the control of cardiac rhythm (see Chapter 8). Mechanical responses include contractile responses in the heart and in coronary arteries. An increase in myocardial contraction is positive inotropy. An increase in myocardial relaxation is positive leusitropy. Likewise, an increase in heart rate is positive chronotropy. In the coronary vasculature, vasodilation and vasoconstriction are possible. These tissue responses are relevant to heart failure, angina, and other diseases (see Chapter 8).

Secretory responses are more complex, and include secretion of vasoactive substances from coronary endothelium and endocardium, secretion of immunoactive substances from specialized cardiac cells, and secretion of neurotransmitters.

LUNGS

Drugs with a tissue mechanism of action restricted primarily to the lung act either on:

- The airways.
- The pulmonary vasculature.
- The immune system in the lung.

Part of the treatment of asthma is the prevention or reversal of the bronchospasm (bronchoconstriction) of airway smooth muscle, which causes the wheezing in asthma. This can be achieved at a number of different levels, including:

- Moderation of the immune process at a fundamental level as occurs with corticosteroids.
- At the level of the autacoids that mediate the allergic response (muscarinic antagonists, H_1 antihistamines to some extent, and leukotriene antagonists).
- Direct relaxation of the smooth muscle of the airways (see Chapter 11).

Relaxation of bronchial smooth muscle in asthma can be achieved indirectly by preventing the action of bronchoconstrictor substances at their receptors or by producing direct relaxation of the smooth muscle.

BRAIN

Mechanisms of drug action on the brain can involve many cell types, cellular organizations, and transmitter substances. The function of the brain arises from its structure at a cellular and molecular level, with specific areas having a specific function, but connected to all other parts of the brain. Each neuron also has the potential for both releasing and sensing a variety of neurotransmitters. There are many brain neurotransmitters, including acetylcholine, catechol and other amines, amino acids, and polypeptides, and they act upon many different types and subtypes of receptor.

One class of drugs that act in the brain is the general anesthetics (see Chapter 7). These compounds share a common tissue mechanism of action despite possessing a range of different molecular and cellular mechanisms of action. As indicated in Chapter 2, these drugs are grouped together only because they share the common property of being able to produce a general loss of consciousness that allows surgery to be performed.

Loss of consciousness with anesthetics is associated with the same tissue response, a reduction in the bioelectric activity in the brain.

In the case of other drugs, relatively discrete regions of brain tissue are affected. This is a consequence of the molecular mechanim of action of such drugs—modulation of receptors and ion channels that are discretely expressed in specific brain regions.

GASTROINTESTINAL TRACT

Drugs used on the gastrointestinal tract have secretory and motility tissue actions, or actions on microflora.

Stomach

One of the most common disorders of the stomach and the proximal portion of the small intestine, the duodenum, is peptic ulceration. This is generally associated with a pathogenic bacterium, *Heliobacter pylori*, the necrotizing actions of which are exacerbated by gastric acid and possibly by stomach hypermotility. Acid secretion by the stomach is controlled by the vagus nerve and hormones such as gastrin.

The tissue mechanism of action of the drugs used to treat peptic ulcer is thus 'antacid,' although the molecular mechanism of actions of antiulcer drugs can vary:

- Antibiotic therapy involves agents that have lethal actions on the causative organism.
- Acetylcholine and histamine antagonists and the selective muscarinic, pirenzepine, reduce acid secretion, but not to the same degree as can be achieved with H_2 antagonists such as cimetidine and ranitidine. More effective than either of these is the inhibitor of the K^+/H^+ transporter, omeprazole.

Small intestine

The major function of the small intestine is absorption (e.g. of amino acids, sugars, and fats). It is controlled by the vagus nerve. It is not an important tissue target for therapeutic drugs.

Large intestine

The major function of the large intestine is to prepare solid waste for excretion in the form of feces. The water content of the material in the large intestine is controlled by water absorption, and a well-coordinated nervous system coupled to the inherent automaticity of the colonic smooth muscle ensures the orderly and appropriate expulsion of feces. The large colon also contains many commensal bacteria.

The main disorders of the large intestine concern the transit time of gastrointestinal contents , which is either too rapid, causing diarrhea, or too slow, resulting in constipation. These problems can arise from inappropriate motility or excessive secretions.

PERIPHERAL AUTONOMIC NERVOUS SYSTEM

The peripheral autonomic nervous system is responsible for interacting with and regulating various body systems. The action of drugs on the autonomic nervous system may be considered mainly in terms of the subsequent influence on the cardiovascular system.

The autonomic nervous system is composed of three major elements:

- The afferent limb.
- The central integrated elements.
- The efferent limb.

The afferent limb carries information from sensors (neuronal receptors sited at the ends of afferent nerves) to the spinal cord and the rest of the CNS. Most of this information is then processed within the hypothalamus and other parts of the lower brain. After processing, appropriate signals are passed from the CNS and down the efferent nerves to the effector organs (Fig. 3.31), which are so named because they produce the responses to activity in the CNS.

Although the autonomic nervous system is considered in detail in Chapter 7, the actions of some drugs on the autonomic nervous system are discussed here to illustrate drug mechanisms of action.

The efferent part of the autonomic nervous system is divided into three separate types on the basis of its anatomy and neurotransmitters:

- The parasympathetic (cholinergic) system.
- The sympathetic (adrenergic) system.
- The nonadrenergic and noncholinergic (NANC) system.

A cholinergic system is one in which the primary neurotransmitter is acetylcholine

Acetylcholine is the neurotransmitter released from presynaptic terminals in the autonomic ganglia and from the prejunctional nerve endings at the effector organ (Fig. 3.32). The receptors of the cholinergic system that bind acetylcholine are cholinoceptors. Cholinoceptors include those classified as muscarinic and nicotinic receptors.

An adrenergic system is one in which the neurotransmitter is related to certain products of the adrenal medulla (epinephrine and norepinephrine)

The other major limb of the autonomic nervous system is the adrenergic system. The nomenclature is an historical accident, as when the system was first described, there was no clear separation between two possible transmitters, namely epinephrine and norepinephrine. It is now known that apart from the special case for the adrenal glands, which secrete epinephrine (adrenaline), the neurotransmitter is always norepinephrine.

The preganglionic transmitter for both the cholinergic and the adrenergic systems is acetylcholine

The efferent nerves for both the cholinergic and the adrenergic systems arise from the appropriate parts of the brain stem and the spinal cord. These efferent nerves then synapse at ganglia situated throughout the body.

- In the adrenergic system, the ganglia lie mainly in a chain close to the spinal cord, known as the paravertebral sympathetic chain.
- In the cholinergic system, the ganglia are usually situated close to or on their effector organ.

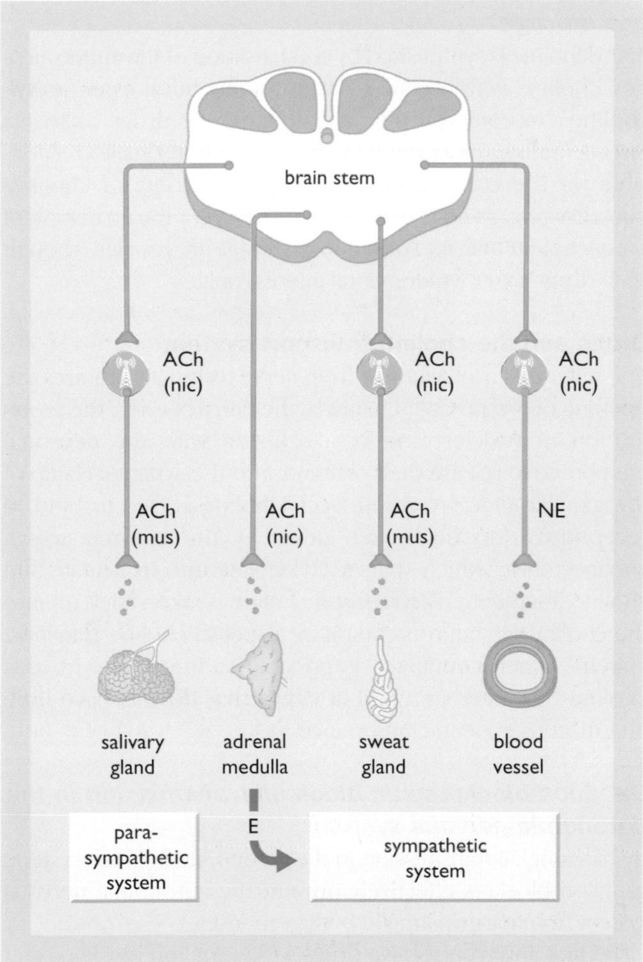

Fig. 3.31 Acetylcholine (ACh) and norepinephrine (NE) are the major neurotransmitters in the peripheral autonomic nervous system. ACh acts on peripheral tissues via two types of receptor, nicotinic (nic) or muscarinic (mus), depending on the tissue. NE acts on peripheral tissues via at least two types of receptors, α and β, depending on the tissue. (E, epinephrine)

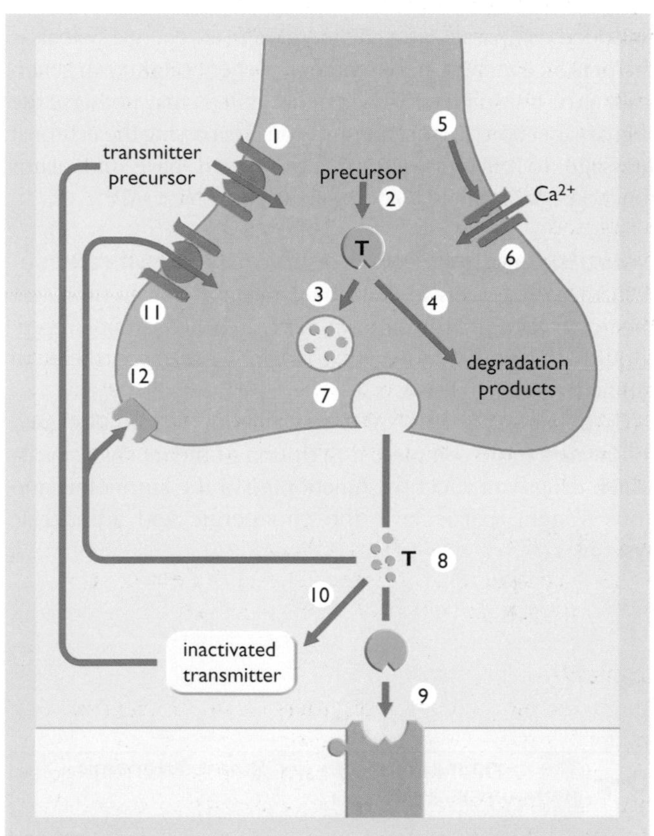

Fig. 3.32 Processes generally involved in the synthesis, storage, and release of neurotransmitters. 1 = uptake of precursors; 2 = synthesis of transmitter; 3 = storage of transmitter in vesicles; 4 = degradation of surplus transmitter; 5 = depolarization by prolonged action potential; 6 = influx of Ca^{2+} through N-type Ca^{2+} channels in reponse to depolarization; 7 = release of transmitter by exocytosis; 8 = diffusion to postsynaptic membrane; 9 = interaction with postsynaptic receptors; 10 = inactivation of transmitter; 11 = reuptake of transmitter or degradation products; 12 = interaction with presynaptic receptors. These processes are well characterized for many transmitters (e.g. acetylcholine, norepinephrine, dopamine, 5-hydroxytryptamine), but may well differ by omission of some of the processes for other transmitters (e.g. amino acids, purines, peptides). (Adapted with permission from *Pharmacology, 3rd edn*, by Rang, Dale, and Ritter, Churchill Livingstone, 1995.)

Despite this clear anatomic distinction, both types of ganglia use acetylcholine as the principal ganglionic transmitter.

The nonadrenergic, noncholinergic system is a third component of the autonomic system

In addition to the cholinergic and adrenergic system, it has been recognized over recent decades that parts of the autonomic nervous system are neither cholinergic nor adrenergic. This section of the autonomic nervous system is therefore known as the nonadrenergic, noncholinergic (NANC) system. It is not clear which neurotransmitters act in this system, although nitric oxide has recently been suggested to be the major neurotransmitter in NANC nerves in various parts of the body.

Co-transmitters add complexity to the cholinergic and adrenergic systems

An added complication for cholinergic and adrenergic systems is the presence in these nerve endings of chemicals known generically as co-transmitters. These co-transmitters may not serve the primary function of neurotransmission (i.e. passing the neuronal message to effector tissue), but instead have modulator functions. An example is adenosine triphosphate (ATP).

Neurotransmitters can modulate their own release

A further complexity is that neurotransmitters can modulate their own release. Neurotransmitters can act back upon receptors on the nerve ending that originally released them, to inhibit their own release.

(Co-transmission and NANC transmission will be discussed following a more complete description of the mechanisms by which drugs can affect the functioning of the autonomic nervous system, particularly the cholinergic and adrenergic systems.)

The components of the peripheral autonomic nervous system

- The autonomic nervous system is composed of an afferent limb, an efferent limb, and central integrating elements
- The efferent limb divides into the parasympathetic (cholinergic) system, the sympathetic (adrenergic) system, and the nonadrenergic noncholinergic (NANC) system
- In the cholinergic system the neurotransmitter is acetylcholine
- In the adrenergic system the neurotransmitter is norepinephrine; epinephrine is released primarily from the adrenals

Cholinergic and adrenergic ganglia cannot be differentiated from each other pharmacologically

Both cholinergic and adrenergic ganglia are considered together in the following discussion since they cannot be differentiated from each other by pharmacologic means, despite their different anatomic locations.

The term 'preganglionic fibers' refers to neuronal axons that arise in the CNS and terminate on cell bodies in the ganglia; they are primarily cholinergic. Axons arising from the cell bodies in the ganglia and terminating at the effector tissue are known as postganglionic fibers. Some postganglionic adrenergic fibers have been found to innervate cholinergic ganglia, adding further complexity to the two systems.

Drugs and ganglionic transmission

Given that transmission in ganglia is primarily cholinergic, it is possible to understand the mechanisms by which drugs may interfere with ganglionic transmission, either to accentuate or to block transmission.

Drugs can interfere with acetylcholine synthesis and storage

Acetylcholine is synthesized by condensation of the amino alcohol, choline, with acetate to form the chemical ester, acetylcholine. No common pharmacotherapeutic drugs or toxins directly inhibit the enzyme (acetylcholine transferase) responsible for the condensation. However, a variety of cholinomimetics (e.g. analogs of choline) can prevent the formation of acetylcholine and its subsequent storage in vesicles, though such drugs are of experimental interest only.

Drugs and the choline transport system

The release of acetylcholine from nerve terminals requires the opening of N-type Ca^{2+} channels, the entry of Ca^{2+}, the mobilization of vesicles, and vesicle fusion with the neuronal membrane to release their contents into the synaptic clamp of the ganglia. Once released, acetylcholine is free to bind to receptors or to be broken down by the enzyme acetylcholinesterase, which splits acetylcholine into its acetate and choline fragments. The released choline is taken back up into the cholinergic neuron ending by a special choline transport system. Experimentally, it is possible to interfere with this choline transport system, but drugs that do this have little pharmacotherapeutic importance.

Ganglion blockers can block all transmission in the autonomic nervous system

By blocking all transmission in the autonomic nervous system, ganglion blockers effectively prevent the autonomic nervous system from participating in body responses.

The first antihypertensive drugs were ganglion blockers, and when they were given in effective doses the resulting wide range of signs and symptoms gave a clear insight into the importance of the autonomic nervous system to humans. A full ganglion-blocking dose of the drug produces a variety of signs and symptoms, including the following:

- Inability to accommodate vision for near sight.
- Drying of secretions in the mouth, stomach, and eyes.
- Constipation.
- Difficulty with urination.
- Loss of sexual function in the male.
- Orthostatic hypotension.

These symptoms emphasize the importance of resting tone in the autonomic nervous system. Both parasympathetic and sympathetic ganglia are blocked by ganglion blockers because these drugs are not selective for different ganglia.

The molecular mechanism of action of ganglion blockers, which is not relevant to this section, is nicotinic antagonism.

Adrenergic nervous system

The adrenergic nervous system innervates many parts of the body, but particularly:

- The gut.
- The heart.
- The lungs.
- Blood vessels.

The adrenergic system innervates some tissues (e.g. the gut) via the cholinergic ganglia. This means that the role of the adrenergic nervous system in the gut and, to a lesser extent, in the lung, is to control activity in the parasympathetic cholinergic ganglia.

The three adrenergic neurotransmitters of interest are norepinephrine, epinephrine, and dopamine

Two of the three adrenergic neurotransmitters are found in the peripheral nervous system and in the CNS, whereas the third, dopamine, is found primarily (although not exclusively) in the CNS.

Norepinephrine, epinephrine, and dopamine are all formed from the same precursor essential amino acid, tyrosine. Tyrosine is exposed to a cascade of enzymes in the adrenergic nerve ending (Fig. 3.33) where synthesis stops at norepinephrine in noradrenergic neurons or dopamine in dopaminergic neurons. Very little of the tyrosine is metabolized to the *N*-methyl product of norepinephrine (epinephrine) in neurons. However, the adrenal gland, which is a very discrete organ lying above the kidney, is an exception. The outer part (cortex) of the gland is

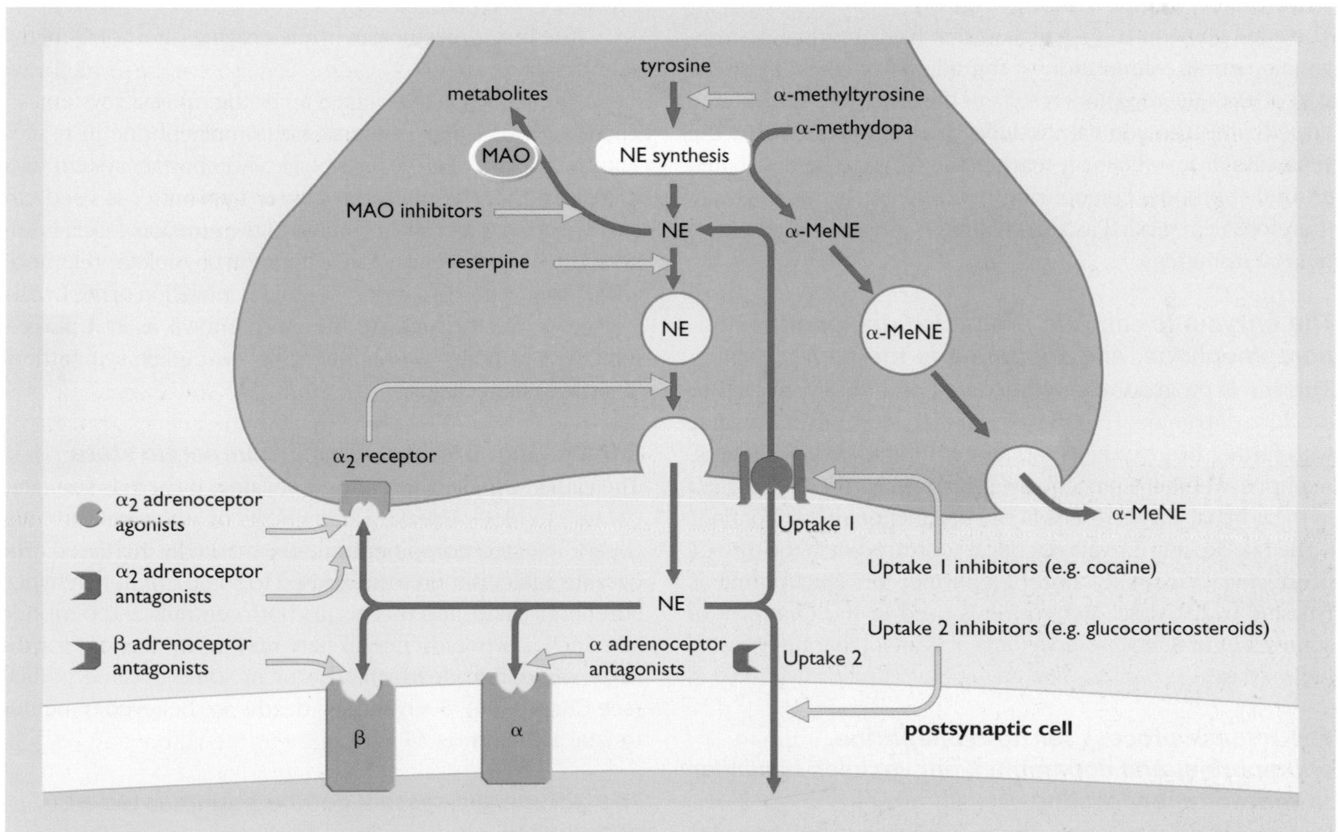

Fig. 3.33 Drug actions on the noradrenergic (sympathetic) nervous system. The molecular actions shown here, at the nerve terminal, affect the noradrenergic system throughout the body. Drugs may affect synthesis, storage, release, uptake, and receptors. (MAO, monoamine oxidase; α-MeNE, α-methylnorepinephrine; NE, norepinephrine) (Adapted with permission from *Pharmacology, 3rd edn*, by Rang, Dale, and Ritter, Churchill Livingstone, 1995.)

involved in the synthesis of steroid hormones, particularly glucocorticosteroids and mineralocorticoids, whereas epinephrine is synthesized in the center of the gland (medulla). High concentrations of cortisol activate expression of phenylethanolamine *N*-methyl transferase, the enzyme catalyzing the conversion of norepinephrine to epinephrine.

> **The three important adrenergic neurotransmitters**
>
> - **Norepinephrine, which is found in the peripheral nervous system and in the CNS**
> - **Epinephrine, which is found predominantly in the adrenal medulla and in the CNS**
> - **Dopamine, which is found primarily in the CNS**

The adrenal medulla is effectively a highly specialized sympathetic ganglion

The adrenal medulla is a ganglion that has a residual postganglionic neuron. Stimulation of the adrenal medulla by activation of nicotinic receptors results in the release of epinephrine directly into the adrenal medullary veins and then into the vena cava, from whence it reaches the heart to be distributed around the body. Epinephrine released in this manner can therefore be regarded as a circulating hormone, rather than a neurotransmitter.

The enzymatic cascade producing epinephrine, norepinephrine, and dopamine is the same

Tyrosine is progressively hydroxylated and decarboxylated to produce dopamine. The process can then stop, or can continue with further hydroxylation and methylation to produce norepinephrine, where the process can again stop. Further methylation in the adrenal glands results in the production of epinephrine.

The rate-limiting enzyme or critical control point in the cascade producing dopamine, norepinephrine, or epinephrine is tyrosine hydroxylase. Metyrosine is used in the treatment of some cases of pheochromocytoma; it is an inhibitor of tyrosine hydroxylase.

The release process for norepinephrine, epinephrine, and dopamine from vesicles is similar to that for acetylcholine

Once synthesized, norepinephrine, epinephrine, and dopamine are packaged into vesicles where they are complexed to ATP and a special vesicular protein. Release of the contents of such vesicles is by the same type of process as for acetylcholine. The arrival of an action potential at the postganglionic nerve ending results in the opening of N-type Ca^{2+} channels, which allow the intracellular flow of Ca^{2+}. The elevation of Ca^{2+} in the nerve endings results in the subsequent mobilization of the vesicles, which fuse with the membrane of the nerve ending. As a result the released norepinephrine diffuses across the junctional cleft to bind to adrenoceptors. Postjunctional adrenoceptors, the molecular targets, are discussed in subsequent chapters.

As with acetylcholine, there is a highly effective system for re-using norepinephrine

Once norepinephrine has acted upon the postjunctional receptor:

- Some diffuses from the junctional cleft.
- Some acts upon prejunctional receptors on postganglionic nerve endings to inhibit the release of more norepinephrine. The receptor here is the α_2 subtype.
- Most is taken back into the nerve terminal. This reuptake requires a special process involving a norepinephrine transporter located in the cell membrane. This transporter carries norepinephrine back into the nerve ending where it is either broken down by the enzyme monoamine oxidase located on mitochondria or it is repackaged into vesicles. Thus, with acetylcholine and the cholinergic system, there is a highly effective system for reusing the transmitter substance.

Any norepinephrine that escapes from the junctional cleft is exposed to two possible fates.

- The first is metabolism by the enzyme catechol-*O*-methyl transferase.
- The second is to be taken up by the Uptake 2 system.

There are two Uptake systems for norepinephrine in tissues. The first, Uptake 1, is the physiologically important system since it ensures that the neurotransmitter transmitter is used efficiently and that its residence time in the junctional cleft is limited. The second, Uptake 2, is of doubtful physiologic relevance.

The major action of a variety of drugs is inhibition of the Uptake 1 process. Such drugs are therefore known as as Uptake 1 inhibitors. Uptake 1 inhibition has complex sympathetic nervous system effects.

Cocaine can produce a hyperadrenergic state

The classic Uptake 1 inhibitor is cocaine. If there is sufficient cocaine to block Uptake 1, the effects of adrenergic stimulation or injected norepinephrine are markedly increased. The cocaine addict is therefore exposed to some extent to a hyperadrenergic state, and this occurs both centrally and peripherally. Such a hyperadrenergic state may partly account for the cases of sudden death that occur in some cocaine addicts (see Chapter 30). Such sudden deaths are believed to be due to fatal arrhythmias.

The adrenergic system can be manipulated at different levels

It is apparent that the adrenergic system can be manipulated at a number of different levels:

- By sympathomimetic drugs, which are agonists.
- By inhibiting Uptake 1 or the enzyme monoamine oxidase.
- By interfering with the storage of norepinephrine in vesicles.

- By disrupting the process that results in the release of vesicles.

Drugs that reduce norepinephrine storage and release affect the adrenergic system to reduce the level of activity. Therapeutically, this can be advantageous (e.g. in the treatment of hypertension).

Drugs interfering with the adrenergic system innervating blood vessels may cause postural hypotension

One adverse system effect of adrenergic neuron blockers is postural hypotension (dramatic fall in blood pressure on rising to a standing position from a previous sitting or supine position). The fall in blood pressure can be profound and cause dizziness or even fainting. This is because normally there is increased activation of the adrenergic system innervating veins and arteries on standing up, resulting in:

- Vasoconstriction (a squeezing action on capacitance veins), which ensures an adequate venous return to the heart and sufficient cardiac output to maintain blood pressure.
- Vasoconstriction of arteries to maintain the blood pressure.

As a result of these two system mechanisms, blood flow in the cerebral arteries is maintained. Impairment of these mechanisms impairs the ability of patients to stand up.

Cholinergic system

The mechanisms of synthesis and release of acetylcholine in the cholinergic autonomic nervous system are similar to those that occur in the parasympathetic and sympathetic preganglionic neurons of the autonomic nervous system. However, the postsynaptic receptors are muscarinic (not nicotinic) (Fig. 3.34).

The system responses to acetylcholine are diverse, and depend on the type of muscarinic receptor mediating the molecular response (M_1, M_2, and M_3).

The prejunctional or presynaptic neuronal membranes contain autoreceptors of the M_2 subtype, and stimulation of these receptors inhibits the release of acetylcholine and possibly other neurotransmitters. The sites at which parasympathetic transmission may be modulated are shown in Fig. 3.34.

Types of muscarinic (M) receptor in different tissues

- M_1 receptors predominate on exocrine secretory cells and postganglionic nerves
- In the heart the receptor is M_2
- M_2 receptors predominate on presynaptic nerve endings
- M_3 receptors predominate on the smooth muscle of gut and bronchi

Nonadrenergic and noncholinergic systems

There are components of the peripheral autonomic nervous system that use neither acetylcholine nor norepinephrine for neurotransmission. In these nerves a variety of substances may be neurotransmitters. Of particular interest is the recent observation that the gas nitric oxide (NO) acts as a neurotransmitter in a number of tissues (e.g. airways smooth muscle and gastrointestinal smooth muscle). NO is synthesized in nerve endings from the precursor amino acid L-arginine by the enzyme nitric oxide synthase. Well-delineated nerves have been identified as innervating certain tissues anatomically and are increasingly referred to as nitrergic nerves.

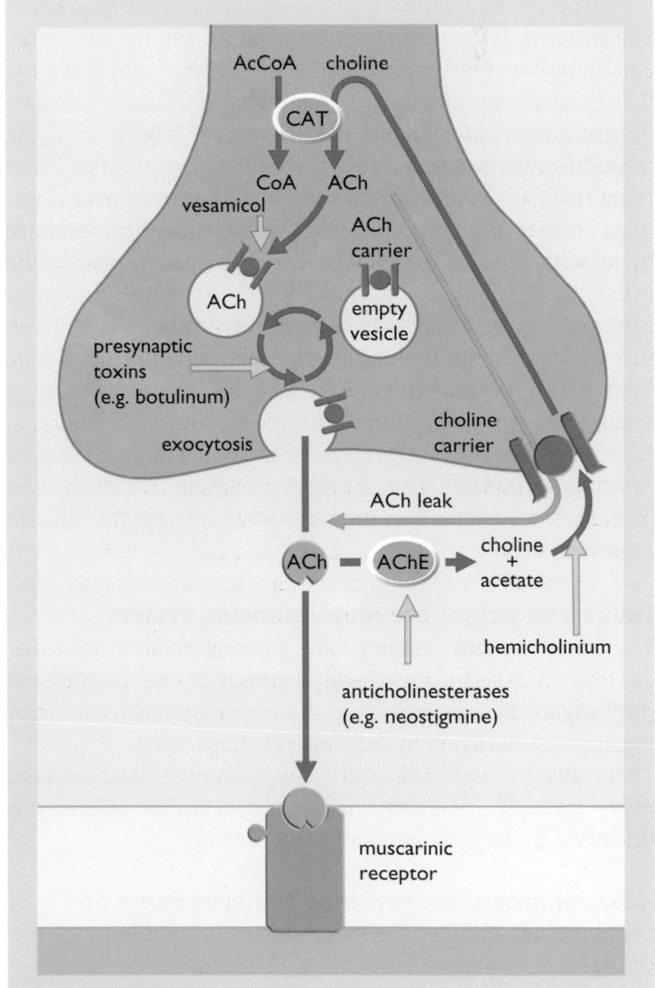

Fig. 3.34 Sites of drug action at a cholinergic nerve terminal. Drugs can interfere with cholinergic transmission in a variety of ways, including effects on synthesis, storage, release, and uptake, and postjunctional effects. (Adapted with permission from *Pharmacology, 3rd edn*, by Rang, Dale, and Ritter, Churchill Livingstone, 1995.)

MOTOR NERVOUS SYSTEM

Control of skeletal muscle system activity by the motor nervous system is complex and involves complex CNS regulation. The afferent limb of the system carries information from a variety of sources, including:

- Stretch receptors in the joints and limbs.
- Muscle spindles in the body of skeletal muscles.
- Proprioceptors in joints.
- Labyrinth receptors in the ear.

Information arriving at the CNS from these afferent sources is integrated at various levels of the CNS with the cerebellum playing a major role. The voluntary aspects of skeletal muscle control arise in the cerebral cortex. Within the CNS there is a comprehensive interplay between information derived from the cortex (the voluntary component) and that derived from the cerebellum, midbrain nuclei, and spinal cord (the involuntary component).

Efferent motor nerves have myelinated axons and generally one axon supplies one muscle fiber

The focus of this section is the efferent limb of the motor nervous system. Efferent motor nerves arise from the brainstem and at various levels of the spinal cord. Once they leave the CNS there are no ganglia and the motor nerve axons thus conduct impulses rapidly from the CNS to skeletal muscle. These axons are myelinated and so allow rapid propagation of action potentials along them. Each axon normally innervates a single muscle fiber. Multiply innervated muscles are rare and are found in the muscle spindle and the extraocular muscles of the eye.

Once the axon reaches the skeletal muscle fiber it terminates in a highly discrete region. The axon abuts onto the muscle fiber at the neuromuscular junction,and, at this site, the nerve ending sits within the 'cup' of folded endplate membrane. Here, acetylcholine mediates its molecular action (activation of nicotinic receptors). This, through a cascade of transduction mechanisms, elicits a system response in skeletal muscle (contraction).

Drugs that act on the motor nervous system

The motor nervous system can be interfered with in ways that are exactly analogous to those discussed above for pre- and postganglionic cholinergic axons. However, there are also drugs that act specifically on the nicotinic cholinoceptor.

Acetylcholine synthesis and the uptake of choline into the nerve ending can be disturbed by drugs in the same way as described above for other cholinergic nerves.

Anticholinesterase reverses the symptoms of myasthenia gravis, a motor nervous system disease

Acetylcholine released from motor nerves acts upon skeletal muscle nicotinic receptors. Myasthenia gravis is an autoimmune disease in which antibodies are produced against these nicotinic receptors, and as a result the number of these receptors at the endplate is reduced by over 90%. Since normal neuromuscular transmission requires activation of 5–10% of the total number of receptors in the neuromuscular junction (i.e. the junction has a 90% reserve), the condition causes muscle weakness. However, neuromuscular transmission can be dramatically improved by inhibiting acetylcholinesterase. An injection of the short-acting anticholinesterase, neostigmine, produces a short-lasting improvement in muscle strength in myasthenia gravis and can be used as a diagnostic tool for myasthenia gravis.

Drugs that act on the motor nervous system

- **Blockers of the neuronal Na^+ channel, such as local anesthetics, interfere with transmission down the nerve**
- **Drugs, such as vesamicol, interfere with acetylcholine synthesis**
- **Drugs, such as hemicholinium, interfere with the uptake of choline into the nerve ending**

THE BLOOD SYSTEM

The blood can be divided into coagulation and hematopoietic systems.

The coagulation system

The coagulation system is essential for ensuring that ruptured vessels do not bleed excessively. It has two components:

- The clotting system, which causes blood to clot.
- The fibrinolytic system (Fig. 3.35), which keeps clotting in check and brings about the dissolution of clots not serving a hemostatic function.

The activation mechanisms of both the clotting and the fibrinolytic systems are analogous in that both require the formation of essential factors by means of a complex cascade from precursor proteins in the blood. Each of these systems is considered in terms of the mechanism of action of the drugs that act upon it.

Plasma proteins

Another component of the blood is the plasma proteins. They are not a conventional target for drugs, but since they can interact with drugs they can be used to explain the mechanisms of action of drugs on their target tissues or target organs within the body. Some plasma proteins bind drugs avidly and reversibly, and sometimes in a saturating manner. The plasma proteins, particularly the albumin fractions, therefore serve as reservoirs for holding drugs within the blood or vascular system.

There are a variety of mechanisms by which drugs bind to plasma proteins, but the number of different types of sites they can bind to is limited. There are, therefore, no unique binding sites for a single drug or even for a single type of drug.

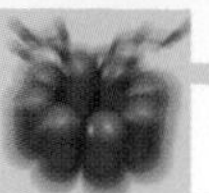

Some drugs displace other drugs from plasma protein binding sites

One consequence of the plasma protein binding of drugs is that some drugs are able to displace each other from plasma protein binding sites. As a result, a second drug given in the presence of a first drug that is heavily bound to plasma protein can displace the first from its binding sites and thereby increase the plasma, and therefore effector, concentrations of the first drug.

The hematopoietic system

The role of the hematopoietic system is the synthesis of blood cells and their precursors in the bone marrow and their subsequent distribution to the body. It is also concerned with the scavenging of red cells by organs such as the spleen, when such cells are defective or have exceeded their normal life span.

For convenience, the cellular elements are divided into red and white cells and platelets. Platelets and mature human red blood cells do not contain a nucleus or the appropriate machinery for *de novo* protein synthesis.

The white cells of the blood have many important functions, in terms of the immune system, producing antibodies and destroying invading organisms, as well as removing dead or dying cells and parasites. These functions will be considered later (see Chapter 15) when discussing drugs with mechanisms of action involving the immune system.

The other major cellular components of the blood, namely the red blood cells, are formed in the blood and often appear initially as reticulocytes, which are an immature form of red blood cell containing the vestiges of a nucleus. Mature red blood cells do not contain a nucleus or other organelles, but are full of the oxygen-carrying molecule hemoglobin. The action of drugs on hemoglobin will be considered in Chapter 9. It is sufficient at this point to remember that such drugs reduce the oxygen-carrying capability of hemoglobin and so reduce the oxygen-carrying capacity of the blood.

Drugs and toxins can affect the integrity of the red blood cell membrane

The ability of drugs to interfere with the integrity of the red cell membrane varies with the status of the membrane and the cell it surrounds. For example in sickle cell anemia a specific genetic defect in the hemoglobin molecule changes the shape of the cell and makes the cell membrane more prone to damage.

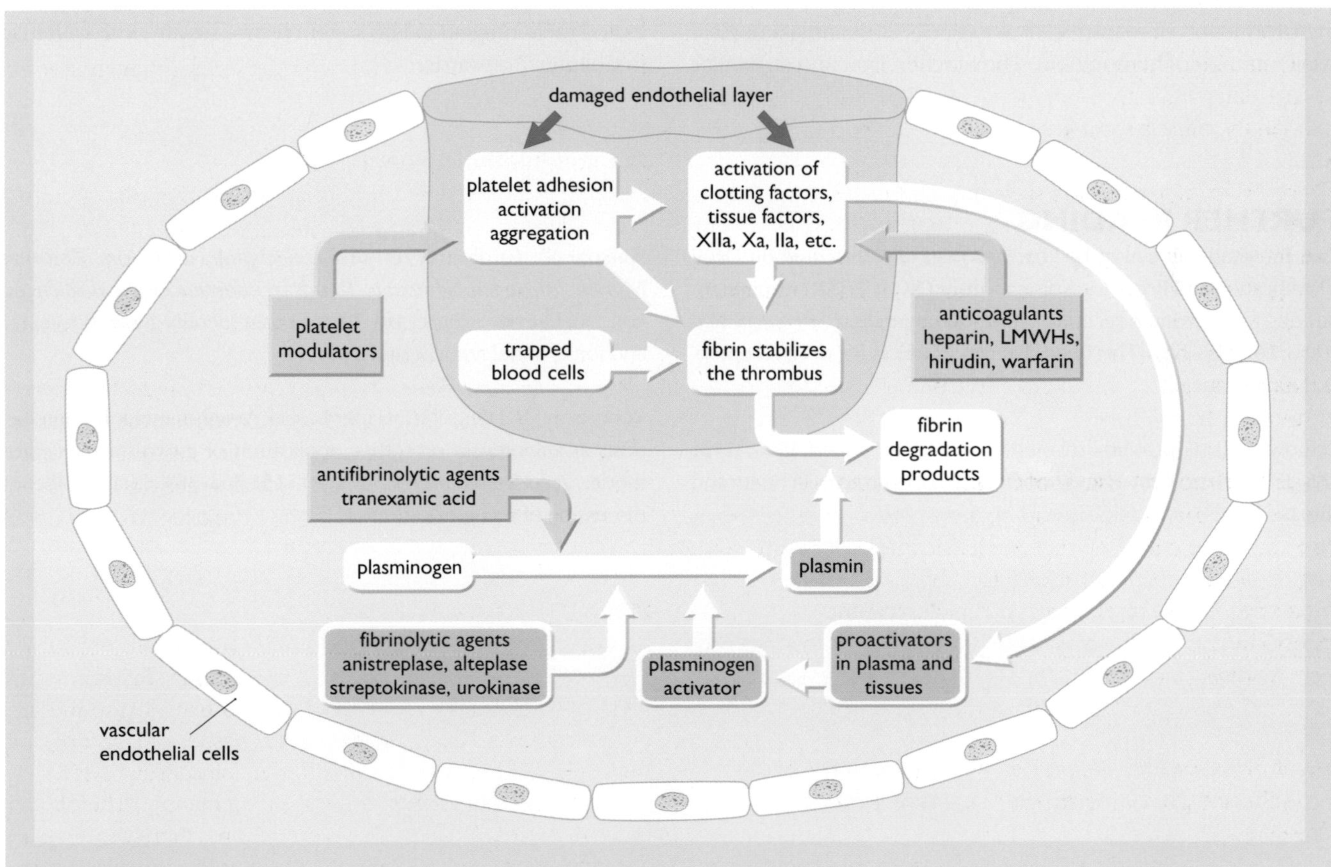

Fig. 3.35 Thrombus formation in a blood vessel, showing the coagulation mechanism and platelet-activation system, and the drugs that act on these systems. Drugs can modify the formation of thrombi at a number of levels by interfering with either the coagulation cascade or platelet activation. Drugs can also modify the fibrinolytic pathway. (Adapted with permission from *Pharmacology, 3rd edn*, by Rang, Dale, and Ritter, Churchill Livingstone, 1995.)

As with other cellular membranes, the red cell membrane can be disrupted by a variety of drugs, and such disruption can account for the toxicity of some drugs.

In addition to drugs, various toxins can disrupt red cell membranes and the membranes of other cells. One example is saponin, a group of toxins found in a wide variety of plants and even in some animals. These toxins have basic steroid structure and can locate within the cell membrane, resulting in its disruption.

Iron, vitamin B_{12} and folic acid deficiencies impair hemoglobin formation

The production of red blood cells and their growth, formation, and maturation are critically dependent on the existence of specific elements and cofactors in the bone marrow. The most obvious such element is iron, which is critical to the functioning of hemoglobin. If there is a low body concentration of iron, hemoglobin formation will be impaired and the size of red blood cells will tend to be smaller. Although this change in color cannot easily be visualized, it can readily be detected using appropriate techniques. Iron deficiency anemia is a classic deficiency disease that can usually be reversed by the addition of adequate iron to the diet.

Vitamin B_{12} and/or folic acid deficiency are other deficiency diseases that result in anemia. Both these vitamins are essential for the production of mature red blood cells containing a normal concentration of hemoglobin. The biochemistry and molecular mechanisms underlying the role of these vitamins in red cell production are described in Chapter 27.

Drugs can irreversibly affect the protein content or protein structure of platelets

Another cell type in the hematopoietic system that can be targeted by drugs is the platelet. Platelets can be considered as fragments of cells that have budded off from megakarocytes. They are therefore organelles rather than true cells. Megakarocytes are formed in the bone marrow and, once mature, can undergo fission to give rise to platelets. Once formed, the platelets have a life span in the blood of approximately 40 days. As they are unable to synthesize proteins, their behavior can be altered by drugs that irreversibly affect their protein content or protein structure. A most important example of this is the unique action of acetylsalicylic acid (ASA) on platelet function.

OTHER TISSUES AND SYSTEMS

The principles of tissue and system mechanisms of action can be applied throughout the body. The principal tissue responses that can be modified are mechanical (i.e. contraction), electrical (excitability and propagation of action potentials), secretory (i.e. release of hormones and neurotransmitters), and related to cell division (miosis, mitosis, and apoptosis). These tissue responses and their integration into system responses are dealt with fully in Chapter 7 onwards.

FURTHER READING

The International Union of Pharmacological Committee on Drug Classification and Receptor Nomenclature (NC-IUPHAR) recommendations for individual receptors and ion channels. *Pharmacol Rev* 1991; **16:** 119–229. [The definitive classification for drug receptors and ion channels.]

Lefkowitz RJ. G-proteins in medicine. *N Engl J Med* 1995; **332:** 185–187. [An excellent overview of the role of G proteins in health and disease.]

Watson S, Girdleston D (eds) *Receptor and Ion Channel Nomenclature Supplement to Trends in Pharmacological Sciences.* London, Elsevier Sciences Ltd, 1995. [A user-friendly guide to receptor and ion channel nomenclature.]

Robertson MJ, Dougall IG, Haper D et al. Agonist–antagonist interactions at angiotensin receptors: application of a two-state receptor model. *Trends Pharmacol Sci* 1994; **15:** 364–369. [State-of-the-art discussion of receptor activation.]

?

Indicate which is the correct answer for each question.

1. A full agonist is
a) a drug with no intrinsic activity
b) a drug with an intrinsic activity of 1
c) a drug that blocks ion channels
d) a β receptor antagonist
e) an inverse agonist

2. An inverse agonist is
a) an antagonist
b) a muscarinic receptor antagonist
c) a drug that antagonizes a symporter
d) a drug that interacts with a receptor to reduce any resting level of molecular activity
e) a drug with an intrinsic activity of 1

3. Receptor antagonists bind to
a) the nucleus
b) membrane proteins
c) lipids
d) oxygen
e) enzymes

4. G proteins are
a) part of the cellular transduction system
b) ion channels
c) found in the nucleus
d) plasma proteins
e) clotting factors

5. Tyrosine kinases are
a) ion channel proteins
b) receptors for growth factors
c) part of the Krebs cycle
d) nucleic acids
e) molecular targets for drugs

6. Ion channels
a) are molecular targets for drugs
b) gate the passage of ions across nuclear membranes
c) gate the passage of ions across lipid bilayers
d) are enzymes
e) are plants

7. Glucocorticosteroids interact with
a) ion channels
b) tyrosine kinases
c) G proteins
d) intracellular receptors
e) lipids

8. β_2 Agonists bind to
a) lipids
b) nucleic acids
c) G proteins
d) seven transmembrane-spanning proteins
e) enzymes

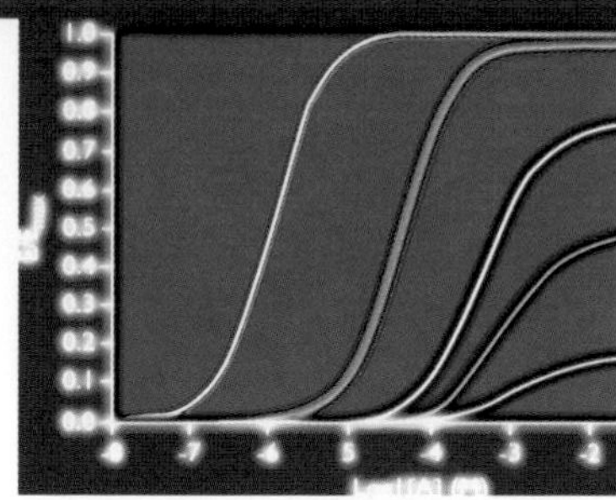

4. Quantification of Drug Action

PRINCIPLES OF DRUG ACTION

THE RECEPTOR

Many drugs must attach to receptors to produce their actions

From the first studies of the effects of drugs on animal tissues in the late nineteenth century, it became evident that many drugs have specific effects on specific tissues. That is:

- A drug that has profound effects on one tissue may have little or no effect on another.
- The same drug may have quite different effects on different tissues.

For example, the alkaloid pilocarpine, like the neurotransmitter acetylcholine, induces intestinal smooth muscle contraction and slows the heart rate. To account for such differences, Langley (1852–1926) proposed in 1878, on the basis of studies of the effects of the alkaloids pilocarpine and atropine on salivation, that 'there is some "receptor" substance ... with which both ... are capable of forming compounds....' Later, in 1905, when studying the action of nicotine and curare on skeletal muscle, he found that nicotine caused contractions only when applied to certain small regions of the muscle and concluded that the 'receptive substance' for nicotine was confined to these regions and that curare worked by blocking the combination of nicotine with its receptor.

Paul Ehrlich (1854–1915) appears to have independently developed the receptor concept, starting from the observation that many organic dyes selectively stain cell constituents. In 1885 he proposed that cells have 'side chains' or 'receptors' to which drugs or toxins must attach to produce their actions. Ehrlich had a huge influence in his time and is still remembered for his idea of the 'magic bullet,' a chemical compound constructed for its selective toxicity to, for example, an infectious organism, as well as for the synthesis of organic arsenicals that were effective in the treatment of syphilis. In Ehrlich's later development of receptor theory he was the first to point out that the rapid reversibility of the actions of alkaloids implied that the 'combination' of such drugs with receptors did not involve strong (covalent) chemical bonds, but the chemical nature of this kind of combination is only now being clarified. Today, the receptor is regarded as one of several important molecular targets for drugs (see Chapter 3).

Whether all drugs have receptors is still a matter of debate or semantics

With drugs that target a known enzyme, the molecular target is the enzyme, and biochemical methodology can serve to characterize drug action. With some drugs, their actions are easily explained without using the molecular target concept, for example, buffers that reduce stomach acidity or bulk laxatives. At the other extreme are agents with obscure mechanisms of action characterized by the virtual absence of strict chemical specificity. The prime example of this is the gas and volatile anesthetic group of drugs, which includes the inert gas xenon. For this group there is no evidence for a molecular target *per se*, but on the other hand they might owe their anesthetic actions to their interference with some as yet undiscovered membrane system (perhaps one type of voltage-gated ion channel) critical to normal neural function. This system would then be the molecular target.

The receptor concept is most important for the drugs that mimic or antagonize hormones, neurohormones, neurotransmitters, and autacoids

Drugs that mimic or antagonize the effects of hormones, neurohormones, neurotransmitters, and autacoids include plant alkaloids such as nicotine, curare, and atropine, which first led Langley to the idea of a receptor. With such drugs, experimental study of how they act has historically been limited to measuring their effects in whole animals and isolated tissues, for example, on blood pressure, heart rate, secretion, or commonly, contraction of intestinal, bronchial, vascular, or uterine smooth muscle. Such effects have long been recognized as indirect reflections of the interaction of drug and receptor, as are most drug effects in the human. The receptor concept has led to the development of methods to use such data to classify drugs in terms of the receptors upon which they act, and to develop new drugs targeted to specific receptors.

Receptors are often large proteins containing a 'lock' (recognition site) and regions linked to transduction systems

Relatively recently there has been great progress in the isolation and chemical characterization of receptors. It has become clear that many receptors are large proteins containing at least one distinct region that constitutes the 'lock' at which the 'key,' a molecule of agonist (i.e. something that induces a biologic response), fits in and binds. Other regions of the receptor are linked to the transduction system(s) that produce(s) the cellular response to the agonist. In addition, regions other than the agonist binding site(s) can be drug targets (e.g. some antagonists and inverse agonists, see Chapter 3). The biochemical approach promises to provide an improvement in the present understanding of how receptors work and for drug development.

Drugs and receptors

- **Many drugs must attach to a receptor to produce their actions**
- **The active agonist–receptor complex produces a response through an 'effector' or 'transduction system'**
- **Tissue responses are generally not directly proportional to the fraction of receptors combined with agonist**

The active agonist–receptor complex produces a cellular response through an 'effector' or 'transduction system'

In modern receptor theory the basic receptor concept has been extended by a new emphasis on the 'effector' or 'transduction system,' through which the active agonist–receptor complex works to produce a cellular response. Examples of such transduction systems are given in Chapter 3. It also seems to be generally accepted that, at least in most cases, the combination of an agonist with a receptor must lead to a conformation change to produce the active complex. This provides an easy explanation for the different actions of agonists, partial agonists, and antagonists.

Generally, any of many drugs may combine with a given receptor. These drugs are 'ligands,' and may act as an agonist, an antagonist, a partial agonist, or an inverse agonist:

- If the ligand produces a molecular response (conformational change in the receptor) the ligand may produce a cellular response. The ligand is then an agonist.
- If the ligand–receptor complex is unable to elicit a cellular response, the ligand will produce no tissue response, but as the ligand ties up receptors in a form incapable of binding with other ligands, including agonists, it will be an antagonist.
- Partial agonists are ligands which cause the receptor to undergo a conformational change capable of causing a cellular response, but so infrequently that even high concentrations of drug produce too few molecular responses to cause a maximum cellular or tissue response. The maximum tissue response to the drug is less than to a 'full' agonist. Such a drug is an agonist and at the same time an antagonist with respect to a full agonist.

Tissue responses are generally not directly proportional to the molecular responses

The relationship between the tissue response and drug concentration (dose) is commonly called the dose–response curve. It is the most important consequence of the transduction system, which typically involves a series of biochemical/biophysical steps. In many cases, tissue responses close to the tissue's maximum response are produced when only a tiny fraction of its receptors are in the active conformation. For example, at the skeletal neuromuscular junction histologic staining shows the presence of about 30 million nicotinic acetylcholine receptors, but simultaneous activation of only about 40,000 of these receptors is enough to elicit an action potential followed by a full twitch of the muscle fiber.

The use of irreversible antagonists to render receptors permanently inoperative has led to the conclusion that some tissues commonly have a 'receptor reserve' of a factor of more than 100 and up to 1000. That is, although elimination of functional receptors always leads to the need for more agonist to produce a given response, the maximal response to an agonist can remain virtually undiminished until only a few of the original receptors remain. It is, therefore, generally incorrect to suppose that tissue responses are directly proportional to the fraction of available receptors combined with agonist, although this false assumption is found throughout the literature before 1956.

The practical consequence of 'receptor reserve' is that, for many agonists, the amounts used clinically (or produced endogenously) activate only a very small fraction of receptors, even when the tissue response is quite large. As a result, the presence or absence of agonist scarcely changes how many receptors are occupied by a competitive antagonist. The effect of an antagonist and how well it can be surmounted by increasing the dose of agonist is therefore essentially the same for an irreversible or a reversible antagonist. For example, blocking acetylcholinesterase at the skeletal neuromuscular junction with a drug such as neostigmine effectively increases the amount of acetylcholine in the synaptic cleft and is equally effective in opposing the neuromuscular blockade produced by:

- Myasthenia gravis, in which immune mechanisms destroy a large fraction of nicotinic receptors.
- A competitive nicotinic antagonist such as pancuronium.

As another example, α adrenoceptor antagonism may be produced clinically with:

- Phenoxybenzamine, whose actions are only overcome with the synthesis of new receptors.
- Phentolamine, which is a rapidly reversible competitive antagonist.

The decision as to which type of antagonist to use depends upon considerations such as the time course of action and adverse effects of the drugs, rather than theoretical differences between competitive, irreversible, or noncompetitive antagonism. With these agents, theory predicts that a dose or concentration of the drug that effectively occupies or renders inactive, say, 90% of the receptors will reduce responses to endogenous or exogenous norepinephrine by about 90%, and the original response to exogenous norepinephrine may be obtained by increasing its dose tenfold. However, this will not be the case if there is little or no tissue reserve.

The quantitative analysis of mechanisms of drug action consists largely of interpreting dose–response curves

The quantitative analysis of mechanisms of drug action is important in the development of new drugs, where the aims are:

- To discover chemical agents that are specific in terms of the receptors with which they interact.
- To discover agents that are selective by virtue of their interaction with only one kind of receptor.

There are several principles fundamental in the understanding of drug–receptor interaction and dose–response curves. They apply to the majority of drugs used clinically and experimentally and are as follows:

- On any one cell in a tissue there are generally numerous receptors of any one type, and most cells express many different types of receptor.
- When drug is present, new drug–receptor complexes are continually created as the random movement of drug molecules leads to their collision with receptors that are not already occupied. The drug–receptor complexes are also continually breaking down randomly, thereby freeing receptors to combine again with drug.
- Agonist–receptor complexes continually fluctuate between inactive and active conformations (the molecular response). The latter induce biophysical events such as the opening of ion channels or biochemical events such as G protein-mediated sequences (transduction, the cellular response), which lead to a tissue response.
- The numbers of receptors expressed on a cell may change in pathologic conditions and with chronic drug administration.

Two rough but near-true and useful rules of thumb that may be added to these fundamental principles are:

- Submaximal tissue responses to agonists are proportional to the product of agonist dose and the number of available receptors.
- Pharmacologic antagonists, in effect, reduce the amount of available receptors to an extent that does not much depend upon how much agonist is present.

The four fundamental principles listed above represent a view of how drugs act that links empirical observations and experimental results to fundamental chemical and physicochemical considerations. The quantitative consequences are in many respects manifested in the measurable association of radioactively labeled ligands with receptors in isolated tissue preparations. As this kind of experiment is relatively easy to understand it is convenient to consider 'receptor binding,' before considering dose–response curves.

RECEPTOR BINDING

The receptor can usually be considered as an entity that binds a variety of ligands

In the context of binding studies it is usually sufficient to think of the receptor in simplistic terms, namely as an entity that can bind a variety of ligands. In addition, at least to begin with, it must be imagined that the ligand binds selectively only to one recognition site and not to other potential binding sites. This should not only be imagined for a preparation of pure receptors, but also for the wide variety of complex macromolecules present in whole-tissue or broken-cell preparations.

The simplest model for reversible ligand binding to receptor

The simplest possible model for reversible ligand binding to receptor is one in which each molecule of ligand (L) can randomly collide with a molecule of receptor (R) in such a way as to form a ligand–receptor complex (LR). This can then break down at any moment to produce a free molecule of ligand and an unoccupied receptor. From basic kinetic theory (i.e. the law of mass action), the rate at which new LRs are formed at any given time is proportional to the concentration of L (i.e. [L]) and the concentration (or amount) of free R (i.e. [R]). At the same time the rate at which LRs break is proportional to the concentration of LR (i.e. [LR]).

At equilibrium, K_L[LR] = [L] [R] where K_L is the dissociation constant

At equilibrium, the rate at which new LRs are formed and the rate at which LRs break is equal and

$$K_L[LR] = [L]\,[R]$$

where K_L is the dissociation constant. K_L depends upon physical factors such as temperature and, most importantly, the chemical nature of the interacting substances. In this simple model K_L will be the ratio of off- to on-rate constants, but it is worth noting that the same simple equation applies with more complicated models in which R and LR can have multiple conformations, in which case K_L depends upon all the rate constants needed to describe the system. Nevertheless, however many conformations of R or LR exist, receptors may be considered in the two forms, R and LR, with $[LR] = [L]\,[R]/K_L$.

[LR]+[R] is a constant

Because the total number of receptors is limited, the total of [LR]+[R] is a constant, designated $[R_t]$. Therefore:

$$[R_t] = [R]+[LR] = [R]\,(1+[L]/K_L)$$

when [LR] is substituted with $[R]\,[L]/K_L$ (see above), combining this with $K_L[LR] = [L]\,[R]$ gives either:

$$[LR] = [R_t]\,[L]/([L]+K_L)$$

or, $$[LR]/[R_t] = ([L]/K_L)(1+[L]/K_L)$$

with $[LR]/[R_t]$ being the chance that any one R will at any moment be combined with L.

Except for notation, the equation:

$$[LR] = [R_t]\,[L]/([L]+K_L)$$

is identical to that describing the adsorption of gases on surfaces (the Langmuir isotherm) and that describing the association of enzyme with substrate.

> **Reversible ligand binding to a receptor**
>
> - Each molecule of ligand (L) can randomly collide with a molecule of receptor (R) in such a way as to form a ligand–receptor complex (LR)
> - LR can then break down at any moment to produce a free molecule of ligand and an unoccupied receptor
> - At equilibrium, K_L[LR] = [L] [R] where K_L is the dissociation constant

Semilogarithmic plots are usually used for both binding studies and dose–response curves

The linear plots of [LR] versus [L] for two ligands with very different K_L values are shown in Fig. 4.1. It is notable that although both plots show the same features (i.e. an initial linear rise with gradual flattening as the maximum is approached) it is rather inconvenient to have both plots on the same *x* axis. In Fig. 4.2 the same information is plotted semilogarithmically ([LR] versus log [L]). Besides allowing both sets of data points to be plotted on the same axis, such a graph makes it evident that both plots are essentially the same, differing only by their position relative to the *x* axis. Such semilogarithmic plots are now usually used for both binding studies and dose–response curves, purely for convenience, although it is only with experience (or separate plots) that it can be seen that the beginning portions of the rising curves in Fig. 4.2 actually represent [LR] rising in proportion to

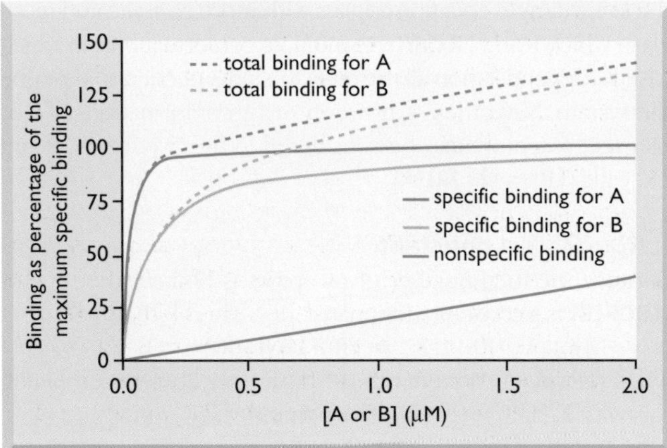

Fig. 4.1 Linear plots for specific and nonspecific receptor binding for two ligands, A and B with K values of 0.01 and 0.1 μM with the assumption that nonspecific binding is proportional to [A] or [B] and that the maximum specific binding is 100. Note the equal spacing on the concentration axis (i.e. it is linear). *y* axis = [LR], *x* axis = [L].

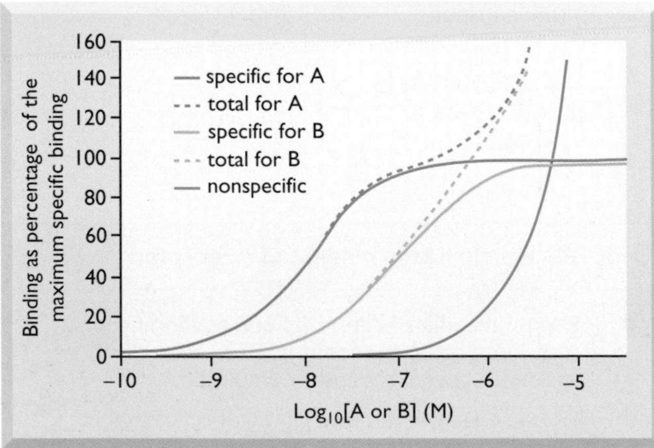

Fig. 4.2 Semilog plot of Fig. 4.1. Higher concentration of A and B for specific and nonspecific binding for two ligands with K_A = 0.01 μM and K_B = 0.1 μM. Note that the x axis is a $\log_{10}$ scale and the concentration ranges from 10^{-10} M to $>10^{-5}$ (i.e. 100,000-fold concentration).

[L]. From the equation $[LR] = [R_t]\,[L]/([L]+K_L)$ given above, it follows that K_L is given by the [L] at which [LR] is just one half of $[R_t]$; the separation between the two parallel curves in Fig. 4.2 is simply the logarithm of the ratio of K_L values.

In a study of 'saturation binding,' tissue (or isolated receptor) samples are incubated with various [L], that are radioactively labeled (usually with ^3H), and then rapidly filtered and 'washed' to remove unbound ligand. The subsequent count of radioactivity in and on the filter gives the total of how much ligand remains. Some of this is, however, simply ligand stuck in the interstices of the filter or between cells or, perhaps, dissolved in the tissue lipid. This nonspecific and specific binding is represented at the cellular level in Fig. 4.3. Nonspecific binding, in contrast to specific binding, is unaltered by a relatively high concentration ('excess') of the same 'cold' (unlabeled) ligand in the incubation medium. Therefore, parallel experiments with excess 'cold' ligand allow subtraction of nonspecific from total binding to give specific binding. A plot of specific 'bound' ('B,' which is the same as [LR]) versus log 'free' ('F,' which is the same as [L]) then gives a characteristic sigmoid curve as in Fig. 4.2. Statistical curve-fitting procedures then show whether the data fit the theoretical form of the plot and, if so, give B_{max} (maximum possible B), which reflects R_t, the amount of receptors in the tissue and K_d (i.e. the dissociation constant of the ligand), which is here the same as K_L.

In much of the older literature on binding, before inexpensive computers became available, such results were often plotted in terms of the 'Scatchard relation' from the equations $K_L[LR] = [L]\,[R]$ and $[R_t] = [R]+[LR]$ given above, to give:

$$K_L[LR] = [L]\,[R] = [L]\,([R_t]-[LR])$$
$$[LR]/[L] = ([R_t]-[LR])/K_d$$
$$B/F = (B_{max}-B)/K_d).$$

Therefore, a plot of B/F versus B produces a straight line that extrapolates to the *x* axis at B_{max} and has a slope of $1/K_d$. The problem with this approach is, in retrospect, twofold:

- Rather esoteric considerations of how to deal statistically with experimental errors.
- More importantly, insensitivity of this plot to any failure of data to fit the theoretical binding curve.

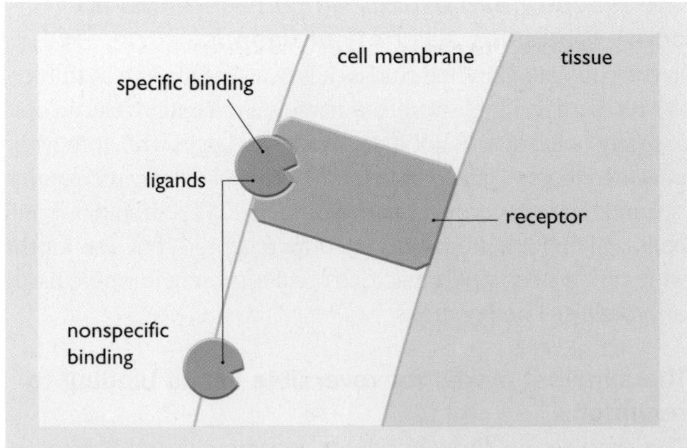

Fig. 4.3 Diagram showing the specific and nonspecific binding of ligands described in Fig. 4.1.

Binding studies do not produce the expected binding curve if the receptor preparation contains more than one kind of binding site for the ligand

The primary hazard of binding studies has been, and still is, the situation in which the tissue or receptor preparation contains more than one kind of binding site for the chosen ligand. Then, total binding fails to fit the theoretical binding curve for a single receptor (equation $[LR] = [R_t]\ [L]/([L]+K_L)$) and is instead given by the sum of two or more expressions of the same form as on the right-hand side of the equation $[LR] = [R_t]\ [L]/([L]+K_L)$ with different $[R_t]$ and K_L values. It is also not uncommon for binding curves to not fit this theoretical equation (i.e. $[LR] = [R_t]\ [L]/([L]+K_L)$) with ligands that are agonists when whole-tissue or -cell preparations are used, presumably because the cellular response elicited affects the molecular interaction between agonist and receptor, changing agonist–receptor affinity.

Binding studies are more complicated if more than one ligand is present

Suppose that a receptor can bind either a molecule of first ligand (L) or second ligand (C), but not both at the same time (Fig. 4.4). Receptors now become partitioned between three forms:

- Free R, with a concentration of [R].
- LR with a concentration of $[LR] = [R][L]/K_L$.
- CR, with a concentration of $[CR] = [R][C]/K_C$ (where K_C is the dissociation constant of CR).

In this situation:

$$[R_t] = [R]+[LR]+[CR] = [R]\ (1+[L]/K_L+[C]/K_C)$$
$$[LR] = [R_t]\ [L]/([L]+K_L(1+[C]/K_C))$$
$$[CR] = [R_t]\ [C]/([C]+K_C(1+[L]/K_L)).$$

The critical feature of this system is that if [L] is raised high enough, most of the receptors will be in the form LR, despite C being present, and if [C] is made high enough most of the receptors will be in the form CR, despite L being present. Therefore C is said to 'compete' with L, and L with C. The mutual competition arises simply because the receptor cannot bind both ligands simultaneously.

It is very important to notice that the equation:

$$[LR] = [R_t]\ [L]/([L]+K_L(1+[C]/K_C$$

is exactly the same as the equation:

$$[LR] = [R_t]\ [L]/([L]+K_L)$$

except for the substitution of the term $K_L(1+[C]/K_C)$ for K_L.

That is, competition is mathematically equivalent to multiplying the dissociation constant by (1+c) where c is the concentration of the competitor divided by its dissociation constant (here $[C]/K_C$). In other words, the equation:

$$[LR] = [R_t]\ [L]/([L]+K_L(1+[C]/K_C))$$

can be written as:

$$[LR] = [R_t]\ [L]/([L]+L50b)$$

which is just the same as the equation:

$$[LR] = [R_t]\ [L]/([L]+K_L)$$

but with K_L replaced by *L50b,* which is an *apparent* K_L with a value given by $K_L(1+c)$. This is of course the [L] at which half the receptors are occupied by L. Also, since the equation:

$$[LR] = [R_t]\ [L]/([L]+K_L(1+[C]/K_C))$$

can be written as:

$$[LR] = [R_t]\ \{[L]/(1+c)\}/([L]/(1+c)+K_L)$$

competition is also mathematically equivalent to dividing each [L] by the factor (1+c).

From the equation:

$$[LR] = [R_t]\ [L]/([L]+K_L(1+[C]/K_C))$$

it follows that the effect of any given concentration of competitor is to shift the plot of [LR] versus log[L] in parallel to the right on the *x* axis, by log(1+c), where c is $[C]/K_C$ (Fig. 4.5). This provides a method for experimentally determining the dissociation constant of the receptor for a substance that is not available with a radioactive label. At any given [C], the dose ratio (DR) (i.e. the ratio of [L] values producing the same [LR] in the presence and absence of C) should be given by:

$$DR = 1+[C]/K_C$$

and, therefore:

$$(DR-1)/[C] = 1/K_C.$$

This method has little importance in binding studies, but is of great importance in quantitative studies of agonist–antagonist–receptor interactions using dose–response curves, for which instead of measuring [LR] a response to an agonist is measured.

Fig. 4.4 If two ligands can bind to the specific binding site of the receptor, the ligands 'compete' with each other.

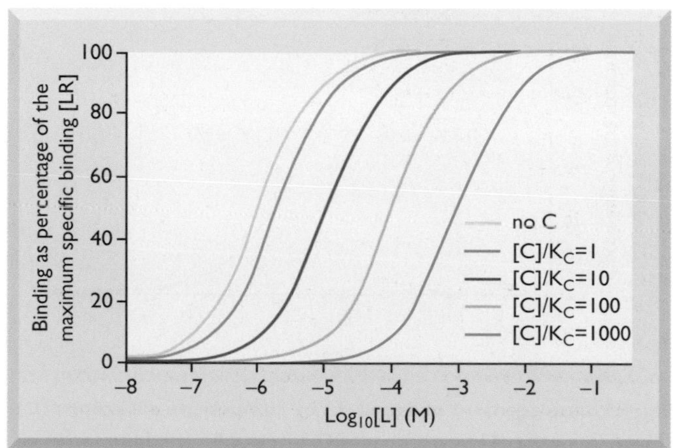

Fig. 4.5 Specific binding of ligand (L) in the presence of competitive antagonist (C) at $[C]/K_C$ = 1, 10, 100, 1000 (a semilogarithmic plot).

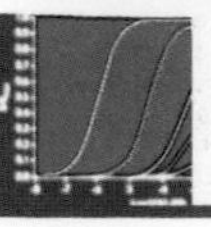

Adding a competitive antagonist such as C is equivalent to reducing agonist concentration by the factor $(1+[C]/K_C)$ which shifts the response–log[agonist] curve in parallel to the right. That is, original responses are restored by multiplying agonist doses by the DR, which is equal to $1+[C]/K_C$.

In practice, there is an easier way, using binding studies to obtain dissociation constants for ligands that are not available in a radiolabeled form. All that is required is one radioactively labeled ligand. This arises from rearrangement of:

$$[LR] = [R_t]\,[L]/([L]+K_L(1+[C]/K_C))$$

to:

$$[LR]/[LR]_{C=0} = 1/(1+[C]/C_{50})$$

where $C_{50} = K_C(1+[L]/K_L)$.

In other words, [LR] follows a smooth displacement curve relative to what it is with no C ($[LR]_{C=0}$) (Fig. 4.6), with a 50% reduction at a certain value of [C], C_{50}, which gives K_C once K_L is known. To find K_L, C can simply be the same ligand as L, but in unlabeled form, so that K_C is the same as K_L (Fig. 4.7). The added concentration of C that displaces 50% of the label, C_{50}, is $K_L+[L]$ and $K_L = C_{50}-[L]$, [L] being the (constant) concentration of labeled ligand.

In the last 25 years since binding studies were begun, numerous experiments similar to that described above have been performed. Saturation binding curves have been used to establish the amount of receptor in a tissue, while displacement curves have been used to establish the dissociation constants of many series of compounds. In general, displacement curves correspond fairly exactly to the theoretical, as pictured in Fig. 4.6. Deviations sometimes occur with ligands that are agonists and the reasons for these are subject to ongoing investigations. Displacement curves also differ from the theoretical if the labeled ligand binds to more than one kind of receptor in the tissue preparation.

Not all antagonists are competitive

Not all substances modify binding in a competitive manner. This occurs because the receptor contains more than one ligand-recognition site and binding at one site alters the affinity at the other. This is called an allosteric interaction. It is characterized in saturation binding experiments by half-maximal binding occurring at an *L50b* (or *apparent* K_L) value that can be varied continuously between two limits, from one extreme in the absence of the allosteric agent to another extreme reached when virtually all receptors are bound to the allosteric agent. When the antagonist binds in this manner it is said to be noncompetitive.

Another theoretical scenario is one where the antagonist can bind only to the LR complex; this can occur only if L causes a conformation change in the receptor (Fig.4.8). In such a case the substance may be termed an uncompetitive ligand (U), and the relevant equation for binding can easily be shown to be much as before, that is:

$$B = [LR]+[LRU] = [R_t]\,[L]/([L]+L50b)$$

where $L50b = K_L/(1+[U]/K_U)$.

That is, the apparent affinity of the receptor for L is increased in the presence of U. This occurs because the form UR cannot exist and LRU must first dissociate to form LR and U before breaking down to form free R, so in effect L tends to be trapped in the LRU form.

If a drug (D) can combine with both the free receptor and LR, then the net result is mathematically the same as a combination of competitive and uncompetitive inhibition. The same general

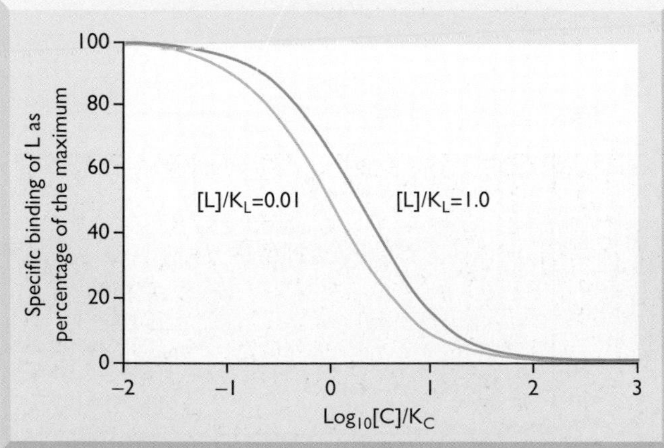

Fig. 4.6 Displacement of ligand (L) by competitive antagonist (C) shown in a case of low occupancy $[L]/K_L = 0.01$ and high occupancy $[L]/K_L = 1.0$ so the curves show specific binding for two levels of $[L]/K_L$.

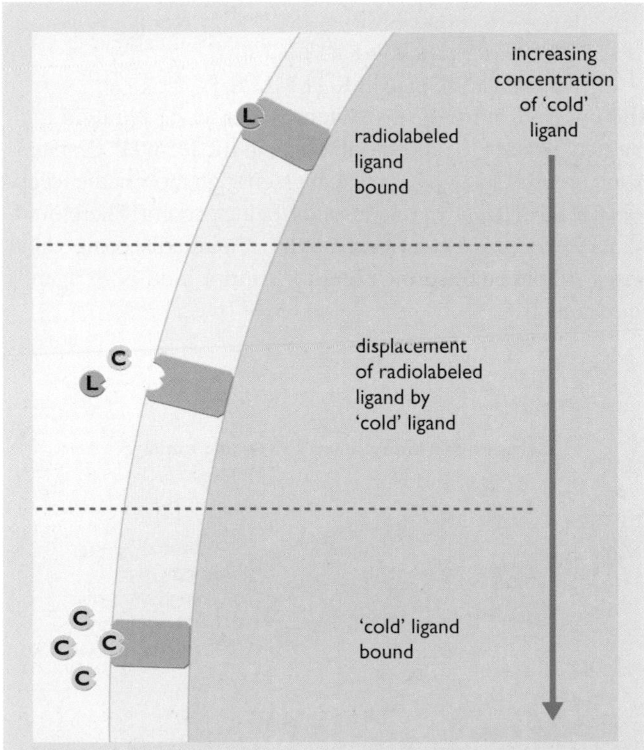

Fig. 4.7 A bound radiolabeled ligand (L) is displaced in an environment of increasing competitive antagonist (C), which is the same ligand in an unlabeled form. This concept is used to find K_L (see Fig. 4.6).

equation applies, that is:

$$B = [LR]+[LRD] = [R_t][L]/([L]+L50b)$$

but in this case:

$$L50b = K_L(1+[D]/K_{Dc})/(1+[D]/K_{Du})$$

where K_{Dc} is the dissociation constant of DR and K_{Du} is the dissociation constant of LRD. In fact, this situation is exactly the same as what was previously termed an allosteric (noncompetitive) interaction; $L50b$ varies between K_L (when $[D]=0$) and $K_L K_{Du}/K_{Dc}$ (when [D] is very large). A displacement type experiment will show that L can at most be partially displaced by D (Fig. 4.9).

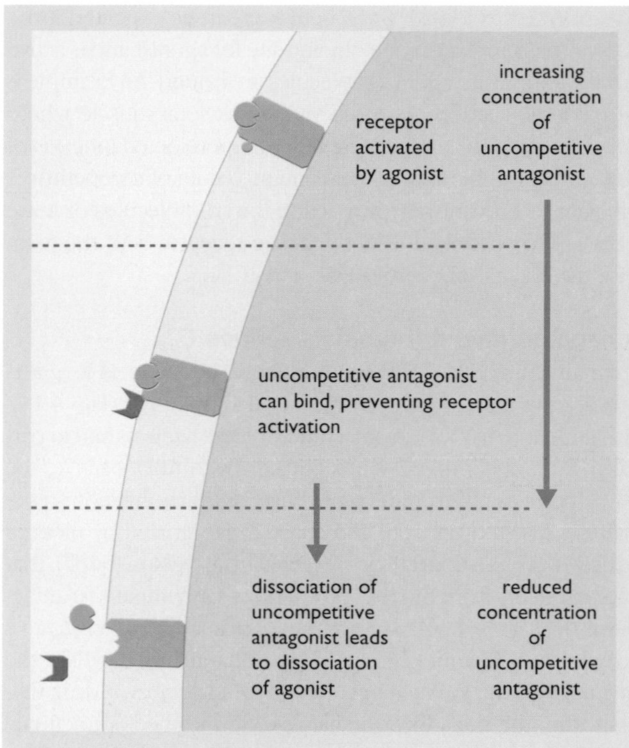

Fig. 4.8 This figure is analogous to Fig. 4.7, but in this case the antagonist is uncompetitive.

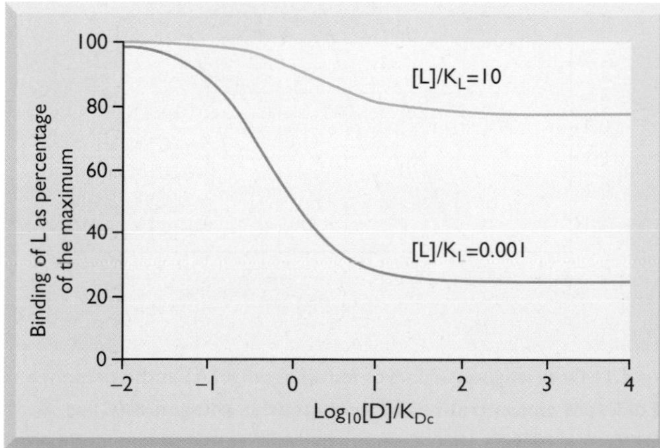

Fig. 4.9 Displacement curves for combined uncompetitive and competitive allosteric systems for two levels of $[L]/K_L$ (0.001 and 10).

DOSE–RESPONSE CURVES

The relationship between the dose (or concentration) of an agonist drug administered and the tissue response (effect) that is obtained invariably follows a curve similar to those shown in Fig. 4.10, which in turn closely resemble the ligand–receptor binding curve shown in Fig. 4.2. The effect (E) might be either a tissue response itself or, less usually, the inhibition of spontaneous activity (e.g. slowing of the pulse rate by acetylcholine). Below a certain concentration of agonist ([A]), E is too low to measure, but at higher concentrations it becomes appreciable and rises with increasing drug concentration ([D]) until at sufficiently high concentration it can no longer be increased by raising [D] and asymptotes to a maximum (E_{max}). Each curve can be conventionally (although perhaps not completely) characterized by three measures:

- E_{max}.
- The [A], here termed A_{50}, at which E is half E_{max}.
- The so-called slope parameter, which describes the steepness of the curve and is obtained by (rather arbitrarily) fitting the E–[A] curve to the 'logistic' function, $E/E_{max} = [A]^p/([A]^p+A_{50}^p)$.

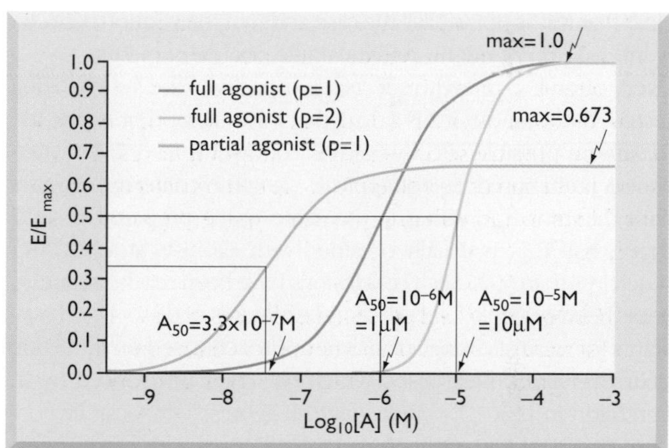

Fig. 4.10 Dose–response curves for agonists (A) with different A_{50} values, maxima, and slopes (p).

Dose–reponse curves

- The relationship between the tissue response and drug concentration is commonly called the dose–response curve
- The quantitative analysis of the mechanism of drug action consists largely of interpreting dose–response curves
- Semilogarithmic plots are usually used for dose–response curves
- Competitive antagonists shift dose–response curves to the right

It should be noted that sometimes an agonist that is closely related chemically to another agonist and is known to be acting through the same receptor (on the basis of antagonism by competitors) can have an E_{max} less than that of a full agonist and in such a case is termed a partial agonist.

POTENCY, INTRINSIC ACTIVITY, AND EFFICACY

Technically, the term potency is used to refer only to the A_{50} (the lower the A_{50} the higher the potency), while E_{max} is referred to as intrinsic activity, or effectiveness. Therefore, one agonist might be more potent than another even if it falls short of the other's effectiveness (i.e. E_{max}). The term efficacy is often used loosely to mean effectiveness, but has also been given a technical meaning that is quite different and is explained below.

The relation between tissue response and concentration of agonist–receptor complex is often nonlinear

Because of the resemblance of the typical E–log[A] curve to a theoretical [LR]–log[L] curve it was in the past (before 1956) commonly assumed that a response E directly reflected the amount of agonist–receptor complex (AR). In particular, it was assumed that E/E_{max} was therefore equivalent to $[AR]/[R_t]$. However, it is now clear that this is not usually the case and that the relation between E and [AR] is commonly nonlinear and may be complex.

Very often E_{max} merely reflects the capacity of the system being tested. For example, if A is a drug that lowers blood pressure, the maximum possible effect would be to lower it to 0. Even when such a limitation does not apply, as shown by different agonists with different E_{max} values in the same tissue preparation, an E that is half E_{max} is usually obtained with agonists at a $[AR]/[R_t]$ much less than 50%. Such conclusions have been reached because it has been possible to obtain good estimates of dissociation constants for agonists using an analytic approach based on the action of irreversible antagonists, which was first introduced by R. Furchgott in 1966. Of course, once an agonist's dissociation constant (K_A) has been obtained, a graph of E versus [A] can be translated into a graph of E versus $[AR]/[R_t]$, yielding information about the transduction system (cellular response) linking [AR] to E.

COMPETITIVE ANTAGONISTS FOR ENDOGENOUS AGONISTS SUCH AS NEUROHORMONES AND AUTACOIDS

Competitive antagonists shift dose–response curves to the right

Reversible competitive antagonists are usually more simply termed competitive, the reversible aspect being understood, since there is no difficulty in distinguishing between drugs whose effects disappear when the drug is removed (i.e. reversible) and those whose effects are maintained indefinitely (i.e. irreversible). These drugs are characterized by producing parallel shifts, to the right, of plots of E versus log[A], where A is an agonist (Fig. 4.11). Such a relation arises automatically from the equation:

$$[LR] = [R_t]\,[L]/([L]+K_L(1+[C]/K_C))$$

given on p. 55 since, whatever the relation between E and [AR], the inhibitory effect of a competitor (C) at any given [A] can always be nullified by increasing [A] by the factor $(1+[C]/K_C)$, which is the DR. In other words the inhibition is surmountable at any level of response and E_{max} is not reduced. That everything works according to theory can be checked graphically since:

$$DR = 1+[C]/K_C$$

and

$$\log(DR-1) = \log[C]-\log(K_C).$$

A plot of the latter equation is known as a Schild plot and is illustrated in Fig. 4.12. An alternative (Fig. 4.13) is to plot (DR–1)/[C] versus log[C] to check that this ratio is, in fact, constant ($=1/K_C$).

Sometimes the equation $DR = 1+[C]/K_C$ given above does not hold for some agonists even though antagonists are clearly competitive in that they produce parallel shifts to the right of plots of E versus log[A]. Such behavior can be expected if the receptor has more than one binding site for agonist and is active only if two or more agonist molecules are bound. An example is the nicotinic acetylcholine receptor in skeletal muscle where the active receptor (associated with an open ion channel) is of the form A_2R. If binding of only one molecule of competitor is sufficient to prevent receptor action, but n molecules of A are necessary to produce E (i.e. the active receptor is of the form A_nR), the equation becomes $DR^n-1 = [C]/K_C$.

Noncompetitive antagonists reduce E_{max}

When an antagonist (D) does produce a reduction of E_{max} it is usually (and inaccurately) termed noncompetitive (Fig. 4.14). Such an action may arise from a variety of mechanisms and in particular from uncompetitive antagonism (with ARD inactive, see p. 4.6), perhaps mixed with competitive, or from inhibition somewhere within the transduction chain. It is signaled by plots of log(DR–1) versus log[D] or of (DR–1)/[D] versus log[D] that differ markedly from the theoretical plots for competitive antagonism (Figs 4.15, 4.16). An example of primarily uncompetitive antagonism is channel blockade (see Chapter 3) in which the drug target is the ion channel opened by an agonist. A drug that acts within the transduction chain is often termed a functional antagonist.

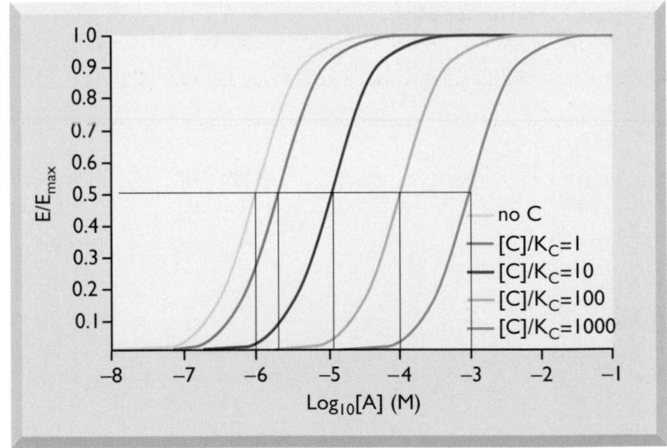

Fig. 4.11 Dose–response curves for an agonist (A) in the presence of different concentrations of a competitive antagonist (C) at $[C]/K_C$ = 1, 10, 100, 1000. Compare this with Fig. 4.5 and note that the x axes are the same; however, the y axis here is the ratio of the effects (E) produced by different concentrations of agonist over the maximum effect (E_{max}).

Many clinically useful drugs are competitive antagonists for endogenous agonists such as neurohormones and autacoids, for example:

- Propranolol (β adrenoceptors).
- Haloperidol (dopamine receptors).
- Naloxone (opioid receptors).
- Phentolamine (α adrenoceptors).
- Cimetidine (histamine H_2 receptors).
- Atropine (muscarinic receptors).
- Curare-like compounds (skeletal muscle nicotinic receptors).

In each of these cases the nature of the antagonism and effectiveness of the compounds (and K_d values) were established using the methods outlined above.

When a dose–response curve is obtained clinically for a competitive antagonist, the effect observed actually represents inhibition of the response to an exogenous or endogenous agonist. An example is the depression of spontaneous histamine-mediated acid secretion in the stomach by cimetidine. Again, the dose–response curves are similar to those shown in Fig. 4.10 and, in the same way as E–[A] curves, are characterized by an E_{max}, a value of drug concentration where the effect is half maximum (usually termed EC_{50}), and a slope parameter. As with dose–response curves for agonists, the exact form of such curves depends critically on the transduction system that links the active agonist–receptor complex (AR^*) to the tissue response, since for competitive antagonists each concentration

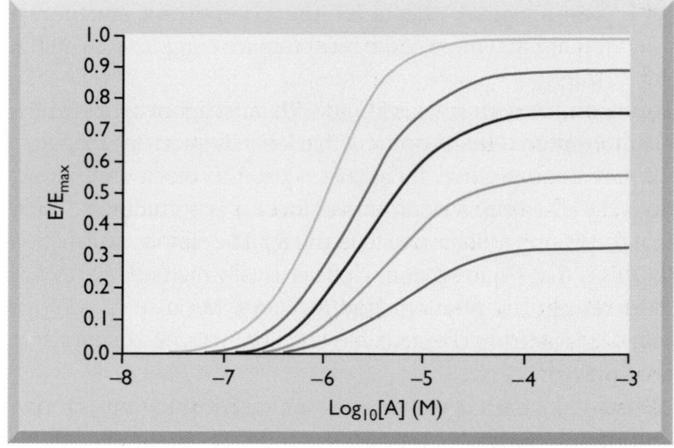

Fig. 4.14 Dose–response curves for an agonist (A) in the presence of different concentrations of a noncompetitive antagonist (D).

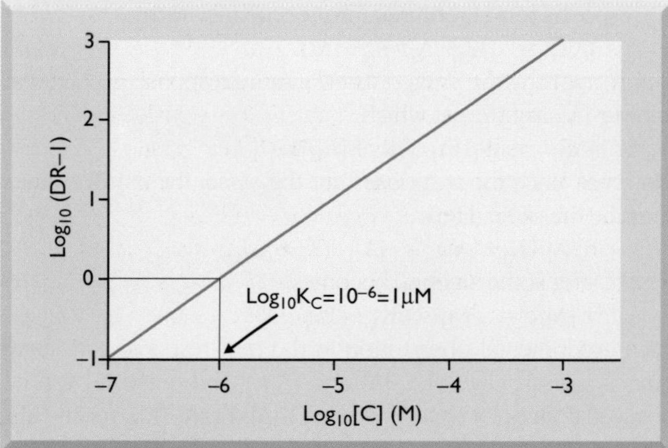

Fig. 4.12 Schild plot for a competitive antagonist (C).

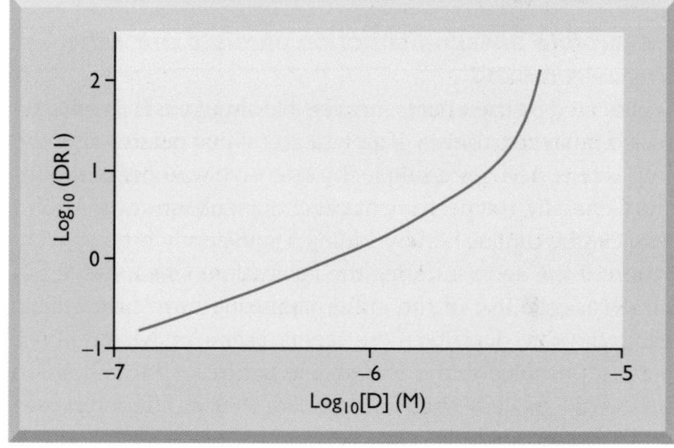

Fig. 4.15 Schild plot for a noncompetitive antagonist (D).

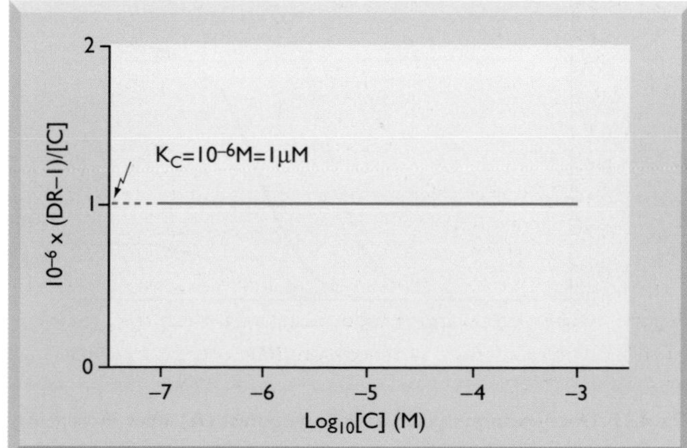

Fig. 4.13 Modified Schild plot for a competitive antagonist (C).

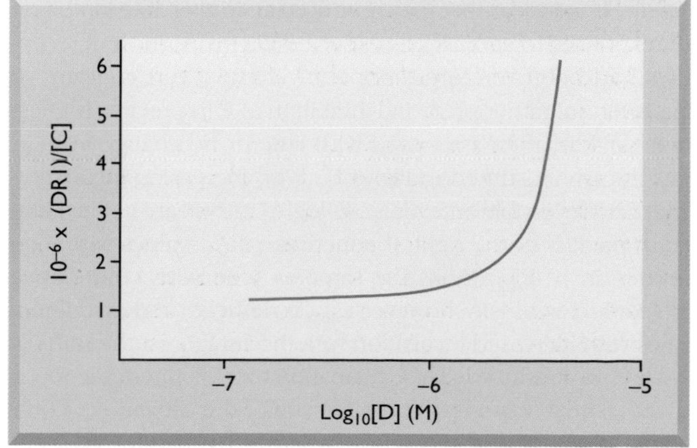

Fig. 4.16 Modified Schild plot for a noncompetitive antagonist (D).

of antagonist corresponds to a reduction of [A]. Nevertheless, it can be shown that the EC_{50} is generally close to the dissociation constant, K_d multiplied by $(1+[A]/A_{50})$. That is, the EC_{50} is much the same provided that the responses to the agonist are well below the maximum ($[A]<A_{50}$). In general:

- Half blockade of the agonist effect is associated with at least half occupancy of receptors.
- Near-maximal effects of the competitive antagonist require that most of the receptors are complexed with the drug.

This contrasts with what is found with most agonists, for which near-maximum effects occur with a low receptor occupancy.

When a competitive antagonist is used to block an endogenous agonist (e.g. a neurotransmitter) it is sometimes found that the EC_{50} is much more than the K_d. The simple explanation for this is that [A] in synaptic clefts is usually high relative to A_{50}. Alternatively, the phenomenon may arise because physiologically [A] is far from constant and equilibrium-type equations do not apply.

Dose–response curves for noncompetitive antagonists representing inhibition of response to endogenous or exogenous agonist also resemble those shown in Fig. 4.10. Since these agents can act by a variety of mechanisms the only generalization that can be made is that, in contrast to competitive antagonists, the EC_{50} fails to rise in proportion to $1+[A]/A_{50}$.

Irreversible antagonist action persists after the drug is removed

As indicated by their name, irreversible antagonists are characterized by an antagonism of agonist action that persists after the drug is removed, for example, by extensive washing of the tissue. Generally, the permanent effect of incubation with such a drug can be diminished by adding a sufficiently high concentration of the agonist during the incubation, which has led to the occasional use of the rather confusing term 'irreversible competitive' to describe these agents. However, what is of primary importance is the irreversible nature of the inhibition caused by covalent chemical bonding that in effect removes functional receptors.

When irreversible antagonists were first developed, their effects on E–[A] curves were a surprise. Previously, pharmacologists had assumed that E was proportional to [AR]. With these agents, it was clear that they produced an irreversible inhibition of responses to agonists, as expected if a proportion of receptors had been rendered inoperative. However, contrary to expectation, rather profound inhibition of E to previously effective [A] was often associated with little or no change in E_{max}. Results are illustrated in Fig. 4.17. With increasing incubation with an irreversible antagonist, E–log[A] curves are at first shifted in parallel to the right; the increase of A_{50} values without a reduction of E_{max} looks the same as seen with competitive blockade! Eventually, however, E_{max} is reduced, and as it diminishes with increased incubation with the antagonist the shifts of A_{50} are also reduced. The explanation for this phenomenon is that maximal responses normally require the activation of only a small minority of receptors. This has been referred to as 'receptor reserve.'

Receptor reserve implies that A_{50} is less than K_A and it varies among agonists acting on the same receptor

Receptor reserve implies that A_{50} (the [A] giving a half-maximum response) is less than K_A (the [A] at which receptors are half occupied). The ratio K_A/A_{50} is a kind of measure of receptor reserve, which varies among agonists acting on the same receptor. Therefore, the change in receptor reserve with variation of the chemical structure of the agonist provides yet another method of characterizing receptors.

The simplest and most generally accepted explanation for the difference between agonists (of what is technically called 'intrinsic efficacy') is that it is only a particular conformation of AR, say AR^*, that is 'active.' Agonists with low intrinsic efficacy (A_{50} close to K_A and little or no receptor reserve), which include partial agonists, have an AR that is seldom in the form AR^*, while agonists with high intrinsic efficacy ($A_{50}<<K_A$) have an AR that is in the AR^* form most of the time.

It was first recognized by Furchgott that data such as those illustrated in Fig. 4.17 contain the information needed to obtain the K_A of an agonist. The logic goes like this. Suppose that an irreversible antagonist has been applied for a period of time sufficient to reduce E_{max}. The change in the dose–response curve has occurred because $[R_t]$ has been reduced to a new value, say, $q[R_t]$. Now consider any level of response on the new curve. It corresponds to a certain receptor occupancy with:

$$[AR] = q[R_t]\,[A]/(K_A+[A]).$$

Before applying the antagonist, the same response occurred at a lower [A], say $[A]_O$ at which:

$$[AR] = [R_t]\,[A]_O/(K_A+[A]_O).$$

However, since the responses are the same, these [AR] values must be the same. Hence:

$$q\,[A]/(K_A+[A]) = [A]_O/(K_A+[A]_O)$$

which, after some algebra, becomes:

$$1/[A]_O = (1/q-1)/K_A+(1/q)/[A].$$

Each experimental observation in the new response–[A] curve gives a pair of values (i.e. [A] and $[A]_O$), and q and K_A can be obtained from a plot of $1/[A]_O$ versus $1/[A]$ (or $[A]/[A]_O$ versus [A]).

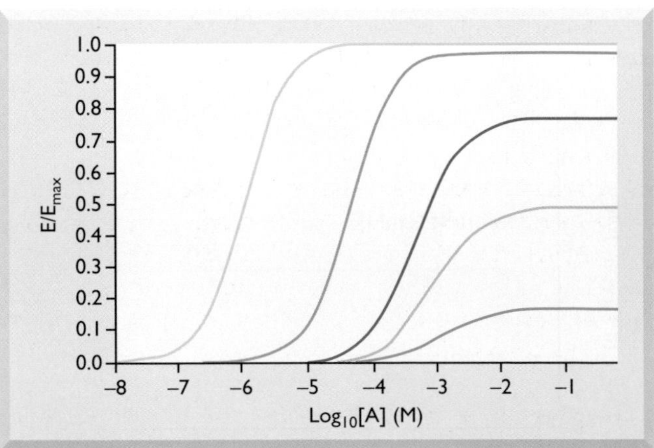

Fig. 4.17 Dose–response curves for an agonist (A) after increasing times (right shift) of exposure to an irreversible antagonist showing responses to an agonist following inactivation of receptors.

A very simple mathematical model introduced by Stephenson is useful for seeing how results such as those in Fig. 4.17 can arise. Suppose that AR produces a stimulus (S) proportional to [AR] and that response (E) is a simple saturating function of S. Then:

$$S = e[AR]/[R_t]$$

where e is a proportionality constant, called efficacy, that can vary from one agonist to another, and

$$E = E'S/(1+S)$$

where E' represents a hypothetical maximum that would occur if S could be made infinite. If agonists vary in the fraction (f) of AR that is in an active conformation (AR^*), e will be proportional to f. Also, with e defined as above it must be proportional to $[R_t]$ (or $q[R_t]$ if some receptors are made inoperable). Intrinsic efficacy is $e/[R_t]$.

Combining the above two equations with that for agonist binding:

$$[AR]/[R_t] = [A]/([A]+K_A)$$

and rearranging gives:

$$E = E_{max}[A]/([A]+A_{50})$$

with $E_{max} = E'e/(e+1)$

and $A_{50} = K_A/(e+1)$.

Therefore, if e is initially large, say 1000, it can be greatly diminished by an irreversible antagonist 'removing' receptors before E_{max} is much diminished—all that is seen is an increase in A_{50}. However, once e is not much more than 1, or if e started low, any (further) reduction of e causes E_{max} to diminish with relatively little increase in A_{50}, which can become, at most, the same as K_A.

On the basis of this model, agonists may be compared in terms of their relative e values, which are the same as relative intrinsic efficacies. The problem here is that the actual values of e obtained depend on the particular relationship assumed between E and S ($E=E'S/(1+S)$), which might or might not be true of any particular transduction system.

A partial agonist is an agonist of low intrinsic efficacy, with an e not much more than 1

From the above discussion it should now be clear that, in terms of the above theory, a partial agonist is simply an agonist of low efficacy, with an e not much more than 1. Experiments with irreversible antagonists have shown that, in agreement with this theory, partial agonists are characterized by having A_{50} values close to K_A values and no receptor reserve, in the sense that any reduction in the amount of functional receptor results in a reduction of E_{max}. As already pointed out, the low e of a partial agonist, relative to a full agonist, may be explained simply on the basis that with a partial agonist only a small fraction of ARs are in the active conformation (i.e. AR^*).

The practical importance of partial agonists is that because any response is associated with a high receptor occupancy they are also competitive antagonists of full agonists. Therefore, a partial agonist can be used therapeutically to block the effect of an endogenous agonist (e.g. epinephrine), while at the same time producing a steady low level of receptor activation.

Physiological antagonists oppose the actions of agonists by mechanisms independent of the agonist receptor

In the previous section antagonist drugs that inhibited the actions of agonists were considered to produce their inhibition by virtue of acting in some manner on the receptors for the agonists. However, drugs may antagonize the actions of agonists by other mechanisms.

Drugs can oppose the action of other drugs by action on other receptors

It often happens that two drugs that have independent molecular targets elicit opposing actions on a tissue or organ. When this occurs, the drugs can be called physiologic antagonists of one another. Obvious examples of such physiologic antagonism are epinephrine and acetylcholine, which respectively raise and lower heart rate, and glucagon and insulin, which respectively raise and lower blood glucose level.

A more subtle example is the antagonism of neuromuscular blockade due to a nondepolarizing neuromuscular blocking drug, such as pancuronium, by an anticholinesterase, such as neostigmine. The dose–response curve for the degree of neuromuscular block versus dose of pancuronium is shifted by neostigmine in a noncompetitive fashion because the two drugs are acting on quite different molecular targets: the nicotinic receptor for pancuronium and the enzyme acetylcholinesterase for neostigmine. Block of the activity of the enzyme can do no more than about double the height of endplate potentials and, as a result, an anticholinesterase cannot reverse neuromuscular blockade due to an excessive dose of pancuronium.

MEASURING RESPONSES AND THE PRACTICAL APPLICATION OF DOSE–RESPONSE CURVES

Responses may be measured in many different ways

Drugs have their initial actions at a molecular level and this results in cellular, tissue, organ, body system, whole body and even population responses, all of which can be measured. Biochemical techniques are used to measure cellular responses, whereas the response of tissues and organs to drugs can also be measured using physical (electrical, optical, mechanical) techniques. When tissues and organs are examined in isolation from the body, such studies are called *in vitro* studies. When studies are made in intact animals and humans they are referred to as being *in vivo*.

In all of the above discussions the terms 'effect' and 'response' have been used synonymously but left undefined because there are innumerable ways in which drugs act and their effects can be defined. However, it should always be borne in mind that, if given at sufficiently high concentrations, drugs have many measurable effects which may not be relevant to the clinical action of the drug.

Dose–response curves almost always appear similar to those shown in Fig. 4.10, the exceptions being those where the drug acts on more than one type of receptor. Below a certain dose or concentration an effect is undetectable and as dose is increased the effect increases until a maximum effect is reached. The dose at which the effect is half maximal is usually called the ED_{50} (effective dose 50%, i.e. that dose which produces a response equal to 50% of the maximum response to that drug). Similarly, the ED_{10} is at 10% of maximum, ED_{25} is at 25%, ED_{75} is at 75%, etc. If drug concentration [C] is known, the corresponding terms EC_{10}, EC_{25}, EC_{50}, etc. may be used.

The ratio ED_{75}/ED_{25} or EC_{75}/EC_{25} provides a simple measure of the steepness of the dose–response relationship which reflects p in the equation

$$E = E_{max}[A]^p/(EC_{50}^p + [A]^p),$$

in which [A] is drug concentration. It is notable that for drugs with a p more than 1.0 (EC_{75}/EC_{25} less than 9), effects increase steeply with drug dose and this is sometimes dangerous. For example, in general anesthesia, the depth of anesthesia may increase alarmingly with only a relatively small increase in dose of the volatile anesthetic being used.

Sometimes effects are all-or-nothing quantal dose response curves

In certain contexts the effect measured is 'quantal' rather than graded. That is, the response either occurs or it does not. In such cases the response axis for the dose–response curve is percentage of people or animals or cells that are affected and give the quantal response. Thus for any drug there is an LD_{50} (dose that is lethal to 50% of animals) that depends upon the route of administration and species tested and an ED_{50} (dose that has a desired effect in 50% of animals).

Drugs are judged according to both their beneficial and adverse effects

The 'therapeutic ratio' which is an index of the safety of the drug is sometimes defined as the ratio LD_{50}/ED_{50}, but this may be misleading if the response–log dose curves for desired effect and death are not parallel and many prefer LD_{25}/ED_{75} or LD_{10}/ED_{90}, reflecting Ehrlich's early suggestion (about 1900) that a drug be judged by the ratio between its maximal tolerated dose and minimal curative dose. Ratios involving estimation of lethal doses can only be determined using animals but at a clinical level it is useful to compare dose–response curves for beneficial effects with those for adverse effects. Unfortunately this information is often not available for drugs.

With quantal responses the steepness of the dose–response curve arises from the variability in the population being tested—if all animals were the same, all would die at the same drug dose—and there exists extensive statistical theory concerning how data of this kind should be treated (such as 'probits') and the reliability of estimates of ED_{50}, LD_{50}, etc. However, conventional fitting of results to the formula:

$$E = E_{max}D^p/(K^p + D^p)$$

where K is ED_{50} or LD_{50} and D is dose, with $E_{max} = 100\%$, will give the same ED_{50} or LD_{50} as the statistical method.

Occasionally, what appear to be graded responses in a tissue actually represent hidden quantal responses — what one measures is the sum of responses of many individual cells which each respond in an all-or-none fashion. This may sometimes provide an explanation of steep dose–response curves, an example being the effect of neuromuscular blocking drugs to inhibit contractions in a skeletal muscle. Here individual neuromuscular junctions on skeletal muscle fibers are either blocked or not blocked by a given concentration of the drug, and single muscle fiber contractions are either present or absent. This contrasts with smooth muscle where contraction in each fiber is continually graded with the dose of a drug.

Therapeutic index

- **The median lethal dose (LD_{50}) is the dose of a drug that kills 50% of a group of animals**
- **The median effective dose (ED_{50}) is the dose that produces the desired pharmacologic effect in 50% of animals**
- **The ratio of LD_{50} versus ED_{50} is a measure of the therapeutic index of that drug (i.e. an estimation of the therapeutic usefulness of a drug)**

Dose–response relationships in a variety of tissues and organs are fundamental to the discovery of receptors and development of new drugs

In research and drug development the primary aim is to characterize chemical compounds in terms of the receptors and biological systems with which they interact, and how they interact with receptors; that is, whether they are agonists, partial agonists, or competitive, noncompetitive or irreversible antagonists. Here, the approach is to measure effects on a variety of enzyme systems and tissue preparations that contain receptors of different types. Thus a compound may be identified as an H_1 agonist if it acts in the same way as histamine in a preparation that both responds to histamine, and has its actions inhibited by an H_1 competitive antihistamine competitively and with the same potency that it blocks the action of histamine. The unidentified active compound in a tissue extract *is* epinephrine if its potency relative to epinephrine is the same in preparations containing different proportions of α and β adrenoceptors and appropriate competitive antagonists shift dose–response curves to the unknown agent in the same way as they shift dose–response curves to epinephrine. Conversely, if a chemical compound has effects that cannot be explained in terms of action on known receptors one has a new receptor, and if the compound occurs naturally in tissues it may be a new autacoid. Historically, such work has led to most of our present understanding of how drugs act as well as the discovery of autacoids and their receptors.

It is still common in research that the measured *in vitro* effect is the contraction of a smooth muscle preparation such as a piece of intestine, artery, vein, bladder, uterus, etc. Such preparations characteristically respond to a variety of agents by contraction or relaxation, the response being graded with dose and fairly fast in onset and offset when the drug is added or removed, respectively. It is therefore possible to determine a dose–response relationship and its alteration by another drug in a matter of hours. Using biochemical indications of drug–receptor interaction, such as accumulation or turnover of a second messenger, can often be even more efficient and is essential in cases when the drug being studied acts on receptors that are not present in tissue preparations that provide an easily measured response.

CLINICAL RESPONSES

Clinical responses to drugs are measured by a wide variety of techniques. These range from simple measurement of physiologic function (heart rate, blood pressure) to cure rates in populations of patients. In some cases the direct effects of a drug cannot be measured and therefore surrogates have to be used (see below). However, since the true aim of drug therapy is to improve both the quality and duration of life, increasingly attempts are being made to measure these directly. However, as noted previously, large numbers of patients are required to obtain such data. Clinical trials of new drugs are now sometimes designed to collect such data. An alternative approach for new drugs entering the market is to monitor all prescriptions (up to some realistic limit) for fatal and adverse events.

Clinically, the use of any drug depends absolutely upon knowing the appropriate dose, which depends upon dose–response curves with respect to both the desired effect and to undesired effects (adverse effects). These have been established in the past, first in isolated tissue preparations, then in experimental animals, and finally in humans. Generally, such determinations become more difficult and time-consuming the closer one approaches clinical reality. For example, the effect of a drug at a certain dose to diminish pain in people can be assessed using the visual analog pain scale in which a subject indicates the subjective pain experienced on a scale of 0 (no pain) to 10 (or 100), the latter being maximal imaginable pain. Because people vary, pain often fluctuates, and pain can arise from a variety of pathologic processes. The determination of full dose–response curves for a new analgesic, versus various kinds of pain, would require hundreds of subjects and many person-years of investigator time. Such extensive studies are generally impractical. On the other hand, using experimental animals (rats or mice), pain reduction can be measured from the average time animals devote to licking a foot that has been injected by an agent that causes temporary inflammation. To obtain a dose–response relationship in this way may require 100–200 animals and several person-days of observation. Such an experiment would typically follow 'screens'—rather rough dose–response curves obtained with a variety of tissue preparations—to establish the absence of pharmacologic actions that could preclude the clinical use of the drug.

In view of the difficulty in obtaining *any* true dose–response relationship in the human, recourse is often made to 'surrogate' measures. For example, essential hypertension is statistically associated with increased mortality. Therefore, the proper measure of response to an antihypertensive drug is the extent to which it reduces mortality, providing it does this without causing negative adverse effects that make a longer life not worthwhile. To assess an antihypertensive in this manner would require a prospective clinical trial involving thousands of subjects, followed over many years. Antihypertensive drugs are therefore usually assessed in terms of their effectiveness and potency with regard to a surrogate, blood pressure reduction, which is fairly easy to measure. A dose–response relationship for true clinical effectiveness has not yet been obtained for most antihypertensives in common use although increasing attention is being paid to whether they reduce mortality.

POPULATION EFFECTS

Different people respond in different ways to drugs. Therefore mechanisms are needed to acquire data on the effects of drugs in the population, and experience has shown that data should be gathered according to some protocol rather than during routine care.

Data gathered during phases II and III of clinical trials are an important source of information for assessing the effect of drugs in the population; they can be used not only to determine toxicity but also to maximize efficacy. One major problem associated with information obtained from premarketing studies, however, can be a lack of heterogeneity among the pool of patients taking the medication. This problem can be confounded further by differences in the severity of disease between different patients. However, these problems can be partly overcome by designing studies to incorporate a large patient base. Certainly in the long term, a continuous gathering of information about the actions of drugs in the population will serve a useful purpose in optimizing the dose to reduce toxicity and maximize the pharmacotherapeutic benefit.

Lifestyle needs to be taken into account when studying the effects of drug in population. For example, a patient who is a smoker defines a different population. In effect, this could mean that a physician prescribing a drug may need to shift from the population mean to accommodate individual patients. Therefore, such scenarios play an important role in the decisions that are made by physician in writing prescriptions.

FURTHER READING

Black JW, Leff P. Operational models of pharmacological agonism. *Proc R Soc Lond [Biol]* 1983; **220:** 141–162. [Gives different perspectives on agonist–receptor dynamics.]

Kenakin T. The classification of drugs and drug–receptor antagonism. *Pharmacol Rev* 1984; **36:** 165–222. [Classification of receptors based on affinity of drugs.]

Pratt WB, Taylor P. *Principles of Drug Actions: The Basis of Pharmacology.* New York: Churchill Livingstone; 1990. [Introduction to the fundamentals of drug–receptor dynamics.]

Schild O. pA_x, and competitive drug antagonism. *Br J Pharmacol* 1949; **4:** 277–280. [Analysis of dose–response curves in the presence of antagonists.]

Stephenson RP. A modification of receptor theory. *Br J Pharmacol* 1956; **11:** 379–393. [An introduction of the concept of a responser being a function of the stimulus.]

?

Indicate which is the correct answer for each question.

1. When the contractile response of a smooth muscle preparation to an agonist for which the receptor reserve ('e') is 1000 is recorded, all of the following are true, except
- a) a competitive blocker will cause a parallel shift of the response–log dose curve, with an increase in the agonist's EC_{50} and no change in the maximum response to agonist
- b) an irreversible receptor blocker will depress the maximum response to this agonist less than it blocks the maximal response to a partial agonist at the same receptor
- c) an irreversible receptor blocker will shift the response–log dose curve in much the same way as a competitive blocker until dose ratios of about 100 or greater are produced
- d) a noncompetitive blocker will reduce the maximum response to the agonist, without changing its EC_{50}
- e) the half-maximal response of the tissue will occur at a concentration of the agonist about equal to 1/1000 (10^{-3}) of the agonist–receptor dissociation constant

2. Chemical groups or sites on the surface of or within the cell, with which drugs combine to produce an effect, are called
- a) autacoids
- b) antagonists
- c) agonists
- d) molecular targets (e.g. receptors)
- e) placebos

3. An agent that interferes with the action of a hormone by binding to the hormone receptor is referred to as
- a) an agonist
- b) an antagonist
- c) an enzyme inhibitor
- d) a modulator
- e) a competitor

4. In the absence of other drugs, pindolol increases heart rate by activating β adrenoceptors. However, when the heart rate has been increased by epinephrine, pindolol causes a dose-dependent reversible decrease in heart rate. From this information, pindolol is probably
- a) a noncompetitive antagonist
- b) a physiologic antagonist
- c) a chemical antagonist
- d) a partial agonist
- e) a spare receptor agonist

5. In a test preparation acetylcholine (ACh) is a full agonist that produces a half-maximum response at a concentration that occupies only 0.1% of the ACh receptors. The maximum response is 100 units. At a certain 'low' dose ACh produces a response of 10 units. An irreversible blocker is applied long enough to inactivate 90% of the receptors. After this treatment, responses to the 'low' dose of ACh and the maximum response to ACh will be close to
- a) 1 unit and 10 units
- b) 10 units and 100 units
- c) 5 units and 50 units
- d) 1 unit and 100 units
- e) none of the above

6. Partial agonist drugs
- a) reduce the apparent potency of a full agonist acting on the same receptor
- b) act at sites on the receptor remote from the agonist binding site
- c) increase the apparent potency of a full agonist drug acting on the same receptor
- d) are always less potent than full agonists at the same receptor
- e) reduce the maximum effect produced by the combination of the partial agonist and the full agonist at the same receptor

7. Which of the following class/classes of antagonist drug produce a block that can *always* be overcome by increasing doses of agonist drug?
- a) irreversible competitive antagonists
- b) irreversible noncompetitive antagonists
- c) reversible competitive antagonists
- d) physiologic antagonists
- e) chemical antagonists

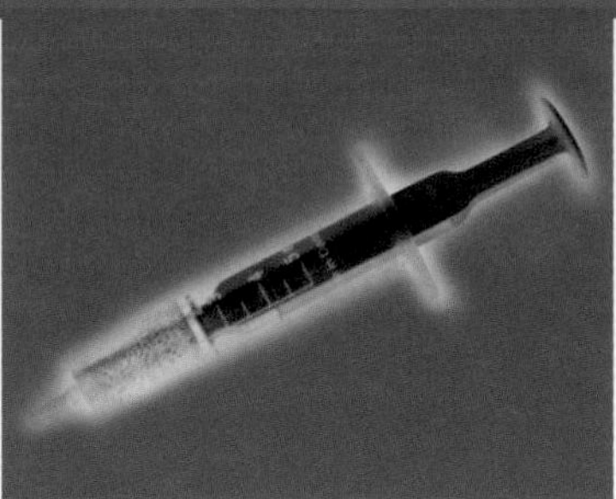

5. Factors Influencing the Action of Drugs

Drugs are given by a variety of routes (e.g. oral, intravenous, inhalation) and must be produced in an appropriate form for a particular route. All drugs, other than those that act locally (topically), are absorbed into the blood from their site of administration. They then are distributed throughout the body. Simultaneously and subsequently, they are metabolized and excreted either changed or unchanged. Alteration of any of these processes (i.e. absorption, distribution, metabolism, and excretion) can modify a drug's effect.

DRUG DELIVERY

Drugs are used in a variety of forms, including tablets, capsules, solutions, suspensions, modified release products, injectables, ointments, creams, and suppositories. In addition, they may be given as prodrugs (precursors), which use the biologic characteristics of the host to liberate the pharmacologically active substance(s) *in vivo*.

DRUG FORMULATION

Depending on its formulation, the drug delivery system can allow selective targeting of a tissue site or avoid systemic drug delivery. Some drug forms deliver the drug only into the gastrointestinal tract in a convenient physical form (e.g. tablets, capsules, solutions, suspensions). Liquid formulations are useful for individualizing the dose and for people who have difficulty swallowing solids.

A strategy for extending the activity of drugs with a brief persistence in the body is to use a drug formulation that releases the drug slowly as it passes through the gastrointestinal tract. Tablets coated with a semipermeable membrane are an example of a newer controlled-release delivery system (Fig. 5.1). Several other formulation strategies can also be used, and plasma concentrations over time after dosing will be influenced by the design of the drug form. Such products include:

- Controlled-release theophylline for asthma.
- Controlled-release verapamil for hypertension.

Drug absorption through the skin can also be used to produce systemic effects

An example of such a delivery system is shown in Fig. 5.2. Ideal compounds for this type of delivery include potent molecules that have a relatively brief persistence in the body, for example:

- The scopolamine skin patch to prevent motion sickness.
- The fentanyl skin patch for chronic severe pain.
- The nicotine skin patch to help people stop smoking tobacco.

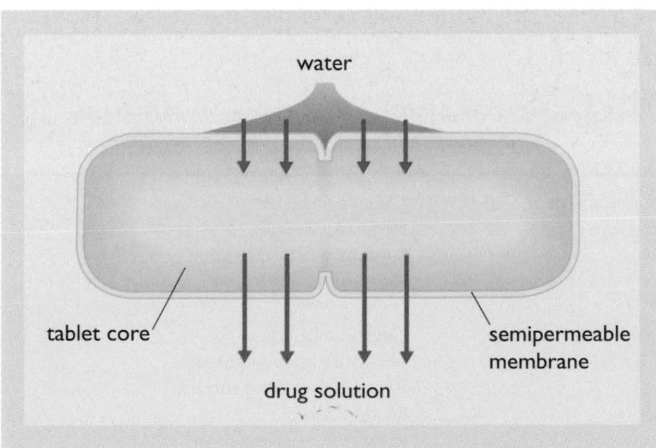

Fig. 5.1 Diagram of a modified-release tablet. This tablet is coated with a membrane that is selectively permeable for water. Water passes into the core of the tablet and releases the drug solution through small holes cut in the membrane.

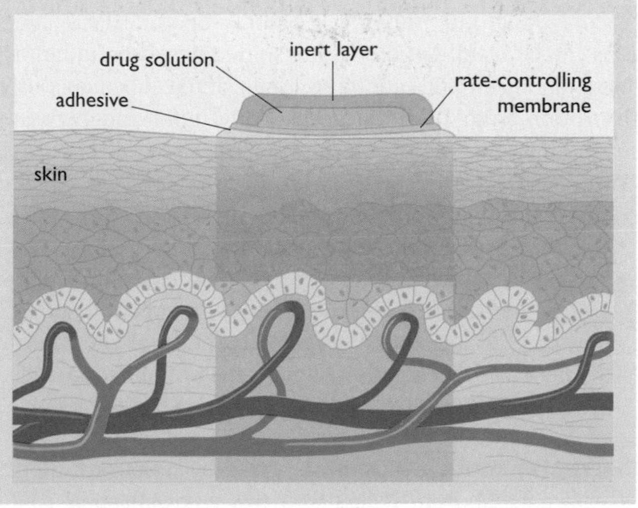

Fig. 5.2 Diagram of skin patch drug delivery. In this formulation, drug solution diffuses through a rate-controlling membrane, which limits the drug absorption by the skin.

Topical products are usually used to produce a local therapeutic effect

Topical products include solutions, ointments, creams, and suppositories, and sites for such applications include the eye, ear, skin, mouth, throat, lung, rectum, and vagina. However, the skin and mucous surfaces provide only a relative barrier to the systemic absorption of drug applied to them.

ROUTES FOR ADMINISTERING DRUGS

Most drugs are given by mouth. Routes other than the oral route (e.g. rectal, sublingual, injection, application to the skin or mucosal surfaces, and inhalation) should be considered if:

- The drug is unstable or rapidly inactivated in the gastrointestinal tract.
- The efficacy of drug absorption from the gastrointestinal tract is uncertain as a result of variable presystemic elimination due to metabolism by the intestine or liver, vomiting, or a disease state that may affect drug absorption.

Routes other than the oral route

The following routes bypass direct exposure to the gastrointestinal tract:

The sublingual route Drug absorption in the mouth from the buccal or sublingual mucosa bypasses exposure to the gastrointestinal tract and the liver and is useful for potent drugs without a disagreeable taste (e.g. sublingual nitroglycerin to relieve an acute attack of angina).

The subcutaneous route Subcutaneous implantation of a drug can extend its pharmacologic effect. This approach is utilized for contraception using subdermal implants of progestins (e.g. norgestrel).

The parenteral route The most direct route of administration is to inject the drug into the blood stream. This is usually accomplished by an intravenous dose. However, in rare instances intra-arterial injections are used. Alternatively, subcutaneous, intramuscular, epidural, or intrathecal injections can be used. Antibiotics are sometimes given intramuscularly, and hormones are often administered subcutaneously. Absorption from these sites is usually rapid and bypasses presystemic elimination by the upper gastrointestinal tract. However, drug absorption from an injection site can be slowed by using:

- A vehicle that tends to bind the drug.
- A vasoconstrictor in the vehicle to reduce perfusion of the injection site (e.g. the use of an α adrenoceptor agonist, with local anesthetic, to prolong the local anesthetic's effect by reducing blood flow at the site of injection, see Chapters 20 and 21).

The rectal route Drugs can be given by suppository. First-pass liver metabolism is less with this gastrointestinal route since less venous return from the lower gastrointestinal tract passes through the liver than from the upper gastrointestinal tract. However, rectal absorption can be inconsistent.

The nasal mucosa is a useful site for the absorption of drugs that undergo considerable presystemic elimination when given orally. Nasal sprays can be used to deliver potent drugs for their systemic effects (e.g. some hormones and opioid analgesic drugs for the management of severe chronic pain). However, nasal mucosa absorption is irregular.

Inhalation Vapors and gases (e.g. general anesthetics, see Chapter 21) are well absorbed when inhaled. In addition, if the lung is the target of drug therapy, inhalation is often an appropriate method of drug administration. The undesirable systemic effects of oral drug forms used to treat reversible bronchoconstriction can be considerably reduced if the drug is inhaled because the total dose can be reduced and less of the administered dose reaches the systemic circulation. Examples of inhaled drugs include inhaled glucocorticosteroids and β_2 adrenoceptor agonists for the treatment of asthma. The proportion of a dose that reaches the site of action depends on the ability of the patient to coordinate inspiration with triggering of the dose release from the canister.

FACTORS INFLUENCING DRUG ABSORPTION AND DISTRIBUTION

ABSORPTION

Both chemical and physiologic factors influence drug absorption (Fig. 5.3).

The diffusion rate usually determines the rate of drug absorption

Most drugs are small molecules with a molecular weight less than 1000 and pass across biologic membranes by diffusion in their uncharged state. This situation arises because cell membranes are essentially lipid bilayers containing various protein molecules, which regulate cell homeostasis. Some charged molecules can be actively transported across membrane barriers (e.g. 5-fluorouracil and levodopa). As most drugs are either weak acids, bases, or amphoteric, the pH of the environment where the drug form disintegrates and dissolves will determine the fraction in solution

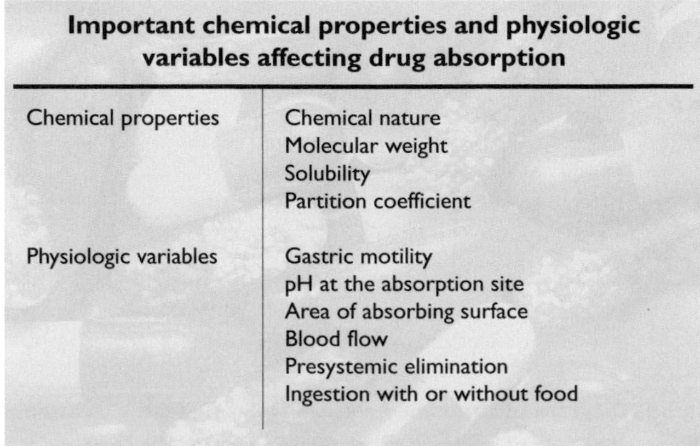

Important chemical properties and physiologic variables affecting drug absorption

Chemical properties	Chemical nature Molecular weight Solubility Partition coefficient
Physiologic variables	Gastric motility pH at the absorption site Area of absorbing surface Blood flow Presystemic elimination Ingestion with or without food

Fig. 5.3 Important chemical properties and physiologic variables affecting drug absorption.

in the un-ionized form that can diffuse across cell membranes. This fraction will depend on the drug's chemical nature, its pKa, and the local pH. The pKa of a drug substance represents the pH at which 50% of the molecules in solution are ionized, and this relationship is described by the Henderson–Hasselbalch equation: for acidic molecules,

$$HA \Leftrightarrow H^+ + A^-$$

and $pKa = pH + \log (HA/A^-)$,

for basic molecules,

$$BH^+ \Leftrightarrow B + H^+$$

and $pKa = pH + \log (BH^+/B)$.

The pKa values and hence fractions of ionized and un-ionized molecules of different drugs at physiological pH (7.4) show considerable differences (Fig. 5.4). A useful concept is that chemicals will tend to exist in the ionized form when exposed to their pH-opposite chemical environment. Therefore, acids are increasingly ionized with increasing pH (basic environment), while bases are increasingly ionized with decreasing pH (acidic environment).

The site of drug administration can alter the rate of drug absorption

The fraction of dissolved drug in the un-ionized form and therefore the rate of drug absorption, but not necessarily its extent, can depend on the site of drug administration. In the stomach, where the pH is approximately 2.0, most acidic drugs in solution will be un-ionized and able to diffuse readily across cell membranes. Conversely, most basic drugs in the stomach will be almost completely ionized and will have little or no ability to diffuse across cell membranes in the stomach.

The rate of diffusion of un-ionized molecules across the membrane lipid bilayer depends on molecular size and lipid solubility

Since the diffusion coefficient is inversely related to the square root of the molecular weight, smaller molecules will diffuse more easily across the membrane than larger molecules. However, the narrow range of molecular weight for most drugs usually means that the diffusion coefficient is rarely a limiting factor in determining the rate of drug absorption.

Lipid solubility, which is often indicated by a parameter termed the partition coefficient, can play an important role in drug absorption. It reflects the solubility of the drug molecule in a lipid solvent relative to its solubility in water or a physiologic buffer. The accuracy of this determination depends on the drug molecule not saturating either of the two liquid phases. The higher the partition coefficient, the more rapidly the drug molecule can diffuse across the lipid membrane. The therapeutic use of the central nervous system (CNS) depressant barbiturates is related to partition coefficient:

- Thiopental, which has a pKa of 7.45 and a high partition coefficient of 580 is used as an anesthetic for inducing anethesia (see Chapter 21) by injection because it rapidly enters brain tissue.
- Phenobarbital, with a similar pKa of 7.20, but a much lower partition coefficient of 3, is used primarily for the chronic treatment of epilepsy.

Drug access to the systemic circulation can be limited by the route of administration

The route of administration can limit drug access to the systemic circulation, for example:

- Drugs in solution administered as eye drops will have primarily local effects, although systemic effects can occur with potent drugs that are subsequently absorbed via the lacrimal ducts.
- Penicillin G is unstable in the acid environment of the stomach and large oral doses are needed to compensate for drug decomposition in the stomach.
- Nitroglycerin is administered sublingually to allow systemic absorption before metabolic hydrolysis terminates its pharmacologic activity.

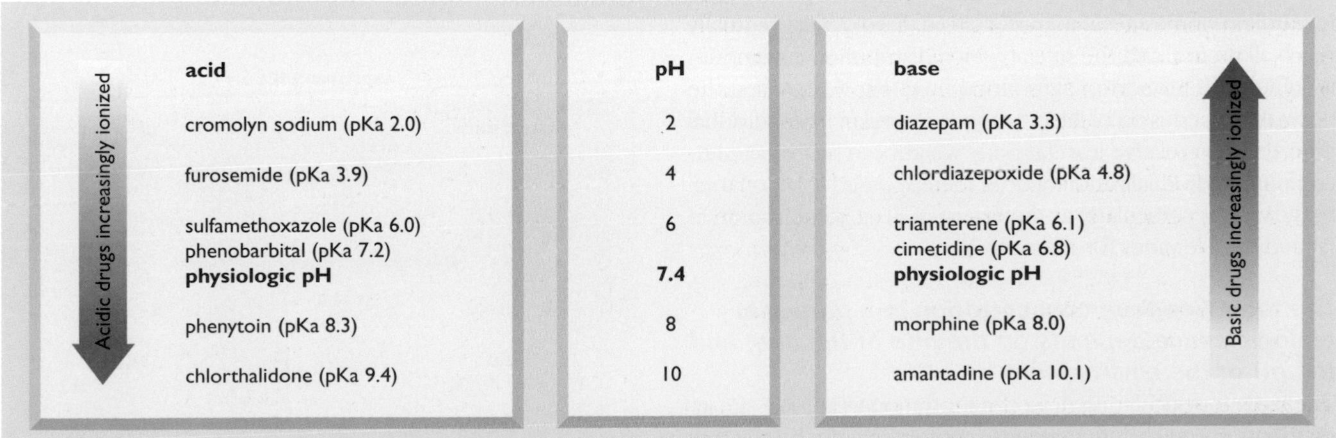

Fig. 5.4 Acidic and basic drugs and their pKa values relative to physiologic pH. The arrows representing fraction ionized indicate only that acidic drugs are increasingly ionized as pH increases. The extent of ionization is calculated with the Henderson–Hasselbach equation, and relates pH of the biologic environment and pKa of the drug of interest.

The rate of drug absorption after an oral dose can be altered by altering the rate of gastric emptying

Ingestion of a solid dosage form with a glass of cold water will accelerate gastric emptying, and exposure of the drug to the upper intestine with a higher pH and a much larger surface area. Accelerated gastric emptying also can be effected pharmacologically by using a drug such as metoclopramide to increase gastric motility. Conversely, ingestion of a drug with a fatty meal, an acidic drink, or another drug with anticholinergic effects will retard gastric emptying.

Drug absorption

- Most drugs are well absorbed from the gastrointestinal tract
- The site of absorption depends on the un-ionized fraction of drug in solution
- Gastric emptying can be accelerated by ingesting the dose with cold water
- Basic drugs ingested by mouth are poorly absorbed until they pass into the duodenum
- Modified-release dose forms prolong the duration of drug effect after a dose and allow for a more convenient dosage regimen

DISTRIBUTION

The molecular size of most commonly used drugs is very small and these drugs readily leave the circulation by capillary filtration, although this may be modified by the extent of drug binding to plasma proteins such as albumin.

Obesity can be expected to influence drug distribution immediately after a dose and at equilibrium

Regardless of the site of administration, a drug will eventually reach all tissues, and the rate at which distribution equilibrium is achieved is proportional to blood flow (Fig. 5.5). At rest the normalized perfusion of fat and muscle is similar. Interindividual differences in relative lean:fat body weight can be expected to confound individualization of drug therapy based solely on total body weight, particularly as the extent of drug accumulation in fat and muscle varies for different drugs.

The total free drug concentration in a particular biologic space depends on the pKa of the drug and the pH of the environment

The basis for calculating drug concentration at a tissue site at - distribution equilibrium depends on the principle that the free concentration of un-ionized molecules will be equal on both sides of the cell membrane. Figures 5.6 and 5.7 illustrate the distribution equilibrium between two biologic environments for an acidic drug (naproxen) and a basic drug (morphine) and demonstrate that:

- Acids are likely to be concentrated in the circulation.
- The concentration of basic drugs in the circulation is much lower than in alternative biologic environments.

It should be noted that these examples refer only to the unbound fraction of drug dissolved in the specific biologic environment. In other words, these examples are highly simplified, especially compared to the body as a whole under nonequilibrium conditions.

Protein binding contributes to the difference in total drug concentration between biologic spaces

Albumin is the most important circulating protein for binding many acidic drugs. Competition for the binding sites on albumin usually becomes important clinically for drugs that are more than 80% bound, and especially if binding exceeds 90%. Small changes in the bound fraction can then lead to large changes in the fraction that is free to exert its pharmacologic effect (Fig. 5.8).

Total and weight-normalized tissue blood flow in an adult

Perfusion	Blood flow (ml/min)	Organ mass (kg)	Blood flow (ml/kg/min)
Cardiac output	5400	–	–
Myocardium	250	0.3	833
Liver	1700	2.5	680
Kidney	1000	0.3	3333
CNS	800	1.3	615
Fat	250	10.0	25
Other (muscle, etc.)	1400	55.0	25
Total		69.4	

Fig. 5.5 Total and weight-normalized tissue blood flow in an adult.

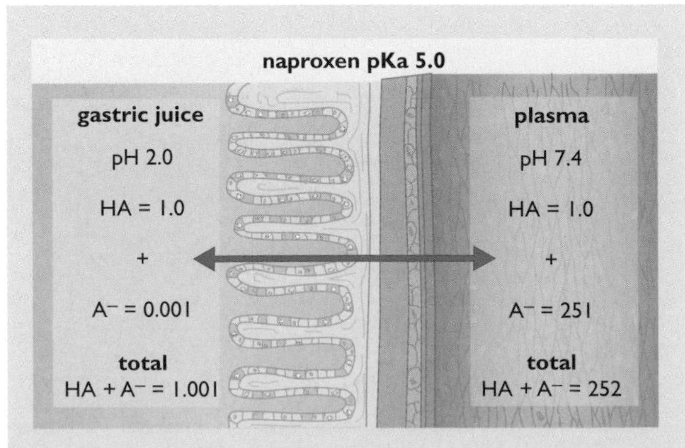

Fig. 5.6 Dissolved drug distribution for an acidic drug. This depicts the dissolved drug distribution at equilibrium between gastric juice and plasma for naproxen. Note acidic drugs concentrate in the circulation.

Many basic drugs are bound to a globulin fraction (i.e. α_1 acid glycoprotein). Interpretation of the clinical importance of this interaction is complicated because this protein is an acute-phase reactant and increases with age and in acute pathologic stress.

In a suspected overdose, the most appropriate site for sampling to identify the drug depends on the drug's chemical characteristics

Acidic drugs will concentrate in the plasma and blood is an appropriate sample site for identifying the drug, while the stomach is a reasonable site for sampling basic drugs regardless of the method of drug administration. Diffusion of basic drugs into the stomach results in almost complete ionization. As a constant gradient remains, basic drugs concentrate in the stomach until there is distribution equilibrium of the un-ionized fraction. The actions of amphetamine can be prolonged by ingesting bicarbonate to alkalinize the urine. As a result of such alkalinization, an increasing fraction of urinary amphetamine is in the un-ionized form and as such is readily reabsorbed across the luminal surface of the kidney.

Anatomic and physiologic factors contribute to drug distribution to different biologic spaces

The anatomic characteristics of the blood–brain barrier affect the ability of drugs to enter the brain. In addition, the intercellular spaces of the brain capillaries are occluded by zonulae, thereby increasing the barrier to drug diffusion into the CNS. However, there are five regions of the brain where this does not occur: the pituitary gland, the pineal body, the area postrema, the median eminence, and the choroid plexus capillaries. The choroid plexus also contains transporters, which remove charged molecules from the cerebrospinal fluid (CSF). Normally, CSF contains no protein, and the drug concentration in this biologic space is similar to the free drug concentration in the blood.

Unless proven otherwise, it should be assumed that all drugs cross the placenta and enter breast milk

Drugs distribute across the placenta, but equilibration between the mother and fetus may be delayed because of the limited placental blood flow from the maternal circulation. Unless proven otherwise, it should be assumed that all drugs cross the placenta and enter breast milk. The clinical importance of drugs in the placenta and in breast milk must be assessed for each drug.

The pharmacokinetic space into which a drug distributes is the 'apparent volume of distribution'

The apparent volume of distribution is a calculated space and does not conform to any actual anatomic space. It is based upon the dose administered and the resulting drug concentration in the circulating plasma. Some molecules (e.g. ethanol) have an apparent volume of distribution that approximates total body water. However, the pharmacokinetic distribution of ethanol does correlate with the distribution of total body water. This is because ethanol is also lipid soluble and is not solely dissolved in water. Some drugs have apparent volumes of distribution that considerably exceed body weight (Fig. 5.9). These drugs are usually basic drugs and their high apparent volume of distribution reflects extensive tissue binding. In this situation, almost all the administered dose will be sequestered outside the circulation. Anatomic studies in animal models demonstrate considerable localization of these drugs, often to specific organs of the body (e.g. the concentration of the antiviral drug amantadine in liver, lung, and kidney is several times that found in the circulation).

The site of action of a drug and the tissue mass in which it concentrates need to be considered to determine the clinical importance of this localization. The cardiac glycoside digoxin concentrates in muscle and its apparent volume of distribution greatly exceeds body weight. Therefore the digoxin dose needed to produce therapeutic plasma concentrations depends on the relative muscle weight to total body weight. In addition, it takes several hours to achieve equilibrium between blood and muscle, and so plasma digoxin concentrations do not readily relate to the inotropic response if distribution equilibrium has not occurred.

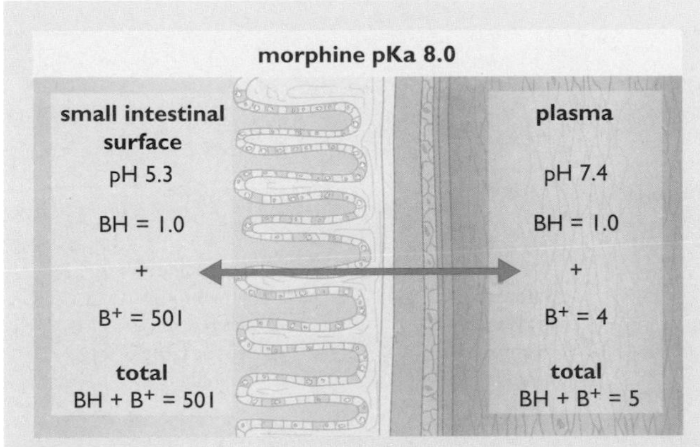

Fig. 5.7 Dissolved drug distribution for a basic drug. This depicts the dissolved drug distribution at equilibrium between the small intestinal surface and plasma for morphine. Note basic drugs generally have lower concentrations in the circulation than in other body compartments.

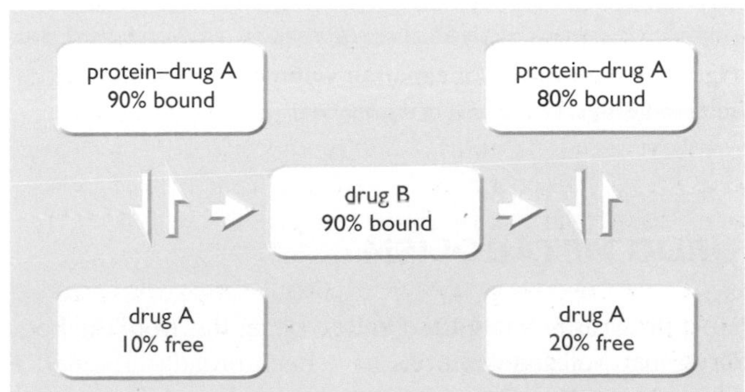

Fig. 5.8 Protein binding and fraction of free drug. This shows the outcome when one drug (A) is displaced from its protein binding site by addition of a second drug (B). The change in free fraction is considerable for highly bound drugs.

Drug distribution

- Drug distribution is based on the principle that the un-ionized concentration is the same throughout the body at equilibrium
- Charged drug molecules are effectively prevented from entering the brain by the blood–brain barrier except when the meninges are inflamed
- Basic drugs concentrate in the stomach because they are mainly ionized

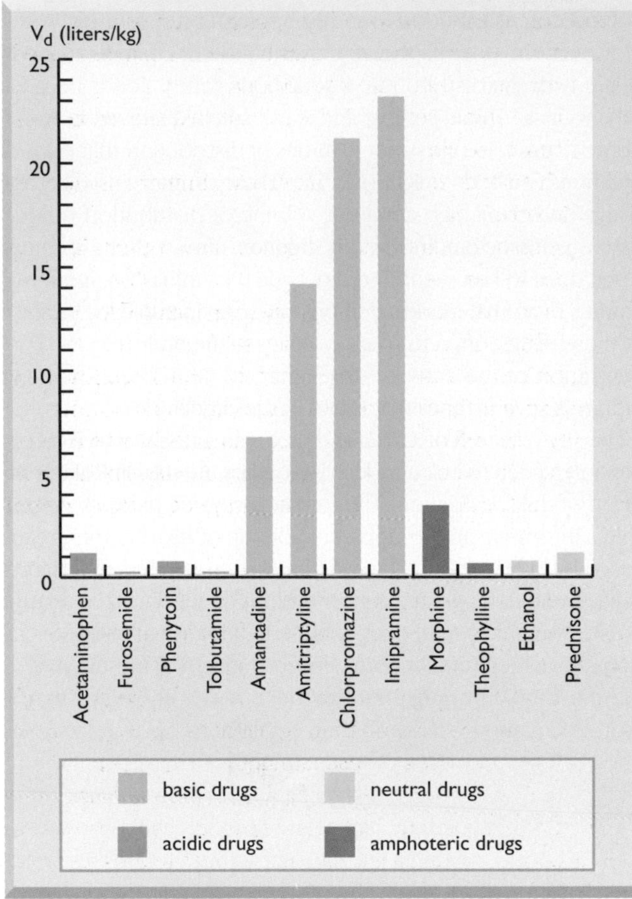

Fig. 5.9 Typical values for apparent volume of distribution of selected drugs. (V_d, volume of distribution)

DRUG METABOLISM

Most drugs are metabolized before being lost from the body. Drug metabolizing reactions have been broadly classified as phase 1 and phase 2 processes.

- Phase 1 processes involve oxidation, reduction, and hydrolysis, reactions that provide a functional group to increase polarity of the drug molecule and a site that is a candidate for phase 2 metabolism.
- Phase 2 processes involve conjugation or synthetic reactions in which a large chemical group is attached to the molecule. This usually increases water solubility and facilitates excretion of the metabolite from the body.

The nature, function, and amount of any drug-metabolizing enzyme can be different, resulting in differing drug disposition among patients

The drug-metabolizing enzymes have broad substrate specificities, and enzyme specificity is relative rather than absolute (e.g. demethylation of theophylline).

Generally, the drug-metabolizing enzymes occur in multiple forms, and interindividual differences in genetic expression can contribute to interindividual differences in drug metabolism. The enzymes have been classified into families, subfamilies, and specific gene products, and their expression can be regulated at many levels. Some enzymes are expressed constitutively. Others are primarily expressed when triggered by an environmental substance. Gene mutations can result in deficient or absent expression of a particular enzyme and unexpected drug toxicity may ensue from administration of a typical drug dose (see Chapter 21). Conversely, redundant genetic code may result in multiple copies of a particular drug-metabolizing enzyme. This is likely to result in resistance to typical therapeutic doses.

The activity of drug-metabolizing enzymes may be increased (induced) or inhibited

Many factors in the diet can affect drug-metabolizing enzymes, including the protein:carbohydrate ratio, plant foods containing flavonoids (e.g. cruciferous vegetables), and barbecued foods, which are usually high in polycyclic aromatic hydrocarbons from burning charcoal.

Increased enzyme synthesis as a result of the presence of an exogenous chemical is referred to as 'induction' (Fig. 5.10). The induction process may be due to a combination of changes in nucleic acid transcription, translational, and post-translational

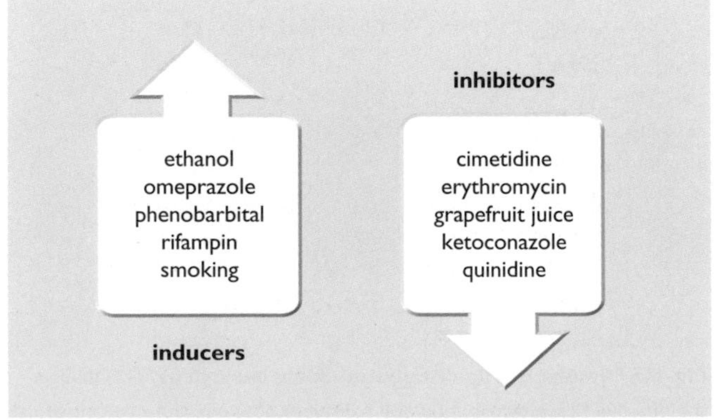

Fig. 5.10 Enzyme inducers and inhibitors. Drugs known to induce or inhibit the metabolism of other drugs administered concurrently.

regulation. Such stimulation can be produced by certain drugs and food constituents, alcohol, and smoking. When chronically ingested, some drugs (e.g. barbiturates, rifampin) induce their own metabolism as well as that of other drugs or endogenous substances.

The tissue site where induction occurs may be determined by the nature of exposure to the chemical responsible. Smokers induce expression of a particular isoform of cytochromes P-450, primarily in the lungs and upper intestine.

Sometimes, two drugs will compete for metabolism by the same enzyme, resulting in a decreased rate of metabolism for one or both drugs. This process is referred to as 'inhibition' (see Fig. 5.10). The cardiac toxicity produced by the nonsedating antihistamine terfenadine, when it is ingested concurrently with the antifungal drug ketoconazole or a macrolide antibiotic such as erythromycin, is a clinically important example of this situation.

Most tissues can metabolize specific drugs

Although the liver is regarded as the major site of drug metabolism, most tissues can metabolize specific drugs. Tissue specificity for drug metabolism depends on the genetic regulation and expression of drug-metabolizing enzyme by particular tissues. Therefore selective tissue effects may result from a unique drug-metabolizing enzyme reaction at the relevant site. For example, the kidney oxidizes the metabolite sulindac sulfide, the active cyclooxygenase inhibitor, back to sulindac, the parent prodrug, thereby protecting the kidney from impaired function due to inhibition of cyclooxygenase by the sulindac sulfide molecule.

The three types of elimination are first order, zero order, and intermediate

The concentration of most drugs in the body is considerably less than that required to saturate the body's eliminating capacity. The rate of removal of such drugs from the body is proportional to their concentration in the plasma (first order elimination), and an effective measure of this process is the plasma half-life. The drug is considered to be essentially completely removed from the circulation in five half-lives.

The concept of half-life is inappropriate for a few drugs (e.g. ethanol) because their rate of elimination does not change with increasing or decreasing circulating concentration, unless the plasma concentration is very low and sometimes pharmacologically ineffective. The metabolism of ethanol is effectively saturated after ingestion of a relatively small dose. Its elimination is best described as removal of a constant amount/unit time (zero order elimination).

Other drugs (e.g. aspirin, phenytoin) show intermediate elimination rates between the two extremes of zero and first order elimination. Owing to this characteristic, the plasma drug concentration increases disproportionately with increasing dose since the elimination rate does not increase as the dose increases. Monitoring of the plasma concentration of such drugs is therefore advisable to avoid toxicity when a dose regimen is changed, since small changes in dose can lead to relatively large changes in plasma concentration.

PHASE I METABOLISM

Oxidation

Cytochromes P-450 form a superfamily of heme protein enzyme isoforms that catalyze oxidative metabolism of many substances, including drugs

Most oxidative metabolism of drugs is catalyzed by cytochromes P-450, though other enzymes are also involved. There are several hundred isoforms of cytochromes P-450. Some are constitutive, while others are present only when synthesized in response to an appropriate signal, usually provided by an exogenous chemical.

Substrate specificity is determined by the isoform of cytochromes P-450, but usually specificity is relative rather than absolute so that the absence of any particular isoform does not necessarily preclude a particular metabolic reaction. Genes for cytochromes P-450 are found on several chromosomes.

A nomenclature for cytochromes P-450 has been developed to help understand their interrelationships:

- The capital letters 'CYP' indicate that the isoform is of human origin.
- CYP is then followed by an Arabic number to indicate the isoform's family.
- Subfamilies are then designated by another capitalized letter of the alphabet.
- Finally there is another Arabic number to designate an individual gene product in the subfamily.

Designation of family and subfamily status relates to the increasing amino acid sequence homology for the various P-450 isoforms. Therefore CYP1A2 is a human cytochrome P-450 isoform and is a member of the first family of enzymes, the A subfamily, and the second gene product assigned to that subfamily.

Only a few members of three families of cytochromes P-450 have been identified as important for the metabolism of a wide variety of drugs

Three families of cytochromes P-450 have so far been identified as important contributors to drug metabolism (Fig. 5.11), and only a few members of these families have been identified as important for the metabolism of a wide variety of drugs.

The CYP3A subfamily has been identified as the major constitutive form in human liver and contributes to the metabolism of a wide variety of drugs. It is also expressed in clinically significant amounts in tissues other than liver. The specific isoform

Cytochrome P-450 families and the isoforms important to oxidative drug metabolism

Family	Isoform	Drug substrate
CYP1	CYP1A2	Theophylline
CYP2	CYP2D6	Codeine
CYP3	CYP3A4	Cyclosporine

Fig. 5.11 Cytochrome P-450 families and the isoforms important to oxidative drug metabolism.

CYP3A4 is thought to be responsible for intestinal presystemic elimination of many drugs showing poor bioavailability.

CYP2D6 has been associated with:

- The oxidative metabolism of many drugs including β adrenoceptor antagonists.
- Demethylation of tricyclic antidepressants.
- Demethylation of codeine to morphine.

Approximately 5–10% of Caucasians have deficient phenotypic expression of this isoform, and this is an autosomal recessive trait. Multiple mutations of CYP2D6 have been described. For example, inability to demethylate codeine is associated with a lack of an analgesic response to codeine.

CYP2E1 is a labile isoform induced by chronic alcohol consumption, while CYP1A2 is important in the metabolism of theophylline and can be induced by flavonoids and polycyclic aromatic hydrocarbons. Knowledge of the metabolic constitution of a patient therefore has potential predictive value in determining whether a particular drug is appropriate. Tests to provide details of the phenotypic expression of drug-metabolizing enzymes in individual patients should be available in the future. Such information will be valuable for determining which specific drugs or drug classes should be free of problems with respect to drug metabolism. Caution is advised, however, in interpreting phenotypic expression of a gene product since the former can be modulated by environmental and physiologic factors.

Cytochromes P-450 require the presence of the mixed function oxidase system

Cytochromes P-450 require the presence of molecular oxygen, NADPH cytochrome P-450 reductase, and NADPH to function. This combination of factors is referred to as the mixed function oxidase system. In this enzyme system, the P-450 isoforms are present in considerable excess relative to cytochrome P-450 reductase, the enzyme that contributes reducing equivalents to the oxidative reaction. The process by which cytochromes P-450 oxidize drug substrates is depicted in Fig. 5.12.

Oxidative reactions usually result in drug inactivation, but the metabolite can be pharmacologically active

Prodrugs are chemicals that are converted into pharmacologically active substances after absorption (e.g. the demethylation of codeine to morphine, Fig. 5.13). Sometimes drug oxidation results in the formation of an active metabolite with a duration of action that exceeds that of the administered drug (e.g. the conversion of diazepam to desmethyldiazepam).

Reduction

This metabolic pathway is used by:

- Sulindac, a prodrug that undergoes reduction of the sulfoxide group to produce sulindac sulfide, which is the active cyclooxygenase inhibitor for the treatment of inflammation associated with rheumatoid arthritis.
- Prednisone, which is administered as a prodrug and undergoes reduction of a ketone to produce the active glucocorticosteroid prednisolone.

Hydrolysis

Hydrolysis can occur spontaneously owing to instability of substituent groups in the drug molecule. Aspirin is therefore hydrolyzed to salicylic acid in the presence of moisture. Some therapeutic agents are administered as prodrugs, which are hydrolyzed after ingestion:

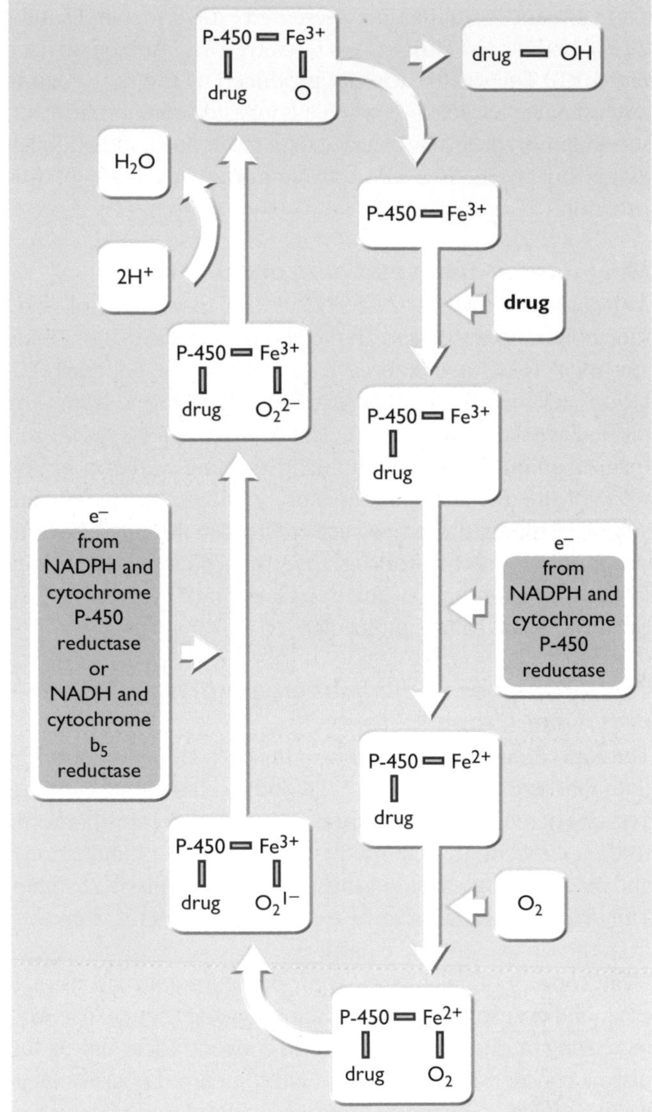

Fig. 5.12 Diagram depicting the oxidation of a drug substrate by the mixed function oxidase system. The drug substrate binds to the oxidized form of a specific cytochromes P-450 isoform. This complex receives a single electron from NADPH via cytochrome P-450 reductase. The reduced complex then reacts with molecular oxygen and a second electron donated either via NADPH and cytochrome P-450 reductase or NADH and cytochrome b_5 reductase. In the process, one atom of oxygen is released as water and the other is incorporated into the drug to produce the hydroxylated metabolite. The metabolic reaction also includes dealkylation reactions in which short-chain alkyl groups, usually methyl, are removed from the drug molecule and combine with oxygen to yield an aldehyde, which can be further oxidized or reduced.

- Sulfasalazine is split into aminosalicylic acid and sulfapyridine by the bacterial flora in the lower gastrointestinal tract.
- Bambuterol, a carbamate ester prodrug of terbutaline, is resistant to presystemic elimination and is absorbed and concentrated in lung tissue where it is hydrolyzed by pseudocholinesterase to release the active β_2 adrenoceptor agonist terbutaline at its desired site of action.

PHASE 2 METABOLISM

Conjugation involves enzyme-mediated attachment of activated moieties to the drug or metabolite generated by phase 1 metabolism

Phase 2 reactions are also referred to as conjugation and occur in a wide variety of tissues. They involve the enzyme-mediated attachment of activated moieties such as glucuronic acid, sulfate, glutathione, and acetate to a functional group on the drug or metabolite generated by phase 1 metabolism. For example, β glucuronic acid is activated by combination with uridine diphosphate (UDP). The activated UDP–glucuronic acid is then transferred to the drug substrate by glucuronosyltransferase.

Other conjugation reactions occur less often with substituents including glycine, methyl groups, and the sugars glucose and ribose. Examples of clinically important conjugation reactions are given in Fig. 5.14. Glucuronide conjugates are quantitatively the most important.

Although conjugation usually increases water solubility, acetylation often results in metabolites with lower water solubility than the unconjugated precursor (e.g. as with the acetylation of sulfonamide antibiotics). Acetylation of a basic amine functional group converts the basic drug to a weak acid (amide). This chemical change has an effect on the distribution and elimination of the resulting metabolite.

Conjugation reactions are usually considered to be inactivation processes. However, there are several notable exceptions, including:

- Acetylation of procainamide to form acetylprocainamide, which is an antiarrhythmic drug in its own right.
- Morphine-6-glucuronide, which is an analgesic with a longer duration of action than its parent molecule morphine.

Impaired renal function has therapeutic and toxic implications for both of these metabolites.

Sulfate conjugation can also be an activation step. Minoxidil, an antihypertensive drug, must be sulfated at the *N*-oxide position in order to produce its vasodilator effect. Promotion of hair growth by minoxidil is less than that of its sulfate metabolite. Variability in hair growth with minoxidil may therefore partly depend on the patient's ability to sulfate minoxidil at the hair follicle.

Multiple isoforms of the conjugating enzymes are being described, with relative specificity for various substrates and metabolites. At least two families and three subfamilies of glucuronyltransferases, and multiple gene products for acetylation and sulfation have been described.

Drug metabolism

- **Most drugs are metabolized before being eliminated from the body**
- **Drug metabolites are generally more polar than their parent compound**
- **The specificity of drug-metabolizing enzymes is relative rather than absolute**
- **The expression of drug-metabolizing enzymes differs between tissues**
- **Concurrent ingestion of two or more drugs can affect the rate of metabolism of one or more of them**

Drugs and prodrugs and their clinically important active metabolites

Drug	Active metabolite
Allopurinol	Oxypurinol
Diazepam	Desmethyldiazepam
Imipramine	Desmethylimipramine
Prodrug	**Active metabolite**
Codeine	Morphine
Prednisone	Prednisolone
Sulindac	Sulindac sulfide

Fig. 5.13 Drugs and prodrugs and their clinically important active metabolites.

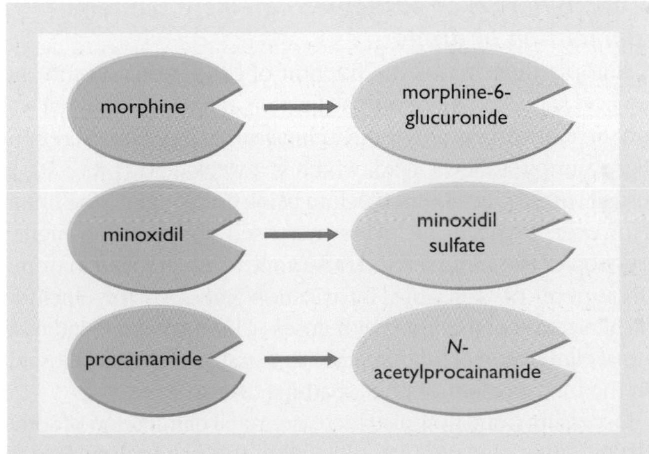

Fig. 5.14 Drug conjugation reactions that result in the production of active metabolites.

The dose of isoniazid, procainamide, and hydralazine depends on a patient's ability to acetylate the drugs. Phenotypic slow acetylators can appear to be rapid acetylators if the above drugs are ingested with ethanol.

Deficiencies of one or more of the isoforms of conjugated enzymes are likely to influence the choice of drugs to treat diseases. Characterizing patients according to their ability to metabolize prototypical substrates has the potential for improving the individualization of drug therapy.

DRUG EXCRETION

Drugs can be excreted by several routes including the kidneys (urine), the intestinal tract (bile and feces), the lungs (exhaled air), breast milk, and sweat. Excretions in the urine and feces are the most important routes for drug elimination.

RENAL EXCRETION

The excretion of some drugs is impaired in the presence of renal disease. Considerable data suggest that renal excretion of drugs correlates with the kidney's ability to excrete creatinine. If it is inconvenient or impossible to assess renal function directly by measuring a 24-hour creatinine clearance, renal function can be estimated using the widely accepted algorithm of Cockroft and Gault. These investigators established the relationship between patient age, weight, serum creatinine concentration ($C_{s,cr}$), and estimated creatinine clearance (Cl_{cr}) by the kidney as:

$$Cl_{cr}\ (\text{ml/min}) = [(140 - \text{age}) \times \text{ideal body weight (kg)}]/[0.8145 \times (C_{p,cr}\ (\mu\text{mol/liter})].$$

This equation applies to males. For females, the derived value for creatinine clearance should be multiplied by 0.85.

Renal creatinine excretion occurs by both filtration and secretion and the fraction excreted by each mechanism changes in favor of secretion as renal function decreases. It is likely that this relationship also applies to drugs that are filtered and secreted by the kidney.

A combination of strategies can increase renal elimination of drugs

Urine pH determines the fraction of drug molecules in the ionized state, and therefore the fraction of filtered drug that will not be reabsorbed across the luminal surface before excretion. For example salicylic acid, which is a weak acid (pKa 3.0), is usually mostly metabolized before being excreted into the urine. However, if the urine pH is increased above 6.0, a higher fraction of the administered dose appears unchanged in urine. Treatment of salicylate intoxication can possibly include alkalinization of the urine with doses of bicarbonate to increase renal elimination of salicylic acid. This strategy can also be useful in the management of phenobarbital overdose.

Increasing urine flow also increases renal elimination of some drugs since the contact time with the luminal surface is decreased, reducing the time for reabsorption of un-ionized molecules.

GASTROINTESTINAL EXCRETION

Drug removal from the gastrointestinal tract can be accelerated by using polyethylene glycol electrolyte lavage solution. Large volumes of this solution can be ingested or placed in the gastrointestinal tract through a gastric tube to increase intestinal peristalsis and hasten excretion of unabsorbed drug via the rectum. However, the decreased transit time through the gastrointestinal tract associated with diarrhea will decrease the absorption of nutrients.

Enterohepatic circulation prolongs the pharmacologic effect

Some drug conjugates excreted in bile are hydrolyzed in the lower intestine to release the original drug substrate for reabsorption and prolongation of effect. This process is referred to as enterohepatic circulation.

LUNG EXCRETION

Excretion of alcohol by the lung is quantitatively unimportant, but provides a noninvasive method for estimating the blood alcohol concentration.

Excretion via the lung also allows monitoring of the end tidal concentration of volatile anesthetic in expired air during anesthesia.

PHARMACOKINETICS

The analysis of all drug disposition factors (absorption, distribution, metabolism, and excretion) is termed pharmacokinetics.

THE ONE-COMPARTMENT MODEL

In its simplest concept, the body is considered to be a single uniform space into which the drug is absorbed and from which it is eliminated (Fig. 5.15). For many drugs, this situation will give rise to a single straight line when the log plasma concentration is plotted against time after a parenteral dose (Fig. 5.16). If the initial

Drug excretion

- **Renal and fecal excretion are the most important routes for drug elimination**
- **Some drug conjugates are hydrolyzed in the lower gastrointestinal tract back to the parent compound and reabsorbed in a process referred to as enterohepatic circulation, which extends the duration of drug action**
- **For some drugs the fraction of the administered dose excreted unchanged by the kidney depends on the urine pH**
- **Creatinine clearance can be used to assess any renal impairment and indicate whether drug doses need to be reduced if renal excretion is an important component of drug elimination**

drug concentration (C_0) in the compartment, assuming its distribution were instantaneous, is divided into the administered dose, the theoretic volume needed to accommodate the drug dose is described. This space is the apparent volume of distribution (V_d).

The time for the drug concentration to decline to 50% of its initial value is its half-life ($t_{1/2}$). Since the decline in logarithmic transformation of drug concentration with time is linear, the $t_{1/2}$ will be constant regardless of the initial drug concentration chosen. The rate of elimination of a drug from the circulation is related to $t_{1/2}$ by the equation:

$$t_{1/2} \times k_{el} = 0.693.$$

Since $t_{1/2}$ is related to the V_d, it may not reflect the ability of the drug to be removed from the body because the two parameters will change in the same direction. The preferred kinetic term to indicate the body's capability to remove a drug from the circulation is plasma clearance (Cl_p), which is calculated as $V_d \times k_{el}$ and will remain constant for most individual drugs if the capacity of the removal mechanisms is not modified by pathologic and/or physiologic factors.

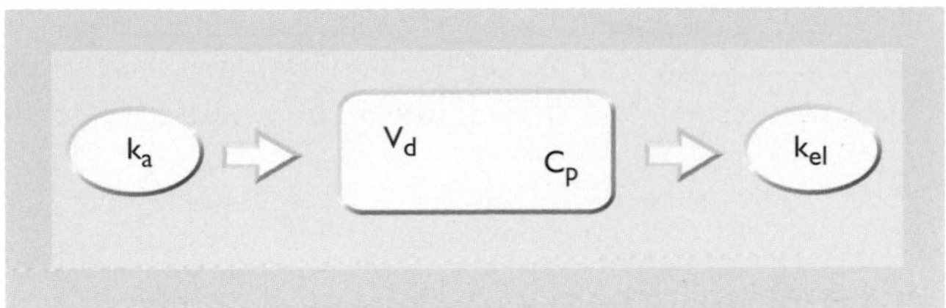

Fig. 5.15 Diagram of the one-compartment open pharmacokinetic model for drug disposition. The plasma concentration of a drug (C_p) is determined by the rate of drug absorption (k_a), the volume of drug distribution (V_d), and rate of drug elimination (k_{el}). When the drug is administered parenterally as a bolus, k_a is instantaneous and is not determined.

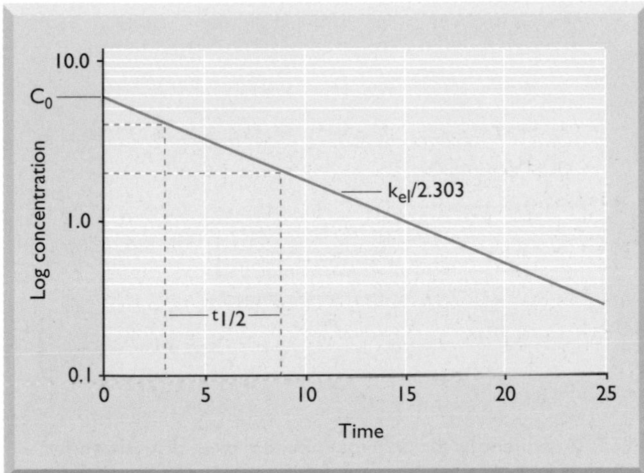

Fig. 5.16 Log plasma drug concentration versus time plot compatible with the one-compartment open pharmacokinetic model for drug disposition after a parenteral dose. Extrapolation of this line (k_{el}) to time 'zero' results in an estimate of the initial drug concentration (C_0) in the compartment if its distribution were instantaneous.

When the drug is administered other than parenterally, the shape of the plasma concentration versus time curve requires the interaction of two log-linear processes to account for both entry (absorption) to and exit (elimination) from the single compartment (Fig. 5.17). Calculation of the disposition parameters is the same as after parenteral dose administration, but some of the derived parameters (V_d and Cl_p) will increase if there is significant presystemic drug elimination. This situation occurs because plasma drug concentrations are lower after an equivalent oral dose and estimation of the initial drug concentration (C_0) is lower. This simple model serves remarkably well for the calculation of most drug dose regimens.

THE TWO-COMPARTMENT MODEL

For some drugs, a plot of the logarithm of plasma concentration versus time results in a curvilinear relationship (Fig. 5.18). In order to explain this observation the simple one-compartment model needs to be expanded to consider the body as two compartments (Fig. 5.19). The greater the discrepancy between β (see Fig. 5.18) and k_{el}, the larger the error in assuming the validity of a one-compartment model. Fortunately, for most drugs, this discrepancy is not as great as the interindividual differences in pharmacokinetic drug disposition. For most drugs, the one-compartment open model can be used as an acceptable clinical approximation for individualization of drug doses.

When a discrepancy in modeling the disposition of a drug becomes clinically evident, the use of the drug is learned as a special case to account for the more complex disposition–effect relationship. Drugs that undergo dose-dependent disposition (e.g. phenytoin, aspirin) belong to this special category of more complicated relationships between dose, concentration, and pharmacologic effects.

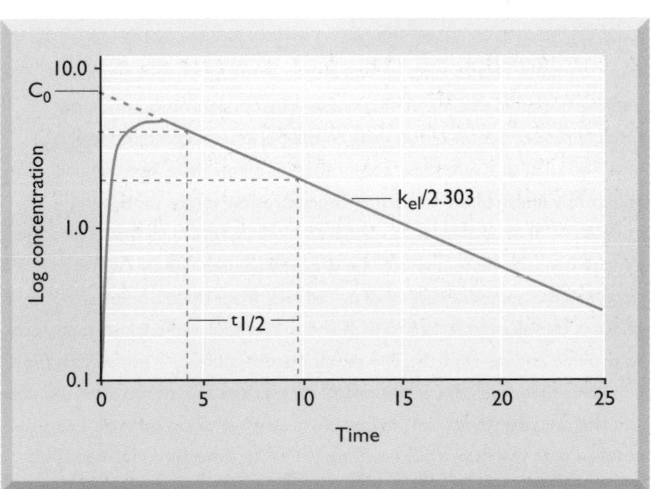

Fig. 5.17 Log plasma drug concentration versus time plot for a drug compatible with the one-compartment open pharmacokinetic model for drug disposition after an oral dose.

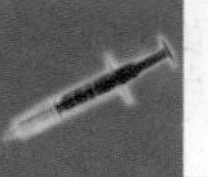

THE MODEL-INDEPENDENT APPROACH

A model-independent approach has been advocated to simplify the determination of pharmacokinetic parameters for drug dose calculation. This approach borrows considerably from the one-compartment open model concept. The relationships between the kinetic parameters are presented in Fig. 5.20. This approach compensates somewhat for the extrapolation of drug concentrations to C_0 in the one-compartment model when no drug has yet been absorbed into the body after an oral dose.

For practical purposes, steady state is assumed to occur four or five terminal half-lives after the start of drug therapy

Most drugs are administered chronically. For drugs with first order disposition the total amount of drug in the body increases until the amount excreted is equal to the dose administered, at which time a steady-state concentration is obtained. The time to steady state for such drugs depends only on the terminal disposition half-life. At the practical level, steady state is assumed to occur four or five terminal half-lives after the start of drug therapy (Fig. 5.21), 94% and 97% of a steady state will have been achieved, respectively. The more frequently the drug dose is administered, the greater the amount of drug in the body at steady state and the less the variation between peak and trough plasma concentrations of the drug. The less frequent the drug dose, the lower the amount of drug in the body at steady state, and the greater the variation between peak and trough plasma drug concentrations. If the dose interval is longer than two terminal disposition half-lives, drug accumulation can be to be clinically unimportant with chronic ingestion.

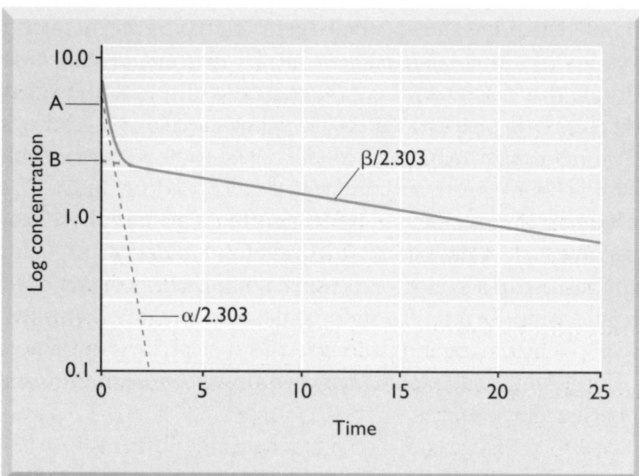

Fig 5.18 Log plasma drug concentration versus time plot that requires a two-compartment open model to account for its disposition after a parenteral dose. The terminal disposition rate constant is not k_{el}, and the decreasing plasma concentration reflects a more complex relationship between drug distribution and elimination. The initial more rapid decline in circulating drug concentration primarily reflects redistribution of the drug to the peripheral compartment (V_p) (see Fig. 5.19) plus a modest component of elimination. The terminal, apparently linear, phase of plasma concentration versus time is a composite of drug elimination buffered by drug returning from V_p to the central compartment in which the drug distributes rapidly (V_c) to decrease the apparent rate of drug removal from the blood plasma. This phase is therefore referred to as β and is extrapolated back to time zero to provide an intercept (B). The extrapolated values of β are subtracted from the observed concentrations of drug at the same time after the dose and the residual values are plotted. A linear regression through these residual data points provides a slope (α) and a time zero intercept (A), which reflects drug distribution to V_p. The greater the discrepancy between β and k_{el}, the larger the error in assuming the validity of a one-compartment model.

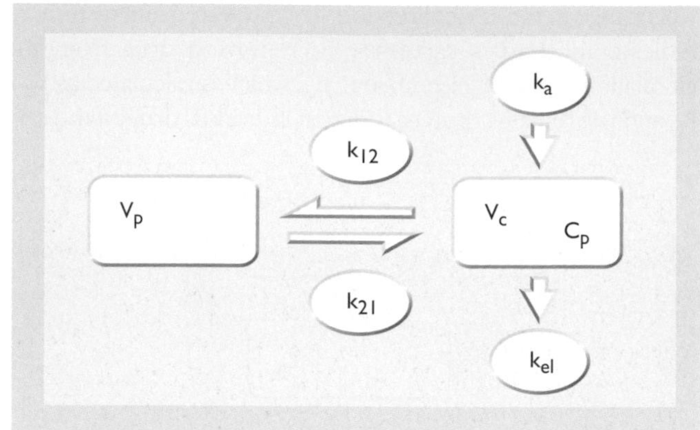

Fig. 5.19 Diagram of the two-compartment open pharmacokinetic model for drug disposition after a parenteral dose. With a bolus dose, k_a is instantaneous and is ignored in solution of the model. When the drug is administered by infusion, k_a is a zero order constant equal to the rate of drug infusion. There is a central compartment in which the drug distributes rapidly (V_c) and from which drug is eliminated, and a peripheral compartment into which the drug can distribute (V_p) and from which it can return to buffer the changing drug concentration in the central compartment when drug is eliminated. (k_{el}, elimination constant)

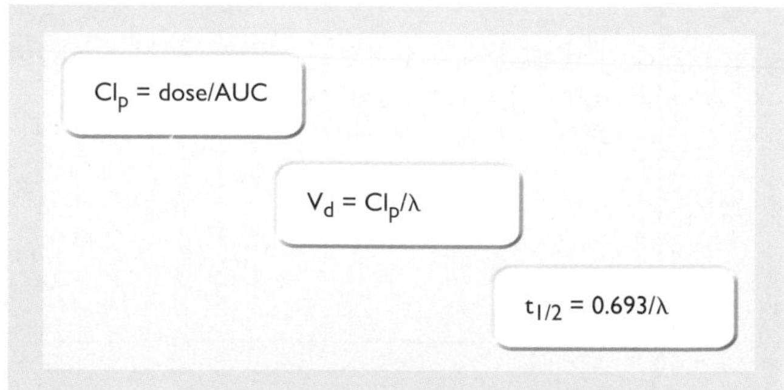

Fig. 5.20 Equations for pharmacokinetic drug disposition for model-independent conditions. The terminal disposition constant is renamed l ('el')so that its interpretation is not prejudiced by either of the two models discussed in Figs 5.15–5.19. A new calculation is introduced which is called area under the plasma concentration versus time curve (AUC). (Cl_p, plasma clearance; V_d, volume of distribution, λ, terminal disposition rate constant)

A loading dose is given to achieve therapeutic drug concentrations rapidly

The dose is calculated on the basis of its V_d and the desired plasma concentration at steady state (C_{ss}):

$$\text{loading dose (mg/kg)} = V_d \text{ (liters/kg)} \times C_{ss} \text{ (mg/liter)}.$$

Usually the loading dose is administered by infusion over a short period of time to reduce the risk of adverse effects associated with the presence of very high drug concentrations in the circulation. Maintenance doses are then based upon the Cl_p and the time interval between doses (τ):

$$\text{maintenance dose (mg/kg)} = Cl_p \text{ (liters/kg/h)} \times C_{ss} \text{ (mg/liter)} \times \tau \text{ (h)}.$$

Pharmacokinetics

- Most drugs are eliminated from the body as a constant fraction of their plasma concentration (first order process)
- Time to steady state depends only on the rate of drug elimination
- Repeated doses result in significant drug accumulation when ingestion is more frequent than twice the terminal disposition half-life
- Practical time to steady state is 4–5 terminal disposition half-lives
- The amount of a drug in the body at steady state depends on the frequency of ingestion and dose
- The plasma half-life of a drug does not reflect metabolic capacity if the apparent volume of distribution changes

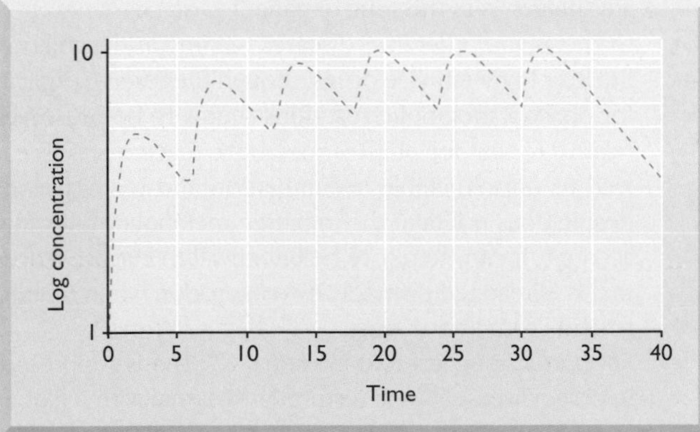

Fig. 5.21 Log plasma concentration versus time plot for a drug administered by mouth every six hours for 6 doses when its terminal disposition half-life is 6 hours. The effective steady state occurs 24–30 hours (4–5 half-lives) after starting the drug.

AGE, SEX, AND RACE

AGE

Drug-metabolizing enzymes are deficient in the fetus and premature infants

The fetus is able to metabolize drugs early in its development, but the expression of drug-metabolizing enzymes differs from that of the adult and is usually less efficient. Drug-metabolizing enzymes are also deficient in premature infants. Drug therapy in these infants is therefore difficult, particularly when more than a single drug dose is administered. In addition, renal function is not fully developed so renal drug elimination is impaired, as with the pharmacologic response to loop diuretics.

Children can metabolize many drugs more rapidly than adults

A few months after birth, oxidative drug-metabolic pathways increase dramatically, and by 2 years of age, children can oxidize many drugs more rapidly than adults. The ability to glucuronidate drugs develops more slowly. As a result, a greater fraction of an administered dose of acetaminophen is sulfate conjugated in children than in adults. The frequency of drug administration may have to be altered to compensate for these special characteristics. As children approach puberty, the rate of drug metabolism approaches that of adults.

Changes that occur with increasing age need to be considered when prescribing for the elderly

Changes that occur with increasing age and affect drug treatment include the following:

- The incidence of chronic diseases increases and therefore the elderly are more likely to be drug consumers than younger people. As a result, competition for cytochrome P-450 isoforms among competing drug substrates is most common in this age group.
- Circulating albumin concentration decreases; therefore protein binding is more likely to saturate, and may result in an increased free fraction of drug in the circulation.
- Lean body mass decreases and so the apparent volume of drug distribution can be expected to change for some drugs and dose adjustment may be necessary.
- Liver weight decreases, thus presystemic elimination of drugs may be reduced.

The expression of cytochrome P-450 isoforms appears to change with increasing age. This change is reflected as a reduced capability to oxidize drugs and this is seen mainly in men. Available data indicate that induction of drug metabolism is both maintained and impaired in the elderly patient, depending on the drug.

SEX

Although some sex differences in drug disposition have been reported (e.g. a lower renal clearance of amantadine in women), the clinical importance of these observations remains to be explored.

RACE

Several racial differences in drug metabolism have been demonstrated (Fig. 5.22). The difference in acetylator phenotype as a characteristic of racial origin is well documented. There are also racial differences in the expression of genetic variation among the cytochrome P-450 isoforms. Racial differences in drug disposition therefore need to be considered when individualizing drug doses.

Drug metabolic pathways affected by racial origin

Metabolic reaction	Caucasian	Asian
Acetylation	50% slow	5–10% slow
CYP2D6 oxidation	5–10% deficient	1% deficient
CYP2C18 oxidation	3–5% deficient	20% deficient

Fig. 5.22 Drug-metabolic pathways affected by racial origin. Deficiency in one metabolic pathway is not predictive for deficiency in other drug-metabolic pathways in the same racial group.

DRUG INTERACTIONS

Some of the many drugs available to treat diseases will interact with other drugs to produce undesirable effects. These interactions can have both a pharmacokinetic and pharmacodynamic basis. Sometimes drug interactions are used intentionally to produce the desired pharmacologic response.

The use of levodopa and carbidopa for patients with Parkinson's disease produces a favorable drug interaction

Carbidopa inhibits the conversion of levodopa to dopamine, but only in the peripheral tissues since carbidopa does not cross the blood–brain barrier. The levodopa can then enter the brain (the site where the pharmacologic effect is desired) where it is converted to dopamine. Carbidopa therefore reduces the severity of adverse effects that would arise from the systemic accumulation of dopamine.

The response of a patient to diuretics used in the control of hypertension is impaired if a nonsteroidal anti-inflammatory is given concurrently

The renal function of many patients receiving diuretics to control hypertension is impaired, but renal blood flow is maintained by renal prostaglandins. Nonsteroidal anti-inflammatory drugs (NSAIDs) block renal cyclooxygenase activity and decrease prostaglandins in the kidney, resulting in decreased renal elimination of waste products and Na^+. One consequence of this interaction is an increase in circulating blood volume resulting in inhibition of the antihypertensive response to the diuretic.

It is more difficult to control coagulation when a patient on oral anticoagulant therapy takes nonsteroidal anti-inflammatory drugs

Two mechanisms contribute to the interaction between anticoagulants and NSAIDs:

- The inhibition of cyclooxygenase by the NSAID.
- Competitive displacement of the oral anticoagulant from plasma protein by the NSAID.

Patients on oral anticoagulants should therefore be advised to use acetaminophen for analgesia instead of an NSAID.

Nutrient–drug interactions can interfere with drug efficacy

Iron in multivitamin preparations will complex with the catechol groups of levodopa to decrease the efficacy of levodopa in the management of Parkinson's disease. Another classical interaction between drugs and nutrients is complex formation of tetracycline antibiotics with Ca^{2+} in milk, resulting in reduced antimicrobial activity.

EFFECT OF DISEASE ON DRUG ACTION

The presence of a disease can have a considerable effect on the choice of drug, its disposition, and the likelihood of increased interindividual variation of responses to drugs. It is therefore important to consider disease–drug interactions when deciding to use drug therapy and choosing a particular drug. For example:

- The choice of diuretic for a patient with cardiovascular disease can depend on whether the patient has osteoporosis. Hydrochlorothiazide is a diuretic that does not increase the renal elimination of Ca^{2+} and therefore is advantageous in this type of patient.
- Cirrhosis and other liver diseases can impair the ability of the liver to metabolize drugs, though the reserve capacity for phase 2 metabolic reactions seems to be preserved relative to that for phase 1 metabolic reactions. This can lead to unpredictable accumulation and toxicity if the dosing does not take the impaired metabolic ability into account. It can therefore be beneficial to choose a drug that is eliminated primarily by conjugation when treating patients with liver disease.
- Recent data suggest that intestinal CYP3A4 is suppressed in celiac disease, but is restored to normal with a gluten-free diet. Intestinal disease might therefore lead to variability in the first-pass elimination of drugs metabolized by this isoform.

- Viral infections appear to suppress hepatic cytochromes P-450, perhaps as a result of interferon induction. A patient with a plasma drug concentration at the upper end of the therapeutic range can therefore suddenly show signs of drug toxicity during a viral infection.
- Achlorhydria is more common in the elderly and may affect the site of absorption of drug formulations with a pH-dependent coating.
- In patients with renal disease, prostaglandins help maintain residual renal function. The use of drugs that inhibit cyclooxygenase (e.g. NSAIDs) can therefore lead to a rapid deterioration of residual renal function.
- β Adrenoceptor antagonists are contraindicated in patients with asthma because they increase bronchoconstriction.
- Anticholinergic drugs can increase cognitive impairment in patients with Alzheimer-type dementia.

Variability of drug disposition

- **The rate of drug disposition is most likely to be impaired in the very young and the very old**
- **Racial differences in the genetic expression of drug-metabolizing enzymes complicate the individualization of drug therapy**
- **Concurrent ingestion of multiple drugs increases the probability of drug interactions owing to the increased likelihood of inducing or inhibiting the drug-metabolizing enzyme systems responsible**
- **Drug doses should be modified if the patient has a disease that impairs the function of organs with an important role in drug metabolism and/or excretion**

FURTHER READING

Benet LZ (ed.) *The Effect of Disease States on Drug Pharmacokinetics*. Washington, DC: American Pharmaceutical Association; 1976. [This monograph provides details on how diseases contribute to altered drug disposition.]

Grymonpre RE, Mitenko PA, Sitar DS, Aoki FY, Montgomery PR. Drug associated hospital admissions in older patients. *J Am Geriatr Soc* 1988; **36**: 1092–1098. [This paper illustrates the role of multiple drug therapy as a contributing factor to hospital admissions.]

Kroemer HK, Eichelbaum M. 'It's the genes, stupid'. Molecular basis and clinical consequences of genetic cytochrome P-450 2D6 polymorphism. *Life Sci* 1995; **56**: 2285–2298. [This review develops the consequences for drug therapy when a single isoform of cytochrome P-450 is altered.]

Sitar DS. Human drug metabolism *in vivo*. *Pharmacol Ther* 1989; **43**: 363–375. [This review evaluates the contribution of factors alleged to cause variation of drug metabolism in man.]

Wood AJJ, Zhou HH. Ethnic differences in drug disposition and responsiveness. *Clin Pharmacokinet* 1991; **20**: 350–373. [This review addresses the contribution of race to variation in drug disposition and efficacy.]

Wrighton SA, Stevens JC. The human hepatic cytochromes P-450 involved in drug metabolism. *Crit Rev Toxicol* 1992; **22**: 1–21. [This review describes the interaction of cytochrome P-450 isoforms in contributing to variation in drug metabolism.]

?

Indicate which is the correct answer for each question.

1. 600 mg of a drug is administered intravenously to a 60 kg patient. The plot of log e plasma concentration of drug versus time (t) is linear and the extrapolated concentration at t = 0 is found to be 1 μg/ml. Based only on this information, which one of the following conclusions can be drawn about the drug in question?
- a) it is extensively bound to plasma proteins
- b) it is largely ionized at physiologic pH
- c) its apparent distribution volume approximates that of total body water
- d) it is extensively accumulated in body tissue
- e) it is likely to show a high first-pass effect following oral administration

2. A drug with an elimination half-life of 7 hours is given as an initial loading dose, followed by repeated maintenance doses to keep the plasma concentration within 80% of the maximal value attained with the loading dose. The maximum allowable dosing interval is
- a) 1/2 hour
- b) 1 hour
- c) 2 hours
- d) 4 hours
- e) 8 hours

3. Based on the knowledge of its half-life, a drug is given as a loading dose of 100 mg followed by daily maintenance doses of 16 mg. What is the assumed half-life?
- a) 2 days
- b) 3 days
- c) 4 days
- d) 5 days
- e) 6 days

4. A drug with a first-order rate constant of elimination equal to 0.3/hour is to be given as an intravenous infusion. Approximately how long would it take for the plasma concentration of this drug to reach a steady state?
- a) one circulation time
- b) 1.5 hours
- c) 3 hours
- d) 6 hours
- e) 12 hours

5. The plasma concentration of a drug showing zero order (saturation) kinetics decreases from 10 mg/liter to 8 mg/liter in 1 hour. How long would it take for the plasma concentration of this drug to fall from 10 mg/liter to 2 mg/liter assuming that zero-order kinetics still apply at this concentration?
- a) 2 hours
- b) 4 hours
- c) 8 hours
- d) 10 hours
- e) none of the above

6. Which one of the following statements is incorrect?
- a) conjugation (phase 2) reactions involving drugs or their metabolites are not mediated by the cytochrome P-450 system in the liver
- b) metabolism of a drug usually decreases its lipid solubility
- c) the extent to which a drug is bound to plasma proteins is not directly predictive of its rate of renal excretion
- d) for drugs with first-order elimination kinetics, a constant amount of drug is lost per unit time
- e) for drugs with zero-order elimination kinetics, the relationship between drug dosage and maximally attained plasma concentration is nonlinear

7. All the following may significantly affect the duration of a drug's effects, except
- a) rate of metabolism to inactive metabolites
- b) rate of absorption into the blood stream
- c) rate of excretion of inactive metabolites
- d) initiation of compensatory reflexes
- e) extensive plasma protein binding of the drug

8. All the following may shorten the duration of a drug's effects, except
- a) extensive plasma protein binding of the drug
- b) compensatory reflexes
- c) redistribution of the drug into skeletal muscle or adipose tissue
- d) renal excretion of the drug
- e) metabolism of the drug

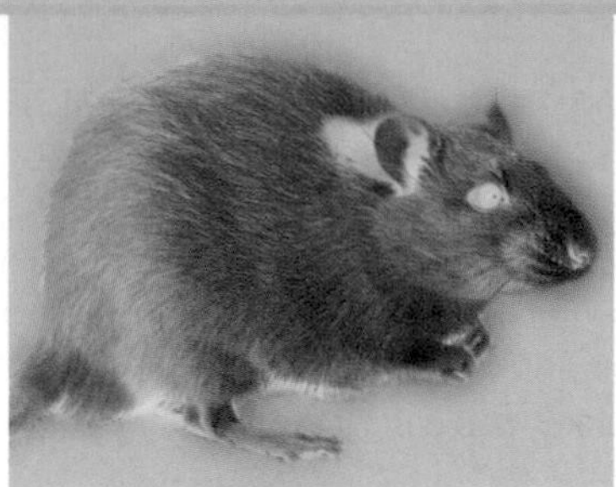

6. Drug Safety and Pharmacovigilance

Drugs can damage health

A drug is a single chemical substance or natural product used to prevent, investigate, or treat disease, or to alter physiologic function (Fig. 6.1). A medicine is a drug or a mixture of drugs combined with other substances to make it stable, palatable, and useful for therapy.

Drugs interact with tissues and organs and alter their function, but their effects are not always desirable. Any drug represents a hazard (i.e. has the potential to cause harm). The probability that a drug will cause some specified harm in any given circumstances is the 'risk' that it will cause that harm. This probability can be estimated by experiment or observation or it can be estimated intuitively. People are generally unable to estimate risk accurately, perceiving new and technical hazards as riskier than they are, while largely ignoring everyday and mundane hazards. Figure 6.2 illustrates the relationship between perceived risk and actual risk for 41 causes of death. The 'perceived risk' determines the way people behave, and can be manifest in what they say (the 'expressed risk') or what they do (the 'revealed risk'). Patients are sometimes fearful of taking medicines (e.g. after a newspaper article discussing one particularly dramatic case of an adverse effect), but will happily continue smoking even though the lifetime risk of fatal illness from tobacco in smokers is about 0.15 (15%). The risks perceived by doctors can also differ markedly from the true risks measured in well-designed studies.

Examples of different uses of drugs	
To prevent disease (for prophylaxis)	Vaccines, such as pertussis vaccine Antimalarial drugs such as chloroquine
To investigate disease	Synthetic adrenocorticotropic hormone (ACTH), to test for adrenal suppression Barium sulfate for gastrointestinal radiology Loxaglate for angiographic radiology
To treat disease	
Symptomatic treatment	Acetaminophen for headache Metoclopramide for nausea
Specific treatment	Penicillin G to treat streptococcal infection
To alter physiologic function	The oral contraceptive pill

Fig. 6.1 Examples of different uses of drugs.

THERAPEUTIC DECISION-MAKING

Therapeutic decisions are among the most difficult decisions in medical practise and are an integral part of medicine.

Why should the patient be treated, and with what drug?

The physician's first therapeutic task is to decide whether the patient has a condition that would benefit from drug treatment. For some illnesses (e.g. coryza) there is no specific treatment for the illness, though symptomatic treatment can be helpful.

If treatment is indicated, the physician then needs to consider its adverse effects and decide whether the treatment should be prescribed. For example, acne can be treated effectively with the

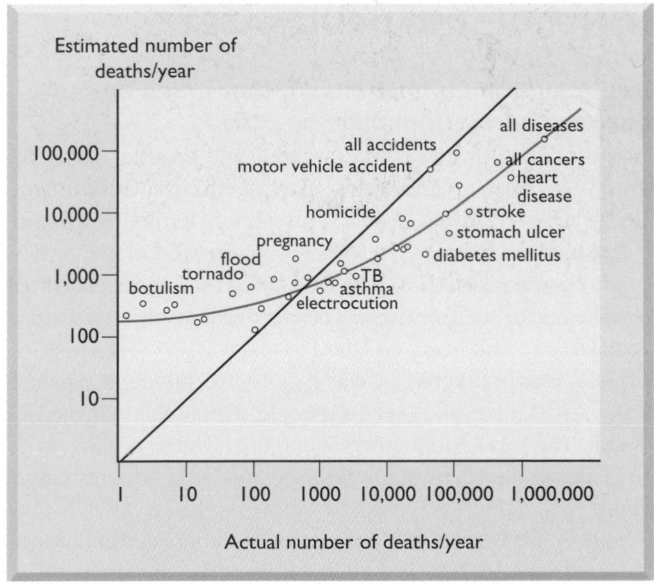

Fig. 6.2 Relationship between perceived frequency and the actual number of deaths/year for 41 causes of death. If the perceived and actual frequencies are equal, the data fall on the straight line. The points and the curved line fitted to them represent the average response. (Adapted with permission from *Judgement Under Uncertainty* by Stone, Cambridge University Press, 1982.)

vitamin A derivative isotretinoin, but this drug can cause serious adverse effects including fetal malformation as a result of exposure *in utero*. It is therefore unsuitable for the treatment of mild acne. Similarly, although the antibiotic chloramphenicol is an effective treatment of bacterial pharyngitis, it is avoided because it carries a risk of causing bone marrow aplasia.

What are the expected costs and benefits of treatment?

The doctor has to weigh up:

- The potential benefits of treatment to the patient.
- The risk of adverse effects.
- The health cost if the treatment produces adverse effects.
- The financial cost.

Usually, the benefits of treatment are benefits for an individual patient, such as freedom from pain. However, there are circumstances where the benefits accrue to society as a whole (e.g. vaccines reduce the prevalence of disease in the community).

The costs fall on:

- The individual, who can suffer adverse effects.
- Society, if the government or insurance schemes pay for expensive drugs.

Recombinant enzymes used to treat the rare hereditary defect in β-glucosidase that causes Gaucher's disease cost around US$100,000 (£65,000)/year/patient. Lipid-lowering drugs, which can significantly reduce the risk of dying from coronary heart disease for mildly hypercholesterolemic men who have never had a myocardial infarct, are also expensive, costing approximately US$600,000 (£400,000) per life saved. Such expense, and limited budgets, mean that a decision has to be made about whether spending so much money to treat a single patient is warranted.

CONTROLLING DRUG SAFETY

Drug regulators aim to ensure that drugs are reasonably free from adverse effects

Before a company can market a medicinal product, it has to demonstrate that it is reasonably safe, and effective. Government regulation is a relatively recent phenomenon. In the US, the current system was set up in the wake of a pharmacotherapeutic disaster. A company called Massengill dissolved the antibacterial drug sulfanilamide in ethylene diglycol (a sweet-tasting solvent) to make it palatable to children, but failed to test the product's toxicity before it was marketed in the late 1930s. Ethylene diglycol causes renal failure, and over 100 people, mainly children, died as a result. The subsequent outcry led to the effective regulation of medicines in the US through the Food and Drug Administration (FDA).

The need for regulation was recognized rather later in Europe. The Medicines Act 1968 in the UK was passed in the aftermath of another drug disaster in 1961 involving thalidomide. Thalidomide was marketed by the German firm Chemie Grünenthal as a safe alternative to barbiturate hypnotics, but had been tested only perfunctorily in experimental animals for safety during pregnancy. It was subsequently found to cause severe fetal deformities when taken during the first trimester of pregnancy. An estimated 10,000 babies were born with phocomelia (a deformity in which the limbs are rudimentary stumps with malformed digits) in countries in which it was widely used. The regulatory authorities in most countries now insist on proof of efficacy, safety, and quality before licensing a drug for use.

The assessment of a new chemical entity that has not previously been used for therapy takes place in the following stages (Fig. 6.3).

- *In vitro* toxicologic studies to test for genetic and biochemical toxicity.
- *In vivo* acute toxicologic studies on a whole animal, physiologic systems, and skin and mucosae (for acute irritancy and sensitization).
- *In vivo* studies of subacute and chronic toxicity in animals.
- *In vivo* studies of oncogenicity in animals.
- *In vivo* studies of developmental and reproductive toxicity in animals.
- *In vivo* studies of genetic toxicity in animals.

The *in vivo* human safety studies that follow comprise four different stages, phases I–IV.

- Phase I studies investigate the pharmacodynamics and pharmacokinetics in healthy volunteers.
- Phase II studies are dose-ranging studies to find safe and effective dosages and to observe the drug's effects and pharmacokinetics in carefully selected patient volunteers. Often, these studies are carried out in special groups of patients, such as those with renal failure.
- Phase III studies are extensive and carefully controlled clinical trials carried out in selected patient volunteers, including trials in special groups such as the elderly.
- Phase IV studies are based on postmarketing surveillance of treated patients and spontaneous adverse reaction reports.

In the UK, the Medicines Control Agency is largely responsible for licensing medicines. However, the European Community countries, including the UK, also allow the marketing of drugs licensed directly by the European Medicines Evaluation Agency (see Chapter 31).

The most important test of a new drug is how safe it is in clinical use

A new chemical entity will usually be given to approximately 1500 patients during the premarketing tests. This number is far too small to detect uncommon or rare adverse events. However, increasing the number of patients studied premarketing would delay marketing of new drugs, thereby delaying the use of the potentially beneficial drugs by ill patients. A useful rule of thumb is the 'rule of three.' This states that if an event has not been observed in n patients, then it is 95% certain that the true frequency of the event in a large population of patients lies somewhere between 0 and $3/n$. Therefore, even if there is no fatal reaction to a drug among 1500 patients, there is still a 5% chance it will cause up to one death among 500 treated patients.

Postmarketing surveillance is extremely important for ensuring drug safety

Rare and even fairly common adverse effects can be detected only after trials involving very large numbers of patients.

Postmarketing surveillance ('pharmacovigilance'), particularly the spontaneous reporting of adverse reactions, is extremely important because many more patients receive a drug after it has been marketed than before marketing. It is inevitable that some drugs are licensed that prove to be less safe than desirable. These drugs can then be removed from the market or their use may be restricted (see Fig. 6.7).

DETECTING ADVERSE DRUG REACTIONS

Adverse drug reactions frequently mimic ordinary diseases. Serious reactions tend to affect:

- Systems in which there is rapid cell multiplication (e.g. the skin, hematopoietic system, and lining of the gut).
- Systems where the drugs are detoxified and excreted (e.g. the liver and kidneys).

Typical examples are adverse effects such as toxic epidermal necrolysis, aplastic anemia, pseudomembranous colitis, hepatitis, and nephritis.

Adverse effects, especially uncommon ones, may be difficult to diagnose. Doctors must always consider whether any effect associated with the use of a new drug is caused by the drug. However, as a general practitioner might work for a lifetime without seeing a case of aplastic anemia, the detection of both common and uncommon adverse drug reactions requires vigilance on the part of the patient, the physician, the pharmacist, and other health professionals.

Adverse reactions are most obvious when they are dramatic, differ from natural disease, and are of rapid onset

An anaphylactic reaction occurring within minutes of a penicillin injection and characterized by tissue edema, bronchospasm, and cardiovascular collapse is obviously an adverse effect. It is much more difficult to detect adverse effects that occur only after prolonged treatment or those with an insidious onset, and even more difficult to detect adverse effects that occur after the drug has been discontinued.

Adverse effects that mimic naturally occurring disease are more difficult to detect than those with unique features, and the commoner the disease, the harder is it to spot any increase due to the drug. The very rare defect phocomelia caused by thalidomide was readily noticed by astute clinicians. In contrast, the increased risk of spina bifida in babies born to women using the antiepileptic drug sodium valproate during pregnancy could be verified only by carefully designed clinical studies.

If the time period between exposure to a drug and an adverse effect is characteristic of a specified reaction, the drug is more likey to be the cause

In deciding whether an adverse effect occurring with treatment is caused by the treatment, its timing must be considered in relation to both its nature and exposure to the drug. An adverse effect occurring before exposure cannot be caused by the drug. Adverse effects may occur:

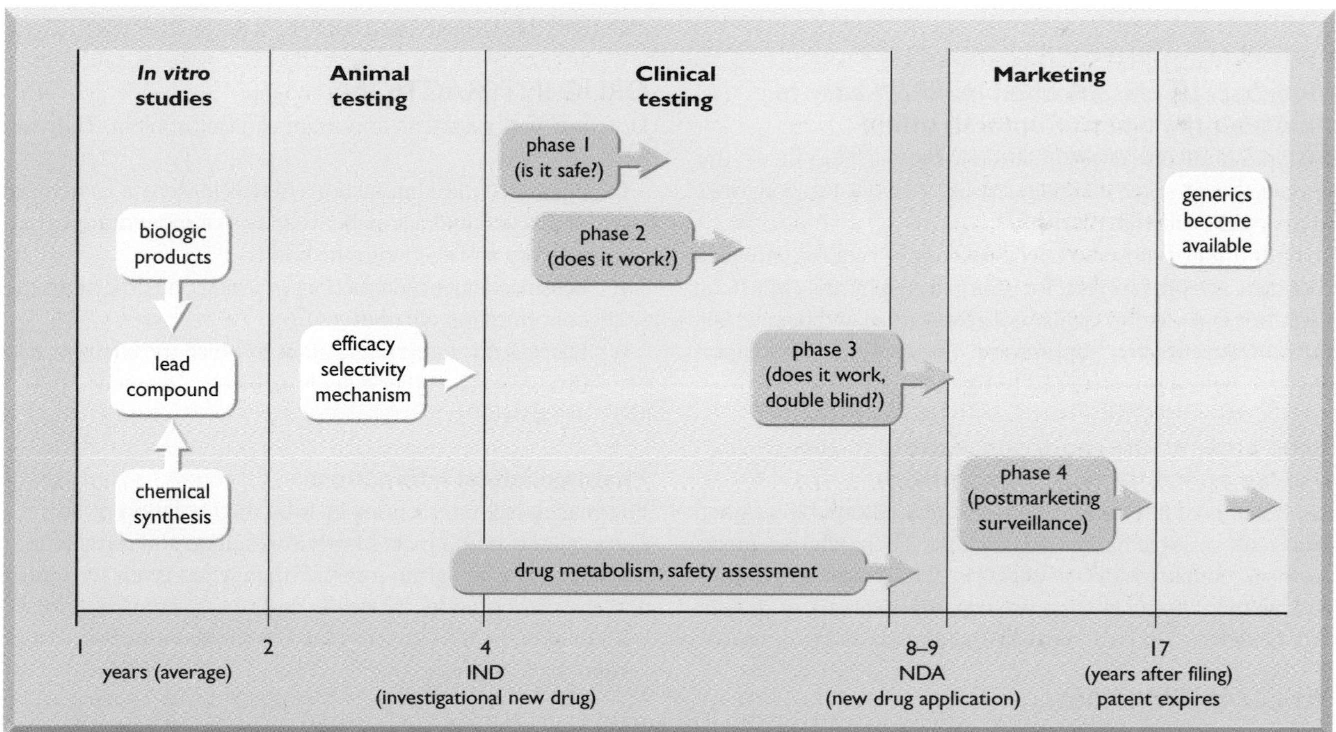

Fig. 6.3 The development and testing process required to bring a drug to market in the US. Some of the requirements may be different for drugs used in life-threatening diseases. (Adapted with permission from *Basic and Clinical Pharmacology, 6e*, by Katzung, Appleton & Lange)

- Shortly after exposure (e.g. anaphylaxis to penicillin, vasodilation and collapse after an injection of vancomycin —'l'homme rouge').
- A few days after exposure (e.g. serum sickness due to equine antirattlesnake antitoxin, an ampicillin rash in patients with infectious mononucleosis).
- After chronic treatment (e.g. iatrogenic Cushing's syndrome after chronic treatment with glucocorticosteroids).
- After cessation of treatment (e.g. withdrawal syndromes from benzodiazepines or 5-hydroxytryptamine reuptake inhibitors).
- In subsequent generations (e.g. phocomelia with thalidomide, retinoid embryopathy).

Certain adverse effects, such as anaphylaxis and bone marrow aplasia, are characteristic adverse effects of drugs.

A drug is more probably the cause of a reversible adverse effect if it disappears after the drug is stopped (de-challenge) and then reappears when the drug is restarted (re-challenge).

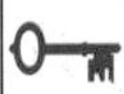 **A drug is more probably responsible for an adverse effect:**

- **If it is well recognized that the adverse effect occurs with the drug**
- **If the adverse effect is recognized as an adverse effect of a class of drugs and the suspect drug resembles this class (e.g. cough is an adverse effect associated with angiotensin-converting enzyme inhibitors)**

An alphabetic classification makes it easy to remember the types of adverse effect

The types of adverse effect are listed in Fig. 6.4. Most fit into this scheme, though some may fit into more than one category, while others can be difficult to classify.

Type B (bizarre) adverse effects are unpredictable, unrelated to dosage, and often severe, for example anaphylaxis (which can result in a fatal cardiovascular collapse), renal and hepatic failure, and bone marrow suppression. Some of the more important Type B reactions are listed in Fig. 6.5.

Some patients are more susceptible to the adverse effects of drugs than others

The benefits of any drug treatment must always be weighed against any possible harm it could cause. Those who are particularly susceptible to adverse effects include the fetuses of pregnant women, patients with pre-existing illnesses or genetic enzyme defects, and patients who are already taking drugs.

PREGNANT WOMEN

Treatment of pregnant (or potentially pregnant) women must take into account the welfare of both the fetus and the mother. Teratogenic drugs (those that are known to cause malformation of the offspring of mothers who take them) must obviously be avoided. However, all drugs are potentially teratogenic. Therefore no drug should be prescribed to a pregnant woman, no matter how innocuous it may seem unless:

- There is a clear need for it and it is believed to be safe for the fetus, or
- The mother is so ill that its use is justified even if the fetus might be harmed.

PRE-EXISTING ILLNESSES

Pre-existing illnesses such as liver or kidney disease can alter the adverse effect profile because a drug may be present in the body in a higher concentration, or for longer as a result of reduced metabolism or excretion, rendering the patient more susceptible to Type A (augmented pharmacologic) adverse effects. The adverse effects of some drugs are also more common in patients with organ failure. For example, the potassium-sparing diuretic amiloride is more likely to cause hyperkalemia in patients with renal impairment, because their K^+ excretion is already compromised. In addition, central nervous system (CNS) depressants, such as diazepam, can precipitate hepatic encephalopathy in patients with severely compromised liver function, and respiratory failure in patients with severe obstructive pulmonary disease who rely on an hypoxic drive to maintain ventilation.

GENETICALLY DETERMINED ENZYME DEFECTS

Genetically determined enzyme defects can make drug therapy hazardous, and sometimes lethal. Such defects include the various forms of glucose-6-phosphate dehydrogenase (G6PD) deficiency, which is an X-linked recessive trait that is therefore manifest in males. Oxidants such as aspirin, primaquine, and dapsone can cause severe hemolysis in people with this defect, who are commonly of Mediterranean, African, or South-East Asian origin.

DRUG INTERACTIONS

Drug interactions are an important clinical problem. They can be classified as:

- Pharmaceutical interactions in which there is a chemical or physical interaction between two or more drugs before they are absorbed into the body.
- Pharmacokinetic interactions in which one drug alters the concentration of another.
- Pharmacodynamic interactions in which the effects of two drugs given together differ from those of either drug given separately.

Pharmaceutical interactions

Pharmaceutical interactions include the chelation of Fe^{2+} by tetracyclines, which makes both iron sulfate and tetracyclines less effective when given together than when given separately, and the precipitation of calcium hydroxide that occurs when calcium gluconate is injected into an intravenous infusion of sodium bicarbonate solution.

Pharmacokinetic interactions

Pharmacokinetic interactions include the important interactions that occur between drugs metabolized by the cytochrome P-450 (mixed function oxidase) enzyme system and drugs that inhibit the enzyme system. For example, the anticoagulant warfarin, theophylline (which is used in the treatment of asthma), and the anti-rejection drug cyclosporine are metabolized by cytochrome P-450. All have a low therapeutic index (i.e. the ratio between toxic concentration and therapeutic concentration is low) and

Alphabetic classification of types of adverse drug effects

Type	Type of effect	Definition	Examples
A	Augmented pharmacologic effects	Adverse effects that are known to occur from the pharmacology of the drug, and are dose-related. They are seldom fatal and relatively common	Hypoglycemia due to insulin injection Bradycardia due to β adrenoceptor antagonists Hemorrhage due to anticoagulants
B	Bizarre effects	Adverse effects that occur unpredictably, are not dose related, and often have a high rate of morbidity and mortality. They are uncommon	Anaphylaxis due to penicillin Acute hepatic necrosis due to halothane Bone marrow suppression by chloramphenicol
C	Chronic effects	Adverse effects that only occur during prolonged treatment and not with single doses	Iatrogenic Cushing's syndrome with prednisolone Orofacial dyskinesia due to phenothiazine tranquilizers Colonic dysfunction due to laxatives
D	Delayed effects	Adverse effects that occur remote from treatment, either in the children of treated patients, or in patients themselves years after treatment	Second cancers in those treated with alkylating agents for Hodgkin's disease Craniofacial malformations in infants whose mothers have taken isotretinoin Clear-cell carcinoma of the vagina in the daughters of women who took diethylstilbestrol during pregnancy
E	End-of-treatment effects	Adverse effects that occur when a drug is stopped, especially when it is stopped suddenly (so-called withdrawal effects)	Unstable angina after β adrenoceptor antagonists are suddenly stopped Adrenocortical insufficiency after glucocorticosteroids such as prednisolone are stopped Withdrawal seizures when anticonvulsants such as phenobarbital or phenytoin are stopped

Fig. 6.4 Alphabetic classification of types of adverse drug effects.

Some important Type B (bizarre) reactions

Adverse effect	Drug causes
Anaphylaxis	Penicillins and other antibacterial agents Foreign protein such as streptokinase or equine antirattlesnake vaccine Iodinated contrast media in radiology
Anaphylactoid reactions (nonimmunologic reactions resembling anaphylaxis, but occurring without prior exposure)	Angiotensin-converting-enzyme inhibitors (angioedema) Intravenous *N*-acetylcysteine (urticaria and anaphylaxis) The solvent polyethoxylated castor oil
Liver disease	Halogenated anesthetic gases such as chloroform, halothane, and enflurane (acute hepatic necrosis) Chlorpromazine, the oral contraceptive pill, and flucloxacillin (intrahepatic cholestasis) Minocycline (chronic active hepatitis)
Kidney disease	Nonsteroidal anti-inflammatory drugs (acute interstitial nephritis) Amphotericin (acute tubular necrosis) Angiotensin-converting-enzyme inhibitors (vascular renal damage)
Bone marrow damage	The antithyroid drugs carbimazole, methimazole, and propylthiouracil Antibacterial agents such as chloramphenicol and co-trimoxazole* Antirheumatic drugs such as gold salts and penicillamine

Fig. 6.5 Some important Type B (bizarre) reactions.

therefore small changes in metabolism can provoke severe Type A adverse effects. Drugs that inhibit cytochrome P-450 include the antibacterial agents erythromycin, co-trimoxazole and ciprofloxacin, the antifungal agents ketoconazole and fluconazole, and the H_2 receptor antagonist cimetidine. A small number of drugs enhance the effects of cytochrome P-450 and therefore reduce the concentration of drugs metabolized by the enzyme. Such enzyme inducers include the anticonvulsants phenobarbital and carbamazepine, and the antituberculous agent rifampin. Women on oral contraception who take these drugs need to take higher doses of estrogens than normal otherwise the enhanced estrogen metabolism will leave them unprotected against pregnancy.

Renal excretion of one drug can be influenced by the presence of another. The classic example is the renal excretion of lithium, another drug with a low therapeutic index, which can be inhibited by thiazide diuretics.

Pharmacodynamic interactions

Anticholinergic drugs and levodopa are used to treat Parkinson's disease, with one drug reducing cholinergic activity and the other increasing dopaminergic activity. Both effects tend to improve the movement disorder, though both can also cause hallucination and delirium.

PHARMACOVIGILANCE

Pharmacoepidemiology is the study of the use and effects of drugs in large numbers of people. Such study uses the methods of epidemiology and is concerned with all aspects of the benefit:risk ratio of drugs. Pharmacovigilance is a branch of pharmacoepidemiology restricted to the epidemiologic study of drug-related events or adverse drug effects. In this context, 'events' are events recorded in the patient's notes during a period of drug monitoring. They may be due to the disease for which the drug is being given, an intercurrent disease or infection, an adverse reaction to the drug being monitored, the activity of a drug being given concomitantly, or a drug interaction.

Pharmacovigilance studies can be:

- Hypothesis generating (e.g. to detect unexpected adverse drug effects of a recently-marketed drug).
- Hypothesis testing (e.g. to prove whether any suspicions raised about a specific drug are justified).
- Both hypothesis generating and hypothesis testing.

Methods of pharmacovigilance

- **Hypothesis generating: spontaneous adverse drug effect reporting (yellow card in the UK)**
- **Hypothesis generating and testing: prescription event monitoring (green form in the UK)**
- **Hypothesistesting: case–control studies, cohort studies, randomized controlled clinical trials**

HYPOTHESIS-GENERATING STUDIES

Spontaneous reporting has led to the identification of many unexpected adverse drug effects

Physicians and, in some countries, other health care professionals as well, are provided with forms for notifying a central authority of suspected adverse drug effects. In the UK, the 'yellow card' has been used since 1964. Similar systems of spontaneous reporting of adverse effects have been established by the FDA in the US (Fig. 6.6), throughout Europe, and by most developed countries.

The great strengths of these schemes are:

- They are operated for all drugs throughout the whole of their lifetime.
- They are an affordable method of detecting rare adverse effects.

Their main weaknesses are:

- Gross underreporting.
- The data provide only a numerator (i.e. the number of reports of each suspected reaction).

Nevertheless, these schemes are invaluable and it is essential that physicians fill in such drug report cards.

Spontaneous reporting has led to identification of many unexpected adverse effects, resulting in the withdrawal of a number of marketed drugs (Fig. 6.7).

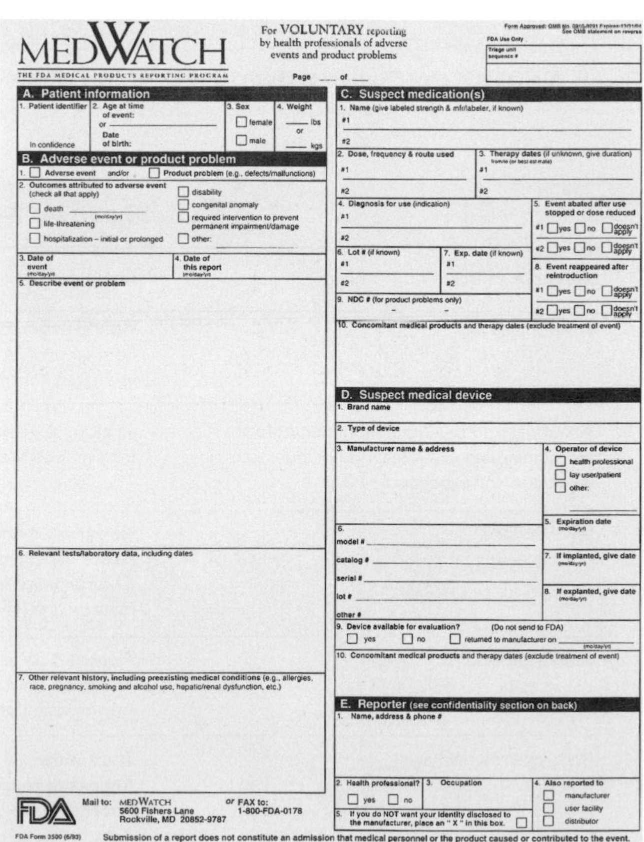

MEDWATCH
THE FDA MEDICAL PRODUCTS REPORTING PROGRAM

For VOLUNTARY reporting by health professionals of adverse events and product problems

Page ___ of ___

FDA Use Only
Triage unit sequence #

A. Patient information
1. Patient identifier — In confidence
2. Age at time of event: or Date of birth:
3. Sex — ☐ female ☐ male
4. Weight — ___ lbs or ___ kgs

B. Adverse event or product problem
1. ☐ Adverse event and/or ☐ Product problem (e.g., defects/malfunctions)
2. Outcomes attributed to adverse event (check all that apply)
☐ death ___ (mo/day/yr)
☐ life-threatening
☐ hospitalization – initial or prolonged
☐ disability
☐ congenital anomaly
☐ required intervention to prevent permanent impairment/damage
☐ other: ___
3. Date of event (mo/day/yr)
4. Date of this report (mo/day/yr)
5. Describe event or problem
6. Relevant tests/laboratory data, including dates
7. Other relevant history, including preexisting medical conditions (e.g., allergies, race, pregnancy, smoking and alcohol use, hepatic/renal dysfunction, etc.)

C. Suspect medication(s)
1. Name (give labeled strength & mfr/labeler, if known) #1 #2
2. Dose, frequency & route used #1 #2
3. Therapy dates (if unknown, give duration) from/to (or best estimate) #1 #2
4. Diagnosis for use (indication) #1 #2
5. Event abated after use stopped or dose reduced #1 ☐ yes ☐ no ☐ doesn't apply #2 ☐ yes ☐ no ☐ doesn't apply
6. Lot # (if known) #1 #2
7. Exp. date (if known) #1 #2
8. Event reappeared after reintroduction #1 ☐ yes ☐ no ☐ doesn't apply #2 ☐ yes ☐ no ☐ doesn't apply
9. NDC # (for product problems only)
10. Concomitant medical products and therapy dates (exclude treatment of event)

D. Suspect medical device
1. Brand name
2. Type of device
3. Manufacturer name & address
4. Operator of device ☐ health professional ☐ lay user/patient ☐ other:
5. Expiration date (mo/day/yr)
6. model # ___ catalog # ___ serial # ___ lot # ___ other # ___
7. If implanted, give date (mo/day/yr)
8. If explanted, give date (mo/day/yr)
9. Device available for evaluation? (Do not send to FDA) ☐ yes ☐ no ☐ returned to manufacturer on ___ (mo/day/yr)
10. Concomitant medical products and therapy dates (exclude treatment of event)

E. Reporter (see confidentiality section on back)
1. Name, address & phone #
2. Health professional? ☐ yes ☐ no
3. Occupation
4. Also reported to ☐ manufacturer ☐ user facility ☐ distributor
5. If you do NOT want your identity disclosed to the manufacturer, place an " X " in this box. ☐

FDA Mail to: MEDWATCH 5600 Fishers Lane Rockville, MD 20852-9787 or FAX to: 1-800-FDA-0178

FDA Form 3500 (6/93) Submission of a report does not constitute an admission that medical personnel or the product caused or contributed to the event.

Fig. 6.6 The FDA MedWatch reporting card.

Drugs licensed since 1972 and withdrawn in the UK owing to toxicity

Product	Therapeutic class	Adverse reaction(s)	Type A/B reaction
Aclofenac	NSAID	Anaphylaxis	B
Polidexide	Hypolipidemic	Impurities	–
Nomifensine	Antidepressant	Hemolytic anemia	B
Fenclofenac	NSAID	Epidermal necrolysis	B
Feprazone	NSAID	Nephrotoxicity, GI toxicity	A
Benoxaprofen	NSAID	Photosensitivity, hepatotoxicity	A
Zomepirac	NSAID	Anaphylaxis	B
Indoprofen	NSAID	GI toxicity	A
Zimeldine	Antidepressant	Guillain–Barré syndrome	B
Suprofen	NSAID	Nephrotoxicity	A
Terodiline	Anti-incontinence	Ventricular tachycardia	A
Triazolam	Hypnotic	Psychiatric reactions	A
Temafloxacin	Antibiotic	Multi-organ toxicity	B
Centoxin	Antibiotic	Increased mortality	B
Remoxipride	Neuroleptic	Aplastic anemia	B
Flosequinnan	Cardiac failure	Increased mortality	B
Metipranolol	Anti-glaucoma	Anterior uveitis	B

Fig. 6.7 Drugs licensed since 1972 and withdrawn owing to toxicity in the UK. This list shows that licensed drugs can be the cause of major unexpected adverse drug reactions and also demonstrates the importance of pharmacovigilance. (NSAID, nonsteroidal anti-inflammatory drug; GI, gastrointestinal)

HYPOTHESIS-GENERATING AND HYPOTHESIS-TESTING STUDIES

Prescription event monitoring is an hypothesis-generating and -testing process

Prescription event monitoring in the UK is an important technique that takes advantage of the way the National Health Service is organized. Dispensed prescriptions written by general practitioners are sent to a central Prescription Pricing Authority, which provides confidential copies of the prescriptions for newly introduced drugs being monitored by a Drug Safety Research Unit. This Unit then sends a 'green-form' questionnaire (Fig. 6.8) to the general practitioner who wrote the original prescription 6 or 12 months after the first prescription. Consequently, the prescriptions provide the 'exposure data,' showing which patients have been exposed to the drug being monitored, and the green forms provide the 'outcome data' detailing any events noted during the period of monitoring. The Drug Safety Research Unit can then follow up pregnancies, deaths, or events of special interest by contacting either the prescribing physician or other holders of the patient's medical record. So far 48 drugs have been studied and the average number of patients included in each study (the cohort size) has been about 10,500.

The great strengths of the 'green form' method are:

- It provides a numerator (i.e. the number of reports) and a denominator (i.e. the number of patients exposed), both being collected over a precisely known period of observation.
- There is no interference with the physician's decision about which drug to prescribe for each individual patient. This avoids selection biases, which can make data interpretation difficult.

The main weakness of prescription event monitoring (PEM) in the UK is that only 50–70% of the green forms are returned. Attempts are now being made to establish PEM outside the UK.

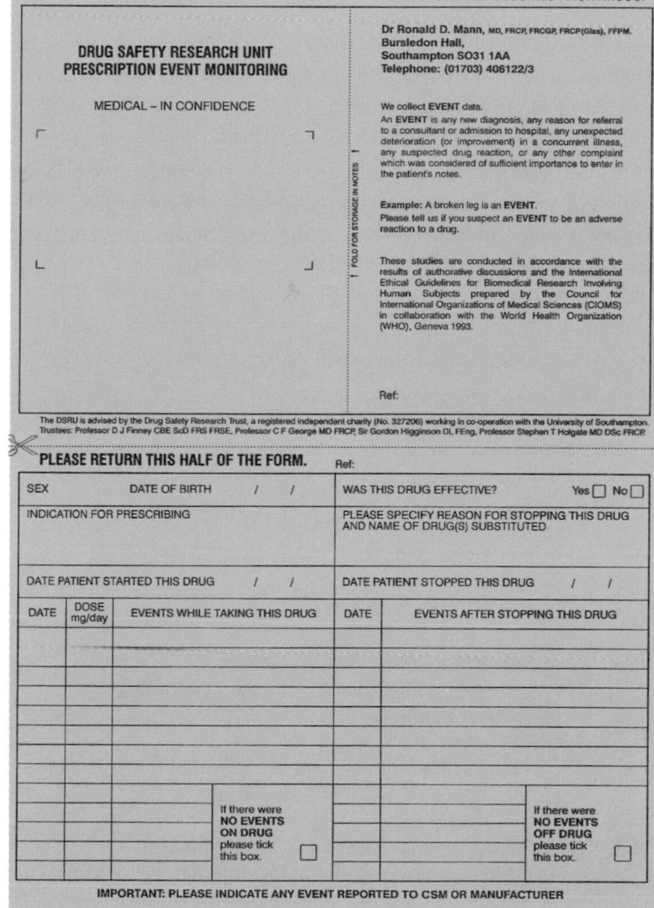

PLEASE REMOVE THIS SECTION OF THE FORM SO THAT THE BOTTOM HALF BECOMES ANONYMOUS.

DRUG SAFETY RESEARCH UNIT
PRESCRIPTION EVENT MONITORING

MEDICAL – IN CONFIDENCE

Dr Ronald D. Mann, MD, FRCP, FRCGP, FRCP(Glas), FFPM.
Bursledon Hall,
Southampton SO31 1AA
Telephone: (01703) 406122/3

FOLD FOR STORAGE IN NOTES

We collect **EVENT** data.
An **EVENT** is any new diagnosis, any reason for referral to a consultant or admission to hospital, any unexpected deterioration (or improvement) in a concurrent illness, any suspected drug reaction, or any other complaint which was considered of sufficient importance to enter in the patient's notes.

Example: A broken leg is an **EVENT**.
Please tell us if you suspect an **EVENT** to be an adverse reaction to a drug.

These studies are conducted in accordance with the results of authorative discussions and the International Ethical Guidelines for Biomedical Research Involving Human Subjects prepared by the Council for International Organizations of Medical Sciences (CIOMS) in collaboration with the World Health Organization (WHO), Geneva 1993.

Ref:

The DSRU is advised by the Drug Safety Research Trust, a registered independent charity (No. 327206) working in co-operation with the University of Southampton. Trustees: Professor D J Finney CBE ScD FRS FRSE, Professor C F George MD FRCP, Sir Gordon Higginson DL FEng, Professor Stephen T Holgate MD DSc FRCP.

PLEASE RETURN THIS HALF OF THE FORM. Ref:

SEX DATE OF BIRTH / /			WAS THIS DRUG EFFECTIVE? Yes ☐ No ☐	
INDICATION FOR PRESCRIBING			PLEASE SPECIFY REASON FOR STOPPING THIS DRUG AND NAME OF DRUG(S) SUBSTITUTED	
DATE PATIENT STARTED THIS DRUG / /			DATE PATIENT STOPPED THIS DRUG / /	
DATE	DOSE mg/day	EVENTS WHILE TAKING THIS DRUG	DATE	EVENTS AFTER STOPPING THIS DRUG
		If there were **NO EVENTS ON DRUG** please tick this box. ☐		If there were **NO EVENTS OFF DRUG** please tick this box. ☐

IMPORTANT: PLEASE INDICATE ANY EVENT REPORTED TO CSM OR MANUFACTURER

Fig. 6.8 The data collection segment of the green form used for prescription event monitoring.

HYPOTHESIS-TESTING STUDIES

Hypothesis-testing studies include case–control and cohort studies. A case–control technique will usually be chosen if there are only a few cases and assembling a large cohort of cases would be impossible. However, some pharmacoepidemiologists believe that the cohort technique provides more convincing results.

Case–control studies compare cases of a disease with controls susceptible to but free of the disease

Case–control studies are technically complex, but have been successfully used by government agencies and many academic units. The final results compare or relate the risks in the cases and controls. The absolute risk can be determined only in very special circumstances. Great care is needed in accurate diagnosis of the cases and in data collection so that potential biases are minimized or excluded, and marginal results must not be overinterpreted. Clearly, a fairly small increase in the risk of a common serious condition such as breast cancer may be of far greater public health importance than a relatively large increase in a small risk, such as primary hepatic carcinoma.

Cohort studies follow up a large group of patients for long enough to assess the outcome of an exposure common to the cohort

Comparative cohort studies include an unexposed control group. Again, potential biases can be a problem, but the method, though usually expensive and time-consuming, has the advantage of revealing the absolute risk and not just relative risk.

Randomized controlled trials avoid biases

In randomized controlled trials one group of patients is divided into two in a strictly random order. One group is then exposed and the other is not exposed to the drug, so that the outcomes can be compared. However, although this method is resistant to biases, it has only a limited, but important, role as a pharmacoepidemiologic tool because most serious adverse effects are relatively uncommon. Appropriate randomized controlled trials can therefore become unmanageably large and expensive.

FURTHER READING

Davies DM (ed) *Textbook of Adverse Drug Reactions 4e.* Oxford: Oxford University Press; 1991. [An extensive, clear account of adverse reactions arranged by disease.]

Dukes MNG, Aronson JK. *Myler's Side Effects of Drugs 12e.* Amsterdam: Elsevier; 1993. [An extensive, clear account of adverse reactions arranged by drugs.]

Faich GA. US adverse drug reaction surveillance 1989–1994. *Pharmacoepidemiology and Drug Safety* 1996 (in press). [This recent paper summarizes the North American experience of pharmacovigilance.]

Ferner RE. Hazards, risks and reality. *Br J Clin Pharmacol* 1992; **33**: 125–128. [A brief account of problems of risk related to pharmaceutical products.]

Rawlins MD. Pharmacovigilance: paradise lost, regained or postponed? *J R Coll Physicians (London)* 1995; **29**: 41–49. [A thoughtful account of the European experience.]

Stockley IH. *Drug Interactions: A Source-book of Drug Interactions, their Mechanisms, Clinical Importance, and Management 3e.* Oxford: Blackwell Scientific Publications; 1993. [An authoritative compendium of drug interactions.]

Indicate whether the following answers are true or false.

1. Anaphylaxis from penicillin ingestion is an adverse drug effect Type
   a) A
   b) B
   c) C
   d) E
   e) D

2. Drug safety is the responsibility of
   a) drug regulatory bodies (e.g. the Food and Drug Administration)
   b) the physician
   c) the pharmaceutical company manufacturing the drug
   d) the American Medical Association

3. For what sort of new medicines is postmarketing surveillance essential in the public interest
   a) medicines intended for widespread long-term use
   b) anesthetic agents
   c) all new drugs
   d) drugs for sexual dysfunction

4. The following patient groups are likely to be more susceptible to the adverse effects of drugs
   a) teachers
   b) neonates
   c) patients with liver disease
   d) athletes
   e) the elderly

5. Drug interactions have important clinical outcomes in
   a) women taking phenobarbital who rely on oral contraceptives
   b) men taking vitamin supplements who are prescribed theophylline
   c) any patient prescribed lithium who is also taking a thiazide diuretic
   d) any patient taking iron sulfate who is then prescribed tetracycline

2

Drugs in Health and Disease

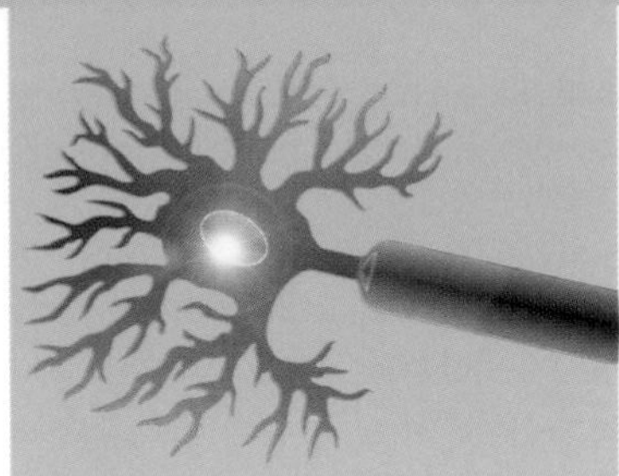

7. Drugs and the Nervous System

PHYSIOLOGY OF THE CENTRAL AND PERIPHERAL NERVOUS SYSTEMS

The nervous system provides for conscious or unconscious control of basic motor and sensory activity, as well as emotional and intellectual functions

The nervous system is organized as a hierarchy.

- Afferent fibers passing from the peripheral tissues to the spinal cord constitute the part of the peripheral nervous system (PNS) that allows perception of external sensation and body function.
- Efferent neurons from the spinal cord constitute the part of the PNS that regulates the activity of peripheral tissues.
- The central nervous system (CNS) starts at the spinal cord and connects the afferent and efferent neurons of the PNS with the brain, which provides higher processing and executive control.

The neuron is the basic unit of both the CNS and PNS

The body contains approximately 10×10^9 neurons (nerve cells) of various types, which differ in length and structure, but are composed of four major areas (Fig. 7.1):

- The cell body, which contains the nucleus and structures concerned with the basic functioning of the cell.
- The axon, which conducts nerve impulses, in the form of an action potential, from the cell body to a distant site, and vice versa.
- Dendrites, which connect neurons with each other and transmit information back to their own cell body.
- Synapses, which are the basis of neurochemical communication.

Axons are either long (as in projection neurons such as peripheral motor and sensory nerves) or short (as in interneurons), and most are covered in myelin. In the PNS this covering (myelin sheath) is provided by Schwann cells, while in the CNS it is provided by neuroglia cells (i.e. oligodendrocytes). At the end of an axon there are usually branches that end in axon terminals or boutons and form synapses with other neurons or tissue cells. Often the connection is with a dendrite from another cell. There are numerous dendrites on most neurons. They have no myelin covering and can be profusely branched. The ends of the axon branches are studded with dendritic spines, which are the points of synaptic connection. The synapse is therefore the point of connection between neurons. Each neuron may have 1000–10,000 synaptic connections with as many as 1000 other neurons.

The synapse comprises the axon terminal of the presynaptic neuron, the dendrite of the postsynaptic neuron, and the gap between them, the synaptic cleft (Fig. 7.2). The numerous types of synapses are named according to which two parts of a neuron are connected (i.e. axoaxonic, axodendritic). In addition there are:

- Electrical synapses or gap junctions, which use ions as a transmitter.
- Conjoint synapses which use both ionic and chemical transmitters.

The general actions of drugs at synapses are listed in Fig. 7.3.

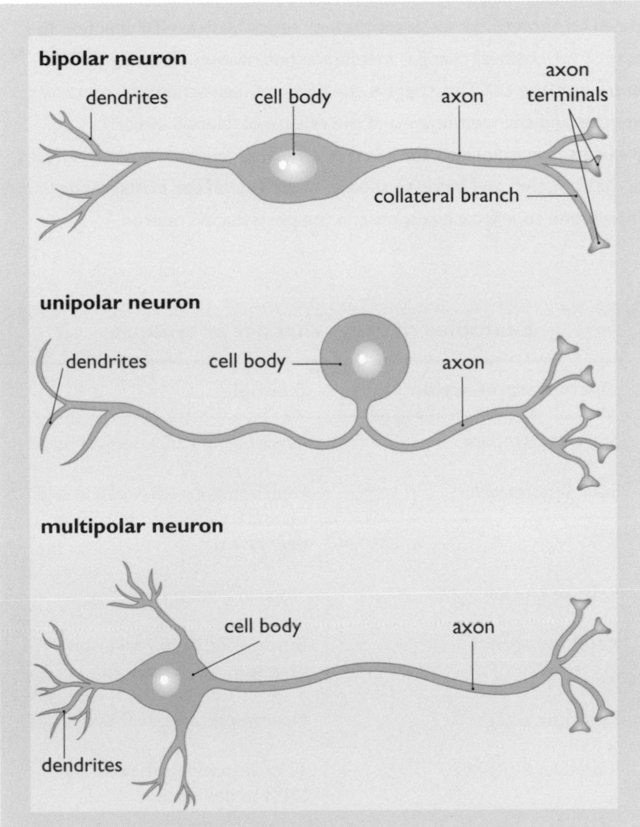

Fig. 7.1 Types of neuron. There are many different types of neuron, which are shaped according to function. Bipolar cells are commonly interneurons, while unipolar cells tend to be sensory neurons and multipolar cells are often motor neurons.

Neurotransmitter release and neurotransmitter effect depend on the neuronal resting membrane potential and action potential

The resting membrane potential of the cell is negative owing to preferential ion distribution across the cell membrane maintained by the membrane ion pumps and ion channels contained within the neuronal phospholipid membrane. The principal ions are Na^+, K^+, Ca^{2+}, and Cl^- (Fig. 7.4).

An action potential is a brief wave of reversal of membrane potential that moves along the axon away from the cell body (Fig. 7.5). During the action potential Ca^{2+} enters the cell and

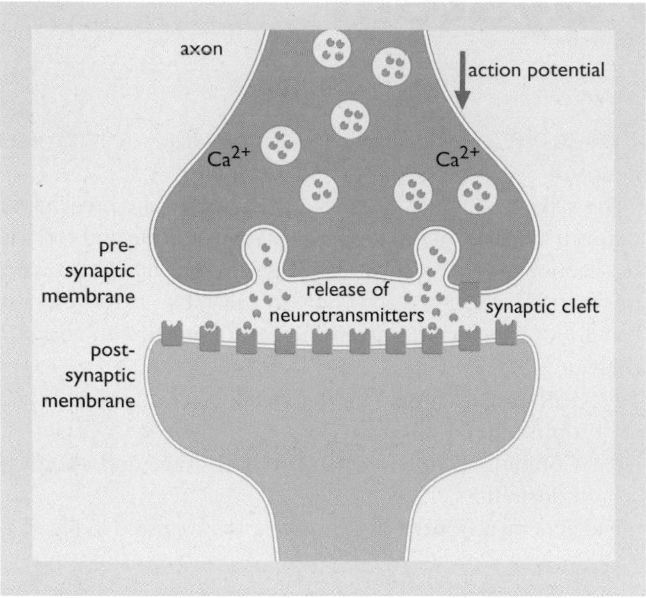

Fig. 7.2 Action potential at the synapse. An action potential passing down an axon to the axon terminal or region with similar function (e.g. axonal varicosities) changes membrane polarization, resulting in Ca^{2+} entry into the cell. This triggers the fusion of neurochemical-containing vesicles and cell membrane and the release of neurochemical (neurotransmitter) into the synaptic cleft. The neurotransmitter diffuses across the cleft and binds to specific receptors on the postsynaptic membrane to initiate a response in the postsynaptic neuron.

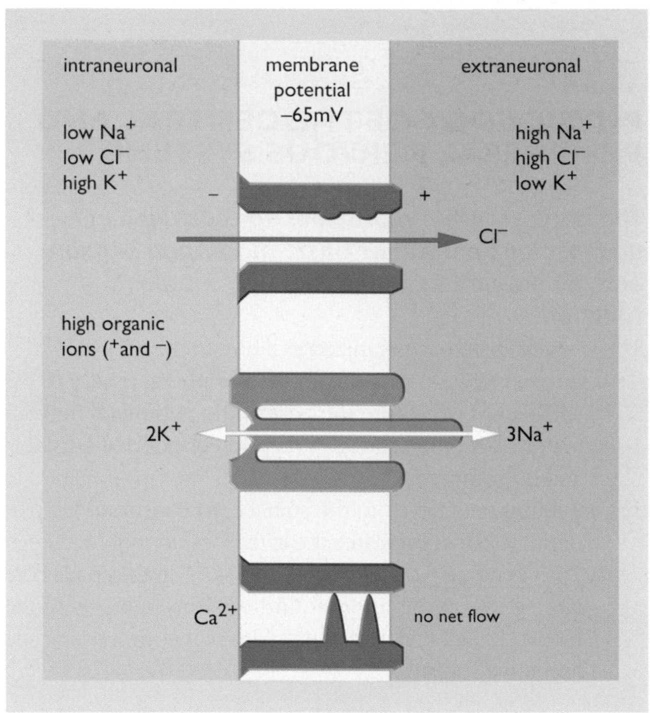

Fig. 7.4 Ion distribution across the neuron membrane at rest. The energy-dependent Na^+/K^+ pump maintains the resting potential by sustaining the Na^+/K^+ concentration gradient across the cell membrane so that the K^+ concentration inside the cell is high. Conversely the Na^+ concentration outside the cell is high.

Examples of drugs that act at synapses

Mechanism of action	Example
Stimulate synthesis	Levodopa in Parkinson's disease
Stimulate release	Fenfluramine in depression and secondary effect of MAOIs in depression
Release blocker	None in clinical use
Receptor agonist	Bromocriptine in Parkinson's disease
Receptor antagonist	Neuroleptic antipsychotic drugs
Reuptake blocker	Tricyclic antidepressants and SSRIs in depression
Degradative enzyme inhibitor	Vigabatrin* in epilepsy

Fig. 7.3 Examples of drugs that act at synapses. (MAOIs, monoamine oxidase inhibitors; SSRIs, selective serotonin reuptake inhibitors)

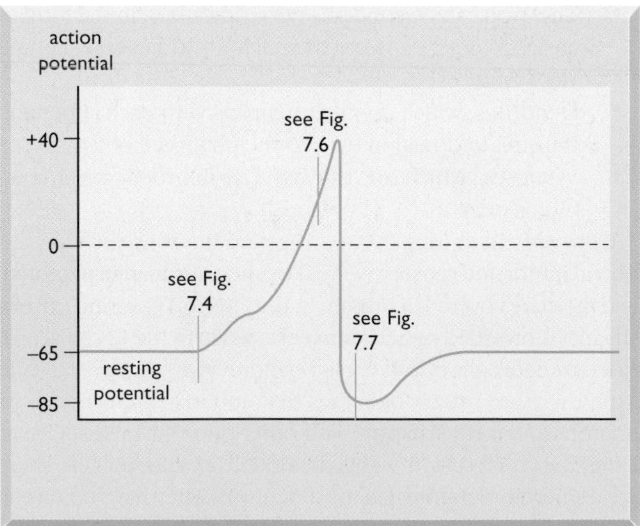

Fig. 7.5 An action potential. This is a brief (0.1–2 msec) wave of reversal of membrane potential (from negative to positive) that moves along the axon away from the cell body.

initiates neurotransmitter release (Fig. 7.6). The action potential is followed by a period of hyperpolarization when the neuron is more negatively charged than at rest (Fig. 7.7). This prevents further action potentials and the degree of hyperpolarization has implications for nerve cell excitability.

Some neurotransmitters inhibit firing of action potentials by hyperpolarizing the neuron

The classic example of a hyperpolarizing neurotransmitter is γ-aminobutyric acid (GABA), which opens Cl^- channels in the cell membrane, thereby increasing the membrane's negative charge. These Cl^- channels are examples of ligand-gated ion channels (i.e. ion channels that change in response to a specific chemical). The other general type of ion channel is a voltage-gated ion channel (e.g. the Na^+ and Ca^{2+} ion channels involved in the generation of the action potential).

There are receptors for 300-plus endogenous molecules that act in the nervous system

Many drugs used to affect the human nervous system exert their actions by altering the function of the receptors for the endogenous molecules that act in the nervous system. The major classes of receptors and transmitters found in the nervous system are listed in Fig. 7.8.

Receptors can be present in the synapse both pre- and postsynaptically. Many presynaptic receptors inhibit further release of the relevant neurotransmitter, though the effect of activating a presynaptic receptor may depend on:

- The number of receptors activated.
- The affinity of the receptor for the transmitter.
- The efficacy with which the receptor modifies transmitter release.

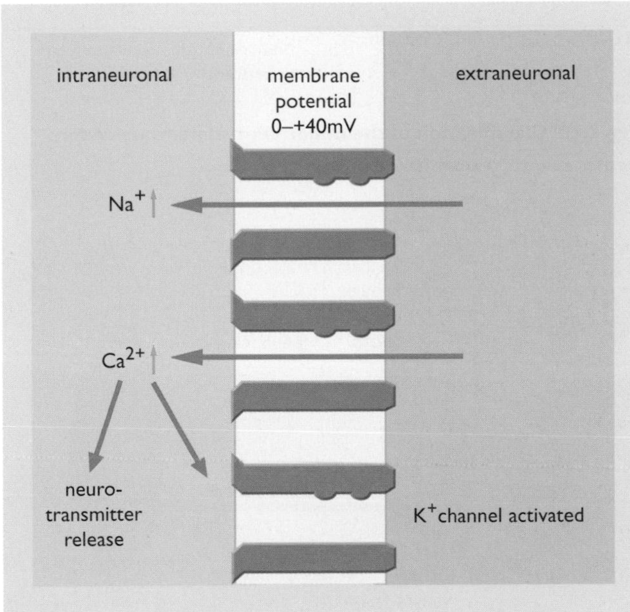

Fig. 7.6 Ion movements during an action potential. An action potential is produced when Na^+ channels open, allowing Na^+ to move along its concentration gradient into the cell. The Ca^{2+} channels then open, allowing Ca^{2+} to enter the cell. Calcium both initiates neurotransmitter release and allows K^+ outflow, which will eventually arrest the action potential.

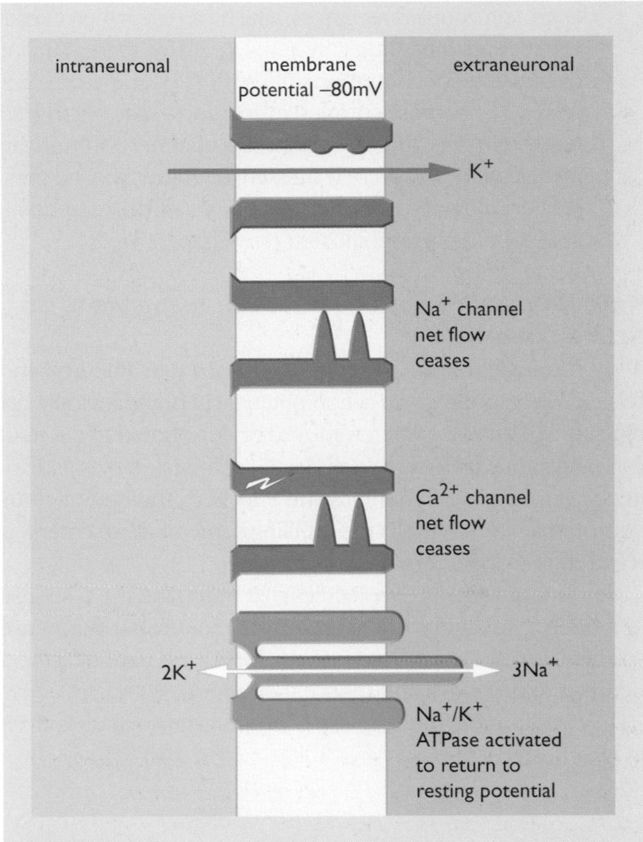

Fig. 7.7 Hyperpolarization. During hyperpolarization, the neuron is more negatively charged than at rest, preventing further action potentials.

The major classes of central nervous system receptors and transmitters

Transmitter	Receptors
Glutamate	NMDA, Non-NMDA
GABA	$GABA_A$, $GABA_B$
Glycine	Glycine (strychnine sensitive)
Acetylcholine	Nicotinic, muscarinic
5-HT	$5\text{-}HT_{1a\text{–}d}$, $5\text{-}HT_{2\text{–}7}$
Norepinephrine	α_1, α_2, $\beta_{1\text{–}3}$
Dopamine	$D_{1\text{–}5}$
Cholecystokinin	CCK_A, CCK_B

Fig. 7.8 The major classes of central nervous system receptors and transmitters. (CCK, cholecystokinin GABA; γ-aminobutyric acid; 5-HT, 5-hydroxytryptamine; NMDA, *N*-methyl D-aspartate)

The two major types of receptor are:

- Those located directly on ion channels such as acetylcholine nicotinic receptors and 5-hydroxytryptamine (5-HT)-3 receptors (both Na^+ and K^+ channels), GABA receptors (Cl^- channels) (Fig. 7.9), and glutamate receptors (*N*-methyl D-aspartate receptors), which are cation channels).
- G protein-coupled receptors, which can exert their effects via second messenger systems (e.g. by increasing or decreasing concentrations of cAMP, see Chapter 3). For some G protein-coupled receptors, the activated G protein acts directly on an ion channel without the involvement of a second messenger. Other second messengers include Ca^{2+} and metabolites of the membrane component phosphoinositol (see Chapter 3).

Neurotransmitters are released in response to an action potential

A neurotransmitter is a molecule synthesized in a neuron and released in response to an action potential in physiologically significant amounts. It is then removed or deactivated in the neuron or synaptic cleft. Such a molecule administered as an exogenous drug typically mimics the effects of the endogenous neurotransmitter. A molecule fulfilling some of these criteria is referred to as a putative neurotransmitter.

Neuromodulators are molecules that modulate the response of a neuron to a neurotransmitter, while neurohormones are substances that are released into the blood and have effects on neurons (e.g. cortisol and tri-iodothyronine).

The classification for the major CNS neurotransmitters is given in Figs 7.8 and 7.10.

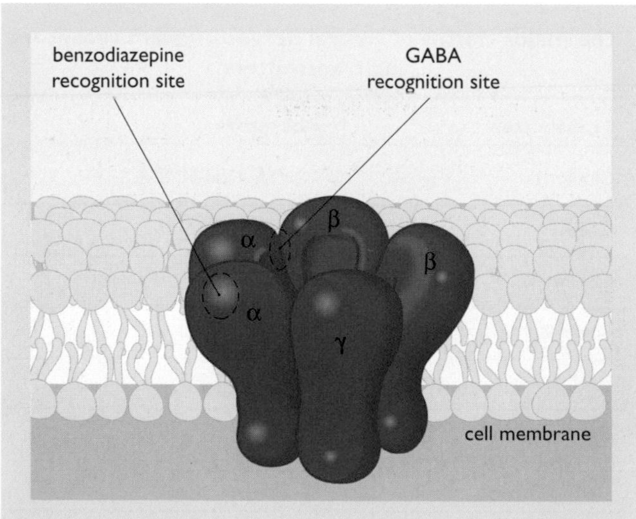

Fig. 7.9 Receptor-gated ionic channels: the γ-aminobutyric acid (GABA) receptor. Each subunit is composed of four protein helical strands. Binding of a benzodiazepine or GABA leads to a conformational change. The channel opens and Cl^- passes down its concentration gradient.

FUNCTIONAL ANATOMY OF THE PERIPHERAL NERVOUS SYSTEM

Motor neurons innervate muscle fibers or intrafusal muscle spindles

Motor neurons send their axons to muscle fibers in the periphery. There are two types of motor neuron:

- α motor neurons are large myelinated fibers and form motor units with the muscle fibers they innervate. The number of muscle fibers innervated by each motor fiber varies with the degree of fine motor control. For fine control only a few fibers are innervated.
- γ motor neurons are much smaller than α motor neurons, have limited myelination, and innervate only intrafusal muscle spindles acting as stretch receptors (Fig. 7.11).

Both α and γ fibers are found in the ventral horn of the spinal cord and synapse with the descending motor tracts within the spinal cord. Interneuronal connection within the spinal cord integrates the fine motor control provided by the extrapyramidal system.

Classification of the major central nervous system peptide neurotransmitters

Family	Examples
Opioid	Endorphins, enkephalins, dynorphins
Neurohypophyseal	Vasopressin, oxytocin
Tachykinins	Substance P, neurokinin
Gastrins	Gastrin, cholecystokinin
Others	Neuropeptide Y, substance P, neurotensin, galanin

Fig. 7.10 Classification of the major central nervous system peptide neurotransmitters.

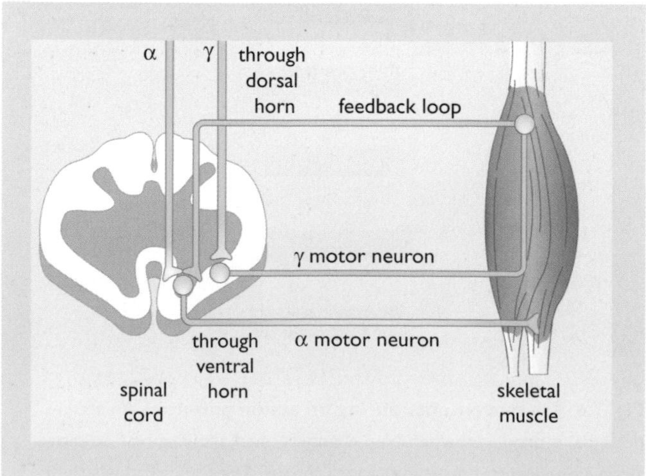

Fig. 7.11 The motor system of the peripheral nervous system. The α and γ neurons provide feedback control of muscle contraction via a loop to the α motor neurons.

Sensory neurons originate in peripheral structures and transduce stimuli into action potentials

The endings of sensory neurons in peripheral structures comprise a highly specialized network of physiologic receptors, which transduce stimuli into action potentials. The sensory fibers pass into the spinal cord through the dorsal root (Fig. 7.12). Some fibers synapse at the level of entry into the spinal cord, while others pass to the brain stem before synapsing and passing to the thalamus. The special sensory systems such as vision and hearing have a highly individualized arrangement and are discussed in Chapters 19 and 22, respectively.

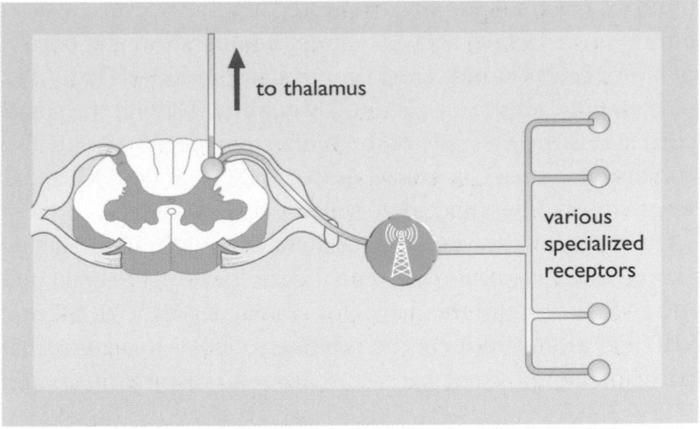

Fig. 7.12 Sensory system of the peripheral nervous system. Sensory neurons originate in peripheral structures and pass into the spinal cord through the dorsal root.

The autonomic nervous system maintains the internal environment of the body

The autonomic nervous system (ANS) controls visceral functions such as circulation, digestion, and excretion, mostly without voluntary or conscious control. It also modulates the function of the endocrine glands, which regulate metabolism. The ANS has both sensory and motor components, and is divided into sympathetic and parasympathetic systems according to its anatomy and physiology. In general the first neurons of the sympathetic system are located in the intermediate horn of the thoracolumbar region of the spinal cord. These synapse with the second neurons in the para- or prevertebral sympathetic ganglia. In the parasympathetic system the first neurons are located either in the cranial nerve autonomic nuclei or in the intermediate horn of the sacral region of the spinal cord. They synapse with the second neurons either in autonomic ganglia in the case of cranial nerves or in the effector tissue itself.

Acetylcholine is the primary neurotransmitter (i.e. in the autonomic ganglia) of both sympathetic and parasympathetic first neurons (preganglionic) and of all parasympathetic second neurons (postganglionic). Norepinephrine is the major neurotransmitter of sympathetic second neurons. Nitric oxide and a variety of peptides may also be important neurotransmitters in the ANS.

Central control of the ANS is from the hypothalamus, the autonomic nuclei of the reticular formation, and the intermediate horn of the spinal cord.

The sympathetic and parasympathetic systems generally antagonize each other

The sympathetic system prepares the body for action (i.e. the 'fear, flight, or fight response'), while the parasympathetic system is generally concerned with the body at rest (Fig. 7.13). Drugs acting in the CNS often produce their adverse effects by changing the activity of the ANS.

FUNCTIONAL ANATOMY OF THE CENTRAL NERVOUS SYSTEM

The spinal cord is part of the CNS and consists of ascending and descending tracts passing information between the brain and

Comparison of sympathetic and parasympathetic autonomic function

Organ (function) effect	Sympathetic effect	Parasympathetic effect
Lens	No effect	Accommodation
Iris	Dilates pupil	Constricts pupil
Salivary glands	Vasoconstriction	Secretion
Sweat glands	Secretion (very localized)	Secretion (generalized)
Heart (rate and force)	Increased	Decreased
Peripheral blood vessels	Constriction	Dilation
Visceral vessels	Constriction	Dilation
Lungs	Vasodilation, bronchodilation	Bronchoconstriction, secretion
Stomach, small intestine, colon	Decreased peristalsis and secretion	Increased peristalsis and secretion
Rectum and anus	Inhibits smooth muscle in rectum and constricts sphincter	Increases smooth muscle tone and relaxes sphincter
Adrenal medulla	No effect	Secretion
Bladder	Relaxation of detrusor muscle and constriction of internal sphincter	Contraction of detrusor and inhibition of internal sphincter
Genitalia	Ejaculation	Penile erection/engorgement of clitoris and labia

Fig. 7.13 Comparison of sympathetic and parasympathetic autonomic function.

the PNS. The tracts are interconnected at various levels by short interneurons, which allow a degree of integration and control of motor function and sensory input at a spinal level (Fig. 7.14).

The medulla oblongata is directly continuous with the spinal cord and is the first part of the brain stem (Fig. 7.15a). It also contains the nuclei for cranial nerves V, IX, X, XI, and XII and is where motor fibers and some sensory fibers cross.

The pons lies between the medulla and midbrain. It can be viewed as a relay station between the cerebellum, the brain, and the PNS. It contains the nuclei for cranial nerves V, VI, VII, and VIII, and motor nuclei in the pontine reticular formation that participate in postural, cardiovascular, and respiratory control (Fig. 7.15b).

The cerebellum lies posterior to the pons (Fig. 7.16) and has incoming and outgoing connections, with sensory and motor tracts ascending and descending the spinal cord. It is the largest motor structure in the brain. Although its function is not entirely clear, the multiplicity of its connections allows the cerebellum to exert fine control over motor functioning and to act as a center for integrating sensory and motor information for performing complex tasks.

Above the pons lies the midbrain (mesencephalon). This is the most primitive part of the human brain and ends in two huge fiber bundles, which form the cerebral peduncles, carrying fibers to and from the thalamus and cerebral hemispheres. It also contains the superior (visual) and inferior (auditory) colliculi (Figs 7.15c, 7.15d), the nuclei for cranial nerves III and IV, two motor nuclei, the red nucleus, and the substantia nigra, which links and acts as a relay between the basal ganglia and the motor system (see Fig. 7.15c).

The diencephalon, the central core of the cerebrum, consists of the hypothalamus, subthalamus, epithalamus, and thalamus (Fig. 7.17):

- The hypothalamus subserves many homeostatic functions such as regulation of the ANS and endocrine function via the pituitary. It also has a role in the control of basic drives such as those involved in hunger, thirst, threat, procreation, and fatigue.
- The subthalamus is involved in motor function and has connections to the basal ganglia, the red nucleus, and the substantia nigra.
- The epithalamus consists of the habenular nuclei and the pineal gland. The habenular nuclei are the center for the integration of olfactory, visceral, and somatic afferent pathways, and are connected to the reticular formation. The function of the pineal gland is unclear, but it contains high concentrations of melatonin and 5-HT and may have a role in circadian rhythm regulation.
- The thalamus is the largest part of the diencephalon and is closely related both functionally and anatomically to the cerebral cortices. Almost all fibers passing to the cerebral hemispheres pass through and synapse within the thalamus. It has outgoing connections with virtually every part of the cerebrum and its function is most likely to be integration of incoming sensory information via its interconnected nuclei. The information is then passed to the cerebral cortex for interpretation.

Basal ganglia is a collective term given to bilateral masses of deeply sited grey matter (Fig. 7.18). They have afferent and efferent connections with the cerebral cortex, the thalamus,

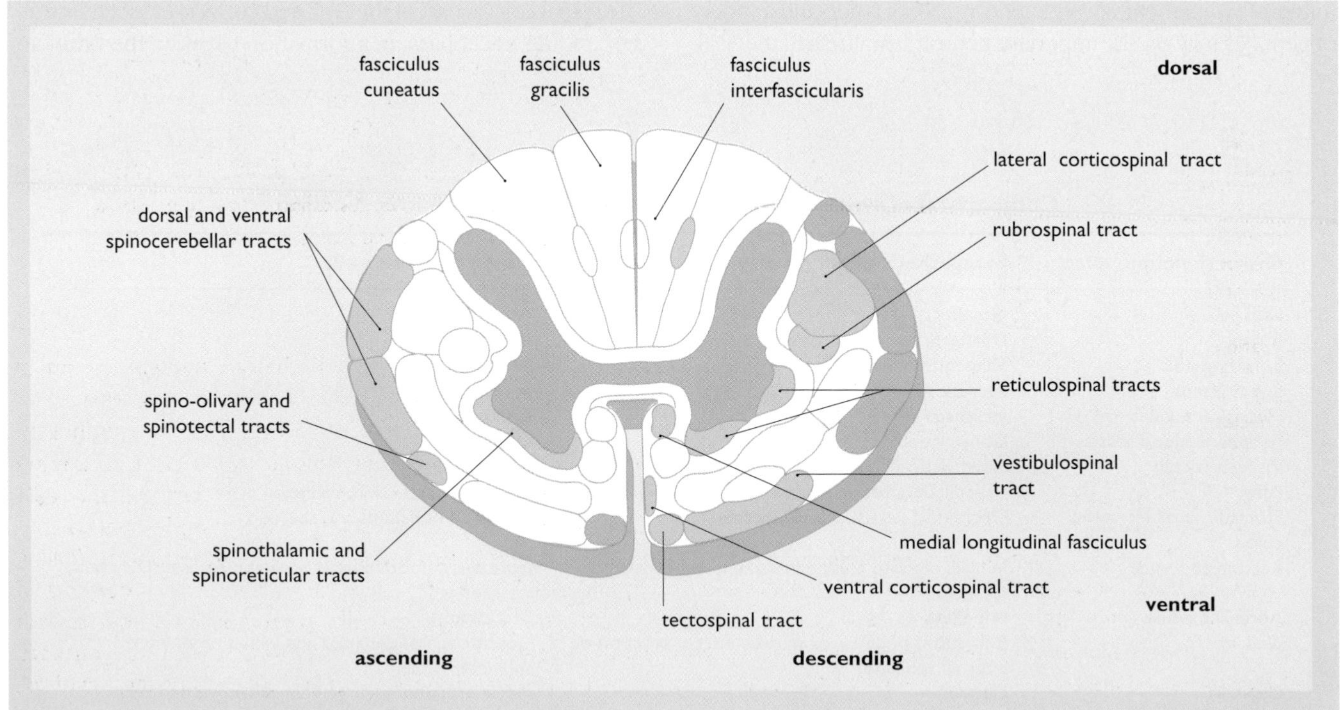

Fig. 7.14 The spinal cord at the midcervical level showing the major tracts of the spinal white matter.

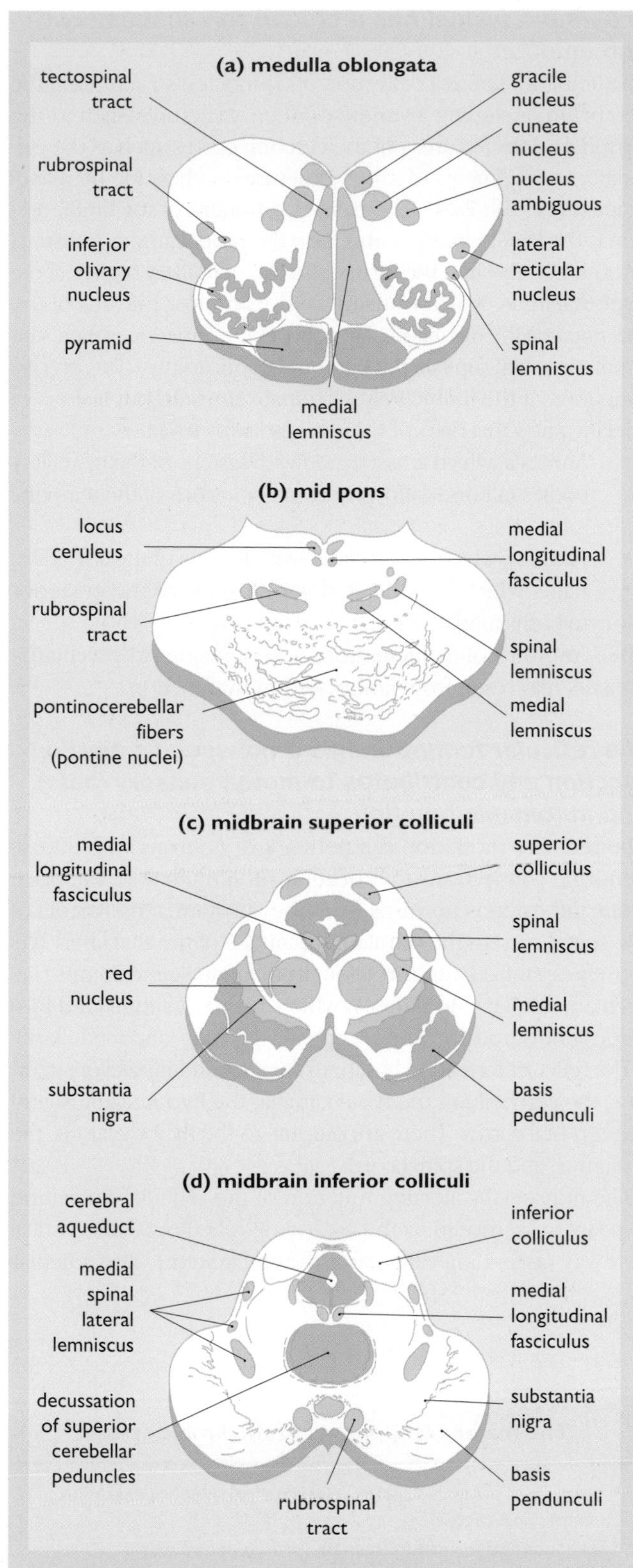

Fig. 7.15 The medulla oblongata, pons, and midbrain. (a) The medulla oblongata is the first part of the brain stem and motor fibers and some sensory fibers cross here. (b) The pons lies between the medulla and midbrain. It can be considered as a relay station between the cerebellum, the brain, and the peripheral nervous sytem. (c) The midbrain superior colliculi allow tracking of visual stimuli. (d) The midbrain inferior colliculi provide selective attention to auditory stimuli.

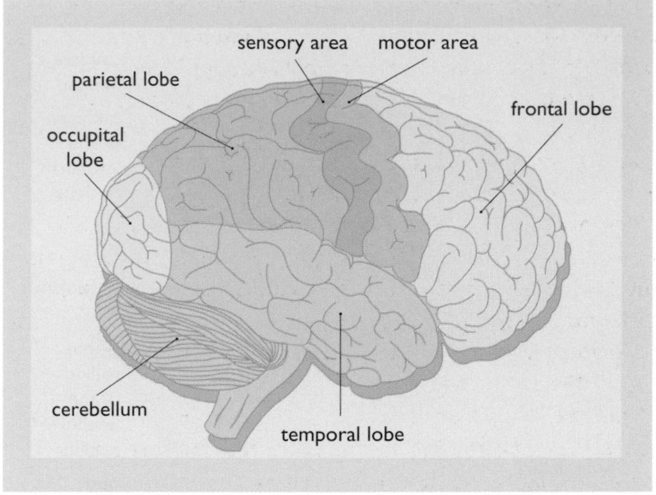

Fig. 7.16 A lateral view of the brain.

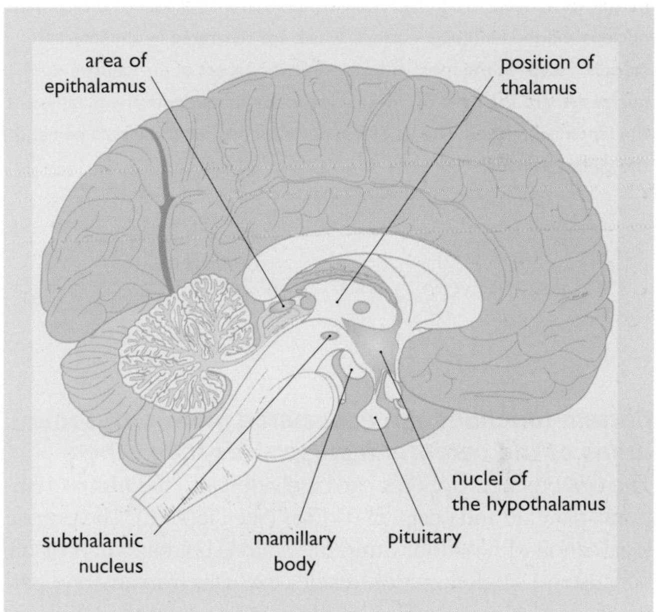

Fig. 7.17 The diencephalon. This consists of the hypothalamus, subthalamus, epithalamus, and the thalamus.

subthalamus, and brain stem, and they are thought to control motor function by an effect on the cerebral hemispheres.

The cerebral hemispheres form the telencephalon. Consciousness and the ability to adapt and react to changing circumstances result from the complexity and size of the right and left hemispheres. The ability to use complex methods of communication is also provided by the telencephalon. These capabilities lead to the capacity for abstract thought and therefore the ability to learn and profit not only from our own experiences but also those of others, and to generate hypotheses. This higher functioning leads to the development of a rich emotional life and therefore the risk of profound mental illness.

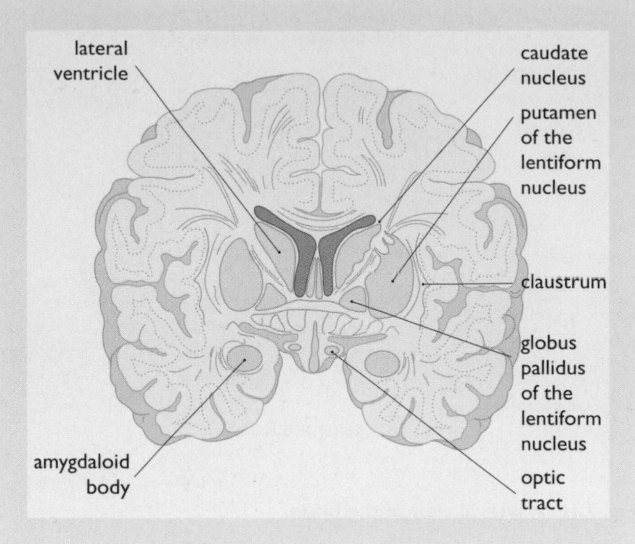

Fig. 7.18 Basal ganglia. The bilaterally represented masses of gray matter form deep structures. The corpus striatum consists of the caudate nucleus and the lentiform nucleus, which are separated by the internal capsule except at the most anterior–inferior aspect of the caudate nucleus where the head of the caudate is continuous with the putamen of the lentiform nucleus. The lentiform nucleus consists of the putamen and the globus pallidus.

Certain functions are associated more with some areas of the cerebral hemispheres than others

The cerebral hemispheres can be divided into the frontal, temporal, parietal, and occipital cortices (see Fig. 7.16). The precise localization of function within the brain is not known, possibly because no single function resides exclusively in any one particular area. However, as with the lower parts of the CNS, certain functions are associated more with some areas than others:

- Voluntary motor function is subserved by the precentral gyrus of the frontal lobe.
- Sensory function lies in the postcentral gyrus of the parietal lobe.
- Part of the dominant frontal lobe appears to have a primary role in the production of speech.
- Part of the frontal lobes bilaterally appear to be involved in the formation of personality, higher reasoning, and intellectual functioning.
- The temporal lobes provide a large proportion of memory function and integration as well as the auditory centers.
- The parietal lobes appear to have a complex integrating function for sensory and motor and, to a lesser extent, emotional functioning. They also allow planning and initiation of complex actions and have a crucial role in topographic, object and word recognition and their association with emotion.
- The occipital cortices receive and process visual input.

The limbic system has a crucial role in memory and emotion

The limbic system is a collection of connected structures in the cerebrum, including a variety of deep structures such as the amygdala, selected areas of the cerebral cortex such as the cingulate, and segments of other structures such as the hypothalamus (Figs 7.19, 7.20). The basic component of the limbic system is the Papez circuit. In this loop the hippocampus transmits information through the fornices to the mamillary bodies of the hypothalamus, which transmit to the anterior nucleus of the thalamus via the mamillothalamic tracts. Information is then sent via the internal capsule back to the hippocampus. The precise functions of the limbic system remain unclear, but lesions of specific parts that disrupt the various loops lead to:

- Amnesia, which is associated with lesions of the mamillary bodies in Korsakoff's syndrome or lesions of the temporal lobes.
- Placidity, which is associated with lesions of the amygdala.
- Rage, which is associated with lesions of the posterior hypothalamus.

The symptoms of hallucinations and delusions in psychiatric patients may result from limbic system dysfunction.

The reticular formation has a nonspecific alerting function and contributes to motor, sensory (pain), and autonomic function

The reticular formation is a network of neurons with diffuse dendritic connections that occupies the midline of the brain stem and extends upwards from the substantia intermedia of the spinal cord to the intralaminar nuclei of the thalamus. It is loosely organized into three longitudinal nuclear columns (i.e. median, medial, and lateral), which are each subdivided into three ventrocaudally (mesencephalic, pontine, and medullary).

The reticular formation has input from ascending sensory neurons, the cerebellum, the basal ganglia, the hypothalamus, and the cerebral cortex. There are outputs to the hypothalamus, the thalamus, and the spinal cord.

The nonspecific alerting function of the reticular formation appears to be related to the ascending reticulothalamocortical pathway (ascending reticular activating system). The reticular

The major components of the limbic system

- Regions of the limbic cortex (cingulate, parahippocampal gyrus, entorrhinal cortex)
- Hippocampal formation (dentate gyrus, hippocampus)
- Amygdala (basolateral complex, centromedial complex, parts of the stria terminalis and the hypothalamus)
- Nucleus accumbens
- Mamillary bodies
- Anterior and dorsomedial nuclei of the thalamus (some authors also include other cortical regions including the orbitofrontal area, the temporal poles and the insula)

Fig. 7.19 The major components of the limbic system.

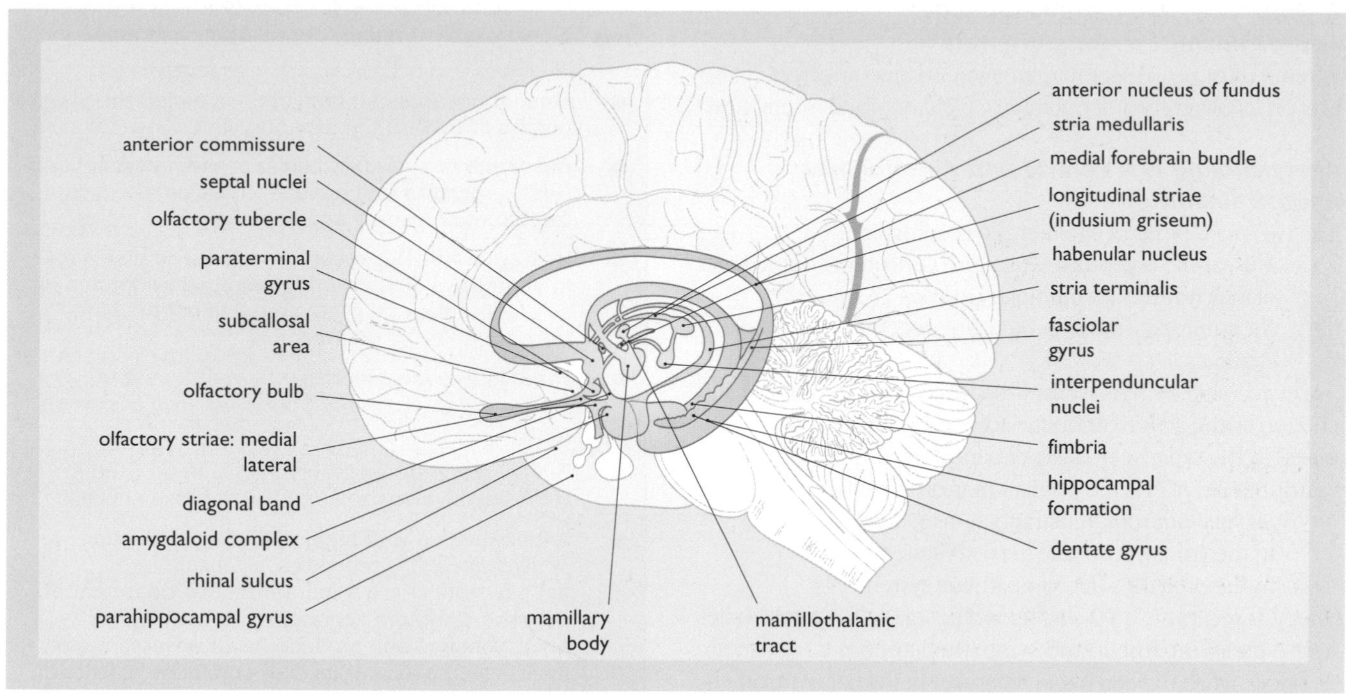

Fig. 7.20 The anatomic relations of the amygdala, the hippocampus, and other components of the limbic system.

formation also makes contributions to motor, sensory (pain), and autonomic function, especially affecting respiration and vasomotor function.

FUNCTIONAL NEUROCHEMISTRY OF THE NERVOUS SYSTEM

The neurotransmitters listed in Figs 7.8 and 7.10 are found within specific regions of the nervous system and together with the complex anatomic arrangement provide for the sophisticated function of the human brain.

Glutamate is the major excitatory neurotransmitter in the CNS

Glutamate is an amino acid and acts on *N*-methyl D-aspartate (NMDA) and non-NMDA receptors. It is the primary neurotransmitter in thalamocortical, pyramidal cell, and corticostriatal projections, and is an important transmitter in the hippocampus. It has been suggested that as some drugs that act on the NMDA receptor produce psychotic symptoms, abnormalities of the glutamate system may have a causative role in psychotic illnesses.

GABA is the major inhibitory neurotransmitter in the nervous system

GABA is also an amino acid and acts primarily on $GABA_A$ and $GABA_B$ receptors. $GABA_A$ receptors are the most common and are present on 40% of neurons. The cortical distribution of $GABA_A$ is shown in Fig. 7.21. $GABA_A$ is a receptor-operated Cl^- channel, while $GABA_B$ receptors are coupled to G proteins.

Benzodiazepines and most anticonvulsants have their effects on the GABA receptor:

- Benzodiazepines act on a specific benzodiazepine receptor on a subunit of the GABA receptor and enhance the effects of GABA on the receptor, thereby acting as neuromodulators.
- Some anticonvulsants have similar effects to benzodiazepines, but most act directly on the GABA receptor.

Abnormalities of the GABA system are thought to be associated with anxiety disorders, and recent work has suggested a role for GABA in the etiology of schizophrenia.

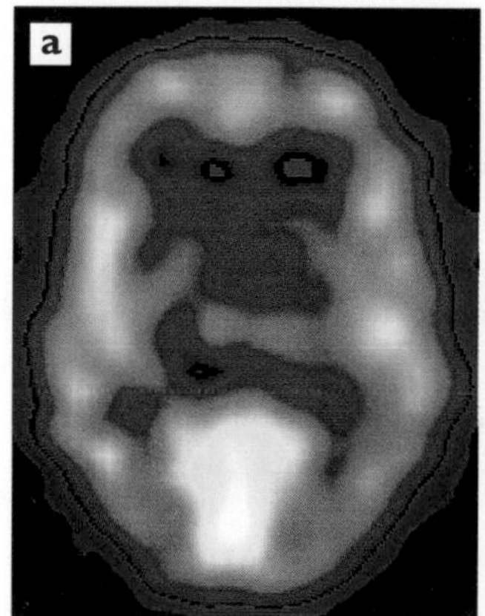

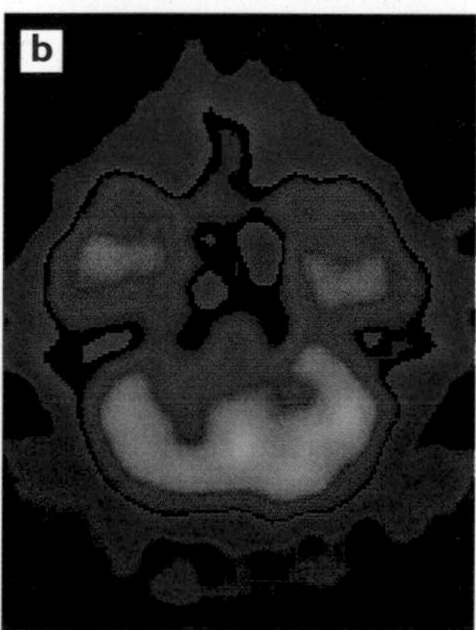

Fig. 7.21 The cortical distribution of γ-aminobutyric acid-A ($GABA_A$) receptors. This is shown using the radioactively labeled benzodiazepine analog lomazenil and single photon emission tomography (SPET). The brightest areas have the highest density of receptors. (a) The image at the level of the midoccipital cortex. (b) The image at the level of the cerebellum.

Glycine is a 'mandatory adjunctive neurotransmitter' for glutamate

Glycine must be present for glutamate to have an effect. It also acts on its own receptor-operated Cl^- channel and is inhibitory.

Acetylcholine is a central and a peripheral neurotransmitter

The two main types of cholinergic receptors are:

- Muscarinic receptors, which are G protein-coupled and of which there are multiple subtypes.
- Nicotinic receptors, which are receptor-operated Cl^- channels.

Acetylcholine (Ach) is synthesized from acetylcoenzyme A and choline by the action of choline acetyltransferase and is metabolized in the synapse by acetylcholinesterase.

Peripherally, ACh is the primary neurotransmitter at:

- Skeletal neuromuscular junctions (NMJs).
- In the parasympathetic nervous system.
- In the preganglionic sympathetic system.

The ACh receptors on the NMJs and postganglionic cell bodies in the parasympathetic and sympathetic nervous system are nicotinic, while the end organ receptors in the parasympathetic system are muscarinic and have a wide distribution.

Centrally, the primary ACh-containing nucleus is the nucleus basalis of Meynert, which is situated in the basal forebrain and has projections to the cerebral cortex and limbic system. Cholinergic fibers in the reticular system project to the cerebral cortex, the limbic system, the hypothalamus, and the thalamus.

5-Hydroxytryptamine, depression, and anxiety

- Most antidepressant medications inhibit the uptake of 5-HT in the synaptic cleft
- Buspirone is a partial agonist of the presynaptic 5-HT_{1A} receptor and appears to be an effective treatment of anxiety and depression
- 5-HT_{2A} and 5-HT_{2c} receptors appear to play a role in depressive illnesses, the negative symptoms of schizophrenia, and protection against the long-term sequelae of neuroleptics
- There is a relative increase in the number of 5-HT_{2A} receptors in the frontal cortices of suicidal patients
- 5-HT_{2A} receptor antagonists have been used to treat negative schizophrenia with some success
- Antipsychotics with high-affinity antagonistic activity at 5-HT_{2A} receptors (atypical antipsychotics) are a more effective treatment of negative symptom schizophrenia than typical antipsychotics and produce fewer adverse motor effects with a similar level of dopamine blockade
- 5-HT_3 receptor antagonists are used in the management of nausea (see p. 132)
- Early and current trials of 5-HT_3 receptor antagonists in schizophrenia are producing equivocal results

Acetylcholine, Parkinson's disease, and Alzheimer's dementia

- The symptoms of Parkinson's disease result from a defect in the balance between acetylcholine and dopamine in the basal ganglia
- Anticholinergic medication is used to treat the parkinsonian adverse effects of antipsychotic medications and idiopathic Parkinson's disease (see p. 107)
- Nicotinic and muscarinic agonists or drugs that enhance endogenous acetylcholine function appear to be beneficial in the treatment of Alzheimer's dementia

More than nine distinct 5-HT (serotonin) receptors have been identified

The 5-HT_{1A}, 5-HT_{2A}, 5-HT_{2C}, and 5-HT_3 subgroups of 5-HT receptors have been most extensively studied. The major site of serotonergic cell bodies is in the area of the upper pons and midbrain. The classic areas for 5-HT-containing neurons are the median and dorsal raphe nuclei. The neurons from the raphe nuclei project to the basal ganglia and various parts of the limbic system, and have a wide distribution throughout the cerebral cortices in addition to cerebellar connections (Fig. 7.22).

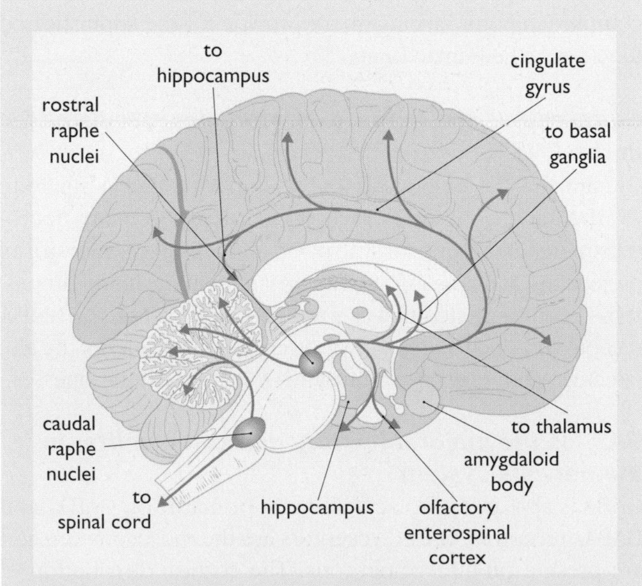

Fig. 7.22 5-Hydroxytryptamine (5-HT) pathways. 5-HT-containing neurons are found in the median and dorsal raphe nuclei, the caudal locus ceruleus, the area postrema, and the interpeduncular area.

All the 5-HT receptors identified so far are G protein-coupled receptors except the 5-HT_3 receptor, which is a receptor-operated Na^+/K^+ channel.

5-HT is synthesized from tryptophan by tryptophan hydroxylase, and the supply of tryptophan is the rate-limiting step in the synthesis of 5-HT. 5-HT is primarily broken down by monoamine oxidase-A to 5-hydroxyindoleacetic acid (5-HIAA).

Norepinephrine is widely distributed

Norepinephrine acts on the adrenoceptors α_1, α_2, β_{1-3}. In the periphery adrenoceptors are mainly found as end-organ receptors in the sympathetic nervous system. The majority of norepinephrine-containing neurons in the CNS are located in the locus ceruleus in the pons/midbrain and their projections to other areas of the brain are shown in Fig. 7.23 (see also Figs 7.15b, 7.15c).

Norepinephrine is synthesized from tyrosine in a common pathway with the other catecholamines, epinephrine and dopamine. The rate-limiting step is the enzyme tyrosine hydroxylase. The first product is dopamine which is then converted into norepinephrine by dopamine decarboxylase. Norepinephrine can then be converted to epinephrine by the action of phenylethanolamine-*N*-methyltransferase. Metabolism is primarily by monoamine oxidase (MAO)-A and the primary metabolite is vanillylmandelic acid (VMA).

In general it seems that:

- Postsynaptic α_1 receptors are linked to stimulation of phosphoinositol turnover.
- α_2 Receptors inhibit the formation of cAMP.
- β Receptors stimulate the formation of cAMP.

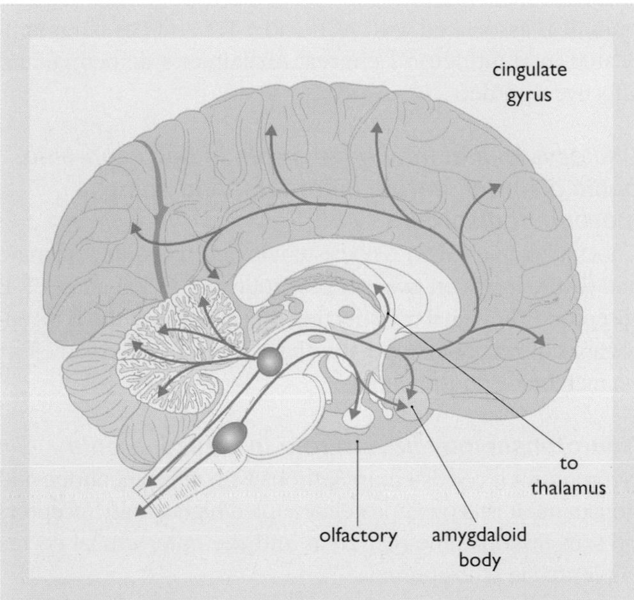

Fig. 7.23 Norepinephrine pathways. Most of the norepinephrine-containing neurons in the central nervous system are located in the locus ceruleus in the pons and midbrain. These neurons project through the medial forebrain bundle to the limbic system, cerebral cortices, the thalamus, and the hypothalamus. A second group of norepinephrine-containing neurons in the ventral tegmental area have projections to the hypothalamus and amygdala.

Norepinephrine and affective and anxiety disorders

- Norepinephrine is thought to play a crucial role in affective disorders, and to a lesser extent in anxiety disorders
- Abnormalities of norepinephrine-containing neurons are incorporated as part of the monoamine theory of depression (see p. 109)
- Most traditional tricyclic antidepressants inhibit the uptake of norepinephrine from the synaptic cleft and thereby increase the availability of synaptic norepinephrine
- Monoamine oxidase inhibitors inhibit the breakdown of norepinephrine
- It is thought that the antidepressant effect of norepinephrine manipulation is mediated by a downregulation in postsynaptic β receptors

Five types of dopamine receptor (D_1–D_5) have so far been identified in the human nervous system

D_1 and D_5 receptors stimulate the formation of cAMP by activating a stimulatory G protein, while D_2, D_3, and D_4 receptors inhibit the formation of cAMP by activating an inhibitory G protein. D_2 receptors are more ubiquitous than D_3 and D_4 receptors. D_3 receptors are primarily located in the nucleus accumbens (one of the septal nuclei in the limbic system) and D_4 receptors are particularly concentrated in the medial frontal cortex.

There are a variety of dopaminergic pathways or tracts (Fig. 7.24):

- The nigrostriatal tract projects from the substantia nigra in the midbrain to the corpus striatum, and has a role in motor control.

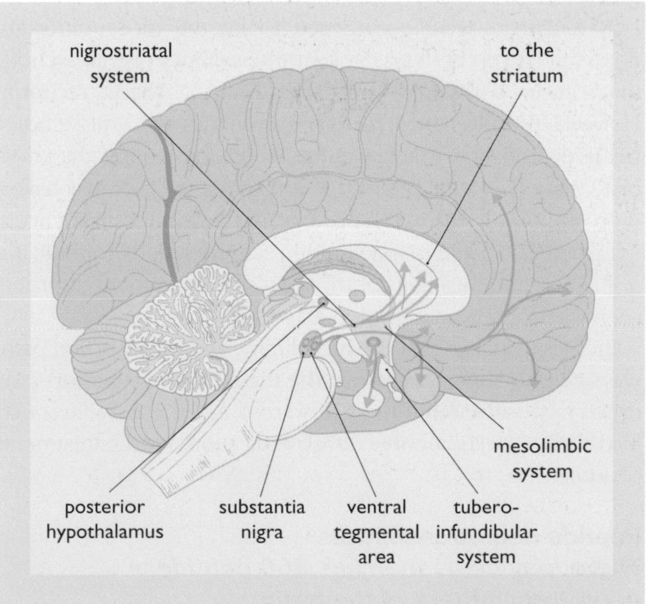

Fig. 7.24 Dopamine pathways. These tracts include the nigrostriatal tract, the mesolimbic/mesocortical tract, and the tuberoinfundular tract.

- The mesolimbic/mesocortical tract has cell bodies in the ventral tegmental area adjacent to the substantia nigra and projects to the limbic system and neocortex in addition to the striatum. It supplies fibers to the medial surface of the frontal lobes and to the parahippocampus and cingulate cortex.
- The third major pathway is the tuberoinfundibular tract. The cell bodies reside in the arcuate nucleus and periventricular area of the hypothalamus, and they project to the infundibulum and the anterior pituitary. Dopamine inhibits the release of prolactin within this tract.

Dopamine, Parkinson's disease, and psychosis

- **Idiopathic Parkinson's disease results from degeneration of cells in the substantia nigra**
- **Parkinsonian adverse effects of typical antipsychotics (e.g. haloperdol, chlorpromazine) result from blocking of dopamine receptors within the nigrostriatal tract**
- **Antipsychotic medications are thought to exert beneficial effects on the mesolimbic and mesocortical tract**
- **The inhibitory drive of prolactin release is removed by dopamine receptor blockade within the tuberoinfundibular tract by antipsychotics and leads to prolactinemia**

Dopamine is synthesized as part of the common pathway for catecholamines (see above), and it is metabolized by two enzymes: MAO-B, which is intraneuronal, and catechol-*O*-methyl transferase (COMT), which is extraneuronal. The primary metabolite of dopamine is homovanillic acid (HVA).

D_2 receptors were considered to be the most important dopamine receptor in psychosis as the potency of antipsychotic medications correlated with their affinity for the D_2 receptor. However, the advent of atypical antipsychotics with equal efficacy, but a relatively low potency at the D_2 receptor, raises the possibility that other subtypes of the dopamine receptor may have a more important role in the etiology and treatment of psychosis.

Chronic blockade of dopamine receptors leads to their upregulation and this may contribute to the movement disorders seen with long-term neuroleptic therapy.

There is evidence that the mesolimbic and mesocortical pathways play an important role in the regulation of behaviors governed by positive reinforcers (rewards), and these findings may lead to the development of novel medications for the treatments of addictions.

Peptide neurotransmitters

There may be as many as 300 peptide neurotransmitters in the brain

A peptide is a short protein consisting of fewer than 100 amino acids. The best-characterized neuropeptides are listed in Fig. 7.10. Often these peptides are synthesized as part of much larger molecules called preprohormones. These are cleaved in the neuronal cytoplasm to prohormones, which are then taken up into vesicles. Within the vesicles the prohormones are further cleaved into the neuroactive peptides. Most peptide neurotransmitters coexist with other neurotransmitters.

Opioids are thought to regulate stress, pain, and mood

The three endogenous opioid groups listed in Fig. 7.10 (i.e. endorphins, enkephalins, and dynorphins) are synthesized from larger precursor molecules. Enkephalin coexists in noradrenergic and serotonergic neurons. Opioids act on three types of receptors:

- μ, where their action is to decrease production of cAMP and increase K^+ conductance.
- δ, where they have a similar action to that on μ receptors.
- κ, where their action is to decrease K^+ conductance.

The neurohypophysial neuroactive peptides vasopressin and oxytocin are thought to be involved in mood regulation

The two neurohypophysial hormones vasopressin and oxytocin are synthesized in the hypothalamus and released in the posterior pituitary. There are three receptors for vasopressin and its actions are mediated either by changes in membrane phospholipids or by increasing cAMP.

Tachykinins include substance P and neurokinin

Substance P is a primary neurotransmitter in most primary afferent sensory neurons and is present in the nigrostriatal tract. It is associated with ACh and 5-HT and has been implicated in Huntington's chorea, Alzheimer's dementia, and affective disorders.

Cholecystokinin may have a role in schizophrenia, panic disorder, eating disorders, and some movement disorders

Cholecystokinin (CCK) is coexistent in neurons with dopamine and GABA. It acts on two receptor subtypes, CCK-A and CCK-B receptors. The signal transduction mechanisms of the B receptor are not yet understood, but the A subtype acts via an effect on membrane phospholipids.

Neurotensin may have a role in schizophrenia

Neurotensin is coexistent in neurons with norepinephrine and dopamine. It acts on G protein-coupled high-affinity receptors present in dopamine-rich areas and the enterorhinal cortex implicated in schizophrenia.

PATHOPHYSIOLOGY AND DISEASES OF THE CENTRAL NERVOUS SYSTEM

PSYCHOSIS

Psychosis describes a mental state characterized by a loss of touch with reality. The patient may describe a variety of abnormalities of perception, thought, and ideas. Psychosis is not a specific illness and psychotic symptoms may occur in depression and other mood disorders and in medical conditions that interfere with brain function. Psychotic illnesses include schizophrenia, schizoaffective disorder, delusional disorders, and some depressive and manic illnesses. The most prevalent psychotic illness that includes all the cardinal psychotic symptoms is schizophrenia.

SCHIZOPHRENIA

Schizophrenia is a psychotic illness characterized by multiple symptoms affecting thought, perceptions, emotion, and volition. Its incidence in industrialized countries is approximately 15 new cases/100,000 population/year. Its prevalence is 0.5–1%, rising to 2.8% in some areas (e.g. Northern Sweden).

Schizophrenia characteristically develops in people aged 15–45 years, but it may occur before puberty or be delayed until the seventh or eighth decade. The typical age of onset for males is 23–28 years and for females, 28–32 years. There is an increased rate among people living in inner cities and those from lower social classes, and in immigrant populations. This appears to be because patients 'drift' down the social ladder into inner cities or overseas as part of their illness during the time before their onset of symptoms or admission into hospital.

Florid symptoms of schizophrenia include delusions, hallucinations, abnormal thought processes, and passivity experiences

The premorbid personality is often described as emotionally and socially detached. Such people have few friends, are often cold and aloof, and engage in solitary occupations. Their behavior may be eccentric and they are indifferent to praise or criticism. People with schizophrenia slowly become more withdrawn and introverted, develop new interests, which are sometimes out of character, and drift away from family and friends. They may begin to fail in their occupation or school work. The onset of overt schizophrenia is commonly slow and insidious, taking weeks to years, but eventually, often with an apparently precipitating event, the symptoms of florid illness appear. The florid symptoms are variable, but usually include delusions, hallucinations, abnormal thought processes, and passivity experiences. In addition there may be formal thought disorder, a flat or inappropriate affect, and abnormal motor signs, which are usually called catatonic symptoms.

Delusions are false personal beliefs held with absolute conviction

The beliefs of delusions are outside the person's normal culture or subculture in spite of what everyone else believes and evidence to the contrary. They dominate the individual's viewpoint and behavior. Delusional disorders are disorders in which delusions are prominent and hallucinations and abnormal thought phenomena are vague or absent.

Hallucinations are false perceptions in the absence of a real external stimulus

Hallucinations are perceived as having the same quality as real perceptions and are not subject to conscious manipulation. Hallucinations in schizophrenia are equally varied and may involve any of the sensory modalities. The most common are auditory hallucinations in the form of voices, which occur in 60–70% of patients diagnosed with schizophrenia. Visual hallucinations occur in about 10% of patients, but should raise the suspicion of an organic disorder. Olfactory hallucinations are more common in temporal lobe epilepsy (TLE) than schizophrenia, and tactile hallucinations are probably experienced more frequently than is reported by patients. No one type of hallucination is specific to schizophrenia and the duration and intensity is probably more important diagnostically.

Thought alienation and disordered thought are common in schizophrenia

Disorders of thought possession in schizophrenia are described as thought alienation. The patient has the experience that his thoughts are under the control of an outside agency or that others are participating in his thinking. Disorders of the form of thought are also characteristic, and as a result the speech is difficult to follow or incoherent and follows no logical sequence.

Catatonic symptoms can occur in any form of schizophrenia

Catatonic symptoms form part of a subtype of schizophrenia. However, these, mainly motor, symptoms can occur in any form of schizophrenia. They include:

- Ambitendence (alternation between opposite movements).
- Echopraxia (automatic imitation of another person's movements).
- Stereotypies (repeated regular fixed parts of movement [or speech] that are not goal directed).
- Negativism (motiveless resistance to instructions and attempts to be moved or doing the opposite of what is asked).
- Posturing (adoption of an inappropriate or bizarre bodily posture continuously for a substantial period of time).
- Waxy flexibility (the limbs can be 'moulded' into a position and remain fixed for long periods of time).

The differential diagnosis of acute schizophrenia includes other psychotic illnesses and organic disorders

The differential diagnosis of acute schizophrenia includes other psychotic illnesses such as schizophreniform disorder, schizoaffective disorder, bipolar affective disorder, paranoid psychosis, and psychotic depression. Certain organic causes must be excluded including drug/substance-induced psychosis, early dementia, some forms of epilepsy, endocrine causes, infections, metabolic disorders, systemic lupus erythematosus (SLE), and the long-term sequelae of head injury.

Approximately 50–65% of patients with acute schizophrenia develop chronic schizophrenia

The symptoms seen in acute schizophrenia are generally termed the positive symptoms of schizophrenia and are characteristic of the acute phase of the illness. In chronic schizophrenia some florid (positive) symptoms may remain, but the predominant negative symptoms are:

- Poverty of speech (a restriction in the amount of spontaneous speech and in the information contained in speech; alogia.
- Flattening of affect (a restriction in the experience and expression of emotion).
- Anhedonia–asociality (an inability to experience pleasure, few social contacts, and social withdrawal).
- Avolition–apathy (reduced drive, energy, and interest).
- Attention impairment (an inattentiveness at work and interview).

Some of these symptoms may also occur as part of a florid psychotic episode. Their presence is associated with a poor prognosis, a poor response to neuroleptics, poor premorbid adjustment, cognitive impairment, and atrophic changes on a CT scan.

Once schizophrenia is diagnosed there are four main outcomes

The clinical course of schizophrenia will usually follow one of the following patterns:

- The illness resolves completely, with or without treatment, and never recurs (pattern A, 10–20% of patients).
- The illness recurs repeatedly with full recovery every time (pattern B, 30–35% of patients).
- The illness recurs repeatedly, but recovery is incomplete and a persistent defective state develops, becoming more pronounced with each successive relapse (pattern C, 30–35% of patients).
- The illness pursues a downhill course from the beginning (pattern D, 10–20% of patients).

There is some debate about the impact of effective treatments for acute schizophrenia on the long-term course and prognosis of the illness. Approximately 55% of schizophrenics now live and work normally. Factors contributing to a poor prognosis include an early onset, an insidious onset, a lack of a prominent affective component, a lack of clear precipitants, a family history of schizophrenia, poor premorbid personality, confusion or perplexity, a low IQ, a low social class, social isolation, and a previous psychiatric history. The converse of these factors usually predicts a better prognosis.

The tendency to develop schizophrenia is genetically transmitted

Although the mode of transmission remains obscure it appears to be polygenic. Twin studies indicate that the genetic contribution to schizophrenia is approximately 50%.

The neurotransmitters dopamine, 5-HT, GABA, and glutamate may have a role in schizophrenia

Many hypotheses have been invoked to explain the manifestations of schizoprenia at the level of neurotransmitters in the brain. The potential pivotal role of excess dopamine in various brain regions has received considerable attention. Although many antipsychotic drugs block dopamine receptors, particularly D_2 receptors, there is little support from current research for a primary dopaminergic abnormality in schizophrenia. Other neurotransmitters that may have a role in schizophrenia include 5-HT, GABA, and glutamate.

The treatment of schizophrenia and all other psychotic illnesses involves the use of antipsychotic medication (the neuroleptic drugs)

Chlorpromazine and other neuroleptics produce a general improvement in all the acute symptoms of schizophrenia, but their efficacy in negative schizophrenia and their ability to affect the course and prognosis of schizophrenia is less clear. The therapeutic effect of these 'typical' antipsychotic drugs was thought to be related to their ability to block dopamine (primarily D_2) receptors (Fig. 7.25). However, the development of newer 'atypical' antipsychotic drugs (e.g. clozapine, risperidone, olanzepine*), which are not very active at the D_2 receptor, but are still clinically effective, has challenged this hypothesis.

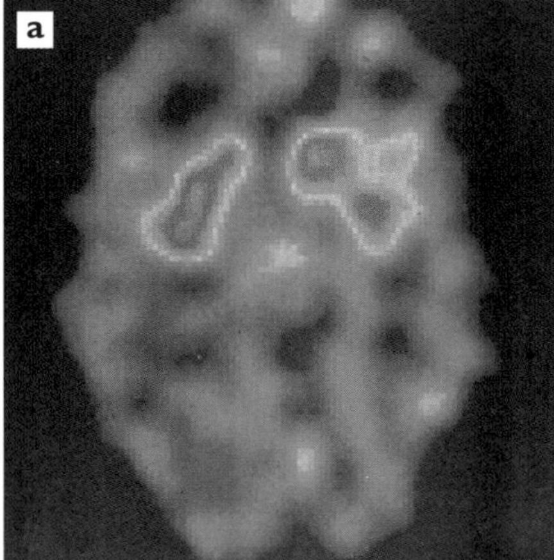

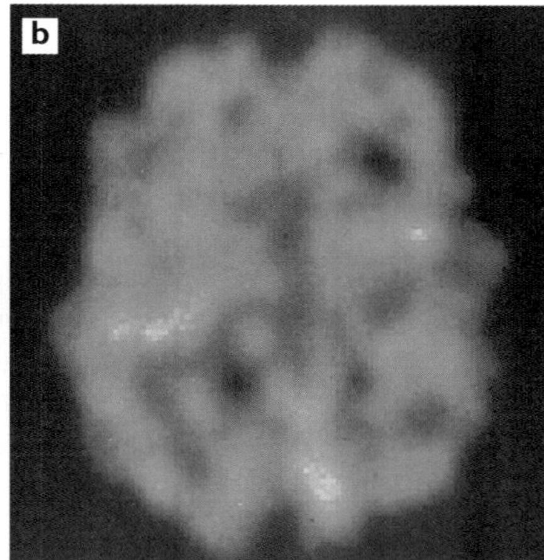

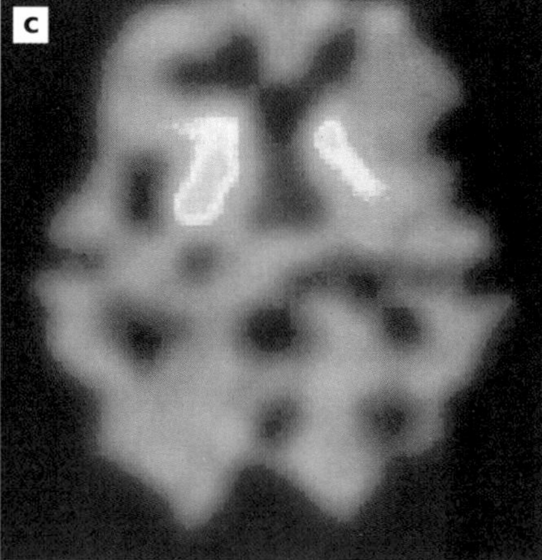

Fig. 7.25 The cerebral distribution of dopamine receptors in treated and untreated schizophrenia. Single photon emission tomography (SPET) scans acquired using the dopamine D_2 ligand I [^{123}I] iodobenzamine. (a) Striatal dopamine receptors in an untreated schizophrenic patient. (b) Complete blockade of the receptors shown in (a) with a typical antipsychotic. (c) Partial blockade of the receptors shown in (a) with an equally effective dose of clozapine, an atypical antipsychotic. (Courtesy of the Institute of Nuclear Medicine, Middlesex Hospital, London, UK.)

Psychotic illness is usually first treated with an oral antipsychotic such as chlorpromazine (sedating), trifluoperazine, or haloperidol

The dose of antipsychotic is titrated against symptoms for a period of 4–6 weeks, which is considered to be necessary for an adequate trial of such a drug. Some authors advocate using the atypical risperidone as the first-line drug because it causes fewer adverse antipsychotic effects at therapeutic doses. If the medication is effective it may then be given as a depot preparation if the patient is poorly compliant, or oral treatment can be continued. If the medication is ineffective an alternative class of typical antipsychotic should be used instead. If the medication is still ineffective, the medication should be changed to an atypical antipsychotic such as clozapine. Approximately 35% of patients do not respond to classic antipsychotics.

The general consensus is that all acute episodes of schizophrenia should be treated with neuroleptics and that the medication should be continued for 1–2 years before being cautiously withdrawn.

Most patients require maintenance therapy after an acute psychotic episode

Generally, the lowest possible dose of neuroleptic should be used for maintenance therapy. In chronic schizophrenia, neuroleptics are used to prevent further acute episodes. Although most studies show a much higher relapse rate for patients whose medication is discontinued, some studies have failed to show a drug/placebo difference. Approximately 16–25% of patients relapse despite the use of medication.

ANTIPSYCHOTIC (NEUROLEPTIC) DRUGS

Antipsychotic drugs are not a homogeneous group, and there are various classes (Fig. 7.26). Typical antipsychotics cause catalepsy in animals via D_2 receptor blockade. Atypical antipsychotics do not. The phenothiazines include:

- Drugs with aliphatic side chains such as chlorpromazine.
- Drugs with piperidine chains such as thioridazine.
- Drugs with piperazine side chains such as trifluoperazine and fluphenazine. Other classes include:
- The thioxanthenes (e.g. flupenthixol* and zuclopenthixol*).
- The dibenzodiazepines (e.g. clozapine and olanzepine*).
- The butyrophenones (e.g. haloperidol and droperidol).
- The diphenylbutylpiperidines (e.g. pimozide).
- The substituted benzamides (e.g. sulpiride*).
- The benzixasoles (e.g. risperidone).

The classes of antipsychotic drugs

Class	Examples
Typical antipsychotics	Phenothiazines (chlorpromazine, fluphenazine, trifluoperazine) Butyrophenones (haloperidol, droperidol) Others (pimozide, thioridazine)
Atypical antipsychotics	Broad spectrum (clozapine, olanzepine) Dopamine/5-hydroxytryptamine blockers (risperidone, sertindole*, ziprasidone*)

Fig. 7.26 The classes of antipsychotic drugs.

Adverse effects of antipsychotics

Acute neurologic adverse effects due to D_2 receptor blockade include acute dystonia. This is characterized by fixed muscle postures with spasm and include clenched jaw muscles, protruding tongue, opisthotonos, torticollis, and oculogyric crisis (mouth open, head back, eyes staring upwards). It appears within hours to days and is most common in young males. It should be treated immediately with anticholinergic drugs (procyclidine 5–10 mg, benztropine intramuscularly or intravenously). The response is dramatic.

Adverse effects of antipsychotics

- Acute neurologic effects: acute dystonia, akathisia, parkinsonism
- Chronic neurologic effects: tardive dyskinesia, tardive dystonia
- Neuroendocrine effects: amenorrhea, galactorrhea, infertility
- Idiosyncratic: neuroleptic malignant syndrome
- Anticholinergic: dry mouth, blurred vision, constipation, urinary retention, ejaculatory failure
- Antihistaminergic: sedation
- Antiadrenergic: hypotension, arrhythmia
- Miscellaneous: photosensitivity, heat sensitivity, cholestatic jaundice, retinal pigmentation

Medium-term neurologic adverse effects due to D_2 blockade include akathisia and parkinsonism.

Akathisia is a motor, generally lower limb, restlessness accompanied by an inner feeling of restlessness. It is usually very distressing to the patient. Treatment primarily involves reducing the drug dose.

Parkinsonism is induced by blockade of D_2 receptors in the basal ganglia. The symptoms appear after a few days to weeks and treatment involves anticholinergic drugs (e.g. procyclidine, orphenadrine), reduction of the neuroleptic dose, or switching to an atypical neuroleptic (e.g. risperidone), which is less likely to produce such extrapyramidal symptoms.

Chronic neurologic adverse effects due to D_2 blockade are tardive dyskinesia and tardive dystonia.

Tardive dyskinesia is usually manifested as orofacial dyskinesia and causes lip smacking and tongue rotating. Tardive dystonia appears as choreoathetoid movements of the head, neck, and trunk. It appears after months to years of drug treatment. There is an increased risk of tardive dyskinesia in older patients, females, the edentulous, and patients with organic brain damage. Approximately 20% of patients who are taking neuroleptics long term will develop tardive dyskinesia, but there is no relationship to duration, total dose of treatment, or class of antipsychotic used. There is no effective treatment, so prevention by limiting the use of neuroleptics and early recognition of symptoms is important. Increasing the dose may temporarily alleviate the symptoms, while reducing the dose may worsen them. Clozapine has been shown to improve symptoms. Newer antipsychotics (e.g. risperidone) may be less likely to induce tardive dyskinesia.

Neuroendocrine adverse effects due to D_2 blockade include hyperprolactinemia by reducing the negative feedback on the anterior pituitary. High serum concentrations of prolactin can produce galactorrhea, amenorrhea, and infertility in some patients.

Neuroleptic malignant syndrome (NMS) is the most life-threatening adverse effect of neuroleptic use. It is thought to be due to deranged dopaminergic function, but the precise pathophysiology is unknown. Symptoms include hyperthermia, muscle rigidity, autonomic instability, and fluctuating consciousness. It is an idiosyncratic reaction that appears from a few days to weeks after beginning treatment, but can occur at any time. The mortality is 20% and immediate medical treatment is required:

- Bromocriptine (a D_1/D_2 agonist) is used to reverse dopamine blockade.
- Dantrolene (a skeletal muscle relaxant) is used for muscular rigidity.
- Dehydration and hyperthermia are managed with supportive treatment.

Renal failure from rhabdomyolysis is the major complication and cause of mortality. NMS can recur on reintroducing neuroleptics. It is therefore recommended to wait at least 2 months before reintroduction and to use a drug of a different class at the lowest recommended dose.

Anticholinergic adverse effects Neuroleptics typically have anticholinergic adverse effects, which include a dry mouth (hypersalivation with clozapine), difficulty urinating or retention, constipation, and blurred vision. Profound muscarinic blockade may produce a toxic confusional state.

Sedative adverse effects of neuroleptics may involve the antagonism of histamine-1 (H_1) receptors by these drugs.

Adverse effects due to α adrenoceptor blockade Many neuroleptics have the capacity to block α adrenoceptors, and this may contribute to postural hypotension.

Adverse effects that may be due to immune reactions include urticaria, dermatitis, rashes, dermal photosensitivity, and a gray/blue/purple skin tinge, which may be autoimmune responses. These are more commonly seen with the phenothiazines, as are conjunctival, corneolenticular, and retinal pigmentation, which are sometimes reported. Cholestatic jaundice due to a hypersensitivity reaction is a rare adverse effect of chlorpromazine. Weight gain is common.

Adverse effects related to individual drugs include neutropenia with clozapine and sudden death secondary to a cardiac arrhythmia with pimozide. It has therefore been recommended that all patients have an ECG before starting pimozide and that it should not be used in patients with a known arrhythmia or a prolonged QT interval.

Atypical antipsychotics

Clozapine has been used since the 1960s for treatment of schizophrenia, but its use has become restricted (see below) since reports of several associated deaths from neutropenia. Clozapine has a low affinity for the D_2 receptor and a higher affinity for the D_1 and D_4 receptors. The low incidence of extrapyramidal adverse effects associated with its use is thought to be due to its low activity at the D_2 receptor. Clozapine also has antagonistic activity at the 5-HT_2 receptor and this may underlie its clinical efficacy in improving positive (and possibly negative) symptoms.

The use of clozapine is restricted because it can cause a fatal neutropenia

In the UK and US clozapine can be used only if a patient:

- Is unresponsive to two other neuroleptics.
- Has tardive dyskinesia or severe extrapyramidal symptoms.

Careful monitoring, especially of the formed elements in blood, is mandatory. Each patient has to be registered and the drug can be dispensed only after the white cell count has been found to be normal. A white cell count is then performed every week for 18 weeks, and then every 2 weeks for the treatment period. Clozapine is contraindicated in patients with a history of neutropenia. The risk of neutropenia is 1–2% and it is usually reversible.

Other adverse effects of clozapine include hypersalivation, sedation, weight gain, tachycardia, and hypotension.

Olanzepine* is a drug similar to clozapine, but does not cause neutropenia.

Risperidone has a high affinity for 5-HT_2 receptors and a lower affinity for D_2 receptors. It appears to be as effective as haloperidol.

Adverse effects of risperidone include the extrapyramidal effects of tremor, rigidity, and restlessness, but these occur less frequently than with 'classic' antipsychotics. Zaprasidone is similar to risperidone, but is not yet in clinical use.

Sertindole is a newly available atypical antipsychotic currently in clinical trials. It has effects at 5-HT and dopamine receptors similar to those of risperidone, but is also a potent antagonist at noradrenergic receptors.

AFFECTIVE DISORDERS

The primary affective disorders are major depressive disorder and bipolar affective disorder.

Major depressive disorder

Major depressive disorder has a lifetime prevalence of approximately 9–15% and perhaps as high as 20% in women. The mean age of onset is 35–40 years, although onset can be at any age. There are no specific correlations with socioeconomic status.

The etiology of major depressive disorder is not clear

Life events (e.g. loss of job, moving house) and environmental stress are associated with an increased risk of developing major depressive disorder, but the precise causal relationship is unclear. The effect may be mediated by changes in the neurochemical environment of the CNS in reaction to stress. There is evidence that major depression also has a genetic component. Although the evidence for this is not as strong as for schizophrenia, the concordance rates are similar in twin studies. There appears to be a genetic factor of approximately 50% in the causation of depression.

Putative neurohormonal and neurochemical causes for depression have received considerable attention. The hypothalamic–pituitary–adrenal axis, which controls much of the body's hormonal equilibrium, has been particularly implicated. It has long been noted that depressed patients have a raised baseline cortisol concentration and that cortisol is not suppressed in response to dexamethasone in approximately 50% of depressed subjects. Fast feedback mechanisms have suggested that the cortisol receptors in the hippocampi of depressed subjects are abnormal. Nonspecific abnormalities have also been noted in thyroid hormone and growth hormone responses.

The most widely accepted neurochemical etiologic theory involves the biogenic amines, norepinephrine, 5-HT (serotonin), and dopamine

The original hypothesis of depression suggested that depression was due to a functional deficit of a transmitter amine (e.g. norepinephrine, dopamine, 5-HT), partly because tricyclic antidepressants (TCA) and monoamine oxidase inhibitors (MAOI) facilitated neurotransmission in aminergic neuron systems. It was also known that drugs that depleted amine stores (e.g. reserpine) could cause depression. Increased numbers of 5-HT receptors in the brains of people who have committed suicide have been attributed to a low 5-HT concentration. Low 5-HT concentration is a relatively consistent finding in studies of cerebrospinal fluid (CSF) 5-HT metabolites in depressed patients. Subsequent work in animal models has shown that all effective antidepressants decrease the sensitivity of β adrenoceptors and 5-HT_{2A} receptors. The delay in treatment response coincides with the time taken for these receptors to downregulate. It is therefore possible that it is the biogenic amine receptors that are related to depression and not the absolute levels of the transmitters themselves.

The dopaminergic system may also be involved in the etiology, since reducing the central dopamine concentration can lead to depression and drugs that increase the central dopamine concentration improve depression.

Other systems that may be involved in depression include the GABA system and some of the neuropeptide systems, particularly vasopressin and endogenous opiates. Second messenger systems may also have a crucial role in the efficacy of some treatments.

> **Evidence for the monoamine hypothesis of depression**
>
> - Drugs that deplete monoamines are depressant
> - Most antidepressants enhance monoaminergic transmission at some point in the synaptic signaling process
> - The concentration of monoamines and their metabolites is reduced in the cerebrospinal fluid of depressed patients
> - In various post-mortem studies, the most consistent finding is elevation in cortical 5-HT_2 binding

The cardinal symptoms of depression are usually divided into emotional/cognitive symptoms and biologic symptoms

In order to make a diagnosis of a major depressive disorder, the symptoms must have been present without a return to normality for at least 2 weeks. The emotional/cognitive symptoms include sadness and misery, decreased pleasure in life, hopelessness, guilt and worthlessness, slowed thinking and speech, and suicidal ideation. These symptoms vary throughout the day, but are characteristically worse in the morning. The biologic symptoms include low energy and fatigue, apathy and poor concentration, a change in appetite (usually decreased, with weight loss), a change in sleep pattern (usually with difficulty getting to sleep), early morning wakening (a change in sleep pattern when the sufferer wakes very early in the morning and cannot return to sleep), low libido, and diurnal variation of mood.

Major depressive disorders can be classified as psychotic depression if they are accompanied by delusions and hallucinations. These are usually consistent with the mood and therefore negative in content.

The differential diagnosis of major depression includes a variety of psychiatric, drug-induced, and medical conditions

The differential diagnosis of major depression includes the depressive phase of bipolar affective disorder, minor depressive disorder, adjustment reaction with depressed mood, anxiety disorders, dementia, and dysthymia. Abuse of various substances (e.g. alcohol, barbiturates, benzodiazepines, cocaine, amphetamines) can produce a depressive syndrome, while certain prescription medications (e.g. some antihypertensives especially reserpine, some antibiotics and analgesics, steroid medications, cimetidine, and some anticonvulsants) can worsen or cause depression. Many medical illnesses are associated with a depressive syndrome, including Parkinson's disease, cerebrovascular disease, Cushing's and Addison's diseases, parathyroid disorders, thyroid disorders, and porphyria.

65% of depressive episodes last 4–6 weeks, provided that the patient is given appropriate treatment

The remaining 35% of depressive episodes have a longer course despite approriate treatment. Untreated depressive illnesses tend to last 6–13 months. Most depressive illnesses relapse at some time, 65% within 5 years.

ANTIDEPRESSANTS

The mechanisms of action of drugs used to treat depression are listed in Fig. 7.27.

Tricyclic antidepressants and related cyclic drugs

TCAs are an effective therapy for depression, but their adverse effects can reduce patient compliance and acceptability.

All TCAs act by preventing 5-HT and norepinephrine uptake into the presynaptic terminal from the synaptic cleft. The potency of different tricyclic antidepressants for blocking uptake varies, and most have some potency for blocking dopamine uptake. All TCAs also have some affinity for H_1 and muscarinic receptors and for α_1 and α_2 adrenoceptors.

TCAs are relatively dangerous in overdose due to cardiotoxicity.

The choice of TCA usually depends on the degree of sedation required:

- Clomipramine is the TCA of choice for obsessive–compulsive disorder.
- Trimipramine is the TCA of choice for agitated states.

Metabolism of TCAs can produce pharmacologically active metabolites (e.g. amitriptyline is metabolized to nortriptyline, imipramine is metabolized to desipramine). Trazodone is a triazolopyridine derivative and is not strictly a tricyclic. It is less anticholinergic and cardiotoxic. Although it is quite sedative it is commonly used in the elderly and may be the antidepressant of choice in epilepsy.

Mechanism of action of drugs use to treat depression

Mechanism of action	Examples
Nonspecific blockers of monoamine uptake	Tricyclic antidepressants (amitriptyline, imipramine, nortriptyline, clomipramine)
Selective serotonin reuptake inhibitors (SSRIs)	Fluoxetine, paroxetine, sertraline, citalopram
Serotonin–norepinephrine reuptake inhibitors (SNRIs)	Venlafaxine
Noncompetitive, nonselective, irreversible blockers of MAO_A and MAO_B	Monoamine oxidase inhibitors (MAOIs) (phenelzine, tranylcypromine)
Reversible inhibitors of MAO_A (RIMAs)	Moclobemide*, brofaramine

Fig. 7.27 Mechanism of action of drugs use to treat depression.

Adverse effects of TCAs The adverse effects due to muscarinic blockade include dry mouth, constipation, urinary retention, and blurred vision. α_1 Adrenoceptor blockade may cause postural hypotension, while histamine blockade leads to sedation. Alterations in serotonergic function lead to sexual dysfunction, including loss of libido and anorgasmia. Generally, tolerance develops to the anticholinergic adverse effects within 2 weeks. These can be minimized by gradually increasing the dose.

Contraindications to TCAs include prostatism, narrow angle glaucoma, recent myocardial infarction, and heart block. Care is needed if the patient has:

- Heart disease (because TCAs increase the risk of conduction abnormalities).
- Epilepsy (because TCAs lower the seizure threshold).

Drug interactions of TCAs TCAs potentiate the effects of alcohol, other anticholinergic drugs, epinephrine, and norepinephrine. A fatal interaction can occur with lignocaine in local anesthetic preparations.

Selective serotonin (5-hydroxytryptamine) reuptake inhibitors (SSRIs)

SSRI mechanism of action After release from nerve terminals, serotonin activates various subtypes of serotonin receptors on nerve cells. Serotonin is inactivated by several mechanisms. The two primary mechanisms are metabolism by MAO to the major inactive metabolite 5-HIAA and reuptake of the transmitter into serotonergic nerve endings (Fig. 7.28). This latter important pathway is a very useful target for the development of antidepressant medications.

Reuptake of serotonin into nerve endings requires a specific transporter expressed on nerve endings. The serotonin transporter is a member of a gene family of neurotransmitter transporters. Transporters for serotonin, as well as for norepinephrine, dopamine, glycine and GABA, have been identified. The overall structure of these transporters involves proteins with 12 putative membrane-spanning domains with *N*-glycosylation sites that are likely to be important for transporter function. There is homology between these transporters and transporters for nutrients such as glucose. The expression of the serotonin transporter has been localized primarily to serotonergic nerves. The specificity with which this transporter is expressed in nerve cells and the selectivity with which it moves serotonin across cell membranes is of major importance in the function of serotonergic nerves. It should be emphasized that the serotonin transporter, as well as transporters for dopamine and norepinephrine, are quite distinct from the vesicular monoamine transporters that concentrate transmitters such as norepinephrine into synaptic granules. Those transporters are inhibited by drugs such as reserpine (see Chapter 3).

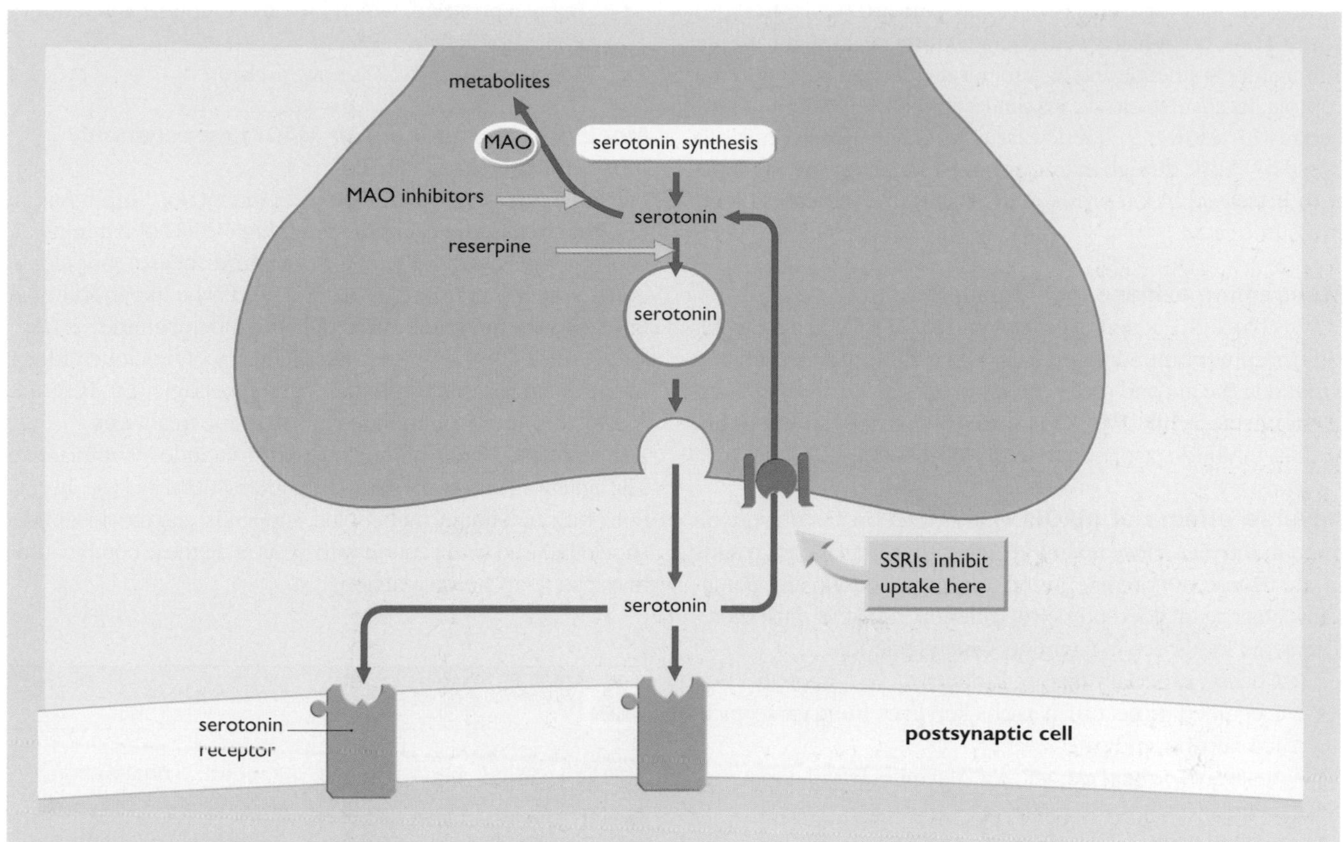

Fig. 7.28 Site of action of specific serotonin reuptake inhibitors (SSRIs) and monoamine oxidase (MAO) inhibitors. Reserpine leads to depletion of serotonin.

The serotonin transporters belong to a class of Na^+/Cl^--coupled transporters. Over-expression of this transporter, as well as very extensive experimentation in serotonergic neuronal preparations, has led to the discovery and development of a novel class of therapeutic agents with high specificity for potent inhibition of serotonin reuptake into nerves while having potentially only minimal effects on reuptake of other neurotransmitters or on other targets. These specific serotonin reuptake inhibitors (SSRIs) are efficacious in the treatment of depression. Some of these drugs also inhibit reuptake of norepinephrine. In some animal models SSRIs have been found to change expression of β adrenoceptors and serotonin receptor subtypes in the brain. The potential clinical significance of these differences between SSRIs in terms of specificity and on effects on receptor expression in the brain is not known.

SSRIs have efficacy similar to that of TCAs. In addition they have clinical advantages:

- They have no anticholinergic activity, thus increasing patient acceptability
- They are not toxic in overdose. This is a major reason for their use.
- They lack cardiotoxic adverse effects and are therefore the drugs of choice in patients also having heart disease.

SSRIs act by inhibiting the uptake of 5-HT from the synaptic cleft and have only a minor effect on noradrenergic uptake. Nefazodone is the newest SSRI and is also a potent 5-HT_{2A} receptor antagonist.

The most potent SSRI is citalopram*, followed in descending order by paroxetine, fluoxetine, sertraline, and fluvoxamine. The half-life of fluoxetine (active metabolite 7–9 days) means that it may take longer to reach steady-state concentrations but may be prescribed on alternate days. The half-lives of the other SSRIs vary from 15 to 24 hours.

Adverse effects of SSRIs include nausea, diarrhea, insomnia, anxiety, and agitation due to their effect on 5-HT receptors throughout the body. Sexual dysfunction may also occur. The adverse effect profile of nefazodone is similar to that of other SSRIs, but the associated incidence of sexual dysfunction may be lower.

Contraindications and interactions are few, but SSRIs should not be used with MAOIs as the combination is likely to produce a serotonergic syndrome, which could be fatal. Care should be taken when prescribing SSRIs concurrently with lithium for similar reasons.

Serotonin (5-hydroxytryptamine) and norepinephrine reuptake inhibitors (SNRIs)

The only drug currently in this new class of antidepressants is venlafaxine, a phenethylamine bicyclic derivative. Its half-life is approximately 5 hours and it has an active metabolite with a half-life of 10 hours.

The pharmacologic effects of venlafaxine are similar to those of the TCAs, but it has fewer adverse effects because it has little affinity for cholinergic and histaminergic receptors or α adrenoceptors. Its adverse effects are similar to those of SSRIs, but they occur with a lower frequency. Drug interactions are similar to those of SSRIs, though extra care must be taken with patients with increased blood pressure as venlafaxine increases blood pressure.

Monoamine oxidase inhibitors

MAOIs block the action of MAO-A and MAO-B, which metabolize norepinephrine, dopamine, and 5-HT. MAO-A is primarily located in the gut and preferentially breaks down 5-HT and norepinephrine, while MAO-B is primarily located in the brain. MAO-A inhibitors are used to treat depression.

Adverse effects of MAOIs Gut MAO-A breaks down tyramine in the diet. Once tyramine enters the circulation it results in the release of norepinephrine, causing a sudden and potentially fatal rise in blood pressure. Patients on MAOIs must therefore avoid foods rich in tyramine, which include:

- Cheese, especially mature varieties.
- Degraded protein such as chicken liver, hung game, pickled herring, and pâté.
- Yeast and protein extract (e.g. Marmite, Bovril, Oxo).
- Beer.
- Chianti wine.
- Broad bean pods.
- Green banana skins.

Drug preparations containing amines to be avoided include:

- Opiates (e.g. meperidine).
- Sympathomimetics, which are often included in cough and cold remedies, nose drops, and laxatives bought over the counter.
- SSRIs.
- Levodopa.
- Some antihistamines.

These restrictions remain for at least 2 weeks after the MAOI is discontinued since MAO blockade is irreversible and requires new protein synthesis to restore function. After ingesting such food or drugs, patients on MAOIs usually experience flushing and a pounding headache, and this may progress to a fatal hypertensive crisis. This so-called 'cheese reaction' is the most important adverse effect of MAOIs.

Other rare adverse effects of MAOIs include hepatotoxicity (especially with phenelzine) and a theoretic risk of precipitating psychosis by increasing the availability of dopamine.

Because of the dietary and drug restrictions, MAOIs are largely reserved for depression resistant to other antidepressants and treatment

Phenelzine has traditionally had a role in treating atypical non-biologic depression with pronounced anxiety and hypochondriac symptoms. It has also been effectively used in the treatment of phobias and panic disorder.

The three irreversible MAOIs currently available are:

- Phenelzine, which is the most commonly used.
- Tranylcypromine, which has amine uptake and amphetamine-like activity.
- Isocarboxazid, which is now rarely used.

Moclobemide is a newer MAOI that reversibly inhibits MAO-A*

Moclobemide* carries the risk of an interaction with tyramine resulting in raised blood pressure if high levels of tyramine are consumed (e.g. more than 50 g of mature cheese), but in general no dietary restrictions are required. The likelihood of an interaction with tyramine is reduced if moclobemide* is taken after a meal. Although the clinical efficacy of moclobemide* is probably similar to that of other antidepressants (i.e. TCAs and SSRIs), it is not recommended as a first-line treatment.

The adverse effects of moclobemide* include insomnia, nausea, agitation, and confusion. Drug interactions include interactions with cimetidine, meperidine, and SSRIs, and moclobemide* should be used with caution with TCAs as all these combinations may lead to a 'cheese reaction.'

Adverse effects of antidepressants

- Tricyclics: blurred vision, dry mouth, constipation, urinary retention, mania, hypotension, arrhythmias
- Serotonin and norepinephrine reuptake inhibitors (SNRIs): sedation, mania
- Selective serotonin reuptake inhibitors (SSRIs): nausea, vomiting, dry mouth, agitation
- Monoamine oxidase inhibitors (MAOIs): as for tricyclics plus sympathetic crisis with dietary tyramine
- Reversible inhibitors of monoamine oxidase (RIMAs): mild agitation

Depression is usually treated with a TCA, provided that there are no medical contraindications and there is no or little risk of suicide

The choice of antidepressant depends on:

- The clinical characteristics of the patient's illness.
- The drug's adverse effect profile.
- The danger of overdose.
- Previous treatments.

Generally, if there are no medical contraindications (e.g. heart disorders) and there is no or little risk of suicide, a TCA can be used. The TCA chosen will depend on whether sedation is required. If there are medical contraindications, or suicide is a risk, or the patient has previously not tolerated the anticholinergic adverse effects of TCAs, then SSRIs are generally used.

Bipolar affective disorder

Bipolar affective disorder (BPAD) is characterized by swings in mood from mania (or hypomania) to depression. There is a high concordance rate of BPAD ranging from 33 to 90% in monozygotic twins, and family studies indicate an 18-fold increased risk for BPAD and a tenfold increased risk for major depression in the first-degree relatives of affected probands. The neurochemical basis for BPAD is unclear.

BPAD is characterized by episodes of depression and mania with periods of normality in between

The cycle of depressive and manic episodes in BPAD may take months or years, but may occur over days or weeks. There is no typical sequence of episodes.

Mania and hypomania are distinguished according to their severity and duration:

- A manic episode usually lasts longer than a week, significantly impairs social and occupational functioning, and may be accompanied by psychotic phenomena such as delusions and hallucinations.
- Hypomania is, by definition, not accompanied by psychotic features.

For ease of explanation, both mania and hypomania are here considered synonymous with the classification manic episode. The signs of a manic episode include an elevated mood, increased motor activity, accelerated thoughts and speech, irritability, decreased sleep, increased or decreased appetite, distractability, grandiose ideas, and delusions and hallucinations, usually of a grandiose nature. Features normally considered to be typical of schizophrenia occur in approximately 10% of patients. Patients with the severest form of manic episode may exhaust themselves, or carry out dangerous plans based on their grandiose ideas.

The depressive episodes in BPAD are clinically identical to depression in the absence of previous manic episodes. The patient may experience several episodes of depression in sequence, or several episodes of mania.

BPAD is treated with a combination of mood stabilizers, antipsychotics, and antidepressants.

MOOD STABILIZERS

Lithium

Lithium is the most widely used mood stabilizer:

- It is used in the prevention of relapse in manic depressive (bipolar) and recurrent unipolar (i.e. no mania) depressive disorders.
- It is an effective treatment in acute mania.
- It can be used in resistant depression to augment antidepressant activity.

Lithium inhibits the scavenging pathway for recapturing inositol for the resynthesis of polyphosphoinositides. Since the entry of inositol into the brain is relatively poor, this action of lithium may diminish the concentrations of lipids important in signal transduction in the brain (see Chapter 3).

Renal and thyroid function must be checked before starting lithium

Owing to adverse effects and contraindications (see below), before starting therapy, renal (urea, creatinine, electrolytes) and thyroid function must be checked. Once treatment is started, plasma lithium concentration should be monitored every 5 days after an increase in dose until the concentration is between 0.6 and 1 mEq/liter (0.6–1.0 mmol/liter). During maintenance, lithium concentration should be measured , with renal function, every 2–3 months. Thyroid function should be measured every 6 months.

Adverse effects and toxicity of lithium In the early stages of lithium therapy patients commonly complain of thirst, nausea, loose stools, fine tremor, and polyuria. These often disappear with continued therapy. Other adverse effects include weight gain, edema, and acne. A long-term adverse effect can be diabetes insipidus leading to polydipsia, which occurs because lithium inhibits vasopressin action in the kidney, leading to obligate water loss, goiter and, less commonly, frank hypothyroidism due to impaired release of thyroid hormone from the thyroid gland.

The first signs of lithium toxicity, which occur at a plasma lithium concentration of 1.5–2 mEq/liter (1.5–2.0 mmol/liter), are anorexia, vomiting, diarrhea, coarse tremor, ataxia, dysarthria, confusion, and sleepiness. Later signs, when the plasma lithium concentration is higher than 2 mEq/liter (2.0 mmol/liter), are impaired consciousness, nystagmus, muscle twitching, hyperreflexia, and convulsions. Coma and death occur at higher concentrations. At the first signs of toxicity the plasma lithium concentration should be measured urgently. If high, the lithium should be stopped and efforts made to increase lithium elimination, possibly involving hemodialysis.

Interactions between lithium and other drugs often lead to a rise in plasma lithium concentration. Such interacting drugs include:

- Antipsychotics (especially haloperidol), which increase neurotoxicity.
- Nonsteroidal anti-inflammatory drugs (NSAIDs) except aspirin, which increase plasma lithium concentration by decreasing excretion.
- Diuretics (especially thiazides), which increase plasma lithium concentration by decreasing excretion.
- Cardioactive drugs (digoxin, angiotensin-converting enzyme inhibitors), which increase the risk of neurotoxicity possibly secondary to membrane effects.

Carbamazepine

Carbamazepine is as effective as lithium in preventing relapses in BPAD and in the treatment of acute mania, and is particularly indicated for rapid cycling bipolar illness.

Carbamazepine is a GABA agonist and this may be the basis of its antimanic properties. It also stabilizes neuronal Na^+ channels and has an effect on Ca^{2+} channels that is currently unclear.

At the start of therapy, carbamazepine induces its own catabolic enzymes in the liver, plasma concentrations therefore should be monitored to establish a maintenance dose.

Adverse effects of carbamazepine include drowsiness, diplopia, nausea, ataxia, rashes, and headache. Hematologic disturbances include agranulocytosis and leucopenia, patients therefore should be warned about fever and infections as these may indicate agranulocytosis and they should be investigated. It is advised that the plasma carbamazepine concentration is measured and a full blood count is obtained every 2 weeks for the first 2 months.

Acute carbamazepine toxicity is associated with diplopia, ataxia, hyperreflexia, clonus, tremor, and sedation.

Interactions between carbamazepine and other drugs

Carbamazepine interacts with:

- Lithium, resulting in CNS adverse effects of carbamazepine and carbamazepine toxicity despite 'normal' plasma carbamazepine concentrations.
- Antipsychotics, resulting in drowsiness and ataxia.
- TCAs, decreasing the plasma TCA concentration as a result of enzyme induction.
- MAOIs, precipitating the cheese reaction.

Carbamazepine is an enzyme inducer (see Chapter 5) and therefore affects the plasma concentrations of many drugs metabolized in the liver.

Sodium valproate

Sodium valproate is an effective third-line mood stabilizer and is worth considering as an adjunct in refractory cases. It has effects on the turnover of GABA, although its precise mechanism of action is unclear. It also appears to enhance GABA-ergic transmission by a poorly understood mechanism.

Adverse effects of sodium valproate include gastrointestinal effects (nausea, vomiting, diarrhea), CNS effects (sedation, ataxia, dysarthria, tremor), and hepatic effects (persistent elevation of liver transaminases). A rare adverse effect is hepatotoxicity leading to death.

Anxiety disorders

The sensation of anxiety is common in all humans. The psychologic symptoms include a diffuse, unpleasant, and vague feeling of apprehension, and this is often accompanied by physical symptoms of autonomic arousal such as headache, perspiration, palpitations, 'upset stomach' ('butterflies'), and tightness in the chest, and in some people restlessness. Anxiety warns of impending danger and enables the individual to take measures to deal with a threat that is usually unknown, internal, vague, or conflictual (stimulatory opposite emotions, e.g. excitement, guilt) in origin. This is in contrast to fear, which is a response to a threat that is known, external, definite, or nonconflictual in origin.

Anxiety is a common symptom in a variety of distinct mental illnesses and is a predominant symptom in phobias, panic disorder, and obsessive–compulsive disorder. Other anxiety disorders include generalized anxiety disorder, post-traumatic stress disorder, and hysterical conversion reactions.

The two neurotransmitters most commonly implicated in the etiology of all anxiety disorders are GABA and 5-HT

Norepinephrine also has a role, particularly in panic disorder. There have been no conclusive studies to confirm the role of these neurotransmitters, but functional imaging of benzodiazepine receptors in the brain has shown differences in receptor binding in the temporal lobes between patients with panic disorder and normal subjects. Benzodiazepines act indirectly on GABA receptors.

Anxiety disorders are treated with anxiolytics and antidepressants.

ANXIOLYTICS

Benzodiazepines

Benzodiazepines (Fig. 7.29) act by potentiating the action of GABA, the primary inhibitory neurotransmitter in the CNS. The

Mechanism of action of drugs use to treat anxiety

Drug	Mechanism of action	Use
Anxiolytics		
Benzodiazepines (diazepam, alprazolam)	Act on GABA receptors	Short-term treatment of anxiety
Buspirone	Acts on 5-HT_{1A} receptor	? Effective in generalized anxiety disorder
Autonomic suppression		
Propranolol	Acts by inhibiting β adrenoceptors	Useful for some social/performance anxiety disorders
Antidepressants		
Imipramine	Tricyclic antidepressant	Most studied biologic treatment in panic disorder
Phenelzine, meclobemide*	MAOIs	Useful for social phobia and panic, may also be useful for PTSD
Fluoxetine, sertraline	SSRIs	Proven efficacy in OCD and panic disorder

Fig. 7.29 Mechanism of action of drugs used to treat anxiety. (GABA, γ-aminobutyric acid; 5-HT_{1A}, 5-hydroxytryptamine-1A; MAOIs, monoamine oxidase inhibitors; OCD, obsessive compulsive disorder; PTSD, post-traumatic stress disorder; SSRIs, selective serotonin reuptake inhibitors)

benzodiazepine receptor lies within the $GABA_A$ receptor complex, and benzodiazepines enhance inhibitory activity (Fig. 7.30). Benzodiazepines reduce anxiety, and the duration of their action will be determined to some extent by their half-lives.

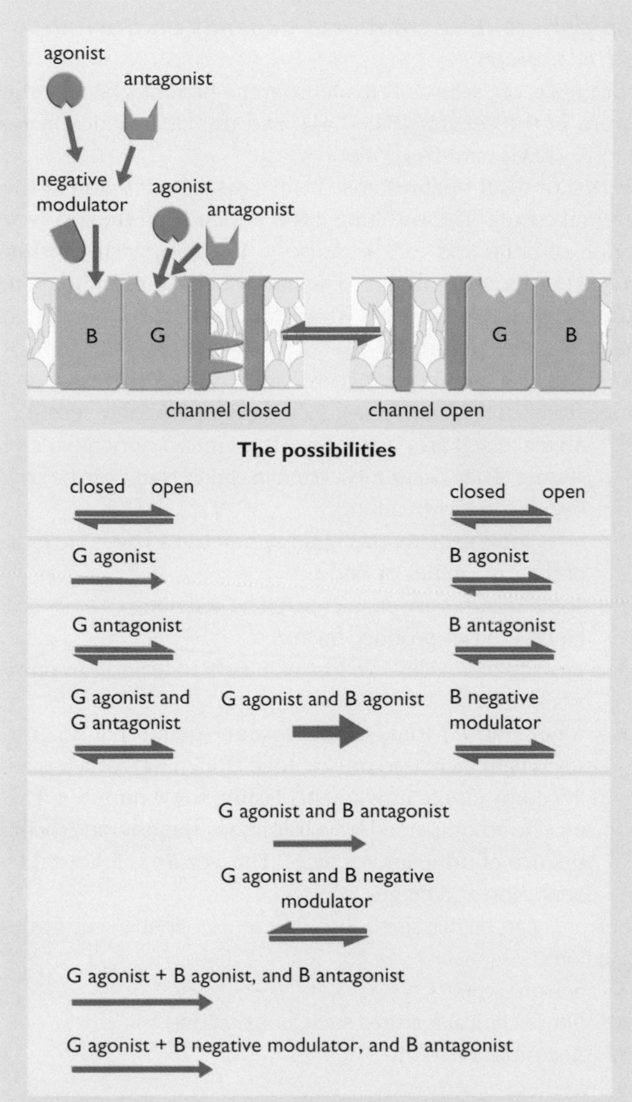

Fig. 7.30 Benzodiazepine agonist and antagonist activity and modulation of γ-aminobutyric acid (GABA) agonist and antagonist activity. A Cl^- channel, part of a receptor-operated channel (ROC), exists in an open and a closed state. This ROC has two distinct ligand-recognition sites, a GABA site (G) and a benzodiazepine site (B). Equilibrium between closed and open states of the Cl^- channel is altered by GABA agonism. The channel, closed at rest, is opened by GABA agonism. Neither benzodiazepine agonism or antagonism on their own affect channel opening. However, GABA agonist-induced channel opening is facilitated by concomitant benzodiazepine agonism. This potentiation is blocked by benzodiazepine antagonism. In addition, benzodiazepine negative modulators reduce the ability of GABA to open the channel, and benzodiazepine antagonists can block the effect of negative modulators. The G and B ligand-recognition sites presumably interact allosterically, with the B site functioning as a modulator of the G site.

Half-lives of benzodiazepines

Diazepam:	14–70 hours (one metabolite is active for up to 200 hours)
Nitrazepam:	15–30 hours
Lorazepam:	8–24 hours
Temazepam:	3–25 hours
Oxazepam:	3–25 hours

Adverse effects of benzodiazepines include dependence and abuse. Generally, tolerance develops within 14 days and their efficacy then declines. Long-term use can result in a withdrawal syndrome characterized by insomnia, anxiety, tremor, loss of appetite, tinnitus, and perceptual disturbances. Benzodiazepine withdrawal is performed by switching to an equivalent dose of a benzodiazepine with a long half-life (e.g. diazepam) and reducing the dose gradually by approximately one-eighth every 2 weeks. This process may take many weeks to 1 year, depending on the severity of tolerance.

The most common adverse effects of benzodiazepines are drowsiness, ataxia, and reduced psychomotor performance, so care should be taken when driving or operating machinery. These effects can become more marked after a few weeks because the long half-life of some benzodiazepines leads to drug accumulation. Disinhibition with aggression may occur, but is rare.

Benzodiazepines are indicated only for short-term relief of severe, disabling, or unacceptably distressing anxiety

Such severe anxiety may occur alone or in association with insomnia or a short-term psychosomatic, organic, or psychotic illness, and diazepam (5–20 mg/day) is the most commonly prescribed anxiolytic. The use of benzodiazepines to treat short-term 'mild' anxiety is inappropriate as dependence and withdrawal are more problematic with benzodiazepines prescribed as anxiolytics than with those prescribed as hypnotics. Alprazolam is effective for panic attacks.

Azapirones

Buspirone is the first of a new class of agents called azapirones. It is thought to reduce 5-HT neurotransmission by acting as a partial agonist at $5\text{-}HT_{1A}$ receptors. $5\text{-}HT_{1A}$ receptors are inhibitory presynaptic receptors and their activation results in decreased firing of 5-HT neurons. Buspirone has no activity at the GABA–benzodiazepine receptor complex and cannot therefore be used to ameliorate the benzodiazepine withdrawal syndrome. It is not an hypnotic.

Adverse effects of buspirone include nervousness, dizziness, headache, and lightheadedness.

Buspirone is indicated for the short-term management of generalized anxiety disorder

The anxiolytic effect of buspirone gradually evolves over 1–3 weeks. In contrast to benzodiazepines, buspirone does not cause significant sedation or cognitive impairment and carries only a minimal risk of dependence and withdrawal. It does not potentiate the sedative effects of alcohol.

β Adrenoceptor antagonists

β Adrenoceptor antagonists such as propanolol reduce heart rate and other manifestations produced by excess catecholamine. Propranolol:

- May ease the somatic manifestations of an anxiety characterized by marked sympathetic autonomic arousal (e.g. palpitations and tremor).
- Is useful for social phobia and may act by reducing the autonomic arousal, thereby preventing amplification of the sufferer's anxiety.
- Reduces performance anxiety in musicians for whom fine motor control may be critical.

Antidepressants

Certain antidepressants have a specific application in particular anxiety disorders:

- Imipramine has been most studied for use in panic disorder and produces a beneficial effect in 60–70% of patients. Generally, the dose used is higher than that for depression and the therapy must be continued for longer before a response is seen.
- MAOIs have uses in several anxiety disorders including panic disorder, agoraphobia, social phobia, and post-traumatic stress disorder, and some studies have indicated benefits over and above regular TCAs.
- SSRIs, especially fluoxetine and the TCA clomipramine, appear to be most effective in the treatment of obsessive–compulsive disorder. The doses must, however, be higher than those used for depression and the therapeutic effect may take 1–3 months to become fully apparent.

Often patients present with a mixed picture of anxiety and depression (agitated depression). Antidepressants are then indicated, and generally a more sedative one is used (see p. 110).

EATING DISORDERS

The two well-defined eating disorders are anorexia nervosa and bulimia nervosa. There is considerable overlap between the two disorders with patients moving from one to the other. Treatment is almost purely with pyschotherapy, though these disorders are often accompanied by depression, which may need pharmacologic treatment (see p. 110).

EPILEPSY

Epilepsy is characterized by recurrent unprovoked seizures. A seizure is a particular behavior produced by an altered neurologic function resulting from a paroxysmal discharge of neurons in the cerebral cortex. Seizures are sometimes called fits. Approximately 10% of the US population experiences one or more seizures during their lifetime, and epilepsy will develop in approximately 1.5% of the population. Behavior during a seizure varies from immobility and slight twitching of a digit through to violent tonic–clonic movements or even purposeful activity, depending on the type of epilepsy.

The cellular mechanisms of epilepsy are not known, but may involve altered GABA metabolism.

Appropriate drug treatment depends on the nature of the epilepsy

A diagnosis of epilepsy is made from the patient's history, the nature of the seizure (Fig. 7.31), and the electroencephalographic (EEG) pattern.

Partial or focal seizures arise from a restricted region of the cerebral cortex. The resulting effect depends on the involved region of brain and can be sensory (including visual disturbances) or motor in nature. The motor behavior can be quite purposeful. Consciousness is variable and usually there is no memory of the seizure.

Generalized seizures are convulsive or nonconvulsive and range from a blank stare to a generalized tonic–clonic seizure:

- Absence seizures are the most common nonconvulsive seizure. They occur most often in children and can be confused with daydreaming.
- Myoclonic seizures are rapid symmetric arrhythmic jerks of the extremities or body.
- Tonic seizures are characterized by stiffening of body and limbs and can produce fractures.
- Atonic seizures involve loss of muscle tone and can cause a fall.
- A generalized tonic–clonic seizure (grand mal seizure) starts with increased muscle tone (stiffening), which is followed by clonic movements lasting a few minutes. This may be accompanied by vocalization, cyanosis, and incontinence of urine and/or feces. The seizure is followed by confusion and fatigue.

Seizures can be classified into different epileptic syndromes based on:

- Seizure type.
- Other clinical features such as age at onset.
- Anatomic location.
- Etiology (e.g. fever).

Status epilepticus describes a state of continuous seizures.

Drug treatment can control, but not cure, 60–90% of recurrences of seizures and treatment is therefore long term

The aim of pharmacologic treatment is to control seizures without producing adverse drug effects, but this is not always accomplished. Partial seizures are controlled in only approximately 45% of cases despite optimum medical treatment. The appropriate drug depends on the nature of the epilepsy (Fig. 7.32).

Treatment should always be initiated with a single drug and its use optimized before adding a second drug

Optimization of drug therapy usually involves increasing the dose of a single drug until toxicity appears. The incidence of

Classification of epileptic seizures
Partial (focal, local) seizures
Simple partial seizures (consciousness not impaired) (motor signs, somatosensory or special sensory signs, psychic symptoms)
Complex partial seizures (consciousness impaired) (simple partial onset followed by impaired consciousness, consciousness impaired at onset)
Partial seizures evolving to generalized seizures (tonic, clonic, or tonic–clonic)
Simple partial seizures evolving to generalized seizures
Complex partial seizures evolving to generalized seizures
Simple partial seizures evolving to complex partial seizures evolving to generalized seizures
Generalized seizures (convulsive or nonconvulsive)
Typical absence seizures (brief stare, eye flickering, no motion)
Atypical absence seizures (associated with movement)
Myoclonic seizures
Clonic seizures
Tonic seizures
Tonic–clonic seizures
Atonic seizures

Fig. 7.31 Classification of epileptic seizures. (From the Commission on Classification and Terminology of the International League Against Epilepsy.)

Drugs used for epilepsy

Seizure type	Primary drugs	Secondary drugs
Partial and/or generalized tonic–clonic seizures	Carbamazepine, phenytoin	Phenobarbital, primidone, valproate
Absence seizures	Ethosuximide, valproate	Clonazepam
Myoclonic seizures	Valproate	Primidone

Fig. 7.32 Drugs used for epilepsy.

adverse drug effects has been reported to be 22% in patients on monotherapy, 34% when two antiepileptic drugs are given, and 44% with three drugs. A single drug is therefore preferable.

The pharmacokinetic properties and adverse effects of any chosen antiepileptic drug must be known to obtain its maximum therapeutic benefit. Monitoring of blood phenytoin concentrations is useful, particularly because of its zero-order pharmacokinetics and a reasonable relationship between its blood concentration and therapeutic or toxic effects (see Chapter 5).

Adverse effects of antiepileptic drugs must be considered when starting treatment because of the long duration of their use. Clinical interactions (see Chapter 5) are common between other drugs and antiepileptic drugs and are particularly important because:

- Antiepileptic drugs are used long term.
- There are small differences between therapeutic and potentially toxic blood concentrations for several antiepileptic drugs.

ANTIEPILEPTIC DRUGS

Barbiturates (phenobarbital and primidone)

Phenobarbital was the first effective antiepileptic drug, and despite the availability of newer agents it can still be useful in reducing the recurrence of tonic–clonic seizures. It is also inexpensive. The antiepileptic dose is limited because phenobarbital produces sedation, but this tends to lessen with continued use. Sometimes phenobarbital produces excitement instead of sedation in children. Primidone is a structural analog of phenobarbital and is converted to phenobarbital in the body.

The cellular mechanism of action of the barbiturates probably involves synaptic inhibition by enhancing the effects of GABA. Phenobarbital and other barbiturates seem to act at $GABA_A$ receptors.

Not all barbiturates can be used as antiepileptic drugs because many produce too much sedation at antiepileptic doses. It is not known why phenobarbital is less sedative.

Phenobarbital is a good inducer of cytochrome P-450 so can be involved in drug interactions (see Chapter 5). Its plasma half-life is 100 hours.

Phenytoin

Phenytoin (diphenylhydantoin) is useful in the treatment of tonic–clonic seizures. At a cellular level it slows the rate of recovery of Na^+ channels from inactivation, thereby reducing neuron excitability, and this may be responsible for its antiepileptic activity. The use of phenytoin is complicated by its characteristic toxicities and zero-order pharmacokinetics, and the necessity for long-term administration. The zero-order pharmacokinetics (see Chapter 5) imply that when blood concentrations of phenytoin approach those that will saturate the systems that metabolize phenytoin, a small increase in dose can produce a disproportionately large increase in its plasma concentration with resulting toxicity. This can be partly prevented by measuring plasma phenytoin concentrations.

Adverse effects of phenytoin may be dose or nondose related:

- The dose-related adverse effects of phenytoin affect the cerebellovestibular system leading to blurred vision, ataxia, hyperactivity, and confusion. Gastrointestinal disturbances also occur.
- The nondose-related adverse effects include skin rashes, gingival hyperplasia, lymphadenomas, and hirsutism.

Phenytoin is also believed to be teratogenic.

Drug interactions Phenytoin is a good enzyme inducer so is liable to produce drug interactions with drugs such as isoniazid, warfarin, chloramphenicol, erythromycin, and cimetidine.

Carbamazepine

Carbamazepine is chemically related to TCAs. Its antiepileptic activity is similar to that of phenytoin, but it is also useful for pain such as that of trigeminal neuralgia and in the treatment of manic depressive illness. Like phenytoin it acts on Na^+ channels at a cellular level, and this may be involved in its antiepileptic activity. Serum concentrations of carbamazepine are not clearly related to its therapeutic effects.

Carbamazepine is a powerful inducer of enzymes, including its own metabolizing enzymes. Its plasma half-life is therefore shortened by chronic administration.

Adverse effects of carbamazepine include drowsiness, vertigo, and ataxia. It is probably as teratogenic as phenytoin.

Sodium valproate

Sodium valproate is useful in reducing the frequency of tonic–clonic and particularly absence seizures. Like phenytoin and carbamazepine it interacts with Na^+ channels. It also increases the GABA content of the brain when given long term. The blood concentrations of sodium valproate do not correlate well with its therapeutic effects.

Adverse effects of sodium valproate include gastrointestinal upset, and more importantly, hepatic failure. Hepatic toxicity appears to be more common when sodium valproate is used with another antiepileptic drug. Tests of liver function do not predict subsequent liver toxicity.

Ethosuximide

Ethosuximide is the agent of choice for absence seizures. It is believed to act by inhibiting low-threshold Ca^{2+} currents (T-currents) in the thalamus, which is currently thought to be the origin of absence seizures. Plasma ethosuximide concentrations do not correlate well with therapeutic effectiveness.

Adverse effects of ethosuximide include gastrointestinal upset, drowsiness, lethargy, euphoria, urticarial skin lesions, and most importantly, leukopenia, and rarely bone marrow depression.

Benzodiazepines

Clonazepam is useful for absence and myoclonic seizures while diazepam and lorazepam are effective in the management of status epilepticus. The benzodiazepines enhance GABA-induced increases in Cl^- conductance and this is probably involved in their antiepileptic activity.

Adverse effects of the benzodiazepines The common adverse effect of the benzodiazepines is sedation. Intravenous diazepam can depress respiration, so resuscitation equipment should be available when treating status epilepticus. Repeated seizures can damage the brain and can be life threatening so status epilepticus should be controlled.

New antiepileptic agents

The exact role of the new antiepileptic agents gabapentin and lamotrigine in the treatment of seizures remains to be defined.

Gabapentin is a highly lipid-soluble molecule and has been designed to mimic GABA in the CNS. It seems to be a useful add-on therapy for patients with partial seizures and is relatively free from adverse effects other than somnolence, dizziness, and fatigue.

Lamotrigine is intended for use in partial seizures and seems to act through Na^+ channels. Reported adverse effects are dizziness, ataxia, blurred vision, and gastrointestinal upset.

Lamotrigine is metabolized by glucuronidation in the liver and concomitant administration of phenytoin, carbamazepine, or phenobarbital decreases the serum half-life of lamotrigine from 24 to 15 hours, presumably by inducing increased hepatic glucuronidation of lamotrigine. In contrast, sodium valproate inhibits lamotrigine metabolism and increases the half-life of lamotrigine to 60 hours.

SLEEP DISORDERS

Normal sleep

Normal sleep is characterized by patterns of electrical activity that can be recorded on an EEG. On the basis of this record sleep is separated into five stages. Stages 1–4 are periods of nonrapid eye movement (NREM) sleep, while stage 5 is the period of rapid eye movement (REM) sleep (Fig. 7.33):

- Stage 1 makes up 5% of total sleep and is the lightest sleep.
- Stage 2 makes up 45% of sleep and is characterized on the EEG by 'sleep spindle' waveforms.
- Stages 3 and 4 are the deepest stages of sleep and make up 12% and 13% of total sleep, respectively. These stages are often classified together on the basis of the EEG as slow-wave sleep or δ wave sleep.
- Stage 5 (REM) sleep makes up 25% of sleep and the EEG record shows low-voltage random sawtoothed waves.

The time between the onset of sleep and the initiation of the first portion of REM sleep is termed REM latency and is usually 90 minutes. NREM is a generally restful state with a regular low blood pressure and heart and respiratory rate; any restless movements are made during these stages and dreaming is lucid and purposeful. Body muscle tone is drastically reduced during REM sleep and the subject is still. However, the blood pressure and heart and respiratory rate are all

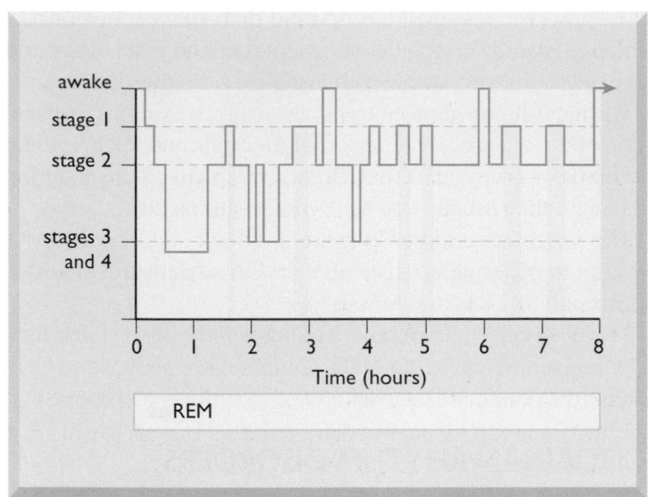

Fig. 7.33 A normal sleep cycle. This shows the normal stages of sleep. (REM, rapid eye movement)

raised, partial or full penile erections occur, and dreams are abstract and surreal.

The central control of sleep is complex and involves:

- Serotonergic neurons in the raphe nuclei.
- Noradrenergic neurones in the locus ceruleus.
- ACh-containing neurones within the pontine raphe nuclei, which have a central role in the production of REM sleep.

The sleep–wake pattern may be governed by melatonin secreted by the pineal gland, which is in turn controlled by the hypothalamus. It is hypothesized that the sleep 'on/off switch' is situated in the hypothalamus and is part of a neuronal circuit connecting the hypothalamus with the reticular activating system.

The normal length of sleep required by an adult is 6–9 hours per night. Deprivation of REM sleep causes irritability and lethargy and a subsequent rebound in REM sleep. Prolonged total sleep deprivation can lead to death.

A variety of sleep abnormalities have been noted in psychiatric illness:

- In depression there is a marked decrease in REM latency and an increase in REM sleep.
- Alzheimer's dementia leads to a decrease in REM and slow-wave sleep.

Various drugs alter sleep patterns:

- Benzodiazepines, and to a lesser extent antidepressants, reduce REM sleep.
- Drugs that increase dopamine release (e.g. amphetamine) increase wakefulness.

Insomnia

Insomnia is a common and nonspecific disorder and may be reported by 40–50% of people at any given time. Of these cases:

- 30–35% are due to psychiatric illness.
- 15–20% are psychophysiologic or primary.
- 10–15% are due to alcohol or drugs.
- 10–15% are due to periodic limb movement disorder.
- 5–10% are due to sleep apnoea.
- 5–10% are due to medical illness.

Among those seeking treatment, the female:male ratio is 2:1 and there appears to be a preponderance of cases in lower socioeconomic groups.

The prognosis, etiology, and treatment of insomnia depend upon the underlying cause

A history should be taken to define the problem (e.g. initial or middle insomnia or early awakening). Is it due to a physical cause (e.g. pain or a cough)? Is it due to environmental factors such as noise?

In many cases, education in 'sleep hygiene' (e.g. reducing caffeine intake, changing sleep habits, or pain relief) might be more appropriate than a sedative medication. Early morning wakening is one of the biologic features of depression, an antidepressant might therefore be appropriate. Generally, treatment should be for the underlying cause. Insomnia without an obvious underlying cause is known as primary or psychophysiologic. Severe psychophysiologic (primary) insomnia is treated with hypnotics.

HYPNOTICS

Benzodiazepines

Benzodiazepines act by potentiating GABA-ergic neurotransmission and therefore enhance inhibitory activity (see p. 118 for adverse effects). The benzodiazepine receptor lies within the $GABA_A$ receptor complex.

Benzodiazepines induce sleep, and their duration of action will be determined to some extent by their half-life.

Benzodiazepines should be used only as hypnotics for severe, disabling, or extremely distressing insomnia, and preferably for only 1 week

Benzodiazepines should never be used as hypnotics for more than 3 weeks and should not be used for chronic insomnia.

Other drugs for insomnia

Chloral hydrate is generally used only in the elderly. Zopiclone* and zolpidem are nonbenzodiazepine hypnotics, but bind to particular subtypes of the benzodiazepine receptor. They are rapidly acting, with a short half-life of approximately 2 hours and minimal hangover effects. Long-term use is not recommended and they should not be used for more than 4 weeks.

NARCOLEPTIC SYNDROME

The narcoleptic syndrome is a relatively rare disorder that occurs in 20–160/100,000 adults. It is characterized by excessive daytime sleepiness and cataplexy, which is characterized by a sudden loss of muscle tone in response to emotional stimuli such as laughter, pain, and fear. Cataplexy affects the jaw, neck, legs, or whole body, leading to collapse. Associated symptoms include sleep paralysis, which is an inability to move any muscles on awakening while apparently conscious. It occurs in 40% of narcoleptics and can last several minutes. Short-duration sleep paralysis lasting seconds can be a normal phenomenon, as can pre-sleep dreaming (sometimes called hypnogogic hallucinations), which occurs in 30% of people with narcolepsy.

The sleep attacks can occur at any time of the day and cannot be avoided. They usually start in the late teens, and almost invariably before 30 years of age. The attacks may progress in severity and frequency or reach a plateau. Spontaneous remission is rare.

The night-time sleep pattern is disrupted, with a markedly reduced REM latency and sleep-onset REM occurring within 10 minutes after the onset of sleep.

Narcolepsy is treated with CNS stimulants

The first management strategy in narcolepsy is to encourage the patient to have regular daytime naps and sometimes this can almost abolish the sleep attacks. However, most patients require medication.

CNS STIMULANTS USED TO TREAT NARCOLEPSY

Methylphenidate hydrochloride and amphetamine

Both methylphenidate hydrochloride and amphetamine are indirectly acting sympathomimetics. Their primary effect is to cause the release of catecholamines from presynaptic neurons. They also inhibit catecholamine reuptake. These actions lead to stimulation of many brain regions, including the ascending reticular activating system and the striatum.

Adverse effects of methylphenidate and amphetamine include anxiety, irritability, insomnia, dysphoria, and an increased blood pressure and heart rate. Long-term effects include a delusional disorder similar to schizophrenia. Overdose leads to pschosis, cardiovascular symptoms, and seizures.

Modafinil

Modafinil is a centrally acting stimulant currently undergoing clinical trials. It is an effective treatment of excessive daytime sleepiness. It may reduce attacks and improve performance in narcolepsy, and is thought to have a better adverse effect profile and less addictive potential than the sympathomimetics. Its mechanism of action is not clear, but it may act as an agonist at α_1 adrenoceptors.

Other drugs used in the treatment of narcolepsy

These include:

- The MAO_B inhibitor selegiline.
- Anticholinergic medications to treat cataplexy.
- SSRIs (e.g. fluoxetine) and SNRIs (e.g. venlafaxine) to improve cataplexy.

SLEEP APNEA

This disorder has been recently recognized and is characterized by disturbed sleep at night and excessive daytime sleepiness. Its prevalence is not yet known, but it appears to be relatively common, particularly in the obese and the elderly, and the apnea is lengthened and made more likely to occur by alcohol.

There is little pharmacologic treatment at this time.

PERIODIC LIMB MOVEMENT DISORDER

Like sleep apnea, periodic limb movement disorder is characterized by disturbed night-time sleep and daytime sleepiness. It is, however, less well understood than sleep apnea or narcolepsy. Possibly up to 30% of patients over 60 years of age and as many as 10% of people with insomnia have this disorder.

The night-time symptoms typically involve a stereotypic extension of the big toes with flexion of the ankle and knee, leading to partial awakening. If they occur more than 30 times during the night they usually lead to daytime somnolence.

The prognosis and etiology are unknown, but the disorder occurs in other sleep disorders and in parkinsonism and is worsened by TCAs and MAOIs.

The most effective treatments to date have been clobazam*, clonazepam, selegiline (a MAO_B inhibitor, see above) and levodopa (the dopamine precursor used in Parkinson's disease).

CIRCADIAN RHYTHM DISORDERS

These are an important group of sleep disorders that affect most people at some time or another. The sufferer has by definition a sleep–wake cycle that is out of step with his or her environment, resulting in impaired social or occupational functioning.

The most common reasons for this disorder include:

- Shift working, and particularly changing shifts to opposite sides of the day/night.
- Jetlag, in which the sufferer has travelled east or west across more than one time zone.
- Delayed sleep phase syndrome, which affects adolescents, particularly males. In this syndrome the sleep onset and awakening times steadily advance by 1–2 hours/day until the sufferer is out of synchrony with his or her environment.

Circadian rhythm disorders are usually self-limiting; however, reestablishment of a normal sleep–wake pattern with a hypnotic and bright light exposure may be helpful. Melatonin is a hormone secreted by the pineal gland and is involved in the sleep–wake cycle experimentally. It is available over the counter and may have some uses in reestablishing a normal sleep–wake cycle in delayed sleep phase syndrome and jet lag.

DEMENTIA

Dementia is defined as a global impairment of higher cortical functions, including memory, of the capacity to solve the problems of day-to-day living, of the performance of learned perceptual–motor skills (e.g. playing an instrument), of the correct use of social skills, and of control of emotional reactions, in the absence of gross clouding of consciousness. The condition is often irreversible and progressive. A shorter definition is

Common causes of dementia

- Alzheimer's disease
- Vascular (multi-infarct dementia)
- Pick's disease
- Dementia of parkinsonism
- Huntington's disease
- Creutzfeldt–Jacob disease

Treatment strategies for Alzheimer's dementia

Strategy	Drug
To increase the concentration of acetylcholine or to stimulate brain cholinergic receptors directly using a precursor	Lecithin
Release enhancers	Hydagine
Cholinesterase inhibition	Tacrine, velnacrine
(None of these are currently licensed in the US or UK)	

Fig. 7.34 Treatment strategies for Alzheimer's dementia.

'Dementia is an acquired global impairment of intellect, memory, and personality, but without an impairment of consciousness.'

Senile dementia of Alzheimer's type (Alzheimer's disease)

Alzheimer's disease (AD) is the most common cause of dementia, accounting for 50–60% of all cases. It is a senile and presenile (i.e. onset before 65 years of age) dementia and women are affected twice as often as men after the age of 70 years, but equally at younger ages. The average duration of the disease is 5–10 years and is increasing as general health improves.

Signs of AD are progressive global memory loss, parietal lobe function abnormalities of spatial orientation, deteriorating social skills, loss of drive, initiative, and intellect, depression, anxiety, aggression, emotional lability, unconcern, agitation, and disruption of the sleep–wake cycle.

Pharmacologic treatments for Alzheimer's dementia target the cholinergic system

Pharmacologic treatments for AD are still being developed and the three approaches (Fig. 7.34) are in use:

- An ACh precursor such as lecithin choline, but while this has been shown to increase CNS ACh concentrations in the rat, there has been no demonstrable improvement in cognition in patients with AD.
- Medications that enhance the release of ACh, such as Hydergine (co-dergocrine mesylate*), which increase ACh release from rat cortical slices. However, there have not yet been any trials of these drugs in humans.
- Cholinesterase inhibitors such as tacrine and velnacrine*, which are significantly better than placebo at increasing short-term memory, selective attention, language abilities, and praxis functions in AD. However, the clinical benefits are generally quite modest.

Adverse effects of tacrine and velnacrine* include abdominal cramps, nausea, polyuria, and diarrhea. Serious adverse effects have been noted with tacrine, including a persistent rise in liver transaminases in 15–30% of patients, as well as severe liver toxicity. This is thought to be due to a mild drug-induced dose-dependent hepatic inflammation.

Vascular dementia (multi-infarct dementia)

Multi-infarct dementia (MID) is traditionally thought to be the second most common dementia, and accounts for 15–30% of all cases of dementia. However, some experts believe that diffuse Lewy body disease is more common, but this remains to be confirmed. MID can coexist with other degenerative dementias and this accounts for 15% of all dementias.

MID is more common in men and in people with a high risk of cardiovascular problems. The onset is usually relatively acute and the progression is typically stepwise as each infarct occurs. The site and extent of the infarcts determines the cognitive deficits. Neurologic signs are generally more common than in AD.

The typical clinical features of MID include an abrupt onset, emotional incontinence, stepwise deterioration, a history of hypertension, a fluctuating course, a history of strokes, nocturnal confusion, atherosclerosis, relative preservation of personality, depression, focal neurologic symptoms and signs, somatic complaints, and patchy cognitive deficits.

Pharmacologic treatments for MID are based on attempting to reduce the risk of further cerebral infarction

Hypertension should be treated with appropriate antihypertensives (see Chapter 8), and any coexisting conditions that predispose to emboli formation (e.g. cardiac arrhythmias, cardiac valve disease) should be treated appropriately. Daily enteric-coated aspirin is indicated for any patient suspected of suffering from MID, because of its antithrombotic activity (see Chapter 9). If there are coexistent features of AD a therapeutic trial of cholinergic medication (see above) may be prescribed.

PARKINSON'S DISEASE

Parkinson's disease is a neurologic disorder characterized by impaired voluntary movements. Voluntary movements are controlled centrally by neuronal pathways that travel in the pyramidal tracts from the motor cortex and down the spinal cord to the lower motor neurons (α motor neurons). The lower motor neurons directly control the activity of voluntary muscle. Although these are the main neuronal pathways, neuronal inputs from other central sources also exert an influence on the pyramidal pathways. These subsidiary pathways provide the extrapyramidal influence, which smoothes voluntary movements. One major extrapyramidal source is the basal ganglia (caudate nucleus, putamen, and pallidum), and disease of these structures (e.g. Parkinson's disease) affects smooth voluntary movements.

Parkinson's disease is characterized by the major symptoms of:

- Bradykinesia (i.e. slow initiation of movements).
- Tremor at rest involving the hands in 'pill-rolling' movements.
- Muscle rigidity, reflected as resistance to passive limb movements.
- Abnormal posture (Fig. 7.35).

The signs include:

- A characteristic shuffling gait.
- A blank facial expression.
- Speech impairment.
- An inability to perform skilled tasks.

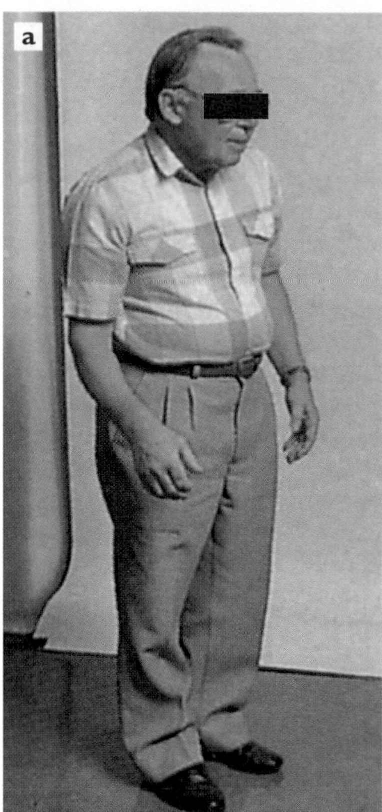

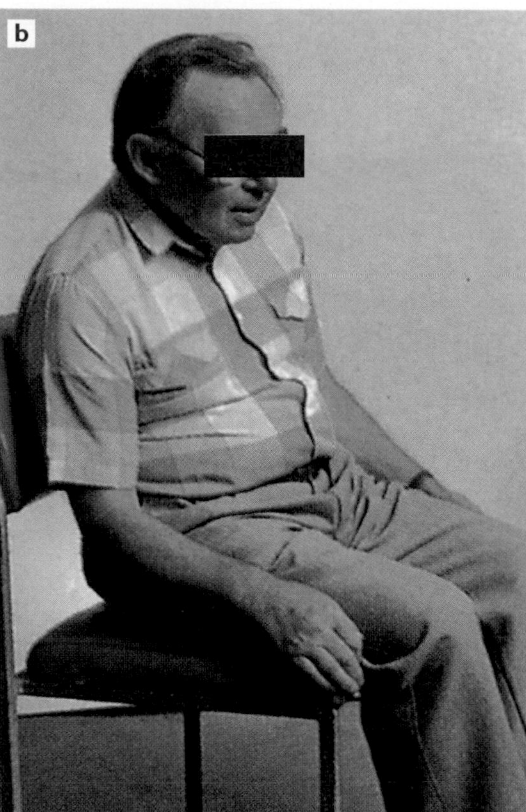

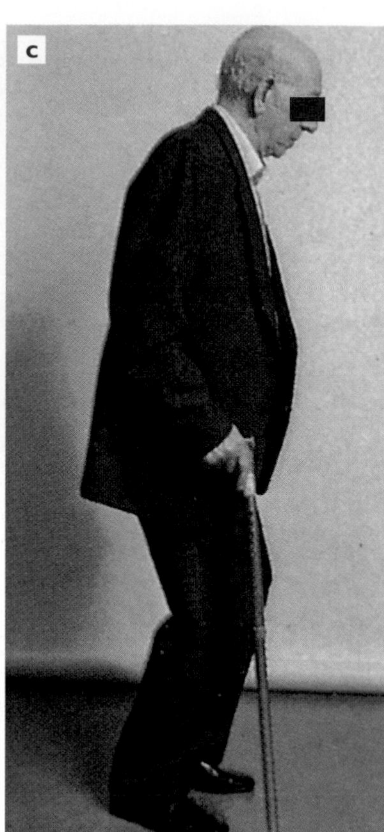

Fig. 7.35 Parkinson's disease. Posture and gait can give important clues to neurologic diagnosis. (Courtesy of Dr R. Capildeo.)

The disease occurs more frequently in the elderly and gets progressively worse with time unless it is treated.

Parkinsonism is usually idiopathic, but can be induced by neuroleptics

Although there is usually no identifiable underlying cause of Parkinson's disease, it has been suggested that it may be caused by an environmental toxin. For example, in primates, 1-methyl-4-phenyl-1,2,3,6-tetrahydropyridine (MPTP), which is a chemical contaminant produced in the synthesis of a heroin substitute, causes irreversible damage to the nigrostriatal dopaminergic pathway that can lead to the development of symptoms similar to idiopathic Parkinson's disease seen in humans. It appears that a metabolite (MPP+) produced from MPTP by MAO_B is actually responsible, and MAO_B inhibitors (e.g. selegiline) can prevent the damage produced by MPTP.

Parkinsonism can be induced by drugs that block striatal dopaminergic receptors (e.g. neuroleptics such as chlorpromazine). Indeed, when such drugs are used in the treatment of schizophrenia, a parkinsonian-like syndrome can occur as an adverse effect. Similarly, drugs such as reserpine, which deplete the nigrostriatal nerves of their dopamine content, also produce a parkinsonian-like syndrome.

At postmortem the brains of parkinsonian patients contain a substantially reduced concentration of dopamine (less than 10% of normal) in the corpus striatum and substantia nigra.

Striatal cholinergic hyperactivity is also associated with the development of Parkinson's disease. Usually, the activity of this neuronal pathway is restrained by inhibition by the dopaminergic pathway that projects from the substantia nigra (Fig. 7.36).

Treatment of Parkinson's disease involves enhancing striatal dopaminergic activity and inhibiting striatal cholinergic activity

The approach to treating Parkinson's disease is based on correcting the imbalance at the basal ganglia between the dopaminergic and cholinergic systems, and two major groups of drugs are used:

- Drugs that increase dopaminergic activity between the substantia nigra and corpus striatum.
- Drugs that inhibit striatal cholinergic activity.

Tissues rich in dopamine (e.g. chromaffin cells from the adrenal medulla) have been surgically implanted into the corpus striatum to improve dopaminergic activity, but the clinical effectiveness of such procedures is uncertain. Gene therapy to increase striatal dopamine content by transfecting the tyrosine hydroxylase gene to the corpus striatum to enhance the rate of synthesis of dopamine has also been considered.

DRUGS THAT INCREASE DOPAMINERGIC ACTIVITY

Levodopa (L-dopa)

Levodopa is used instead of dopamine, which does not cross the blood–brain barrier, to replenish the dopamine content of the striatum. It is a precursor from which dopamine is produced by decarboxylation (Fig. 7.37). Levodopa crosses the blood–brain barrier, undergoes decarboxylation, and increases the content of releasable dopamine, so opposing excessive striatal cholinergic activity and restoring balance between the two systems.

Levodopa is rapidly absorbed from the small intestine by an active transport system for aromatic amino acids. Levodopa absorption can be impaired by dietary aromatic amino acids, gastric juice hyperacidity, delayed gastric emptying, and the presence of food. Peak plasma concentrations are reached 1–2 hours after an oral dose. The plasma half-life is only 1–3 hours, owing to extensive metabolism in the wall of the intestine (Fig. 7.38). Levodopa is also metabolized in the blood and peripheral tissues and only about 1% of the administered dose is left to enter the brain and produce therapeutic effects. Dopamine is the major peripheral product of levodopa metabolism and is responsible for most of the peripheral adverse effects. Other metabolic products derived from levodopa include HVA and 3,4-dihydroxyphenylacetic acid (see Fig. 7.37). The extensive peripheral metabolism of levodopa means that large doses have to be given to produce therapeutic effects in the brain, but such doses produce many adverse effects (see below).

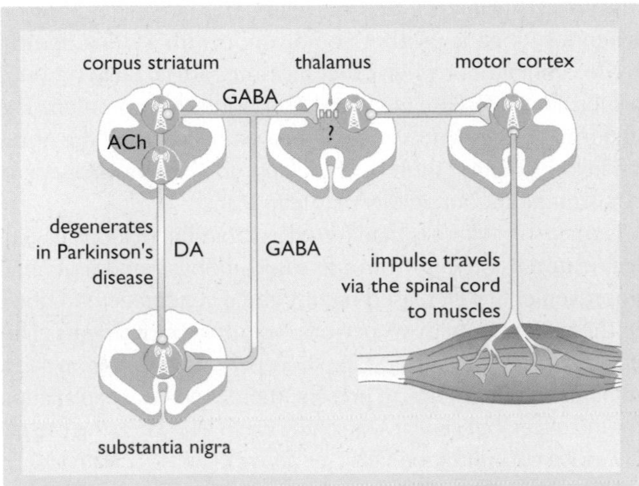

Fig. 7.36 The basal ganglia systems involved in Parkinson's disease. In Parkinson's disease, inhibitory dopaminergic activity of the extrapyramidal pathway from the substantia nigra to striatal cholinergic neurons is considerably depleted (20–40%), usually through neurodegeneration. This results in unrestrained cholinergic overactivity, which contributes to the pathologic features of Parkinson's disease. Normally there is two-way trafficking of nerve impulses between the corpus striatum and the substantia nigra to maintain smooth voluntary movements, but in Parkinson's disease voluntary movements are impaired. (ACh, cholinergic neuron; DA, dopaminergic neuron; GABA, γ-aminobutyric acid neuron)

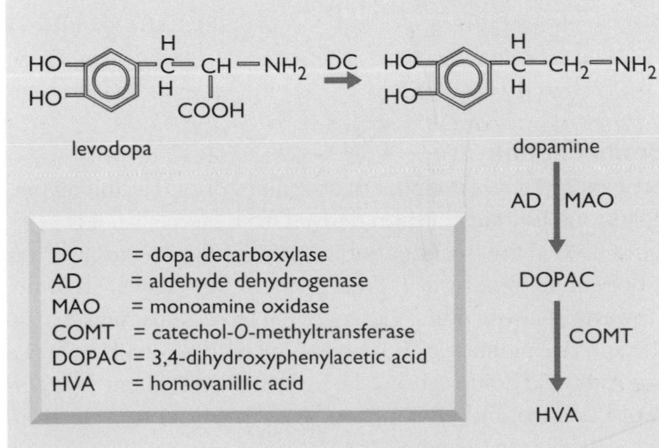

Fig. 7.37 Conversion of levadopa to dopamine and other metabolites.

The peripheral adverse effects of levodopa can be reduced by combining it with a peripheral dopa decarboxylase inhibitor or by co-administering domperidone or selegiline*

These can be reduced by combining levodopa with a peripheral dopa decarboxylase inhibitor such as carbidopa or benserazide*, which reduce the peripheral metabolism of levodopa so that a lower dose of levodopa can be used. Neither carbidopa nor benserazide* cross the blood–brain barrier; consequently, they interfere with levodopa metabolism only in the periphery. However, this drug combination not only maximizes the therapeutic effectiveness of levodopa but also increases the unwanted central effects of dopamine. Additionally, pyridoxine

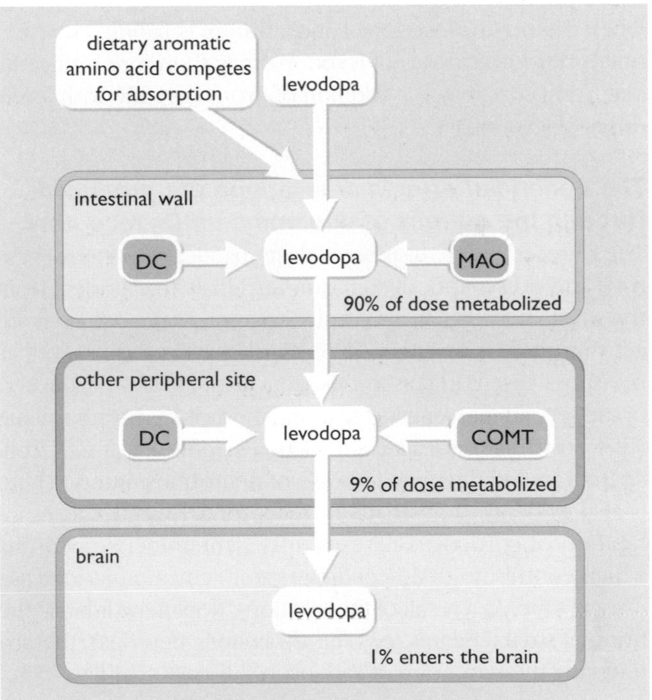

Fig. 7.38 Percentage of levodopa entering the brain after oral administration. There is extensive metabolism in the wall of the intestine by dopa decarboxylase (DC) and to a lesser extent by monoamine oxidase (MAO). Levodopa is also metabolized in the blood and peripheral tissues by catechol-O-methyltransferase (COMT) and DC. The extent of peripheral metabolism is of the order of 99%, leaving only about 1% of the administered dose of levodopa to enter the brain to produce therapeutic effects.

(vitamin B_6), which usually exacerbates peripheral metabolism of levodopa, does not interfere with the therapeutic effectiveness of the drug combination.

Some of the peripheral adverse effects of levodopa can also be decreased by co-administration of the dopaminergic D_2 antagonist domperidone*, which does not cross the blood–brain barrier. Alternatively, selegiline, an MAOI that selectively blocks MAO_B, can be used to inhibit dopamine metabolism selectively in the brain. MAO_B is the predominant MAO isoform responsible for metabolizing dopamine in the brain (MAO_A predominates in the periphery). Unlike the nonselective MAOIs, selegiline does not inhibit the peripheral metabolism of tyramine to produce the 'cheese reaction' (see p. 112).

Effects of levodopa during treatment When levodopa is first used, the parkinsonian symptoms of rigidity, bradykinesia, and motor functions, as well as facial expression, speech, and handwriting, usually improve. However, the effectiveness of levodopa decreases after several years of treatment, possibly owing to a progressive loss of dopaminergic neurons in the nigrostriatal pathway.

The beneficial effects of levodopa can fluctuate suddenly during effective therapy, leading to a worsening of symptoms (e.g. rigidity and bradykinesia). This phenomenon, termed the 'on–off effect' (see below), results in difficulty initiating movement, even while walking or attempting to rise from a chair. The mechanism of this phenomenon is not understood, but sometimes it occurs when the plasma levodopa concentration is falling. More frequent but lower doses of levodopa may therefore reduce its occurrence, as may the addition of bromocriptine with lower doses of levodopa.

The beneficial effects of levodopa are produced through the actions of dopamine on D_2 receptors

The D_2 receptors are distributed postsynaptically on striatal neurons and presynaptically on axon terminals that project from the substantia nigra to the corpus striatum. At the cellular level, activation of D_2 receptors inhibits adenylyl cyclase as well as phospholipase-C and as a consequence decreases production of the second messengers cAMP and inositol 1,4,5-triphosphate (IP_3). Such changes lead to a reduction in intracellular Ca^{2+} concentration and decreased release of neurotransmitters. There is also evidence that striatal D_2 receptor activation causes inhibition of corticostriatal excitatory gentaminergic neurons which contribute to descending motor activation to increase muscle tone. As a result of these actions, dopamine inhibits the firing of striatal nerves (e.g. the cholinergic neurons), thereby reducing the symptoms of Parkinson's disease (see Fig. 7.36).

Adverse effects of levodopa include:

- Nausea, vomiting, and anorexia.
- Hypotension and cardiac arrhythmias.
- Abnormal involuntary movements (dyskinesias).
- The 'on–off' effect.
- Behavioral changes.

Nausea, vomiting, and anorexia result from stimulation of dopaminergic receptors in the chemoreceptor trigger zone of the area postrema. They can be minimized by giving levodopa with either domperidone* or a dopa decarboxylase inhibitor (e.g. carbidopa).

The cardiac effects are usually tachycardia or extrasystoles, both of which are due to increased catecholamine stimulation following the excessive peripheral metabolism of levodopa. Although the explanation for the hypotension is uncertain, there is evidence that central interference with sympathetic activity may be involved. However, the hypotension diminishes with continued levodopa treatment in many patients.

Dyskinesias develop after long-term treatment with levodopa and involve mainly the face and limbs. They are more common when levodopa is used in combination with a dopa decarboxylase inhibitor or when other measures are taken to produce a substantial increase in central dopamine concentration. The abnormal movements can be improved by reducing the doses of levodopa and thereby reducing the central dopamine concentrations, but rigidity may reappear.

The 'on–off' effect is manifested as rapid fluctuations in clinical features, varying from increased mobility and a general improvement to increased rigidity and a general deterioration in the patient's ability to perform voluntary movements. This effect occurs suddenly and for short periods lasting from a few minutes to a few hours. At present, there is no clear explanation for the effect, but similar worsening can occur when the plasma levodopa concentration falls (see above).

Behavioral changes include insomnia, confusion, and other effects that are commonly seen in schizophrenia. Schizophrenia is attributed to increased dopaminergic activity in the mesolimbic area of the brain and can be controlled with a neuroleptic such as clozapine.

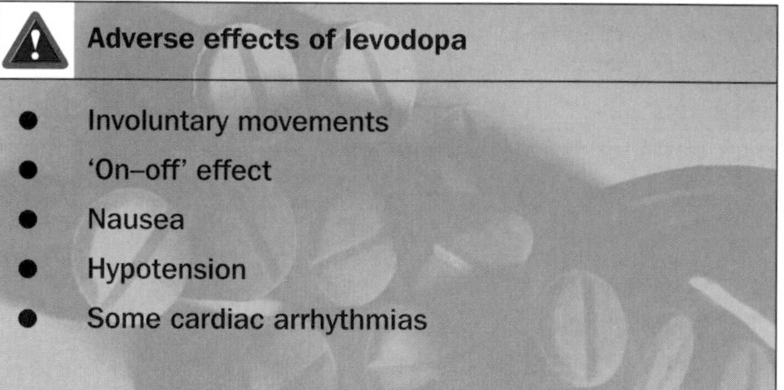
Adverse effects of levodopa

- Involuntary movements
- 'On–off' effect
- Nausea
- Hypotension
- Some cardiac arrhythmias

Bromocriptine

Bromocriptine is a member of a group of drugs (including pergolide and lisuride maleate) derived from ergot alkaloids.

It is used in the treatment of Parkinson's disease because it is a dopamine agonist at D_2 receptors in the corpus striatum. However, it also activates other central D_2 receptor sites (e.g. in the anterior pituitary gland) and D_1 receptors. Members of the ergot alkaloid group can also be used in the treatment of hyperprolactinemia and to suppress growth hormone release in acromegaly (see Chapter 12).

Bromocriptine is often added to levodopa in the treatment of Parkinson's disease when levodopa alone does not adequately control the symptoms or when patients experience severe 'on–off' effects. Usually, the combination consists of submaximal doses of levodopa and bromocriptine, but occasionally full doses of bromocriptine are given alone. Good therapeutic results are obtained with both regimens and the incidence of involuntary movements is reduced. However, it has not been clearly established that bromocriptine is effective in patients who have become refractory to levodopa. The plasma half-life of bromocriptine (6–8 hours) is longer than that of levodopa, although peak plasma concentrations of both drugs are reached over the same period (1–3 hours) following administration.

Adverse effects of bromocriptine are similar to those of levodopa, except that in some patients hypotension can be severe enough to cause fainting after the first dose of bromocriptine. It is therefore recommended that patients should be tested for susceptibility to the hypotensive effect using a 1 mg test dose of bromocriptine after a meal and with the patient lying in bed before full bromocriptine treatment is started. Other unwanted effects include visual and auditory hallucinations and erythromelalgia involving the feet and hands. Dyskinesia occurs much less frequently than with levodopa, perhaps because the agonist effect at the D_2 receptor in the striatum is greater than the partial agonist effect at the D_1 receptor at this site.

Pergolide relieves the symptoms of Parkinson's disease as effectively as bromocriptine

Both pergolide and lisuride maleate are agonists at D_2 receptors and pergolide relieves the symptoms of Parkinson's disease as effectively as bromocriptine. Pergolide also produces less nausea, vomiting, and hypotension, but this drug is still undergoing clinical evaluation.

Amantadine

Amantadine is useful in the treatment of Parkinson's disease because it increases central dopamine release. However, it is less effective than the dopaminergic agonists, possibly because of its mechanism of action, which is thought to be facilitation of neuronal dopamine release and inhibition of its reuptake into nerves. If this were the mechanism of action, the effectiveness of amantadine would be brief, since there is progressive degeneration of the nigrostriatal dopaminergic neurons through which amantadine produces its therapeutic effects in Parkinson's disease. Amantadine is therefore only of short-term benefit, since most of its effectiveness is lost within 6 months of initiating treatment. Nevertheless, addition of amantadine to the levodopa regimen leads to synergistic effects and an improvement in the therapeutic benefits.

Amantadine is usually given orally and is quickly absorbed from the gastrointestinal tract. Its plasma half-life is 2–4 hours, but it can accumulate in the body during renal impairment because it is excreted unchanged in the urine.

Adverse effects of amantadine are similar to, but less severe than, those of levodopa. They include hallucinations, confusion, nightmares, and anorexia. Prolonged use of amantadine may lead to the development of livedo reticularis owing to catecholamine-induced vasoconstriction in the lower extremities.

DRUGS THAT INHIBIT STRIATAL CHOLINERGIC ACTIVITY

Inhibition of striatal cholinergic activity is also a therapeutic strategy used for treating Parkinson's disease. The drugs most commonly used are antagonists at the muscarinic receptors that mediate striatal cholinergic excitation and presynaptic dopaminergic inhibition. Their major function in the treatment of Parkinson's disease is to reduce the excessive striatal cholinergic activity that characterizes the disease.

The prototype of this group of drugs is trihexyphenidyl hydrochloride; other members of the group are benztropine hydrochloride, biperiden, orphenadrine hydrochloride (has antihistamine properties) and procyclidine hydrochloride. As a group, their therapeutic effectiveness is less than that of levodopa and the tremor is reduced more than the rigidity and bradykinesia. They also reduce the excessive salivation associated with Parkinson's disease.

Adverse effects of muscarinic antagonists used in Parkinson's disease The typical peripheral anticholinergic adverse effects (i.e. dry mouth, blurred vision, urinary retention, and constipation) are uncommon. More often, patients

Drug therapy of parkinsonism

- Drugs are used to restore nigrostriatal dopaminergic activity or to inhibit striatal cholinergic overactivity
- Levodopa (L-dopa), a precursor of dopamine, is the major drug used. It can cross the blood–brain barrier and is converted to dopamine centrally
- The effectiveness of levodopa lasts for only about 2 years because its central conversion to dopamine gradually diminishes, owing to progressive degeneration of the dopaminergic neurons
- The therapeutic benefits of levodopa are maximized by giving it in combination with a peripheral dopa decarboxylase inhibitor (e.g. carbidopa) or a selective monoamine oxidase-B (MAO_B) inhibitor (e.g. selegiline) or a catechol-O-methyltransferase (COMT) inhibitor
- Peripheral adverse effects of levodopa can be prevented by combining it with domperidone, a peripheral dopamine antagonist
- Bromocriptine (a dopamine agonist), amantadine (which increases dopamine release), and the anticholinergic drugs (e.g. trihexyphenidyl hydrochloride and benztropine mesilate) are also used to treat Parkinson's disease
- The anticholinergic drugs are more effective in controlling tremor than other symptoms of the disease

experience a variety of CNS adverse effects, including mental confusion, delusions, hallucinations, drowsiness, and mood changes. As parkinsonism can worsen when these drugs are discontinued, any termination of treatment should be gradual.

HUNTINGTON'S DISEASE

Like Parkinson's disease, Huntington's disease is a movement disorder associated with defects in the basal ganglia and related structures but, unlike Parkinson's disease, it is a hyperkinetic disorder characterized by excessive and abnormal movements. The movements are irregular, involve different groups of muscles, and produce a dancing-like appearance. The disorder is also characterized by progressive dementia.

Huntington's disease is hereditary and often appears during adult life. The symptoms are associated with biochemical defects in the basal ganglia that in many ways are the mirror image of the defects that produce the symptoms of Parkinson's disease. For example, increased concentrations of dopamine are found in the putamen of patients with Huntington's disease at postmortem. Reduced glutamic acid decarboxylase (a synthetic enzyme for GABA) and choline acetyltransferase activities have also been demonstrated and correlate with the production of deficient levels of GABA and ACh in the basal ganglia. It is thought that these deficiencies reduce the inhibitory influence on the nigrostriatal dopaminergic neurons and lead to the dopaminergic hyperactivity associated with Huntington's disease. Further evidence for this mechanism of action is provided by the observations that the symptoms of Huntington's disease are suppressed by drugs that block dopaminergic receptors and worsened by drugs that increase basal ganglia dopaminergic activity.

Treatment of Huntington's disease involves the use of drugs to reduce basal ganglia dopaminergic activity

Drugs that deplete central dopamine stores by blocking dopamine entry into the neuronal storage vesicles include reserpine (given in small doses of 0.25 mg daily)—no longer used in the UK—and tetrabenazine*. The adverse effects of these drugs include hypotension, depression, sedation, and gastrointestinal disturbances. These effects occur less frequently with tetrabenazine* than with meserpine.

Drugs that reduce dopaminergic activity by blocking the receptors include the phenothiazines (e.g. perphenazine) and the butyrophenones (e.g. haloperidol), which are neuroleptics. The major adverse effects associated with their use include restlessness and parkinsonism.

NAUSEA AND VOMITING

Nausea frequently precedes the act of vomiting, but either may occur alone

Nausea is a highly subjective and peculiarly unpleasant sensation normally felt in the throat or stomach as a sinking sensation in the epigastrium. Acute nausea is a temporarily unpleasant sensation that precludes other mental and physical activity and is usually relieved by an emetic episode. Chronic nausea severely reduces the quality of life.

Nausea is usually accompanied by a vasomotor disturbance causing pallor, sweating, and relaxation of the lower part of the esophagus and abdominal muscles. The latter tends to increase tension on the gastric and esophageal muscles, stimulating afferent nerve endings that may induce the sensation of nausea. The upper small intestine then contracts and this is closely followed by contraction of the pyloric sphincter and the pyloric portion of the stomach. These changes result in emptying of the contents of the upper jejunum, duodenum, and pyloric portion of the stomach into the fundus and body of the stomach, which are relaxed. The cardiac sphincter, the esophagus, and the esophageal sphincter are also relaxed. The gastrointestinal system is therefore prepared for retching and vomiting, which is reflex in origin and serves to remove the contents of the upper gastrointestinal tract from the body. This is useful for removing toxic material from the gut, but does not provide an adequate explanation for most causes of emesis.

The emetic reflex involves a series of highly coordinated changes in gastrointestinal motility and respiratory movements

Emesis is initiated by a deep and sharp inspiration and is immediately followed by reflex closure of the glottis and a raising of the soft palate, thereby preventing the passage of vomitus into the lungs and nasal cavity (Fig. 7.39). The abdominal muscles then contract in the rhythmic manner of 'retching' movements, which compress the stomach between the contracted diaphragm and abdominal organs. The inevitable increase in intragastric pressure causes evacuation of the stomach contents through the relaxed esophagus; definite antiperistalsis in the stomach itself is rarely observed. This profile of activities varies in the infant, in whom the abdominal muscles and diaphragm do not apparently play a role in, for example, regurgitation of an oversize meal; instead, the reverse peristalsis is produced by contraction of the stomach muscles alone. Reverse peristalsis originating in the upper bowel may itself be a direct cause of nausea and vomiting.

Pivotal events in nausea and emesis

- **Relaxation of the esophagus, esophageal sphincter, cardiac sphincter, and fundus and body of the stomach**
- **Contraction of the upper small intestine and pyloric stomach, emptying their contents into the relaxed stomach**
- **Deep inspiration and closure of the glottis and raising of the soft palate**
- **Rhythmic contraction of the diaphragm and abdominal muscles to compress the stomach and evacuate its contents via the mouth**

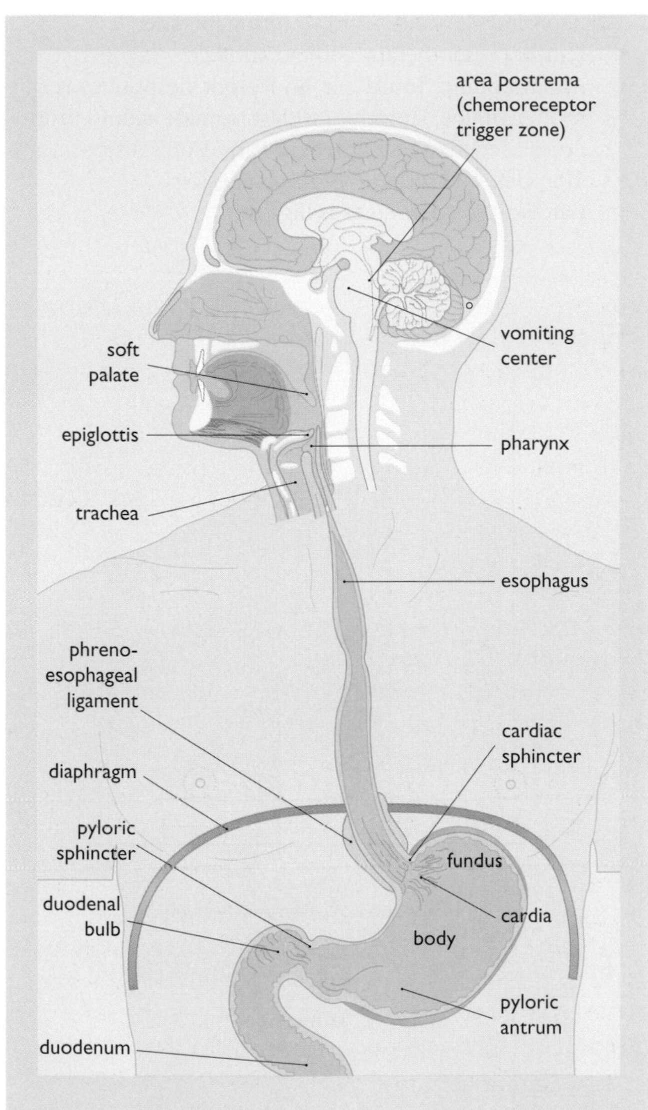

Fig. 7.39 The major visceral and central structures involved in the emetic reflex.

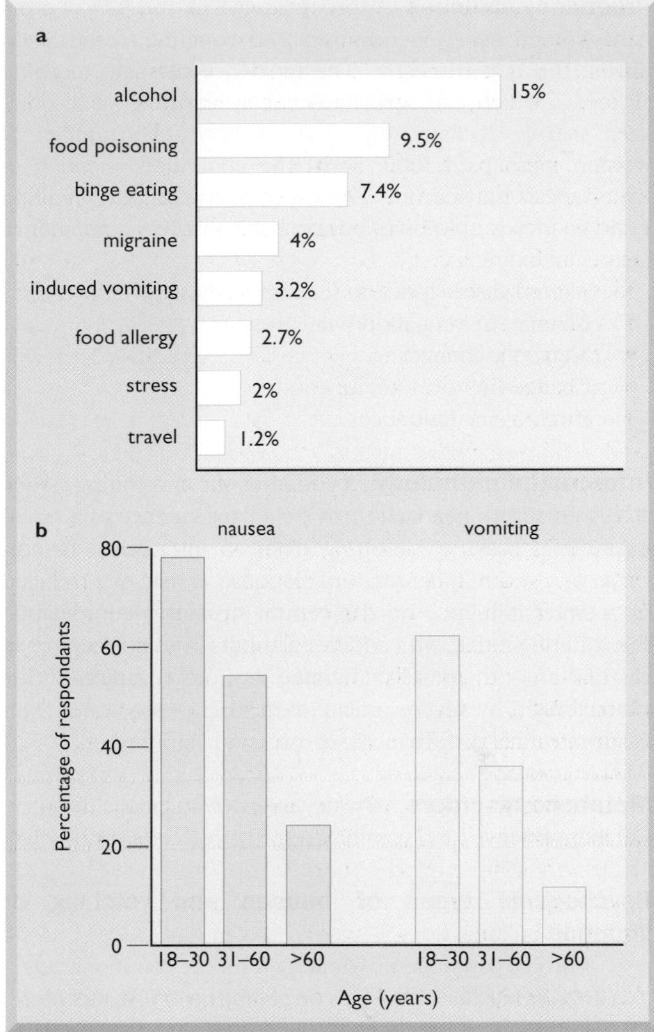

Fig. 7.40 Causes and incidence of nausea and vomiting. (a) The percentage of participants from an otherwise healthy population in the UK reporting vomiting from different causes. (b) The percentage of individuals in each group who reported nausea or vomiting at least once during the previous 12-month period.

Nausea and/or vomiting may result from single or, more usually, multifactorial stimuli

The most frequent causes of nausea and emesis in an otherwise healthy population are shown in Fig. 7.40.

Gastrointestinal irritation is a frequent inducer of nausea and emesis and is produced by:

- Stimulation of mechanoreceptors by distension or obstruction in the gut.
- Stimulation of chemoreceptors responsive to bacterial endotoxins.
- The accidental or deliberate ingestion of toxic materials such as alcohol or a wide range of therapeutic agents (e.g. nonsteroidal anti-inflammatory agents (NSAIDs) and antibiotics).

Projectile vomiting, an unusual type of vomiting of considerable force, may be observed in the infant and results from pyloric stenosis.

Motion sickness Explanations of motion or movement sickness are centered around the sensory conflict that can occur between a discordant visual, vestibular (the semicircular canals and otolith organs), and proprioceptive input. An essential function of the vestibular system is the development of compensatory eye movements to stabilize the retinal image of an earth-fixed visual target in the presence of head movement. This reflex is inappropriate when the visual world shares the same movement as that of the head and generates sensory conflict.

Pregnancy sickness Approximately 85% and 52% of pregnant women experience nausea and vomiting, respectively, during the first trimester. The incidence of such 'morning sickness,' which can actually occur at any time of the day, then sharply declines (Fig. 7.41). A very small number of women, perhaps 1/1000, show the continued vomiting of hyperemesis gravidarum. The cause of nausea and vomiting in pregnancy is unknown, but probably involves a number of factors including:

- Altered gastric function (e.g. delayed gastric emptying).
- Changes in intra-abdominal pressure.
- Metabolic changes.
- Changes in hormone function.
- Psychogenic influences.

Intracranial pathology A sudden bout of vomiting associated with severe headache may be a consequence of a raised intracranial pressure resulting from an intracranial hemorrhage or a severe inflammatory response. It may be produced by a direct influence on the central structures coordinating the vomiting reflex, with additional inputs from nociceptors in vascular smooth muscle. Migraine is more common and is characterized by severe unilateral headaches associated with gastrointestinal disturbances, nausea, and vomiting.

Metabolic disorders A wide variety of metabolic disorders can induce nausea and vomiting (e.g. hypoglycemia or uremia).

Psychogenic types of nausea and retching or vomiting include:

- Chronic psychogenic vomiting (or more commonly retching), which usually occurs on getting up or just after breakfast; it may persist for years.
- Nervous dyspepsia, which describes a feeling of satiety, abdominal discomfort, nausea, and vomiting associated with psychoneurotic features such as anxiety, irritability, and weight loss.
- Anorexia nervosa and bulimia, which have a well-established psychopathology and in which retching and/or vomiting is a symptom of serious psychiatric illness.
- Certain sights, smells, or feelings, which can trigger revulsion or fear that can cause immediate nausea and vomiting.
- Anticipatory nausea and vomiting, which occurs in up to 30% of patients with cancer and results from inadequate control of chemotherapy-induced emesis. It is a learned response and the patients associate their emetic treatment with the hospital and its personnel. Associated 'stimuli' (e.g. the hospital or nurses) can trigger emesis on sight.
- Anxiety, which predisposes to nausea and emesis.

Pain The severe discomfort of somatic or cardiac pain or the intense pain caused by distension of the bile or urethral ducts can induce nausea and vomiting.

Drug- and radiation-induced emesis Many compounds can induce emesis and the major classes of drugs that predictably induce nausea and vomiting include:

- Cancer chemotherapy and radiation.
- Apomorphine, levodopa, and ergot derivatives (e.g. bromocriptine, lergotrile) with dopamine agonist properties used in the treatment of Parkinson's disease.
- Morphine and related opioid analgesics.
- Cardiac glycosides such as digoxin.

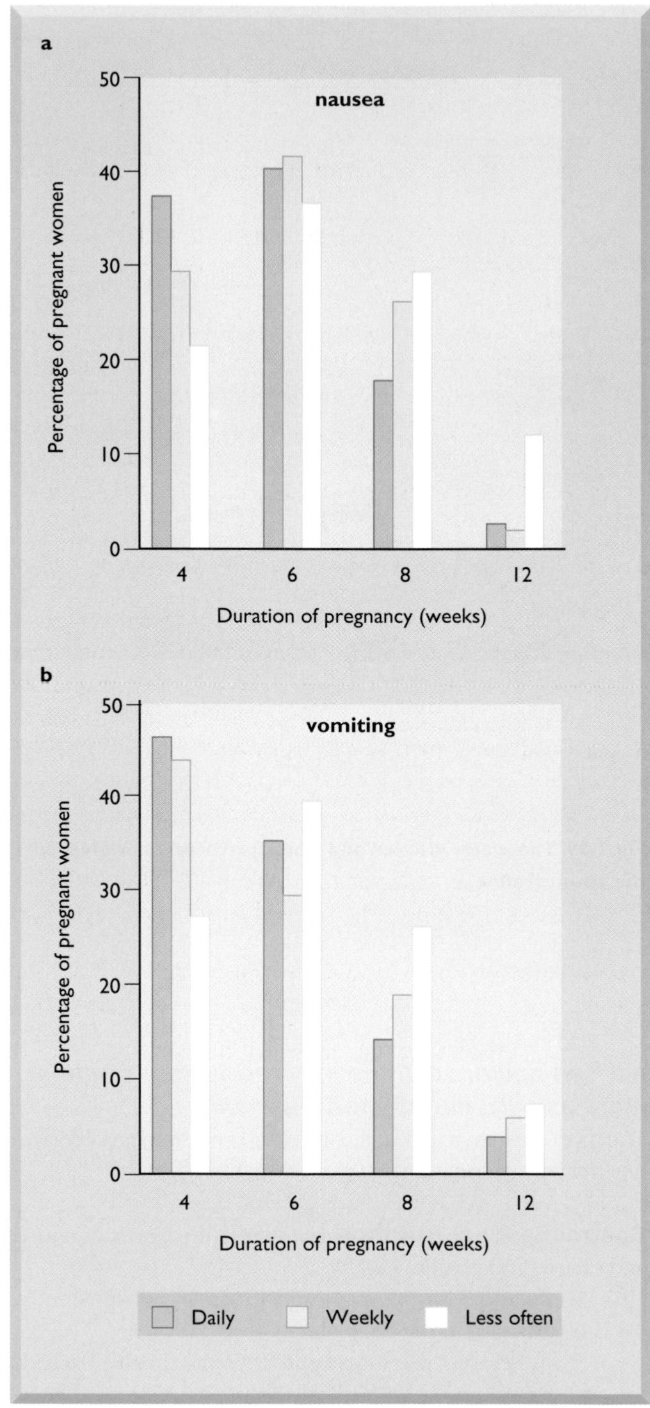

Fig. 7.41 The frequency of sickness in pregnancy during the first trimester. The majority of women who experienced daily symptoms of nausea and vomiting reported that the onset of their symptoms occurred within 4–6 weeks of their last menstruation.

- Drugs enhancing 5-HT function.
- Miscellaneous agents (e.g. heavy metals, ipecacuanha* alkaloids, veratrum alkaloids).

Many cytotoxic treatments cause dose and regimen-related severe nausea and vomiting (Fig. 7.42). Nausea and vomiting induced by radiation is also related to the dose used and to the area and extent of the body irradiated. In addition, cytotoxic or radiation treatment frequently causes severe disruption to the gastrointestinal tract where products of tissue destruction may be released and a local inflammatory response may influence vagal afferent nerve endings within the gut to trigger the emetic reflex. The release of 5-HT from the enterochromaffin cells provides an important example. Such substances may be transported in the blood and, with the cytotoxic agents themselves, directly stimulate the central components mediating the emetic reflex.

Apomorphine, levodopa, and ergot derivatives with dopamine agonist properties used in the treatment of Parkinson's disease act mainly by directly stimulating the central chemoreceptor mechanisms. They also induce gastric stasis.

Morphine and related opioid analgesics have probably the most complex mechanisms of action of any drugs that cause nausea and vomiting. Acute administration of such agents to opioid-naïve patients frequently induces nausea and sometimes vomiting. However, tolerance develops rapidly to such effects and the first treatment antagonizes the emetic effects to a second opioid injection or other emetogens. The emetic potential may be mediated in the chemoreceptor trigger zone (CTZ), whereas the 'broad spectrum' antiemetic effect may be mediated downstream from the CTZ and close to the 'vomiting center.' The antiemetic effect may relate to an endogenous tone exerted by opioids from the enkephalin, dynorphin, or the pro-opiomelanocortin series. The ability of narcotic antagonists such as naloxone to precipitate nausea or vomiting supports this hypothesis.

Cardiac glycosides such as digoxin can induce abdominal pains, nausea, and vomiting. This probably relates to a central action on the chemoreceptor trigger zone and an irritant action within the gastrointestinal tract, which may be worsened by a cardiac arrhythmia.

Drugs enhancing 5-HT function (e.g. 5-hydroxytryptophan*, the precursor of 5-HT, or SSRIs such as fluoxetine and paroxetine) have been reported to induce nausea and occasionally vomiting.

Emetic potential of chemotherapeutic drugs

Severely emetogenic in almost all patients	Moderately emetogenic	Least emetogenic
Cisplatin	Mitomycin C	5-Fluorouracil
Mustine*	Procarbazine	Cytarabine
Cyclophosphamide	Nitrosoureas	6-Mercaptopurine
Dacarbazine		Bleomycin
Doxorubicin		Vinblastine
		Vincristine

Fig. 7.42 Emetic potential of chemotherapeutic drugs.

This may relate to increased 5-HT activity in both the brain and intestine .

When administered orally, heavy metals such as copper sulfate, zinc sulfate, antimony, and mercuric chloride have an irritant action in the gut, triggering the emetic reflex via vagal and splanchnic nerves. Some of these agents may also directly stimulate the central mechanisms. The ipecacuanha* alkaloids also stimulate peripheral and central mechanisms, while veratrum alkaloids stimulate the nodose ganglia of the vagus to trigger the emetic reflex.

Major stimuli of nausea and vomiting

- Gastrointestinal irritation
- Motion sickness
- Hormone disturbance
- Intracranial pathology
- Metabolic disorders
- Psychogenic factors
- Pain
- Drugs and radiation
- Endogenous toxins

Postoperative nausea and vomiting (PONV) provides one of the best examples of the multifactorial nature of nausea and vomiting. It may be triggered by:

- Inhalational agents, particularly nitrous oxide, which are variably associated with PONV.
- Intravenous anesthetics and spinal anesthesia.
- Certain types of surgery, particularly gynecologic, pediatric strabismus, and abdominal surgery. The latter can cause stretching, distension, or tissue damage (i.e. gastrointestinal irritation).
- Pain resulting from surgery or disease.
- Hypoxia, hypotension, and carbon dioxide retention.
- Clumsy movement of the patient in the recovery room or ward or following day-case surgery, causing a labyrinthine disturbance.
- Certain pre- or postoperative drug treatments (e.g. opioid analgesics).
- Psychogenic factors such as anxiety.
- A high body weight.
- Sex and age. The risk of PONV is three times higher in adult females than in adult males, and children are twice as susceptible as adults.

Individual responses to many emetic stimuli vary widely

Even the simple introduction of a spatula into the mouth to facilitate oral examination will immediately provoke a 'gagging' reflex in some people. Approximately 70% of women suffer

PONV following gynecologic surgery, but it is not possible to identify the women at risk. Patients who have had nausea and vomiting following previous surgery are likely to experience it again. Furthermore, women who experience pregnancy sickness are much more likely to develop nausea and vomiting in response to any hormonal disturbance (e.g. the contraceptive pill) or travelling, and with migraine (Fig. 7.43). Also, people who have an emetic response to a first drug challenge are likely to show a similar response to a subsequent challenge (i.e. an individual tends to have a consistent response). A simple enquiry may therefore identify people at greater risk (i.e. those who have a lower emetic threshold). These people are particularly likely to develop nausea and vomiting under emotional strain.

The frequency and intensity of nausea and vomiting vary enormously

A single short-lived bout of emesis induced by a single psychogenic stimulus is quite different to the intense, intractable, and devastating nausea and vomiting caused by highly emetogenic chemotherapy. The first is unpredictable and therefore untreatable by drugs, but the latter can now be efficiently managed in most patients.

The consequences of vomiting pose different problems to both patient and clinician

To the patient, either a brief or persistent period of vomiting is always of concern. However, a brief period of vomiting in an otherwise healthy individual generally poses little medical risk, whereas, in the postoperative patient, even a brief but powerful period of retching or vomiting can cause tissue rupture. Not only will persistent nausea and vomiting incapacitate the patient, but the persistent vomiting may result in the loss of hydrochloric acid, leading to alkalosis and dehydration.

Persistent nausea or vomiting may be symptoms of an underlying disease

Persistent nausea or vomiting may be indicative of gastrointestinal, neurologic, or metabolic disorders that require direct treatment, and it may be desirable to withhold antiemetic therapy until a diagnosis has been made.

The number of women who reported sickness with oral contraceptives, travel, or migraine and the relationship to vomiting in pregnancy

Pregnancy sickness	Oral contraceptive sickness	Travel sickness	Migraine sickness
Vomiting	30 (70%)	77 (63%)	45 (65%)
No vomiting	13 (30%)	46 (37%)	24 (35%)

Fig. 7.43 The number of women who reported sickness with oral contraceptives, travel, or migraine and the relationship to vomiting in pregnancy. There was a higher than expected incidence of vomiting during pregnancy in these groups of women than in women who had no sickness.

Both central and peripheral systems mediate nausea and emesis

The causes of emesis provide vital clues to the stimuli influencing the emetic reflex, although the precise circuitry and transmitter mechanisms mediating the reflex remain largely unknown. However, key structures and pathways are now being identified, based on the results obtained almost exclusively from animals, of central and peripheral nerve lesions, intracerebral injection of drugs into discrete brain regions, and electrophysiologic stimulation of discrete brain regions. Pharmacology is establishing the relevance of specific neurotransmitters (Fig. 7.44).

The chemoreceptor trigger zone (CTZ) is a key structure in mediating nausea and vomiting and is located within the area postrema, a circumventricular organ located at the caudal end of the fourth ventricle. It lacks an effective blood–brain barrier and is therefore ideally suited for detecting emetic agents in both the systemic circulation and the CSF. A lesion of the CTZ abolishes the emetic response to many emetogens. The area postrema has numerous afferent and efferent connections with the underlying structures, the subnucleus gelatinosus and nucleus tractus solitarius. These brain regions are also important structures in the emetic reflex and, with the area postrema, receive vagal afferent fibers from the gastrointestinal tract, which is a major source of emetic stimuli.

The 'vomiting center' is a second major 'structure' mediating nausea and vomiting and is more accurately described as a collection of effector nuclei rather than a discrete brain area. It receives major inputs from:

- The CTZ.
- A vagal and sympathetic input from the gut.
- The cardiovascular system.
- A variety of limbic brain nuclei (e.g. the olfactory tubercle, amygdala, hypothalamus, and ventral thalamic nucleus).

Electrical stimulation of all these structures can induce emesis. The latter nuclei may be involved in olfactory, emotional/anticipatory, hormonal/stress, and pain-induced vomiting, respectively. The location of the visual inputs to the emetic circuitry remains unknown.

The brain regions that produce the sensation of nausea have been difficult to assess, as nausea is a subjective human experience and animal models are not available. However, noninvasive magnetic source imaging has recently revealed that there is neuronal activation in the cortex in the inferior frontal gyrus in volunteers nauseated by ipecacuanha* or vestibular stimulation. The activation caused by ipecacuanha*, but not by vestibular stimulation, was antagonized by ondansetron. This brain area may therefore be important in the perception or sensation of nausea.

Retching, vomiting, or regurgitation occasionally constitute a medical or surgical emergency

Retching, vomiting, or regurgitation occasionally needs emergency treatment for example:

- When it is induced by major intracranial pathology or intestinal obstruction.
- In infants, where fluid loss may cause dehydration.
- When the force of retching or vomiting tears esophageal tissue.
- In emergency surgery, when the patient has recently had a meal and therefore has a high risk of developing aspiration pneumonia. This is an important cause of death in pregnant women.
- In patients with a defective gag reflex, who have a high risk of developing aspiration pneumonia.
- When it is due to hyperemesis gravidarum.

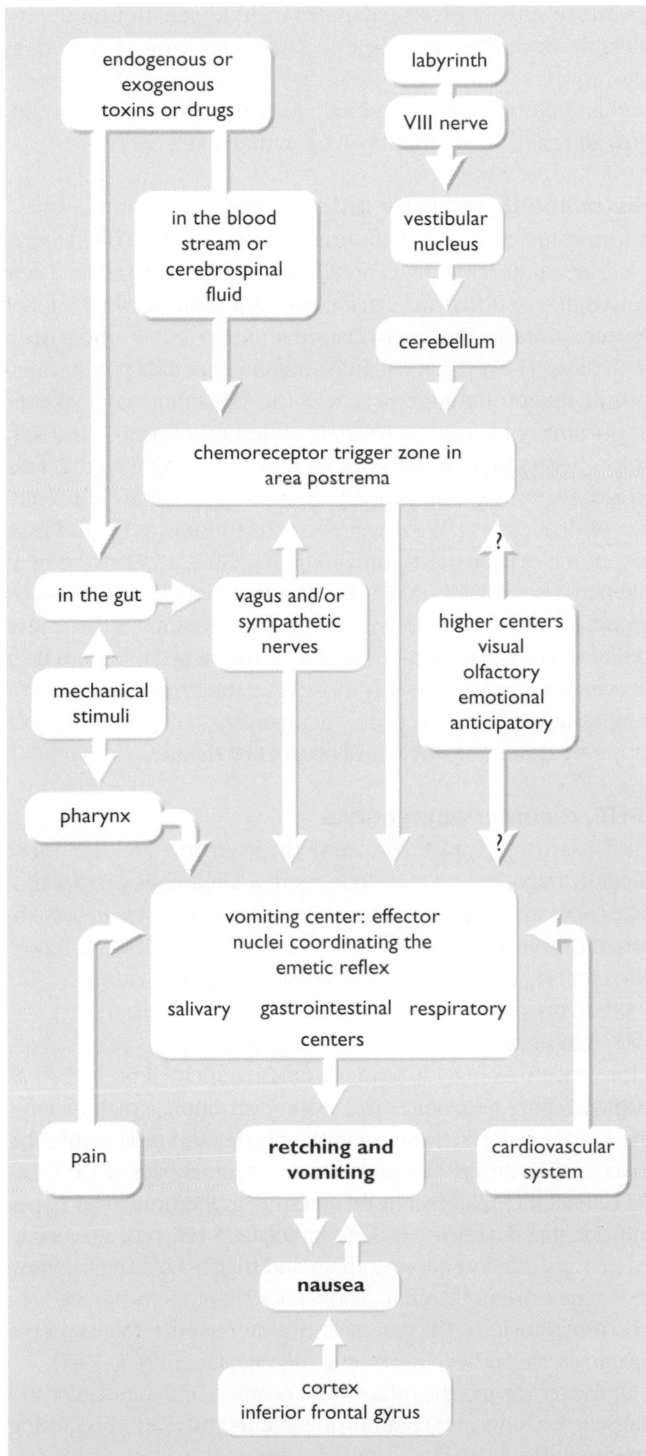

Fig. 7.44 The major emetic stimuli, pathways, and structures mediating the emetic reflex and nausea.

> **Major systems mediating nausea and vomiting**
>
> - The vagus and splanchnic nerves (stimuli from the gut)
> - The cranial nerves (vestibular, olfactory, taste, and visual stimuli, and touch from the oral cavity and pharynx)
> - Forebrain systems (psychogenic stimuli)
> - The chemoreceptor trigger zone in the area postrema (responds to circulating emetogenic neurotransmitters, hormones, toxins, and drugs)
> - The 'vomiting center' in the reticular formation (coordinates the visceral and somatic components of the emetic reflex)

The preferred treatment of nausea and vomiting is removal of the cause

Treatment of the cardiovascular pathology in migraine with sumatriptan will relieve the neurologic manifestations, headache, gastrointestinal effects, and nausea and vomiting. Yet sumatriptan has no direct effect on the emetic reflex.

Antiemetic therapy can be life-saving for patients with cancer

Patients with cancer will more readily accept or continue with what may be a curative course of chemotherapy if they are given effective antiemetic therapy. More aggressive chemotherapy regimens with a greater chance of eradicating the tumor can now be given without producing an unacceptable incidence of nausea and vomiting.

DRUGS USED FOR THE SYMPTOMATIC RELIEF OF NAUSEA AND VOMITING

Symptomatic control of nausea and vomiting involves using drugs and procedures that affect the emetic reflex.

Although acute nausea itself poses no medical problem, it is a very distressing symptom and can cause as much suffering as pain. Indeed, a bout of retching or vomiting may be welcomed by the patient because it terminates the feeling of nausea. Persistent nausea usually leads to a loss of appetite, a reduced food intake, malnutrition, and serious debilitation, requiring prompt medical treatment.

There are now at least four major groups of compounds to control nausea and emesis. Procedures and treatments that alleviate retching and vomiting generally prevent nausea.

Inadequate control of the first bout of nausea and vomiting may compromise the treatment of later episodes.

Drugs used for the symptomatic relief of nausea and vomiting include:

- Dopamine receptor antagonists.
- Muscarinic receptor antagonists.
- Histamine H_1 receptor antagonists
- 5-HT_3 receptor antagonists.
- Sedatives and hypnotics.
- Phenothiazines.

Dopamine receptor antagonists

Apomorphine induces intense nausea and vomiting and has a high affinity for the dopamine receptor. It is antagonized by dopamine receptor antagonists. Dopamine and dopamine receptors are found in high concentrations in the area postrema, the dorsal motor nucleus of the vagus nerve, and the nucleus tractus solitarius. The traditional view has been that apomorphine, levodopa (via dopamine), lergotrile, bromocriptine, and other dopamine agonists used in the treatment of Parkinson's disease induce nausea and vomiting by stimulating dopamine receptors in the CTZ. Dopamine receptor antagonists block such receptors and thereby prevent nausea and emesis.

Specific dopamine receptor antagonists (e.g. haloperidol and fluphenazine) The use of these drugs is limited in two ways:

- First, they do not inhibit nausea and emesis induced by stimuli other than dopamine agonists (although droperidol is used in PONV, see below).
- Second, they have major adverse effects of motor impairment, severe akinesia and muscle rigidity, and dystonias (muscle spasm) caused by striatal dopamine receptor blockade, particularly in young people.

The adverse effects are less with domperidone and sulpiride because they are less able to penetrate the blood–brain barrier in the striatal areas, but can easily access structures such as the area postrema, which lack a blood–brain barrier.

Metoclopramide is a dopamine receptor antagonist that has been widely used as an antinauseant/antiemetic for gastrointestinal disorders and migraine and, in much higher doses, for cancer chemotherapy- and radiation-induced sickness. Its unusual and established ability to facilitate gastric emptying and intestinal activity may contribute directly to its antinauseant/antiemetic actions in gastrointestinal disorders and migraine. However, such actions do not reflect a dopamine receptor blockade, but more probably an agonist action at the 5-HT_4 receptor. Furthermore, its ability to prevent chemotherapy/radiation-induced emesis when used in exceptionally high doses is more readily attributed to its low potency 5-HT_3 receptor antagonism (see below).

Muscarinic receptor antagonists

Scopalamine is the most effective remedy for motion sickness of all types, although nausea and vomiting induced by extreme changes in motion and space travel remains an intractable problem and it fails to control all types of movement sickness (e.g. due to severe vestibular disturbance). Scopalamine has a greater central depressant effect than atropine and its antiemetic action is attributed to a blockade of muscarinic cholinergic receptors in the area postrema or associated nuclei of the dorsal vagal complex. Scopalamine is also a potent inhibitor of gastrointestinal movements and relaxes the gastrointestinal tract and these effects may make a modest contribution to the antiemetic action.

Adverse effects of scopalamine include sedation and predictable autonomic adverse effects with increase of dose (e.g. blurred vision, urinary retention, decreased salivation). The sedation and blurred vision preclude its use in airline pilots, train, bus, and car drivers, and those operating machinery.

Histamine H_1 receptor antagonists

Antihistamines used for motion sickness include buclizine*, cyclizine, dimenhydrinate, meclizine, and promethazine. Their antiemetic actions are attributed to a central blockade of H_1 receptors in the area postrema and possibly underlying structures. However, most antihistamines are also potent muscarinic receptor antagonists, and this behavior may make an important contribution to their antiemetic actions. Indeed, chlorpheniramine, which is an H_1 receptor antagonist that fails to block centrally mediated cholinergic effects, does not inhibit motion sickness. Whatever the contribution of H_1 and ACh receptor blockade to the antiemetic potential, a sedative potential may also contribute to the effect, although this is less or absent for cinnarizine. However, some antihistamines that cause sedation are not antiemetic and in addition sedation can be a dangerous adverse effect in those operating machinery or driving vehicles. The H_1 receptor antagonists may play some role in the treatment of PONV and pregnancy sickness.

5-HT_3 receptor antagonists

Ondansetron, granisetron, and tropisetron* are the most recently introduced antiemetic agents. Their ability to antagonize chemotherapy- and radiation-induced emesis was first established in animal models in 1986. Their efficacy relates to blockade of 5-HT_3 receptors, which are located in high density:

- In the area postrema and nucleus tractus solitarius.
- On vagal afferent nerve endings in the gut.

It is hypothesized that severely emetogenic regimens such as cisplatin cause gastrointestinal tissue disruption, which initiates the release of 5-HT from the enterochromaffin cells within the mucosa. 5-Hydroxyindoleacetic acid, the metabolite of 5-HT, can then be detected in increased amounts in the urine. It is hypothesized that the release of 5-HT stimulates 5-HT_3 receptors located on vagal afferent nerve endings and trigger vagus nerve firing to initiate the emetic reflex. The 5-HT_3 receptors within the area postrema/nucleus tractus solitarius lie on the vagus nerve terminals, since they disappear if the vagus is cut (Fig. 7.45).

Ondansetron and the other 5-HT_3 receptor antagonists control nausea, retching, and vomiting in patients with cancer receiving emetogenic treatments, especially during the acute phase (i.e. day 1 of treatment): the symptoms are completely controlled in 70% of patients and there is reduced vomiting in the others.

However, on the second and subsequent days (i.e. a 'delayed phase') the antiemetic effects are less pronounced and the addition of a glucocorticosteroid is needed to produce a maximally efficacious antiemetic regimen. Dexamethasone or methylprednisolone are now frequently used in combination with ondansetron or other 5-HT_3 receptor antagonists to secure optimal control, even on the first day of treatment. This is vitally important for the patient with cancer, since the development of almost any nausea and vomiting during treatment can lead to a learned 'anticipatory nausea,' which is characterized by nausea and vomiting at all future treatments and even at the sight of the nursing staff or hospital where the treatment was initially given. Such anticipatory nausea is resistant to all drug treatments, including the 5-HT_3 receptor antagonists.

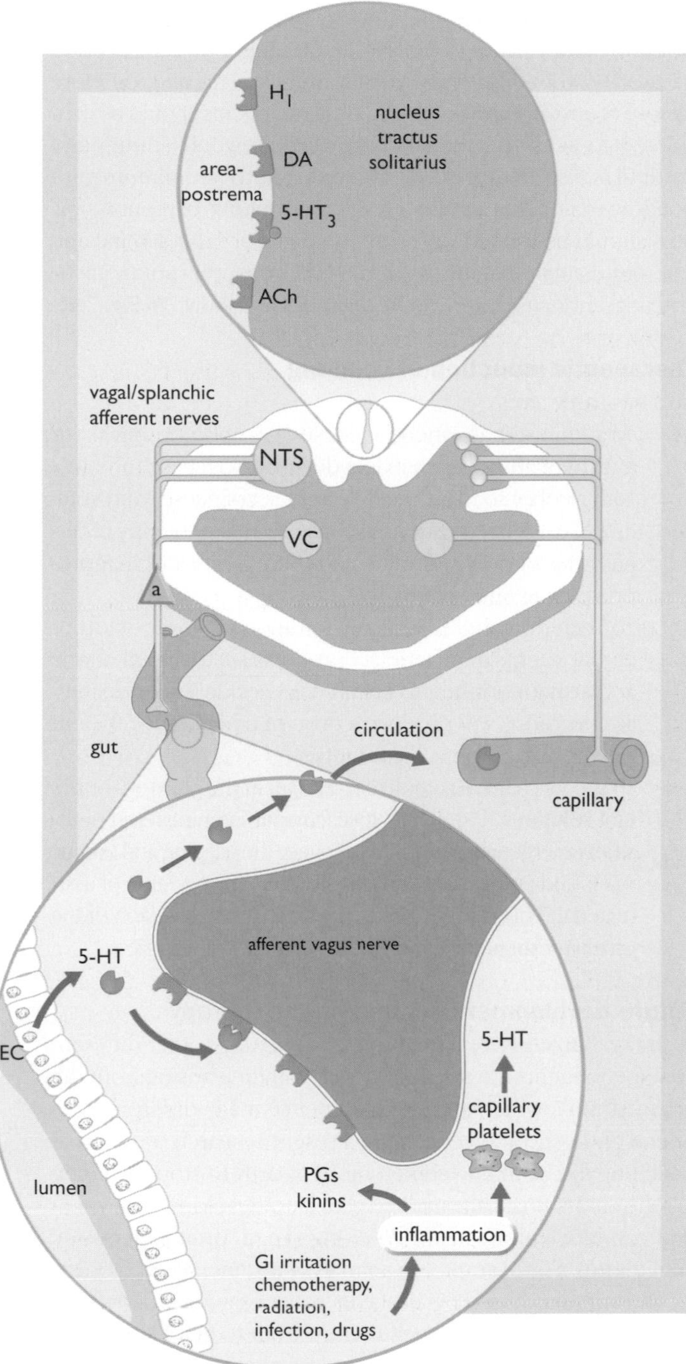

Fig. 7.45 Chemical transmitters mediating emetic stimuli. Stimuli in the gastrointestinal tract cause nausea and vomiting via neuronal (vagus nerve) and bloodborne influences on the central chemoreceptor trigger zone in the area postrema and nucleus tractus solitarius (NTS) and the 'vomiting center' (VC). 5-Hydroxytryptamine (5-HT) released from the enterochromaffin cells (ECs) and possibly platelets acting on 5-HT_3 receptors may play a major role, along with inflammatory mediators released in the vicinity of afferent nerve endings. (GI, gastrointestinal; PGs, prostaglandins)

The 5-HT_3 receptor antagonists have no effect on motion sickness or apomorphine-induced vomiting. They will, however, block the vomiting induced by ipecacuanha. Ondansetron has also been shown to antagonize:

- The nausea induced by morphine.
- The nausea and gastrointestinal adverse effects of SSRIs.

Its use in the treatment of other causes of gastrointestinal irritation is being investigated.

Adverse effects of 5-HT_3 receptor antagonists 5-HT_3 receptor antagonists have a remarkable safety profile, their use being accompanied by a small incidence of headache, constipation, and a sensation of warmth or flushing.

Major advantages of 5-HT_3 receptor antagonists are that they are not sedative, they do not interact with other drugs, and they do not cause generalized autonomic adverse effects, endocrine changes, or motor impairments. This contrasts with the endocrine and motor impairments induced by metoclopramide, which blocks dopamine and 5-HT_3 receptors at the same concentration. Before the availability of ondansetron, the most effective control of chemotherapy- and radiation-induced vomiting had been achieved by the empirical use of exceptionally high doses of metoclopramide.

Ondansetron is the drug of choice in the treatment of PONV

The lack of interaction between 5-HT_3 receptor antagonists and other drugs prompted the use of ondansetron in the treatment of PONV, for which it is as efficacious as any of the existing remedies, (e.g. cyclizine, droperidol), but does not produce their adverse effects. Also, ondansetron does not adversely affect the course of anesthesia or postoperative recovery. It is effective in approximately 60% of patients. Its mechanism of action is thought to relate to a central and peripheral 5-HT_3 receptor blockade to attenuate the overall influence of the many factors triggering PONV.

Sedatives and hypnotics

Vomiting is blocked by anesthesia and lesser degrees of CNS depression, which may attenuate a low emetic threshold that would normally trigger intractable nausea and vomiting. Barbiturates and chloral hydrate have been used, but benzodiazepines are a more contemporary treatment and have the advantage of causing amnesia to prevent recall of a highly distressing event. However, caution is needed as the potential for vomiting or aspiration in the presence of reduced consciousness with a reduction or loss of reflex closure of the trachea can be catastrophic.

Phenothiazines

Agents such as chlorpromazine, promethazine, prochlorperazine, and trimeprazine have a mixed pharmacology as antagonists at muscarinic, histaminergic, dopaminergic, adrenergic, and serotonergic receptors. Nausea and vomiting that fails to respond to specific pharmacologic treatments may sometimes respond to this multireceptor blockade (e.g. pregnancy sickness, PONV). As the mechanisms mediating most types of nausea and vomiting are not clear, but there may be many different contributary stimuli, the use of a 'mixed' pharmacologic approach is logical.

Ancillary treatments of nausea and vomiting

Movement disturbance and visual, olfactory, and emotional psychogenic factors are potent but variable emetic stimuli and can be expected to contribute to the development of nausea and vomiting in many, and perhaps most, patients. For example:

- The residual vomiting of patients with cancer placed on an open ward after 5-HT_3 receptor antagonism could well be partly psychogenic rather than an exclusively chemotherapy-induced vomiting.
- The sight, sound, or smell of just one other patient who is vomiting is sufficient to trigger the same response in others.

Arrangements should therefore be made to avoid, obviate, or reduce such behavior.

The apparent effectiveness of histamine H_1 receptor antagonists in pregnancy sickness in some patients may reflect a vestibular stimulus from disturbed movement. If so, alternative approaches might be considered to reduce movements. This is particularly important in the pregnant patient, in whom drug treatments should not be used unless unavoidable, because of the risk of teratogenicity.

Treating nausea and vomiting

- **Medical, surgical, or psychiatric procedures are used to alleviate the cause**
- **Provide an environment for the patient to adopt a supine position with no visual, olfactory, vestibular, or emotional precipitants of nausea or vomiting**
- **Pharmacologic blockade at specific neurotransmitter receptor sites within the vomiting reflex**
- **Psychologic procedures to offer relaxation and reassurance and relieve anxiety**
- **Advice about modifying eating habits**
- **Acupuncture at the Neiguan point (the sixth point on the pericardial meridian)**

Nausea and vomiting is often best managed using a combination of ancillary and drug treatments

Since individuals have such marked variations in their response to emetic stimuli, and the various stimuli contributing to nausea and vomiting may differ between patients, there is probably no absolute antiemetic regimen for any one clinical presentation (e.g. pregnancy sickness, PONV). Many clinical presentations of nausea and vomiting are potentially multifactorial and therefore the use of ancillary and combined drug treatments should be considered to achieve optimal control. Psychogenic stimuli and vestibular disturbance should be reduced to a minimum with nondrug treatments and then residual symptoms of motion sickness should be treated with antihistamines or scopolamine and gastrointestinal irritation with 5-HT_3 receptor antagonists. Potential antinausea/antiemetic regimens are shown in Fig. 7.46.

Therapeutic induction of vomiting

This has three aims:

- To administer an emetic agent such as apomorphine with a drug of abuse or an aldehyde dehydrogenase inhibitor with alcohol so that the unpleasant act of nausea and vomiting is associated with drug abuse. Aversion therapy of this nature is of doubtful value and there is a risk of inappropriate drug interactions.
- To include subemetic doses of apomorphine or other emetic agents in proprietary products such as methadone and acetaminophen to ensure that accidental or deliberate overdose will produce a dose of emetogen sufficient to empty the stomach contents.
- To use mechanical stimuli (e.g. a finger in the pharynx) or irritant solutions (e.g. saline, ipecacuanha) administered orally as an emergency procedure to trigger the gagging and emetic reflex and empty the stomach following the ingestion of toxic material. This is carried out only if there is no erosion of the gastrointestinal tract and gastric lavage is not feasible.

Future developments in antiemetic therapy

A disadvantage of present antiemetic therapy is that different antiemetic agents are needed to treat vomiting arising from different stimuli, which appear to influence many different peripheral and central mechanisms. Present research is aimed at inhibiting the 'vomiting center' more directly to stop the emetic reflex at its final output. The goal is to develop a treatment that can block all forms of vomiting (i.e. a 'broad-spectrum' antiemetic). For example, in animals, substance P antagonists block vomiting caused by all agents so far examined. However, it will be essential, if any such therapies are to be of significant clinical value, that they also antagonize nausea.

DRUGS AND INFECTIONS OF THE CENTRAL NERVOUS SYSTEM

Infections can occur in every part of the CNS and include:

- Meningitis (inflammation of the meninges).
- Radiculitis (inflammation of the spinal nerve roots).
- Myelitis (inflammation of the spinal cord).
- Encephalitis (inflammation of the brain).
- Brain abscess (a localized collection of pus).

The treatment of nausea and vomiting

Cause of nausea and vomiting	Symptomatic and other treatments	Adverse effects
In all cases reduce psychogenic and vestibular stimuli to a minimum and give appropriate reassurance		
Gastrointestinal irritation	Ondansetron Metoclopramide Phenothiazines	Headache, constipation, and warmth or flushing Extrapyramidal adverse effects Anticholinergic adverse effects and sedation
Motion sickness	Hyoscine or antihistamine	Anticholinergic adverse effects and sedation
Pregnancy sickness	Advice on diet and dangers to the fetus of using drugs	Teratogenicity
If nausea or vomiting remains unacceptable use phenothiazine, antihistamine, or ondansetron		
Chronic psychogenic retching/vomiting	Psychiatric referral: no useful drug treatment	–
Severe pain	Opioid analgesics	Respiratory depression, constipation
Dopamine agonist therapy in the parkinsonian patient	Domperidone, sulpiride; adjust dose of dopamine agonist	–
Parkinsonian patients are exceptionally sensitive to neuroleptic-induced extrapyramidal adverse effects		
Morphine and opioid compounds	Phenothiazine Ondansetron	Anticholinergic adverse effects and sedation Headache, constipation, and warmth or flushing
Cardiac glycosides	Reduce dose of cardiac glycoside	–
Drugs enhancing 5-HT function (e.g. SSRIs)	Ondansetron; adjust dose of 5-HT agonist	Headache, constipation, and warmth or flushing
Cancer chemotherapy/radiation treatment	Ondansetron/granisetron/tropisetron plus glucocorticosteroid	Headache, constipation, and warmth or flushing
Pyloric stenosis	Scopolamine butylbromide before surgery	Anticholinergic adverse effects
Postoperative nausea and vomiting	Ondansetron	Headache, constipation, and warmth or flushing

Fig. 7.46 The treatment of nausea and vomiting. (5-HT, 5-hydroxytryptamine; SSRIs, selective serotonin reuptake inhibitors)

In addition, new imaging techniques such as magnetic resonance imaging (MRI) have revealed that many regions of the CNS show dynamic fluctuating inflammatory processes in unnamed syndromes involving the CNS. The cause of these lesions is unknown, but could be a virus or similar microbiologic agent.

The CNS is protected by the skull, spinal column, and meningeal membranes, but infectious agents can gain access:

- Through any breach in the CNS protection (e.g. a skull fracture).
- Via the blood (e.g. septicemia with subsequent abscess formation).
- Via the nerves (e.g. rabies virus).
- By uncertain means (e.g. herpes simplex virus [HSV]).

The local immune response of the CNS varies with the site and the infecting organism and the degree and nature of the tissue response to different microbial agents is therefore quite diverse.

The biologic agents that infect the CNS range from helminthic parasites (e.g. *Trichinella spiralis*, a nematode), to fungi and bacteria (e.g. *Coccidioides immitis* and *Mycobacterium tuberculosis*) through to viruses (e.g. HSV) and subviral proteins (e.g. prions in Creutzfeldt–Jacob disease).

Diagnosis of a CNS infection is based on findings from the patient's history, physical examination, and laboratory tests

The signs and symptoms vary and depend on the site affected. They include fever, irritability to the extent of convulsions, altered mentation, altered motor function, and lassitude, drowsiness, or coma. As abscesses and parasitic cysts are space-occupying lesions they can produce symptoms and signs resulting from pressure on or destruction of adjacent structures (e.g. visual field defects due to pressure on or destruction of the optic nerve).

Examination of the CSF can be helpful:

- An increased initial pressure and an increased concentration of CSF protein suggest that there is an infection.
- Microscopy may reveal increased leukocytes (bacterial infection), increased lymphocytes (viral infection), or increased eosinophils (parasitic infection).
- A Gram stain may demonstrate meningococcus (*Neisseria meningitidis*) or *Streptococcus pneumoniae* as the infective agent, while India-ink staining may reveal a fungal infection.

- Biochemical examination may reveal the presence of viruses or parasites or their corresponding antibodies.

Special CNS scanning techniques such as computerized axial tomography (CAT) or MRI also help in the diagnosis, especially of an abscess or other space-occupying lesion.

Whenever bacteria enter the blood stream (septicemia) there is a possibility that a cerebral abscess will develop. Although rare, this can occur after staphylococcal skin infections, for example.

Encephalitis can occur without inflammation of the meninges and vice versa, but they often occur together. Meningeal irritation is due to either an infection or the presence of an inflammation-inducing substance in the CSF (e.g. blood). The particular symptoms and signs of meningeal irritation are:

- A stiff neck.
- Pain on neck flexion.
- Pain accompanying limitation of passive straight leg raising.

These physical findings should always lead to further investigations.

The primary use of drugs for CNS infections is to control or eliminate the causative organism

The organism must be identified and the drug most likely to be selectively toxic is chosen. This drug must be able to reach the site of infection in adequate concentration. It must therefore cross the blood–brain barrier at an adequate rate and there must be adequate access of the drug to the infected site (i.e. abscesses must be surgically treated in addition to any pharmacologic treatment).

A secondary use of drugs for CNS infections is to control responses to the infection

Such responses include seizures, which are treated with antiepileptic drugs (see p. 116), and allergic and other immunologic tissue responses, which are treated with glucocorticosteroids (see Chapter 15).

Antibiotics and antiviral agents do not readily penetrate into the CNS, presumably because of the blood–brain barrier

The relative concentration of penicillin G in the CSF compared with that in the serum is 5%, while that for ampicillin is 15%, nafcillin 5%, vancomycin 10%, chloramphenicol 30%, gentamicin 20%, cefotaxime 15%, ceftriaxone 5% and ceftazidime 20%. The tissue distribution of antibiotics and antivirals is discussed in Chapters 23 and 24.

The question whether antibiotics should be given directly into the CSF has not been satisfactorily answered, but the mortality rate of children with meningitis due to Gram-negative bacilli increases when gentamicin is injected into the cerebral ventricles. This suggests that injecting antibiotics into the CSF carries considerable risk.

Viral meningitis and encephalitis

Almost any virus can cause encephalitis accompanied by varying degrees of meningeal inflammation, including rubeola or mumps virus, a variety of herpes viruses, HSV types 1 and 2, Epstein–Barr virus (EBV), cytomegalovirus (CMV), varicella–zoster virus (VZV), coxsackie virus, and human immunodeficiency virus (HIV) (see Chapter 24).

Treatment involves the use of the appropriate antiviral drug, if such a drug exists, and intravenous administration of drug is almost always required:

- Acyclovir is the drug of choice for treating encephalitis due to HSV-1 and its use has reduced the mortality rate due to this infection from 80% to 20%.
- Ara-A or foscarnet are used for acyclovir-resistant HSV-1 encephalitis.
- Sorivudine* is selective for VZV infections.
- Ganciclovir is useful for CMV encephalitis, but must be used with caution because of bone marrow toxicity and, since it is excreted primarily by the kidneys, renal function should be monitored.

The treatment of cerebral disease in patients with HIV is evolving and involves decisions as to whether HIV or some other agent is causing the problem (see fungal and parasitic infections below).

Several viruses that cause encephalitis (e.g. the virus causing eastern equine encephalitis) are not susceptible to antiviral drugs.

Bacterial meningitis and encephalitis

The bacterium most likely to produce meningitis varies with the age of the patient. The commonest bacteria causing meningitis are:

- Gram-negative bacilli and group B streptococci in neonates less than 1 month old.
- *Haemophilus influenzae, N. meningitidis,* and *S. pneumoniae* in children aged 1 month to 15 years.
- *N. meningitidis, S. pneumoniae* and staphylococci in adults (i.e. those over 15 years of age).

A bacterial cause of a CNS infection must be diagnosed as soon as possible so that specific antibiotic therapy can be instituted. The CSF should be cultured to identify which bacteria are present and appropriate sensitivity tests are indicated to guide the choice of antibiotic.

If the etiology of the CNS infection is unknown but believed to be bacterial, the initial antibiotic therapy is listed in Fig. 7.47. If the bacterial etiology is known, the currently recommended antibiotics of choice for beginning therapy are given in Fig. 7.48.

CNS tuberculosis and syphilis

Mycobacterium tuberculosis and *Treponema pallidum,* the cause of tuberculosis and syphilis, respectively, are important causes of CNS infections.

M. tuberculosis can infect the CNS and cause meningitis, tuberculous abscesses, or widespread miliary tuberculosis in the brain and spinal cord. All these are serious diseases and require appropriate therapy with antibiotics (see Chapter 11).

Syphilitic meningitis and neurosyphilis are manifestations of infection with *T. pallidum* during secondary and tertiary syphilis. Neurosyphilis is often accompanied by changes in mental status and can be mistaken for other forms of mental illness. During tertiary syphilis, syphilitic gummas (areas of focal degeneration of brain tissue similar to abscesses) may form in the CNS. All stages

Initial antibiotic therapy for meningitis or encephalitis if the etiology is unknown but believed to be bacterial

Patient group	Antibiotics
Neonates less than 1 month old	Ampicillin plus either gentamicin or ceftriaxone or cefotaxime
Children aged 1 month to 15 years	Ampicillin plus either chloramphenicol or ceftriaxone or cefotaxime
Adults (i.e. those over 15 years of age)	Ampicillin or penicillin G
Immunocompromised adults	Ampicillin plus ceftriaxone or cefotaxime plus gentamicin
Postcraniotomy patients	Nafcillin plus ceftriaxone or cefotaxime plus gentamicin

Fig. 7.47 Initial antibiotic therapy for meningitis or encephalitis if the etiology is unknown but believed to be bacterial.

Currently recommended initial antibiotic therapy for bacterial meningitis or encephalitis if the bacterial etiology is known

Bacterial cause	Antibiotic
S. pneumoniae, streptococcus A and B, *Listeria monocytogenes, N. meningitidis*	Penicillin G
H. influenzae (β lactamase negative)	Ampicillin
Methicillin-sensitive *Staphylococcus aureus*	Nafcillin
Methicillin-resistant *Staph. aureus*	Vancomycin
H. influenzae (β lactamase positive)	Cefotaxime or ceftriaxone
Escherichia coli, Klebsiella, and *Proteus*	Cefotaxime or ceftriaxone with gentamicin
Pseudomonas aeruginosa	Gentamicin plus ceftazidime

Fig. 7.48 Currently recommended initial antibiotic therapy for bacterial meningitis or encephalitis if the bacterial etiology is known.

of syphilis should be treated with penicillin as soon as they are diagnosed; even gummas are reduced by penicillin treatment.

Fungal CNS infections

Several fungi can cause meningitis and/or focal lesions in the brain and spinal cord, particularly in immunocompromised patients (e.g. in people with AIDS or those who have been treated with anticancer or immunosuppressant drugs). Such fungi include *C. immitis* and *Histoplasma capsulatum* (see Chapter 26). The behavior of these organisms resembles that of *M. tuberculosis* in that they are inhaled and the resulting disease usually involves the lungs, but may involve the CNS, presumably because the organism is transported to the CNS in the blood. The CSF contains complement-fixing antibody in 95% of cases of coccidioimycosis, and the demonstration of such antibodies justifies starting antifungal therapy. In approximately 50% of cases *C. immitis* can be found on microscopic examination of CSF. Complement-fixing antibodies are less common in histoplasmosis and its diagnosis depends on isolating *H. capsulatum* in culture.

Treatment of both coccidioimycosis and histoplasmosis is difficult, but centers on amphotericin B.

Protozoal CNS infections

Malaria Worldwide, cerebral malaria resulting from infection by *Plasmodium falciparum* (see Chapter 25) is probably the most serious and common CNS infection. There are approximately two million deaths due to malaria each year. African children with cerebral malaria account for about half a million of these deaths. The death rate of cerebral malaria is approximately 20% despite the best current treatment, which involves intravenous quinine (or quinidine) or *Artemisia* derivatives such as artemether*.

Toxoplasmosis CNS infections with *Toxoplasma gondii* can occur in immunosuppressed patients. If the immunosuppression has a cause other than AIDS, 2–5% of CNS infections are due to this agent, but in patients with AIDS, the incidence rises to 25–80%. In these conditions, there are often cerebral lesions, which are best detected by MRI. Motor weakness, hemiparesis, and convulsions can occur, depending on the location of the lesions.

The drugs of choice in treating toxoplasmosis are pyrimethamine plus a sulfonamide, but bone marrow depression due to the antifolate activity of pyrimethamine can be a problem. Another antifolate, trimethoprim, is of little value in this disease. The macrolide antibiotic clarithromycin may be of use.

Helminthic CNS infections

Three helminths can infect the CNS: *Trichinella spiralis, Taenia solium*, and *Echinococcus granulosis.* The first two are ingested in infected inadequately cooked pork or game (e.g. bear). *E. granulosis* is harbored by dogs and the eggs are excreted in the feces; they can then be ingested by humans. Once in the intestine, all three parasites can be transported in the blood to the brain where they produce space-occupying cerebral lesions that can be seen on CAT or MRI scans. The neurologic signs they produce will depend on the location of the lesions.

Trichinosis involving the CNS is definitively diagnosed by identifying the larvae in the CSF. It is usually treated with prednisone to suppress the CNS immune response to the nematode, which is often accompanied by marked eosinophilia in the CSF. Mebendazole is given to suppress the parasite.

T. solium cysticerci (larvae) develop in the brain. The definitive diagnosis is by biopsying one of the cystic lesions. Drug treatment involves glucocorticosteroids to suppress immune responses plus albendazole or praziquantel.

Echinococcal cysts usually develop in the liver or lungs but, if they rupture, eggs can then be carried to the brain, where new cystic lesions develop. Such cysts are often detected by CAT or MRI scan. Surgical removal of the cyst is the definitive therapy, but the cyst must not be ruptured otherwise eggs will be spread elsewhere by the blood. Giving albendazole during the surgery may reduce this risk of spreading the infection.

PATHOPHYSIOLOGY AND DISEASES OF THE PERIPHERAL NERVOUS SYSTEM

Peripheral nervous system control of skeletal muscle tone is accomplished mainly through the activities of the somatic nerves and afferent influence from sensory receptors on muscles and tendons. The main controlling influence for somatic nerves is the motor cortex via the pyramidal tracts to the lower motor neuron (α motor neuron), which is the final neuronal pathway to the muscle.

SKELETAL MUSCLE DISORDERS

Myasthenia gravis

Myasthenia gravis is an autoimmune disease affecting the NMJ (Fig. 7.49). Characteristic symptoms are skeletal muscle weakness and fatigability after a brief period of repeated activity with recovery after a short period of rest. However, adequate muscle strength may not always return after a period of rest in those patients in whom the disease has progressed to the crisis level. Additionally, about 85% of myasthenic patients experience generalized weakness involving the eyelids, extraocular muscles, limb muscles, diaphragm, and neck extension muscles. Sometimes the weakness is localized to the eyelids and extraocular muscles, but this occurs in only about 15% of patients and is manifest by the characteristic appearance of drooping eyelids (ptosis).

The prevalence of myasthenia gravis is about 100 cases/million of the population and it usually occurs in women under 50 years of age, though it also occurs in a significant number of men over 60 years of age.

The pathophysiologic features of myasthenia gravis result from a deficit in the number of nicotinic cholinergic receptors at the NMJ

The population of nicotinic cholinergic receptors at myasthenic muscle end plates is only about one-third of that at normal muscle end plates. The receptor deficit appears to be linked to an immunologic response involving the thymus gland, since muscle strength usually improves after the thymus has been removed from myasthenic patients. This immunologic link is supported by the finding of cholinergic receptor antibodies in the serum of some myasthenic patients. Furthermore, it appears that the antigen may be located in the thymus (Fig. 7.50), since cholinergic receptors have been demonstrated on the surface of muscle-like cells in the thymus. The triggering mechanism for the immune response is uncertain, but it may be due to a defect in the regulation of the immune response in myasthenic patients, as normal individuals also have thymic muscle-like cells with cholinergic receptors.

In myasthenia gravis, neurally induced somatic muscle contraction is inadequate for sustained physical activities

This is because the magnitude of neurally induced contraction depends on the number of interactions between ACh and

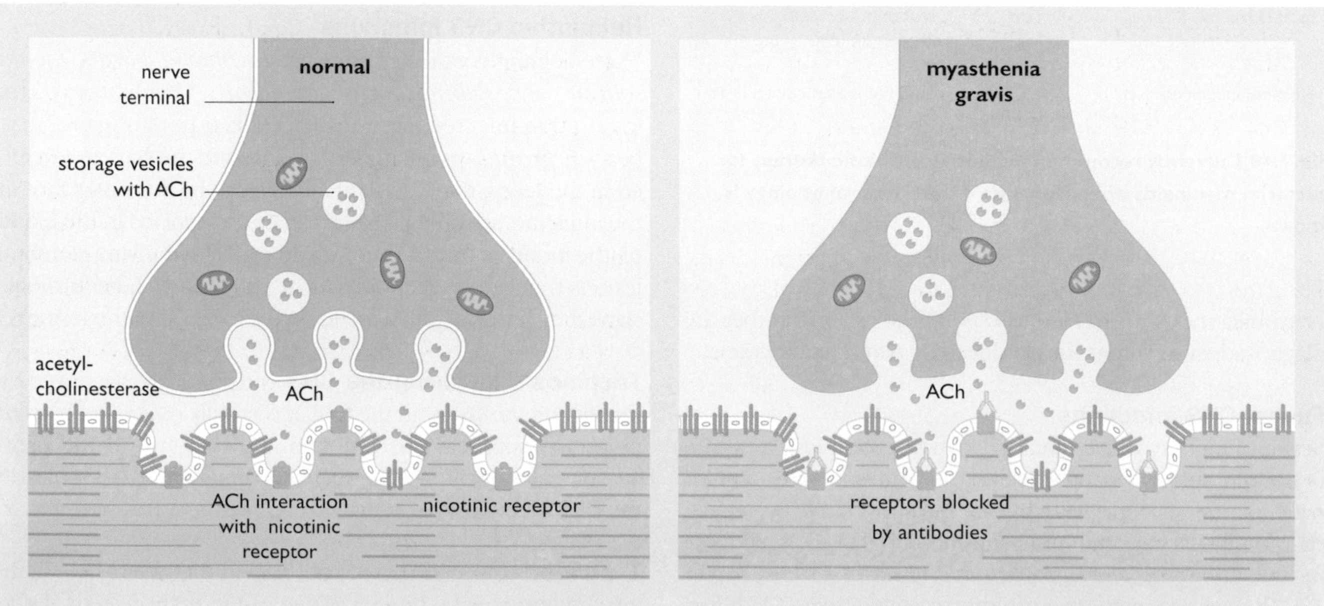

Fig. 7.49 Neurotransmitter release and its interaction with nicotinic receptors at the neuromuscular junction (NMJ). In myasthenia gravis the nicotinic receptors are blocked by antibodies, preventing interaction between the neurotransmitter and the receptor. (ACh, acetylcholine)

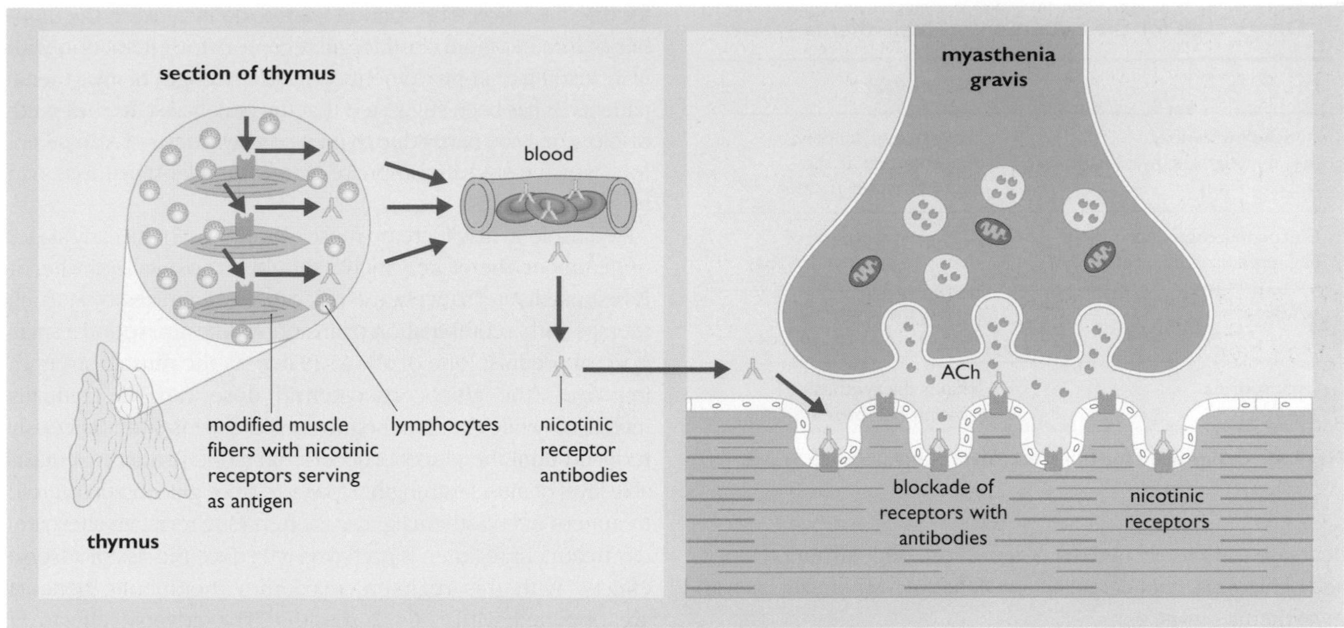

Fig. 7.50 Postulated source of antigen and antibody production in myasthenia gravis. A diagrammatic representation of a section of the thymus gland containing modified muscle cells with nicotinic receptors on the surface. It is suggested that this gland may be the source of the antigen that serves as a template for the production of nicotinic antibodies in myasthenic patients. These antibodies block the nicotinic receptors at the neuromuscular junction and prevent interaction between the neurotransmitter and the nicotinic receptors (see Fig. 7.49). (ACh, acetylcholine)

nicotinic receptors at the NMJ. Normally ACh is released from the nerve terminal and diffuses across the junctional cleft to interact with nicotinic cholinergic receptors on the muscle end plate (see Fig. 7.49). The transmitter–receptor interactions produce a localized end plate potential, mainly due to increased Na^+ permeability (see Chapter 3). If this potential reaches a threshold value, an action potential is produced and invades the muscle fiber, causing contraction. These events are terminated by strategically located acetylcholinesterase enzymes in the synaptic folds, which metabolize ACh. For sustained muscle contraction, this cycle of events must take place in many muscle fibers, which act together to generate muscle power.

In myasthenia gravis, contraction cannot be sustained because the number of transmitter–receptor interactions is lower than normal, owing to the deficit in nicotinic cholinergic receptors at the muscle end plate (see Figs 7.49, 7.50). Furthermore, this subnormal number of transmitter–receptor interactions means that action potentials can be generated only in a small proportion of the muscle fibers. Contraction is therefore likely to fail after a brief period of muscle activity. However, this failure can be prevented by enhancing the number of cholinergic transmitter–receptor interactions.

Effective drug treatment of myasthenia gravis enhances the number of cholinergic transmitter–receptor interactions

Treatment of myasthenia gravis involves procedures that:

- Increase the junctional synaptic concentration of ACh (e.g. anticholinesterase drugs).
- Suppress the immune response.

ANTICHOLINESTERASE DRUGS

ACh is the junctional transmitter that mediates somatic muscle contractions, but it cannot be given effectively as a drug because it is rapidly metabolized by acetylcholinesterase at the NMJ. However, the concentration of ACh at the NMJ can be increased by using anticholinesterase drugs, which inhibit the metabolism of ACh. The peak effects of anticholinesterase drugs are typically obtained promptly during the initial phases of treatment but, after weeks or months of treatment, the drugs often lose their efficacy. It then becomes necessary to add other drugs to the treatment regimen.

Carbamates

The carbamates, particularly neostigmine and pyridostigmine, are among the most widely used anticholinesterase drugs for the treatment of myasthenia gravis (Fig. 7.51). Both drugs reversibly inhibit acetylcholinesterase by binding at its anionic and esteratic sites. During the period of inhibition of 3–6 hours, ACh concentration increases at the NMJ and as a result there are repeated interactions with the reduced number of nicotinic cholinergic receptors. This leads to improved muscle contraction in the myasthenic patient.

Grip strength and vital capacity are usually used for monitoring the improvement in muscle strength produced by anticholinesterases

A short-acting anticholinesterase such as edrophonium chloride is used for this type of monitoring (and for diagnosis of myasthenia gravis). This monitoring procedure is a precautionary measure to prevent excessive dosing, which may

Drugs used for the treatment of myasthenia gravis

Drug	Major effect
Anticholinesterases (e.g. neostigmine, pyridostigmine, ambenonium)	Increase acetylcholine concentration at the neuromuscular junction
Glucocorticosteroids (e.g. prednisolone, prednisone)	Inhibit the synthesis of nicotinic receptor antibody
Azathioprine	Inhibits the synthesis of nicotinic receptor antibody
Cyclosporine	Inhibits the synthesis of nicotinic receptor antibody

Fig. 7.51 Drugs used for the treatment of myasthenia gravis.

decrease muscle strength by ACh-induced depolarization blockade of nicotinic cholinergic receptors at the NMJ of patients with myasthenia gravis.

Longer-acting anticholinesterases

Longer-acting (i.e. over 3–8 hours) anticholinesterases such as ambenonium can also be used in the treatment of myasthenia gravis. However, the organophosphates, which are also long-acting anticholinesterases, are not used because of difficulty in controlling the dose in relation to the patient's need.

Adverse effects of anticholinesterase drugs result from the stimulation of muscarinic receptors and include abdominal cramps, increased salivation, increased bronchial secretion, miosis, and bradycardia. These effects can be controlled with muscarinic receptor antagonists such as atropine, but this is not usually given as it is preferable not to mask the appearance of the muscarinic effects, which are indicative of excessive anticholinesterase treatment. Most patients become tolerant to these adverse effects.

Drug interactions with anticholinesterases The effectiveness of the anticholinesterases is diminished and the symptoms of myasthenia gravis are worsened if the patient is exposed to either tubocurarine (a nondepolarizing neuromuscular blocker) or an aminoglycoside antibiotic, which interferes with neuromuscular transmission.

Drugs that suppress the immune response in myasthenia gravis

Since the effectiveness of anticholinesterase treatment often diminishes within weeks or months, additional therapeutic measures are used. These include the use of immunosuppressant drugs, which are indicated if muscle strength is inadequate.

Glucocorticosteroids

Glucocorticosteroids are used in the treatment of myasthenia gravis because they can inhibit the synthesis of the antibodies to the nicotinic cholinergic receptors at the NMJ (see Fig. 7.51). Prednisolone or prednisone are typical glucocorticosteroids used for this indication. Their action leads to an increase in the number of free nicotinic cholinergic receptors for interaction with ACh, leading to improvement in muscle strength of myasthenic patients. It has been suggested that the beneficial effects of prednisolone may be partly due to increased synthesis of ACh receptors, which would also improve neuromuscular transmission in myasthenia gravis.

Prednisolone may increase muscle weakness in the early stages of treatment, therefore patients should be hospitalized when it is first used. Alternatively, the risk can be minimized by starting therapy with a combination of an anticholinesterase and a small dose of prednisolone of about 20 mg. As the muscle strength improves, the glucocorticosteroid dose can be gradually increased while the anticholinesterase dose is simultaneously reduced until the glucocorticosteroid alone produces a desirable level of muscle strength. However, since glucocorticosteroid treatment of myasthenia gravis is often long term, an alternate-day treatment regimen is preferred to reduce the risk of adverse effects. With this regimen, maximum therapeutic benefits are obtained within 6–12 months. The adverse effects of glucocorticosteroids are described in Chapter 15.

Azathioprine

Azathioprine (see also Chapter 15) is used as an alternative to prednisolone for advanced myasthenia gravis and for myasthenia gravis that does not respond adequately to glucocorticosteroid therapy (see Fig. 7.51). Azathioprine is effective because it suppresses nicotinic cholinergic receptor antibody synthesis by inhibiting T lymphocyte proliferation. However, its therapeutic effectiveness develops slowly, taking up to 1 year to produce satisfactory clinical responses.

Major adverse effects of azathioprine include a reaction similar to influenza, nausea and vomiting, dermatitis, bone marrow depression, and hepatotoxicity.

Cyclosporine

Cyclosporine is another immunosuppressant drug that can be used in the treatment of myasthenia gravis (see Fig. 7.51). Its effectiveness is due to inhibition of the synthesis of nicotinic cholinergic receptor antibody by blocking the activation of T helper cells and, as a consequence, the subsequent events that lead to antibody production are suppressed. The therapeutic benefits of cyclosporine are obtained earlier (within 1–2 months) than with azathioprine.

Major adverse effects of cyclosporine include renal toxicity, hepatotoxicity, hypertension, and tremor (see Chapter 15).

Other approaches to the treatment of myasthenia gravis

Surgical removal of the thymus is often recommended when the dose of immunosuppressant drugs needs to be reduced so as to prevent the development of serious adverse effects. The benefits of surgery include removal of the source responsible for the sustained antigenic stimulation that leads to the production of antibodies to the nicotinic cholinergic receptors at the NMJ.

Plasmapheresis can be used to remove ACh nicotinic receptor antibodies from the circulation, but is used as a short-term therapy only in patients with myasthenia gravis who are experiencing a myasthenic crisis.

SPASTICITY

The major pathophysiologic feature of spasticity is hypertonic muscle contraction. It often occurs as a symptom of neurologic disorders such as cerebral palsy, multiple sclerosis, and stroke. The causes of hypertonia in muscles are:

- Excessive tendon reflexes driven by increased γ neuron activity.
- Flexor muscle spasms, which are due to clonus produced by a volley of discharge from spindle afferents onto several lower motor neurons (α motor neurons).

Spasticity is treated with drugs that reduce excessive afferent stimulation of the α motor neurons innervating the skeletal muscles

Drugs that reduce the excessive afferent stimulation of the lower motor neurons (Fig. 7.52) are preferable to the neuromuscular blockers for treating spasticity because they are more selective. Neuromuscular blockers produce muscle relaxation by disrupting both normal muscle tone and increased tone due to spasm of any etiology.

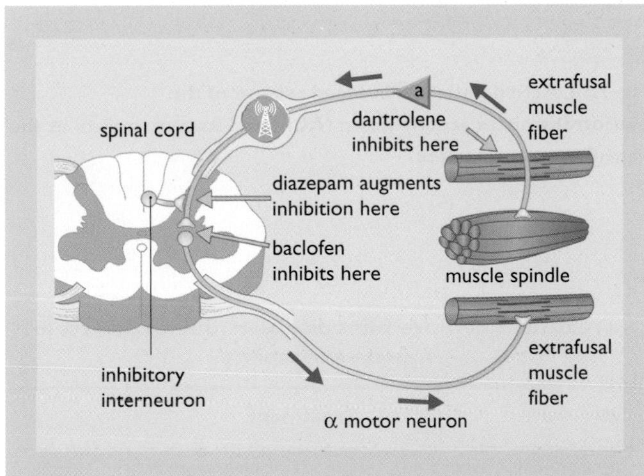

Fig. 7.52 The neuronal pathway that contributes to the development of clonus in spasticity is inhibited by diazepam and baclofen. Stretching the muscle activates the IA afferents from the muscle spindle and sends a flood of impulses to the α motor neuron, triggering contraction of the muscle. This relieves the tension on the spindle and terminates activity in the afferents. However, when the muscle relaxes, the tension on the spindle returns because the sensitivity of the reflex is increased in spasticity and the cycle of events is repeated, giving rise to clonus.

Baclofen

Baclofen is derived from the inhibitory neurotransmitter GABA, and was designed as a source of GABA that could more readily cross the blood–brain barrier.

In the treatment of spasticity, baclofen is most useful for reducing flexor and extensor spasms. These effects are produced at the level of the spinal cord, but are not associated with any interference of voluntary muscle power or normal tendon reflexes. Baclofen produces these effects by inhibiting the afferent input to the lower motor neurons via an interaction with $GABA_B$ receptors on the afferent nerve terminal and the associated interneurons. It is believed that the interaction of baclofen with $GABA_B$ receptors reduces Ca^{2+} influx into the afferent nerve. As a result, less neurotransmitter is released for activating the lower motor neuron, which becomes less active (see Fig. 7.52).

Baclofen is effective for spasticity due to spinal cord lesions and multiple sclerosis, but is ineffective for spasticity due to stroke and other cerebral lesions

Baclofen is usually given orally and it is rapidly absorbed from the gut. It has a plasma half-life of 3–4 hours and is excreted unchanged by the kidneys.

Major adverse effects of baclofen include drowsiness, motor incoordination, mental confusion, and nausea. An overdose may produce seizures, and it is therefore not recommended for patients with epilepsy. Furthermore, baclofen should be withdrawn gradually at the termination of treatment after prolonged use because sudden withdrawal can cause hallucinations, anxiety, and tachycardia.

Diazepam

Diazepam is effective for treatment of spasticity associated with spinal cord lesions, but is less effective than baclofen, especially against flexor spasm

Diazepam is a member of the benzodiazepine group of drugs. It is useful in the treatment of spasticity because it reduces muscle tone by depressing polysynaptic and monosynaptic reflexes. These reflexes help maintain muscle spasticity. Although this action of diazepam can be produced at both spinal and supraspinal levels, it appears that the spinal level is the important site of action in reducing spasticity. To produce this effect in the spinal cord, diazepam binds (via benzodiazepine receptors) to $GABA_A$ receptor complexes on afferent nerve terminals that synapse with lower motor neurons (see Fig. 7.52). It therefore increases presynaptic inhibition mediated by GABA by increasing Cl^- influx (Fig. 7.53).

Dantrolene sodium

Unlike baclofen and diazepam, dantrolene sodium relieves spasticity by a direct action on skeletal muscle (Fig. 7.53).

Dantrolene sodium is a hydantoin derivative that not only relieves spasticity but also produces muscle weakness, which reduces its clinical usefulness. Its mechanism of action involves interference with skeletal muscle excitation–contraction coupling by decreasing the amount of Ca^{2+} released from the sarcoplasmic reticulum. This reduces the tension generated by the muscle.

Dantrolene sodium is mainly used to relieve the spasticity of paraplegia and hemiplegia

Dantrolene sodium is usually given orally, but is not completely absorbed. It has a half-life of 9 hours and is metabolized by the liver.

Adverse effects of dantrolene sodium include muscle weakness and sedation, and sometimes hepatotoxicity.

MOVEMENT DISORDERS RESULTING FROM DEFECTS IN MUSCLE EXCITABILITY

Although many movement disorders are attributed to defects in the basal ganglia, some disorders result from impaired skeletal muscle excitability (e.g. Lambert–Eaton syndrome, McCardle syndrome, congenital myotonia, and tetany).

Lambert–Eaton syndrome (myasthenia syndrome)

Lambert–Eaton syndrome is a syndrome associated with a variety of malignancies, especially lung cancer. As the NMJ is the site of the defect, it resembles myasthenia gravis. However, it differs from myasthenia gravis because the weakness, which particularly affects the limb muscles, does not respond to anticholinesterases. This is because, unlike myasthenia gravis, which results from a reduction in the number of cholinergic receptors at the NMJ, Lambert–Eaton syndrome results from disrupted coupling between nerve terminal excitation and ACh release at the NMJ (Fig. 7.54). In some patients this is associated with autoantibodies directed against neuronal Ca^{2+} channels. Consequently, approaches to treatment involve procedures that increase the release of transmitter at the NMJ. These include:

- Physical exercise, which improves muscle power.
- Ca^{2+} salts, which seem to be beneficial because Ca^{2+} plays an important role in the release of neurotransmitter from nerve terminals (Figs 7.54, 7.55).

McCardle syndrome

Characteristically, the main symptoms of this syndrome are disabling weakness, muscle pain, and stiffness after a brief period of exercise. These symptoms are produced because the muscles fail to relax, owing to inadequate production of ATP, which is necessary for Ca^{2+} sequestration in the sarcoplasmic reticulum to terminate contraction. The underlying cause of inadequate ATP production is an inability to liberate glucose from glycogen due to an inherited deficiency of glycogen phosphorylase in the muscles. These patients have only a limited supply of ATP from blood glucose and fatty acids for muscle activity, which is therefore short.

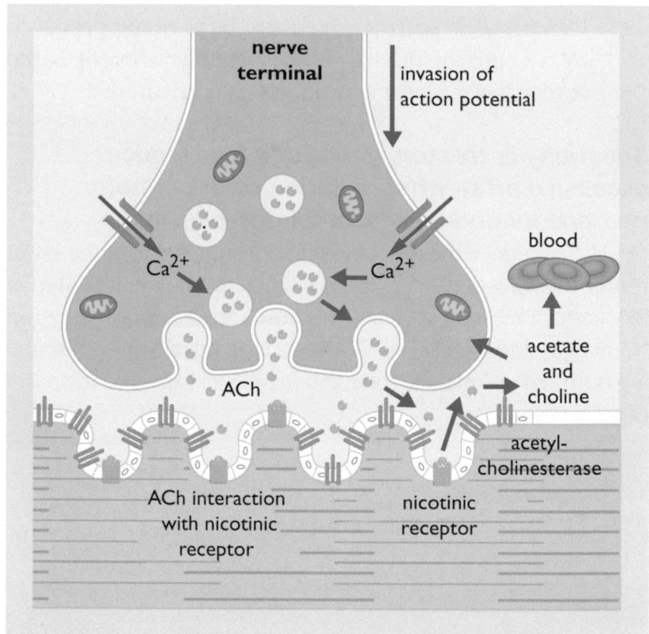

Fig. 7.54 Action potential-induced release of the neurotransmitter acetylcholine (ACh) and its metabolism at the neuromuscular junction.

Drugs used for treatment of spasticity

Drugs	Mechanism of action
Baclofen	Inhibits flexor and extensor muscle spasm via $GABA_B$ receptor-mediated blockade of afferent stimulation of the α motor neuron
Diazepam	$GABA_A$ receptor-mediated presynaptic inhibition of afferent stimulation of the α motor neuron
Dantrolene sodium	Inhibition of skeletal muscle excitation–contraction coupling by decreasing Ca^{2+} released from the sarcoplasmic reticulum

Fig. 7.53 Drugs used for treatment of spasticity. (GABA, γ-aminobutyric acid)

Treatment of movement disorders due to defects in muscle excitability

Disorder	Treatment
Lambert–Eaton syndrome	Ca^{2+} salts, physical exercise
McCardle syndrome	Large doses of glucose, injection of epinephrine or glucagon
Congenital myotonia	Membrane stabilizers such as quinine and phenytoin
Tetany	Normalise plasma Ca^{2+}

Fig. 7.55 Treatment of movement disorders due to defects in muscle excitability.

Treatment of this syndrome includes the administration of large doses of glucose or the injection of epinephrine or glucagon to increase glucose release from the liver (see Fig. 7.55).

Congenital myotonia

Congenital myotonia is an inherited disorder characterized by violent muscle spasm due to irritability of the muscle fiber membrane. The irritability is due to a structural defect in the muscle fiber membrane that renders the fiber hyperexcitable and therefore easily re-excited by the afterpotential that follows an action potential.

Membrane stabilizers such as quinine and phenytoin can be used to reduce the frequency and severity of the spasm.

Tetany

Tetany is characterized by widespread muscular twitching, together with persistent contraction of muscles in the hands and feet, resulting in painful cramps. The cause of tetany is due to hypocalcemia, which increases excitability of the somatic nerves. It is suggested that low extracellular Ca^{2+} decreases the depolarizing current that is required to open Na^{+} channels in somatic nerves and causes repetitive firing, leading to persistent muscle contraction.

Tetany is treated with Ca^{2+} salts (e.g. Ca^{2+} gluconate) to restore extracellular Ca^{2+} concentrations.

PATHOPHYSIOLOGY AND DISORDERS OF THE AUTONOMIC NERVOUS SYSTEM

Dysautonomias are disorders associated with defects in the autonomic nervous system (e.g. familial dysautonomia [Riley–Day syndrome], Shy–Drager syndrome, and Horner's syndrome).

FAMILIAL DYSAUTONOMIA

This is an inherited disorder transmitted as an autosomal recessive trait and characterized by a complex mixture of symptoms. It is more common in Ashkenazi Jewish infants than in any other ethnic group. Manifestations of the disorder are usually present at birth and the child commonly dies during infancy. The major symptoms include an inability to control body temperature and to produce tears, uncontrollable perspiration, hypertension and sometimes postural hypotension, corneal and pain insensitivity, fever, and frequent episodes of pneumonia. These symptoms are associated with defects in both the parasympathetic and sympathetic divisions of the autonomic nervous system as well as defects in some peripheral sensory nerves (Fig. 7.56). The cutaneous nerves contain a decreased number of unmyelinated fibers, which are the neuronal pathways for pain and temperature sensation. Neurons in the vagus and the glossopharyngeal nerves are typically smaller and

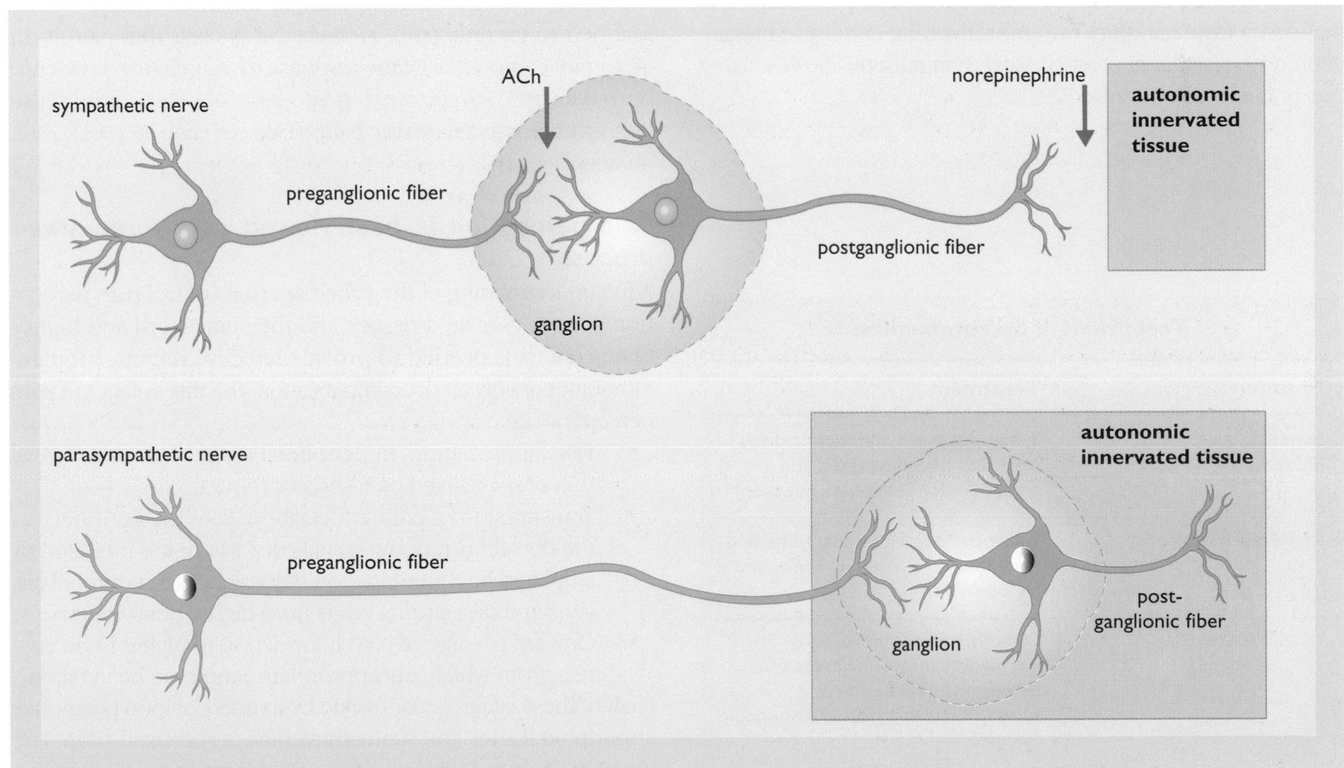

Fig. 7.56 The two major divisions of the autonomic nervous system that may become defective in dysautonomia.

reduced in number. Similarly, there appear to be fewer neurons in the cervical and thoracic sympathetic ganglia.

Treatment is symptomatic as there is no cure (Fig. 7.57). Sedatives and the phenothiazine drugs are often used for gastrointestinal and behavioral symptoms. In addition, antibiotics are used for pulmonary infection, which is quite common.

SHY–DRAGER SYNDROME

This syndrome is also due to autonomic nervous system failure. It is characterized by a complex mixture of symptoms, which include severe postural hypotension, urinary incontinence, male erectile dysfunction, akinesia, tremor, muscle rigidity, and the inability to sweat. Pathologic evidence suggests that the autonomic deficiency is due to a loss of preganglionic sympathetic cells from the intermediolateral column of cells in the spinal cord. There also appears to be CNS motor control involvement with the syndrome, as reflected in the symptoms of akinesia and muscle rigidity.

The most troublesome symptom is postural hypotension, which is treated with small doses of fludrocortisone (0.1 mg). This increases Na^+ and water retention and may increase the sensitivity of blood vessels to catecholamines. α Adrenoceptor agonists are also used, including phenylephrine and ephedrine; however, the disadvantage of these drugs is that they tend to produce hypertension when the patient is supine.

HORNER'S SYNDROME

Horner's syndrome results from a loss of cervical sympathetic control to the head. It is characterized by miosis due to the loss of pupillary dilation, slight drooping of the eyelids (ptosis), recession of the eyeball (enophthalmos), facial vasodilation, and loss of the ability to sweat. These symptoms are often unilateral and may result from an injury or tumor involving either the preganglionic or postganglionic cervical sympathetic nerves. Lung cancer is a common cause.

Treatment of dysautonomias

Disorder	Treatment
Familial dysautonomia (Riley–Day syndrome)	Symptomatic (i.e. autonomic drugs, sedatives, phenothiazines, and antibiotics for pulmonary infection)
Shy–Drager syndrome	Fludrocortisone, phenylephrine, and ephedrine to counteract the postural hypotension
Horner's syndrome	Directly and indirectly acting sympathomimetics for preganglionic lesions and directly acting sympathomimetics for postganglionic lesions

Fig. 7.57 Treatment of dysautonomias.

The location of the lesion must be clearly defined for effective treatment, for example:

- If the lesion is confined to preganglionic fibers, both directly and indirectly acting sympathomimetics (phenylephrine, ephedrine, and cocaine) are effective (e.g. restore a mydriatic response). This is because their effects are mediated via direct action on the tissue receptor and indirectly by the release of stored norepinephrine from the postganglionic nerve terminal, respectively (see Fig. 7.56).
- If the lesion is on the postganglionic fiber, only the directly acting sympathomimetics (e.g. phenylephrine) are therapeutically effective. The indirectly acting agents are ineffective because they act on postganglionic fibers.

PAIN

Pain is a normal manifestation of everyday life and serves a vital defensive function. However, uncontrolled pain can dramatically diminish quality of life. Pain is often associated with a range of other psychologic and central disturbances (e.g. anxiety, depression, insomnia, anorexia) and profound changes in autonomic function (e.g. heart rate, blood pressure, micturition).

Pain can be subdivided into acute and chronic forms.

- Acute pain is short term, generally persisting only for the duration of the tissue damage, and represents a natural, physiologic defense reaction of the body.
- Chronic pain is evident even when the normal healing mechanisms have been completed, and in diseases such as rheumatoid arthritis may persist for weeks, months, or even years.

It is not known what physiologic function, if any, can be ascribed to chronic pain. However, it is clear that pain is an important component of the response to trauma (e.g. accidents, burn damage), surgery (e.g. postoperative pain), and disease (e.g. arthritis, cancer, cardiac pain, sickle cell crisis, herpes zoster, myofascial pain).

Pain perception is best viewed as a three-stage process

A full understanding of the processes that control pain perception in both damaged tissues and the spinal cord and higher brain centers is needed to provide effective therapy for pain. Although possibly an oversimplification, the three stages of pain perception are:

- Pain 'appreciation' in peripheral tissues following activation of specialized pain sensors (nociceptors).
- Transmission of pain information from the periphery to the dorsal horn of the spinal cord where it is inhibited or amplified by a combination of local (spinal) neuronal circuits and descending tracts from higher brain centers.
- Onward passage of pain information to higher brain centers, from which any appropriate action can be initiated.

Each of these stages is controlled by a variety of local hormones at peripheral sites and neurotransmitters at central sites. The interactions between the various neurotransmitters are highly complex and have not yet been clearly defined.

The first step in the perception of pain appears to be activation of pain-specific receptors called nociceptors in the peripheral tissues

Unlike other sensory receptors that detect, for example, mechanical pressure or temperature changes, nociceptors (Fig. 7.58) are poorly defined anatomically. It seems likely that they are simply bare nerve endings in the skin, muscle, and deeper viscera. Exactly how they are activated following, for example, tissue damage, remains a mystery, although a number of chemical mediators known to be present at the site of tissue disease or decay can stimulate nociceptors and therefore promote pain (see Fig. 7.58). Inflammatory mediators included in this group include histamine (also causes itching) and bradykinin (BK). When applied in low doses to an exposed blister base in human volunteers, both histamine and BK are able to trigger a painful response (Fig. 7.59). BK acts via G protein-linked receptors to produce a range of proinflammatory effects including vasodilation and edema. BK receptor stimulation also activates membrane-bound phospholipase A_2 enzyme activity, which in turn causes membrane de-esterification, leading to the release of free arachidonic acid (eicosatetraenoic acid) and the subsequent biosynthesis of prostaglandins (e.g. PGE_2 and prostacyclin, PGI_2) by cyclooxygenase (COX). It is therefore not surprising that there are PGs at the site of the inflammatory response (e.g. PGs are found in synovial fluid aspirated from the joints of patients with rheumatoid arthritis or osteoarthritis). Once synthesized, PGs cause hyperalgesia but not algesia. Physiologic concentrations of PGs (PGE_2, PGI_2) do not cause pain when applied to exposed blister bases in human volunteers or following intradermal injection in animals. However, such concentrations of PGs powerfully accentuate the pain-producing effect of mechanical or chemical stimulation, as well as that resulting from the application of chemical agents such as histamine and BK (see Figs 7.56, 7.57).

5-HT is another local hormone that triggers pain responses from peripheral nociceptors. It is released from degranulating mast cells at the site of tissue damage and triggers a powerful pain response, which is probably greater than that elicited by either BK or histamine. A variety of metabolic substances released from damaged cells (e.g. ATP, lactic acid, K^+) also exhibit algesic activity.

Pain-related definitions

- Pain is an unpleasant sensory and emotional experience associated with actual or potential tissue damage
- Acute pain is pain of recent onset and limited duration. It usually has an identifiable cause relating to injury or disease
- Chronic pain is pain that persists for long periods, usually beyond the time of tissue healing, and for which the cause may not necessarily be easily identifiable
- Hyperalgesia is tenderness and/or pain arising from relatively innocuous stimulation
- A noxious stimulus is a stimulus that damages or is potentially damaging to the tissue
- Nociception is the process of detecting and signalling the presence of a noxious stimulus. This term is frequently reserved to describe the process in experimental animals
- Pain behavior is behavior that leads an informed observer to conclude that a human or an experimental animal is experiencing pain
- An algogen is a chemical mediator that promotes pain behavior and is usually generated within diseased or damaged tissue
- An analgesic drug is a drug or therapy that effectively removes or at least curtails pain sensation in humans
- An antinociceptive drug is a drug or therapy that effectively removes or at least curtails pain behavior

The second step in pain perception is the transfer of information from stimulated nociceptors in the periphery to the spinal cord

Information is transferred from stimulated nociceptors in the periphery to the spinal cord by:

- Myelinated Aδ fibers, which transmit information rapidly at a rate of approximately 15 m/s and appear to produce a sharp and intense pain sensation.

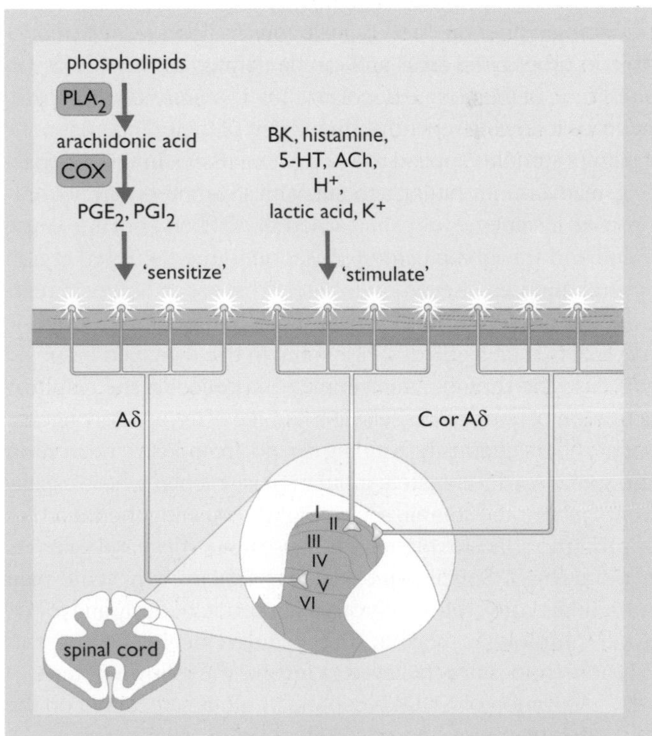

Fig. 7.58 Perception of pain. (ACh, acetylcholine; BK, bradykinin; COX, cyclooxygenase; 5-HT, 5-hydroxytryptamine; PG, prostaglandin; PLA, phospholipase A)

- Unmyelinated C fibers, which transmit information more slowly at a rate of approximately 1 m/s and appear to produce a less well-localized pain that may be described as a dull and throbbing ache.

The cell bodies of both Aδ and C fibers lie within the dorsal root ganglion, from which fibers enter the dorsal spinal cord through the dorsal root to synapse with so-called 'nociresponsive' neurons located in the superficial laminae I and II and to a lesser extent lamina V (Aδ fibers only) (Figs 7.58, 7.60). Excitatory amino acids (EAA) such as glutamate and neurokinins such as substance P and neurokinin A act as neurotransmitters at the junction between primary afferent nerve terminals and spinal cord nociresponsive neurons.

Electrophysiologic analysis of membrane potentials from dorsal horn nociresponsive cells in response to peripheral noxious stimuli reveals a complex pattern of electrical activity

An early rapid membrane depolarization takes place and has been ascribed to activation of AMPA (2-amino-3, 3-hydroxy 5-methlisooxazol-4-yl propionic acid) receptors by glutamate released from primary afferent nerves. This initial response is followed by a more slowly developing secondary depolarization. Glutamate acting on *N*-methyl D-aspartate (NMDA) receptors and substance P are generally considered to be the major neurotransmitters at this site, but other neuropeptides such as vasoactive intestinal polypeptide, somatostatin, and cholecystokinin may also regulate this process.

An additional important role for glutamate acting on NMDA receptors located on the spinal nociresponsive neurons is the induction of a process called spinal 'wind up.' This electrophysiologic phenomenon is analogous to 'long-term potentiation' in other brain areas and can be defined as the increase in amplitude of membrane depolarization in spinal nociresponsive neurons following repetitive stimulation of their C fiber input by a painful stimulus applied to a peripheral tissue. In this way, pain (e.g. inadvertently hitting a thumb with a hammer) may not only provoke instantaneous pain (carried by Aδ fibers) but also cause a dull and throbbing painful sensation in the damaged region several minutes or even hours later. This secondary pain reaction is triggered by the formation of proinflammatory algesic mediators such as BK and histamine in the damaged tissue, in this case the thumb. As inflammation proceeds, the resulting activation of nociceptors sets up a barrage of impulses along sensory C fibers, gradually 'winding up' nociresponsive neurons in the spinal cord. Ultimately, a situation is reached where usually nontroublesome stimuli, such as lightly brushing the thumb or applying an adhesive plaster, can cause tenderness and pain (i.e. hyperalgesia). Spinal 'wind up' may explain why acute pain sometimes converts into chronic pain spontaneously and for no good physiologic reason. The cellular mechanism of this phenomenon is now believed to involve the following steps:

- Activation of NMDA receptors by glutamate, either on the nociresponsive neuron itself or on adjacent neurons.
- Opening of NMDA-linked Ca^{2+} channels in these neurons.
- Activation of Ca^{2+}–calmodulin-dependent nitric oxide synthase (NOS) to yield nitric oxide (NO).

NO is a freely diffusible and highly lipid-soluble mediator and rapidly passes retrogradely to the primary afferent nerve terminal to increase efflux of glutamate (and perhaps also substance P). In this way, the initial release of even a very small amount of glutamate from sensory C fiber terminals is able to trigger the efflux of larger and larger quantities of glutamate, enhancing depolarization of the nociresponsive neuron and ultimately completing the 'wind up' process. It might therefore be predicted that breaking this 'circle' by administering NOS inhibitors such as L-N^G-nitro-arginine methyl ester (L-NAME) in experimental animals will relieve pain. Whether such drugs will be effective for chronic pain awaits the identification of novel NOS inhibitors with fewer adverse effects that can be studied in humans.

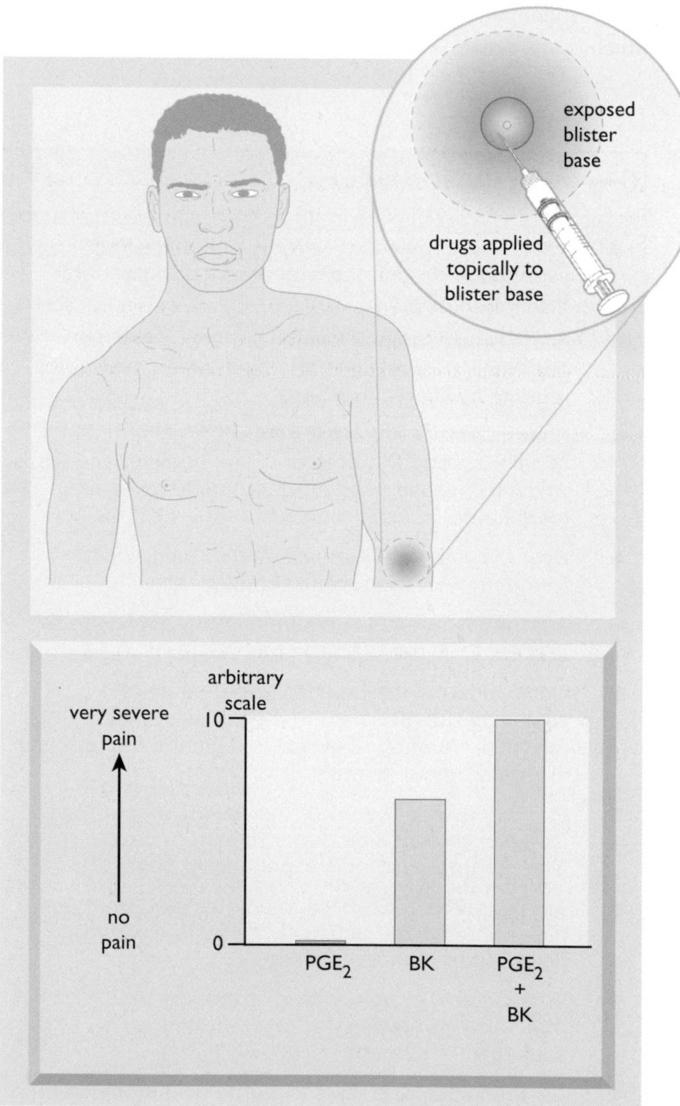

Fig. 7.59 The role of bradykinin (BK) and prostaglandin (PG) in pain. In low doses BK is algesic (i.e. causes pain), whereas PGE_2 is hyperalgesic (i.e. not painful by itself, but potentiates BK-induced algesia).

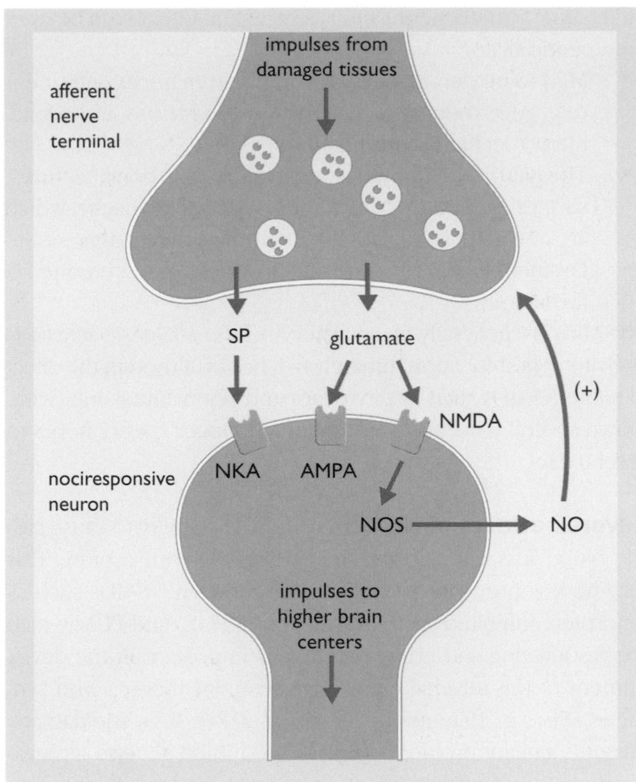

Fig. 7.60 Mechanism of pain perception. Activation of nociceptors in damaged, diseased, or inflamed tissues by a range of algesic and hyperalgesic chemical mediators stimulates Aδ and C sensory afferent nerves, which terminate in the superficial laminae (I and II) and lamina V of the spinal cord. Nitric oxide (NO) is the retrograde transmitter increasing substance P (SP) and glutamate release to cause 'wind-up.' (AMPA, 2-amino-3, 3-hydroxy-5-methylisooxazol-4-yl propionic acid ; NKA, neurokinin A; NMDA, *N*-methyl D-aspartate receptors; NOS, nitric oxide synthase)

Electric activity of spinal nociresponsive neurons is 'fine tuned' by neurotransmitters released from spinal neurons and major supraspinal descending nerve bundles

Perhaps the greatest local control over spinal cord pain sensitivity is provided by opioid peptides, particularly Met-enkephalin and β-endorphin, and perhaps to a lesser extent Leu-enkephalin and dynorphin. Each of these peptides is located within neurons of laminae I and II of the dorsal spinal cord and each provokes analgesia by interacting with specific opioid receptors (i.e. μ, δ, and κ).

As intrathecally applied opioids such as morphine are analgesic their site of action must be spinal, but systemically administered opioids may also influence pain perception by an effect on higher brain centers. The mechanism of action of opioids at the spinal level involves inhibiting the release of substance P and glutamate from C fiber terminals, but the cellular mechanism of action is not clear.

Opioid receptors have been cloned and belong to the G protein-coupled family of receptor proteins

Activation of opioid receptors has a number of cellular consequences, including inhibition of adenylyl cyclase activity leading to a reduction in intracellular cAMP concentration. This fall in neuronal cAMP was believed to account entirely for the analgesic effect of opioids. However, more recent studies indicate that other cellular results of opioid receptor activation are also important including:

- Opening of K^+ channels to cause hyperpolarization of the nociresponsive neuron, thereby reducing excitability.
- Blocking the opening of voltage-gated Ca^{2+} channels to inhibit glutamate and substance P release from primary afferent terminals.

Other neurotransmitters that play a part in controlling the function of nociresponsive neurons include GABA, which has also been detected by mapping the synthetic enzyme glutamic acid decarboxylase (GAD) in the dorsal spinal cord. Like opioids, GABA acting on $GABA_B$ receptors located presynaptically on primary afferent nerve fibers is believed to reduce the release of glutamate and substance P. In this way, baclofen, which is a GABAB agonist, produces behavioral antinociception in experimental animals.

The third step in the perception of pain is the onward passage of pain information to higher brain centers

The plethora of excitatory and inhibitory neuronal inputs acting on nociresponsive neurons in the dorsal spinal cord highlights the major importance of these neurons in transferring information from nociceptors in the tissues to the brain. This function underlies the 'gate control' theory of pain put forward by Melzack and Wall in the mid-1960s, according to which nociresponsive neurons of lamina I and II act as intelligent 'gatekeepers' between damaged tissues and the brain. The information they receive is modified by both spinal and supraspinal influences before being transmitted as a 'package' of knowledge about the painful stimulus to higher centers. The ascending nociceptive pathways involved in this final stage of the process travel in the ventrolateral and dorsolateral funiculi of the spinal cord and terminate mainly in the thalamus and reticular formation. Further ascending tracts terminate in the cerebral cortex and limbic systems where the cognitive and emotional aspects of pain are coordinated.

TESTING ANALGESIC DRUGS

A wide variety of procedures are available to assess analgesic drugs. Tests used in human volunteers include:

- Application of a tourniquet to the upper arm, measuring the length of time the volunteer can bear the resulting ischemia-induced discomfort. This is probably the best-characterized human model of pain.
- Application of radiant heat or pressure to the skin.
- Electric shock stimulation of the skin or tooth pulp.
- Cold pressor tests in which the arm or hand is placed in ice-cold water and the time to removal recorded.
- Intraperitoneal injection of BK.

Experimental subjects use a variety of techniques to quantify their perception of the level of pain

Objective measurement of pain is not usually possible. Experimental subjects (volunteers or patients) are therefore required to express an opinion on their perception of the level of pain. This is commonly obtained using a sliding scale, which can either be verbal (e.g. 0 for no pain to 10 for worst possible pain) or visual (e.g. placing a mark on a 10 cm line graded from no pain to the worst possible pain). Occasionally such a system cannot be used. For example, assessing pain in young children is difficult, using such scales. The children can then be asked to draw a face that can be graded between a happy face to indicate no pain and a sad face to indicate intense pain. Clearly, all these measurements are highly subjective and properly trained personnel and rigorous statistical evaluation of the results are needed to avoid misleading or biased conclusions. Furthermore, the personality of the individual and other factors such as the nature of the environment in which testing takes place and the general attitude of the investigator can markedly affect the response of individuals to pain. There is therefore a need for randomization, allocating subjects to control and test groups. Despite these problems, however, each of the tests described above has been used with varying degrees of success to demonstrate drug-induced analgesia.

DRUG THERAPY OF PAIN

Nonsteroidal anti-inflammatory drugs (NSAIDs)

The NSAIDs inhibit the biosynthesis of hyperalgesic and proinflammatory PGs and form a chemically disparate group of drugs. Pharmacologically, NSAIDs exhibit anti-inflammatory, antipyretic, and mild analgesic activity.

Tissue damage and the accompanying plasma membrane distortion activate phospholipase A_2 enzyme activity, which cleaves free arachidonic acid from its binding sites in membrane phospholipids and renders it susceptible to attack by cyclooxygenase (COX or PGH synthase). All NSAIDs inhibit COX activity and this effect underlies their analgesic activity. Two separate isoforms of COX have been identified:

- COX-1 is a constitutive enzyme found in a wide variety of cells throughout the body; it maintains the formation of PGs involved in 'housekeeping' (i.e. control of vascular flow through individual organs).
- COX-2 is synthesized *de novo* in inflammatory cells such as neutrophils and mast cells following exposure to bacterial endotoxins and/or cytokines (e.g. tumor necrosis factor [TNF] and interleukin 1β). It is responsible for generating PGs at the site of inflammation and/or tissue damage.

Most NSAIDs show little or no selectivity as inhibitors of the two COX isoforms with the exception of meloxicam*, which is a relatively selective inhibitor of COX-2 and combines anti-inflammatory and antinociceptive activity in experimental animals.

There are numerous NSAIDs and each can be used to treat mild to moderate pain with an inflammatory component

Aspirin is the archetypal NSAID and was first used clinically in 1899. Since then numerous other NSAIDs have been developed including acetaminophen, ibuprofen, naproxen, fenoprofen, mefenamic acid, tolmetin, and piroxicam, and each can be used therapeutically for:

- Mild to moderate pain with an inflammatory component (e.g. gout, rheumatoid arthritis, osteoarthritis, toothache, ultraviolet light-induced sunburn).
- The pain of cancer metastases, injury (e.g. bone fractures, surgical procedures), and some types of headache, which are also associated with an inflammatory reaction.
- Dysmenorrhea, which results from increased uterine PG formation.

NSAIDs are generally given orally and the analgesic activity is likely to persist for approximately 6–8 hours, although the effect of some NSAIDs such as piroxicam and phenylbutazone (withdrawn several years ago) can last much longer (i.e. 12 hours to several days).

Adverse effects of NSAIDs include the ability to cause gastric blood loss and ulceration, particularly with aspirin. This may be less prevalent with the more modern NSAIDs such as ibuprofen. Inhibited gastric formation of PGE_2 and PGI_2, which are vasodilating and cytoprotective, is important in the development of this adverse effect. Replacement therapy with synthetic PG (e.g. 15-methyl PGE_2) is available if gastric damage presents a major problem. NSAIDs also inhibit platelet aggregation and accelerate bleeding time as a result of inhibiting platelet formation of thromboxane A_2 (TxA_2), which is vasoconstricting and proaggregatory. Other adverse effects include dizziness, headache, and water and sodium chloride retention (all adverse effects of piroxicam). Finally, large doses of aspirin (1000–1500 mg/day) and other NSAIDs can cause auditory and visual disturbances accompanied by fever and changes in blood pH, and sometimes coma.

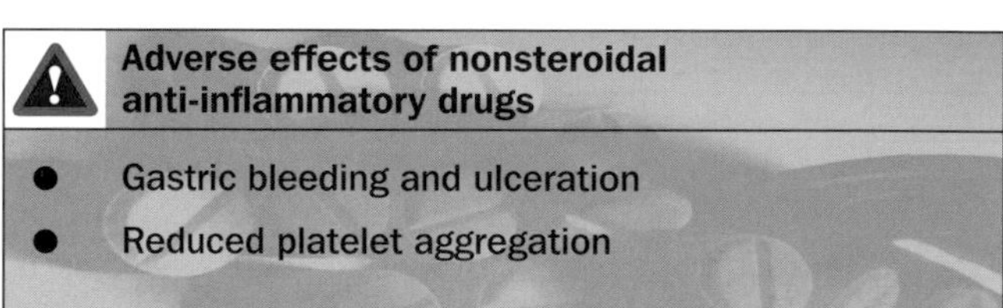
Adverse effects of nonsteroidal anti-inflammatory drugs

- Gastric bleeding and ulceration
- Reduced platelet aggregation

Opioids

All opioid drugs, whether naturally occurring like morphine or chemically synthesized, interact with specific opioid receptors to produce their pharmacologic effects. The three major classes of opioid receptors are μ, δ, and κ. A fourth opioid receptor (σ) was suggested, but a variety of other nonopioid drugs also appear to act as ligands at this site so it is doubtful whether the σ receptor should now be considered a true opioid receptor. Further subclassification of some opioid receptors (e.g. into μ_1 and μ_2) has been suggested on the basis of ligand binding and other experiments, but their pharmacologic and clinical significance remains obscure. Drugs interact with opioid receptors as either full agonists, partial agonists, mixed agonists (full agonist on one opioid receptor, but partial agonist on another), or antagonists (see Chapter 3 for definitions). Opioids include morphine, codeine phosphate, meperidine hydrochloride, papaveretum, heroin hydrochloride, etorphine*, methadone hydrochloride, and fentanyl.

Opioids are useful for most moderate to severe pain, and particularly postoperative or cancer-related pain

Opioids have less effect against nerve pain (neuropathic pain) such as trigeminal neuralgia or phantom limb pain. In addition to their analgesic effect, opioid drugs have a variety of other actions within the CNS, but not all are beneficial. For example, opioids cause euphoria accompanied by a general sense of peace and contentment, which accounts for the illicit use of such drugs by addicts. This calming activity undoubtedly contributes to their analgesic efficacy by helping to relieve the anxiety and distress associated with pain, and this can be important in the treatment of acute myocardial infarction, for example. Morphine-induced euphoria appears to be mediated by activation of μ and/or κ receptors, which are presumably located within the limbic system.

Opioid analgesics are administered systemically (oral, intramuscularly, or subcutaneously) or directly into the spinal cord (intrathecally). Usually a loading dose is given, followed by maintenance dosing to ensure steady-state plasma concentrations.

Tolerance and dependence Tolerance develops rapidly to the analgesic effect of opioids and can often be detected within 12–24 hours of administration. As a result, larger and larger doses of the drug are needed to achieve the same clinical effect, leading to an increased severity and incidence of adverse effects. Physical dependence may develop and is characterized by a definite abstinence syndrome following drug withdrawal. This syndrome comprises a complex mixture of irritable and sometimes aggressive behavior coupled with extremely unpleasant autonomic symptoms such as fever, sweating, yawning, and pupillary dilation.

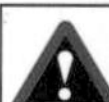 **Adverse effects of opioid drugs**

- Respiratory depression (μ, δ, and κ receptors)
- Constipation (variable, μ, and κ receptors)
- Nausea and vomiting
- Pupillary constriction (μ/δ receptors)
- Rapid development of tolerance
- Physical dependence and abstinence syndrome

Adverse effects of opioids tend to limit the dose that can be given and the analgesia that can be maintained. They are all direct consequences of opioid receptor activation and relate largely to the preponderance of opioid receptors in the medulla and peripheral nervous system. They can therefore be inhibited by opioid receptor antagonists such as naloxone. The most serious adverse effect is probably respiratory depression, which results from reduced sensitivity of the medullary respiratory centers to carbon dioxide. It is the most common cause of death from opioid overdose. Another common adverse effect is constipation due to changes in lower gastrointestinal smooth muscle tone resulting in decreased propulsion. Other adverse effects include pupillary constriction (miosis) and vomiting via an action on the CTZ in the medulla (see p. 130). The antitussive activity of opioids is an adverse effect that has been exploited clinically and as a result codeine and dextromethorphan are frequently included in proprietary cold medicines (see Chapter 11).

Pharmacologic adjuncts to analgesia

Benzodiazepines Severe pain can lead to intense emotional distress and therefore drug therapy of the associated anxiety is frequently considered to be helpful. The benzodiazepines are often used for this purpose. Diazepam and lorazepam are usually the drugs of choice, providing effective anxiolytic cover over a long period coupled with a mild amnesic effect which, although beneficial in some patients, can cause distress and confusion, particularly in older patients.

Nitrous oxide (N_2O) is another adjunct to analgesia. It is a useful analgesic in its own right for acutely painful procedures of short duration (e.g. dental procedures, childbirth) and the analgesia it provides when inhaled (sometimes as a 50% mixture in air i.e. entonox) is rapid in both onset and offset.

Ketamine was originally introduced as a dissociative anesthetic, but can also provide useful short-term analgesia, although unpleasant adverse effects such as delirium and bizarre hallucinations limit its widespread use.

Opioids and NSAIDs are the mainstay of pain relief, but cannot be considered to be 'ideal' analgesics

Both opioids and NSAIDs are relatively effective against different types of pain, but the relatively high incidence of adverse effects and other problems associated with their clinical use means that neither group can be considered to be the 'ideal' analgesic. It is hoped that the continually improving understanding of the physiologic basis of pain will ultimately be translated into the development of more powerful and safer analgesic drugs.

FURTHER READING

Hornykiewicz O, Kish SJ. Biochemical pathology of Parkinson's disease. *Adv Neurol* 1986; **45**: 19–34, 183–190. [Recommended for better understanding of the neurochemical basis of Parkinson's disease.]

Kaplan HI, Sadock BJ, Grebb JA. *Synopsis of Psychiatry: Behavioral Sciences, Clinical Psychiatry, 7e.* Baltimore: Williams & Wilkins; 1994. [An excellent general psychiatry text with coprehensive coverage of biology and psychopharmacology.]

Kenny GNC. Risk factors for postoperative nausea and vomiting. *Anaesthesia* 1994; **49** (Suppl): 6–10. [Illustrates the different stimuli that may trigger emesis.]

Kopin IJ. The pharmacology of Parkinson's disease therapy: an update. *Annu Rev Pharmacol Toxicol* 1993; **32**: 467–495. [Recommended for a better understanding of the basis for the therapeutic regimens used in the treatment of Parkinson's disease.]

Millar AD. Physiology of the brain stem emetic circuitry. In: Bianchi AL, Grélot L, Miller AD, King GL (eds) *Mechanisms and Control of Emesis, Vol. 223.* Colloque INSERM: John Libbey Eurotext Ltd; 1992, pp. 41–50. [Indicates the brain systems mediating emesis.]

Naylor RJ, Rudd JA. Emesis and antiemesis. In: Hanks GW, Sidebottom E (eds) *Cancer Surveys: Palliative Medicine – Problem Areas in Pain and Symptom Management, Vol. 21.* Cold Spring Harbor Laboratory: Cold Spring Harbor Laboratory Press; 1994, pp. 117–135. [A review of drug-induced emesis and its treatment.]

Pleuvry BJ, Lauretti GR. Biochemical aspects of chronic pain and its relationship to treatment. *Pharmacol Ther* 1996; **71**: 313–324. [A good general overview of the role of neurotransmitters in acute and chronic pain and of analgesic drugs.]

Stot JRR. Prevention and treatment of motion sickness in man. In: Bianchi AC , Grélot L, Miller AD, King GL (eds) *Mechanisms and Control of Emesis, Vol. 223.* Colloque INSERM: John Libbey Eurotext Ltd; 1992, pp. 203–211. [A review of the prevention and treatment of motion sicknes.]

Whitehead SA, Holden WA, Andrews PLR. Pregnancy sickness. In: Bianchi AL, Grélot L, Miller AD, King GL (eds) *Mechanisms and Control of Emesis, Vol. 223.* Colloque INSERM : John Libbey Eurotext Ltd; 1992, pp. 297–306. [An account of the factors contributing to pregnancy sickness.]

Make a provisional diagnosis and determine a rational pharmacologic treatment for the following hypothetical case.

A 27-year-old man attends the emergency room. He complains of feeling down and having suicidal thoughts for 6 months and finds it difficult to get to sleep. He also reports that other people can hear his thoughts and that words of songs on the radio refer to him. He says that he hears voices telling him he is a bad person and is responsible for a recent disaster. His friends say that he has become increasingly reclusive and has stopped attending work. When he speaks, there often seems to be little logical sequence to his thoughts and his personal hygiene is poor.

1. How would you manage this patient in the short term?
2. What are the two most likely diagnoses? List three additional features for both diagnoses that would help clarify the diagnosis.
3. Which drugs would you use for these two most likely diagnoses? In each case give the name of the class of drug and say which drug you would use and for how long, what the endpoints of therapy are, and what adverse effects might be expected.

?

Indicate which of the following are true and which are false.

1. Primarily inhibitory neurotransmitters include
- a) dopamine
- b) glutamate
- c) glycine
- d) acetylcholine
- e) γ-aminobutyric acid (GABA)

2. The following are examples of G protein-coupled receptors
- a) $GABA_A$ receptors
- b) dopamine D_2 receptors
- c) 5-hydroxytryptamine-3 ($5\text{-}HT_3$) receptors
- d) muscarinic acetylcholine receptors
- e) β adrenoceptors

3. The following statements are true
- a) the nucleus basalis of Meynert is the primary acetyl-choline-containing nucleus
- b) the tuberoinfundibular dopamine tract is involved in the regulation of prolactin release
- c) 5-HT is the principal neurotransmitter in the locus ceruleus
- d) the amygdala has input from both noradrenergic and dopaminergic tracts
- e) the raphe nuclei are the origin of most norepinephrine-containing neurons

4. Components of the limbic system include
- a) mamillary bodies
- b) olivary nuclei
- c) cingulate gyrus
- d) locus ceruleus
- e) amygdala

5. In major depressive disorders
- a) diurnal variation of mood and early morning awakening are common
- b) cortisol concentration is sometimes raised
- c) selective serotonin reuptake inhibitors are a more effective treatment than tricyclic antidepressants
- d) lithium is contraindicated
- e) one-third of cases relapse within 5 years

6. Characteristic symptoms of schizophrenia include
- a) auditory hallucinations in the second person
- b) thought withdrawal
- c) mood congruent delusions
- d) pressure of speech
- e) 'knight's move' thinking

7. Adverse effects of typical neuroleptics include
- a) cogwheel rigidity
- b) hair loss
- c) sedation
- d) hiccoughs
- e) akathisia

8. The following are true
- a) patients taking monoamine oxidase inhibitors should not eat fava beans with Chianti
- b) lithium can cause diabetes mellitus
- c) tricyclic antidepressants can cause cardiac arrhythmias in overdose
- d) the most common adverse effect of selective serotonin reuptake inhibitors is a dry mouth
- e) clozapine can cause agranulocytosis

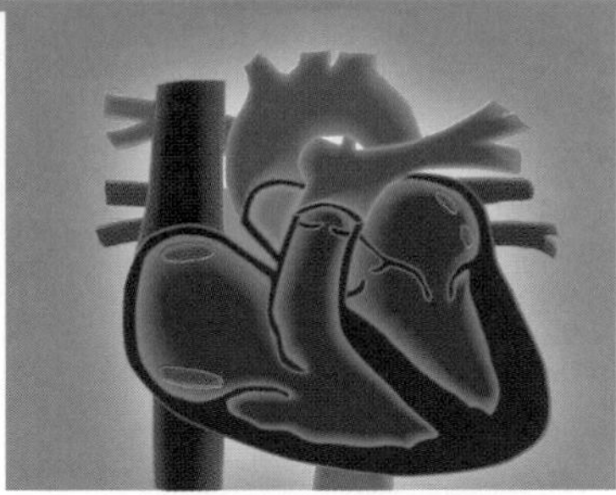

8. Drugs and the Cardiovascular System

PHYSIOLOGY OF THE CARDIOVASCULAR SYSTEM

The cardiovascular system is composed of the heart and the blood vessels

The heart is a pump that supplies the body with blood, which is distributed around the body by blood vessels. The blood vessels are collectively known as the vascular system. Together with the blood vessels, the heart provides a blood supply that maintains an optimal environment for the body tissues by supplying oxygen and nutrients and removing waste products. The normal partial pressures of oxygen and carbon dioxide in oxygenated blood are:

- pO_2 105 mmHg.
- pCO_2 40 mmHg.

On average the heart contracts about 70 times every minute and pumps approximately 7000 liters of blood every day.

Fig. 8.1 The heart consists of four chambers and is located in the chest cavity. The direction of blood flow through the heart is shown.

The heart is a hollow muscular organ

In adults, the heart weighs approximately 300 g. It has four chambers: two smaller chambers located towards the base called the atria and two larger chambers called ventricles located towards the apex (Fig. 8.1). The wall of the heart is made up of three layers: the epicardium (outer layer), the myocardium (the middle layer), and the endocardium (the inner layer).

A series of valves ensures that blood flows only in one direction

The right atrium and ventricle receive used, deoxygenated blood from the body and pump it out of the heart through the pulmonary artery to the lungs. The left atrium and ventricle receive the re-oxygenated blood via the pulmonary veins and pump it out through the aorta to the rest of the body.

> **Heart valves**
>
> - Valves prevent the backward flow of blood through the heart
> - Atrioventricular valves are sited between the atria and the ventricles
> - Backflow into arteries is prevented by semilunar valves
> - Artificial valves can replace valves damaged by diseases such as rheumatic fever

VASCULAR TREE

The body's vascular system consists of a series of components with different properties and is often referred to as a vascular tree. The two main types of blood vessel are arteries and veins. In a typical artery, the layer that lines the lumen and is in contact with the blood is the endothelium. For many years the endothelium was considered to be a simple barrier between the blood and the surrounding vessel, but it is now known to release many important vasoactive substances (e.g. nitric oxide) that help regulate blood flow and blood clotting (Fig. 8.2).

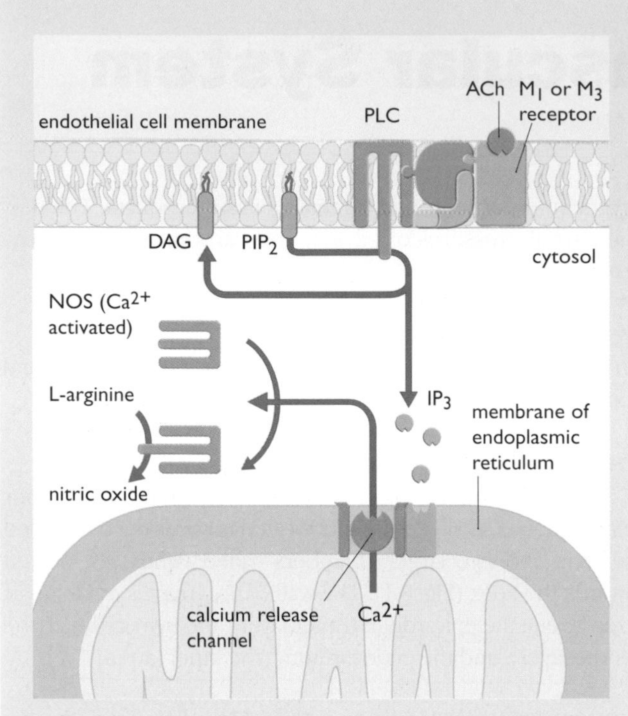

Fig. 8.2 Example of release of vasoactive substance (here, nitric oxide) from endothelim. Acetylcholine (ACh), bradykinin, thrombin, serotonin, shear stress, and other substances can release nitric oxide. ACh utilizes numerous untermediates in the cellular response that ultimately facilitates nitric oxide release. (DAG, diacylglycerol; NOS, nitric oxide synthase; IP_3, inositol-1,4,5-triphosphate; PIP_2, phosphatidylinositol)

Normal blood pressure is 120/80 mmHg

As blood flows through the body's circulatory system from the aorta, blood pressure falls from approximately 90 mmHg in the aorta, to almost zero in the veins. Blood pressure is intermediate in the capillaries, which are small vessels that connect arterioles and venules. Nutrients and metabolites leave and enter the vasculature through capillary membranes.

Blood pressure in a vessel is generated by, and is proportional to, the output of the heart (cardiac output) and the resistance to flow, which in turn depends on factors such as vessel caliber, elasticity, geometry, and blood viscosity. Blood pressure is expressed as systolic pressure/diastolic pressure and the normal value is 120/80 mmHg. Peak blood pressure occurs during systole as the left ventricle pumps blood into the aorta. The trough occurs during diastole as the ventricles relax (Fig. 8.3).

CARDIAC ELECTROPHYSIOLOGY

The distribution of K^+, Na^+, Cl^- and Ca^{2+} across the ventricular cell membrane results in a resting membrane potential of around –85 to –90 mV (calculated using the Nernst equation). In sinoatrial (SA) and atrioventricular (AV) nodal tissue the value is more positive. Membrane potential stays at these levels because of the high concentration of K^+ inside the cell, which is maintained by the Na^+/K^+ pump (also known as Na^+/K^+ ATPase, see Chapter 3) and because the membrane is more permeable to K^+ than to other ions. The Na^+/K^+ pump moves three Na^+ ions outward in exchange for two K^+ ions inward (i.e. it is an electrogenic pump, Fig. 8.4).

An action potential is generated when the cell is depolarized to around –75 mV

The upstroke of the action potential (Fig. 8.5) is due to opening of Na^+ channels with voltage-dependent gates, with channel opening being triggered by depolarization (see Chapter 3).

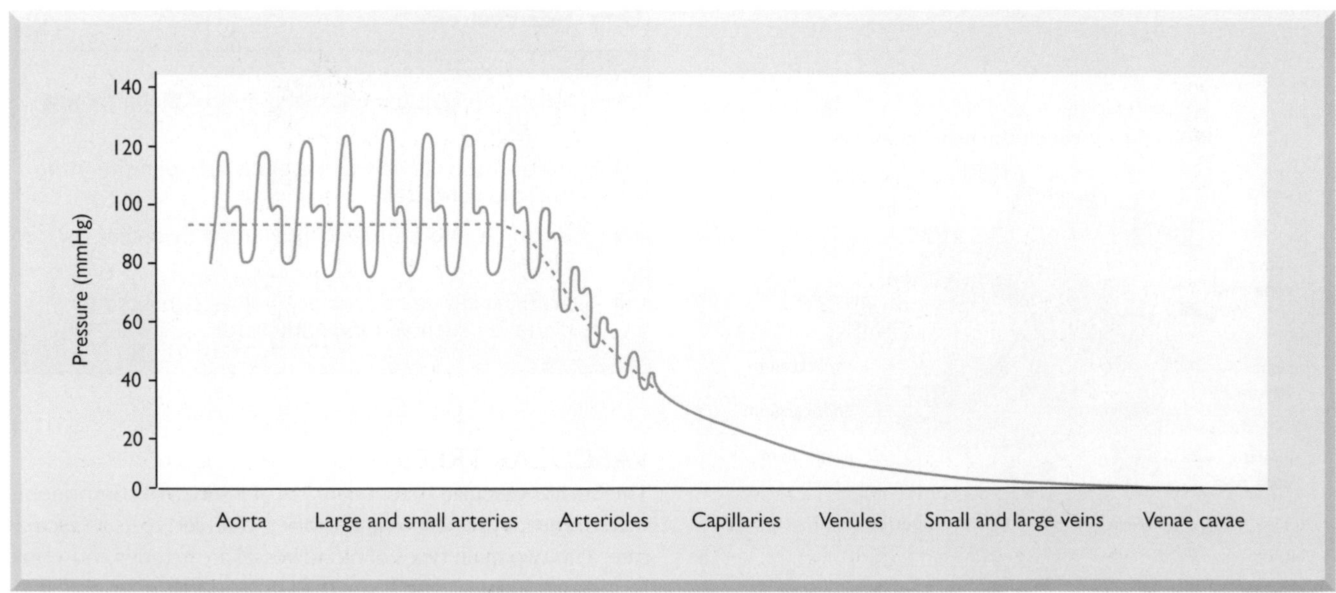

Fig. 8.3 Blood pressure in various blood vessel types. Systolic and diastolic blood pressures are shown, as well as mean arterial pressure. (Adapted with permission from *Principles of Anatomy and Physiology* by Tortora and Grabowski, HarperCollins.)

Activation of these Na^+ channels is transient and, if the membrane remains depolarized for more than a few milliseconds, the channel inactivates and the inward current stops. Such inactivation results in a period during which a second action potential cannot be triggered. This is known as the effective refractory period.

During the rapid depolarization phase of the action potential, other voltage-dependent channels are activated, particularly a variety of K^+ channel subtypes. These carry K^+ ions in the outward direction, so leading to repolarization of the action potential.

The characteristic plateau of the cardiac ventricular action potential results from an influx of Ca^{2+} through L-type Ca^{2+} channels. These channels, like the Na^+ channels, are voltage dependent, but the resulting current has a much slower time course. The resulting currents are therefore often referred to as:

- The fast inward Na^+ current (I_{Na}).
- The slow inward Ca^{2+} current (I_{Ca} or I_{si}).

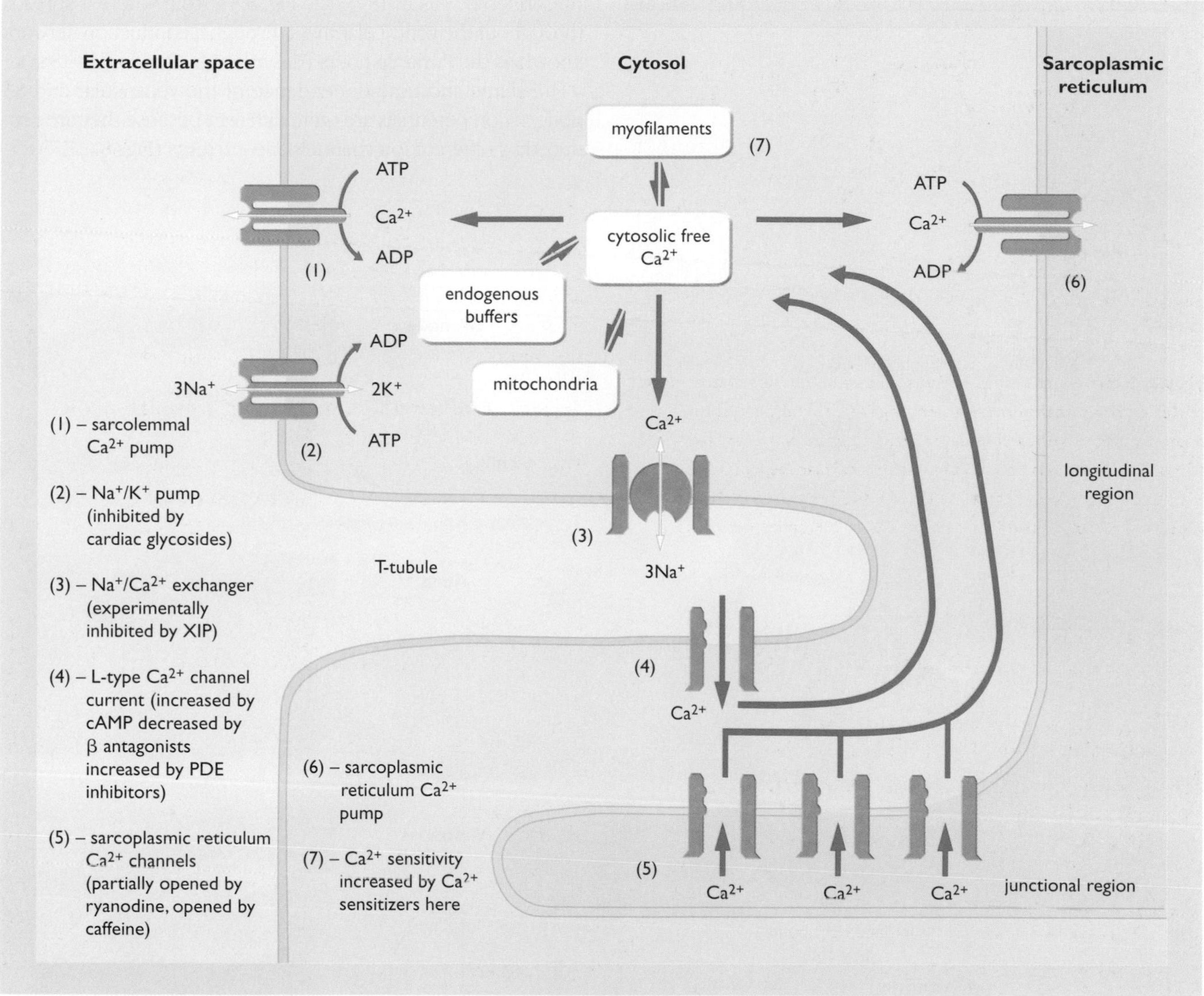

Fig. 8.4 Ion transport pathways in the heart, focusing on Ca^{2+} movements during the cardiac cycle. Membrane depolarization at the start of the action potential is the trigger for the opening of Ca^{2+} channels which span the surface membrane (sarcolemma). The local increase in Ca^{2+} concentration in the interior of the cell (cytosol) causes further release of Ca^{2+} from the intracellular stores (sarcoplasmic reticulum). Some Ca^{2+} may also enter the cell via the Na^+/Ca^{2+} exchanger. Once inside the cytosol, Ca^{2+} is bound to endogenous buffers, which include the inner surface of the sarcolemma and the contractile machinery (myofilaments; not shown functioning in this mode), which are activated by the presence of Ca^{2+}, leading to contraction. At the end of the action potential, Ca^{2+} leaves the cell by the Na^+/Ca^{2+} exchanger, and is also taken up again into the sarcoplasmic reticulum by ATP-driven Ca^{2+} pumps. (PDE, phosphodiesterase; XIP, exchanger inhibitory peptide)

Cardiac K^+ currents

- Delayed rectifier current (I_K), which is activated by depolarization
- Transient outward current (I_{to}), which causes the initial repolarization phase, referred to as the 'notch' of the action potential, which is important in some, but not all, regions of the heart
- Inward rectifier current (I_{K1}), with a main role of stabilizing the resting membrane potential
- ATP-sensitive current ($I_{K(ATP)}$), which is blocked by basal levels of ATP, and is therefore important when ATP is reduced (e.g. in disease conditions such as ischemia)

Heart beats start as a result of spontaneous depolarization of specialized cells in the sinoatrial node

The SA node (Fig. 8.5) rhythmically fires impulses approximately 80 times/min, a rate that is faster than that for any other region of the heart. The node is innervated by autonomic nerves, and release of acetylcholine from the vagus nerve can decrease the rate of firing.

The impulse from the SA node is conducted rapidly through the atria, and then delayed at the AV node for about 70 mseconds because of the small diameter of the fibers here. The AV node is the only electrical connection between the atria and the ventricles; it sorts and controls the movement of impulses from the atria to the ventricles. The impulse is then rapidly conducted through the left and right branches of the bundle of His (described by His in 1893; see Fig. 8.5), from where it spreads throughout the ventricular mass through a conduction network known as the Purkinje fibers (described by Purkinje in 1845).

The shape and time dependence of the ventricular and SA node action potentials are quite different because they are produced by different ion channels and currents (Figs 8.6, 8.7).

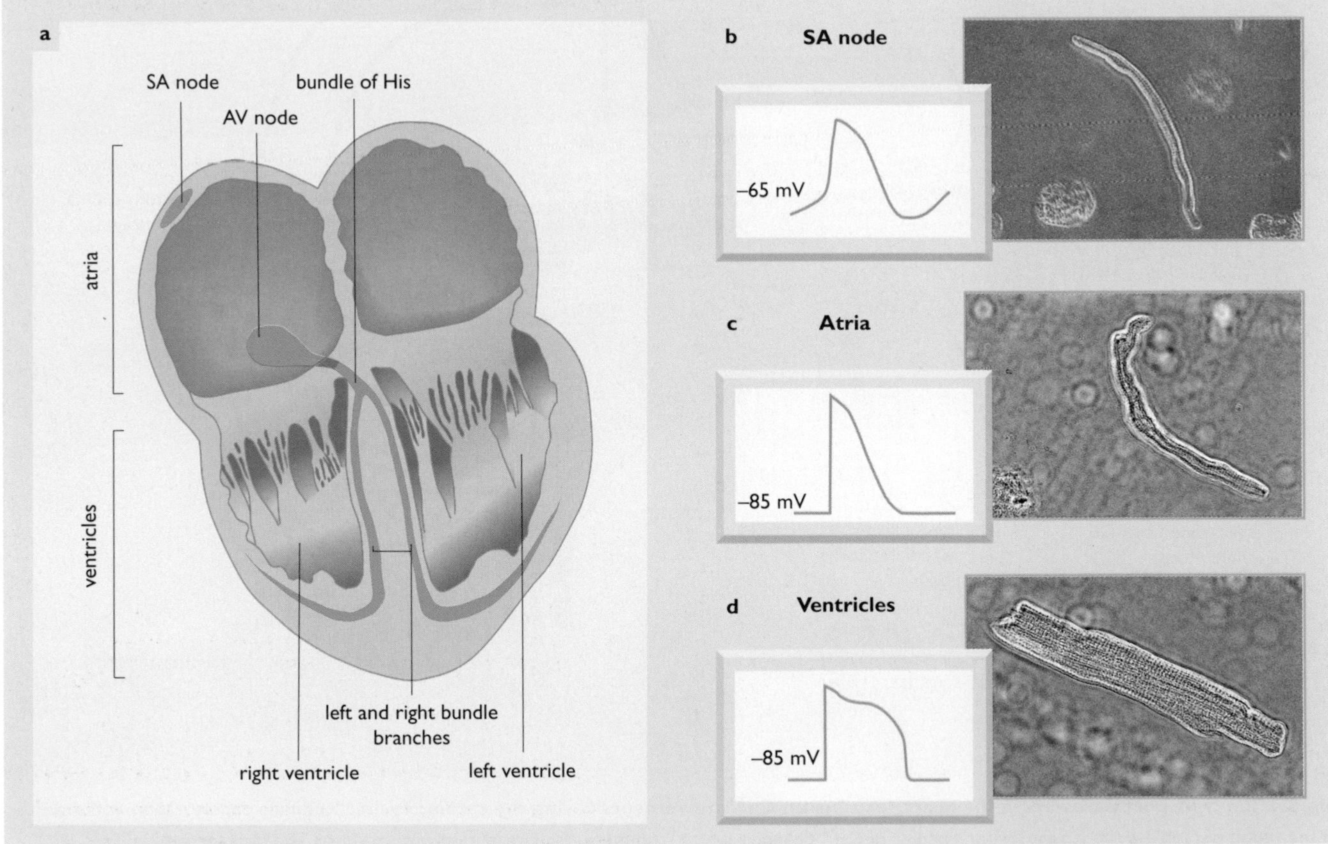

Fig. 8.5 Regional variation in cell structure and action potential configuration throughout the heart. Action potentials from different heart regions are quite different due to differences in the ion channels that underlie action potentials in these regions. (a) Location of the sinoatrial (SA) node, the atrioventricular (AV) node, and the bundle of His. (b) An action potential from the SA node and an SA node cell. (Courtesy of Dr Hilary F. Brown.) (c) An action potential from the atria and an atrial cell. (d) An action potential from the ventricles and a ventricular cell.

Excitation is coupled to contraction

One of the most important events in the cardiac action potential is the voltage-dependent opening of L-type Ca^{2+} channels (see Chapter 3). This leads to a relatively small inward movement of Ca^{2+} ions across the sarcolemmal membrane, which in turn activates a process known as Ca^{2+}-induced Ca^{2+} release, leading to the release of much larger amounts of Ca^{2+} from intracellular stores (i.e. sarcoplasmic reticulum). As a result, intracellular Ca^{2+} rises from 100 nM at rest to 10 μM during contraction. As the cytosolic Ca^{2+} concentration rises, Ca^{2+} binds to troponin C, which regulates the position of actin and myosin filaments, causing them to slide past one another, leading to contraction.

After contraction, the Ca^{2+} is re-sequestered into the stores by an adenosine triphosphate (ATP)-dependent Ca^{2+} pump, whereupon it is ready to take part in the next cycle. In addition, Ca^{2+} is pumped out of the cell via the electrogenic Na^+/Ca^{2+} exchanger. This pumps one Ca^{2+} ion out of the cell in exchange for three Na^+ ions moving inward, thereby generating an inward current (note, however, that the direction of exchange can change during the action potential and also depends on the internal concentrations of Na^+ and Ca^{2+}). Figure 8.4 shows schematically how cell Ca^{2+} is controlled, as well as how drugs may modulate the processes involved.

The sequence of events during one heart beat, also known as the cardiac cycle, takes place in the following order:

- Depolarization of the atria.
- Right atrial contraction.
- Left atrial contraction.
- After a short interval, ventricular contraction, with left ventricular contraction preceding right ventricular contraction.
- When the pressure in the ventricles is great enough, the pulmonary valve and the aortic valve open, accompanied by ejection of blood from the ventricles.

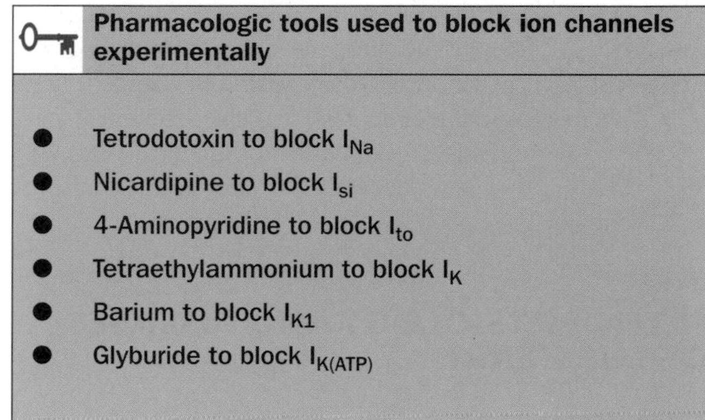

Pharmacologic tools used to block ion channels experimentally

- Tetrodotoxin to block I_{Na}
- Nicardipine to block I_{si}
- 4-Aminopyridine to block I_{to}
- Tetraethylammonium to block I_K
- Barium to block I_{K1}
- Glyburide to block $I_{K(ATP)}$

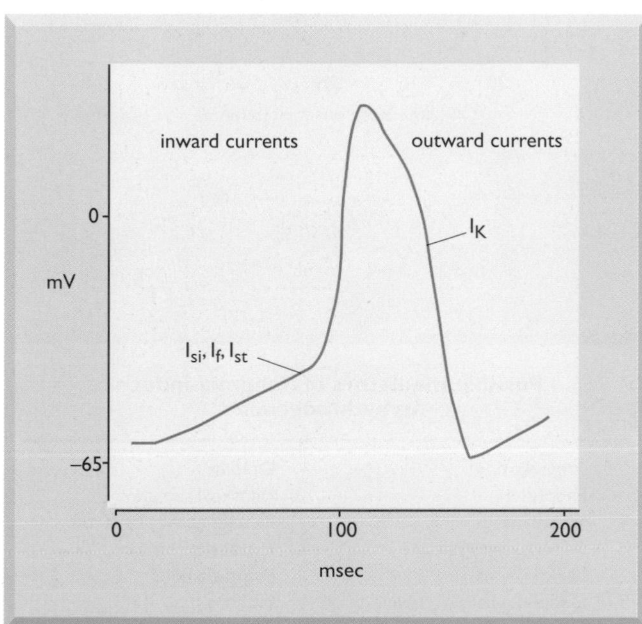

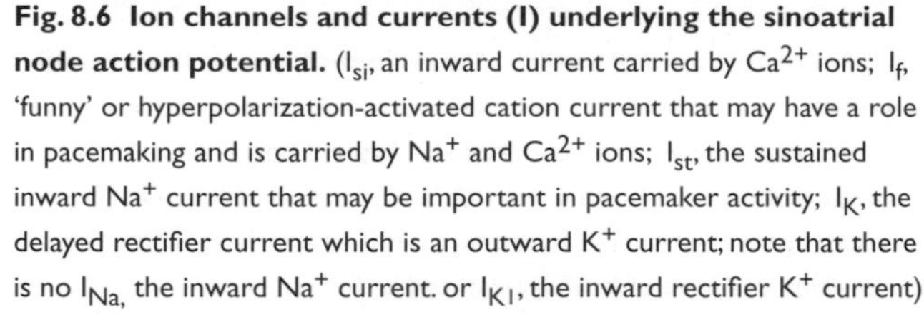

Fig. 8.6 Ion channels and currents (I) underlying the sinoatrial node action potential. (I_{si}, an inward current carried by Ca^{2+} ions; I_f, 'funny' or hyperpolarization-activated cation current that may have a role in pacemaking and is carried by Na^+ and Ca^{2+} ions; I_{st}, the sustained inward Na^+ current that may be important in pacemaker activity; I_K, the delayed rectifier current which is an outward K^+ current; note that there is no I_{Na}, the inward Na^+ current. or I_{K1}, the inward rectifier K^+ current)

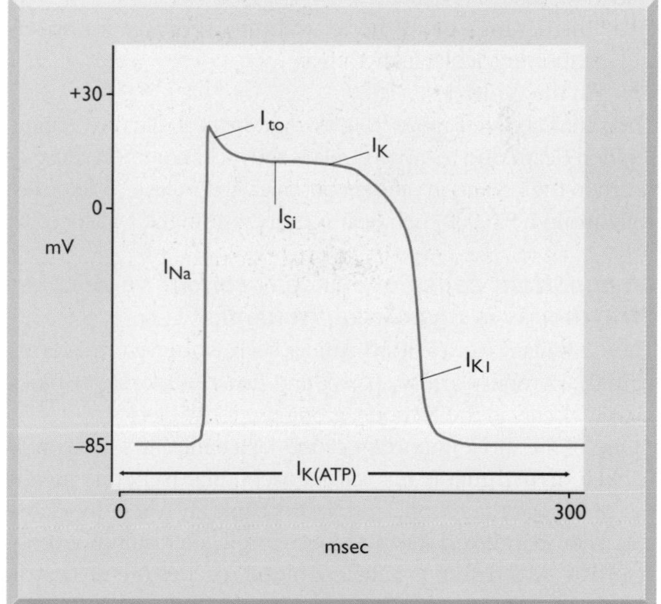

Fig. 8.7 Configuration of a typical ventricular action potential showing the activation of the most important ionic currents. (I_{Na}, fast inward Na^+ current; I_{si}, slow inward Ca^{2+} current; I_{to}, transient outward K^+ current; I_K, delayed rectifier K^+ current; I_{K1}, inward rectifier K^+ current; $I_{K(ATP)}$, ATP-sensitive K^+ current; note, the last of these is activated only during ischemia or hypoxia)

The electrocardiogram is an electrical recording of the changes that occur during a single cardiac cycle

The electrocardiogram (ECG) records the average signal of the depolarizations and repolarizations occurring in all the cardiac myocytes. It can be recorded on the surface of the body using electrodes and is generally recorded at rest and during stress.

An understanding of the normal ECG (see Fig. 8.9a) is essential before considering the different types of arrhythmia:

- The PR interval is the time from the beginning of the P wave to the beginning of the QRS complex. It is equivalent to the time taken for electrical activity to propagate through the AV node.
- The QRS complex represents ventricular depolarization; atrial repolarization is hidden beneath this large complex.
- The ST segment is the time between the QRS complex and the T wave, and its level is characteristically changed during ischemia (elevation or depression of the segment).
- The QT interval is the time from the start of the QRS complex to the end of the T wave and represents ventricular depolarization and repolarization.

PATHOPHYSIOLOGY AND DISEASES OF THE HEART

ARRHYTHMIAS

Arrhythmia (a- rhythm) means no rhythm, whereas dysrhythmia (dys- rhythm) means an abnormal heart rhythm. In practice, both terms are used interchangeably to mean an abnormal or irregular heart beat.

Arrhythmias may originate:

- In the atria or AV node, whereby they are known as supraventricular arrhythmias.
- In the ventricles.

Their clinical effects range from asymptomatic to life threatening. Sudden death due to arrhythmia is the most common cause of death in the US and in other economically developed countries, with around 350,000 such deaths every year in the US alone.

An important cause of clinically serious ventricular arrhythmias is myocardial ischemia

There are many causes of arrhythmia, such as arteriosclerosis (see p. 190), coronary artery spasm, and heart block. Heart block usually occurs in the AV node, giving rise to 'AV block.'

One of the most important causes of a clinically serious ventricular arrhythmia is myocardial ischemia. Ischemia means 'holding back the blood,' and occurs clinically when, for example, a coronary artery becomes obstructed as a result of arteriosclerosis. As a result, insufficient blood reaches the myocardium to meet the tissues' needs for oxygen and nutrients, and removal of metabolic waste. If the region of myocardium (especially within the ventricles) rendered ischemic is sufficiently large, an arrhythmia may occur, with the time-course shown in Fig. 8.8a. The molecular and cellular causes of an ischemia-induced arrhythmia are not clear, but there are a variety of possibilities. These include accumulation of extracellular K^+ (Fig. 8.8b) and activation of cyclic adenosine monophosphate (cAMP) production and can occur in response to a variety of mediators.

Reperfusion, which means re-admission of coronary flow to the ischemic region, is essential if the tissue is to recover and cell death (infarction) is to be avoided. However, spontaneous reperfusion carries the risk of inducing an arrhythmia. In animal models, reperfusion after ischemia causes serious ventricular arrhythmias, including ventricular fibrillation. In humans, clinically serious reperfusion-induced arrhythmias may be avoided:

- If reperfusion is achieved deliberately (e.g. by using thrombolytic or fibrinolytic drugs, see Chapter 9).
- If the rate of reperfusion is carefully controlled (e.g. following coronary artery surgery) and monitored.

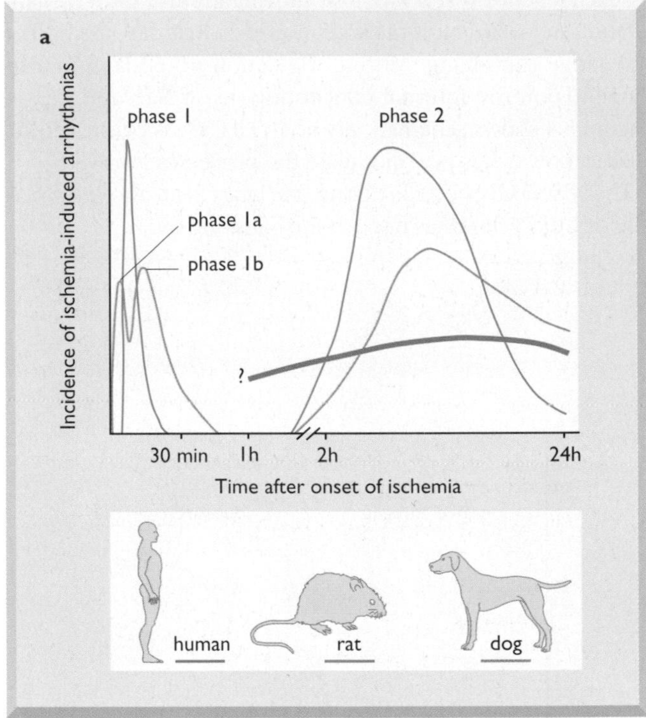

b **Possible mediators of ischemia-induced arrhythmogenesis**

Angiotensin II	Opioids
Endothelin	Palmitoyl carnitine
Histamine	Platelet activating factor
5-Hydroxytryptamine	Extracellular K^+
Leukotrienes	Prostaglandins
Lysophosphatidyl choline	Protons
Norepinephrine	Thromboxane A_2

Fig. 8.8 Time course of ventricular arrhythmias due to ischemia in mammalian hearts. (a) There are two main phases of arrhythmias, phase 1 and phase 2. In the dog, phase 1 arrhythmias may be further subcategorized into phase 1a and 1b arrhythmias. Very little is known about phase 1 arrhythmias in the human, but they are thought to exist. (b) Possible mediators of ischemia-induced arrhythmogenesis.

However, the underlying causes of clinically serious ventricular arrhythmias in humans are not entirely clear in the majority of cases, making treatment difficult and hampering research efforts.

Ischemia

- **Ischemia resulting from a reduced blood flow is associated with contractile failure, ECG abnormalities, and chest pain**
- **Silent ischemia is characterized by contractile failure and ECG abnormalities without chest pain**
- **Myocardial infarction occurs if sustained ischemia results in cell death**
- **Stunning is a reversible impairment of cardiac or vascular function that is detectable during the first few hours or days after the start of reperfusion**
- **Hibernating myocardium occurs if the myocardial function is depressed during relative ischemia. It preserves energy substrates, thereby aiding recovery when reperfusion occurs**
- **Preconditioning is caused by a short period of ischemia and describes the resulting protection (from arrhythmias and contractile dysfunction) afforded to the heart against the effects of a longer period of ischemia**

Arrhythmias are defined according to their electrocardiographic configuration

Arrhythmias are defined on the basis of their ECG configuration using guidelines known as the Lambeth Conventions drawn up by researchers in the field:

- Ventricular premature beats (VPBs, Fig. 8.9b) are sometimes referred to as ventricular ectopic beats, and are defined as discrete and identifiable premature QRS complexes.
- Ventricular tachycardia (Fig. 8.9c) is defined as a run of four or more consecutive VPBs.
- Ventricular fibrillation (Fig. 8.9d) is a lethal arrhythmia if it lasts for more than a few minutes, and is defined as a signal from which individual deflections vary in size and frequency on a cycle-to-cycle basis.
- Torsades de pointes, a French term meaning 'twisting of points,' is a syndrome characterized by a clinically serious ventricular arrhythmia similar to fibrillation, with rapid asynchronous complexes and an undulating baseline on the ECG, which is always spontaneously reversible (unlike ventricular fibrillation which usually is not). It is usually associated with a prolonged QT interval in the ECG, which may be congenital (in congenital long QT syndrome) or drug induced (e.g. by Class Ia and Class III antiarrhythmics, see p. 162).
- In parasystole, any part of the heart may compete with the SA node for the pacemaking role, thereby creating a focus for arrhythmias. It is recognizable from the ECG as an abnormal complex, which is coupled at varying intervals to the sinus-initiated complex.
- Atrial premature beats appear on the ECG as abnormal P waves and are usually symptomless.
- Atrial flutter is a condition in which the atria beat rapidly (>300 beats/min) and is often complicated by AV block so that not every atrial beat is conducted to the ventricles.
- In atrial fibrillation, the atria beat asynchronously so that the active pumping function of the atria is reduced (often to zero). It is a relatively common arrhythmia in the elderly.

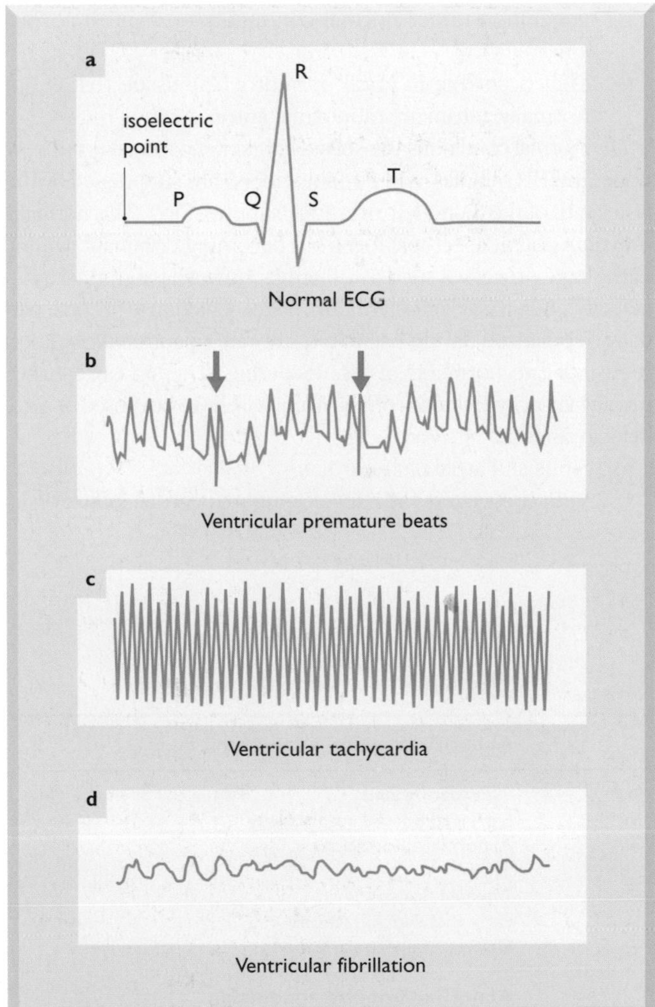

Fig. 8.9 Electrocardiograms (ECGs). (a) The normal ECG. (b) Ventricular premature beats. (c) Ventricular tachycardia. (d) Ventricular fibrillation. Note that in (a), the P wave represents depolarization of the atria, the QRS complex reflects depolarization of the ventricles, and the T wave, repolarization of the ventricles. Arrhythmias are manifest as abnormalities in the configuration of the ECG. Arrhythmias are defined according to the Lambeth Conventions.

- Wolff–Parkinson–White syndrome is an inherited condition in which there is an abnormal connection between the atrium and the ventricle known as the bundle of Kent. This connection allows impulses to be conducted quickly from the atria to the ventricles and bypass the AV node. It is recognizable on the ECG by a short PR interval followed by a wide QRS complex, and it is frequently associated with atrial fibrillation.

Mechanisms for arrhythmias

The two main mechanisms for arrhythmias are abnormal impulse generation and abnormal impulse conduction. Abnormal impulse generation can be automatic or triggered (Fig. 8.10).

Automatic abnormal impulse generation Automaticity describes the development of a site of premature beat generation and there are two types:

- That occurring in tissues capable of automatic impulse generation under normal conditions (enhanced normal automaticity).
- That occurring in atrial or ventricular tissue that is not normally automatic (abnormal automaticity).

Under normal conditions the subsidiary (slow) pacemakers (the AV node, the His bundles, and Purkinje fibers) are suppressed by the faster rate of the SA node ('overdrive suppression'). This normally prevents potential ectopic foci from becoming dominant. During pathologic processes such as ischemia, however, abnormal automaticity often arises in the Purkinje fibers, which may become partially depolarized, giving rise to a faster rate of automaticity. Local release of catecholamines, as occurs during ischemia, can enhance this automaticity. Examples of arrhythmias likely to be caused by automaticity are:

- Sinus and atrial tachycardias.
- VPBs associated with developing myocardial infarction.

Mechanisms of arrhythmogenesis
Abnormal impulse generation
Automatic rhythms Enhanced normal automaticity Abnormal automaticity
Triggered rhythms Early afterdepolarizations Delayed afterdepolarizations
Abnormal impulse conduction
Conduction block First-, second-, or third-degree block
Re-entry Circus movement Reflection

Fig. 8.10 Mechanisms of arrhythmogenesis.

Triggered abnormal impulse generation Triggered activity is a form of abnormal automaticity and can also be of two types:

- Early afterdepolarizations (EADs).
- Delayed afterdepolarizations (DADs, Fig. 8.11).

Impulses are triggered by the previous 'normal' impulse. EADs occur during the repolarization phase of the action potential (i.e. during phase 2 or 3), whereas DADs occur after the action potential has ended (i.e. during phase 4).

Early afterdepolarizations are associated with an abnormally prolonged action potential

EADs are frequently associated with an abnormally prolonged action potential and are therefore more likely to occur during bradycardia or treatment with compounds that prolong the action potential (see Class III antiarrhythmics, p. 163). The mechanism of such EADs is not known, but they may result from a decrease in the repolarizing delayed rectifier K^+ (I_K) current. Clinically there is some evidence that EADs cause torsades de pointes and reperfusion-induced arrhythmias.

Delayed afterdepolarizations typically occur as a result of cellular Ca^{2+} overload

DADs typically occur as a result of cellular Ca^{2+} overload, as may occur during ischemia, reperfusion, or digitalis intoxication. It is believed that such Ca^{2+} overload leads to an oscillatory release of Ca^{2+} from the sarcoplasmic reticulum. This then leads to the production of an inward current (resulting in the DAD), which may be due to current associated with the Na^+/Ca^{2+} exchanger (the transient inward current, I_{TI}).

Abnormal impulse conduction Arrhythmias occurring as a result of abnormal conduction may be caused by a conduction block (heart block) or by re-entry.

The most common site of heart block is the AV node, and the block is first-, second-, or third-degree, as follows:

- In first-degree AV block, conduction through the AV node is slowed. This is manifested on the ECG as a prolonged PR interval.
- In second-degree AV block some of the impulses generated in the SA node are not conducted to the ventricles (i.e. a beat is missed) and, on the ECG, no QRS complex follows the P wave.
- In third-degree AV block, which is clinically the most serious type, there is a complete block of conduction through the AV node, with no impulses being conducted to the ventricles. Abnormal conduction of this type can lead to premature beats (VPBs) via automatic or re-entry mechanisms.

Re-entry is a probable cause of ventricular tachycardia and ventricular fibrillation. As early as 1914, Mines established the criterion for re-entry in excised rings of cardiac tissue as an area of unidirectional block of the impulse that can allow reverse (retrograde) conduction, which then re-excites the tissue beyond the block; this is known as circus movement re-entry. The following criteria must be fulfilled to provide proof of a circus movement mechanism:

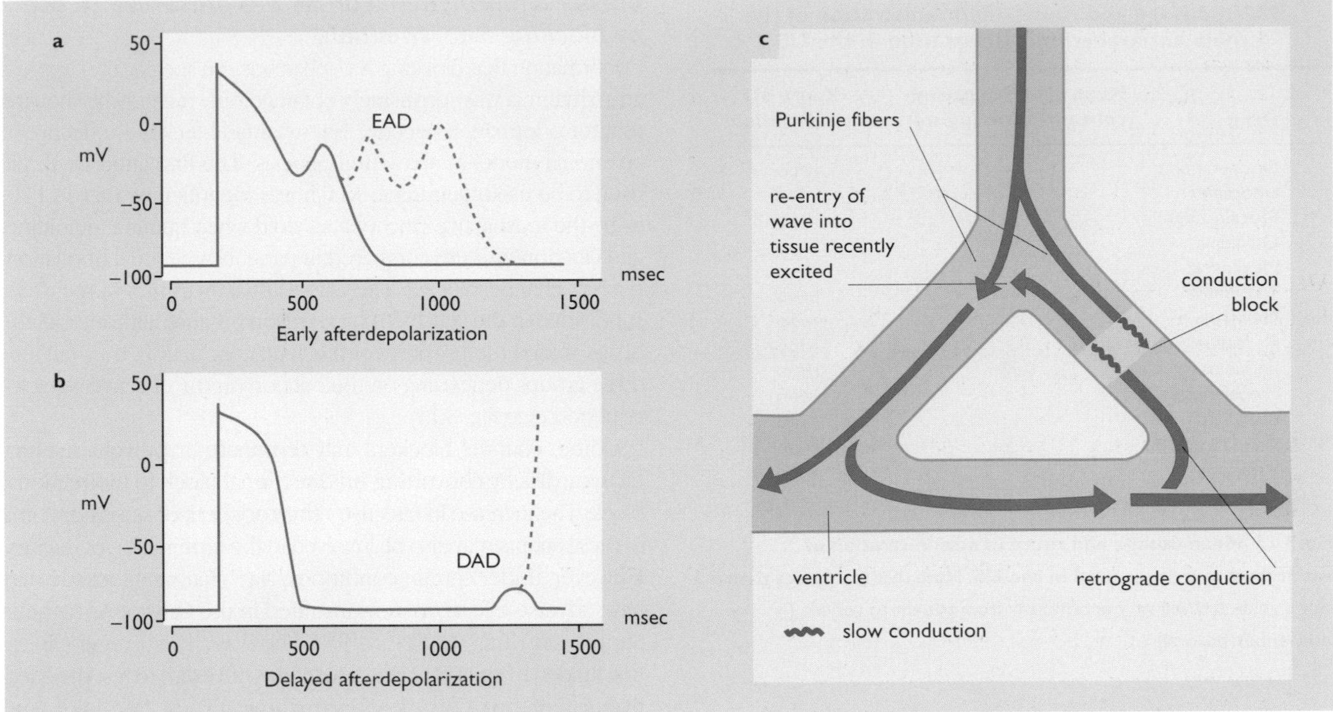

Fig. 8.11 Main mechanisms of arrhythmogenesis. (a) Early afterdepolarizations (EADs) occur during the repolarization phase of the action potential. The dotted line indicates repetitive EADs. (b) Delayed afterdepolarizations (DADs) occur after repolarization of the action potential, during diastole. The dotted line shows an action potential generated from a DAD. (c) Unidirectional block. The impulse moves from the sinoatrial node to the atrioventricular node and then into the Purkinje fibers, from where it passes into the mass of ventricular tissue. However, conduction is blocked in an area of ischemia in a unidirectional fashion; this allows retrograde conduction of an impulse from the ventricle back into the Purkinje fibers, hence re-exciting tissue that has passed through its refractory period and is excitable once more.

- The path for circus movement must have adequate boundaries to prevent short circuiting.
- The length of the path must be greater than the wavelength (W) determined by the effective refractoriness of the path (ERP) and conduction velocity (CV), and described by the equation, W = ERP × CV.
- The presence of a unidirectional block.

The area of unidirectional block may be anatomic (as in the tachycardia resulting from Wolff–Parkinson–White syndrome), or functional (e.g. prolonged refractoriness resulting from ischemia or the arrhythmia itself), or both. Based on the second criterion, re-entry may be due to slowed conduction which may occur during myocardial ischemia. Re-entry can be terminated by interrupting the circuit by premature activation, by overdrive pacing, and by some drugs (see Treatment of arrhythmias, below).

A second type of re-entry is known as reflection. It occurs in non-branching bundles in which an impulse can return over the same bundle owing to electrical dissociation within the bundle.

Re-entry is believed to be involved in atrial tachycardia, atrial fibrillation, atrial flutter, AV nodal re-entrant tachycardia, Wolff–Parkinson–White syndrome, ventricular tachycardia, and ventricular fibrillation.

There are many other putative arrhythmogenic mechanisms and details will be found in the 'Further reading' list at the end of this chapter.

Treatment of arrythmias

The objective of treating an arrhythmia is to provide an effective drug at an appropriate concentration that can be tolerated by the patient and is free of adverse effects. The concentration needed will depend on the patient and, in particular, on their particular arrhythmia profile, but the mean dosages for most of the compounds in use in the US are shown in Fig. 8.12.

The Vaughan Williams classification of antiarrhythmic drugs Antiarrhythmic drugs can be classified according to their mechanism of action at the molecular, cellular, or tissue level. Since the first antiarrhythmic drug, quinidine, was discovered in 1914 by chance by Wenckebach, the list of antiarrhythmic drugs has grown. A system of classification became necessary because of their diverse pharmacologic properties and their large number. Vaughan Williams devised the first antiarrhythmic classification in 1970, and this was later modified by Harrison (Fig. 8.13).

Mean dosage and route of administration of the main antiarrhythmic drugs used in the US

Drug	Mean effective plasma concentration (μg/ml)	Route of administration
Disopyramide	3	iv/po
Lidocaine	3	iv
Procainamide	7	iv/po
Quinidine	4	iv/po
Mexiletine	1	iv/po
Tocainide	7	iv/po
Phenytoin	15	iv/po
Flecainide	0.7	iv/po
Encainide	0.75	iv/po
Propafenone	1.5	iv/po
Bretylium	1	iv/po
Amiodarone	1.5	iv/po
Verapamil	0.1	iv/po

Fig. 8.12 Mean dosage and route of administration of antiarrhythmic drugs used in the US. Note that the dosage given is only a guide and will vary enormously from patient to patient. (iv, intravenous; po, oral)

Class I antiarrhythmic drugs are presumed to act by blocking Na+ channels

Confirmation that blocking Na^+ channels can specifically suppress an arrhythmia was surprisingly obtained only recently by showing that tetrodotoxin, a selective Na^+ channel blocker, is effective in an animal model of arrhythmogenesis. The first antiarrhythmic drug to be used, quinidine, which was identified by Frey in 1918 to be the most active cinchona alkaloid when quinine, quinidine, and cinchonine were compared in patients with atrial fibrillation, is a Na^+ channel blocker. The Class I antiarrhythmics were further subdivided in the late 1970s by Harrison because, although all the drugs shared the property of blocking conduction, they fell into three groups depending on their action on the effective refractory period (see Fig. 8.13).

Sodium channel blockers may terminate or prevent re-entry tachycardias by converting unidirectional block to bidirectional block. The increase in effective refractory period caused by some of these agents may also be involved in the termination of re-entry. However, under certain conditions, Na^+ channel blockade may have adverse effects, as demonstrated in the Cardiac Arrhythmia Suppression Trial (CAST) in 1989. This was a multicenter clinical trial funded by the US National Institutes of Health to test the effectiveness of two Class I antiarrhythmic drugs, flecainide and encainide. The surprising result was that mortality in patients treated with flecainide/encainide was higher than that of those who received placebo (4.5% versus 1.2 %, respectively, Fig. 8.14). The CAST study clearly showed that treatment with antiarrhythmic drugs can carry with it a considerable risk of proarrhythmia (increased occurrence of arrhythmias).

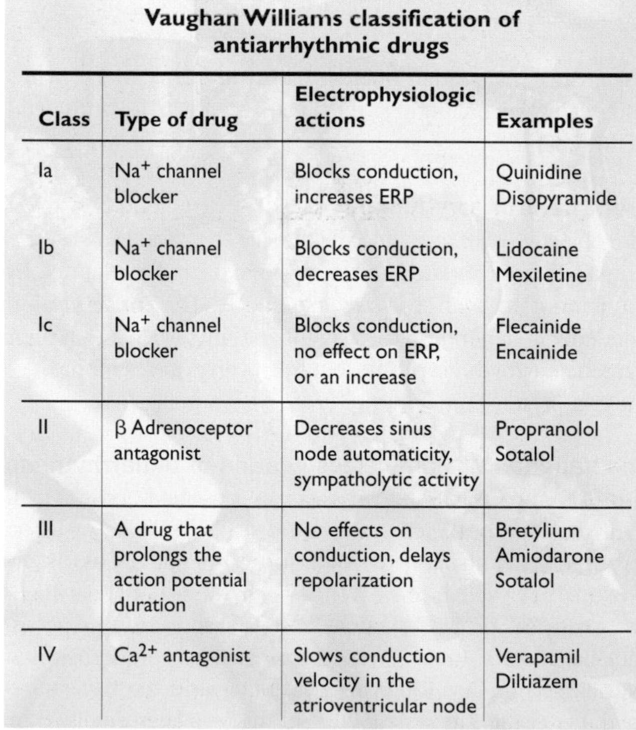

Vaughan Williams classification of antiarrhythmic drugs

Class	Type of drug	Electrophysiologic actions	Examples
Ia	Na^+ channel blocker	Blocks conduction, increases ERP	Quinidine Disopyramide
Ib	Na^+ channel blocker	Blocks conduction, decreases ERP	Lidocaine Mexiletine
Ic	Na^+ channel blocker	Blocks conduction, no effect on ERP, or an increase	Flecainide Encainide
II	β Adrenoceptor antagonist	Decreases sinus node automaticity, sympatholytic activity	Propranolol Sotalol
III	A drug that prolongs the action potential duration	No effects on conduction, delays repolarization	Bretylium Amiodarone Sotalol
IV	Ca^{2+} antagonist	Slows conduction velocity in the atrioventricular node	Verapamil Diltiazem

Fig. 8.13 Vaughan Williams classification of antiarrhythmic drugs. (ERP, effective refractory period)

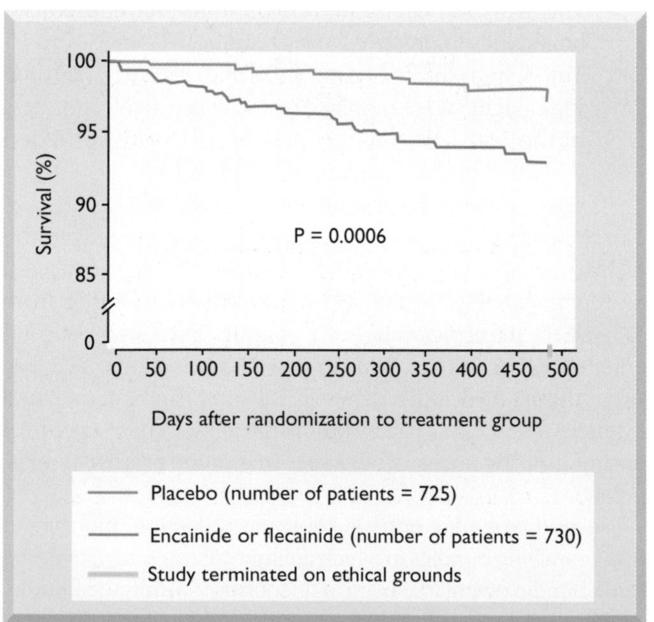

Fig. 8.14 Survival of patients in the Cardiac Arrhythmia Suppression Trial. Note that patients were allocated to groups in a randomized blinded fashion and that the cause of death in each case was cardiac related.

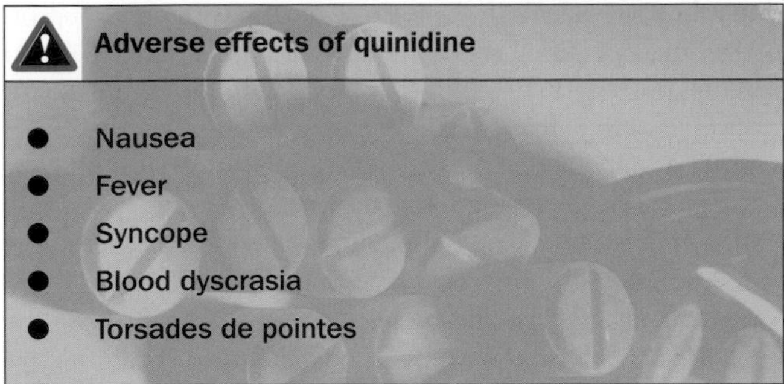

Adverse effects of quinidine

- Nausea
- Fever
- Syncope
- Blood dyscrasia
- Torsades de pointes

Class II antiarrhythmics act by reducing sympathetic activity

An increase in sympathetic tone can stimulate myocardial β_1, β_2, or α_1 adrenoceptors and precipitate or aggravate arrhythmias. However, whether the contribution of adrenoceptor stimulation to arrhythmogenesis is clinically important (e.g. in ischemia) remains controversial. The prototype of this class of drug is propranolol, which is a nonselective β_1 and β_2 antagonist, but conventionally Class II antiarrhythmic actions are attributed to β_1 antagonism.

Several β adrenoceptor antagonists have been shown to reduce the mortality of patients with myocardial infarction, a benefit that has not been reproducibly demonstrated for any other antiarrhythmic drug class. Suppression of arrhythmias that occur during exercise or mental stress is particularly successful.

β Adrenoceptor antagonists should be avoided in patients with

- Asthma
- Diabetes mellitus with hypoglycemic reactions
- Severe intermittent claudication

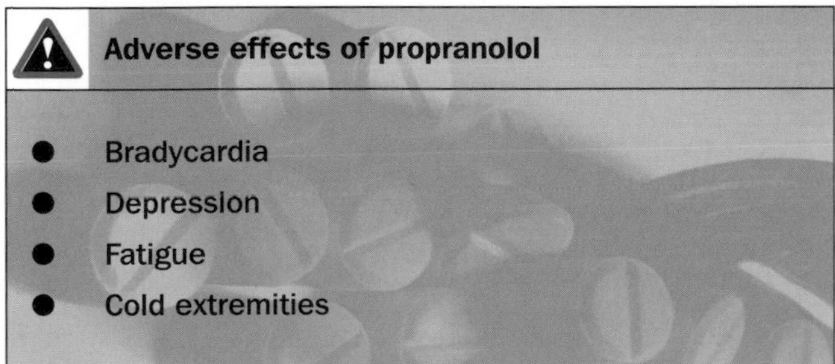

Adverse effects of propranolol

- Bradycardia
- Depression
- Fatigue
- Cold extremities

Class III antiarrhythmics act by prolonging the action potential

Prolongation of the action potential by Class III antiarrhythmics is manifest on the ECG as an increase in QT interval. This third class of antiarrhythmic drug was introduced when amiodarone and sotalol, drugs that prolong the action potential, were found to possess antiarrhythmic activity. Amiodarone is an effective drug, which unfortunately has some clinically serious adverse effects.

Although amiodarone is generally referred to as a Class III antiarrhythmic, it also blocks Na^+ and Ca^{2+} channels and α and β adrenoceptors. This poor molecular selectivity means that its molecular mechanism of action is unclear, and its classification as a Class III agent is questionable. Its onset of action is quite fast when given intravenously, but the loading oral dose must be given for up to three weeks to achieve a pharmacotherapeutic effect. It also has a very long half life of over 50 days. It has been shown to be effective against both atrial and ventricular arrhythmias.

Until recently, the Class III drugs used clinically have all been K^+ channel blockers, even if some may be rather unselective. However, other molecular actions can lead to the tissue response characteristic of Class III drugs (i.e. action potential prolongation). These include α_1 adrenoceptor agonism and inhibition of Na^+ channel inactivation. The latter is believed to contribute to the molecular mechanism of action of ibutilide, a newly introduced Class III agent that has been approved for the treatment of supraventricular tachycardia. Bretylium is the least effective of this class.

Class III drugs and the QT prolongation they induce have been associated with proarrhythmia, and particularly torsades de pointes. This is most common in the presence of factors such as hypokalemia, bradycardia, or the concomitant administration of other drugs such as α_1 agonists, antibiotics, and certain antihistamines.

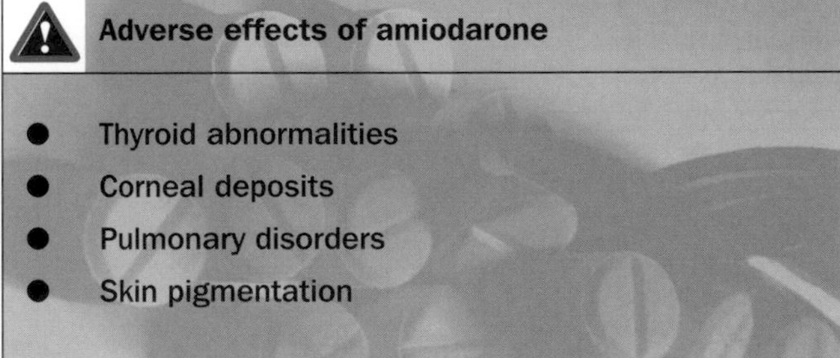

Adverse effects of amiodarone

- Thyroid abnormalities
- Corneal deposits
- Pulmonary disorders
- Skin pigmentation

Class IV antiarrhythmics are Ca^{2+} antagonists

Verapamil (a papaverine derivative) is the prototype of Class IV antiarrhythmics. It:

- Decreases sinus rate.
- Decreases AV nodal conduction velocity.
- Causes negative inotropy.
- Causes coronary and peripheral vasodilatation.

These drugs are mainly used for the treatment of supraventricular arrhythmias. In studies in rats and dogs it appears that, during acute ischemia, ventricular arrhythmias may be suppressed by verapamil. However, clinical trials of Ca^{2+} antagonists in patients with coronary artery disease have rarely demonstrated any useful suppression of ventricular arrhythmias. One reason for this may be that, as a result of the vasoselective nature of these drugs, the maximum safe doses used are insufficient to act in the ventricles to inhibit arrhythmias.

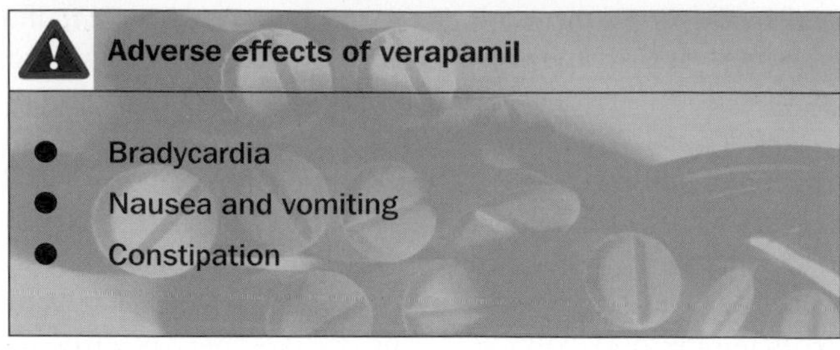

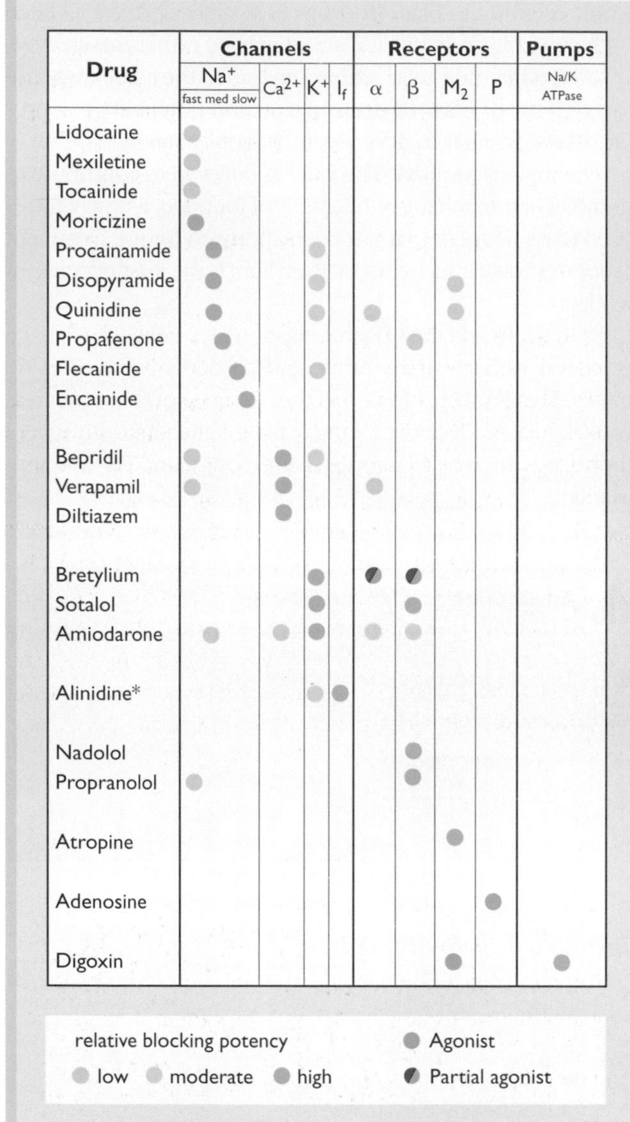

Drug	Channels: Na^+ fast	Na^+ med	Na^+ slow	Ca^{2+}	K^+	I_f	Receptors: α	β	M_2	P	Pumps: Na/K ATPase
Lidocaine	●										
Mexiletine	●										
Tocainide	●										
Moricizine	●										
Procainamide		●			●						
Disopyramide		●			●				●		
Quinidine		●			●		●		●		
Propafenone		●						●			
Flecainide			●		●						
Encainide			●								
Bepridil	●			●	●						
Verapamil	●			●			●				
Diltiazem				●							
Bretylium					●		◐	◐			
Sotalol					●			●			
Amiodarone		●		●	●		●	●			
Alinidine*					●	●					
Nadolol								●			
Propranolol	●							●			
Atropine									●		
Adenosine										●	
Digoxin									●		●

relative blocking potency: ● low ● moderate ● high; ● Agonist; ◐ Partial agonist

Fig. 8.15 The Sicilian Gambit approach to antiarrhythmic drug classification. This is a new approach to antiarrhythmic drug classification introduced by the Task Force of the Working Group on Antiarrhythmias of the European Society of Cardiology. This scheme summarizes the actions of a variety of antiarrhythmic drugs on ion channels, drug receptors, and ion pumps. I_f, hyperpolarization activated current; M_2, muscarinic subtype 2 receptors; P, purinergic receptors; Na/K ATPase, Na^+/K^+ pump. (Reproduced with permission from *Circulation* 1994, **84**, 1848. Copyright 1994 American Heart Association.)

The 'Sicilian Gambit' (Task Force of the Working Group on Arrhythmias of the European Society of Cardiology, 1991) is a recently proposed approach to the classification of antiarhythmic drugs (Fig. 8.15). In this scheme, classification is based on both a consideration of a drug's action at the molecular and cellular level and its action at the tissue level on certain 'vulnerable parameters.' This reappraisal of antiarrhythmic classification is welcome since there are possibly some disadvantages with the Vaughan Williams classification, such as:

- It is a hybrid, with Class I and Class IV representing a molecular mechanism (ion channel blockade), Class II representing a molecular mechanism (blockade of receptors), and Class III representing a tissue mechanism (prolongation of action potential).
- It does not take into account the fact that drugs may act differently in normal and diseased tissue.
- It may oversimplify the situation, so that it is assumed that all members of one class are the same (although, for example, different Class III antiarrhythmics act via blockade of different K^+ channel subtypes).
- Antiarrhythmic drugs may act on pumps, carriers, exchangers, and second messenger systems, as well as on receptors and ion channels, and so it is difficult to use this system to classify new compounds.

However, the Vaughan Williams classification does have the advantages of being physiologically based, and easily learnt and recalled. The Sicilian Gambit approach to classification is still new and has not been readily accepted everywhere, but there is no doubt that such a reappraisal was necessary.

Non-pharmacologic ways of treating arrhythmias include electrical defibrillation, surgery, and implantation of artificial pacemakers.

ANGINA PECTORIS

Angina pectoris produces a sensation of throttling and pressure in the chest region. It is a syndrome involving radiating chest pain associated with acute myocardial ischemia. It is often worsened by exercise and alleviated by rest, so may be regarded as an expression of a coronary blood supply–demand mismatch. The various possible reasons for this are listed in Fig. 8.16.

Crescendo angina or unstable angina is angina that occurs

Diseases that cause unstable angina

- Coronary arteriosclerosis
- Transient platelet aggregation and coronary thrombosis
- Coronary artery spasm
- Coronary vasoconstriction following adrenergic stimulation
- Accumulation of potent vasoconstrictors at sites of endothelial injury

Fig. 8.16 Diseases that cause unstable angina.

suddenly at rest or with limited physical activity and increases in frequency and severity.

Variant angina pectoris or Prinzmetal's angina occurs at rest and is associated with ST segment elevation and coronary artery spasm. The clinical features of variant angina differ from those of typical angina (Fig. 8.17).

Clinical features of variant angina pectoris
• Chest pain at rest
• Pain at the same time of day (early morning)
• ST segment elevation during chest pain
• Chest pain accompanied by ventricular arrhythmias
• Nitroglycerin relieves chest pain and ST segment elevation

Fig. 8.17 Clinical features of variant angina pectoris.

Treatment of angina

The approaches to treatment depend on the type of angina:

- For attacks of acute angina, sublingual nitrates and nifedipine provide rapid relief by reducing preload and afterload.
- For stable angina, several different classes of drug may be used and include long-acting nitrates, β adrenoceptor antagonists, and Ca^{2+} antagonists. Each of these differ in their molecular, cellular, and tissue mechanisms of action, but all affect one or more of preload, afterload, myocardial oxygen consumption, and heart rate.
- For unstable angina it is common to use aspirin to reduce the likelihood of platelet aggregation, which may precipitate an acute attack.
- Acute angina pain, especially when caused by coronary thrombosis, may be treated with morphine.

Types of angina

- **Angina pectoris presents as a radiating chest pain, is due to insufficient oxygen supply to the myocardium, and can occur during exercise and stress**
- **Chronic stable angina is caused by a fixed coronary stenosis (narrowing)**
- **Unstable angina occurs at rest or with physical activity and has a crescendo pattern**
- **Variant angina or Prinzmetal's angina occurs at rest and is caused by coronary vasospasm**

Nitrates dilate the systemic veins and large and medium-sized coronary arteries

Nitrates may relieve angina within a few minutes, and several preparations are available, including:

- Erythrityl tetranitrate.
- Isosorbide dinitrate.
- Nitroglycerin.
- Pentaerythritol tetranitrate.

The tissue mechanism of action is dilation of the systemic veins. This decreases the venous return to the heart, which in turn reduces myocardial wall tension and oxygen demand.

Nitrates also cause vasodilation of large and medium-sized coronary arteries, thereby increasing coronary blood flow and oxygen delivery to the subendocardial region of the myocardium. The molecular mechanism of action for this coronary vasodilator effect is associated with an increase in vascular guanylyl cyclase activity, which increases cyclic guanosine monophosphate (cGMP) levels (Fig. 8.2). cGMP is an important transduction component (see Chapter 3). Most nitrates are prodrugs, and decompose to form nitric oxide (NO), which then activates guanylyl cyclase (Fig. 8.18).

Nitrate tolerance is associated with continuous nitrate administration

Long-acting nitrates such as isosorbide dinitrate are usually given at 6–8-hour intervals during the day, whereas the shorter-acting drug, nitroglycerin, may be applied as a patch preparation on the chest overnight. These treatment regimens minimize the effect of nitrate tolerance, which is associated with repeated nitrate administration over time. The patient must be free of nitrate for at least eight hours of the day to prevent development of tolerance. As a general principle, tolerance is avoided by careful planning of dosing in relation to the drug's pharmacokinetics to ensure that a steady-state plasma concentration is not sustained over a 24-hour period.

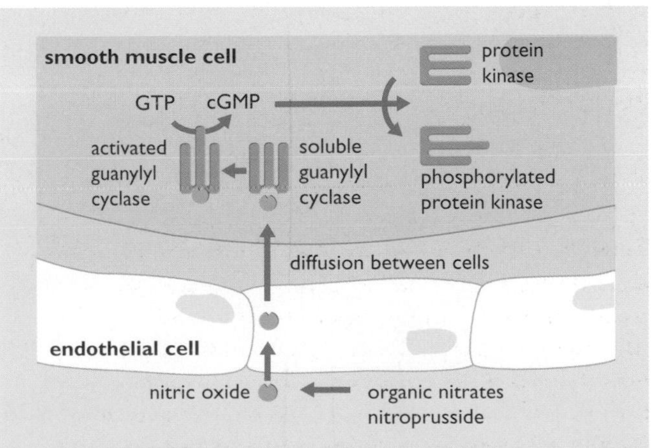

Fig. 8.18 Molecular and cellular mechanisms of action of nitrate and nitrite vasodilators. The product, phosphorylated protein kinase, causes vascular smooth muscle relaxation by an unknown mechanism.

β Adrenoceptor antagonists reduce myocardial oxygen demand

β Adrenoceptor antagonists (also known as β blockers):

- Decrease heart rate.
- Decrease systolic blood pressure.
- Decrease cardiac contractile activity.

As a result β adrenoceptor antagonists reduce myocardial oxygen demand. The details of their molecular mechanisms of action are shown in Fig. 8.19. Their pharmacology is discussed further in the section on hypertension in this chapter (see pp. 179–190). Drugs in this class include those listed in Fig. 8.20.

At low doses, β_1 selective agents such as metoprolol reduce heart rate and myocardial contractile activity without affecting bronchial smooth muscle. However, at higher doses, selectivity is lost and the effects resemble those of nonselective β adrenoceptor antagonists, such as propranolol, which may exacerbate bronchospasm in some asthmatics.

β Adrenoceptor antagonists cause a variety of adverse effects including fatigue, insomnia, dizziness, male sexual dysfunction, bronchospasm, bradycardia, heart block, hypotension, and decreased myocardial contractility. They may also worsen coronary artery spasm. β Adrenoceptor antagonists should not therefore be used in patients with bradycardia (heart rate less than 55 beats/min), bronchospasm, hypotension (systolic pressure less than 90 mmHg), AV block, or severe congestive heart failure.

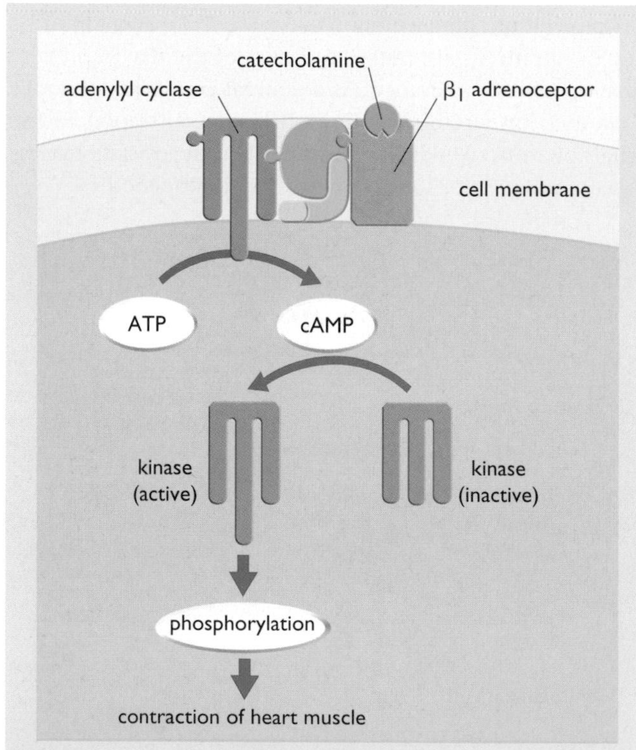

Fig. 8.19 Molecular mechanism of action of β adrenoceptor antagonists. Stimulation of β adrenoceptors by catecholamines leads to activation of adenylyl cyclase and an elevation of cAMP. This process is inhibited by β adrenoceptor antagonists.

Calcium antagonists modulate L-type Ca^{2+} channel activity

Calcium antagonists are effective in angina because they have the following three tissue mechanisms of action:

- They reduce venous pressure (preload).
- They reduce arteriolar pressure (afterload).
- They reduce myocardial oxygen consumption.

Each of these effects occurs as a result of the same molecular mechanism of action, which is modulation of L-type Ca^{2+} channel activity. This reduces Ca^{2+} entry into vascular and cardiac cells, and so reduces the concentration of intracellular Ca^{2+} (the cellular mechanism of action), resulting in reduced contractile activity in vascular and cardiac muscle.

Verapamil and diltiazem reduce cardiac contractility and in high doses affect atrioventricular conduction

Calcium antagonists include verapamil, nifedipine, and diltiazem. Some of the pharmacotherapeutic and adverse effects of verapamil and diltiazem result from their ability to affect L-type Ca^{2+} channels in cardiac tissue itself. Nifedipine does not do this at therapeutic doses. These drugs therefore possess slightly different tissue and system mechanisms of action, despite having similar molecular and identical cellular mechanisms of action.

Both verapamil and diltiazem reduce myocardial oxygen consumption at rest and during exercise by reducing heart rate and cardiac contractile activity, increasing coronary blood flow, and reducing preload and afterload. High doses of verapamil and diltiazem may affect conduction through the AV node (see section on antiarrhythmic drugs, pp. 161–164).

Nifedipine neither affects atrioventricular conduction nor reduces cardiac contractility

The 1,4-dihydropyridines such as nifedipine do not affect AV conduction and do not reduce cardiac contractility. Indeed, nifedipine may indirectly increase heart rate as a reflex response to the associated systemic arterial vasodilation. Nifedipine's beneficial actions

β Adrenoceptor antagonists used in patients with angina

Drug	Selectivity	Classification
Acebutolol	β_1 Selective	Partial agonist
Alprenolol	β_1 Selective	Partial agonist
Atenolol	β_1 Selective	Antagonist
Metoprolol	β_1 (low doses)	Antagonist
Oxprenolol	β_1, β_2 Nonselective	Partial agonist
Pindolol	β_1, β_2 Nonselective	Partial agonist
Propranolol	β_1, β_2 Nonselective	Antagonist
Sotalol	β_1, β_2 Nonselective	Antagonist
Timolol	β_1, β_2 Nonselective	Antagonist

Fig. 8.20 β Adrenoceptor antagonists used in patients with angina.

are attributed to increases in coronary blood flow to the epicardial regions of the myocardium and peripheral vasodilation.

Calcium antagonists can be used in patients with chest pain following exercise or stress, either alone or in combination with nitrates and/or β adrenoceptor antagonists. If nifedipine is combined with a β adrenoceptor antagonist there is only a low risk of AV block and of impairing cardiac output as a result of reduced ventricular contractility, which are potential problems if the patient has congestive heart failure or AV conduction abnormalities. Nifedipine can therefore be used in patients with these conditions. However, this risk is higher if verapamil or diltiazem are combined with a β adrenoceptor antagonist. Since verapamil and diltiazem have negative inotropic effects they should not be given to patients with severe heart failure.

Calcium antagonists have several adverse effects, with nifedipine being the least well tolerated. The systemic vasodilating effects of nifedipine may cause dizziness and palpitations. Nifedipine also causes venodilation, which may explain the peripheral edema that occurs in some patients.

The main adverse effect of verapamil is constipation, but bradycardia, hypotension, and heart failure may also occur. Verapamil in combination with a β adrenoceptor antagonist results in a marked bradycardia and should not be used in patients with heart failure, bradycardia, hypotension, or AV block. Diltiazem is associated with bradycardia. It may be useful as an alternative to β adrenoceptor antagonists for treating stable angina.

Treatment of unstable angina

Platelet function modulators Certain drugs may reduce the platelet aggregation that is initiated by coronary endothelial injury and can participate in the etiology of unstable angina. If platelets aggregate they can occlude severely narrowed coronary arteries and release potent vasoconstrictors, which worsen the angina. These vasoconstrictors include thromboxane A_2, serotonin, adenosine diphosphate (ADP), thrombin, and platelet activating factor.

Aspirin is a potent inhibitor of cyclooxygenase

Aspirin is a potent inhibitor of cyclooxygenase, which is an enzyme with a pivotal role in the biosynthesis of thromboxanes in platelets and prostacyclin in vascular endothelium (Fig. 8.21):

- Platelet-derived thromboxane is a potent vasoconstrictor, so aspirin may reduce coronary occlusion by inhibiting its synthesis.
- Endothelium-derived prostacyclin is a potent vasodilator and inhibits platelet aggregation, so inhibition of its synthesis is potentially hazardous.

Aspirin's molecular mechanism of action is acetylation of the α amino group of the terminal serine residue of the cyclooxygenase enzyme. This irreversibly inhibits the activity of the enzyme.

Adverse effects of Ca^{2+} antagonists

Nifedipine
- Dizziness
- Flushing
- Hypotension
- Skin rash
- Peripheral edema
- Tachycardia

Verapamil/diltiazem
- Bradycardia
- Hypotension
- Congestive heart failure
- Heart block
- Skin rash
- Constipation

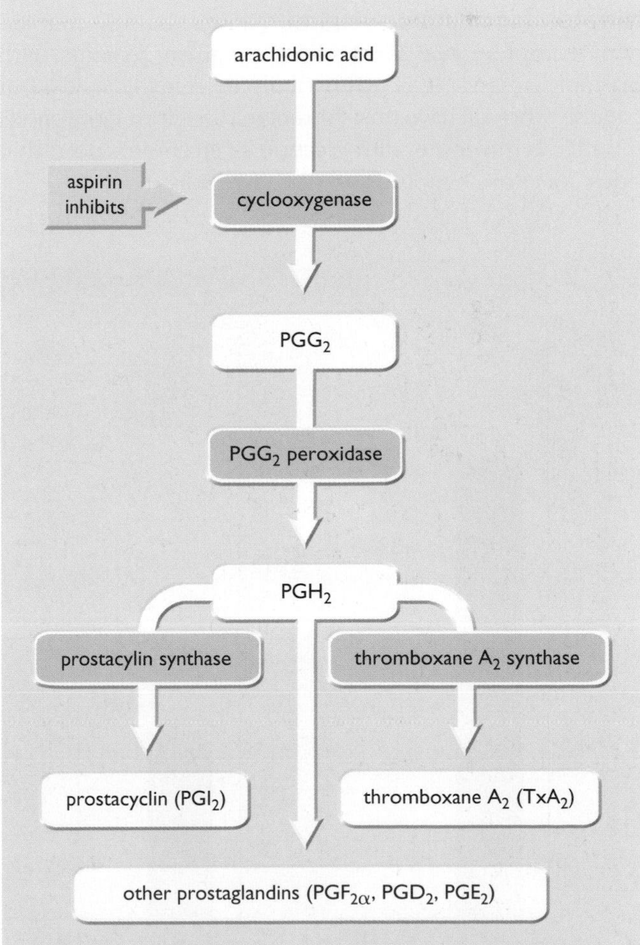

Fig. 8.21 Mechanism of action of aspirin. Aspirin blocks the activity of cyclooxygenase and reduces the formation of prostacyclin and thromboxane A_2. PGG_2 and PGH_2 are both prostaglandin cyclic endoperoxides and are unstable intermediates.

Aspirin reduces the incidence of myocardial infarction and death in patients with unstable angina

The pharmacotherapeutic mechanism of action of aspirin is a selective inhibition of thromboxane synthesis. This is achieved because platelets do not possess a cell nucleus and are therefore unable to resynthesize cyclooxygenase, whereas endothelial cells can resynthesize cyclooxygenase within a few hours. Low-dose aspirin (30 mg/day) is insufficient to block the activity of cyclooxygenase completely, so its use can achieve a maintained suppression of thromboxane synthesis with only a transient inhibition of prostacyclin synthesis and an overall effect of reduced platelet aggregation. Aspirin (325 mg twice daily) has been shown to reduce the occurrence of myocardial infarction and death in patients with unstable angina (Fig. 8.22).

Adverse effects related to aspirin use include:

- Gastrointestinal bleeding, which is common.
- Possible gastric ulceration, especially with overdosage.
- Reduced renal function as a result of a reduction in renal blood flow with inappropriately high doses.
- Occasional bronchospasm with inappropriately high doses.

Nitrates for unstable angina Nitrate therapy coupled with complete bed rest relieves pain in patients with unstable angina. It is given orally or transdermally, but patients who still have unstable angina are given intravenous nitrates. Intravenous nitroglycerin is given at a dose that does not cause hypotension or tachycardia.

Calcium antagonists or β adrenoceptor antagonists can be given if unstable angina persists. β Adrenoceptor antagonists may be preferred for patients with angina at rest and ST segment elevation during the pain without an elevated heart rate or blood pressure.

Thrombin modulators are given to patients with persistent angina despite bed rest or drug therapy (i.e. nitrates, Ca^{2+} antagonists, or β adrenoceptor antagonists) to reduce the risk of myocardial infarction by reducing the likelihood of coronary thrombosis.

Intravenous heparin reduces the incidence of unstable angina and myocardial infarction

Heparin is a thrombin inhibitor that inhibits blood clotting by preventing fibrin formation and platelet aggregation, probably as a result of its thrombin inhibitory effects since thrombin is a potent platelet aggregator. Intravenous heparin has been shown to relieve unstable angina and reduce the incidence of myocardial infarction and subsequent death (Fig. 8.23).

Heparin's molecular mechanism of action involves binding to the lysine site on antithrombin III, which accelerates the rate of reaction of antithrombin III, the endogenous inhibitor of thrombin. Antithrombin III also inhibits the other serine proteases in the coagulation cascade—XIIa, XIa, IXa, and Xa. The arginine site on antithrombin III interacts with the serine site on thrombin, thereby rendering it inactive.

These interventions increase the risk of bleeding disorders so should be avoided if there is a history of a preexisting bleeding disorder (e.g. peptic ulceration).

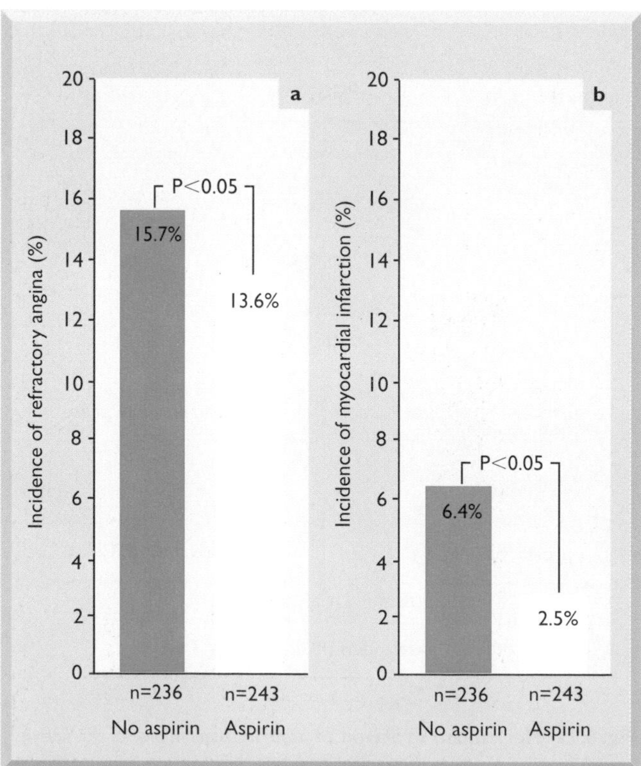

Fig. 8.22 Effect of aspirin (325 mg twice daily) on incidence of (a) angina and (b) myocardial infarction.

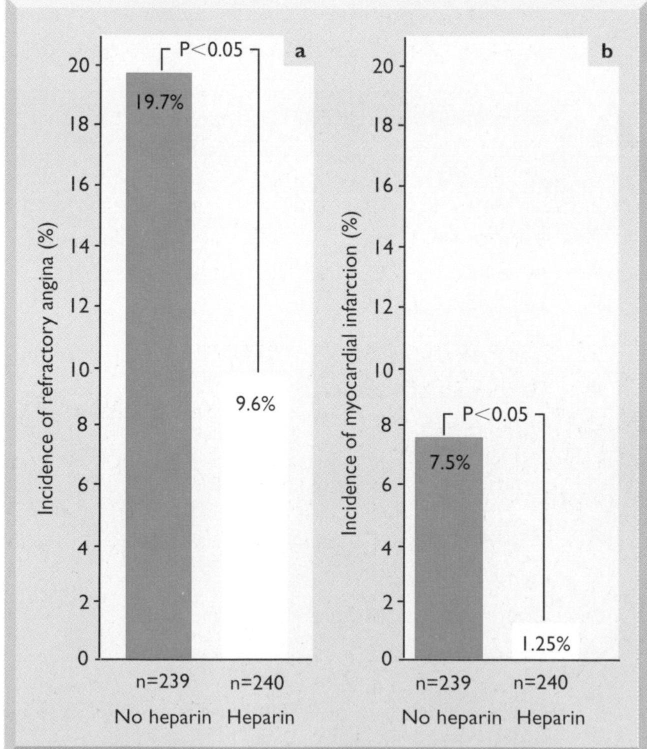

Fig. 8.23 Effect of heparin (1000 units/hour) on the incidence of (a) angina and (b) myocardial infarction.

Intravenous morphine is an opioid analgesic that alleviates the chest pain of unstable angina in patients at risk of sudden cardiac death.

Morphine reduces preload and afterload in agitated patients with raised sympathetic tone

Morphine has two beneficial actions:

- Its analgesic properties, discussed in Chapter 7, relieve chest pain.
- It has a relatively selective ability to reduce preload (venous tone) and afterload (arterial tone) in the agitated patient with raised sympathetic tone.

This second action results from the activation of opioid receptors on the presynaptic sympathetic terminal, which leads to a reduced release of neural norepinephrine. This reduces myocardial oxygen demand and so relieves chest pain, and possibly the progression of ischemia to infarction. However, although this has been demonstrated in animal models, it is not well established in patients. In addition, morphine releases histamine from mast cells, and this action may contribute to the vascular dilatation.

In the absence of a raised sympathetic tone, morphine does not have a clinically relevant effect on cardiovascular variables, so a degree of disease selectivity is exhibited.

Surgical intervention Cardiac catheterization or coronary artery revascularization is necessary for patients with unstable angina that persists despite pharmacologic intervention. Coronary arteriography is:

- Recommended for patients with unstable angina and no other severe medical conditions following successful control of their angina by drug intervention.
- Essential for patients with recurring unstable angina, even after drug treatment.

Coronary artery bypass graft surgery (CABG), percutaneous transluminal coronary artery angioplasty (PTCA), or the insertion of a stent are advised for this second group of patients.

Coronary artery revascularization extends life for patients with left main coronary stenoses, or with three-vessel coronary stenoses and depressed left ventricular function.

Drug therapy for angina

- Nitrates are effective because they decrease oxygen demand. The principal tissue mechanism of action is a reduction in preload
- β Adrenoceptor antagonists decrease heart rate, systolic blood pressure, and cardiac contractile activity
- Calcium antagonists reduce preload and afterload and may increase coronary flow
- Aspirin inhibits platelet and endothelial cyclooxygenase and reduces the incidence of coronary thrombosis

Treatment of variant angina

Variant angina is caused by coronary vasospasm and is also known as Prinzmetal's angina (after the physician who first characterized it).

Variant angina is treated with drugs that dilate the coronary arteries

Variant angina is the only form of angina in which dilatation of coronary arteries is the principal tissue mechanism of action of the drugs used to treat it. It should initially be treated with nitrates, either alone or with a Ca^{2+} antagonist:

- Nifedipine (40–160 mg/day) may be sufficient alone to prevent variant angina in up to 75% of patients. Its effectiveness is not modified by the presence of concurrent partially obstructive coronary arteriosclerosis.
- Verapamil (Fig. 8.24) and diltiazem may also be used, as well as the newer agents nicardipine, israpidine, and amlodipine.

Despite differences in tissue selectivity (vasculature versus AV node, see section on treatment of supraventricular tachycardia, p. 163), all these Ca^{2+} antagonists appear to be equally effective, although individual patients may respond better to one drug than another. For unknown reasons the combination of diltiazem and nifedipine may be beneficial if the agents are less than completely effective when used alone.

β Adrenoceptor antagonists are not recommended in these patients because they are often ineffective and may increase the frequency and severity of spasm.

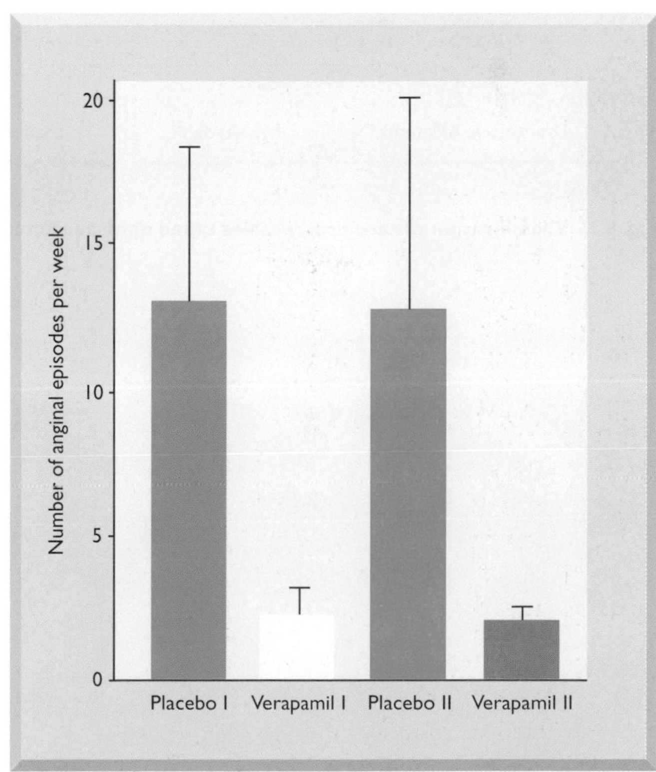

Fig. 8.24 Effect of verapamil in patients with variant angina. I and II refer to two different patient populations.

CONGESTIVE HEART FAILURE

Congestive heart failure (CHF) is the most common reason for hospitalization of people over 65 years of age in the US, where over 400,000 new cases are reported each year. Diagnosis is made on the basis of cardiac function and impaired tolerance to exercise.

The forms of CHF that are amenable to drug treatment are in most cases the result of cardiomyopathy. Heart failure resulting from arterial hypertension also responds to drug treatment.

Cardiomyopathies are primarily disease processes of the myocardium, which result from both known and unknown etiologies. Categorization of these diseases is based upon physiologic and anatomic characteristics (Figs 8.25, 8.26). Myocarditis resulting from bacterial infection is discussed on p. 194. Regardless of the type of cardiomyopathy, the common endpoint is a gradual reduction in heart function and precipitation of CHF. The failure may be acute or chronic and usually involves both ventricles. CHF occurs if the heart does not supply sufficient oxygenated blood to the organs of the body.

The reasons for CHF may involve a failure in cardiac excitation–contraction coupling processes. In CHF there is progressive systolic and diastolic ventricular dysfunction, which is characterized by structural and metabolic changes to cardiac muscle that can be acute or chronic, with a spectrum of symptoms depending upon the severity of heart failure (Fig. 8.27):

- Acute CHF can result from exposure of cardiac muscle to toxic levels of drugs or as a result of coronary artery occlusion.
- Chronic CHF occurs when the heart is damaged by conditions such as primary hypertension or myocardial ischemia and infarction.

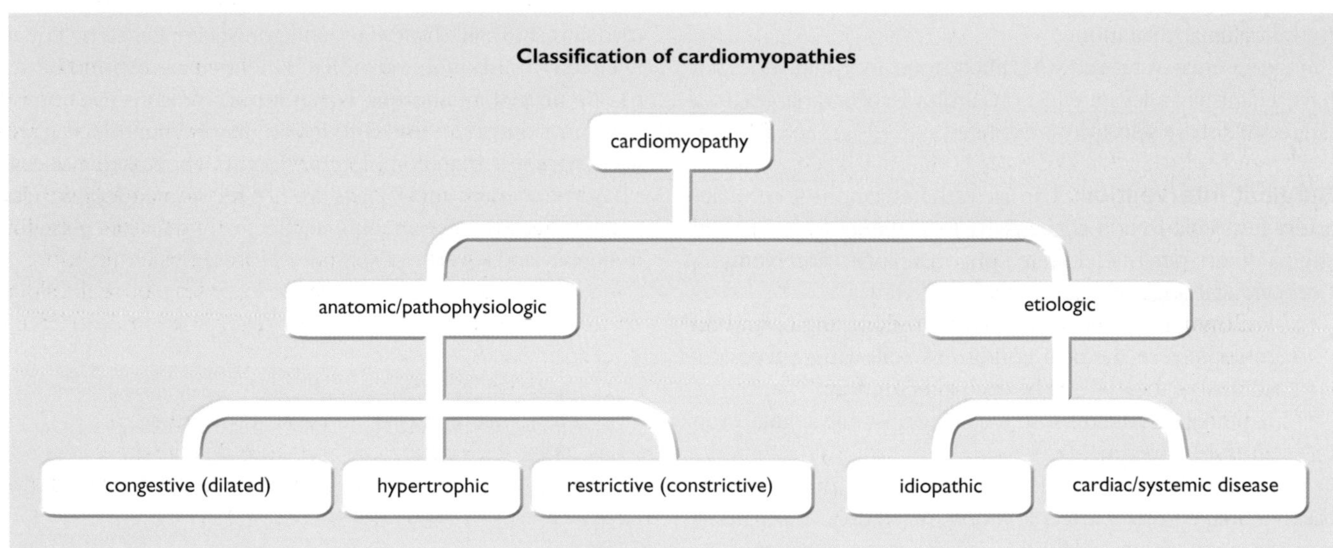

Fig. 8.25 Classification of cardiomyopathies based upon anatomic, pathophysiologic, and etiologic considerations.

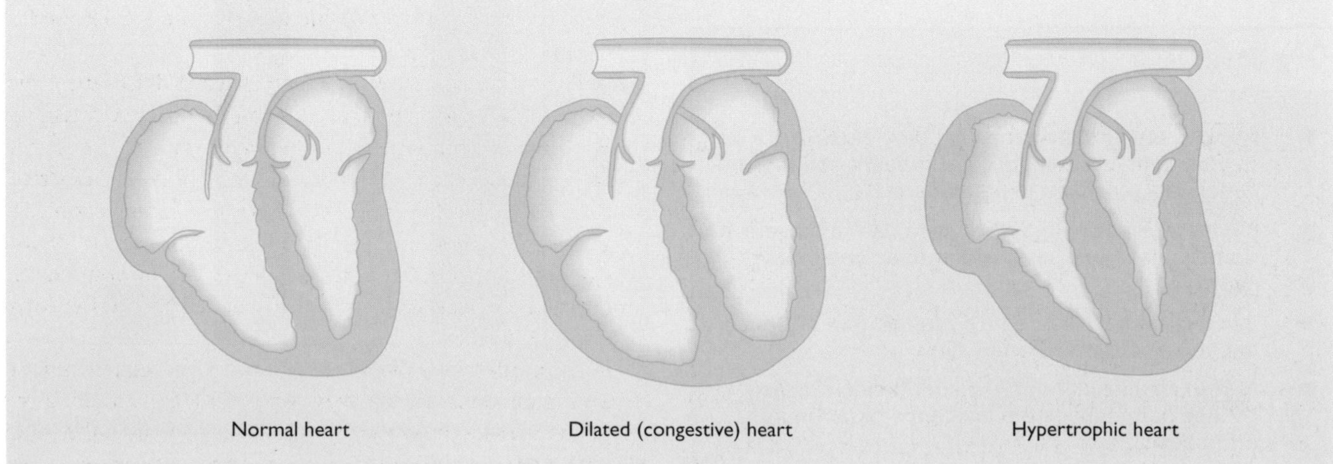

Fig. 8.26 Types of cardiomyopathies involving both the right and the left ventricle.

Symptoms associated with congestive heart failure

Acute	Chronic
Tachycardia	Various arrhythmias
Shortness of breath	Hypertension
Edema (peripheral/pulmonary)	Cardiomegaly
Decreased exercise tolerance	Edema (peripheral/pumonary)

Fig. 8.27 Symptoms associated with congestive heart failure. The severity of the symptoms depends upon the degree of heart failure.

Clinical features of congestive heart failure

- Reduced force of cardiac contraction
- Reduced cardiac output
- Reduced tissue perfusion
- Increased peripheral vascular resistance
- Edema

Right ventricular heart failure is characterized by dyspnea, edema, and fatigue

The characteristics of right ventricular heart failure (dyspnea, edema, and fatigue) result from 'backward failure.' In this condition central venous and right atrial pressures are both high, producing general venous congestion. Any obstruction to right ventricular inflow or excessive load imposed on the right ventricle can precipitate this condition.

Left ventricular heart failure is characterized by reduced cardiac output and blood pressure, and pulmonary congestion

Left ventricular heart failure produces 'forward failure,' with reduced cardiac output and blood pressure, and the associated backward failure due to pulmonary congestion.

Regardless of the type of heart failure, both cardiac output and blood pressure are reduced. The cardiovascular system compensates for these decreases, initially maintaining adequate organ and tissue perfusion. Two processes usually occur:

- Activation of extrinsic neurohumoral reflexes.
- Intrinsic cardiac compensation.

Both work in conjunction, improving cardiac function.

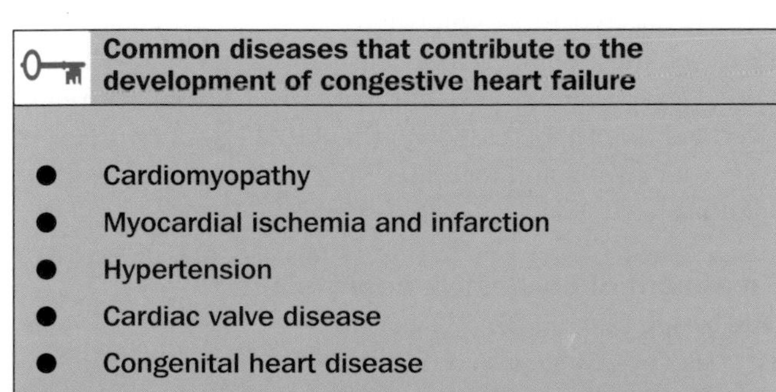

Common diseases that contribute to the development of congestive heart failure

- Cardiomyopathy
- Myocardial ischemia and infarction
- Hypertension
- Cardiac valve disease
- Congenital heart disease
- Coronary artery disease

Extrinsic neurohumoral reflexes help to maintain cardiac output and blood pressure

Hypotension activates baroreceptors, which increase the activity of the sympathetic nervous system, leading to an increased heart rate and vasoconstriction. Cardiac contractility and the vascular tone of the blood vessels therefore increase, and the latter increases cardiac 'afterload.'

Cardiac afterload is defined as the resistance against which the cardiac muscle must pump to expel blood from the ventricles. When it increases, the ejection fraction (the amount of blood ejected from the ventricles) is reduced, and perfusion to organs such as the liver and kidneys is reduced. A reduction in renal perfusion activates the renin–angiotensin system, leading to renin secretion, which increases plasma angiotensin II and aldosterone levels.

Angiotensin II causes peripheral vasoconstriction while aldosterone increases Na^+ retention leading to the following sequence of events:

- Increased water retention.
- Increased venous and arterial blood pressures.
- Increased vascular and interstitial fluid volume.
- Congestion and edema both systemically and in the lungs.
- Increased cardiac preload (Fig. 8.28).

Intrinsic cardiac compensatory mechanisms are activated by an increase in cardiac preload

The cardiac changes that occur include:

- Ventricular dilatation.
- An increase in the volume and pressures generated by the ventricles.

As preload increases, there is incomplete emptying of the ventricles and a resulting increase in end-diastolic pressure, which initially maintains cardiac output by increasing the muscle tension. In cardiac muscle the tension depends on the degree of stretch of the muscle fiber (i.e. preload at the onset of contraction).This relationship is described by the behavior of cardiac muscle length–tension curves, which parallel the output–volume relationship of the heart (Frank–Starling ventricular function curve, see Fig. 8.32).

The hypertrophy and dilatation that develop as a consequence of CHF increase cardiac muscle mass, which facilitates ventricular systole and increases the efficiency of blood ejection from the ventricles. It is also an adaptive mechanism which reduces ventricular wall stress.

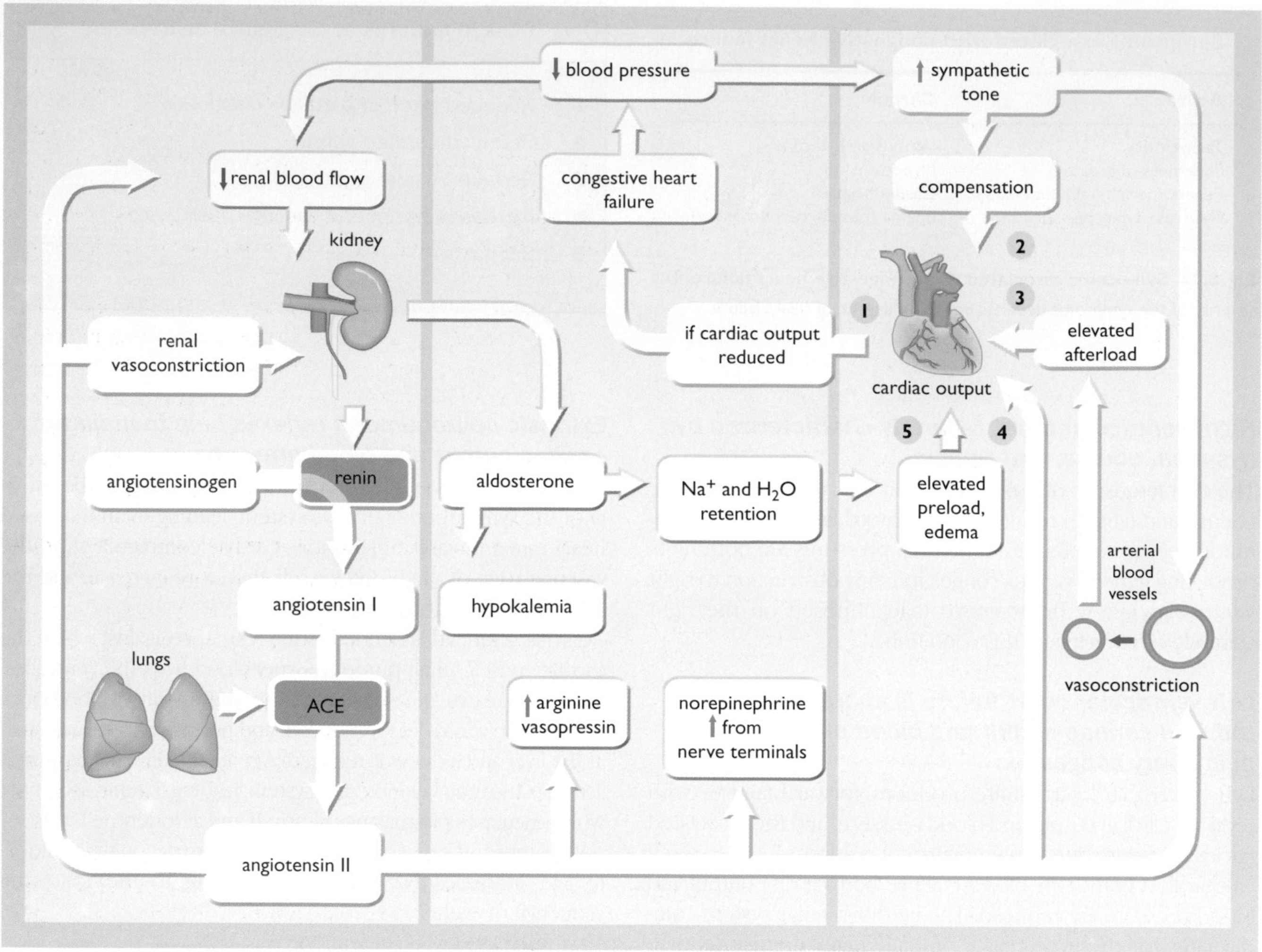

Fig. 8.28 The major extrinsic neurohumoral compensatory mechanisms involved in congestive heart failure. (CHF). (1) Cardiac output is reduced in CHF. (2) Reflex sympathetic compensation can increase cardiac output, but (3) an associated increase in afterload can reduce cardiac output. The cascade of other events can lead to hypertrophy (4) owing to actions of angiotensin II on the heart, which increases cardiac output and Na^+ retention. This may increase cardiac output (5) by raising preload and left ventricular end-diastolic pressure, but this may cause death by initiating pulmonary edema.

Heart wall tension is directly related to ventricular chamber pressure by the relationship known as Laplace's law ($T = (P \times r)/w$, where T is the tension developed in the heart muscle wall, P is the transmural pressure, r is the radius of the ventricle, and w is wall thickness).

If ventricular wall stress were not relieved, severe damage would result. With Laplace's law, however, ventricular wall tension varies inversely with wall thickness, and the ventricular hypertrophy may reduce the developing wall stress as preload increases. However, this adaptive process cannot compensate for CHF indefinitely, and with time the ventricles usually become much less compliant than normal and cardiac output falls.

Compensatory mechanisms activated during CHF result in positive inotropism

The compensatory mechanisms activated during CHF result in positive inotropism:

- An increase in the rate of contractility $[(+dP/dt)_{max}]$.
- Increased efficiency in systolic emptying.
- Reduced diastolic emptying.

However, these compensatory mechanisms are not well maintained and progressively fail. Failure results from ventricular overload due to increased ventricular filling pressures, systolic wall stress, and increased myocardial energy requirements.

Treatment of congestive heart failure

The basic treatment for CHF aims to:

- Reduce congestion (edema).
- Improve cardiac systolic and diastolic function (contraction and relaxation, Fig. 8.29). Many drugs can be used to achieve this purpose (Fig. 8.30).

Pharmacotherapeutic approach to congestive heart failure

Problem	Approach
Fatigue	Rest, positive inotropes
Edema	Diet (salt restriction), diuretics, digitalis
Poor cardiac contractility	Positive inotropes
Dyspnea	Diuretics (thiazides/loop)
Congestion	Nitrovasodilators
Increased cardiac preload and afterload	Angiotensin-converting enzyme inhibitors, venodilators, vasodilators
Irreversible heart failure	Heart transplantation

Fig. 8.29 Pharmacotherapeutic approach to congestive heart failure. The most important approach is to reduce congestion (edema) and improve cardiac contractility.

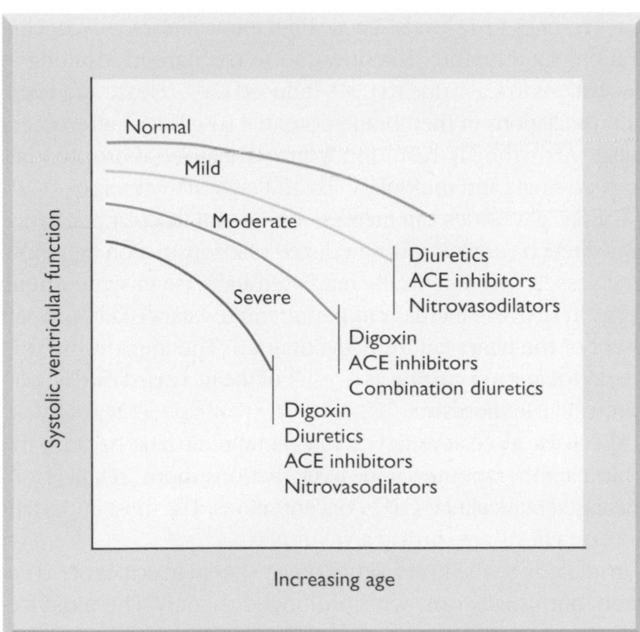

Fig. 8.30 Drugs used in the treatment of the various stages of congestive heart failure. The slow decline in ventricular function with age is exacerbated by disease. (ACE, angiotensin-converting enzyme)

Cardiac glycosides Digoxin is the prototype cardiac glycoside and is extracted from the purple (*Digitalis purpurea*) and white (*D. lanata*) foxglove. Although there are several other cardiac glycosides, digoxin has the most widespread clinical use. An endogenous digitalis-like factor has been detected in mammals, but its pharmacology is still being determined.

All cardiac glycosides share a similar chemical structure. Digoxin, digitalis, and ouabain all possess an aglycone steroid nucleus where the pharmacologic activity of the compound is found. An unsaturated (C17-linked) lactone ring is present, which conveys cardiotonic activity, and C3-linked sugar moieties alter potency and the pharmacokinetic distribution of the compound.

Cardiac glycosides inhibit membrane-bound Na^+/K^+ ATPase

Cardiac glycosides improve cardiac contractility at the molecular level by inhibiting membrane-bound Na^+/K^+ ATPase (Fig. 8.31). This enzyme is involved in establishing the resting membrane potential of most excitable cells. The energy to pump three Na^+ ions actively out of the cell and two K^+ ions into the cell against their concentration gradients is derived from the hydrolysis of ATP. Inhibition of the pump results in an increased cytoplasmic Na^+ concentration.

The increase in Na^+ concentration leads to a marked increase in Ca^{2+} concentration as a result of the inhibition of another membrane-bound ion exchanger (Na^+/Ca^{2+} exchanger). The direction in which this transports Na^+ and Ca^{2+} depends upon the membrane potential and the concentrations of ions across the membrane. It is an ATP-dependent antiporter (see Chapter 3) that normally causes a net extrusion of Ca^{2+} from cells. The increased intracellular Na^+ concentration passively reduces the exchange function so that less Ca^{2+} is extruded. The raised intracellular Ca^{2+} concentration is then actively pumped into the sarcoplasmic reticulum and becomes available for release during subsequent cellular depolarizations, thereby enhancing excitation–contraction coupling. The resultant tissue mechanism of action is a greater force of contractility, known as positive inotropism (Fig. 8.31).

In the failing heart, the positive inotropic actions of the cardiac glycosides produce changes in the Frank–Starling ventricular function curve. Figure 8.32 outlines the actions of positive inotropic agents on cardiac output.

Despite widespread use, there is no convincing evidence that digitalis, the most commonly used cardiac glycoside, has a beneficial effect on the long-term prognosis of patients with CHF. The symptoms are improved, but digitalis is not a cure for the underlying dysfunction.

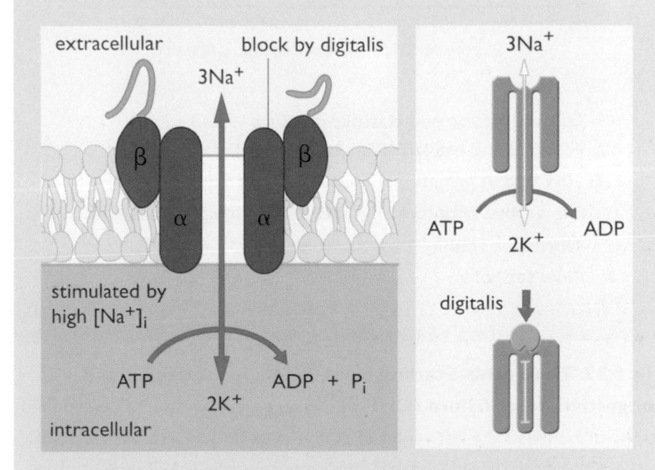

Fig. 8.31 Mechanism of action of digitalis glycosides. The binding site for digitalis is on the extracellular aspect of the α–β heterodimer structure of the Na^+/K^+ ATPase enzyme. Inhibition of this enzyme raises intracellular Na^+ concentration, which raises intracellular Ca^{2+}, and mediates the positive inotropic actions of cardiac glycosides.

Positive inotropes that improve cardiac contractility

- Cardiac glycosides (e.g. digoxin)
- Phosphodiesterase inhibitors (e.g. amrinone)
- β_1 Agonists (e.g. dobutamide)

Cardiac glycosides alter the electrical activity in the heart

In addition to improving the force of contraction, cardiac glycosides alter the electrical activity in the heart both directly and indirectly.

At pharmacotherapeutic doses cardiac glycosides indirectly alter the heart rate by increasing vagal (cranial nerve X) tone, which results from stimulation of paravertebral ganglion reflex arcs. The vagal actions predominate in the supraventricular regions and include:

- Slowing of the SA node firing rate.
- Slowing of AV node conduction velocity.
- Shortening of the atrial action potential.

At toxic doses, cardiac glycosides increase the heart's sympathetic tone. However, the rate of neural discharge is not uniform and can result in non-uniform myocardial excitability and arrhythmias including AV node block, AV junctional tachycardia, and VPBs.

The direct effects of cardiac glycosides on cardiac tissue are most marked at high doses and relate to the loss of intracellular K^+ due to inhibition of Na^+/K^+ ATPase. The continued loss of intracellular K^+ to the extracellular space reduces the resting membrane potential of the cell, resulting in:

- Enhanced automaticity.
- Decreased cardiac conduction velocity.
- Increased AV node refractory period.

Owing to the increase in cytosolic Ca^{2+} concentration, eventually the sarcoplasmic reticulum (SR) may become overwhelmed. With increasing cardiac glycoside concentrations, free Ca^{2+} reaches toxic levels. These high intracellular Ca^{2+} concentrations saturate the SR sequestration mechanism resulting in oscillations in Ca^{2+} due to Ca^{2+}-induced Ca^{2+} release and resultant oscillations in membrane potential (oscillatory afterpotentials). Arrhythmias resulting from oscillatory afterpotentials include single and multiple VPBs and tachyarrhythmias.

Cardiac glycosides can increase peripheral vascular resistance by a direct α adrenoceptor-mediated vasoconstriction in peripheral vessels and a centrally mediated increase in sympathetic tone. In CHF the increase in peripheral resistance falls as treatment of the heart failure is maintained. The improvement in hemodynamics occurring as a result of the increased cardiac output results in diuresis.

All cardiac glycosides have a low therapeutic ratio because the pharmacotherapeutic and toxic actions both result from increased intracellular Ca^{2+} concentrations. The most important adverse effects are cardiac arrhythmias.

In addition to the heart, other organ system toxicities are common, but usually only with prolonged therapy. The most frequent non-cardiac adverse effects of cardiac glycosides involve:

- Actions on the gastrointestinal tract.
- Central nervous system (CNS) effects due to stimulation of the vagal system and chemoreceptor trigger zone resulting in nausea, vomiting, diarrhea, and anorexia. Other CNS effects include visual disturbances, headaches, dizziness, fatigue, and hallucinations, which are especially common in the elderly.

Rare adverse effects include eosinophilia and a skin rash. Gynecomastia may occur in men and is thought to be due to either hypothalamic stimulation or peripheral estrogenic actions of cardiac glycosides.

Plasma monitoring of cardiac glycoside concentrations is important since the pharmacotherapeutic window is so narrow.

In Europe, attempts have been made to identify drugs that may be used with digitalis to alleviate its tendency to evoke cardiac arrhythmias, but as yet none has been introduced for widespread use.

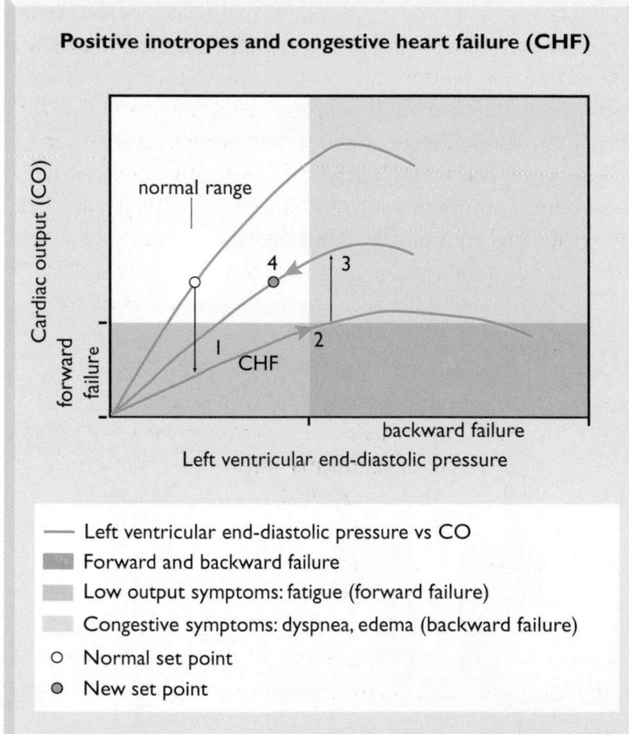

Fig. 8.32 The Frank–Starling curve, positive inotropes, and congestive heart failure (CHF). Normal cardiac output is determined by the pressure in the left ventricle at end-diastole. In CHF, the set point for cardiac output is reduced and cardiac output falls (1). Compensatory neurohumoral responses become activated which increase end-diastolic pressure and improve cardiac output; however, this can give rise to backward failure (2). Positive inotropic agents increase cardiac output. (3). The improved cardiac output reduces the drive for a high end-diastolic pressure, and decompensation occurs to a new set point (4).

The pharmacokinetics of individual cardioglycosides varies according to lipophilicity of the compound.

Cardiac glycoside toxicity can be treated

Cardiac glycoside toxicity may be worsened by hypokalemia associated with the use of diuretics and secondary aldosteronism. Cardiac glycosides and K^+ ions compete for a common binding site on Na^+/K^+ ATPase. Hypokalemia facilitates cardiac glycoside binding to the enzyme, thereby enhancing the toxic effects.

Treatment includes:

- Oral administration of K^+ supplements to raise serum K^+ concentration.
- Antiarrhythmic drugs such as procainamide and phenytoin to reverse cardiac glycoside-induced arrhythmias.
- Monoclonal antibodies specific to cardiac glycosides if the arrhythmias are refractory to antiarrhythmic treatment.
- Intravenous digoxin-immune fragment for antigen binding (Fab) derived from specific antibodies to digoxin for patients with life-threatening intoxication. The high affinity of cardiac glycosides for the antibody prevents binding to Na^+/K^+ ATPase and the drug can be cleared from the circulatory system.

Although these treatments are available to reverse cardiac glycoside toxicity, it should be minimized or prevented by careful monitoring of serum electrolytes and cardiac glycoside blood levels. A very important element in the risk of developing digoxin toxicity is renal function. Since digoxin is primarily excreted unchanged by the kidneys, maintenance doses of digoxin must be adjusted in patients with renal insuffficiency.

 **Adverse effects of cardiac glycosides**

- Toxicity because the therapeutic dose ratios are narrow
- May promote cardiac K^+ loss and hypokalemia which precipitate life-threatening arrhythmias when used with diuretics
- Abdominal discomfort, emesis, and anorexia
- Arrhythmias with cardioversion, which should therefore be used with extreme caution

The phosphodiesterase inhibitors are a group of agents used in patients with CHF refractory to other treatment. These agents predominantly inhibit the F-III isoform of the enzyme (PDE-3) found in myocardial and vascular smooth muscle. Their cellular mechanism of action is a cascade that begins with inhibition of cAMP degradation and ends with an elevation of intracellular Ca^{2+} content.

There are many tissue-specific phosphodiesterase isoforms. Inhibitors such as amrinone, milrinone, and recently vesnarinone, are bipyridines that increase cAMP levels by inhibiting PDE-3. Inhibition results in a more prolonged influx of Ca^{2+} during the cardiac action potential and increases contractility. cAMP breakdown is also inhibited in arterial and venous smooth muscle, resulting in marked vasodilation.

These agents increase cardiac output, decrease pulmonary capillary wedge pressure, and reduce total peripheral resistance, without producing any significant changes in heart rate or arterial blood pressure.

Amrinone is a PDE inhibitor useful for short-term treatment of CHF

Amrinone is used clinically for the short-term treatment of patients with CHF that is refractory to digitalis and diuretic therapy. It can be used alone or in conjunction with β_1 agonists to:

- Improve cardiac output.
- Increase stroke volume.
- Reduce right atrial and pulmonary capillary wedge pressures.

Prolonged intravenous use does not result in tachyphylaxis, but can cause adverse effects. There is a high incidence of nausea and vomiting in patients treated with amrinone, but liver function abnormalities and thrombocytopenia cause most concern. These adverse effects can be remedied by stopping the drug. Amrinone can also cause supraventricular and ventricular arrhythmias and can therefore only be used clinically if the ECG is frequently monitored.

Milrinone is a potent PDE-3 inhibitor that must not be used in long-term therapy

Milrinone is an amrinone analog, but is a more potent inhibitor of PDE-3. It has a similar spectrum of dose-limiting toxicities to that of amrinone, but is rarely associated with thrombocytopenia. There is less gastrointestinal upset if it is used orally. Its use is limited, however, because it can precipitate arrhythmias and increase death rate; it is not, therefore, used for chronic therapy. Similar findings have limited the use of a similar agent, enoximone.

Vesnarone is a PDE inhibitor with additional potentially useful molecular actions

Studies suggest that vesnarinone may increase cardiac contractility by additional mechanisms such as activation of the Na^+/Ca^{2+} exchange antiporter, which:

- Increases intracellular Ca^{2+}.
- Prolongs the cardiac action potential duration.
- Increases the L-type Ca^{2+} current (I_{si}).

The major limiting adverse effect is agranulocytosis, which occurs in 1–3% of patients. However, this is reversible when the drug is stopped. Its effectiveness in the long-term therapy of heart failure is unknown.

β_1 Adrenoceptor agonists selectively increase cardiac contractility through β_1 receptor activation in the heart with less of the undesirable peripheral α adrenoceptor activity associated with the use of nonselective sympathomimetics. The β_1 adrenoceptor is predominantly found in cardiac tissue and selective agonism (the molecular action of the β_1 adrenoceptor agonist) results in elevated intracellular Ca^{2+} concentrations (cellular action), which increases the strength of cardiac contractility (tissue action).

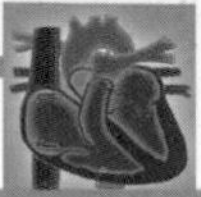

Dobutamine and dopamine are the two most widely used β_1 agonists, but their use is limited to emergency intravenous therapy.

Dobutamine (a racemate) is a relatively selective cardiac β_1 adrenoceptor agonist, although the optical enantiomers differ in their selectivity for the various adrenoceptors. At doses less than 5 µg/kg/min it is a selective β_1 agonist, while higher doses result in actions on β_2 and mild effects on α adrenoceptors. Less peripheral vasoconstriction is therefore produced than if epinephrine were administered. Dobutamine improves many indices of cardiac function that are impaired in CHF:

- Cardiac output is increased.
- Mean arterial pressure is decreased.
- Systemic vascular resistance is decreased.
- Ventricular filling pressure is reduced.

Dobutamine is therefore the most widely used β_1 agonist in the treatment of both right and left ventricular dysfunction associated with treatable acute CHF. A short half-life means that it is unsuitable to be given orally or chronically. It does not increase renal blood flow.

Dopamine is a widely used β_1 agonist that also possesses dopamine receptor agonist activity. It is actually an endogenous neurotransmitter and has actions on the peripheral and central nervous systems. When given as a slow intravenous infusion it has a positive inotropic effect on cardiac muscle as a result of:

- Directly stimulating β_1 adrenoceptors.
- Release of endogenous norepinephrine.

Dopamine produces renal arteriolar vasodilation and therefore increases urinary output and relieves edema. It is useful when there is cardiogenic, traumatic, and hypovolemic shock where blood pressure is low and renal blood flow is poor.

Other β_1 agonists such as isoproterenol, norepinephrine, and epinephrine are never used in CHF because of their chronotropic and α adrenergic agonist properties. These agents are all notorious for their ability to waste myocardial oxygen, which precludes their use in CHF.

The use of β_1 agonists in CHF must be considered in terms of the pharmacodynamic events that occur at the receptor level. In CHF, the high cardiac sympathetic tone produces $\beta_1$adrenoceptor downregulation. Therefore, repeated exposure of cardiac muscle to β_1 agonists may result in tachyphylaxis or a loss of β_1 function in the failing heart, which may be a result of receptor uncoupling to the second messenger system. So, paradoxically, the long-term use of selective β_1 agonists may enhance receptor downregulation and worsen myocardial function in CHF.

Additional drugs used in CHF to reduce edema and cardiac preload and afterload

- Diuretics (e.g. thiazides, furosemide)
- Angiotensin-converting enzyme (ACE) inhibitors (e.g. captopril)
- Nitrovasodilators (e.g. intravenous nitroprusside, oral hydralazine, topical nitroglycerin)

Diuretics are routinely used with digitalis glycosides to treat congestive heart failure

Diuretics reduce cardiac preload by inhibiting Na^+ and water retention in the kidney. Cardiac pump efficiency increases with the resulting reduction in venous pressure, and so the signs and symptoms of edema decrease (Fig. 8.33). Thiazide (e.g. chlorothiazide) and loop diuretic (e.g. furosemide) therapy reduce intravascular and extravascular fluid accumulation in CHF and have beneficial effects in both acute and chronic CHF.

Diuretics are also discussed in Chapter 10 and again in this chapter in the section on hypertension (see p. 181).

Adverse effects resulting from diuretic therapy are usually only seen with long-term use. They include:

- Activation of hormone pathways.
- Changes in electrolyte balance.
- Changes in metabolic processes.

Electrolyte imbalances occur for serum Na^+, Mg^{2+}, Ca^{2+}, and K^+ ions. The loss of K^+ ions from serum (hypokalemia) is especially serious and may precipitate ventricular arrhythmias. Potassium-sparing diuretics such as spironolactone or triamterene can be used to reduce K^+ loss.

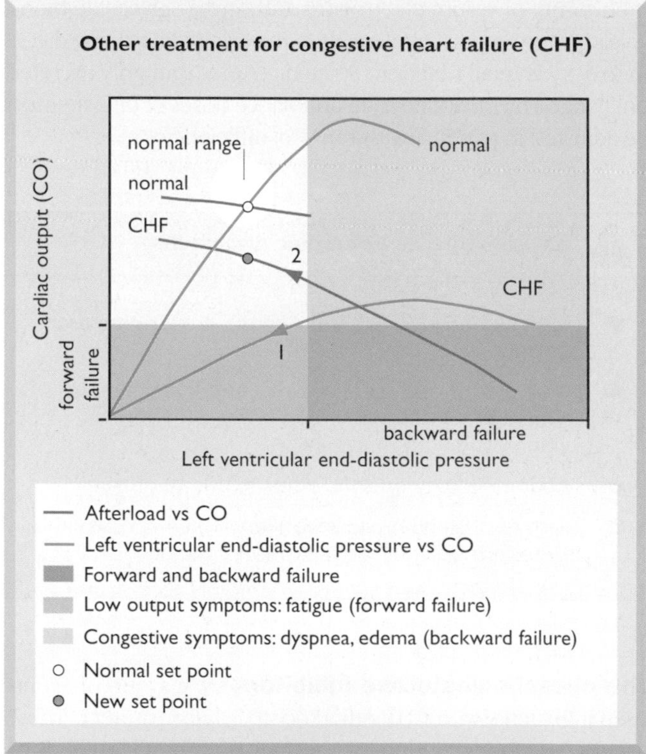

Fig. 8.33 The mechanism of action of other drugs used to treat congestive heart failure (CHF). Venodilation, diuretic therapy, and angiotensin-converting enzyme (ACE) inhibitors reduce backward failure and the symptoms of edema and congestion by reducing end-diastolic pressure. However, when used alone they may precipitate forward failure by this mechanism. (1). Vasodilators and ACE inhibitors improve cardiac output by reducing cardiac afterload resulting from increased peripheral vasoconstriction and pulmonary congestion, thus providing a new set point out of the forward and backward failure domains (2).

The main metabolic changes that can occur include increased concentrations of glucose and uric acid in some patients. Diuretic use should be carefully considered in the elderly where reduced renal function may predominate and in whom azotemia, urinary incontinence, hypovolemia, and dizziness may occur with therapy.

Drug interactions with diuretics are rare. However, the diuretic action of loop diuretics such as furosemide may be reduced when used concomitantly with aspirin-like non-steroidal anti-inflammatory agents (NSAIDs). The mechanism probably involves NSAID inhibition of renal prostaglandin (PG) synthesis, especially PGI_2 and PGE_2, which are endogenous vasodilators.

Ototoxicity and nephrotoxicity can result when loop diuretics are used with aminoglycoside antibiotics.

Angiotensin-converting enzyme inhibitors are first-line therapy for congestive heart failure

Angiotensin-converting enzyme (ACE) inhibitors were first used in CHF after it was found that neurohumoral systems are activated during periods of reduced organ perfusion and increased ventricular volume. The renin–angiotensin cascade decreases cardiac performance by producing angiotensin II, which increases systemic vascular resistance (cardiac afterload) and aldosterone, which causes edema. Inhibition of this system by ACE inhibitors such as captopril, enalapril, and lisinopril therefore reduces circulating angiotensin II levels. This in turn reduces peripheral vascular resistance (cardiac afterload) and prevents aldosterone-mediated Na^+ retention (i.e. reduces cardiac preload) (see Fig. 8.33). The increase in sympathetic tone is also reduced, allowing for a reduction in circulating epinephrine levels and an increased efficiency in systolic emptying, or an increase in cardiac output. ACE inhibitors may also reduce angiotensin II-induced cardiac hypertrophy.

ACE inhibitors are the only agents that have been shown to prolong life in CHF patients, and are therefore major therapeutic agents in this syndrome.

The ACE inhibitors have few clinical adverse effects. Hypotension is common as a result of the reduced arterial pressure and may cause dizziness and lightheadedness. Renal dysfunction and hyperkalemia occur, but are reversible if the drug is stopped. Approximately 10% of patients develop cough.

Less frequent adverse effects include skin rashes, gastrointestinal upset, altered taste, and angioneurotic edema, which may occur as a result of bradykinin accumulation.

Toxicity occurs when ACE inhibitors are used with NSAIDs. Concomitant use of these agents prevents the autoregulatory mechanism of PG-mediated efferent arteriolar vasodilatation and results in renal hypertension.

Nitrovasodilators This group of drugs consists of a variety of chemically diverse agents that mediate a potent vasodilating action on both arterial and venous smooth muscle. The molecular mechanism of action remains poorly characterized. However, these agents:

- Are thought to produce relaxation at the cellular level by nitrosothiol intermediate enhancement of cGMP activity.
- May regulate intracellular Ca^{2+} release from the sarcoplasmic reticulum, alter sympathetic tone, and produce smooth muscle relaxing autacoids such as PGI_2 and PGE_2.
- Reduce diastolic pressure and improve diastolic function in the heart (see Fig. 8.33).

Nitroprusside is a standard first-choice nitrovasodilator in the treatment of acute CHF because it reduces both cardiac preload and afterload. It reduces left ventricular filling pressures by reducing venous tone, and by doing so increases venous capacitance and produces a shift in blood volume distribution. The reduced intracardiac pressure and volume reduce the myocardial hypertrophy that can develop in CHF.

Since nitroprusside has no direct effect on ventricular contractility, the increase in cardiac output and stroke volume occur as a result of a reduction in cardiac afterload. The increase in cardiac output is not accompanied by a reflex increase in blood pressure or heart rate, and nitroprusside lowers myocardial oxygen consumption.

Nitroprusside must be given intravenously at 0.10–0.20 μg/kg/min with dose titration, and is used as an acute short-term treatment of CHF.

Liver metabolism results in the production of cyanide, which is then cleared by the kidney. Cyanide can accumulate in patients with renal insufficiency, resulting in nausea, confusion, and convulsions. Nitroprusside can also be metabolized to prussic acid, which avidly binds hemoglobin.

The major adverse effect of nitroprusside is hypotension, which may be severe.

Nitroglycerin (glyceryl trinitrate) and isosorbide dinitrate predominantly decrease cardiac preload, but produce a slight reduction in cardiac afterload. Tolerance develops rapidly and so administration has to be intermittent. A high first-pass metabolism can be avoided by sublingual administration or topical application.

Hypotension is the most common adverse effect.

Adverse effects of drugs used in the treatment of congestive heart failure

- Cardiac glycosides have a narrow therapeutic index and may precipitate arrhythmias
- Short-term treatment with phosphodiesterase inhibitors can cause thrombocytopenia and arrhythmias
- β_1 Agonists may precipitate tachyarrhythmias, and long-term use may worsen myocardial function
- Diuretics produce serious electrolyte imbalances such as hypokalemia, which may produce ventricular arrhythmias
- Angiotensin-converting enzyme (ACE) inhibitors produce few adverse effects, and generally only hypotension
- Nitrovasodilators have few adverse effects

Concomitant use of hydralazine and nitrates is a life-saving alternative first-line therapy for congestive heart failure

In addition to reducing cardiac afterload, hydralazine has an indirect positive inotropic effect on cardiac muscle action resulting from enhanced sympathetic nervous system activity due to arterial vasodilation. It is therefore useful when withdrawing dobutamine or β_1 agonist treatment. Hydralazine also increases renal blood flow. Hydralazine alone is insufficient to reduce vascular congestion adequately, and is therefore used with topical nitroglycerin or oral isosorbide dinitrate to induce venodilation.

Hydralazine used in combination with nitrates has been shown to increase the life expectancy of patients with CHF. This combination is therefore an alternative first-line therapy to ACE inhibitors, especially for patients who are unable to tolerate ACE inhibitors. The adverse effects of hydralazine include:

- Those associated with nitroprusside and nitroglycerin.
- Drug-induced systemic lupus erythematous, which is rare with doses of hydralazine less than 200 mg/day.

Since myocardial oxygen consumption increases with hydralazine, this drug is contraindicated in patients with CHF who have ischemic coronary artery disease unless nitrates are used at the same time.

Emerging drugs Several studies are currently examining the following drugs for use in the treatment of moderate to severe CHF:

- Novel phosphodiesterase inhibitors (OPC-18790).
- Mixed α and β adrenoceptor antagonists (carvedilol).
- Potent angiotensin II receptor antagonists (losartan).

Although there are many drugs that relieve the signs and symptoms of CHF, they do not prevent the underlying deterioration of cardiac function. Valve surgery (if valve insufficiency is the cause) or heart transplantation (if a major myocardial infarction or viral myocarditis are the cause) may be required if drugs fail to relieve the symptoms.

HYPERTENSION

Hypertension is a condition of increasing blood pressure associated with an increased risk of other diseases. It is a sign rather than a disease itself, and the underlying cause is rarely diagnosed. It is defined arbitrarily as sustained diastolic arterial pressure greater than 90 mmHg (Fig. 8.34).

Blood pressure is controlled by an integrated system, and the major elements that regulate it are shown in Fig. 8.35. The main elements that contribute to hypertension are:

- Blood volume.
- Cardiac output.
- Peripheral vascular resistance.

The factors that contribute to the maintenance of normal blood pressure can be manipulated by drugs to treat hypertension.

The system mechanism of action for reducing hypertension is reduction of the sign itself (the hypertension), while the tissue mechanisms of action are altered blood volume, altered cardiac output, and altered peripheral vascular resistance.

Classification of blood pressure based on the 1993 Joint National Committee

Category	Systolic (mmHg)	Diastolic (mmHg)
Normal†	<130	<85
High normal	130-139	85–89
Hypertension		
Stage 1 (mild)	140-159	90–99
Stage 2 (moderate)	160-179	100–109
Stage 3 (severe)	180-209	110–119
Stage 4 (very severe)	≥210	≥120

†Optimal blood pressure with respect to cardiovascular risk is less than 120 mmHg systolic and less than 80 mmHg diastolic

Fig. 8.34 Classification of blood pressure based on the 1993 Joint National Committee. Values are from the 5th report of the JNC on detection, evaluation, and treatment of high blood pressure. Isolated systolic hypertension is defined as a systolic blood pressure of 140 mmHg or more and a diastolic blood pressure of less than 90 mmHg and staged approximately.

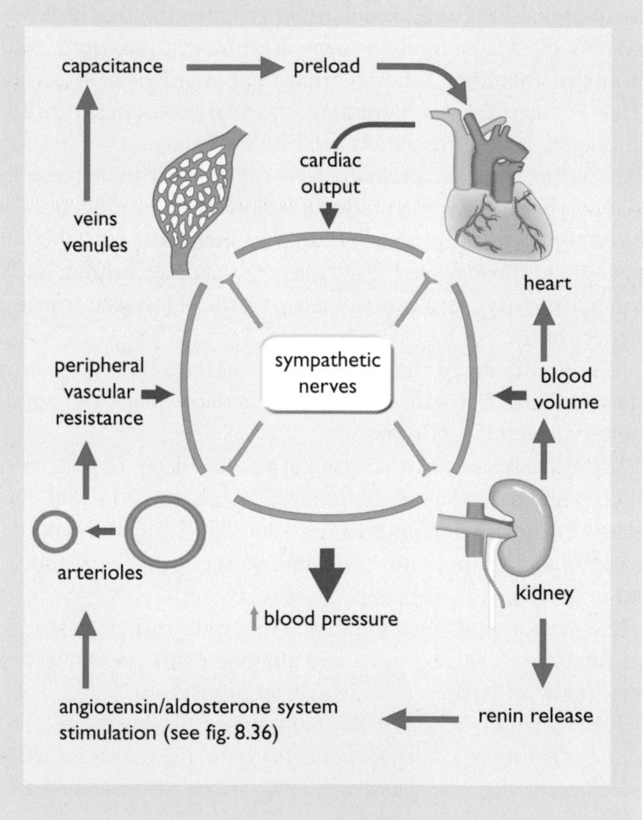

Fig. 8.35 Factors involved in blood pressure control. Determinants of blood pressure are cardiac output, which is determined by heart rate and stroke volume. Cardiac output depends on the amount of blood returning to the heart, which in turn depends on vein and venule capacitance (preload) and blood volume (under the control of the kidneys). Peripheral vascular resistance is determined by the arterioles.

The tissue targets for antihypertensive drugs are:

- The sympathetic nerves, which release the vasoconstrictor norepinephrine.
- The kidney, which regulates blood volume.
- The heart (the output of which can be altered).
- The arterioles, which determine peripheral vascular resistance.
- Endothelial cells, which regulate circulating levels of the endogenous hypertensive agent, angiotensin II.
- The CNS, which determines the blood pressure set point and regulates some systems involved in blood pressure control.

Hypertension can be classified into primary (or essential) hypertension and secondary hypertension

Primary hypertension is an elevation of blood pressure with no apparent cause. It accounts for 90–95% of all cases and usually occurs in adulthood, typically at ages above 40 years. Several risk factors are associated with primary hypertension including a genetic predisposition, obesity, high alcohol consumption, and physical inactivity. Some of these may represent additional systems targets for antihypertensive drugs.

Secondary hypertension accounts for 5–10% of all cases and is due to an identifiable cause, usually renovascular disease, which elevates blood pressure by activating the renin–angiotensin–aldosterone system (Fig. 8.36). A variety of endocrine diseases (e.g. pheochromocytoma, an adrenal medulla cancer that secretes excessive epinephrine) may also cause secondary hypertension.

Both primary and secondary hypertension can be classified as mild, accelerated, or emergency

In mild hypertension the blood pressure increases progressively over many years. As a result, the blood-vessel changes (i.e. thickening of the intima due to increased migration of smooth muscle cells from the media) develop slowly in response to the increase in blood pressure (Fig. 8.37). It is a chronic condition requiring long-term control of blood pressure.

In accelerated hypertension there is a larger increase in blood pressure over a shorter period of time and the destructive changes in the blood vessel walls develop rapidly (Fig. 8.38). In this situation the pharmacotherapeutic objective is to control the blood pressure (particularly the diastolic pressure) over a period of days to weeks.

A hypertensive emergency occurs when the patient's life is immediately at risk and blood pressure control is required within minutes or hours.

Treatment of hypertension

Nondrug treatment is the ideal first-choice therapy

All antihypertensive drugs have adverse effects, as do most pharmacotherapeutic drugs. However, in the case of hypertension, adverse effects are particularly important since most hypertensive patients do not have symptoms. It is only when secondary complications such as a stroke ensue that the disease becomes symptomatic. Therefore, any drug with an adverse effect will

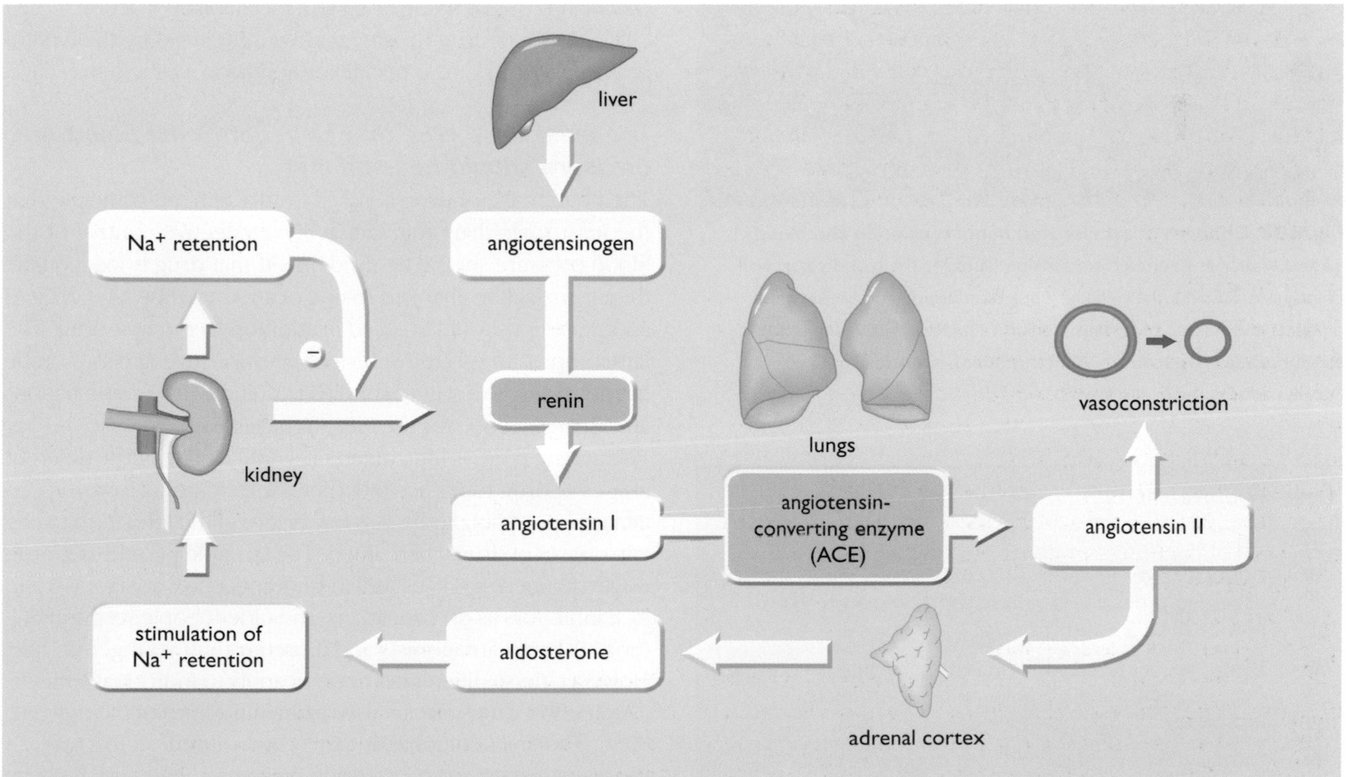

Fig. 8.36 Renin–angiotensin–aldosterone system. Release of renin stimulates conversion of angiotensinogen (from the liver) to angiotensin I, which in turn is converted to angiotensin II under the influence of angiotensin-converting enzyme. Angiotensin II leads to vasoconstriction, release of aldosterone (adrenal cortex), and Na^+ retention. The latter increases blood pressure but reduces renin release, so the system is a homeostatic process.

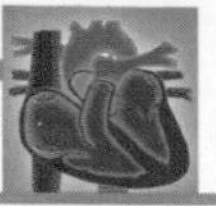

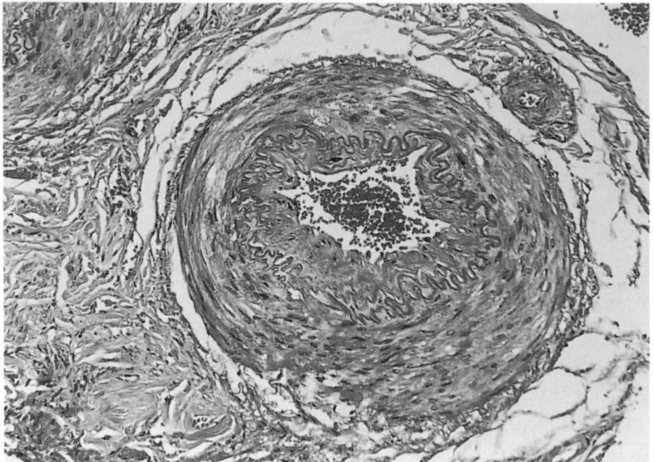

Fig. 8.37 Changes of chronic hypertension in the blood vessel wall. These occur slowly over time. Medial smooth muscle cells migrate into the intima so that the intima becomes thicker. (Courtesy of Dr Alan Stevens and Professor Jim Lowe.)

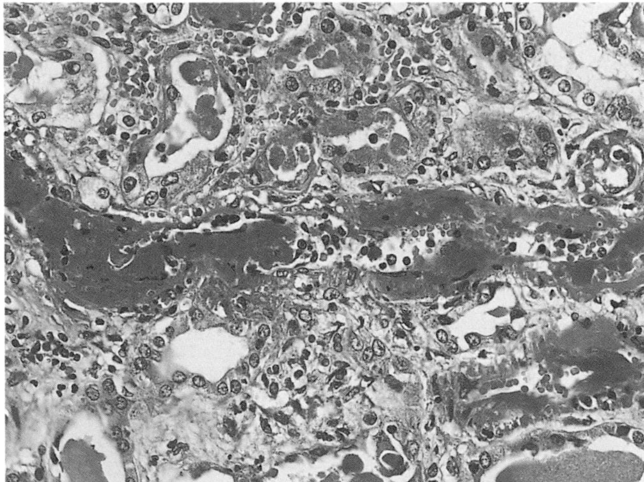

Fig. 8.38 Changes of accelerated hypertension in the blood vessel wall. Accelerated hypertension damages the blood vessel wall. Damage to the endothelial lining leeds to adhesion and activation of platelets and release of various mediators (platelet activating factor, thromboxane A_2, serotonin, ADP, thrombin). (Courtesy of Dr Alan Stevens and Professor Jim Lowe.)

Hypertension

- Hypertension is commonly diagnosed when the diastolic pressure is consistently found to be higher than 90 mmHg
- Blood pressure can be raised by increased cardiac output, increased peripheral resistance, or increased blood volume
- Primary hypertension has no apparent cause
- Secondary hypertension results from another disease such as pheochromocytoma

Classes of drugs used for treating hypertension

- Diuretics
- Sympatholytics
- Direct-acting vasodilators
- Calcium antagonists
- Renin–angiotensin cascade inhibitors (including the angiotensin II receptor antagonist, losartan)

make the patient feel worse and compliance is then often poor.

Patients with hypertension are advised to avoid activities that may predispose to cardiovascular disease. The major recommendations are:

- To exercise.
- To reduce body weight.
- In some cases, to restrict dietary salt intake.

The pharmacotherapeutic response in the treatment of hypertension is a reduction in blood pressure to an acceptable level (typically a diastolic blood pressure ≤ 90 mmHg). This can be achieved by diverse system, tissue, cellular, and molecular mechanisms of action.

Five classes of drug are currently used, but the classification is heterogeneous since some of the classes comprise drugs grouped in terms of their molecular mechanism of action, and others in terms of tissue or system mechanism of action.

The choice of drug therapy may be influenced by the type of hypertension and any other clinical condition a patient may have.

The least toxic drug that can control the blood pressure should be used first

The first choice of drug is based on the general principle that the least toxic drug that can achieve effective control of the blood pressure should be used first. If that drug is inadequate, then it should be changed to one of another class, or a drug of another class should be used in addition to the first drug. The latter approach is often sufficient because several class combinations produce a synergistic effect. Multiple drug combinations are usually needed for the most intractable cases.

Generally, there is little difference in the ability of the different classes of drug to reduce blood pressure acutely. However, certain groups of people are less responsive in the long term to certain classes of drugs than others. For example people of African origin do not respond as well to β adrenoceptor antagonists and ACE inhibitors as do Caucasians, and older people respond better to calcium antagonists and diuretics than younger people. However, these differences may not apply to individual patients.

A variety of drugs may be used as an initial form of therapy (Fig. 8.39). The first additional drug may be a diuretic, if this was not the drug of first choice, or a β adrenoceptor antagonist. Calcium antagonists such as nifedipine or an ACE inhibitor such as lisinopril are increasingly used as an alternative to diuretics or β adrenoceptor antagonists.

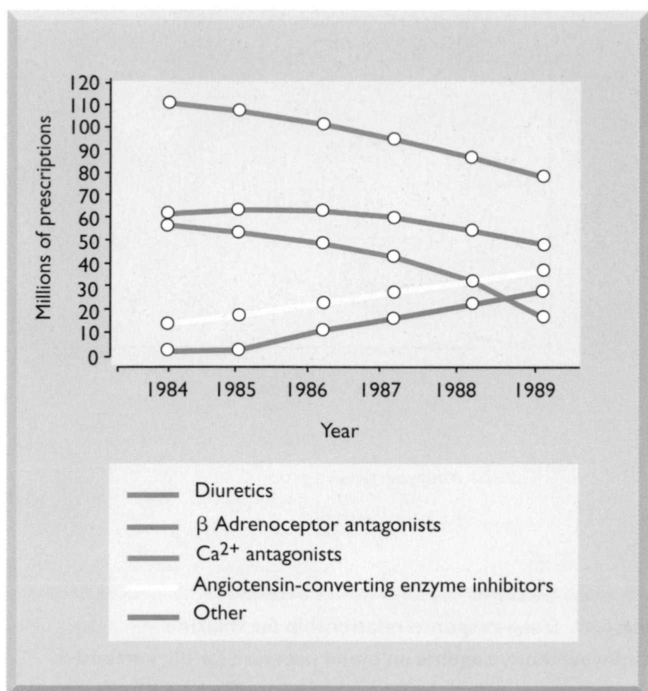

Fig. 8.39 Number of antihypertensive prescriptions in the US, 1984–1989.

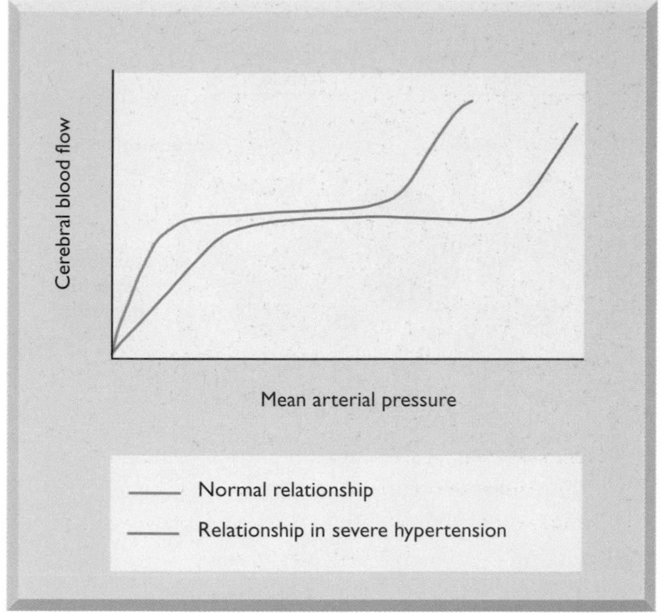

Fig. 8.40 The relationship between cerebral blood flow (CBF) and mean arterial pressure (MAP). In severe hypertension, particularly in emergency hypertension, a rapid reduction of MAP may cause an excessive reduction in CBF, cerebral ischemia, and possibly stroke.

A hypertensive emergency may occur if the therapy is inadequate or if patients stop taking their medication because they falsely think they are 'well.' If this occurs it is important to reduce the blood pressure quickly by intravenous drug administration, but carefully and in stages (usually chosen arbitrarily) to avoid low cerebrovascular pressure and cerebral ischemia (Fig. 8.40)

Diuretics The pharmacology of diuretics is discussed in some detail in Chapter 10. Diuretics were once thought to lower blood pressure at the tissue level because they increase Na^+ excretion in the kidney, which leads to a reduction of plasma volume, extracellular fluid volume, and cardiac output. However, there are several reasons for questioning this (see below).

Diuretics used in hypertension are subclassified into three groups:

- Thiazides.
- Loop diuretics.
- Potassium-sparing agents.

Although diuretics may share a common system mechanism of action (i.e. reduction of blood volume) and tissue mechanism of action (i.e. enhancement of water excretion by the kidney), they differ in terms of their cellular and molecular mechanisms of action, and therefore their site of action within the kidney (Fig. 8.41). More importantly, their action as antihypertensive agents is poorly related to their diuretic activity:

- Loop diuretics are moderate antihypertensive agents, yet powerful diuretics.
- Thiazides are powerful antihypertensive agents, but moderate diuretics.

So, although diuresis has been the conventional explanation for the beneficial effect provided by diuretics in hypertension, there is increasing awareness that the molecular and tissue mechanism of action is not well understood. The only certainty is that a site of action does appear to be the kidney, but other possible sites such as resistance arterioles may also be involved.

Thiazide diuretics act on the distal convoluted tubule

Thiazide diuretics (e.g. bendrofluazide, hydrochlorothiazide) and thiazide-like drugs, which are sulfonamide derivatives, such as chlorthalidone, are actively transported by a probenecid-sensitive secretory mechanism into the proximal renal tubule. As diuretics, this group of agents acts on the luminal membrane of the cortical diluting segment of the distal convoluted tubule:

- At the molecular level they modulate ion transport function in the tubule.
- The cellular response is impaired movement of sodium chloride from the lumen to the distal tubule and a resultant reduction in the passive reabsorption of water, which is determined by the osmotic gradient between the lumen and its tissue environment.

The diuretic effect of thiazides is not responsible for their antihypertensive effect

If the diuretic effect of thiazides was responsible for their antihypertensive effect, the dose–response relationship for these two effects would be superimposable. This is not the case (Fig. 8.42), reinforcing the concept that another action is responsible for the antihypertensive effect. On the other hand, thiazides lose efficacy in patients with moderate renal insufficiency.

Recently, it has been suggested that diuretics (especially the thiazides) may produce their effects in hypertension by

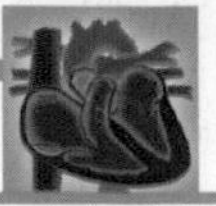

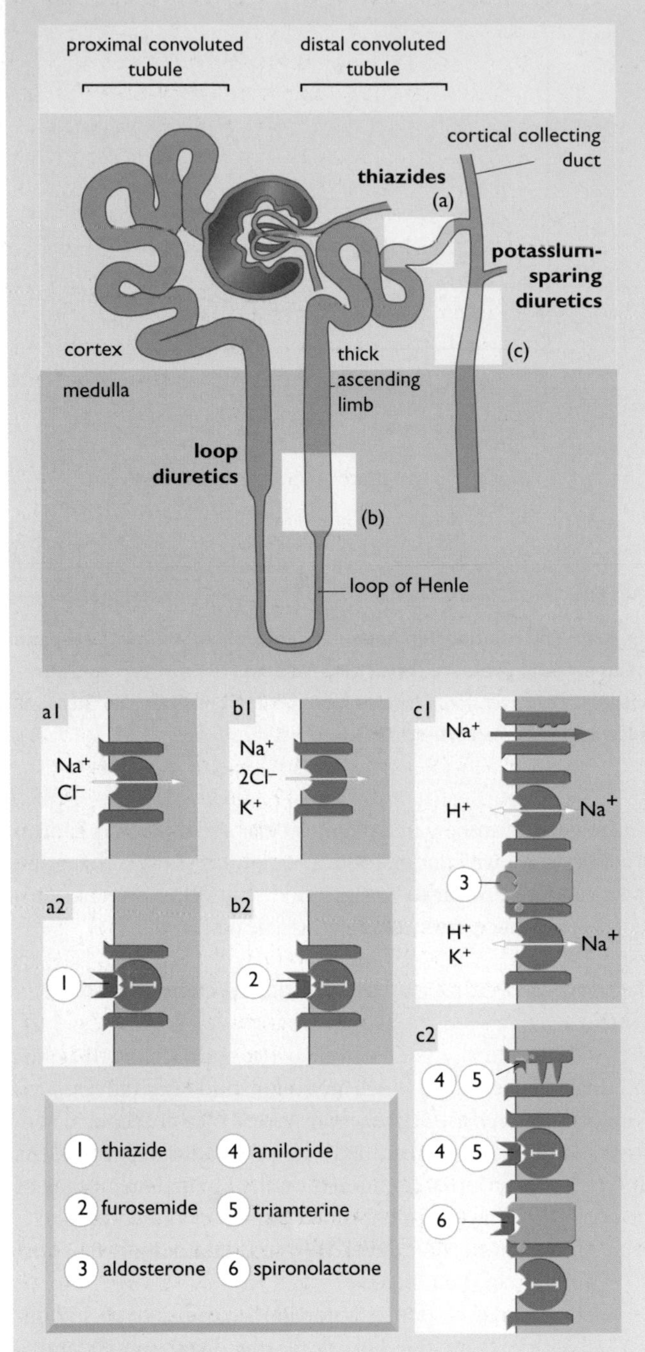

Fig. 8.41 Sites of action of thiazides, loop diuretics, and potassium-sparing diuretics in the kidney. Loop diuretics are generally not effective antihypertensive agents except in patients with renal insufficiency. The possible action of thiazides on K^+ channels is not shown, nor is their secondary cellular action on K^+ reabsorption. Parts a1, b1, and c1 refer to sites in the top panel; a1 is the drug target and a2 is the modulated target, etc. Note that for aldosterone and spironolactone, there is an intracellular molecular target and transduction is more complex than illustrated.

modulating the activity of K^+ channels. ATP-regulated K^+ channels in resistance arterioles may be activated by thiazides. This molecular action leads to membrane hyperpolarization, which opposes smooth muscle Ca^{2+} entry and contraction and, at the system level, reduces peripheral vascular resistance.

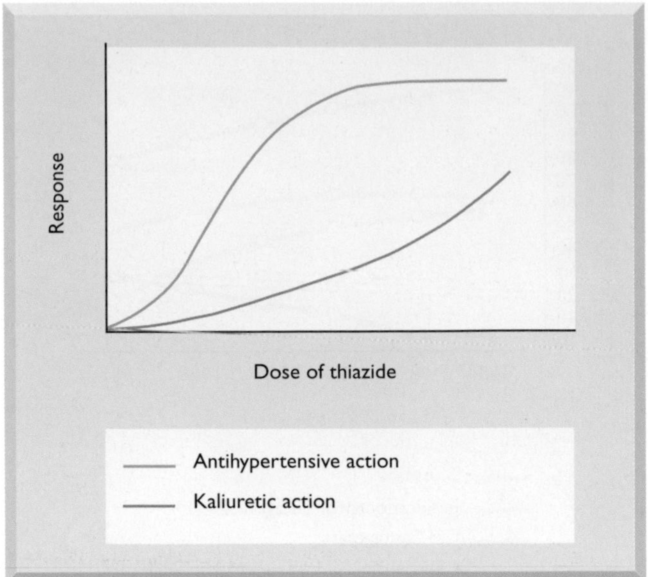

Fig. 8.42 Dose–response relationship for thiazide antihypertensive agents on blood pressure (antihypertensive action) and as a diuretic (shown here as effect on K^+ excretion, the kaliuretic action). The lack of overlap of the curves suggests that the two effects may not be related.

Hypokalemia may occur as an adverse effect of long-term thiazide treatment

One cellular response of thiazides is associated with a characteristic adverse effect: an increase in Na^+ concentration in the distal convoluted tubule. This impairs K^+ reabsorption, since K^+ reabsorption is mediated here by the Na^+ pump and therefore depends on an appropriate Na^+ gradient to allow Na^+/K^+ exchange. This may result in an increase in K^+ excretion (kaliuresis) and hypokalemia. However, if appropriately low doses of thiazides are used in the treatment of hypertension, these potential changes may not be clinically significant. Hypokalemia may give rise to ventricular ectopic beats. Potassium supplements (oral potassium chloride) may be used to avoid this. Alternatively, potassium-sparing drugs may be given in combination with thiazides.

Thiazides may induce an increase in plasma renin (owing to reduced blood Na^+ concentration) and therefore angiotensin II and aldosterone. As aldosterone contributes to K^+ loss from the kidney, this action therefore contributes to the hypokalemic effect of thiazides. Concomitant use of a β adrenoceptor antagonist or an ACE inhibitor reduces plasma renin activity and plasma angiotensin II activity, respectively. This can ameliorate the aldosterone-dependent component of the hypokalemic effect of thiazides. In addition, ACE inhibitors potentiate the hypotensive effects of thiazides.

Another adverse effect of thiazides is male sexual dysfunction.

Loop diuretics act on the thick main ascending loop of Henle

Loop diuretics (furosemide and bumetanide) act primarily on the thick main ascending loop of Henle, with some action on the proximal tubule and cortical diluting segment. Their molecular mechanism is impairment of the $Na^+/K^+/2Cl^-$ cotransporter molecule for Na^+, K^+, and Cl^- reabsorption, which is located mainly in the loop of Henle. Approximately 25% of Na^+ in the glomerular filtrate is reabsorbed in the ascending loop. Loop diuretics have a higher ceiling of natriuretic action compared with the thiazides and are particularly effective in patients with renal failure.

Hypokalemia may be avoided using potassium-sparing diuretics

Secondary hypokalemia is a potential adverse effect of these diuretics, as for thiazides, and K^+ supplementation may be needed in some patients. Avoidance of hypokalemia may be achieved by using so-called potassium-sparing diuretics. These act at the cortical collecting duct, where exchange of Na^+ for K^+ and H^+ ions occurs via an exchanger that is regulated by endogenous aldosterone:

- Drugs such as amiloride and triamterene act at the luminal membrane. Their molecular mechanism is blockade of Na^+ channels and noncompetitive antagonism of aldosterone.
- Spironolactone is a reversible competitive antagonist of aldosterone at its receptor in the luminal membrane of the cortical collecting duct.

Potassium-sparing diuretics have a weak natriuretic and diuretic action. However, when drugs in this class are combined with thiazides or loop diuretics, there is a synergism at the level of the tissue response (i.e. the maximum level of diuresis achievable with either class alone is increased). However, triamterene is not an antihypertensive drug.

In general, when predictable adverse effects are anticipated and avoided, diuretics are well tolerated, with only 10% of patients stopping therapy during long-term treatment.

Sympatholytics The tissue mechanism of action of sympatholytics is a direct or indirect reduction of activity at the sympathetic neuroeffector junction or at sites where circulating epinephrine acts. This tissue mechanism of action is the basis for their definition and may be achieved in a variety of different ways according to the site of action:

- Some drugs act on the vasomotor center in the brain to reduce sympathetic tone centrally.
- Other drugs act peripherally on adrenergic neurotransmission at pre- or postsynaptic sites or on receptors activated by circulating epinephrine.

Many of these agents possess both a direct and an indirect tissue mechanism of action, since they may act in nervous tissue and reduce responses in cardiac, vascular, or other tissue. The molecular and cellular mechanisms of action are also diverse, involving a variety of different receptors and transduction components. Below, the sympatholytics are described in an order that reflects their selectivity of action as sympatholytics and not in relation to the frequency of their use, which is described for each type of drug within each subsection.

Drugs in this class are rarely used today because of their adverse effects, which are described below. Two examples are reserpine and guanethidine, which act through different molecular and cellular mechanisms to achieve a similar tissue response.

Reserpine produces arteriolar vasodilatation and reduces cardiac output

Reserpine is transported into peripheral sympathetic nerve terminals by Uptake-1 (a mechanism for norepinephrine re-uptake into nerves) and its mechanisms of action are as follows:

- Its molecular mechanism of action is inhibition of the norepinephrine pump (an ATP and Mg^{2+}-dependent uptake molecule) located on the storage vesicles for norepinephrine in the neuronal cytoplasm.
- Its cellular mechanism of action is a reduction of the norepinephrine content of neuronal storage vesicles.
- Its direct tissue mechanism of action is a reduction of nerve action potential-mediated release of norepinephrine from sympathetic nerve terminals.
- Its indirect tissue mechanism of action is arteriolar vasodilatation and reduced cardiac output.

Reserpine can reduce blood pressure effectively. However, a percentage of patients experience severe psychologic depression, and so use of this drug has declined. This adverse effect is dose dependent so can be avoided by careful titration of dosage, starting from 0.1 mg/day or less.

Guanethidine has two molecular and cellular mechanisms acting in parallel

Guanethidine and related guanidine compounds including guanadrel, bethanidine, and debrisoquine are, like reserpine, transported into peripheral sympathetic nerve terminals by Uptake-1. However, their molecular and cellular mechanisms of action differ from those of reserpine. In fact, two molecular and cellular mechanisms act in parallel:

- One molecular mechanism is competition with norepinephrine for the norepinephrine pump (an ATP- and Mg^{2+}-dependent uptake molecule). The drugs are actually taken up and stored in the adrenergic vesicles in preference to norepinephrine. The associated cellular mechanism of action is a reduced content of norepinephrine in the storage vesicles, while the direct tissue mechanism of action is a reduction of nerve action potential-mediated release of norepinephrine from sympathetic nerve terminals.
- The second molecular mechanism is binding to the inner surface of the neurolemma. The associated cellular mechanism is reduction of the fusion between storage vesicles and the neurolemma, known as the 'adrenergic neuron blocking' mechanism. The associated tissue mechanism of action is a reduction of nerve action potential-mediated release of norepinephrine from sympathetic nerve terminals, while the secondary tissue mechanism is a reduction in cardiac output as a result of a reduction in heart rate.

Reserpine and the guanidine analogs share two common adverse effects:

- Postural hypotension.
- A generalized block of sympathetic neurotransmission.

Postural hypotension is a sudden fall in blood pressure on suddenly standing up. It results from a loss of the sympathetic-mediated reflex arterial and venous constriction in the lower body that normally occurs on standing. There is venous pooling of blood in the lower limbs (giving a reduction in preload) and a fall in cardiac output via the Starling mechanism (see section on heart failure, p. 170), which may cause fainting. Because of this and the availability of newer safer drugs, guanethidine is now used only for patients with severe hypertension who are unresponsive to other drugs.

Ganglion blocking drugs are used only for emergency hypertension

Trimethaphan is a nicotinic receptor antagonist with relative selectivity for the nicotinic receptors found in autonomic ganglia. It is used only for emergency hypertension associated with a dissecting aortic aneurysm. When given intravenously it produces generalized antagonism of both parasympathetic and sympathetic ganglia and is therefore unsuitable for maintenance therapy of hypertension.

α_2 Adrenoceptor agonists are second or third choices for treating hypertension

Centrally acting α_2 adrenoceptor agonists such as clonidine and α methyldopa are second or third choices for the treatment of hypertension. These agents mimic the autoinhibitory effects of norepinephrine on sympathetic activity without producing sympathomimetic effects (Fig. 8.43). The reason for this is their relative selectivity for α_2 receptors rather than α_1 and β adrenoceptors. The mechanisms of action are as follows:

- The molecular mechanism of action is α_2 adrenoceptor agonism (Fig. 8.44).
- The direct tissue mechanism of action is a reduction in the activity of the vasomotor center in the brain, leading to a fall in sympathetic nervous activity.
- The secondary tissue mechanism of action is a reduction in peripheral resistance as a result of arteriolar relaxation. However, with maintained therapy, a reduction in heart rate and cardiac output appear to be the predominant effects, especially with clonidine.

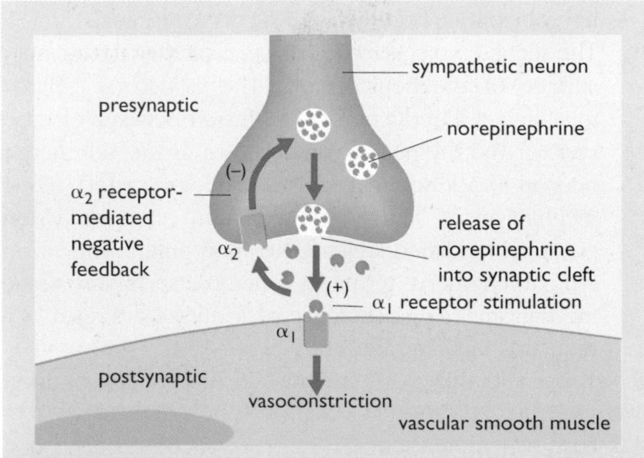

Fig. 8.43 Autoinhibition of norepinephrine release. This is mediated by presynaptic α_2 receptors, which prevent the release of norepinephrine and postsynaptic α_1 agonism. If the postsynaptic receptor is β_1, this, in the heart, mediates tachycardia.

Clonidine is a a widely used α_2 agonist, while α methydopa is a prodrug which is metabolized to α methylnorepinephrine in the CNS via a two-step enzymatic process (Fig. 8.45). α Methylnorepinephrine is an α_2 agonist in the CNS and stimulates the vasopressor centers in the brain stem to inhibit sympathetic outflow. Because renal blood flow is well maintained with α methyldopa, it has been widely used in hypertensive

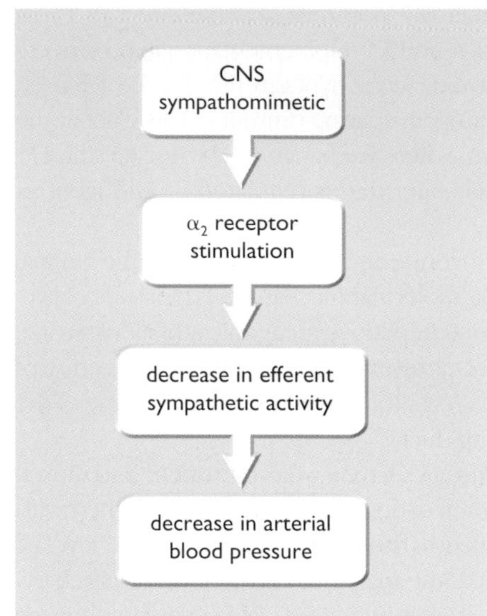

Fig. 8.44 **α_2 Agonism decreases sympathetic activity and consequently reduces blood pressure.**

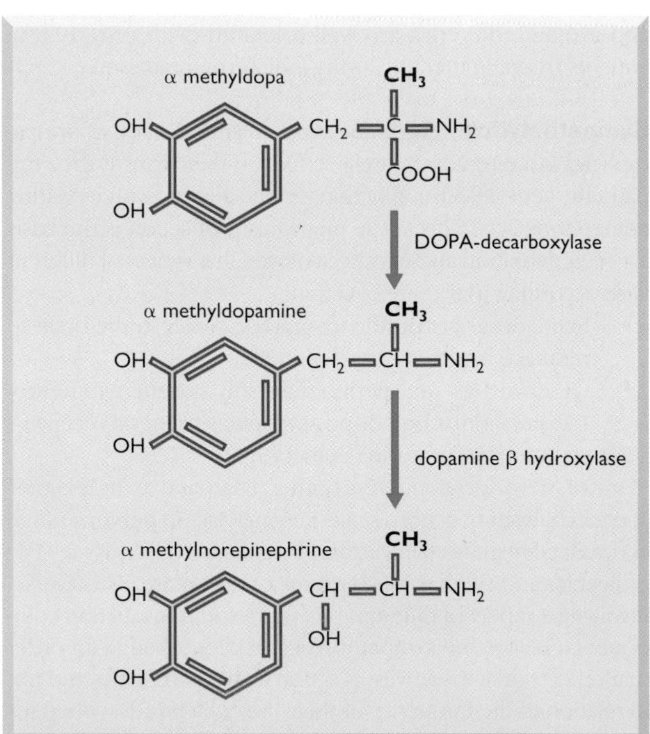

Fig. 8.45 Metabolism of α methyldopa to α methylnorepinephrine. Note that CH_3 is absent in DOPA, the endogenous precursor to dopamine, which is metabolized by the same enzymes to norepinephrine.

patients with renal insufficiency or cerebrovascular disease. α Methyldopa is also recommended for use in hypertensive pregnant women because it has no adverse effects on the fetus despite crossing the blood–placenta barrier. Similar, but direct acting, α_2 agonists include guanabenz and guanfacine.

Adverse effects of this group of drugs are dry mouth, sedation, orthostatic hypotension (particularly in the elderly), male sexual dysfunction, and galactorrhea. α Methyldopa also causes diffuse parenchymal injury in the liver resembling the effects of viral hepatitis and, rarely, fever and hemolytic anemia. Owing to adverse effects, α methyldopa is now used very infrequently.

The use of clonidine in hypertensive patients has been associated with a rapid rebound of blood pressure to pretreatment levels when the treatment is stopped abruptly. This can cause withdrawal symptoms, including tachycardia, restlessness, and sweating. The rebound of blood pressure may be treated by reintroducing the drug or using a peripherally acting α_1 adrenoceptor antagonist to prevent sympathetic nervous-mediated peripheral vasoconstriction. The risk of this withdrawal syndrome is probably related to the severity of underlying hypertension and the dose of clonidine. These adverse effects can be avoided by gradually decreasing the dose of clonidine over time.

Clonidine is available as a transdermal preparation that may provide control of blood pressure for up to seven days with the potential for fewer adverse effects. However, adverse effects of the patch on the skin may be troublesome.

α_1 Adrenoceptor antagonists are potentially beneficial in hypertensive patients with congestive heart failure or prostate hyperplasia

Prazosin was the first selective agent with the molecular mechanism of postsynaptic α_1 adrenoceptor antagonism. Prazosin and newer analogs such as terazosin and doxazosin are sympatholytics that act directly on the effector component of the sympathetic neuroeffector junction as antagonists. Their tissue mechanism of action is therefore inhibition of α_1 adrenoceptor-mediated blood vessel constriction. This reduces peripheral resistance and venous pressure. So, unlike the sympatholytics described above, the direct tissue mechanism of action is not on sympathetic nerves, but on the nerves' target tissue. Since presynaptic α_2 receptors are not blocked, the negative feedback loop for inhibiting norepinephrine release remains intact, and this may explain the lack of tachycardia due to stimulation of β adrenoceptors seen with nonselective α (α_1 and α_2) antagonists (Fig. 8.46).

α_1 Adrenoceptor antagonists can modify plasma lipid levels

α_1 Adrenoceptor antagonists can modify the plasma levels of low density lipoprotein (LDL) cholesterol, and apoprotein B, so that overall LDL cholesterol levels are reduced as well as very low density lipoprotein (VLDL) levels and total triglyceride levels. These agents also increase high density lipoprotein (HDL) cholesterol levels and therefore reduce one of the risk factors associated with coronary artery disease (see Chapter 12), though the relevance of this is unknown.

α_1 Adrenoceptor antagonists are also of benefit in hypertensive patients with CHF or prostate hyperplasia.

- In CHF, prazosin's tissue mechanism of action is a reduction in peripheral resistance, leading to reduced left ventricular filling pressure and therefore improving the symptoms of heart failure. However, this effect is short-lived and does not contribute significantly to relieving the heart failure symptoms. Angiotensin-converting enzyme inhibitors are preferred in this setting.
- In prostate hyperplasia these agents have beneficial effects by reducing resistance in the bladder sphincter and prostate, facilitating voiding.

Doxazosin and terazosin require only once-daily administration because of their long plasma half-life, an advantage over prazosin, with respect to compliance, which is given twice a day.

Adverse effects of this group of drugs include postural hypotension, dizziness, weakness, fatigue, and headaches, but little sedation, dry mouth, or ejaculation failure.

β Adrenoceptor antagonists are the second most widely used group of antihypertensive drugs after diuretics.

Their mechanisms of action are as follows:

- The molecular mechanism of action is generally regarded to be competitive antagonism of β_1 adrenoceptors, although β_2 adrenoceptor antagonism may be important, but this is not clear.
- The cellular mechanism is not known, largely because controversy still exists with respect to the tissue and molecular mechanisms of action.
- β Adrenoceptor antagonists may act in the CNS to reduce sympathetic tone (see Fig. 8.46), in the heart to reduce heart rate and cardiac output, and in the kidney to reduce renin production. However, a common feature of their action in hypertension is a reduction in peripheral resistance, but it is not clear how this effect occurs.

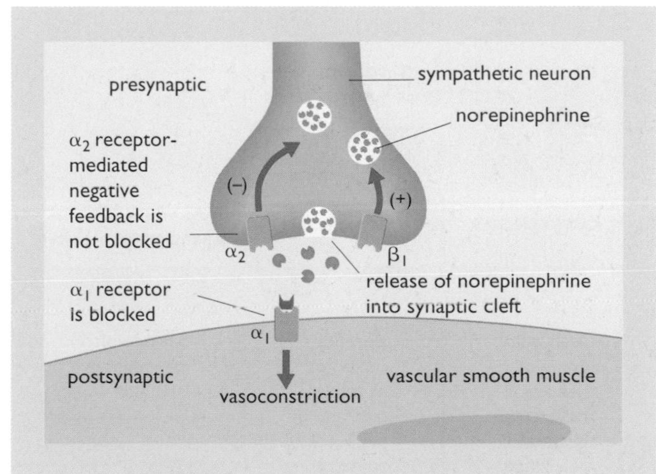

Fig. 8.46 Antagonism at postsynaptic α_1 adrenoceptors. Prazosin prevents vasoconstriction by norepinephrine. Further effects of norepinephrine are reduced by the feedback mechanism since presynaptic α_2 adrenoceptors are not blocked by prazosin and so the α_2 receptors can be occupied by norepinephrine, thereby activating the negative feedback pathway.

There is a wide variety of β adrenoceptor antagonists (Fig. 8.47). They differ in their ability to block β_1 adrenoceptors in the heart and CNS versus β_2 receptors in the bronchi and peripheral blood vessels.

Atenolol and metoprolol are selective β_1 adrenoceptor antagonists

Historically, the term 'cardioselective' has been used to describe β_1 adrenoceptor antagonists, although these agents will affect any tissues that express β_1 adrenoceptors. Cardioselective β adrenoceptor antagonists such as atenolol and metoprolol antagonize the effects of norepinephrine and epinephrine on heart rate, but have less effect on the the airways than nonselective β adrenoceptor antagonists. Nonetheless, these drugs are not safe enough to use in asthmatics, except under special circumstances.

Pindolol is a partial adrenoceptor agonist

Some partial agonists at β_1 adrenoceptors are used in the treatment of hypertension (e.g. pindolol). These drugs inhibit sympathetic hyperactivity, but partially stimulate β receptors if the sympathetic tone is low. Historically these drugs have been described as 'β blockers with intrinsic sympathomimetic activity.' However, this description is vague as the agents are partial agonists, as defined in Chapter 3. The β_1 adrenoceptor partial agonists reduce blood pressure to a similar degree as β_1 adrenoceptor antagonists, but cause less reduction in heart rate. These drugs are probably likely to elevate concentrations of VLDL more than nonselective antagonists do.

Labetalol and carvedilol are dual-acting α_1 and β_1 adrenoceptor antagonists

Drugs such as labetalol and carvedilol are known as dual-acting β_1 adrenoceptor antagonists since they block both β_1 and α_1 receptors, with a greater ratio of β_1 to α_1 antagonism (β_1:α_1 blockade: 10:1 for carvedilol; 4:1 for labetalol). These drugs, like pindolol, lower blood pressure via a reduction in peripheral vascular resistance with no change in heart rate or cardiac output.

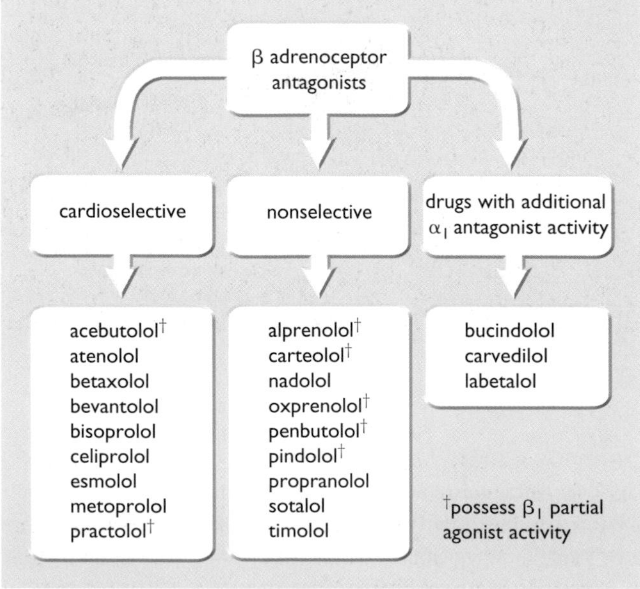

Fig. 8.47 **β Adrenoceptor antagonists classified according to cardioselectivity and partial agonist activity.**

β Adrenoceptor antagonists have few adverse effects

Although β adrenoceptor antagonists do not usually have serious adverse effects (see Chapter 19), they may be sufficient to impair compliance:

- β_1 Adrenoceptor antagonism can exacerbate CHF by reducing cardiac output.
- β_2 Adrenoceptor antagonism (the basis for 'non-cardioselective' actions) may lead to poor tissue perfusion, especially in peripheral vascular disease, and bronchospasm, especially in asthmatics.

These drugs are therefore contraindicated in patients with bronchospasm. While carvedilol may be useful in the treatment of CHF in carefully selected patients, this is best undertaken by specialists.

It has been reported that β adrenoceptor antagonists reduce renal blood flow and so hypertensive patients with renal disorders should be given lower doses of lipid-insoluble drugs such as atenolol and nadolol.

Sudden discontinuation of β adrenoceptor antagonists can cause angina pectoris and myocardial infarction

Discontinuation of some β adrenoceptor antagonists can cause rebound sympathetic stimulation of the heart, leading to angina pectoris and myocardial infarction. It is recommended that if the β adrenoceptor antagonist is ineffective or poorly tolerated, the patient should be gradually weaned off it, rather than abruptly transferred to other agents.

Calcium antagonists Drugs that act at the molecular level by interfering with the opening or closure of L-type Ca^{2+} channels (i.e. Ca^{2+} antagonists) are increasingly used in hypertension. They fall into three main groups based on their chemical structure:

- The 1,4-dihydropyridines are the most vascular-selective group. The prototype is nifedipine, which is the most effective antihypertensive of the Ca^{2+} antagonists and generally has little effect on cardiac conduction.
- The phenethylalkylamines (e.g. verapamil) and benzothiazepines (e.g. diltiazem) are less vascular selective and may also affect the AV node, causing AV block. Verapamil and diltiazem are therefore associated with cardiac conduction problems, especially when given to patients receiving β adrenoceptor antagonists.

Elderly hypertensive patients respond well to calcium antagonists. However, people of African origin are less responsive.

In general, Ca^{2+} antagonists have a rapid onset of action and reduce blood pressure within half an hour of administration.

Occasional adverse effects include a throbbing headache, palpitations, sweating, tremor, and flushing. The main adverse effect with verapamil is constipation, but more importantly both verapamil and diltiazem can have negative inotropic effects in patients with pre-existing cardiac failure, and are therefore contraindicated in such patients. Nifedipine does not do this.

Direct-acting vasodilators Agents that dilate arterioles by a molecular mechanism that is not α_1 adrenoceptor antagonism or L-type Ca^{2+} channel modulation have traditionally been called 'direct-acting vasodilators.' This was once a convenient shorthand for indicating that at the time the molecular (and often the cellular) mechanism of action was unknown. Although this has now largely been resolved, the term 'direct-acting' has been retained.

These agents are increasingly used for the treatment of emergencies.

Sodium nitroprusside is used in hypertensive emergencies

Sodium nitroprusside is given intravenously to produce a rapid reduction in blood pressure during a hypertensive emergency. It has a short half-life of 30–40 seconds.

Sodium nitroprusside causes vasorelaxation by increasing cGMP in vascular smooth muscle cells by stimulating cytosolic guanylyl cyclase activity and thereby lowers blood pressure (see Chapter 3). The molecular mechanism of action for this effect is brought about by nitric oxide (NO, see Fig. 8.3). Sodium nitroprusside is a prodrug that spontaneously degrades to NO inside smooth muscle cells.

Hydralazine is a third-line drug for mild to moderate hypertension

Hydralazine is the only direct-acting vasodilator used in treating mild to moderate hypertension, usually as a second- or third-line drug. It is also still used as a parenteral treatment in hypertensive emergencies and in hypertensive pregnant patients.

The molecular and cellular mechanisms of action of hydralazine are to increase cGMP following activation of guanylyl cyclase, resulting in relaxation of smooth muscle in precapillary resistance vessels and thereby reducing blood pressure by a reduction in peripheral resistance (see Fig. 8.3).

Hydralazine, in doses in excess of 200 mg/day, is associated with a lupus-like syndrome in some patients.

Minoxidil is useful for severe hypertension with renal failure

Minoxidil is highly effective in reducing blood pressure, especially in severe hypertension and if there is renal failure. Diazoxide is similar to minoxidil, but is rarely used except in emergencies because of its adverse effects.

Minoxidil is a more efficacious vasodilator than hydralazine and produces dilatation of resistance vessels. It works at the molecular level by activating ATP-sensitive K^+ channels. Consequently, the smooth muscle membrane is hyperpolarized and Ca^{2+} influx via the L-type Ca^{2+} channel is reduced. Minoxidil is given once or twice a day and is more effective than hydralazine. It is very effective in patients with severe hypertension and renal insufficiency. Like hydralazine, it should also be given in combination with diuretics and adrenoceptor antagonists to prevent reflex increases in cardiac output and fluid retention.

A common adverse effect of minoxidil is facial hair growth, which limits the use of this drug in women.

Renin–angiotensin cascade modulators The inactive decapeptide angiotensin I is converted to the active octapeptide angiotensin II by ACE (see Fig. 8.36). A reduction in blood pressure may be achieved by blocking ACE activity or angiotensin II receptors. ACE inhibitors have the following mechanisms of action:

- The molecular mechanism of action is inhibition of ACE activity.
- The resultant cellular mechanism of action is reduced angiotensin II synthesis and reduced metabolism of some vasodilating kinins.

ACE inhibitors are useful for all severities and types of hypertension and are widely used.

Captopril is the prototype ACE inhibitor

Angiotensin II has a variety of effects that contribute to elevating blood pressure (Fig. 8.48). It constricts arterioles and stimulates aldosterone release from the adrenal cortex; in turn, aldosterone stimulates Na^+ reabsorption in the kidney (see use of spironolactone, p. 182). As a result of reducing the synthesis of angiotensin II, captopril has two main tissue mechanisms of action: it causes vasodilatation and reduces Na^+ retention.

Angiotensin-converting enzyme inhibitors

- Alacepril
- Benazepril
- Cilazapril
- Perindopril
- Quinapril
- Ramipril
- Zofenopril
- Delapril (clinical trials)
- Moexipril (phase III clinical trials)
- Spirapril (US new drug application)
- Trandolapril

Other commonly used ACE inhibitors are enalapril and lisinopril

Enalapril and lisinopril have similar mechanisms of action to captopril, but a slower onset and longer duration of action. Many ACE inhibitors are prodrugs. The suffix '-at' is used to denote the active metabolite of ACE inhibitors. For example, enalapril is metabolized to its active metabolite, enalaprilat.

ACE inhibitors may alter the balance between the actions of angiotensin II and bradykinin

Surprisingly, chronic use of ACE inhibitors is associated with a recovery in angiotensin II concentration, but blood pressure levels remain low. This suggests that additional cellular mechanisms may be responsible for the antihypertensive effects. One possibility is an alteration of plasma bradykinin concentration. ACE catalyzes the inactivation of bradykinin, which is an endogenous vasodilator. The pharmacotherapeutic effects of ACE inhibitors may therefore be related to altering the balance between the actions of angiotensin II, bradykinin and other kinins (see Fig. 8.48).

The tissue responses to ACE inhibitors are:

- A reduction in peripheral resistance with little change in heart rate or cardiac output.
- A reduction in Na^+ retention secondary to altered aldosterone levels.

This group of drugs are as effective as diuretics or β adrenoceptor antagonists in treating hypertension. However, concomitant use of a diuretic enhances their effectiveness, probably because the diuretic activates the renin–angiotensin system.

Inhibition of angiotensin II may cause a substantial reduction in renal perfusion pressure

Experimental and clinical evidence suggests that the reduction in efferent arteriolar resistance as a consequence of angiotensin II reduction that results from treatment with ACE inhibitors may be useful in patients with renal dysfunction, particularly those with diabetic nephropathy or a reduced renal functional mass. This is because inhibition of angiotensin II may cause a substantial reduction in perfusion pressure. As a result, renal failure may develop in these patients.

ACE inhibitors are associated with few adverse effects. One unusual adverse effect is a characteristic cough (see Chapter 11).

Angiotensin II receptor antagonists were discovered two decades ago. The prototype was saralasin, but since it is a peptide it is not orally active, and when administered intravenously it is immunogenic. More recently, compounds that are not peptides and are orally active have been developed. Such novel nonpeptide angiotensin II antagonists include losartan and EXP3174.

Losartan is a drug that has recently been approved for use in the treatment of hypertension in the US. It differs from ACE inhibitors in that it does not directly affect bradykinin degradation. It is not yet known whether this confers advantages in terms of effectiveness and adverse effect profile against those of ACE inhibitors. However, the incidence of cough is less compared to that with ACE inhibitors.

Emerging therapy Renin inhibitors are a new class of drugs that reduce angiotensin II levels. Several renin inhibitors have been developed with high potency and long duration of action. However, the oral bioavailability of currently available agents is too low to achieve effective plasma concentrations in humans.

Endopeptidase-24.11 is an enzyme that hydrolyzes the polypeptide atrial natriuretic peptide (ANP). ANP has diuretic, natriuretic,

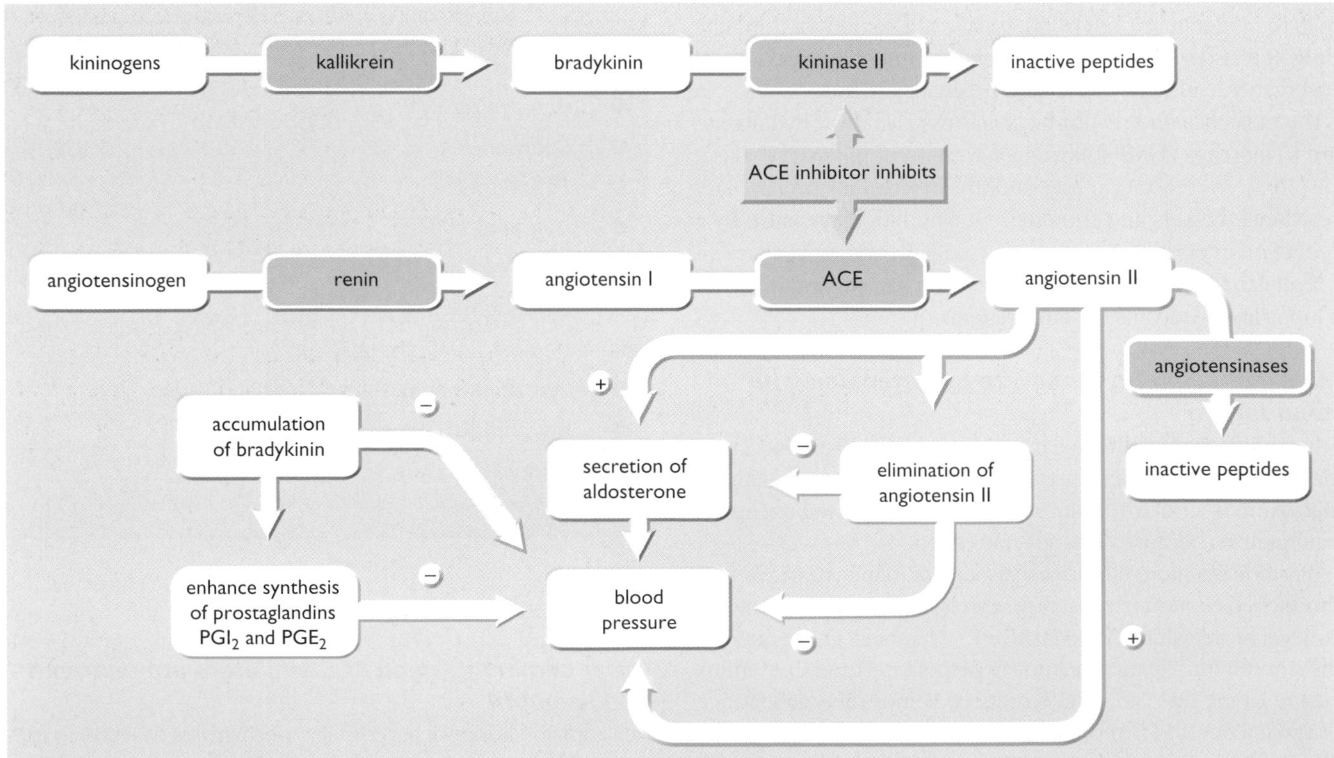

Fig. 8.48 Effects of angiotensin-converting enzyme (ACE) inhibitors. ACE inhibitors reduce angiotensin II (vasoconstrictor) concentrations and elevate bradykinin (vasodilator) concentrations. The accumulation of bradykinin shown in the lower part of the figure results from the action of the ACE inhibitors on kininase II. Note, kininase II and ACE are actually the same enzyme (peptidyl-dipeptidase).

and vasodilator properties; it is released following changes in atrial volume or pressure, and therefore plays a role in regulating blood pressure.

Theoretically, inhibition of endopeptidase-24.11 should reduce ANP degradation and thereby increase circulating levels of ANP.

This form of drug treatment may prove beneficial in patients with hypertension. However, there are few clinical data to support the proposal that drugs of this group are effective antihypertensive agents. This is probably due to their poor bioavailability or the low potency of agents tested so far. Recent data suggest that this group of drugs may have most benefit in patients with volume-dependent hypertension or low-renin hypertension.

Mechanisms of action of the major classes of antihypertensive drugs

- Thiazide diuretics increase Na^+ excretion and transiently reduce blood volume, but the mechanism by which they lower blood pressure is uncertain
- Sympatholytics reduce the ability of sympathetic nervous system to raise blood pressure
- Vasodilators relax vascular smooth muscle and reduce peripheral resistance
- Angiotensin-converting enzyme (ACE) inhibitors reduce peripheral resistance and blood volume with no effect on heart rate

Combination treatment A useful pharmacotherapeutic approach for controlling elevated blood pressure is to use two or more drugs in combination.

The β adrenoceptor antagonist–diuretic combination is the most common combination strategy. By combining drugs with different mechanisms of action the doses may be reduced, thereby reducing the adverse effects.

β Adrenoceptor antagonists and Ca^{2+} antagonists (dihydropyridine Ca^{2+} antagonists only) are usually well tolerated when used in combination, provided that care is taken with the dosage. Occasionally, the combination of nifedipine with β adrenoceptor antagonists is associated with bradycardia and heart failure owing to synergism of their negative inotropic effects (one mediated via cardiac β adrenoceptors and the other via venous L-type Ca^{2+} antagonism).

Using Ca^{2+} antagonists other than the dihydropyridines with β adrenoceptor antagonists is dangerous

Using Ca^{2+} antagonists (e.g. verapamil) other than the dihydropyridines in combination with β adrenoceptor antagonists is dangerous since such combinations have been reported to cause asystole, severe bradycardia, and hypotension because of the combination of molecular mechanisms described above. Each lowers cardiac intracellular Ca^{2+}, an effect that reduces myocardial contractility. Nifedipene does not do this.

Diuretics and ACE inhibitors (e.g. hydrochlorothiazide and perindopril) provide an effective combination for treating arterial hypertension that is well tolerated in many patients with mild to moderate hypertension. The advantage of combining diuretics and ACE inhibitors is an additive effect in reducing blood pressure.

The combination of ACE inhibitors and Ca^{2+} antagonists is also effective at lowering blood pressure and is usually well tolerated.

Calcium antagonists and diuretics in combination do not usually have additive effects.

Treatment for hypertensive emergencies Hypertensive emergencies are situations in which the blood pressure is so high that the patient's life is in immediate jeopardy. There is no particular level of blood pressure that provides the diagnosis but this depends on the clinical presentation. Without emergency treatment the patient has a high risk of cerebrovascular hemorrhage, left ventricular heart failure, or myocardial ischemia and infarction.

Hypertensive emergencies

- Occurs when mean arterial pressure is an immediate threat to life
- Intravenous nitroprusside is an efficacious drug in this setting

Intravenous nitroprusside is generally the drug of choice for life-threatening hypertension

Intravenous nitroprusside is often used in the treatment of life-threatening hypertension on account of its rapid onset of action and efficacy. It is a profound arterial and venous dilator (Fig. 8.49). An infusion of nitroprusside can be used to reduce blood pressure rapidly, but it is important to monitor the blood pressure constantly. This is because nitroprusside can cause an

Drugs used in hypertensive crises

Vasodilators	Onset of action (min)
Nitroprusside	Immediate
Diazoxide	2–4
Hydralazine	10–20
Enalaprilat	15
Nicardipine	10
Sympatholytics	
Trimethaphan	1–5
Esmolol	1–2
Labetalol	5–10

Fig. 8.49 Drugs used in hypertensive crises. The drugs are shown in order of preference based on their rapidity of action.

abrupt fall in blood pressure, resulting in hypoperfusion of vital organs; dose must be titrated carefully, depending on the blood pressure response.

A very high blood pressure on its own, in the absence of acute illness, does not usually require parenteral therapy, which can be dangerous. Patients with a less severe emergency can be given oral drug treatment. Any class of drug may be used, but the four classes most commonly used are:

- Diuretics.
- β Adrenoceptor antagonists.
- Ca^{2+} antagonists.
- ACE inhibitors.

PATHOPHYSIOLOGY AND DISEASES OF BLOOD VESSELS

A variety of diseases involve a generalized or localized impairment of blood flow to specific tissues or organs and are grouped together here as peripheral vascular disease.

In most cases the specific molecular, cellular, and tissue mechanisms of action of the drugs used to treat peripheral vascular diseases are described elsewhere in this book. Specifically, the pharmacology of agents that dilate arterioles (e.g. Ca^{2+} antagonists) is described in the section on hypertension (see pp. 178–190) and antithrombotic drugs are described in the section on angina pectoris (see pp. 164–169).

Principles of treatment of peripheral vascular disease

- **Drugs are targeted at the perfusion deficit and at the underlying cause (e.g. vasospasm) if known**
- **Thrombolytics are used if thrombosis has impaired perfusion**
- **Arteriodilators are used if vasospasm has impaired perfusion**

Arterial disease

Peripheral vascular disease affecting the arteries can be caused by a number of pathologic processes:

- Arteriosclerosis is one of the pathologic processes that leads to peripheral vascular disease (Fig. 8.50).
- Dystrophic calcification of the media is observed in Mönckeberg's sclerosis, which is common in the major lower limb arteries of the elderly and is more common in people with diabetes mellitus.
- Cystic medial necrosis or degeneration describes mucoid degeneration of the collagen and elastic tissue of the media, often with cystic changes, and occurs predominantly in elderly patients with hypertension. Indeed, peripheral vascular disease is a common feature associated with longstanding hypertension.

In patients with pre-existing peripheral vascular disease, aspirin and dipyridamole are effective in delaying the progression of the disease to thrombosis so may be used as prophylaxis. It is presumed that:

- Aspirin prevents thrombosis.
- Dipyridamole prevents thrombosis and dilates arterioles.

Chronic ischemia of the legs and intermittent claudication (limping) may arise as a consequence of atheromatous disease involving the aorta, iliac arteries, and/or any other peripheral vessels.

Treatment of chronic ischemia is with low-dose aspirin therapy and surgery

Treatment is directed towards prophylaxis against thrombosis and comprises low-dose aspirin therapy (325 mg/day) and surgery. The molecular mechanism of action of aspirin is through cyclooxygenase inhibition and has been described in Chapter 3. The cellular mechanism of action is inhibition of the prothrombotic products of cyclooxygenase, especially thromboxane A_2, and the tissue response is inhibition of platelet aggregation.

Acute ischemia of the legs can be caused by arterial thrombi, but also occurs when stasis thrombi dislodge from the atria when atrial fibrillation is terminated. The only treatment is surgery, but prophylaxis with heparin or other anticoagulants is advisable before any elective termination of atrial fibrillation.

Aortic aneurysm is most commonly abdominal, but can also be thoracic, and is usually a result of arteriosclerosis. Emergency surgery is required if it is symptomatic. Aortic aneurysms can also be dissected.

Thromboangiitis obliterans (Buerger's disease) involves the small vessels of the lower limbs and occurs in young male smokers. Patients are advised to stop smoking since drug therapy is usually ineffective.

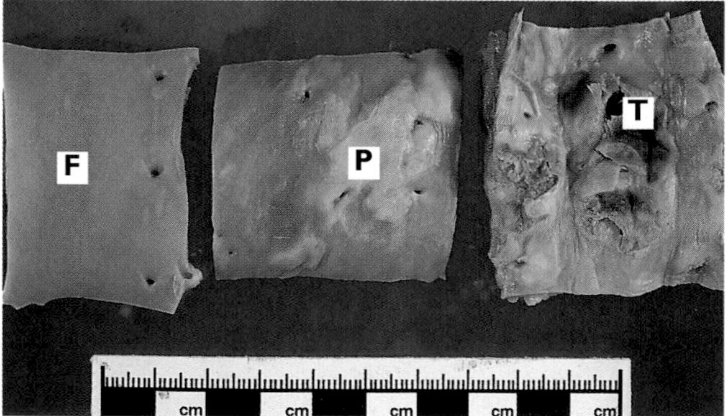

Fig. 8.50 Arteriosclerosis is characterized by thickening and hardening of walls of arteries and arterioles. The earliest changes are small fatty streaks (F), which are visible as pale areas beneath the endothelium in the aortic segment on the left. The central segment shows pearly white fibrolipid plaques (P), and the segment on the right shows advanced ulcerated plaques with adherent fibrin–platelet thrombus (T). (Courtesy of Dr Alan Stevens and Professor James Lowe.)

Vasculitis is a broad term signifying inflammation within and surrounding blood vessels caused by immune complex deposition. Arteries, venules, or capillaries affected by inflammation show necrosis and infiltration by lymphocytes and eosinophils, resulting eventually in ischemia of the related tissue. The different forms of vasculitis include systemic necrotizing vasculitis (e.g. polyarteritis nodosa, allergic angiitis), hypersensitivity vasculitis (e.g. serum sickness, Henoch–Schönlein purpura), and those associated with cardiac transplant rejection. These diseases are discussed in Chapter 17.

Takayasu's syndrome is a rare condition, except in Japan. It is characterized by a vasculitis involving the aortic arch as well as other major arteries. Although glucocorticosteroids are used to treat this disease, heart failure and cerebrovascular accidents may eventually supervene. The molecular and cellular mechanisms of action of glucocorticosteroids are described in Chapter 3.

Raynaud's disease is an isolated condition in which bouts of intense arteriolar vasoconstriction occur in the arteries supplying the fingers or toes and is usually precipitated by cold or vibration.

Initially, treatment includes avoidance of exposure to cold and stopping smoking. More severe symptoms may require vasodilator treatment. In each case the tissue response of the drugs discussed below is to cause arteriolar vasodilation, although their efficacy may be modest for this disease.

α_1 Adrenoceptor antagonists such as prazosin may be used to reduce the vasospasm, but are not selective in their action on the vessels in spasm and can adversely lower blood pressure. The molecular mechanism of action of α_1 antagonists is antagonism of α_1 adrenoceptors and the cellular mechanism is the same as for the treatment of hypertension (see p. 181).

Direct-acting vasodilators (e.g. nitroglycerin and nitrates) are also used. These prodrugs are converted to NO, which activates guanylyl cyclase leading to an elevation in cGMP (the cellular response; see Fig. 8.3).

Calcium antagonists such as diltiazem and nifedipine are also used. The molecular mechanism of action of diltiazem and nifedipine is blockade of L-type Ca^{2+} channels, and the cellular response is a reduction in Ca^{2+} entry and the cascade of events that leads to vasoconstriction (see section on treatment of hypertension, pp. 178–190).

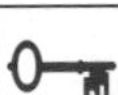

Local treatment is needed for peripheral vascular disease

Drugs that prevent or disperse thrombosis or relieve vasospasm to treat peripheral vascular disease act locally. This is in contrast to the treatment of coronary artery disease in which vessel dilatation at distant sites is effective by reducing preload or afterload

In four separate clinical trials investigating the use of nifedipine in Raynaud's phenomenon, the majority of patients improved symptomatically. Nifedipine is more effective than prazosin and can be given by mouth before cold exposure to avoid attacks.

ACE inhibitors are also used. Their molecular mechanism of action is to inhibit the conversion of angiotensin I to angiotensin II, and the cellular mechanism of action is to prevent the formation of the vasoconstrictor substance, angiotensin II (see Fig. 8.36).

Prostacyclin may also be a beneficial treatment of Raynaud's disease because it causes vasodilation.

Venous disease

The two main peripheral vascular diseases affecting the veins are varicose veins and venous thrombosis (including thrombophlebitis).

Varicose veins develop when veins lose their elasticity and become engorged with blood. They are treated by injection or surgery. Sodium tetradecyl sulfate is injected into the vein as sclerotherapy. It causes inflammation of the intima and thrombus formation, which usually occludes the vein. The subsequent formation of fibrous tissue results in complete occlusion and subsequent loss of the vein.

Venous thrombosis consists predominantly of coagulated blood with a small component of platelet aggregation. There are two types: superficial thrombophlebitis and deep vein thrombosis.

Superficial thrombophlebitis is a local superficial inflammation of the vein wall with secondary thrombosis

Superficial thrombophlebitis is treated with NSAIDs, including aspirin, because the inflammatory process rather than the tendency for thrombosis is the primary tissue target.

Hyaluronidase is used to improve the circulation in superficial thrombophlebitis. It is a spreading or diffusing enzyme that modifies the permeability of connective tissue by hydrolyzing hyaluronic acid. This temporarily decreases the viscosity of the cellular cement and promotes the diffusion of injected fluids or of localized transudates or exudates.

Deep vein thrombosis occurs when a thrombus forms in a vein and any inflammation is secondary

In deep vein thrombosis a thrombus forms in a vein, commonly deep in the leg. It is necessary to inhibit formation of the thrombus rather than direct therapy towards the secondary inflammation. The important secondary aim of treatment is to prevent pulmonary embolism resulting from entrapment of the dislodged venous thrombus in the pulmonary circulation (a goal similar to that in the ancillary treatment of atrial fibrillation).

Large doses of heparin are given as prophylaxis

Large doses of the anticoagulant heparin (or low molecular weight fragments) can be given as prophylaxis for one week to three months. Heparin initiates anticoagulation, but has a short duration of action. It inhibits the reactions that lead to the clotting of blood and formation of fibrin clots and, in combination with antithrombin III, inhibits thrombosis by inactivating activated factor X and inhibiting the conversion of prothrombin to thrombin. Heparin will not disperse an established thrombus.

Oral anticoagulants are given if the thrombus remains localized

Oral anticoagulants such as warfarin are given if the thrombus remains localized. Warfarin, another prophylactic agent, antagonizes the ability of vitamin K to facilitate the synthesis of clotting factors II, VII, IX, and X. However, it takes at least 49–72 hours for these anticoagulant effects to develop.

Heparin and warfarin can cause inappropriate bleeding, so careful titration between effective and adverse doses is required.

Streptokinase is used for established thrombi

Streptokinase is used in the treatment of established thrombi, and is followed by anticoagulant prophylaxis to prevent recurrence. It acts with plasminogen to produce an 'activator complex,' which converts plasminogen to plasmin. Plasmin degrades fibrin clots as well as fibrinogen and other plasma proteins.

The section on blood clotting (see Chapter 9) may be read for further details.

Venous thrombosis and its treatment

- Venous peripheral vascular disease is characterized by vascular inflammation and thrombosis
- Treatment of superficial thrombophlebitis is targeted towards inflammation using nonsteroidal anti-inflammatory drugs
- Treatment and prophylaxis of deep vein disease is directed towards the thrombosis
- Heparin and warfarin are used as prophylaxis against thrombosis
- Streptokinase is used to disperse established thrombi

INFECTIONS OF THE CARDIOVASCULAR SYSTEM

The general principles of treatment of infections are discussed in Chapters 23–26. Here, attention is drawn to the aspects of treatment of infection that are particular to the cardiovascular system.

Myocarditis

Myocarditis is an acute illness characterized by fever and heart failure. A leukocytic infiltrate in the myocardium can be observed followed by resultant non-ischemic necrosis or degeneration of myocytes. Most cases are thought to be caused by enteroviruses (coxsackie, influenza, rubella, polio, adenovirus, echovirus) and are difficult to treat with drugs. However, myocarditis may also be caused by bacterial infection (exotoxin produced by *Corynebacterium, Rickettsia, Chlamydia, Coxiella*) and protozoa (*Trypanosoma cruzi, Toxoplasma gondii*).

Chagas' disease

Chagas' disease (American trypanosomiasis) is a protozoal infection that causes myocarditis. It is caused by the intracellular protozoan parasite, *T. cruzi*, and is the most frequent cause of heart failure in Brazil and neighbouring Latin American countries. The parasite is transmitted by various insects including *Triatoma infestans, Rhodnius prolixus,* and *Panstrongylus megistus*. There is an initial local lesion at the site of entry, followed by bouts of parasitemia and fever. Damage to the heart is caused by the toxins released by the parasite and by inflammatory cells.

There are two clinically distinct presentations of this disease:

- Acute Chagas' disease, which mainly affects children and is mild in most individuals. Damage to the heart results from a direct invasion of the myocardial cells by the parasite and the subsequent inflammatory events.
- Chronic Chagas' disease, which is characterized by damage to the heart muscle resulting from an autoimmune reaction induced by *T. cruzi* parasites and is mediated by cytotoxic T cells.

Treatment Any treatment used is directed at the infective organism (see Chapters 23–26). However, there is no really effective treatment, although primaquine, puromycin, nifurtimox, and benznidazole are used, the latter two only being used in acute disease. Over 80% of patients with the acute form and slightly more with the chronic form are cured of the infection.

Nifurtimox exerts its trypanocidal action by forming free radicals

Nifurtimox is the drug of choice, with benznidazole as an alternative drug that is effective against nifurtimox-resistant *T. cruzi*. Nifurtimox and benznidazole are not available in the UK. Nifurtimox exerts its trypanocidal action by forming free radicals. The free radicals react with molecular oxygen to form superoxide anions, hydrogen peroxide, and hydroxyl free radicals. Trypanosomes are susceptible to these reactive intermediates, which cause lipid and DNA peroxidation, because these organisms contain no catalase or glutathione peroxidase to inactivate the toxic products. Primaquine eliminates tissue infection and prevents the development of the blood (erythrocytic) forms of the parasite.

Adverse effects of benznidazole and nifurtimox include gastrointestinal upsets and rashes. Nifurtimox is highly toxic to human cells, but limited selectivity is achieved because the rates of radical formation are much lower in human cells than in trypanosomes. Nifurtimox may also cause anorexia, tremors, paresthesia, polyneuritis, and transient leukopenia. The adverse effects of primaquine are predominantly gastointestinal.

Pericarditis

Pericarditis is an infection of the pericardium, which surrounds the epicardial surface of the heart. Inflammation of the pericardium is usually secondary to a variety of cardiac diseases, systemic disorders, or metastases from neoplasms arising in remote sites. Pericarditis has numerous etiologies, but coxsackie viral infections are the commonest cause.

Treatment Anti-inflammatory medication such as oral aspirin, naproxen, or indomethacin is used to treat pericarditis. However, if it is severe or recurrent, systemic glucocorticosteroids may be necessary.

Infective endocarditis

Infective endocarditis is an infection of the endocardium or vascular endothelium. Occasionally it occurs as an acute infection, but more commonly it runs an insidious course and is known as subacute bacterial endocarditis (Fig. 8.51).

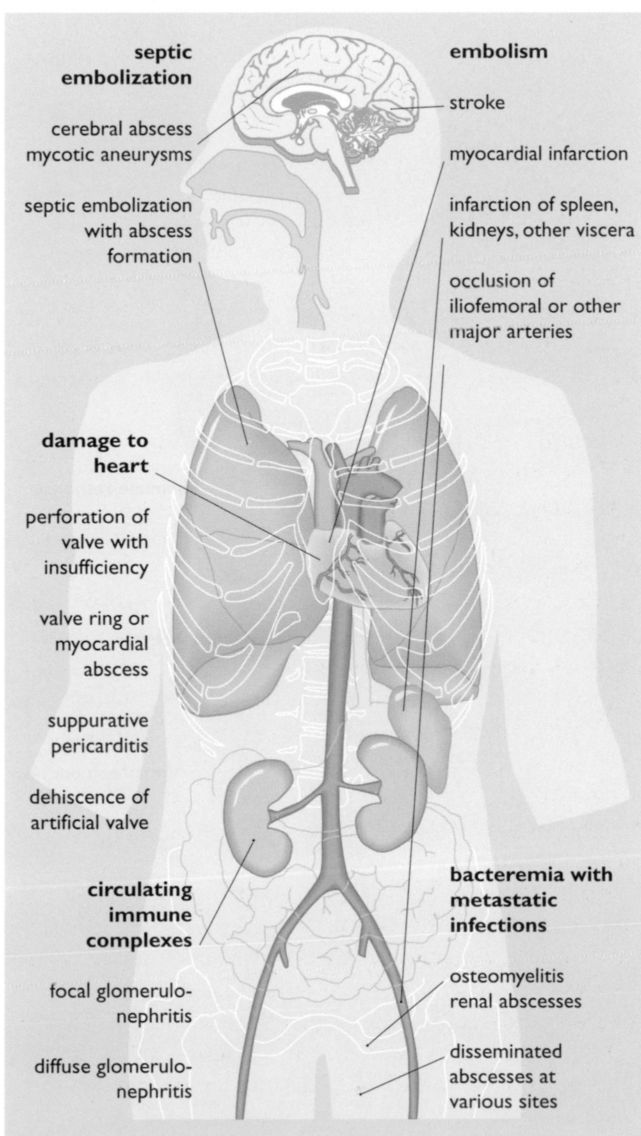

Fig 8.51 The potential complications of infective endocarditis. (Modified from Bisno et al., *Hospital Practice* 21, **139**, 1986.)

Infective endocarditis is rare in the UK and US (6–7/100,000), but more common in developing countries. It occurs most commonly on rheumatic or congenitally abnormal valves as well as on a prolapsed mitral valve and in calcified aortic valve disease. However, normal valves may be involved, particularly after injection by addicts of nonsterile drugs. Virtually every form of microbiologic agent, including fungi, rickettsiae, and chlamydiae, have been shown to cause infective endocarditis. Most cases are, however, bacterial in origin with *Streptococcus viridans*, *Strep. faecalis*, and *Staphylococcus aureus* being the most common organisms.

Treatment If infective endocarditis is caused by *Strep. viridans* or *Strep. faecalis*, treatment is with penicillin G and gentamicin. If *Staph. aureus* is responsible, flucloxacillin* and either fusidic acid or gentamicin are used.

Infective endocarditis may occur following dental surgery as a result of bacteria from the oral cavity entering the blood stream, and so penicillin prophylaxis is used and started seven days before surgery (see Chapter 20).

Kawasaki's disease

Kawasaki's disease is a generalized vasculitis causing extensive damage to the vessels of the heart, which can be fatal. Although the etiology is unknown, current evidence suggests that it is probably not an autoimmune disease, but may be triggered by a virus.

During the acute phase, Kawasaki's disease may be characterized by medium and large vessel arteritis, arterial aneurysms, valvulitis, and myocarditis. Of particular concern are coronary artery aneurysms, which may precipitate thrombosis.

Lymphocyte and macrophage activation is evident in this disease. Experimental studies have shown the presence of antibodies that can kill endothelial cells previously treated with interleukin-1 or tumor necrosis factor. The function of these antibodies in the disease process is unknown: they may simply be a marker of the disease or they may have a pathogenic role.

Patients with Kawasaki's disease can be classified according to their relative risk of myocardial ischemia on a scale of 1–5. No therapy is recommended until level 3, at which small- to medium-sized solitary coronary artery aneurysms are observed. Aspirin is then prescribed.

Level 4 is characterized by the presence of one or more giant coronary artery aneurysms or multiple small- to medium-sized aneurysms without obstruction, and is treated with aspirin with or without the addition of warfarin.

Patients considered to have the highest risk of myocardial infarction have evidence of coronary artery obstruction and are classified as level 5. They are treated with aspirin with or without the addition of warfarin, as well as Ca^{2+} antagonists to reduce myocardial oxygen demand.

Use of intravenous gammaglobulin before the tenth day of the illness can reduce the morbidity

Recent studies have found that the use of intravenous gammaglobulin therapy before the tenth day of the illness has reduced the morbidity from Kawasaki's disease and the apparent incidence of coronary artery abnormalities. Gammaglobulin contains antibodies against various viruses present in the population. The antibodies are directed against the virus envelope and can 'neutralize' some viruses and prevent their attachment to host cells.

Rheumatic fever

Rheumatic fever is an inflammatory disease that occurs in children and young adults and is common in the Middle East, Far East, and Eastern Europe. It occurs in a small proportion of individuals (those who have a significant antibody response to streptococcal proteins) several weeks after a pharyngeal infection with group A streptococcus, at which stage autoantibodies against the heart can be detected (Fig. 8.52). There is evidence to suggest that carbohydrate antigens on the streptococci crossreact with an antigen on the heart valves and myocardium. Rheumatic fever is therefore thought to develop as a result of an abnormal host immune response, both cellular and humoral, triggered by streptococcus A. It is likely that the disease is due to a complex interrelationship between the genetics of the host's immune system and the streptococcus bacillus.

The treatment of rheumatic fever initially involves eradication of residual streptococcal infections with a single intramuscular injection of benzathine penicillin or oral phenoxymethylpenicillin four times daily for one week. High-dose salicylate therapy inhibits cyclooxygenase activity and is given to the limit of tolerance determined by the development of tinnitus. If there is carditis, systemic glucocorticosteroids can be given.

Recurrences are prevented by continued treatment until 20 years of age or for five years after the last attack

Recurrences are common if there is persistent cardiac damage and are prevented by the continued use of oral phenoxymethylpenicillin daily or by monthly injections of benzathine penicillin until the age of 20 years or for five years after the last attack.

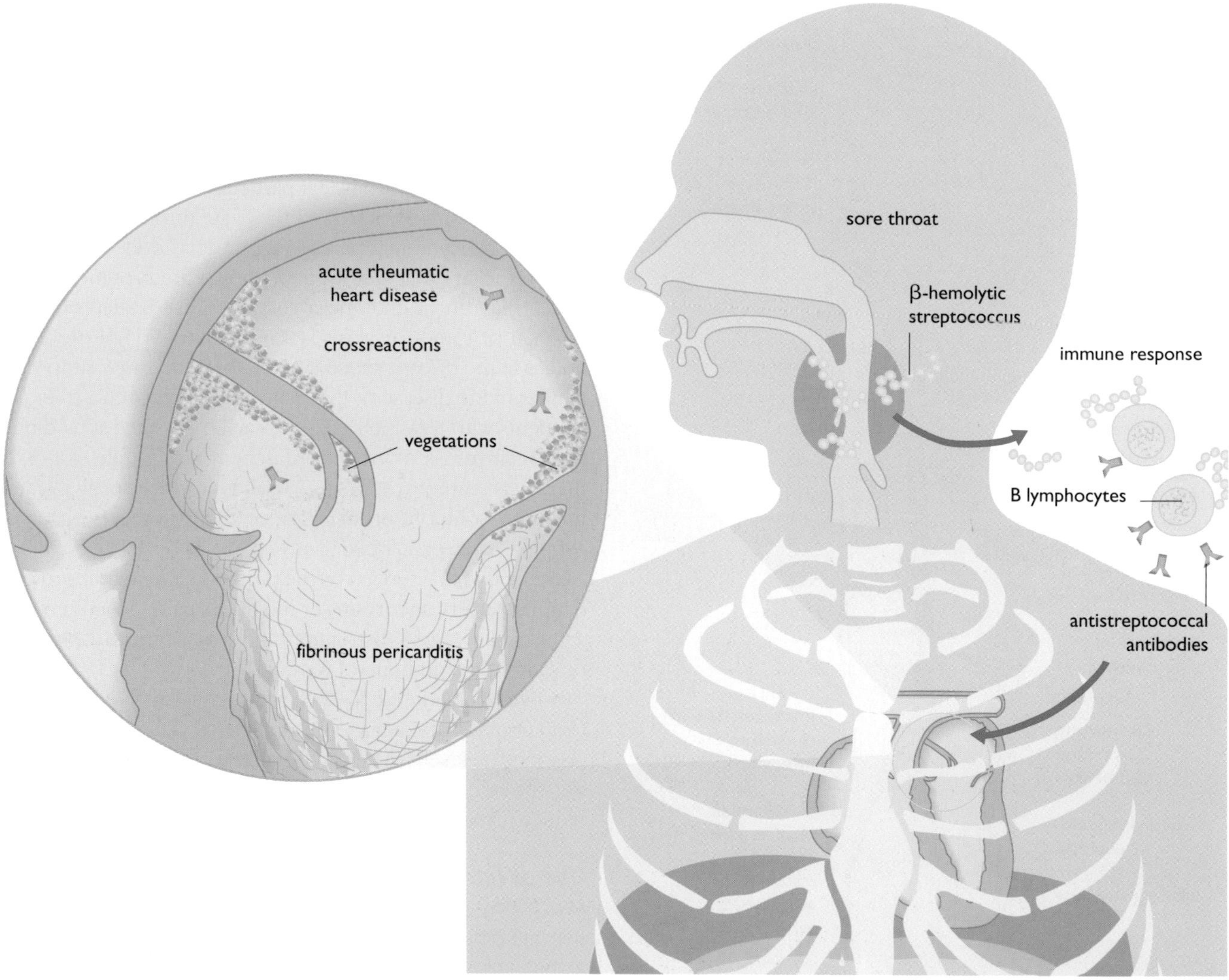

Fig 8.52 Pathogenetic sequence and main morphologic features of acute rheumatic heart disease. Acute rheumatic fever often causes mitral valvulitis characterized by a linear arrangement of vegetations along the line of closure of the leaflets.

FURTHER READING

Fozzard HA, Haber E, Jennings RB, Katz AM, Morgan HE (eds) *The Heart and Cardiovascular System*. New York: Raven Press Ltd; 1995. [This two-volume book contains some excellent chapters written by researchers who are at the forefront of their field.]

Hosenpud JD, Greenberg BH (eds) *Congestive Heart Failure: Pathophysiology, Diagnosis and Comprehensive Approach to Management*. New York: Springer Verlag; 1994. [An excellent textbook that details the basic pathophysiology, pharmacologic therapy, and clinical approach to management of congestive heart failure.]

Levi AJ, Boyett MR, Lee CO. The cellular actions of digitalis glycosides on the heart. *Prog Biophys Mol Biol* 1994; **62**: 1–54. [A comprehensive review that discusses the actions of cardiac glycosides at the membrane level of cardiac cells.]

Noble D. The surprising heart: a review of recent progress in cardiac electrophysiology. *J Physiol* 1984; **353**: 1–50. [This is an excellent review of cardiac electrophysiology written in an accessible style.]

Rees SA, Curtis MJ. Which cardiac potassium channel subtype is the preferable target for suppression of ventricular arrythmias? *Pharmacol Therapeutics* 1996; **69**: 199–217. [An up-to-date summary of Class III antiarrhythmics, their uses, and adverse effects.]

Task Force of the Working Group on Arrhythmias of the European Society of Cardiology. The Sicilian Gambit: A new approach to the classification of antiarrhythmic drugs based on their actions on arrhythmogenic mechanisms. *Circulation* 1991; **84**: 1831–1851. [This is a reappraisal of the state of antiarrhythmic therapy after a landmark clinical trial.]

Make a provisional diagnosis and determine a rational pharmacologic treatment for the following hypothetical case.

A 53-year-old man with a history of severe hypertension for at least 20 years which was generally well controlled by medication, tended to stop taking his drugs from time to time, occasionally for extended periods. Several weeks before admission he had stopped taking his medications, which included lisinopril, nifedipine, and atenolol. Several days before admission he had a headache and was noted by his wife to be confused. On admission he was obtunded with multifocal neurological findings. His blood pressure was 240/135 mmHg, he had papilledema, and rales in both lungs, and his urine contained multiple red blood cells.

1. Is his clinical condition immediately life threatening?
2. Which additional diagnostic tests might be indicated immediately?
3. What properties would an ideal drug have in this setting? Give an example of such a drug.
4. What is the target goal for blood pressure?
5. After this man's blood pressure has been sufficiently lowered, what would be the long-term plan for him?

Indicate which is the correct answer for each question.

1. An asymptomatic female patient with mild hypertension (140/95 mmHg) should be treated with which of the following regimens or drugs?
a) guanethidine
b) nifedipine
c) hydrochlorothiazide, exercise and reduced salt intake
d) prazosin
e) clonidine

2. Drug X is used in the treatment of cardiac arrhythmias. It is not used as an anticonvulsant and is not recommended for use in asthmatic subjects because of effects on certain adrenoceptors. It is probably:
a) procainamide
b) propranolol
c) quinidine
d) disopyramide
e) lidocaine

3. In the management of cardiac arrhythmias that result from the appearance of an ectopic focus (as opposed to re-entry), the Class I antiarrhythmic agents are effective because they
a) inhibit voltage-sensitive Ca^{2+} channels
b) decrease phase 4 depolarization
c) increase atrioventricular conduction velocity
d) have negative inotropic actions
e) increase sinoatrial node automaticity

4. All of the following antiarrhythmic drugs are incorrectly matched with a statement regarding their properties and uses, except
a) amiodarone is used as an oral treatment of ventricular arrhythmias; severe adverse effects are common.
b) bretylium stabilizes heart rhythm in the majority of patients with resistant ventricular fibrillation that has not responded to other treatment
c) tocainide is a new orally effective congener of lidocaine
d) acebutolol is a β_1 selective adrenoceptor antagonist
e) disopyramide is reserved by most consultants for patients not in heart failure who cannot tolerate quinidine, procainamide, or tocainide

5. All of the following antiarrhythmic drugs are correctly classified with their principal mechanism of action, except
a) quinidine: Na^+ channel blockade
b) verapamil: Ca^{2+} antagonism
c) bretylium: delays repolarization
d) amiodarone: Na^+ channel blockade
e) tocainide: Na^+ channel blockade

6. A frequency-dependent blockade of Na^+ channels is the principal mechanism of action of which of the following antiarrhythmic drugs?
a) verapamil
b) quinidine
c) propranolol
d) sotalol
e) lidocaine

7. An increase in cardiac output is associated with which one of the following drugs?
a) clonidine
b) α methyldopa
c) hydralazine
d) propranolol
e) guanethidine

8. If daily maintenance doses of digoxin are given without an initial loading dose, the maximal effect on the heart will be achieved in about
a) seven days
b) 24 hours
c) two weeks
d) five days
e) five weeks

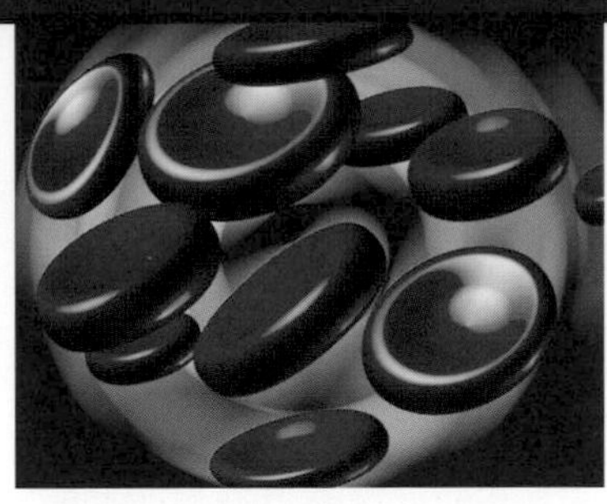

9. Drugs and Blood

PHYSIOLOGY OF THE HEMATOPOIETIC SYSTEM

Blood is a suspension of cells in plasma, which is a solution of proteins and salts. The cells of the blood are red blood cells (erythrocytes), white blood cells (leukocytes) and platelets.

- Erythrocytes are anuclear cells containing hemoglobin and carry oxygen from the lung to all the tissues where it is exchanged for carbon dioxide.
- Leukocytes (neutrophils, monocytes, lymphocytes, and others) defend the body against microorganisms that enter the body from the environment.
- Platelets form plugs with coagulation proteins in the plasma to stop leaks from the blood vessels (Fig. 9.1).

All blood cells are derived from the hematopoietic stem cell

Blood cells originate in the bone marrow (except during an early part of fetal life) and are derived from the hematopoietic stem cell. This stem cell self-replicates and exists in very small numbers in the bone marrow and blood. Although it has a great capacity for self-renewal, as a group hematopoietic stem cells are relatively quiescent and only a minuscule fraction are proliferating and differentiating at any one time to replenish the lost blood elements.

Hematopoietic stem cells give rise to hematopoietic progenitor cells. Compared with stem cells, these cells have a decreased capacity for self-renewal and are more committed to differentiating into a particular blood cell type. With each generation, the descendents of the progenitor cells differentiate further into more mature cells with a more limited life span and become restricted to a particular blood cell lineage. Ultimately, the process ends with mature cells, which have no further capacity to divide and give rise to red cells, leukocytes, and platelets. This maturation process is controlled by hematopoietic growth factors. Many of these have been purified and cloned, and some have been produced by recombinant technology and are used pharmacotherapeutically, as discussed later (Fig. 9.2).

PATHOPHYSIOLOGY AND DISEASES OF THE BLOOD

This chapter describes the pharmacologic agents that are useful in the treatment of four important dysfunctions of the blood: anemia, neutropenia, thrombosis, and bleeding.

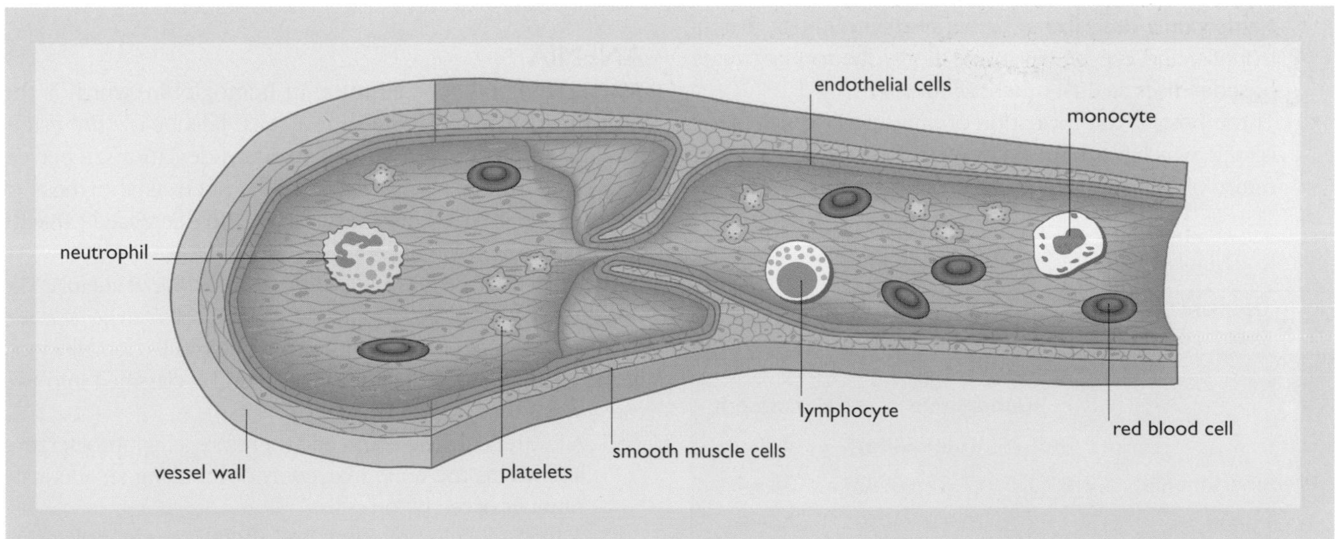

Fig. 9.1 Blood vessel and the blood cells. The blood vessel wall and its surrounding smooth muscle cells are lined by endothelial cells, which provide a nonthrombotic surface for smooth blood flow. White blood cells, including neutrophils, monocytes, and lymphocytes interact with the blood vessel cells to defend the body against microbial invasion. Red blood cells carry oxygen to end organs. Platelets plug leaks in the blood vessels to prevent blood loss.

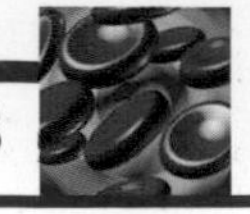

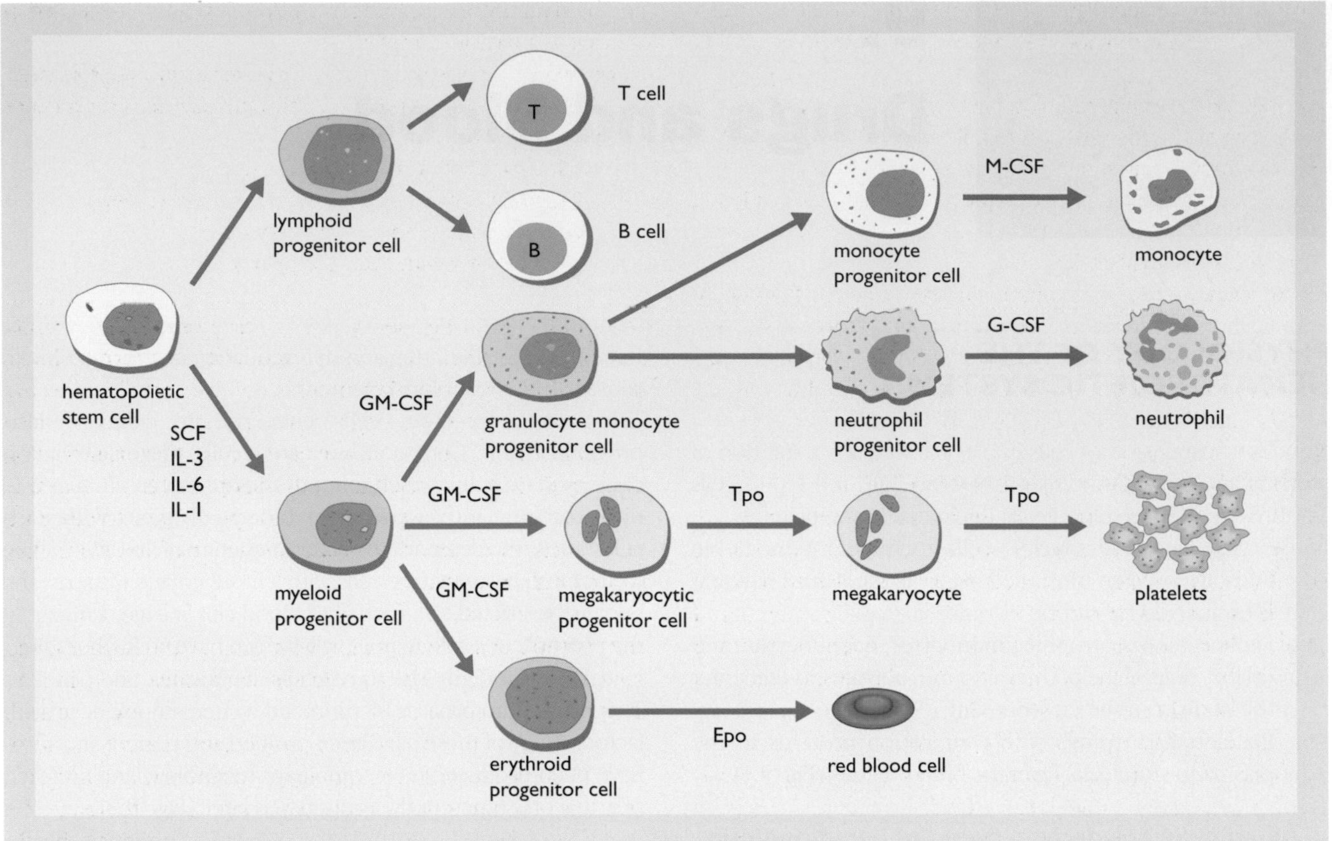

Fig. 9.2 Hematopoiesis and hematopoietic growth factors. Hematopoietic stem cells have a high regenerative potential, but with each generation the descendent cells acquire lineage-specific characteristics and decreased proliferative capacity. Growth factors Epo, G-CSF, GM-CSF, IL, M-CSF, SCF, and Tpo are needed for regulating each step of hemopoiesis. (Epo, erythropoietin; G-CSF, granulocyte colony stimulating factor; GM-CSF, granulocyte–macrophage colony stimulating factor; IL, interleukin; M-CSF, macrophage colony stimulating factor; SCF, stem cell factor; Tpo, thrombopoietin)

- Anemia describes a below normal concentration of circulatory hemoglobin and symptoms due to the decreased oxygen-carrying capacity can result.
- Neutropenia describes a below normal number of neutrophils, and can result in infections due to inadequate host defenses against microbial invasion.
- Thrombosis is the formation of unwanted clots in blood vessels, which block the delivery of blood to end organs or return of blood to the heart.

Normal concentrations (mean ± SD) of hemoglobin and hematocrit

	Hemoglobin		Hematocrit
	g/dl	(mmol/liter)	%
Prepubertal child	12.5±1.5	(7.37±0.93)	38±4
Male adult	15.4±1.8	(9.56±1.12)	44±5
Female adult	13.5±2.0	(8.38±1.24)	38±5

Hematocrit in third trimester for pregnant women may be as low as 30%

- Bleeding disorders result from failure of the hemostatic system to form clots and stop leaks in the blood vessels. Drugs used to treat these disorders are shown in (Fig. 9.3).

ANEMIA

When the blood concentration of hemoglobin, which is the oxygen-carrying molecule in red cells, falls below the established mean by more than two standard deviations, a person is anemic. Anemia causes symptoms such as shortness of breath and fatigue, which result from the decreased capacity to carry oxygen.

Treatment must be tailored to the specific cause of anemia. The bone marrow's ability to produce red blood cells can be assessed by measuring the number of young red blood cells (reticulocytes) in the blood. Causes of anemia can then be classified into two categories:

- A low reticulocyte count and therefore a hypoproliferative anemia, as the bone marrow is not making an adequate number of red blood cells.
- A high reticulocyte count and therefore a hemolytic anemia, in which there is increased peripheral destruction of red blood cells despite increased production by the bone marrow.

Hypoproliferative anemias can be further subdivided according to the size of the red blood cells as seen under the microscope, as follows:

- Microcytic (small red blood cells).
- Normocytic (normal size red blood cells).
- Macrocytic (large red blood cells).

Figure 9.4 lists the etiologies of anemia according to these criteria.

Iron-deficiency anemia

Iron deficiency is the most common cause of anemia. In women, it is usually due to blood loss from menstruation and pregnancy; in men and postmenopausal women, iron-deficiency anemia is often a clue to pathologic blood loss and warrants a search to discover the source of bleeding.

Two-thirds of body iron is in hemoglobin

Iron is needed to form the complex molecule, heme, which is the oxygen-carrying component of hemoglobin. When aging red cells are destroyed, almost all the iron is salvaged to form new red blood cells. However, a small but critical fraction of red blood cell iron is obtained from the diet. Dietary iron is absorbed mostly in the duodenum as part of heme and in elemental forms by the intestinal epithelial cell through cell surface receptors. Heme iron is readily absorbed and released in the cell from the porphyrin ring by heme oxygenase. However, non-heme iron absorption is highly variable. Many foods such as tea, egg yolk, and bran interfere with iron absorption. Excess iron is stored in the cell as a ferritin complex.

Iron enters the plasma by binding to transferrin, and iron transport between the absorptive cells and the plasma is via another receptor (Fig.9.5).

Physiologic loss of iron is approximately:

- 1 mg/day in men and non-menstruating women.
- 2–3 mg/day in menstruating women.
- 500–1000 mg with each pregnancy.

Diagnosis Iron deficiency can be diagnosed by measuring serum ferritin levels. It is associated with low ferritin levels unless there is a concurrent process that abnormally raises the level, such as infection or liver disease. Iron deficiency also results in a low serum iron level and a high total iron binding capacity (TIBC). Microcytosis on the peripheral blood smear is a late finding. The most sensitive and specific test to diagnose iron deficiency is a bone marrow examination of iron stores, but is not usually needed.

Treatment Supplementation with oral ferrous sulfate is the standard treatment for iron deficiency anemia. Iron is best absorbed when taken on an empty stomach with ascorbic acid, which binds to iron and facilitates iron transport into the intestinal cell. At the acid pH of the stomach, mucin binds to inorganic iron and enhances its absorption, which may therefore be impaired by antacids or medications that reduce stomach acid production. Commercial preparations of ferrous sulfate usually contain 60 mg of elemental iron, and only 10–20% of ingested

Drugs used to treat blood disorders

Drugs for anemia	Iron Vitamin B_{12} Folate Erythropoietin
Drugs for neutropenia	Granulocyte colony stimulating factor (G-CSF) Granulocyte–macrophage colony stimulating factor (GM-CSF)
Antiplatelets	Aspirin Ticlopidine Dipyridamole
Anticoagulants	Heparin Warfarin Hirudin* Hirulog
Thrombolytics	Streptokinase APSAC Urokinase Tissue plasminogen activator
Antifibrinolytics	Factor concentrates Vitamin K Desmopressin ϵ Aminocaproic acid

Fig. 9.3 Drugs used to treat blood disorders. (APSAC, anisoylated plasminogen–streptokinase activator complex)

Causes of anemia

	Hypoproliferative
Microcytic	Iron deficiency Anemia of chronic disease Sideroblastic anemia
Normocytic	Anemia of chronic disease Endocrine anemia Bone marrow failure
Macrocytic	Vitamin B_{12} deficiency Folic acid deficiency Myelodysplastic syndrome
	Hyperproliferative
Hemolytic	Hemoglobinopathies Autoimmune Membrane disorder Drug-induced Metabolic abnormalities Glucose-6-phosphate dehydrogenase deficiency Infections

Fig. 9.4 Causes of anemia.

iron is absorbed by iron-deficient patients. The hemoglobin concentration of patients who are optimally treated with 180 mg/day of elemental iron increases by about 1 g/dl/week (mass concentration 10 g/liter/week; substance concentration 0.62 mmol/liter/week). Iron supplementation should continue for 6 months after the hemoglobin level has normalized, to replenish the body's iron stores.

The most common complaint of patients taking iron is gastrointestinal irritation. Sometimes this can be very bothersome. A polysaccharide–iron complex preparation is available that may cause less gastrointestinal irritation, but is much more expensive. If oral supplementation is not tolerated despite careful counseling, iron can be administered parenterally. The intramuscular route is painful and may cause skin discoloration at the injection site. Alternatively, iron dextran can be slowly infused intravenously, but this must only be carried out with close monitoring as there is a high incidence of anaphylactic reactions.

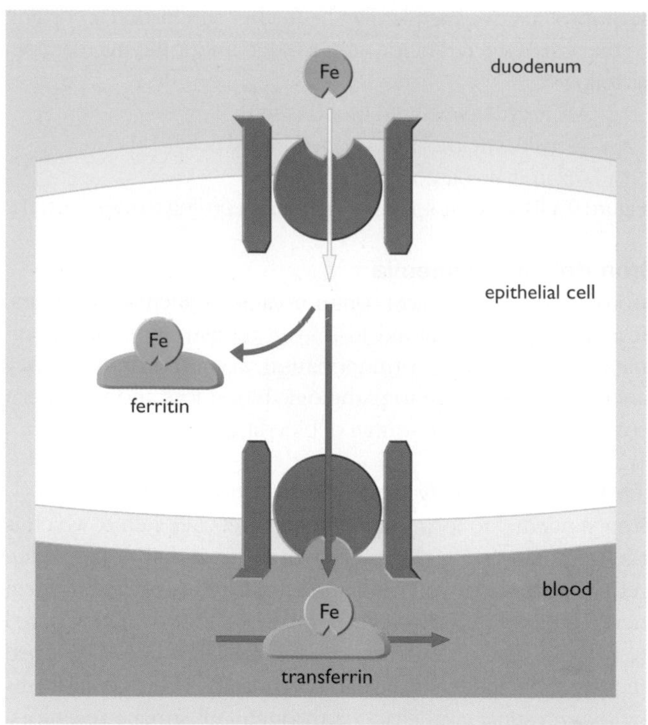

Fig. 9.5 Iron absorption by the gastrointestinal epithelial cell. Iron is absorbed via a cell surface transporter on the epithelial cell. Some of the iron passes through the cell and is carried in the blood by transferrin. Excess iron is stored as ferritin.

Vitamin B_{12} and folate-deficiency anemia

Deficiency of vitamin B_{12} (cobalamin) and folate causes megaloblastic anemia (see also Chapter 24), and can lead to macrocytic changes in the red blood cells and hypersegmented (more than five lobes) neutrophils. Both cobalamin and folate are critical cofactors in enzymatic reactions required for deoxyribonucleic acid (DNA) synthesis (Fig. 9.6). The interdependency of cobalamin and methylfolate may explain the similar morphologic changes observed when either cobalamin or folate is deficient. Unlike folate

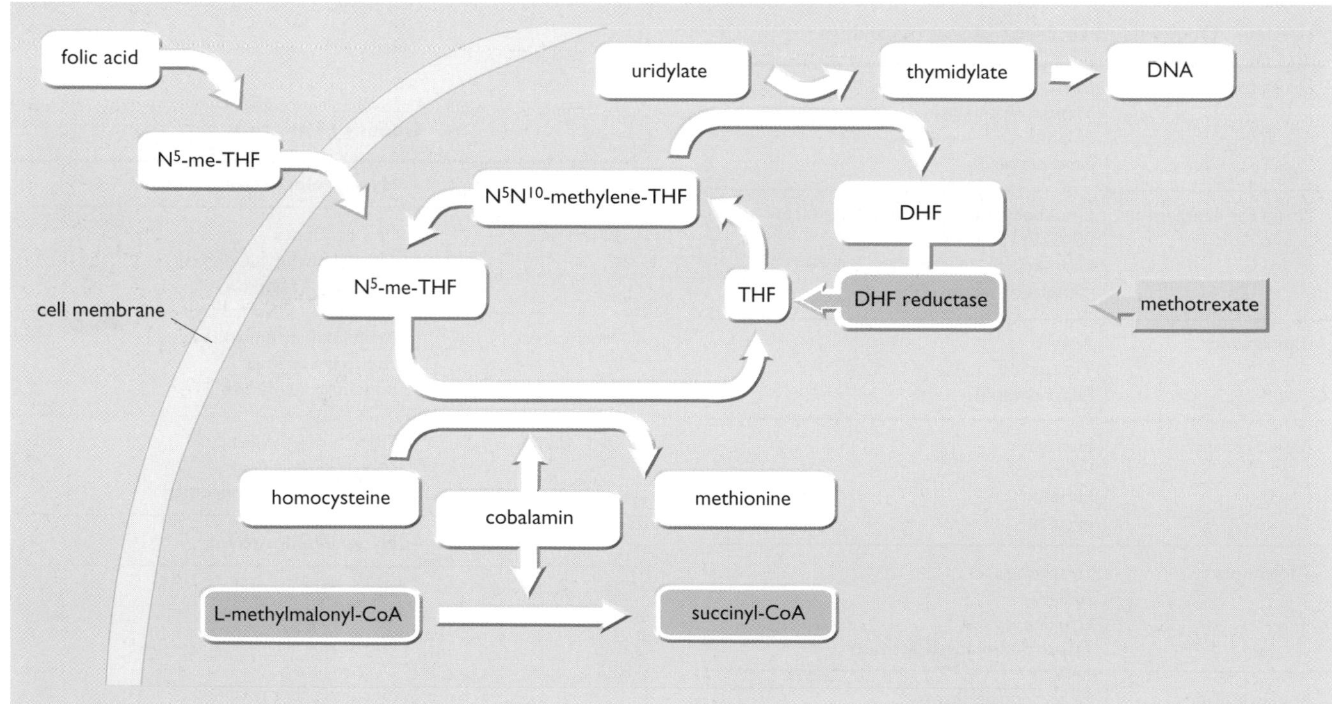

Fig. 9.6 Role of folate and vitamin B_{12} in DNA synthesis. Folate compounds are required as carbon donors in the conversion of deoxyuridine to dexoxythymidine. Cobalamin is a cofactor for homocysteine–methionine methyltransferase, which transfers a methyl group from methyltetrahydrofolate to homocysteine to make methionine. Cobalamin is also required for methylmalonyl coenzyme A mutase, which converts methylmalonyl coenzyme A to succinyl coenzyme A. Methotrexate inhibits DNA synthesis by inhibiting DHF reductase which converts DHF to THF. (DHF, dihydrofolate; N^5-me-THF, N^5-methyltetrahydrofolate; THF, tetrahydrofolate)

deficiency, however, vitamin B_{12} deficiency can also cause neurologic deficits: paresthesias are the earliest symptom and are then followed by loss of vibratory sense, ataxia, dementia, and coma.

The most common cause of vitamin B_{12} deficiency is pernicious anemia.

The daily requirement of vitamin B_{12} is 0.6–1.2 mg, and the biologic half-life of vitamin B_{12} stored in the liver is about one year. Therefore, more than two years must elapse after a complete cessation of vitamin B_{12} intake before clinical manifestations of deficiency become apparent.

Vitamin B_{12} is readily absorbed from the gastrointestinal tract with the aid of intrinsic factor secreted by the parietal cells of the stomach, and the intrinsic factor–cobalamin complex is absorbed via receptors on the ileal cell surface (Fig. 9.7).

As vitamin B_{12} is widely available in animal products, dietary deficiency is an uncommon cause of vitamin B_{12} deficiency except in the strictest vegetarians/vegans. The most common cause of B_{12} deficiency is pernicious anemia, a form of gastric secretory failure with gastric atrophy and a consequent failure to secrete intrinsic factor. It is strongly suspected that pernicious anemia results from an autoimmune destruction, and antiparietal cell and anti-intrinsic factor antibodies are detected in many patients.

Diagnosis of vitamin B_{12} deficiency involves measuring serum vitamin B_{12} levels, although a significant minority of deficient patients have normal levels. Vitamin B_{12} deficiency leads to increased serum and urine concentrations of methylmalonic acid, and these are a sensitive index of vitamin B_{12} deficiency. A two-stage test, first with radiolabeled vitamin B_{12} alone and then radiolabeled B_{12} with intrinsic factor (Schilling test), can be performed to determine whether a vitamin B_{12} deficiency is due to pernicious anemia.

Treatment of vitamin B_{12} deficiency should be started with parenteral cyanocobalamin (the form available in the US). The recommended maintenance treatment of pernicious anemia is monthly injections of 1 mg cyanocobalamin. However, oral therapy with 1 mg vitamin B_{12} five times a week has been shown to be equally effective. Despite the lack of intrinsic factor, absorption by passive diffusion still functions and can fulfill the 2–5 μg/day requirement. The application of a vitamin B gel intranasally (ENER-B gel) has been approved by the Food and Drug Administration (FDA) for dietary supplementation, but not for the treatment of pernicious anemia, although it does consistently raise serum vitamin B_{12} levels. The serum K^+ concentration may fall after initial treatment with vitamin B_{12} owing to an increased need for intracellular K^+ to support new cell synthesis.

Megaloblastic anemia due to folate deficiency may respond to supraphysiologic doses of vitamin B_{12} therapy. Conversely, large doses of folic acid can reverse megaloblastic anemia due to vitamin B_{12} deficiency. Importantly, however, the neurologic damage due to vitamin B_{12} deficiency is not reversed by folate.

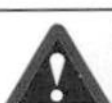

Warning about using folic acid

Large doses of folic acid can reverse the megaloblastic anemia caused by vitamin B_{12} deficiency, but do not reverse the neurologic damage of vitamin B_{12} deficiency.

Causes of folate deficiency include pregnancy, alcohol abuse, and drugs

Folates are found in a wide variety of fresh foods, but are rapidly destroyed by heating during food preparation. Folic acid is widely distributed in nature as a conjugate with one or more molecules of glutamic acid. Naturally occurring folates must be reduced to mono- and diglutamates by conjugases in the stomach before they can be efficiently absorbed from the proximal small intestine. Folates are then transported to the liver where they are stored and transformed into 5-methyltetrahydrofolate, which is the form that enters tissue cells. In the cell, 5-methyltetrahydrofolate is converted into the metabolically active tetrahydrofolate by vitamin B_{12}-dependent methyltransferase.

The normal daily requirement of folate is about 100 μg, and tissue stores of folate are estimated at 10 mg. Inadequate dietary

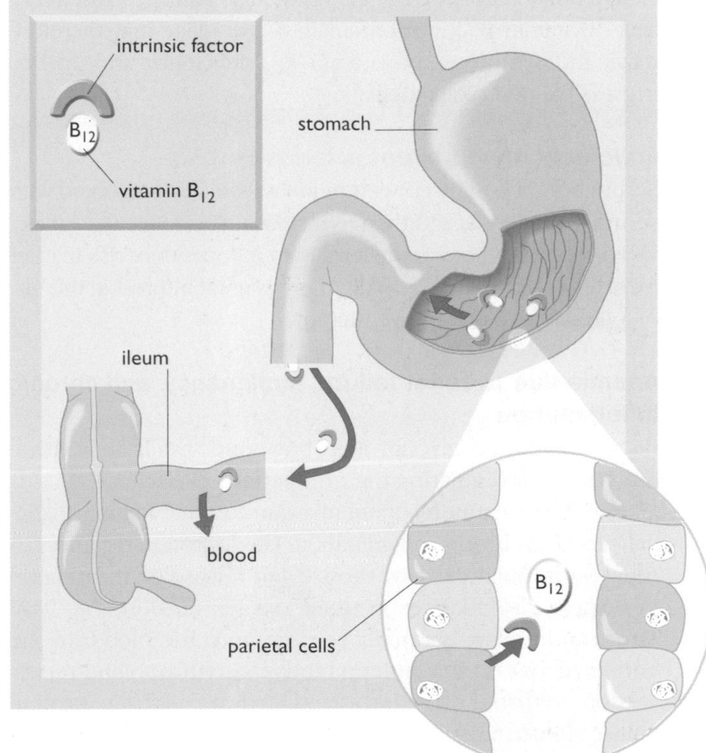

Fig. 9.7 Absorption of vitamin B_{12}. Intestinal absorption of vitamin B_{12} requires intrinsic factor, which is secreted by parietal cells in the stomach, and occurs in the distal ileum via cell surface receptors.

folate intake, therefore, will lead to megaloblastic anemia much sooner than will vitamin B_{12} deficiency.

During pregnancy, the need for folates is markedly increased and folate deficiency during this period is associated with congenital neural tube defects. Folate supplementation is recommended for all pregnant women or those who are likely to get pregnant.

Alcohol abuse is a common cause of folate deficiency anemia as a result of reduced folate intake and diminished folate absorption.

As the concentration of folate in bile is several times that in plasma, biliary diversion will reduce the plasma concentration of folate. Patients with prolonged biliary drainage should therefore be given oral folate supplementation.

People taking phenytoin and related anticonvulsants tend to have lower serum folate levels than controls, but rarely have megaloblastic anemia. Antifolates such as methotrexate are widely used to treat hematologic and inflammatory diseases. Methotrexate competes with dihydrofolate for the enzyme dihydrofolate reductase and, even at the relatively low doses used in the treatment of rheumatoid arthritis, there is evidence of red blood cell macrocytosis (see Fig. 9.6 and Chapter 17).

Diagnosis of folate deficiency is obtained by measuring serum or red blood cell folate levels.

Treatment of folate deficiency Folate deficiency responds promptly to treatment with 1 mg/day of oral folate. An injectable form is available for patients who are unable to take anything orally or have poor enteric absorption. As previously stated, folate may correct the megaloblastic anemia of vitamin B_{12} deficiency, but will not correct the neurologic damage caused by a lack of vitamin B_{12}. Indiscriminate use of folate may therefore mask the symptoms of vitamin B_{12} deficiency and lead to irreversible neurologic deficits.

Folic acid may prevent arteriosclerosis

Serum homocysteine concentration is inversely correlated with serum folate levels, and there is increasing evidence that an elevated serum homocysteine level is an independent risk marker for arteriosclerosis. As a result, there is great interest in the use of folic acid as a preventive therapy.

Anemia due to renal failure, malignancy, and chronic inflammation

Erythropoietin, a glycoprotein hormone that is the critical growth factor regulating the production of red blood cells, is an effective treatment of anemia due to renal failure, malignancies, and chronic inflammation. Hemoprotein receptors in renal peritubular cells synthesize and release erythropoietin in response to changes in tissue oxygen tension (Fig. 9.8). After synthesis, it is rapidly released into the blood. In the bone marrow, erythropoietin binds to erythropoietin receptors on erythroid progenitor cells, activates tyrosine protein kinase signal transduction pathways, and thereby stimulates cell proliferation and differentiation into red blood cells (Fig. 9.9).

The anemia of chronic renal failure results from a loss of the renal cells that produce erythropoietin. Recombinant human

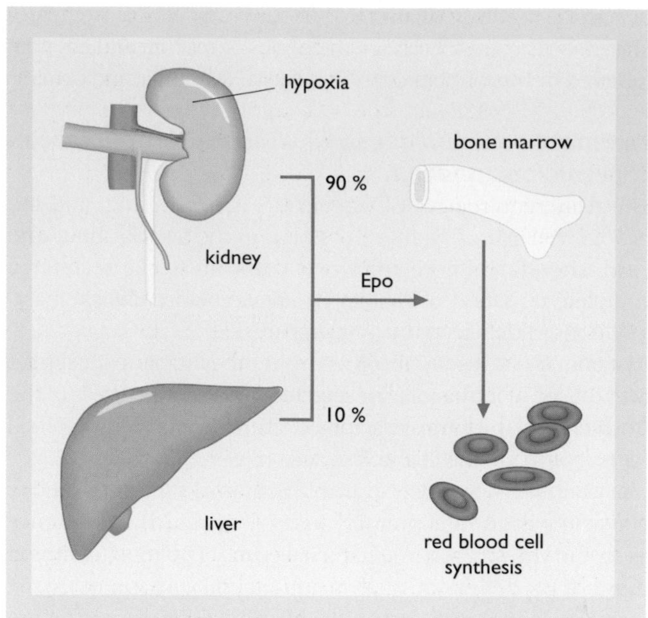

Fig. 9.8 Stimulation of erythropoietin (Epo) synthesis by hypoxia. Low oxygen tension, 'sensed' by renal peritubular cells, induces these cells to produce Epo, which stimulates the bone marrow to produce red blood cells. The liver also produces a small amount of Epo, which can therefore still be detected in anephric patients.

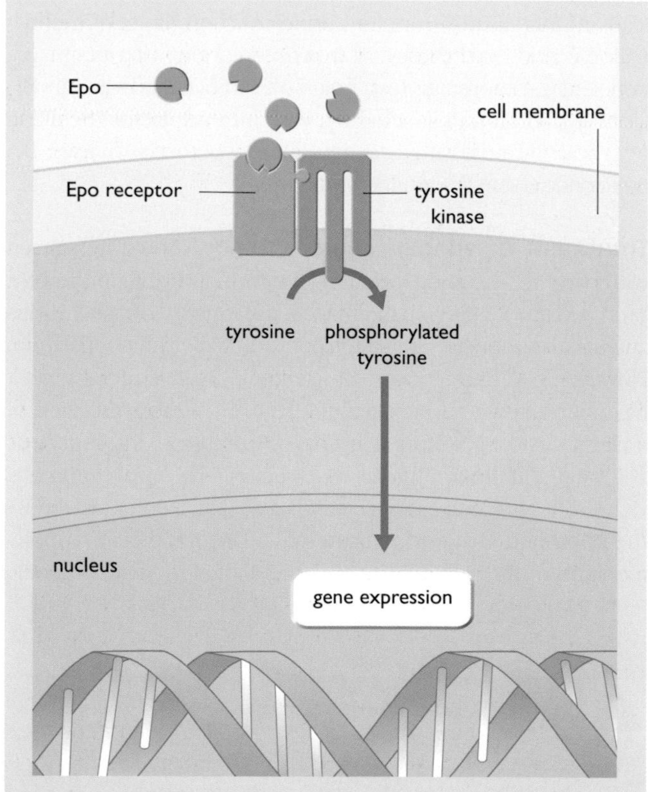

Fig. 9.9 Erythropoietin (Epo) receptor signal transduction. Stimulation of Epo receptors on erythroid progenitor cells activates tyrosine protein kinases and receptor tyrosine phosphorylation leading to the transcription of genes related to growth and differentiation.

erythropoietin is now a standard treatment for the anemia of chronic renal failure, and subcutaneous or intravenous erythropoietin (150 units/kg three times a week) will correct the anemia of 80% of such patients. The reticulocyte response to erythropoietin can develop within 3 days of starting treatment, with a significant rise in hematocrit occurring at 1 week. Maximum effects are achieved after 4–8 weeks.

The plasma half-life of intravenously administered erythropoietin is approximately 8 hours, and it is primarily metabolized by the liver.

Complications of erythropoietin treatment include hypertension and thrombosis, which may occur if the hematocrit rises too rapidly. Seizures have been reported in patients with a pre-existing history of seizure disorder.

The iron stores of patients with anemia of renal failure are often rapidly depleted during erythropoietin treatment owing to active erythropoeisis. As it may be difficult to supplement with oral iron alone in these patients owing to continued iron loss secondary to bleeding, treatment with parenteral iron may be required.

Erythropoietin is also an effective treatment of zidovudine-induced anemia in patients with human immunodeficiency virus and in cancer patients receiving chemotherapy.

NEUTROPENIA

Neutrophils are the principal defense cells against bacterial and fungal infections. Their continuous turnover and replenishment in the tissues are critical for maintaining an uninfected state. Unlike other blood cells, they and the precursor cells committed to become neutrophils spend most of their relatively brief life span (15 days) in the bone marrow. Normal granulopoiesis must support a cell population in the blood and tissue compartments that rapidly turns over. The numbers of neutrophils in the blood and tissue are therefore highly susceptible to rapid depletion when the marrow storage pool is compromised.

Drugs are the most common cause of neutropenia

The most common cause of neutropenia is myelosuppression by cancer chemotherapy, but many commonly prescribed medications can also cause neutropenia. Other causes include congenital, autoimmune, and infectious disorders (Fig. 9.10). The proliferation and maturation of myeloid progenitor cells are regulated in part by specific hematopoietic hormones called colony stimulating factors.

Treatment

Recombinant granulocyte colony stimulating factor (G-CSF) and granulocyte–macrophage colony stimulating factor (GM-CSF) have dramatic stimulatory effects on neutrophil production when administered pharmacotherapeutically. However, their specific physiologic roles in the normal regulation of myelopoiesis are not clearly defined. G-CSF and GM-CSF also enhance the functional responsiveness of mature neutrophils to inflammatory signals and may increase neutrophil-dependent host defenses by enhancing the function of neutrophils. G-CSF acts only on hematopoietic cells that are committed to become neutrophils, so it is relatively more lineage specific than GM-CSF, which also stimulates macrophages. Recombinant G-CSF or GM-CSF given intravenously or subcutaneously raises the absolute neutrophil count within 24 hours. When the drug is stopped, the absolute neutrophil count decreases by half within 24 hours and returns to baseline in 1–7 days. The response to these factors is decreased in patients who have been extensively treated with radiation or chemotherapy because they have a reduced number of progenitor cells that can respond to the growth factors.

Adverse effects of G-CSF and GM-CSF Treatment with G-CSF is better tolerated than treatment with GM-CSF. Although administration of both may cause bone pain, GM-CSF therapy can also cause a pulmonary capillary leak syndrome with pulmonary edema and heart failure. Treatment with GM-CSF, unlike G-CSF, may also cause constitutional symptoms including fever, headache, and malaise.

HEMOSTATIC DISORDERS

Normal hemostasis is a delicate balance between procoagulant, anticoagulant, and fibrinolytic processes in the blood vessel. Damage to the blood vessel wall initiates a complex series of events involving platelets, endothelial cells, and coagulation proteins that result in the formation of a platelet–fibrin clot. At the same time, physiologic anticoagulants and the fibrinolytic systems are activated by the products of the coagulation cascade to prevent the formation of unwanted clots (i.e. thrombosis).

Platelet adhesion, activation, and aggregation are some of the earliest events in hemostasis

Platelets are formed in the bone marrow from the cytoplasm of large multinucleated cells called megakaryocytes, which, like other hematopoietic cells, are derived from hematopoietic stem cells. Thrombopoietin is the primary growth factor that regulates platelet production. Recent molecular cloning of this factor has shown that thrombopoietin promotes both the proliferation of megakaryocyte progenitor cells and their maturation into platelet-producing megakaryocytes. This discovery holds the promise of the use of recombinant thrombopoietin pharmacotherapeutically to hasten the recovery of platelet counts following bone marrow suppressive chemotherapy.

Drugs and disorders that can cause neutropenia

- Myelosuppressive chemotherapy
- Analgesics and anti-inflammatory drugs
- Antibiotics: sulfonamides, semisynthetic penicillins, chloramphenicol, cephalosporins
- Antipsychotics
- Anticonvulsants
- H_2 antagonists
- Autoimmune disorders: systemic lupus erythematosus, rheumatoid arthritis
- Malignancy
- Viruses: human immunodeficiency virus, Epstein–Barr virus
- Tuberculosis

Fig. 9.10 Drugs and disorders that can cause neutropenia.

Platelet adherence to the damaged site of a vessel wall occurs through the interaction of integrin glycoprotein receptors with matrix proteins such as collagen. Following injury to an artery or arteriole, circulating von Willebrand factors (vWF) bind to the exposed collagen matrix and the matrix–vWF allows binding to platelets through the platelet membrane receptor glycoprotein GPIb-IX. Aggregation of platelets then requires the binding of fibrinogen to the platelet–receptor complex GPIIb-IIIa. Novel antiplatelet agents that block this receptor and thereby decrease platelet aggregation are currently undergoing clinical trials for the treatment of thrombotic diseases such as myocardial infarction.

Activated platelets release the contents of their granules during aggregation, and stimulate procoagulant activity by providing the phospholipid binding surfaces for the enzyme complexes in the coagulation cascade.

The platelet plug is reinforced by fibrin formed from activation of the coagulation cascade

In vivo, the tissue factor–factor VIIa complex plays a key role in initiating coagulation. After vascular injury, factor VII binds to exposed tissue factor and converts factor X to Xa, which in turn activates factor II (prothrombin) to IIa (thrombin). Thrombin then cleaves fibrinogen to fibrin, which stabilizes the primary platelet plug into a permanent plug (Fig. 9.11). The tissue factor–factor VIIa complex also activates factor X indirectly by activating factor IX to IXa. Continued activation of factor X requires the factor IXa–factor VIIIa complex (Fig. 9.12). This explains why hemophiliacs with factor VIII or IX deficiency have a bleeding disorder.

Physiologic anticoagulants

Hemostasis is regulated by specific inhibitors of the activated factors. The tissue factor–factor VIIa complex is inhibited by a protein called tissue factor pathway inhibitor (TFPI). TFPI first binds to factor Xa and then inactivates tissue factor–factor VIIa by forming a quaternary complex. Administration of heparin releases endothelium-associated TFPI into the circulation.

Anticoagulant-activated protein C with its cofactor protein S (both vitamin K-dependent proteins) is the major inhibitor of factor Va and VIIIa. Thrombin activates the protein C pathway by first binding to thrombomodulin, which activates protein C on endothelial cell surfaces. Another physiologic anticoagulant is antithrombin III (ATIII). Heparin, as a cofactor for ATIII, greatly increases the ATIII inactivation of factor Xa and thrombin. The physiologic relevance of ATIII, protein C and protein S is underscored by the greatly increased risk of venous thrombosis in people who have deficiencies of these natural anticoagulants (Fig. 9.13).

Replacement therapy with recombinant ATIII is available to prevent thrombosis in hereditary or acquired (nephrotic syndrome) ATIII-deficient patients.

The fibrinolytic system also regulates hemostasis

In addition to the physiologic anticoagulant, the body also uses the fibrinolytic system to regulate hemostasis by lysing established fibrin clots. Fibrinolysis is mainly regulated by the enzyme tissue-type plasminogen activator (t-PA). Circulating t-PA is relatively inactive. Once incorporated into the fibrin clot, it actively converts fibrin-bound plasminogen to plasmin, which degrades the fibrin clot. Inhibitors of the fibrinolytic system are plasminogen activator inhibitor (PAI-1) and α_2 antiplasmin (Fig. 9.14).

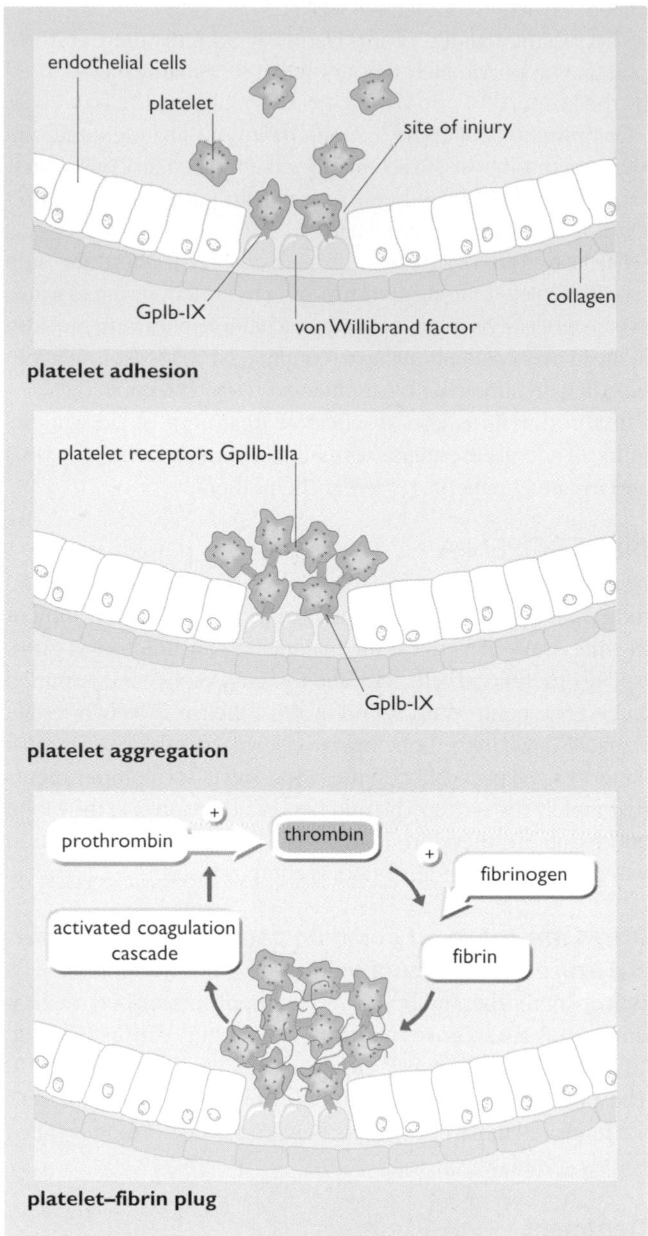

Fig. 9.11 Platelet function in hemostasis. There are three steps in the formation of the platelet–fibrin plug. The first step is platelet adhesion: vascular injury damages the endothelial cells and exposes the underlying collagen matrix. Platelets adhere to the exposed collagen after von Willebrand factors sitting on the collagen have bound to platelet receptors, GPIb-IX. The second step is platelet aggregation: activation of platelets by local factors such as thromboxane A_2, thrombin, and collagen, attracts other platelets, which aggregate through platelet receptors GPIIb-IIIa. The third step is the formation of the platelet–fibrin plug: the platelets provide a phospholipid surface for the activated coagulation cascade to activate thrombin which cleaves fibrinogen to produce fibrin to consolidate the initial platelet plug.

Thrombosis

Thrombosis is a major cause of death and disability as a result of:

- Arterial occlusion leading to myocardial infarction, stroke and peripheral ischemia.
- Venous occlusion causing deep venous thrombosis and pulmonary embolism.

Disabling or fatal thrombotic disease may stem from the formation of thrombi within arteries at the sites of arterial endothelial damage or in veins as a consequence of stasis or increased systemic coagulability. Thrombi may also form within the chambers of the heart, on damaged or prosthetic heart valves, or within the microcirculation as the result of disseminated intravascular coagulation (DIC).

Endothelial injury is the main cause of arterial thrombosis

In the high-flow arterial system, endothelial injury is the dominant influence in thrombogenesis. Arterial thrombi form only at sites with underlying arterial wall pathology (e.g. damage caused by arteriosclerosis, trauma following balloon angioplasty, or autoimmune vasculitis). Arterial thrombosis due to an increased concentration of plasma homocysteine, probably results from its toxic effect on endothelial cells and damage to the arterial wall.

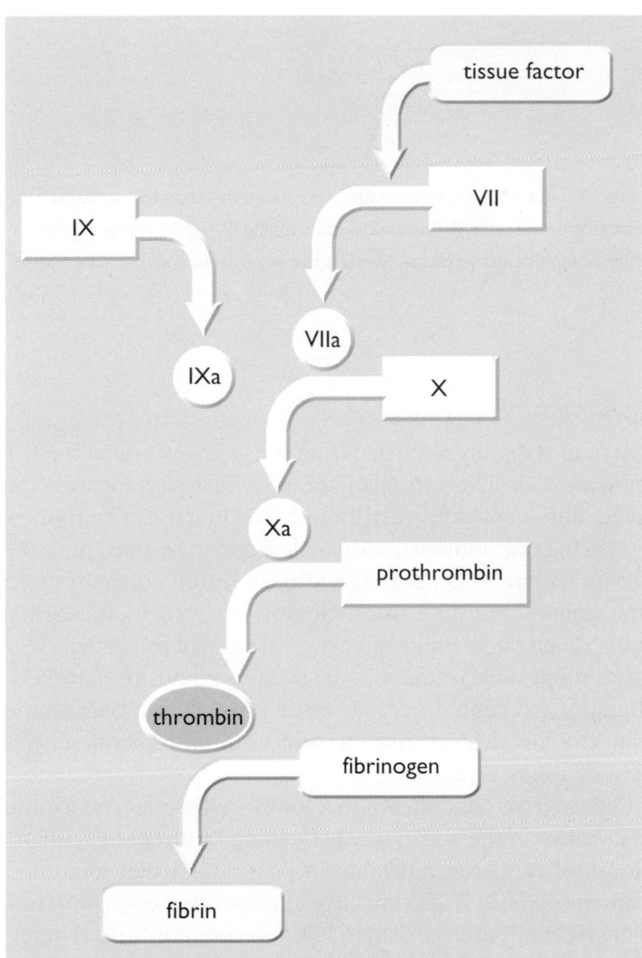

Fig. 9.12 The coagulation cascade. Initiation of coagulation by tissue factor activates factor VII, which activates both factor X and IX. Factor IX in turn activates factor X to Xa. Factor Xa cleaves prothrombin to thrombin, which cleaves fibrinogen to fibrin. Factors in squares are inhibited by warfarin. Factors in circles are inhibited by heparin.

Stasis and hypercoagulability are the main causes of venous thrombosis

In contrast, in venous thrombosis the vessel wall is frequently intact. Stasis plays a more dominant role and permits the build-up of platelet aggregates and nascent fibrin in areas of sluggish flow. Hypercoagulability is also an important contributor.

The best-understood and prototypic hypercoagulable states are associated with hereditary deficiencies of the natural anticogulants antithrombin III, protein C, or protein S. The recent discovery of a relatively common hereditary mutation of factor Va, which is much more resistant to inactivation by activated protein C, greatly increases the number of patients with diagnosable hypercoagulable states.

Lifelong anticoagulation Patients with an underlying hypercoagulable abnormality should be treated with lifelong anticoagulation once they have had a thrombotic event. In addition, hypercoagulability may also be an important mechanism for the pathogenesis of a thrombotic diathesis in several more common clinical settings such as nephrotic syndrome, following severe trauma or a burn injury, and in disseminated cancer.

Antiplatelet agents

There are many physiologic activators of platelets including thrombin, adenosine diphosphate (ADP), epinephrine, collagen, arachidonic acid, and thromboxane A_2, which promote platelet aggregation. There are also physiologic platelet inhibitors such as prostacyclin and nitric oxide. Intact undamaged endothelium secretes these inhibitors to prevent platelet activation and aggregation. However, with vessel injury, the damaged endothelium produces less prostacyclin and therefore promotes platelet activation. Furthermore, collagen and locally generated thrombin stimulate platelets to release arachidonic acid from its membrane phospholipids. Arachidonic acid is first converted to prostaglandin H_2 by cyclooxygenase. Prostaglandin H_2 is then metabolized to thromboxane A_2, which further activates surrounding platelets (Fig. 9.15).

Aspirin blocks thromboxane A_2 synthesis from arachidonic acid in platelets by irreversibly acetylating and thereby inhibiting cyclooxygenase, a key enzyme in prostaglandin synthesis. The aspirin-induced inhibition of thromboxane A_2 and the resulting suppression of platelet aggregation last for the approximately 7–10-day life span of the platelet. Aspirin also blocks the synthesis of the platelet inhibitor prostacyclin in endothelial cells. However, this effect is short-lived compared with that on thromboxane A_2 synthesis in platelets because endothelial cells can re-synthesize cyclooxygenase. Aspirin's physiologic effect on platelet aggregation is demonstrated by prolonged bleeding times in patients taking aspirin.

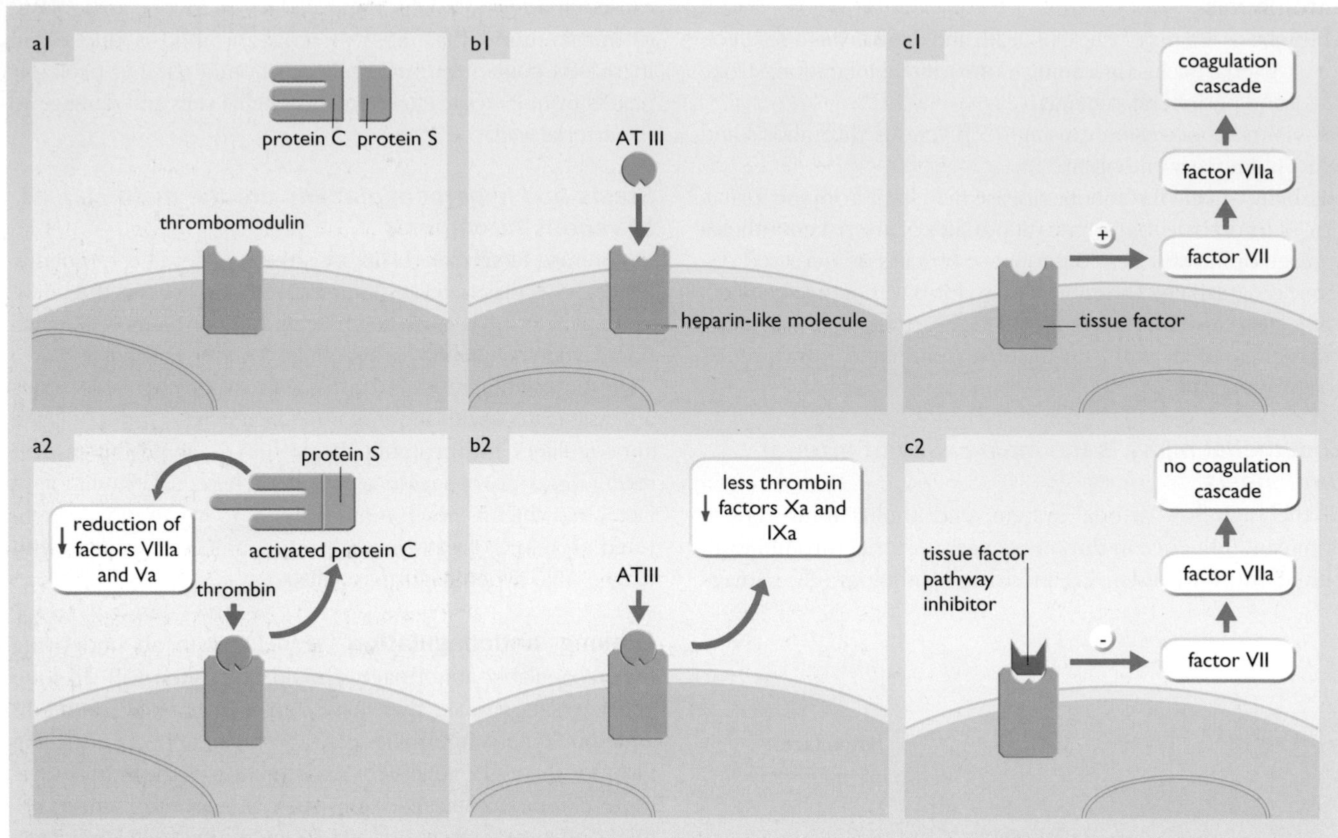

Fig. 9.13 Natural anticoagulants. Three physiologic anticoagulation systems exist. (a1 and a2) Thrombomodulin stimulated by thrombin activates protein C, which with its cofactor protein S, inhibits cofactors Va and VIIIa in the coagulation cascade. (b1 and b2) Antithrombin III (ATIII) stimulated by heparin inhibits thrombin, factor Xa and IXa. (c1 and c2) Tissue factor pathway inhibitor inhibits tissue factor, which is the key activator of the coagulation cascade.

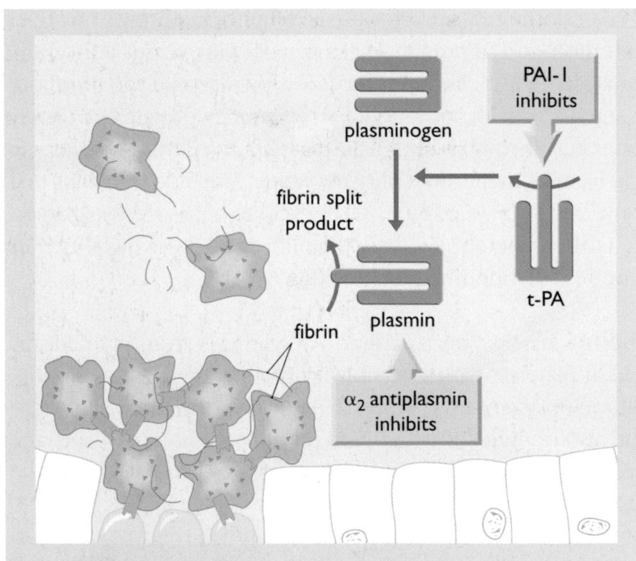

Fig. 9.14 The fibrinolytic system. Fibrin-bound tissue plasminogen activator (t-PA) changes fibrin-bound plasminogen to plasmin, which cleaves fibrin. Physiologic inhibitors are plasminogen activator inhibitor (PAI-1) and α_2 antiplasmin.

Aspirin is rapidly absorbed from the gastrointestinal tract, is partially hydrolyzed to salicylate on its first pass through the liver, and is widely distributed into most body tissues. Following oral administration, salicylate can be present in the serum within 5–30 minutes and peak serum concentrations are attained within 1 hour. Hemostasis returns to normal approximately 36 hours after the last dose of the drug.

Gastrointestinal irritation is the most common adverse effect. Tinnitus and central nervous system toxicity are uncommon with the low dosages used to achieve antithrombotic effects (see Chapters 17, 20, and 22).

Clinical trials have shown that low-dose (80 mg/day) aspirin is effective in the secondary prevention of myocardial infarction and reducing mortality in post-myocardial infarction patients. Aspirin is also effective in preventing recurring transient ischemic attacks (TIAs). It is also commonly used in settings where there is an increased risk of arterial thrombosis such as coronary catherization, balloon angioplasty, and the post-operative period following vascular surgery. Aspirin is often used in conjunction with other anticoagulants, heparin, or warfarin.

Ticlopidine interferes with the ADP-induced binding of fibrinogen to the platelet membrane receptors. Platelet adhesion and aggregation are therefore inhibited, and the inhibitory effects on platelet aggregation are irreversible.

Ticlopidine is rapidly and well-absorbed through the gastrointestinal tract. Peak plasma concentrations are achieved within approximately 2 hours, but the inhibitory effect on platelets is not attained until after approximately 4 days of regular dosing. Steady-state concentrations are achieved in 14–21 days. Ticlopidine is extensively metabolized and is excreted mainly through the kidney. Renal impairment significantly increases the plasma concentrations.

Ticlopidine is indicated to prevent a recurrence of thrombotic stroke. In clinical trials it has been shown to be more efficacious than aspirin. However, serious adverse effects such as neutropenia and agranulocytosis have limited its use to patients who are intolerant or unresponsive to aspirin.

Dipyridamole was approved by the FDA as an antiplatelet agent in 1986. However, it will not inhibit platelet aggregation when used alone but, in conjunction with warfarin therapy, it has been shown to prolong the survival of platelets in patients with valvular heart disease and to maintain platelet counts in patients undergoing open heart surgery.

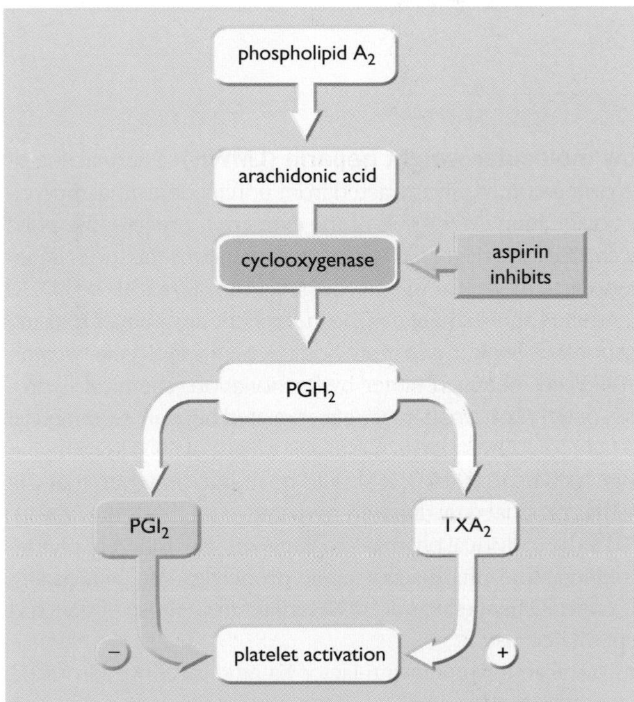

Fig. 9.15 Effects of antiplatelet agents on platelet activation. Thromboxane A_2 (TXA_2) activates and prostacyclin (PGI_2) inhibits platelet activation. Aspirin's effect on the production of PGI_2 in endothelial cells is relatively short-lived compared with its effect on TXA_2 production. (PGH_2, prostaglandin H_2)

Novel antiplatelet agents Many promising novel antiplatelet agents (Fig. 9.16) are currently undergoing clinical trials to determine their role in the management of thrombotic diseases.

Anagrelide High platelet counts due to myeloproliferative diseases such as essential thrombocythemia, unlike the relatively benign reactive thrombocythemia, may have thrombotic consequences. Conventional treatment of these disorders has been with lineage-nonspecific chemotherapeutic agents such as hydroxyurea. Anagrelide, an orally active quinazolin, has a high specificity against megakaryocytes and therefore selectively lowers the platelet count. If long-term trials confirm that anagrelide does not have a leukemogenic potential, this agent may become the treatment of choice for thrombocythemia.

Anticoagulants

Heparin is a glycosaminoglycan composed of chains of alternating residues of D-glucosamine and a uronic acid. Standard heparin is a heterogeneous preparation with molecular weights ranging from 5000 to 30,000 kD. As a result, the anticoagulant activity is variable because the chain lengths of the molecules affect the activity and clearance. The higher molecular weight molecules are cleared from the circulation more rapidly than the lower molecular weight species. Furthermore, there is differential activity, with lower molecular weight species being more active against factor Xa than against thrombin.

Heparin primarily exerts its anticoagulant effect through binding to ATIII, thereby greatly altering the conformation of ATIII and accelerating its inhibition of thrombin, factor Xa, and factor IXa. ATIII is an α-globulin that inhibits serine proteases, including several of the clotting factors, by binding in a 1:1 ratio to the serine residue in the reaction center of coagulant factors, leading to the inactivation of these factors. Heparin participates in these reactions as a catalytic agent, catalyzing the inactivation of thrombin by ATIII by acting as a template to which both ATIII and thrombin bind to form a ternary complex. In contrast, ATIII inactivation of factor Xa does not require the formation of a ternary complex. Low molecular weight species of heparin that contain fewer than 18 polysaccharide chains are unable to serve

Novel antiplatelet agents

Drug	Mechanism
C7E3	Monoclonal antibody against GPIIb–IIIa (fibrinogen receptor)
SC-5486A	Synthetic GPIIb-IIIa antagonist
Indobufen	Reversible cyclooxygenase inhibitor
Ridogrel	Thromboxane A_2 synthase and receptor antagonist

Fig. 9.16 Novel antiplatelet agents.

as a template for ATIII inactivation of thrombin, but retain the ability to inactivate factor Xa (Fig. 9.17).

Heparin is poorly absorbed after oral administration and must therefore be given either subcutaneously or intravenously. It is often given intravenously in a bolus loading dose to achieve rapid anticoagulation and then maintained with a continuous infusion. Alternatively, subcutaneous boluses two or three times a day are equally effective. If immediate anticoagulation is needed, however, the intravenous route is preferred because there is a 1–2-hour delay with subcutaneous heparin. Treatment with heparin requires close laboratory monitoring. Heparin dosages need to be titrated to achieve an activated partial thromboplastin time (aPTT) that is 1.5–2.5 times the normal control.

Heparin binds to a variety of plasma proteins such as platelet factor 4, fibronectin, and von Willebrand factor. This property contributes to its reduced bioavailability at low concentrations.

The pharmacokinetic properties of heparin are complex. It binds to receptors on macrophages and endothelial cells, where it is rapidly internalized and degraded. However, this is a dose-dependent saturable mechanism. Heparin is also cleared more slowly with first-order kinetics, mostly through the kidney. As a result, the biologic half-life of heparin depends on the dose. With an intravenous bolus of heparin at 25 units/kg, the biologic half-life is 30 minutes, but this increases to 60 minutes with 100 units/kg and 150 minutes at 400 units/kg.

Heparin is effective for:

- Preventing venous thrombosis.
- Treating deep venous thromboembolism.
- The early treatment of patients with unstable angina and acute myocardial infarction.
- Preventing clotting in catheters used to cannulate blood vessels.
- Anticoagulating extracorporeal devices, as in cardiac bypass surgery and hemodialysis.
- Treating arterial thrombosis, as in acute myocardial infarction, in conjunction with antiplatelet and thrombolytic agents.

The pharmacotherapeutic range of heparin is relatively narrow and bleeding is the major complication. Not surprisingly, bleeding occurs much more frequently when heparin is given in large doses pharmacotherapeutically than when it is used in small doses prophylactically. A less common but serious complication is heparin induced thrombocytopenia. The platelet counts of patients receiving heparin should therefore be monitored, and heparin therapy should be stopped if heparin-induced thrombocytopenia is suspected. Paradoxically, thrombocytopenia due to heparin can be a highly prothrombotic disorder. Long-term heparin therapy (usually longer than 3 months) is also associated with osteoporosis.

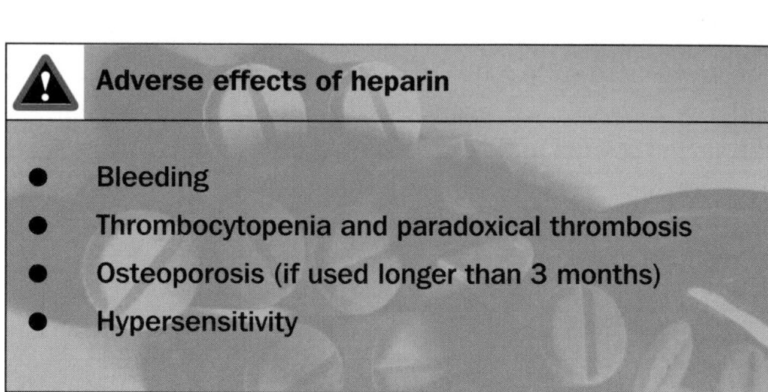

Adverse effects of heparin

- **Bleeding**
- **Thrombocytopenia and paradoxical thrombosis**
- **Osteoporosis (if used longer than 3 months)**
- **Hypersensitivity**

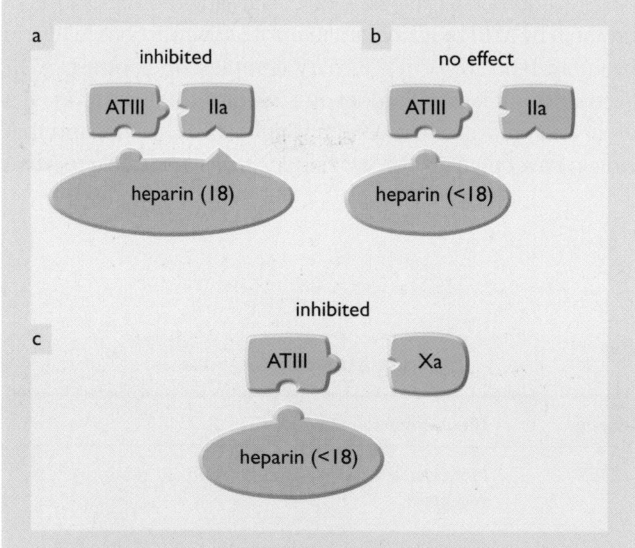

Fig. 9.17 Anticoagulation mechanism of heparin. Binding of heparin with antithrombin III (ATIII) greatly facilitates its inhibition of thrombin (IIa) (a). However, this requires heparin molecules longer than 18 polysaccharide residues (b). Inhibition of factor Xa is not dependent on the size of the heparin molecule (c).

Low molecular weight heparin (LMWH) Pharmaceutical heparin is commonly extracted from porcine intestinal mucosa or bovine lung. As a result of the extraction process, the polysaccharides are degraded into a heterogeneous mixture of fragments with molecular weights ranging from 300 to 30,000 kD. As mentioned above, there may be therapeutic advantages to using fractionated heparin of a more homogeneous molecular weight. LMWHs are obtained either by fractionation, chemical hydrolysis, or depolymerization of unfractionated heparin. Commercial preparations have a mean molecular weight of 5000 kD, ranging from 1000 to 10,000 kD. It should be noted, however, that the LWMHs produced by different preparative methods are considered to be individual pharmacologic agents with different pharmacokinetic and pharmacodynamic properties. Mechanistically, the anticoagulant effects of LMWHs differ from those of standard heparin because:

- The antithrombin/anti-factor Xa ratio is reduced from 1:1 to 1:4.
- The pharmacokinetic properties are improved owing to reduced protein binding.
- There is reduced interaction with platelets.

LMWHs have a number of advantages over heparin. Maximum plasma levels after subcutaneous injections of LMWHs are reached within 2–3 hours. In comparison, the half-life of LMWHs is about 4 hours (i.e. twice as long as the half-life of standard heparin). In addition, the bioavailability of LMWHs is about 90%, whereas that of standard heparin is only in the range of 20%. LMWHs have a more predictable anticoagulant response based on a weight-adjusted dose, which means that they can be given subcutaneously once or twice a day without laboratory monitoring. Clinical trials have shown that LMWHs are as effective as standard heparin in the prevention and treatment of venous thrombosis and may be associated with fewer bleeding complications.

Hirudin and hirulog While multiple other factors may contribute to the pathogenesis of thrombotic disorders, thrombin plays a central role. Hirudin, a 65 amino acid (7 kD) protein originally purified from the salivary glands of the leech, *Hirudo medicinalis*, is now available as a recombinant protein. Hirudin and hirulog, a synthetic analog, are both potent direct inhibitors of thrombin and have shown promise as novel antithrombotic agents. Unlike heparin, which needs ATIII to inhibit thrombin, hirudin and hirulog directly inhibit thrombin independent of ATIII. Theoretically, these direct thrombin inhibitors should be safer than heparin because they selectively inhibit thrombin and do not affect platelet function. Furthermore, these agents are not associated with thrombocytopenia. Clinical trials are in progress to determine whether hirudin and hirulog have a role in the management of thrombotic diseases.

Warfarin, a vitamin K antagonist, is widely used clinically as an oral anticoagulant. The synthesis of several coagulation factors (factors II, VII, IX, and X) in the liver is dependent on vitamin K, the post-translational carboxylation of the glutamic acid residues of these coagulation factors to γ-carboxyglutamic acid requiring vitamin K as a cofactor in the enzymatic reaction. In the presence of calcium ions, the γ-carboxyglutamyl residues allow the coagulation factors to undergo a conformational change, which is necessary for their biologic activity. Warfarin inhibits vitamin K epoxide reductase, leading to depletion of reduced vitamin K (KH) and decreased γ-carboxylation (Fig. 9.18), and thereby indirectly impairs the function of coagulation factors.

Warfarin does not directly inhibit vitamin K-dependent coagulation factors, and the anticoagulant effects of warfarin result from disappearance of γ-carboxylated coagulation factors. Prothrombin has the longest elimination half-life of 60 hours; therefore 5 days of treatment are required if warfarin is to be fully antithrombotic. This is the rationale for overlapping heparin therapy with warfarin therapy for at least 5 days in the treatment of thrombotic diseases, even if the INR (international normalized ratio of prothrombin times) reaches the therapeutic level before 5 days.

The anticoagulant effects of warfarin can be partially reversed by low doses of vitamin K acting through a warfarin-resistant pathway. Patients also become warfarin resistant if large doses of vitamin K are given. Fresh frozen plasma or prothrombin complex concentrate can be infused if a rapid reversal of the warfarin effect is needed, as in bleeding.

Warfarin is indicated in many clinical settings. Clinical trials have shown that warfarin is effective for:

- The prevention and treatment of venous thromboembolism.
- The prevention of thrombotic and embolic strokes and of recurrence of infarction in patients with acute myocardial infarction.

Patients with mechanical prosthetic heart valves should be anticoagulated. A combined regimen of warfarin and low-dose aspirin seems to be superior to warfarin alone. There are now convincing data that most patients with atrial fibrillation should be on lifelong anticoagulation with warfarin (Fig. 9.19).

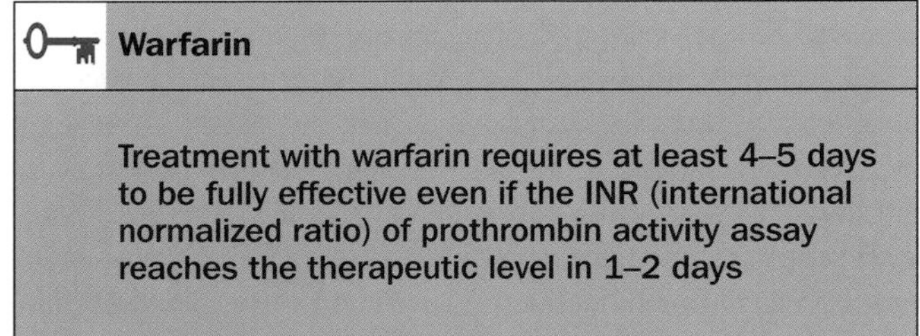

Warfarin

Treatment with warfarin requires at least 4–5 days to be fully effective even if the INR (international normalized ratio) of prothrombin activity assay reaches the therapeutic level in 1–2 days

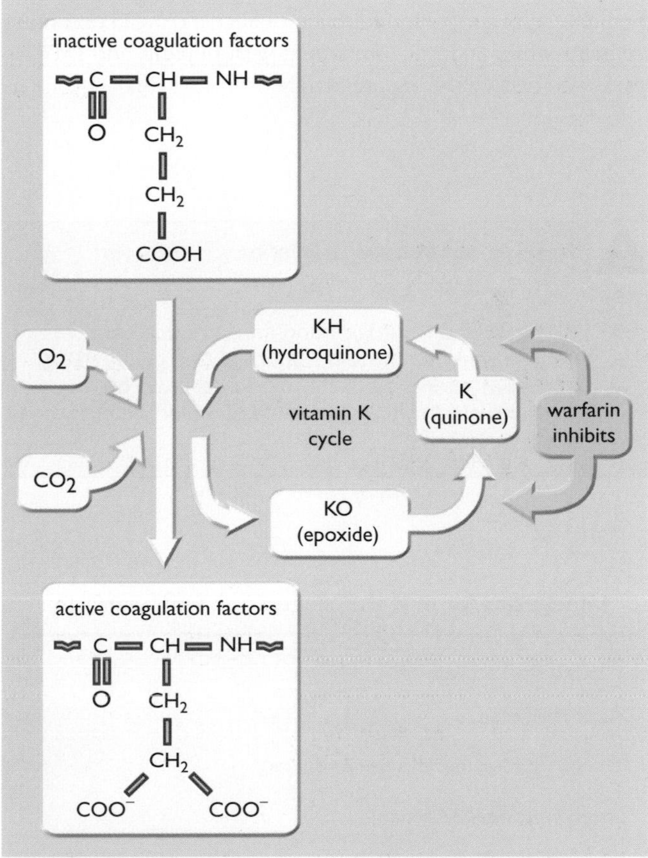

Fig. 9.18 Vitamin K-dependent synthesis of coagulation factors. Warfarin inhibits production of the reduced form of vitamin K (KH), which is required for γ-carboxylation of glutamic acids on factors II, IX, and X, protein C, and protein S.

Warfarin is well absorbed orally and has excellent bioavailability. It is highly bound to plasma proteins and accumulates in the liver.

Many clinical conditions and drug interactions may potentiate or attenuate the anticoagulant effects of warfarin (Fig. 9.20). Fluctuating levels of dietary vitamin K can be an important factor in causing variations in anticoagulation in patients on long-term warfarin therapy.

The major adverse effect of warfarin is bleeding, and this risk is correlated with the intensity of treatment and the concomitant use of antiplatelet agents such as aspirin. The risk of clinically important bleeding is reduced by lowering the INR therapeutic range from 3.0–4.5 to 2.0–3.0.

The most important nonhemorrhagic adverse effect of warfarin therapy is skin necrosis caused by extensive thrombosis of the microvasculature within the subcutaneous fat. This phenomenon seems to be associated with protein C and S deficiency. (Proteins C and S are vitamin K-dependent anticoagulants as discussed on p. 205.) The thrombotic tendency may be due to a transient procoagulant state during the initial treatment period with warfarin. Proteins C and S have much shorter elimination half-lives than prothrombin. The fall in protein C and S levels, therefore, occurs before there is a reduction in the prothrombin level. Skin necrosis can be avoided by using concurrent therapeutic doses of heparin when starting warfarin therapy.

Warfarin crosses the placenta and is teratogenic, so it must not be given to pregnant women. Women receiving warfarin should be informed of its teratogenic effect and avoid becoming pregnant while taking it. Treatment with heparin and LMWHs appears to be safe during pregnancy.

Thrombolytic agents

The use of thrombolytic agents to dissolve pathologic thrombi has become a standard therapy in acute myocardial infarction. Thrombolytics also appear to be beneficial in the initial treatment of acute peripheral vascular occlusion, deep venous thrombosis, and massive pulmonary embolism. Clinical trials are in progress to determine the role of these agents in the treatment of acute thrombo-embolic strokes.

Currently, four thrombolytic agents are commercially available for clinical use (Fig. 9.21). Their thrombolytic activity is based on the ability to enhance the generation of plasmin from its precursor plasminogen.

- Streptokinase (SK) is derived from group A β-hemolytic streptococci and is therefore highly antigenic. It has no intrinsic enzymatic activity. Following intravenous infusion, it combines with plasminogen to form a complex that activates plasminogen to plasmin.
- Anisoylated plasminogen–streptokinase activator complex (APSAC) is a modified SK that is pre-bound to a plasminogen molecule. However, it is also without enzymatic activity until its active site is deacylated following administration. It has a fourfold longer half-life than SK and can therefore be given as an intravenous bolus. Like SK, it is also highly antigenic.
- Urokinase (UK) is purified from human kidney cells and recombinant tissue plasminogen activator (rt-PA) is produced by recombinant techniques. Both UK and rt-PA are enzymes that convert plasminogen to plasmin by cleaving the arginine–valine bond in plasminogen. They do not

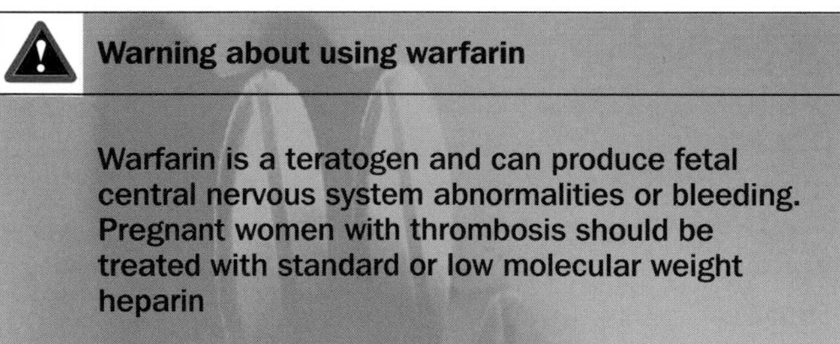
Warning about using warfarin

Warfarin is a teratogen and can produce fetal central nervous system abnormalities or bleeding. Pregnant women with thrombosis should be treated with standard or low molecular weight heparin

Indications for oral anticoagulation with warfarin

Indications
Mechanical prosthetic heart valves
Atrial fibrillation
Treatment of venous thromboembolism
Acute myocardial infarction
Prevention of venous thromboembolism
Episodic systemic embolism

Fig. 9.19 Indications for oral anticoagulation with warfarin.

Drugs and conditions interacting with warfarin

	Activity
Antibiotics	+
Amiodarone	+
Cimetidine	+
Clofibrate	+
Fluconazole	+
Metronidazole	+
Phenytoin	+
Barbiturates	–
Carbamazepine	–
Griseofulvin	–
Nafcillin	–
Rifampin	–
Sucralfate	–
Age	+
Biliary disease	+
Congestive heart failure	+
Hyperthyroidism	+
Hypothyroidism	–
Nephrotic syndrome	–

Fig. 9.20 Drugs and conditions interacting with warfarin. (+, increased activity; –, decreased activity)

Pharmacologic properties of thrombolytics				
	Streptokinase	**Urokinase**	**rt-PA**	**APSAC**
Source	Streptococcal culture	Mammalian tissue culture	Mammalian tissue culture	Streptococcal culture
Molecular weight (kD)	47	32–54	70	131
Half-life (min)	12–18	15–20	2–6	40–60
Systemic fibrinolytic activation	Yes	Yes	Yes	Yes
Fibrin specificity	1+	2+	3+	1+
Antigenic	Yes	No	No	Yes

Fig. 9.21 Pharmacologic properties of thrombolytics. (APSAC, anisoylated plasminogen–streptokinase activator complex; rt-PA, recombinant tissue plasminogen activator)

induce an antigenic response. Unlike UK or SK, the enzymatic activity of rt-PA depends on the presence of fibrin and theoretically should cause less systemic fibrinolytic activation. In therapeutic use, at doses sufficient to be clinically effective, rt-PA also induces a systemic lytic state and an increased bleeding tendency.

BLEEDING DISORDERS

Therapeutic approaches to hemorrhagic disorders are formulated after determining whether the problem is acquired or hereditary (Fig. 9.22).

- Von Willebrand's disease (vWD) is the most common inherited coagulopathy. Patients typically present with abnormal bruising and mucosal bleeding such as epistaxis and melena. In contrast, soft tissue bleeding and spontaneous hemarthroses are more characteristic of hemophilias (factor VIII or IX deficiency).
- Acquired bleeding disorders include secondary deficiencies of coagulant factors such as a deficiency of vitamin K, which can be treated by replacement of vitamin K, increased fibrinolysis in DIC, and platelet disorders.

Bleeding disorders
Hereditary
Hemophilia A (factor VIII deficiency)
Hemophilia B (factor IX deficiency)
Von Willebrand's disease
Platelet disorders (e.g. Glanzmann's thrombasthenia)
Acquired
Vitamin K deficiency
Liver disease
Disseminated intravascular coagulation
Thrombocytopenia (immune, infection, splenic sequestration)
Platelet disorder (uremia)

Fig. 9.22 Bleeding disorders.

Coagulation factor concentrates

Factor VIII concentrates with varying degrees of purity are commercially available for prophylactic and therapeutic use in patients with hemophilia A. In the past, transmission of viral infections, including human immunodeficiency virus (HIV), has been the major cause of morbidity and mortality in these patients. Since 1985, all factor VIII concentrates have been treated with effective virus attenuation procedures, and the risk of HIV and hepatitis C transmission has essentially been eliminated. Recombinant factor VIII generated from genetically engineered mammalian cells is also now available (Fig. 9.23). The introduction of highly purified factor IX concentrate treated with viral attenuation procedures since 1991 has greatly improved the treatment of hemophilia B patients.

Factor VIII concentrates	
Product name	**Purity**
Recombinate	Recombinant
Monoclate-P	High
Koate-HP Humate-P	Intermediate Intermediate
Hyate-C	Porcine

Fig. 9.23 Factor VIII concentrates.

The development of alloantibodies that inhibit factor VIII or factor IX can be a severe problem in the treatment of hemophilias with factor concentrates. Patients with high levels of factor VIII inhibitor can be treated with porcine factor VIII if the antibodies do not strongly cross react with the porcine protein. Other options include using factor IX complex concentrates or recombinant factor VIIa concentrates.

Desmopressin

An infusion of desmopressin, 1-deamino-(8-D-arginine)-vasopressin (DDAVP), a synthetic analog of vasopressin, causes the release of von Willebrand factor (vWF) and factor VIII from body storage sites such as endothelial cells. DDAVP is used in patients with mild factor VIII deficiency (>5%) prophylactically before minor surgical procedures. DDAVP cannot be used in patients with severe hemophilia A because they do not have any stored factor VIII.

DDAVP is also indicated for the prevention and treatment of bleeding in patients with vWD. vWF is needed to mediate the formation of the platelet plug and also for factor VIII activity by forming a factor VIII–vWF complex. Patients with vWD subtypes that are quantitatively deficient in vWF may respond to DDAVP treatment. Patients with qualitatively defective vWF or a severe deficiency of vWF should be transfused with intermediate-purity factor VIII concentrates which contain functional vWF. Recombinant factor VIII is not an appropriate treatment for these patients.

Vitamin K

Vitamin K is used to reverse anticoagulation and bleeding caused by the vitamin K antagonist warfarin. Vitamin K deficiency may also occur in patients with biliary obstruction and liver diseases, and after prolonged treatment with oral antibiotics, owing to suppression of the intestinal bacteria that synthesize vitamin K.

Natural vitamin K derived from green leafy vegetables is vitamin K_1 (phytomenadione). Vitamin K_2 (menaquinone) is synthesized by intestinal bacteria. Vitamin K_1 and K_2 are fat-soluble vitamins and therefore bile salts are required for their gastrointestinal absorption. Synthesized vitamin K_3 (menadione sodium bisulfite) is water soluble and can therefore be injected. The body converts vitamin K_4 to an active form, vitamin K_4 (menadione diacetate) (Fig. 9.24).

A major therapeutic application of vitamin K is to prevent hypoprothrombinemia in the newborn. Vitamin K levels in the newborn are quite marginal and may be exacerbated by inadequate nutritional intake in the first few days of life. The

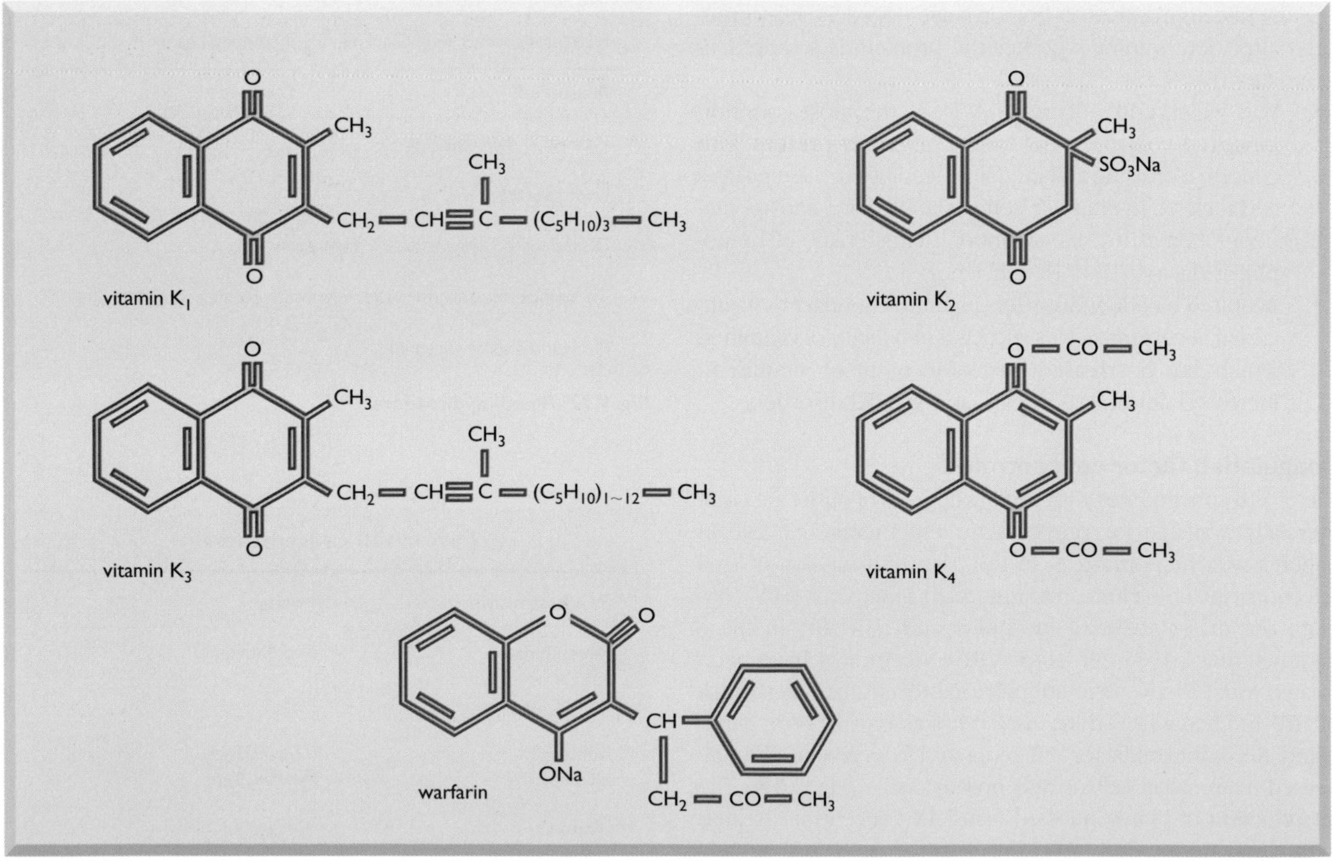

Fig. 9.24 Chemical structures of vitamin K and the antagonist warfarin.

concentration of factors II, VII, IX, and X in newborn infants is approximately 20 to 50% of adult plasma levels; premature infants have even lower concentrations. Trace amounts of vitamin K will prevent hypoprothrombinemia by attenuating the decline in concentrations of vitamin K-dependent coagulation factors although this treatment will not raise concentrations of these coagulation factors to adult levels. Prophylactic administration of small doses of vitamin K to the newborn infant is routinely recommended and considered safe. Excessive dosages can provoke hemolytic anemia, hyperbilirubinemia, and kernicterus in the newborn infant. Premature infants and newborn infants with a congenital deficiency in erythrocyte glucose-6-phosphate dehydrogenase are particularly sensitive to administration of vitamin K. There are several synthetic analogues of vitamin K, including phytonadione (mephyton), menadione, and menadiol. Phytonadione is the drug of choice for prophylactic treatment in newborn infants since it can be safely administered by oral or parenteral ways. Although menadione and menadiol do not require the presence of bile for gastrointestinal absorption, they can provoke toxic effects in the newborn and are contraindicated in newborn infants and during later pregnancy. An alternative way to give prophylatic phytonadione to newborn infants is to administer it to mothers prior to delivery.

Vitamin K is an essential cofactor for the liver synthesis of prothrombin, as well as of factors II, VII, IX, and X. These coagulation factors are synthesized in the liver in a process that requires an adequate dietary intake of vitamin K. Lack of vitamin K or the presence of competitive inhibitors such as warfarin causes the production of non γ-carboxylated prothrombin, which is activated by factor Xa at only 1–2% of the normal level, as discussed on p. 209.

ε Aminocaproic acid

ε Aminocaproic acid (EACA) acts as a hemostatic agent by inhibiting the fibrinolytic system. It interferes with lysine-binding sites on plasminogen, blocking plasminogen association with fibrin, and thereby inhibiting the activation of plasminogen to plasmin. The elimination half-life of EACA is approximately 2 hours. It is available in both oral and parenteral formulations, and has been used in the treatment of many bleeding conditions, but most commonly urinary tract bleeding.

Antifibrinolytic agents may exacerbate the thrombotic component of DIC and should be avoided in this condition.

FURTHER READING

Dalen JE, Hirsh J (eds) Fourth ACCP consensus conference on antithrombotic therapy. *Chest* 1995; **108** (supplement): 225S–522S. [An excellent collection of up-to-date reviews on antithrombotic agents.]

Wallerstein RO. Laboratory evaluation of a bleeding patient. *West J Med* 1989; **150**: 51–58. [A classic review on the evaluation of bleeding patients.]

Colman RW, Hirsh J, Marder VJ, Salzman EW (eds) *Hemostasis and Thrombosis: Basic Principles and Clinical Practice 3e*. Philadelphia: JB Lippincott; 1992. [An excellent textbook covering all aspects of hemostasis from molecular mechanism to clinical application.]

Handin RI, Lux SE, Stossel TP (eds) *Blood: Principles and Practice of Hematology*. Philadelphia: JB Lippincott; 1995. [A well-written textbook covering all aspects of clinical hematology by authoritative authors.]

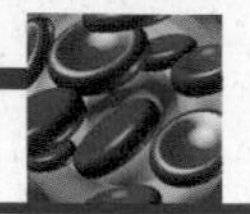

Make a provisional diagnosis and determine a rational pharmacologic treatment for the following hypothetical case.

A 54-year-old man complains of excessive fatigue and unsteadiness when walking. He has a history of alcoholism. The physical examination is essentially normal except that he appears pale and vibratory sense is absent in both lower extremities.

1. Would you reassure the patient and urge him to stop drinking alcohol? Explain your answer.
2. Would you encourage better dietary intake and prescribe vitamin supplementation? Explain your answer.
3. Would you order a complete blood count and start him on an oral folate and vitamin B_{12} supplement right away? Explain your answer.
4. Would you order a complete blood count and serum folate and vitamin B_{12} levels? Explain your answer.

The patient returns the next day and his symptoms and examination remain the same. Laboratory tests show that his hemoglobin concentration is 10 g/dl (6.21 mmol/liter) and mean cell volume is 110 μm^3 (110 fl).

5. Would you call a family meeting to discuss the patient's alcohol problem? Explain your answer.
6. Would you wait for serum vitamin B_{12} levels and if low, start him on oral vitamin B_{12}? Explain your answer.
7. Would you wait for the serum folate level and if low, prescribe 1 mg/day of folate? Explain your answer.
8. Would you start the patient on ferrous sulfate and continue another 6 months after his hemoglobin level has normalized? Explain your answer.

Indicate which is the correct answer for each question.

1. A 73-year-old man with a history of congestive heart failure and thrombotic stroke who has been on ticlopidine is admitted for shortness of breath and atrial fibrillation. Initial laboratory evaluation shows a white blood cell count of 1.0 K (1.0×19^9/liter) and platelet count of 250 K (250×10^9/liter). What is the best treatment option?
- a) continue ticlopidine since it is indicated for the prevention of thrombotic stroke
- b) discontinue ticlopidine and treat with aspirin
- c) discontinue ticlopidine and treat with lifelong heparin
- d) discontinue ticlopidine and treat with warfarin
- e) continue ticlopidine and add warfarin

2. Which of the following is a correct description of vitamin K deficiency?
- a) directly inhibits synthesis of coagulation factors II, VII, IX, and X
- b) commonly due to inadequate dietary intake
- c) may be caused by prolonged antibiotic use
- d) diagnosis is provided by prolongation of prothrombin time alone

3. Which of the following statements is incorrect regarding iron absorption?
- a) absorption of iron in the gastrointestinal tract requires intrinsic factor
- b) ascorbic acid facilitates iron absorption
- c) many foods such as eggs interfere with iron absorption
- d) an acidic environment in the intestine increases iron absorption

4. A 24-year-old woman with von Willebrand's disease has persistent bleeding following a dental procedure. In the emergency room, she has received desmopressin (DDAVP) intravenously, but she continues to bleed. Her hemoglobin level is 8 g/dl (4.96 mmol/liter). Which of the following treatment options is inappropriate?
- a) repeat treatment with DDAVP until the bleeding stops
- b) use a recombinant factor VIII concentrate to minimize risk of viral transmission
- c) use a high purity factor since it is as good as recombinant factor VIII
- d) use an intermediate purity factor VIII concentrate

5. A 54-year-old man is brought to the emergency room with an acute myocardial infarction. Two weeks ago, he was prescribed penicillin to treat a streptococcal sore throat. Which of the following treatment options is inappropriate?
- a) aspirin and streptokinase
- b) aspirin, heparin, and anisoylated plasminogen streptokinase activator complex (APSAC)
- c) aspirin, heparin, and recombinant tissue plasminogen activator (rt-PA)
- d) aspirin and APSAC

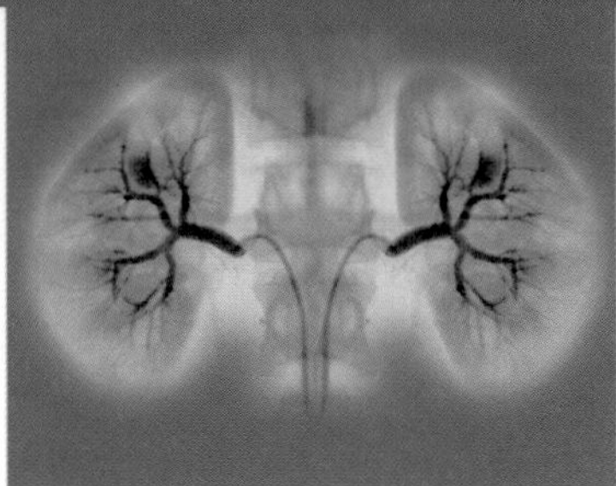

10. Drugs and the Renal System

PHYSIOLOGY OF THE KIDNEY

Functions of the kidney include:

- Excretion of nitrogenous waste products of metabolism such as urea and creatinine in the urine.
- Regulation of the volume of extracellular fluid.
- Regulation of the concentration of various ions in the body.
- Regulation of the pH of body fluids.

The renal system includes the bladder where urine is temporarily stored before final excretion through the urethra (see Chapter 16).

The kidney has two distinct regions: the outer cortex and the inner medulla

Two distinct regions can be identified in the kidney: a dark outer region, the cortex, and a paler inner region, the medulla. The medulla is further divided into a number of conical areas, the renal pyramids (Fig. 10.1).

The basic functional unit of the kidney is the nephron and each kidney contains approximately one million nephrons. The nephron is a blind-ended tube with the blind end forming a capsule, Bowman's capsule, which surrounds a knot of capillaries, the glomerulus. The glomerular capillaries are supplied with blood by the afferent arteriole, while blood leaves the

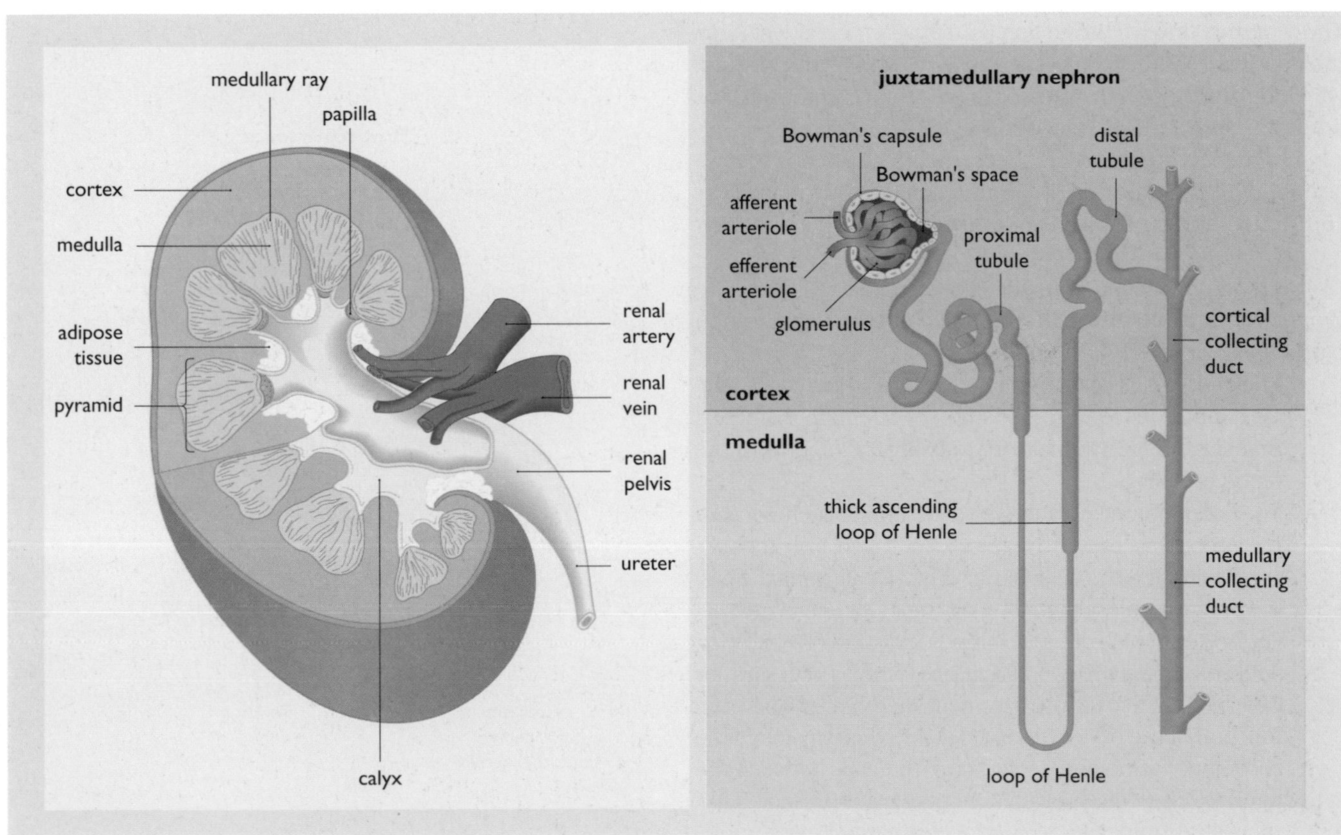

Fig. 10.1 The structure of the kidney. The kidney consists of two regions, the cortex and medulla, with the latter being divided into the renal pyramids. The basic functional unit of the kidney is the nephron, which filters plasma at the glomerulus. The resulting ultrafiltrate is modified by a series of reabsorptive and secretory processes as it passes along the nephron before draining into the renal pelvis.

glomerulus not in a vein but in a second resistance vessel, the efferent arteriole. The other parts of the nephron are the proximal tubule, the loop of Henle, the distal tubule, and the collecting duct (see Fig. 10.1). Many distal tubules join each collecting duct which then merges into larger ducts, which drain into a renal calyx and then into the renal pelvis.

There are two populations of nephron: cortical nephrons and juxtamedullary nephrons

The nephrons form two distinct populations:

- Cortical nephrons have glomeruli in the outer two-thirds of the cortex with short loops of Henle, which either extend a short distance into the medulla or do not reach the medulla. These account for 85% of nephrons. The efferent arteriole of cortical nephrons forms a network of peritubular capillaries that encircles all sections of the nephron.
- Juxtamedullary nephrons (15% of nephrons) have glomeruli in the inner third of the cortex with long loops of Henle, which extend deep into the medulla (Fig. 10.1) and are responsible for generating medullary hypertonicity. The efferent arteriole of juxtamedullary nephrons gives rise to some peritubular capillaries, but also forms a series of vascular loops termed the vasa recta, which descend into the medulla and surround the loop of Henle.

Urine is a modified ultrafiltrate of plasma produced by three filtration barriers

The force that drives ultrafiltration (i.e. filtration dependent upon molecular size) is the glomerular capillary hydrostatic pressure, which depends upon the ratio of the resistance in the afferent arteriole compared with that of the efferent arteriole.

In contrast to other vascular beds, the presence of a second arteriole, the efferent arteriole, ensures that the hydrostatic pressure in glomerular capillaries declines very little along their length.

Ultrafiltration occurs from the glomerular capillaries into Bowman's capsule through the following three filtration barriers:

- The endothelial cells of glomerular capillaries, which contain numerous fenestrations (pores 60 nm in diameter) that act as a filtration barrier to cellular elements of the blood only (Fig.10.2).
- The basement membrane, which lies immediately beneath the endothelial cells and consists of collagen and other glycoproteins. It is the main filtration barrier allowing the passage of molecules depending on their size and charge.
- Podocytes, which are specialized cells of Bowman's capsule with numerous projections (foot processes or pedicels) that cover the basement membrane. The main function of the podocytes is to lay down and maintain the basement membrane. In addition, the gaps between the interlocking pedicels of adjacent podocytes presents a further filtration barrier to negatively charged macromolecules (see Fig.10.2).

Ultrafiltration prevents molecules with a relative molecular mass of 70 kDa from passing into the proximal tubule and so they remain in the glomerular capillaries. In contrast, molecules of less than 7 kDa (such as glucose, amino acids, Na^+ and K^+) are freely filtered and enter the proximal tubule in a similar concentration to that in blood entering the glomerulus. Molecules of 7–70 kDa are retarded by the filter to an extent proportional to their molecular mass. The charge of the molecule may also influence the degree of filtration because the basement membrane and podocytes have a negative charge and this repels anionic macromolecules. This is relevant to the filtration of albumin (69 kDa), which is filtered to a much smaller extent than would be anticipated on the basis of molecular mass alone because it has a net negative charge at physiologic pH.

The ultrafiltrate is modified in the tubules

The ultrafiltrate produced at the glomerulus enters the proximal tubule and is modified by a series of reabsorptive and secretory processes occurring along the length of the nephron (Fig. 10.3). These involve the following transport mechanisms:

- Active transport directly coupled to adenosine triphosphate (ATP) hydrolysis.
- Simple diffusion using transcellular (across cells) or paracellular (across the tight junctions between cells) routes.
- Movement via ion channels.
- Cotransport (symport), which is carrier-mediated transport with substances transported in the same direction.

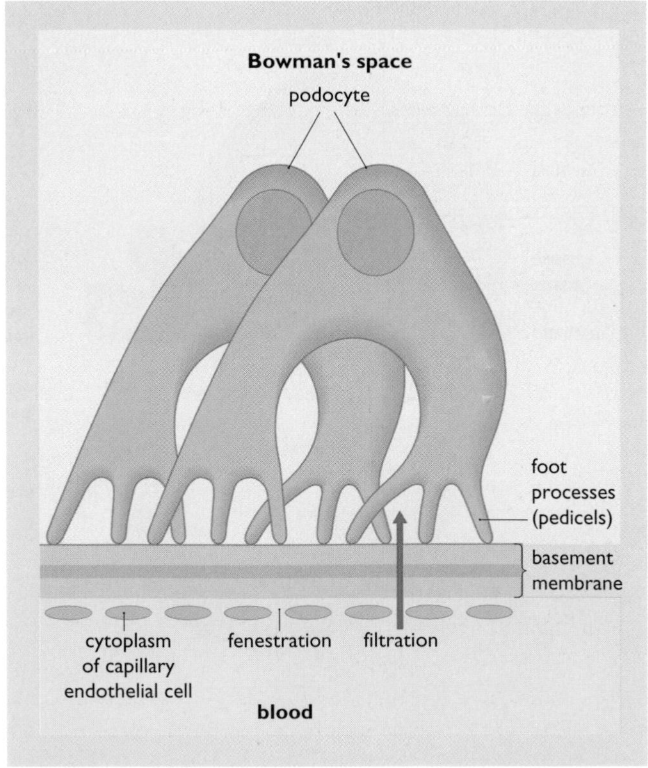

Fig. 10.2 Structure of the glomerular filter. The barriers to ultrafiltration are the capillary endothelium, the basement membrane, and the gaps between the foot processes of the podocytes.

- Countertransport (antiport), which is carrier-mediated transport with substances transported in opposite directions.

Many transport mechanisms are not directly linked to ATP hydrolysis, but indirectly depend on electrochemical gradients established by the active transport of Na^+ and K^+ across the basolateral membrane. These are mediated by Na^+/K^+ ATPase, which moves three Na^+ ions out of the cell while transporting two K^+ ions into the cell (see Chapter 3). The activity of Na^+/K^+ ATPase drives Na^+ reabsorption and cotransport of solutes such as glucose across the luminal membrane. The details of the transport mechanisms of particular sections of the nephron are described in relation to the mechanism of action of different diuretic drugs (see below).

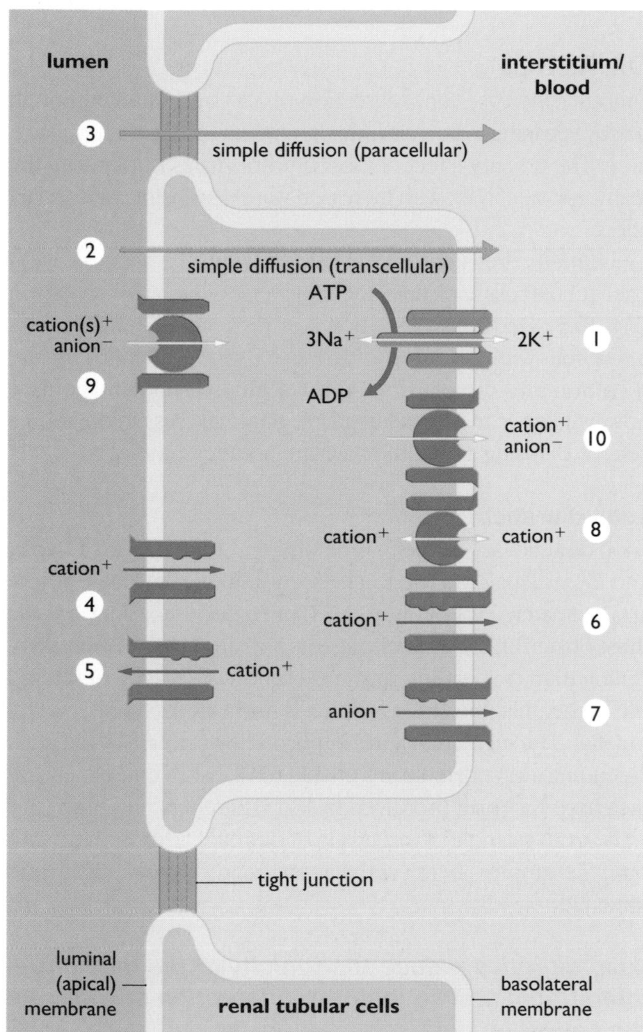

Fig. 10.3 Transport mechanisms in renal tubule cells. Solutes are transported across renal tubular cells by active transport (a process involving hydrolysis of ATP) (1), diffusion (2–3), ion channels (4–7), countertransport (transport of solutes in opposite directions across a membrane) (8) and cotransport (transport of solutes in the same direction across the membrane) (9–10).

PATHOPHYSIOLOGY AND DISEASES OF THE RENAL SYSTEM

EDEMA

Edema is an increase in the volume of interstitial fluid resulting in tissue swelling

Edema results from an imbalance between the rate of interstitial fluid formation and reabsorption. Interstitial fluid formation depends upon capillary hydrostatic pressure and the oncotic pressure (protein osmotic pressure) of interstitial fluid, while reabsorption depends upon the hydrostatic pressure of the interstitial fluid and capillary oncotic pressure (Fig. 10.4).

Edema

- Edema is an increase in the volume of interstitial fluid resulting in tissue swelling
- A decrease in plasma protein concentration and an increase in venous pressure reduce the reabsorption of interstitial fluid back into the capillaries, thereby increasing the volume of interstitial fluid
- Activation of the renin–angiotensin system plays an important role in the development of edema by increasing the blood volume, which in turn increases venous pressure and reduces the concentration of plasma proteins
- Edema develops in patients with the nephrotic syndrome, liver disease, and congestive heart failure

The nephrotic syndrome is the most common kidney disorder producing edema

Edema in the nephrotic syndrome results from increased permeability of the glomerular basement membrane to proteins, particularly albumin. This leads to heavy proteinuria (protein in the urine) and a reduced plasma protein oncotic pressure, which results in edema. In addition, the increase in interstitial fluid volume decreases the effective circulating volume and therefore activates the renin–angiotensin system (see Chapter 8). This activation increases Na^+ and water retention, thereby increasing the blood volume and venous and capillary pressures, which in turn lead to further edema formation. In addition, the nephrotic kidney may avidly retain Na^+ by other mechanisms. An expansion of blood volume also reduces the concentration of plasma proteins and plasma oncotic pressure (see Fig. 10.4).

Most patients with the nephrotic syndrome are children and it is usually attributable to minimal change nephropathy. This is glomerulopathy in which the glomeruli appear normal, but the negative charge on the basement membrane is

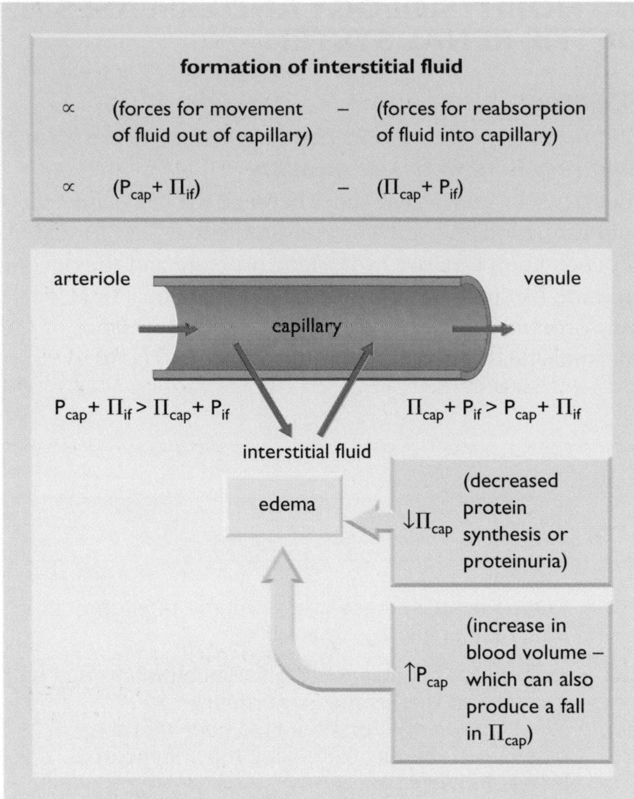

Fig. 10.4 Factors that govern the formation of interstitial fluid. Edema (an increase in the volume of interstitial fluid that results in tissue swelling) occurs as a result of either a fall in capillary oncotic pressure or an increase in capillary hydrostatic pressure. (P_{cap}, capillary hydrostatic pressure; P_{if}, interstitial fluid hydrostatic pressure; Π_{cap}, capillary oncotic pressure; Π_{if}, interstitial fluid oncotic pressure)

diminished. In adults, a multitude of glomerular lesions may cause nephrotic disease.

Treatment of nephrotic syndrome may be symptomatic or involve treating the renal lesion.

There are two modes of therapy for the nephrotic syndrome:

- Symptomatic, which aims to correct the disturbances that originate from the kidney disease and, in particular, to reversing the edematous state with diuretic drugs.
- Treatment of the underlying renal lesion may reverse or delay progression of nephrotic syndrome. Glucocorticosteroids and immunosuppressant drugs, such as cyclophosphamide, are frequently required.

Congestive heart failure and liver disease are other causes of edema

The nephrotic syndrome is an example of a disorder of the kidney that directly results in edema, but edema can also arise indirectly from diseases of other systems.

In congestive heart failure there is a reduction in cardiac output with consequent renal hypoperfusion. This results in activation of the renin–angiotensin system with retention of Na^+ and water by the kidney, and the development of edema due to increased venous and capillary pressure, together with a reduction in plasma protein oncotic pressure as outlined above. A rise in pulmonary venous pressure leads to pulmonary edema, which causes breathlessness, while an increase in central venous pressure causes edema in peripheral tissues such as the legs.

Liver disease may also cause edema, particularly in the peritoneal cavity where it is called ascites. In this situation it results from increased hydrostatic pressure in the hepatic portal vein together with decreased albumin synthesis. Loss of fluid from the capillaries into the peritoneal cavity decreases circulating blood volume, which activates the renin–angiotensin system, leading to increased Na^+ and water absorption in the kidney, which further contribute to the edema.

Diuretics will relieve edema

Edema can be relieved by appropriate use of diuretic drugs, which promote the loss of fluid without appreciably reducing the plasma volume. However, excessive use of diuretics can decrease the effective circulating volume and reduce organ perfusion.

DIURETICS

Diuretics increase renal excretion of Na^+ and water, although strictly speaking a diuresis only signifies an increase in urine volume. The primary effect of most diuretic drugs is to reduce the reabsorption of Na^+, with increased water loss being a secondary effect.

All diuretic drugs other than osmotic diuretics act directly on renal tubule cells at distinct anatomic regions within the nephron (Fig. 10.5). Generally this action is at sites on the luminal membrane following filtration of the drug at the glomerulus and secretion into the proximal tubule. Aldosterone antagonists, however, act at an intracellular site, gaining access to the tubule cells by diffusing across the basolateral membrane.

Loop diuretics

Loop diuretics act, as their name suggests, on the loop of Henle, and in particular, on the thick ascending loop of Henle where approximately 25% of filtered Na^+ is reabsorbed. They are the most powerful of all diuretic agents and are referred to as high-ceiling diuretics leading to the excretion of 15–25% of filtered Na^+ rather than the 1% or less that is normally excreted on a typical diet. The segments of the nephron downstream of the thick ascending loop of Henle are unable to reabsorb completely the increased Na^+ load produced by loop diuretics.

The main example of this group of diuretics is furosemide with other examples being ethacrynic acid, bumetanide, and torsemide.

Loop diuretics reduce the tonicity of the medullary interstitium and so inhibit reabsorption of water in the collecting duct

The loop diuretics molecular mechanism of action is an inhibitory action on the $Na^+/K^+/2Cl^-$ cotransporter in the luminal membrane of the thick ascending loop of Henle (see Fig. 10.6). This portion of the nephron is impermeable to water and provides the kidney with the ability to concentrate urine by producing a hypertonic medullary interstitium (the high osmotic pressure in the medulla is responsible for water reabsorption from the collecting tubules in the presence of vasopressin). Loop diuretics reduce the tonicity of the medullary interstitium and therefore inhibit reabsorption of water in the collecting duct. This results in a profuse diuresis.

The reabsorption of Ca^{2+} and Mg^{2+} is also inhibited by loop diuretics since absorption of these ions is driven by a luminal positive potential produced by recycling of K^+ across the luminal membrane (see Fig. 10.6).

Loop diuretics increase the delivery of Na^+ to the collecting duct, which increases K^+ and H^+ secretion, leading to a hypokalemic alkalosis (see below).

Loop diuretics also have an indirect venodilator action and increase renal blood flow

In addition to their diuretic properties, loop diuretics have an indirect venodilator action as a result of the release of a renal factor (most probably prostaglandins). This action leads to a fall in left ventricular filling pressure and helps relieve pulmonary edema before the onset of the diuretic effect.

Loop diuretics also increase renal blood flow by a mechanism also thought to involve the production of prostaglandins.

The clinical indications for loop diuretics include:

- Acute pulmonary edema for which they are administered intravenously to ensure a rapid onset of action (this is a major use).
- Other edematous states such as the nephrotic syndrome, ascites of liver cirrhosis, and chronic renal failure.
- Hypertension in patients who have not responded to other diuretics or antihypertensive drugs, usually in the presence of renal insufficiency.
- Acute renal failure, when they are given to increase urine production (see below).

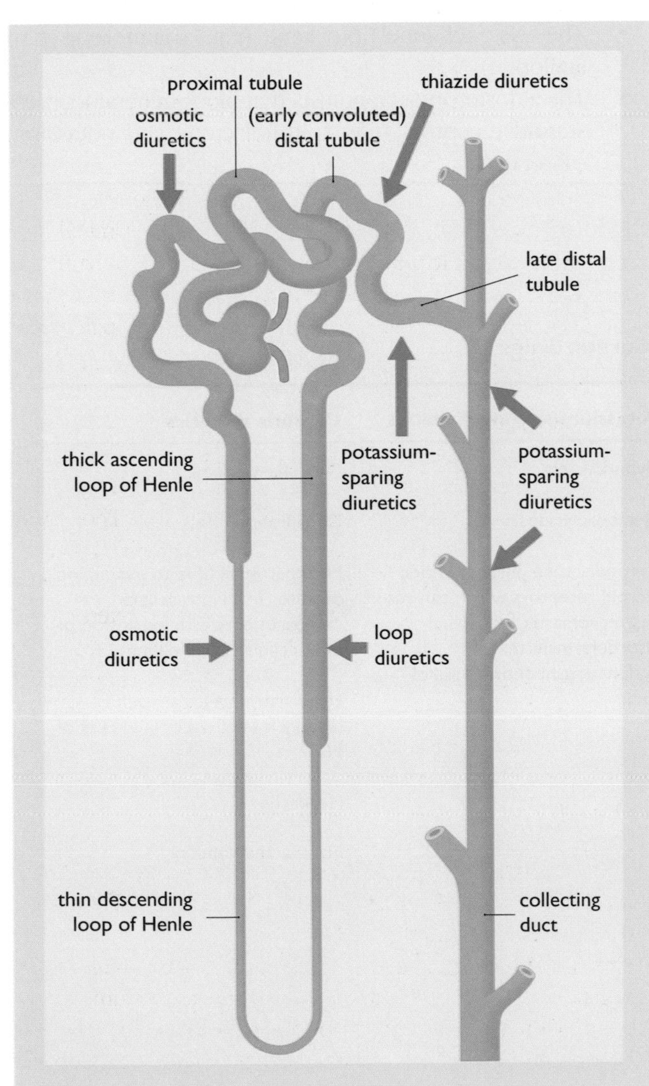

Fig. 10.5 Sites of action of diuretic drugs.

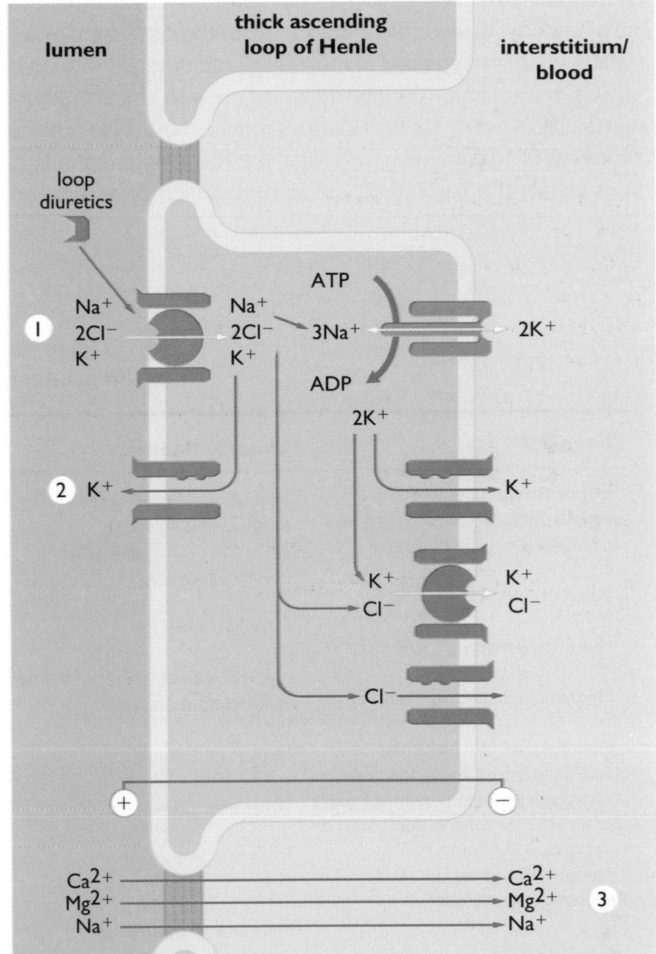

Fig. 10.6 Transport mechanism in the thick ascending loop of Henle. Loop diuretics block the $Na^+/K^+/2Cl^-$ cotransporter (1) thereby increasing the excretion of Na^+ and Cl^-. These drugs also decrease the potential difference across the tubule cell, which arises from the recycling of K^+ (2), and this leads to increased excretion of Ca^{2+} and Mg^{2+} by inhibiting paracellular diffusion (3).

The main adverse effects and principal drug interactions that occur with the use of loop diuretics are listed in Figs 10.7 and 10.8.

Thiazide diuretics

Thiazide diuretics inhibit the Na^+/Cl^- cotransporter in the distal tubule

The molecular mechanism of action of thiazide diuretics is inhibition of the Na^+/Cl^- symporter in the distal convoluted tubule (Fig.10.9). In comparison to loop diuretics, thiazides produce a moderate diuresis excreting a maximum of 5% of filtered Na^+ since 90% of filtered sodium is reabsorbed before reaching the distal tubule. Examples of thiazide diuretics include bendroflumethiazide, chlorothiazide, hydrochlorothiazide, indapamide and metolazone.

Thiazide diuretics increase K^+ and H^+ secretion into the collecting duct, but decrease Ca^{2+} excretion

Like loop diuretics, thiazide diuretics increase K^+ and H^+ secretion into the collecting duct. However, in contrast to loop diuretics, they decrease the excretion of Ca^{2+}, although the exact mechanism underlying this effect is uncertain. In the distal tubule Ca^{2+} is reabsorbed via a channel in the luminal membrane followed by Na^+/Ca^{2+} exchange (countertransport) across the basolateral membrane (see Fig. 10. 9). Thiazides reduce the tubule cell concentration of Na^+, thereby increasing the Na^+ concentration gradient across the basolateral membrane, which may stimulate Na^+/Ca^{2+} exchange. A decrease in intracellular concentration of Ca^{2+} will promote Ca^{2+} influx via the luminal membrane channels, resulting in increased Ca^{2+} reabsorption from the tubule lumen.

Thiazide and loop diuretics can cause metabolic alkalosis

Thiazide and loop diuretics increase the lumen-negative potential as a result of increased Na^+ reabsorption in the late distal tubule and collecting duct, which promotes H^+ secretion with the consequent risk of metabolic alkalosis.

The pharmacotherapeutic indications for thiazide diuretics include:

- Edema associated with congestive heart failure, hepatic cirrhosis, and the nephrotic syndrome.
- Hypertension (see Chapter 8), where they are used either alone or in combination with other antihypertensive drugs.

Potassium-sparing diuretics

Potassium-sparing diuretics act on the late distal tubule and collecting duct

Potassium-sparing diuretics can be divided into two groups:

- The Na^+ channel blockers (e.g. triamterene and amiloride).
- The aldosterone antagonists that block mineralocorticosteroid receptors (e.g. spironolactone and potassium canrenoate.

Adverse effects of diuretic drugs

Loop diuretics	Thiazide diuretics	Potassium-sparing diuretics	Osmotic diuretics
Hypokalemia (corrected by K^+ supplements or combination with potassium-sparing diuretics)	Hypokalemia (corrected as for loop diuretics)	Hyperkalemia	Pulmonary edema
Metabolic alkalosis	Metabolic alkalosis	Metabolic acidosis	Dehydration
Hyponatremia	Hyponatremia	Spironolactone binds to other steroid receptors which can result in: gynecomastia, menstrual disorders, male sexual dysfunction, hirsutism, loss of libido	Hyponatremia (due to extraction of water from intracellular compartments with expansion of extracellular fluid volume)
Hypovolemia and hypotension	Hyperuricemia (same mechanism as for loop diuretics)		Hypernatremia (as a result of urinary loss of water in excess of Na^+)
Hyperuricemia, which may precipitate gout (enhanced uric acid absorption in proximal tubule as a result of volume depletion or decreased secretion due to competition at organic acid secretory mechanism)	Hypomagnesemia		Headache
Hypocalcemia	Hypercalcemia		Nausea and vomiting
Hypomagnesemia	Increases in glucose and cholesterol in some patients		
Ototoxicity (hearing loss, tinnitus more likely with ethacrynic acid)	Male sexual dysfunction		

Fig. 10.7 Adverse effects of diuretic drugs.

Diuretic drug(s)	Drug(s) interacting	Consequence	Comment
Thiazide and loop diuretics	Cardiac glycosides	Increased risk of cardiac glycoside-induced arrhythmias	Hypokalemia potentiates action of cardiac glycosides
Thiazide and loop diuretics	Lithium	Increased plasma levels of lithium with risk of lithium toxic effects	Increased tubular reabsorption of lithium
Thiazide and loop diuretics	Uricosuric agents	Reduced effect of uricosuric agents	Decreased tubular secretion of uricosuric agents
Thiazide and loop diuretics	Nonsteroidal anti-inflammatory drugs	Reduced diuretic response	Interaction is a result of inhibition of prostaglandin synthesis
Loop diuretics	Aminoglycosides and cisplatin	Increased risk of ototoxicity	Synergism of ototoxicity
Potassium-sparing diuretics	Angiotensin-converting enzyme inhibitors and K^+ supplements	Increased risk of hyperkalemia	Additive hyperkalemic effects

Fig. 10.8 Drug interactions with diuretic drugs.

Both types of potassium-sparing diuretic drug have a mild diuretic action resulting in the excretion of 2–3% of filtered Na^+, although the magnitude of the diuresis produced by aldosterone antagonists depends on the levels of aldosterone.

There are two types of cells in the late distal tubule and collecting duct:

- Principal cells, which are sites for Na^+, K^+, and water transport.
- Intercalated cells, which are sites for H^+ secretion.

The late distal tubule and collecting duct are the major locations for K^+ secretion in the kidney, and the transport of both K^+ and Na^+ across the luminal membrane occurs via ion channels rather than transporters (Fig. 10.10). The concentration gradient for the movement of Na^+ into the principal cells is greater than that for the movement of K^+ out of the cells and as a result a lumen-negative potential difference is established. Na^+ that enters the principal cell is transported across the basolateral membrane by Na^+/K^+ ATPase with the subsequent movement of K^+ into the cell. K^+ then moves out of the cell into the lumen of the tubule driven by the lumen-negative potential difference.

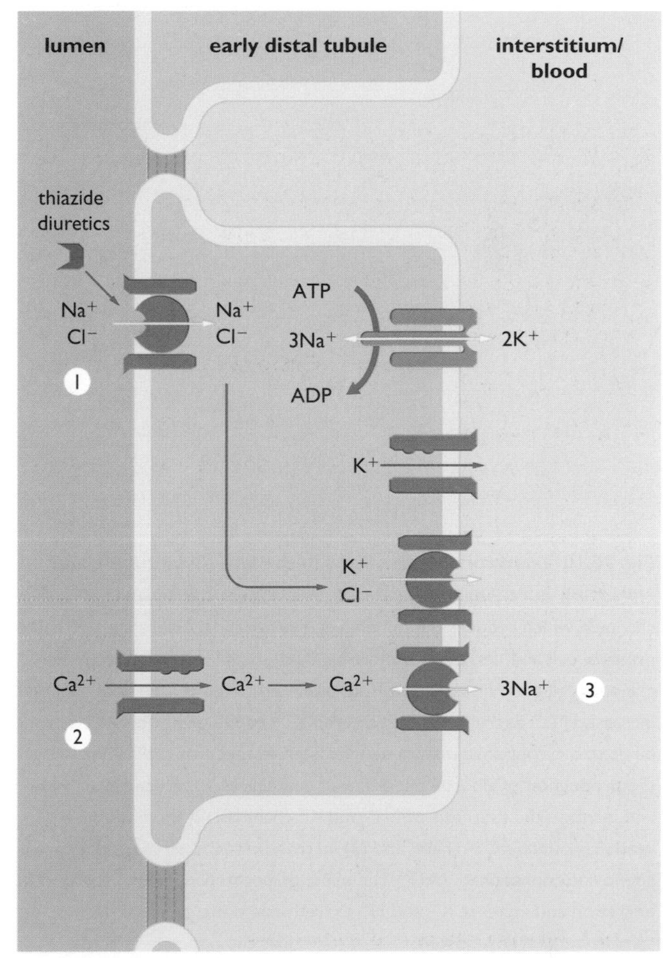

Fig. 10.9 Transport mechanisms in the early distal tubule. Thiazide diuretics increase the excretion of Na^+ and Cl^- by inhibiting the Na^+/Cl^- cotransporter (1). The reabsorption of Ca^{2+} (2) is increased by these drugs by a mechanism that may involve stimulation of Na^+/Ca^{2+} countertransport (3) due to an increase in the concentration gradient for Na^+ across the basolateral membrane.

Amiloride and triamterene block the luminal Na^+ channels

Blockade of the luminal Na^+ channels by amiloride or triamterene reduces the luminal potential difference and consequently decreases the driving force for K^+ secretion. The net effect of these drugs is therefore to reduce Na^+ reabsorption and decrease K^+ secretion, hence the term potassium-sparing diuretics. The latter effect can result in the development of hyperkalemia. In contrast, increased Na^+ delivery to the collecting duct by the action of loop and thiazide diuretics will promote K^+ secretion, which may result in hypokalemia.

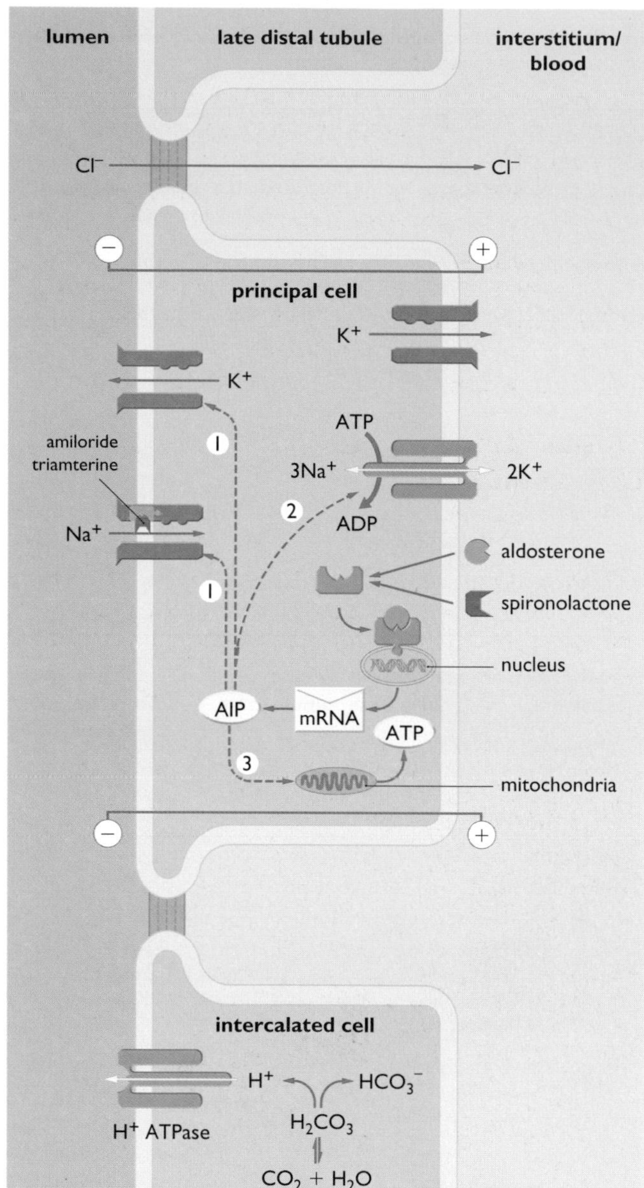

Fig. 10.10 Transport mechanisms in the late distal tubule and collecting duct. Amiloride and triamterene block the luminal Na^+ channels, which reduces the lumen-negative potential difference across the principal cell and decreases the driving force for K^+ secretion from the principal cell and H^+ secretion from the intercalated cell. The net effect is increased Na^+ excretion and decreased K^+ and H^+ excretion. Aldosterone binds to a cytoplasmic mineralocorticosteroid receptor (MR) stimulating the production of aldosterone-induced proteins (AIP), which (1) activate and increase the synthesis of Na^+ and K^+ channels; (2) increase the synthesis of Na^+/K^+ ATPase, and (3) increase mitochondrial production of adenosine triphosphate (ATP). The effect of aldosterone is to decrease Na^+ excretion and increase K^+ and H^+ excretion in urine, whereas spironolactone, an aldosterone antagonist, has the opposite effects.

Amiloride and triamterene can cause metabolic acidosis

Amiloride and triamterene also indirectly decrease H^+ secretion via H^+ ATPase in the intercalated cells since H^+ secretion is aided by the lumen-negative potential, which is reduced by the action of amiloride and triamterene. The reduction in H^+ secretion can cause metabolic acidosis.

Aldosterone increases Na^+ reabsorption and K^+ and H^+ secretion

The cells of the late distal tubule and collecting duct contain cytoplasmic receptors for mineralocorticosteroids which, when bound to aldosterone, migrate to the nucleus and initiate DNA transcription, translation, and production of specific proteins (aldosterone-induced proteins). These proteins:

- Activate silent Na^+ and K^+ channels and increase the synthesis of these channels.
- Increase the synthesis of Na^+/K^+ ATPase.
- Increase mitochondrial production of ATP (see Fig. 10.10).

As a result of these actions, the net effect of aldosterone is to increase Na^+ reabsorption and K^+ and H^+ secretion.

Spironolactone reduces Na^+ reabsorption and K^+ and H^+ secretion

Spironolactone competitively inhibits the binding of aldosterone to its receptor (see Fig. 10.10), thus blocking stimulation of the

Mechanisms of action of diuretic drugs

- Loop diuretics block the $Na^+/K^+/2Cl^-$ cotransporter in the thick ascending loop of Henle, resulting in the excretion of 15–25% of filtered Na^+
- Thiazide diuretics block the Na^+/Cl^- cotransporter in the distal convoluted tubule, resulting in the excretion of 5% of filtered Na^+
- Potassium-sparing diuretics increase the Na^+ excretion by 2–3% and decrease K^+ excretion by acting on the late distal tubule and collecting duct
- Potassium-sparing diuresis is produced by blockade of luminal Na^+ channels (e.g. with amiloride or triamterene) or by blockade of cytoplasmic mineralocorticosteroid receptors (e.g. with spironolactone)
- Osmotic diuretics reduce water reabsorption resulting in a subsequent decrease of Na^+ reabsorption in the proximal tubule and descending limb of the loop of Henle

synthesis of proteins that modify the transport functions of the collecting duct. The effects of spironolactone are therefore to reduce Na^+ reabsorption and K^+ and H^+ secretion. The latter actions can lead to hyperkalemia and metabolic acidosis.

Clinical indications Triamterene, amiloride, and spironolactone are rarely used alone. Instead they are used in combination with potassium-losing diuretics (i.e. thiazides and loop diuretics) to preserve K^+ balance. To facilitate patient compliance with diuretic therapy, there are tablets combining potassium-sparing diuretics with a thiazide or a loop diuretic. The inclusion of potassium-sparing diuretics in diuretic treatment is an alternative to the use of K^+ supplements with potassium-losing diuretics.

Aldosterone antagonists potentiate the diuretic actions of thiazide and loop diuretics since the blood pressure lowering effect of thiazide and loop diuretics activate the renin–angiotensin system resulting in increased aldosterone secretion. Aldosterone opposes the diuretic-induced increase in Na^+ excretion.

Aldosterone antagonists are useful in the treatment of:

- Primary aldosteronism.
- Edema associated with secondary aldosteronism that can occur in congestive heart failure, the nephrotic syndrome, and hepatic cirrhosis.

Adverse effects A disadvantage to the use of aldosterone antagonists is their range of adverse effects, which occur as a consequence of their binding to other steroid receptors (see Fig. 10.7).

Osmotic diuretics

Osmotic diuretics reduce water and Na^+ reabsorption and increase extracellular fluid volume

Osmotic diuretics such as mannitol (given intravenously) and isosorbide (given orally) are freely filtered at the glomerulus and undergo little, if any, reabsorption. They increase the osmotic pressure of tubular fluid, thereby reducing the reabsorption of water and lowering luminal Na^+ concentration, with a subsequent decrease in Na^+ reabsorption in the proximal tubule and descending loop of Henle. Osmotic diuretics increase the extracellular fluid volume by increasing water loss from intracellular compartments, and this increase inhibits renin release and decreases blood viscosity, effects that increase renal blood flow. In addition, renal vasodilation produced by osmotic diuretics may involve the release of prostaglandins. The increase in medullary blood flow contributes to the overall diuretic effect by reducing medullary hypertonicity.

Clinical indications Osmotic diuretics are sometimes used in the treatment of oliguria (see p. 224), but not in the treatment of edema. If given to patients with heart failure, they may cause pulmonary edema as a result of extracting water from intracellular compartments and expanding the extracellular fluid volume.

POLYURIA

Polyuria is excessive production of a dilute urine and is usually accompanied by polydipsia (increased fluid intake). The main causes of polyuria are:

- Diabetes mellitus.
- Diabetes insipidus, which is caused either by a failure to produce sufficient vasopressin (central diabetes insipidus) or because the collecting ducts fail to respond to vasopressin (nephrogenic diabetes insipidus).

Vasopressin increases the water permeability of the collecting duct

Vasopressin (antidiuretic hormone) increases the water permeability of the collecting duct, which in the absence of vasopressin is impermeable to water. Vasopressin binds to V_2 receptors on the basolateral membrane of principal cells of the collecting duct. These receptors are G protein coupled and when stimulated activate adenylyl cyclase (see Chapter 3). The resultant increase in cyclic adenosine monophosphate (cAMP) activates protein kinase A. This in turn leads to fusion of intracellular vesicles containing preformed water channels with the luminal membrane, thereby increasing the permeability to water (Fig. 10.11).

Desmopressin is the drug of choice for central diabetes insipidus

Central diabetes insipidus can be treated with synthetic arginine vasopressin or its lysine and desamino analogs. Desamino vasopressin (desmopressin), a selective V_2 agonist, is the drug of choice because it has the longest duration of action, and unlike arginine and lysine vasopressin, it has no vasoconstrictor effect resulting from stimulation of V_1 receptors.

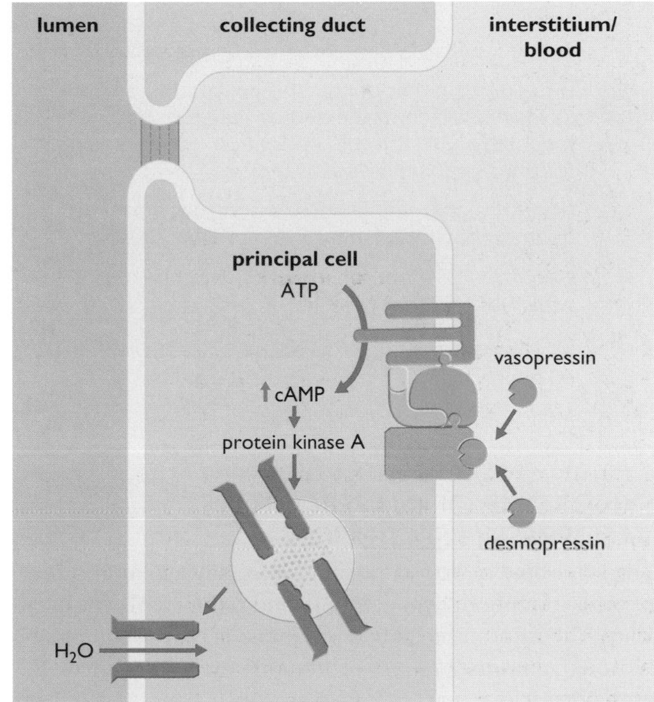

Fig. 10.11 The mechanism for controlling water permeability of the collecting duct. Vasopressin or its analog (e.g. desmopressin) bind to V_2 receptors in the basolateral membrane of principal cells. This leads to the fusion of vesicles containing preformed water channels with the luminal membrane, thereby increasing the permeability to water.

The polyuria of partial central diabetes insipidus in patients who are unable to tolerate vasopressin peptides, can be controlled using either chlorpropamide or carbamazepine. Both drugs potentiate the antidiuretic effect of residual vasopressin, but the underlying mechanism for this action is unclear.

Nephrogenic diabetes insipidus is treated with a long-acting thiazide and indomethacin

Nephrogenic diabetes insipidus can be controlled using a long-acting thiazide diuretic (e.g. chlorothiazide) in combination with the cyclooxygenase inhibitor indomethacin. The antidiuretic action of both drugs is poorly understood:

- Thiazides reduce the effective circulating fluid volume and this may increase the oncotic pressure of plasma proteins and reduce the hydrostatic pressure of the peritubular capillaries of the proximal tubule. This would then favor Na^+ and water reabsorption from this region of the nephron, resulting in decreased fluid delivery to the collecting ducts with a consequent reduction in the polyuria.
- Indomethacin has been reported to decrease glomerular filtration rate and enhance fluid reabsorption from the proximal and distal tubules. In addition, it potentiates the effect of vasopressin on the principal cells of the collecting duct.

Diabetes insipidus

- **This condition is characterized by polyuria**
- **It is due to either decreased production of vasopressin (central diabetes insipidus) or insensitivity to the renal effects of vasopressin (nephrogenic diabetes insipidus)**
- **Central diabetes insipidus is controlled by desmopressin (desamino vasopressin)**
- **Nephrogenic diabetes insipidus can be treated with thiazide diuretics**

SYNDROME OF INAPPROPRIATE VASOPRESSIN SECRETION

The syndrome of inappropriate vasopressin secretion consists of water retention, hyponatremia, and reduced plasma osmolality. The urine osmolality often exceeds that of the plasma. Although plasma Na^+ concentrations are diminished, Na^+ excretion in urine may be normal, and the patient is neither edematous nor dehydrated. The causes of inappropriate (excess) vasopressin secretion include:

- Some tumors.
- Pulmonary infections such as tuberculosis.
- Head injuries.

Treatment is with demeclocycline

Treatment is with the tetracycline demeclocycline, which blunts the action of vasopressin on the collecting ducts, possibly by inhibiting vasopressin-induced increases in cAMP. This reduces water permeability and increases urine flow.

OLIGURIA

Oliguria is a clinical feature of acute renal failure

Oliguria describes a reduced urine volume. In normal adults, urine output is about 1.5 liters/24 hours, but in oliguric patients urine volume is inappropriately low, generally less than 400 ml/24 hours. When urine production falls to less than 50 ml/24 hours, the patient is said to be anuric.

Oliguria is a clinical feature of acute renal failure. Renal function depends on:

- Adequate perfusion of glomeruli to produce an ultrafiltrate.
- Modification of the ultrafiltrate by tubule cells to produce urine.
- Drainage of urine by the ureters, bladder, and urethra.

A disturbance of any of these functions can cause acute renal failure. For instance, severe hypoperfusion of the kidneys, acute damage to the tubules, or blockage of the urinary tract can individually cause acute renal failure. Hypoperfusion of the kidney can be corrected by restoring the effective circulating volume and obstruction of the urinary tract can often be rectified by surgery. In both situations, renal function usually returns to normal. If the tubule cells have been damaged, oliguria persists for 2–4 weeks before there is a recovery phase and a gradual return to normal renal function, which occurs in most patients.

No drugs prevent or treat acute renal failure, but mannitol or furosemide may be useful

At present, there are no satisfactory drugs for preventing or treating acute renal failure. However, diuretic therapy with either mannitol or furosemide may be of value if intratubular obstruction plays a role in the pathogenesis of renal dysfunction. These drugs increase renal blood flow and the diuresis they evoke helps to maintain tubule patency by eliminating debris from the tubule lumen.

Many organs or body systems are adversely affected by acute renal failure and drugs may be used in the management of such secondary effects. For example:

- Antihypertensive drugs are used for hypertension.
- Anticonvulsant drugs are given to patients who develop seizures.
- H_2-antagonists have proved beneficial in preventing gastric ulceration.

CHRONIC RENAL FAILURE

Chronic renal failure describes deteriorating renal function due to a loss of functional nephrons and is common to the later stages of all chronic renal disease. Common causes include:

- Severe hypertension.
- Diabetes mellitus.
- Glomerulonephritis.
- Obstruction of the urinary tract.

Drugs are used to treat the symptoms of chronic renal failure

The only effective treatments for chronic renal failure are dialysis and transplantation. However, drugs can be used to aid patient management and these include:

- Loop diuretics, which can be used to increase urine volume and Na^+ excretion.
- Antihypertensive drugs (see Chapter 8) to control the hypertension of chronic renal failure since they have been shown to reduce the rate of decline in renal function; angiotensin-converting enzyme inhibitors are particularly effective. Most patients with chronic renal failure have hypertension, which can damage the kidney, leading to proteinuria and hyperfiltration with subsequent loss of glomeruli.
- Antiemetics (see Chapter 7) to control the symptoms of nausea and vomiting experienced by many patients with late renal failure.
- Recombinant human erythropoietin to treat the anemia that develops following the loss of the major source of erythropoietin from the peritubular cells in the renal cortex. Erythropoietin stimulates the production of red blood cell precursors in the bone marrow.
- Hydroxylated derivatives of vitamin D (1α-hydroxycholecalciferol and 1,25-dihydroxycholecalciferol) to maintain plasma Ca^{2+} and prevent hyperparathyroidism. In chronic renal failure vitamin D metabolism (see Chapter 27) is abnormal because there is impaired hydroxylation of 25-hydroxycholecalciferol to 1,25-dihydroxycholecalciferol within the kidney. As a result, absorption of dietary Ca^{2+} is reduced and plasma Ca^{2+} is low. Secondary hyperparathyroidism (see Chapter 12) then develops, which can lead to bone disease.

RENAL STONE DISEASE (NEPHROLITHIASIS)

Renal stones develop when poorly soluble substances crystallize in the urine and the crystals aggregate to form particles large enough to lodge within the urinary system.

Thiazide diuretics prevent Ca^{2+} stone formation

Most renal stones are composed of calcium oxalate and/or calcium phosphate. Management consists of removing the stones and preventing further stone formation. Thiazide diuretics can be used to prevent stone formation because in the long term they diminish urinary excretion of Ca^{2+} (see above).

Allopurinol prevents uric acid stone formation

Renal stone disease also results from precipitation of uric acid. In this case treatment with allopurinol, an inhibitor of xanthine oxidase, is beneficial because this drug reduces urinary uric acid levels and the incidence of stone formation. Oxalic acid stones can be a complication of ingesting polyethylene glycol (antifreeze).

D-penicillamine prevents cystine stone formation

There are some rare inherited disorders associated with stone formation. Cystinuria is an autosomal recessive condition that impairs cystine, ornithine, arginine, and lysine transport in the proximal renal tubules. Cystine is much less soluble than the other dibasic amino acids whose transport is affected, and renal stones develop in homozygous individuals. These can be prevented by D-penicillamine, which by thiol exchange reacts with cystine to form a soluble penicillamine–cysteine product.

URINARY TRACT INFECTION

Urinary tract infections are common and can be associated with underlying renal disease. They are more prevalent in women than men owing to the short length of the female urethra and its site of opening, which is more readily contaminated with fecal organisms. Apart from gender, several other factors predispose to urinary tract infections and these are listed in Fig. 10.12.

Bacterial infections may be localized to the lower urinary tract or affect the kidney to produce tubulointerstitial disease (i.e. pyelonephritis, Fig. 10.13). The most common acute infection is cystitis, an infection localized to the bladder.

Typical symptoms of a urinary tract infection include:

- A burning sensation when passing urine (dysuria).
- Increased frequency of micturition.
- Increased nocturnal micturition.
- Pyrexia.
- Loin pain if the infection is in the upper urinary tract.

Predisposing factors for urinary tract infections

Factor	Comments
Pregnancy	Estrogens cause dilation of the ureter and reduce urine flow. This may be made worse by the gravid uterus
Childhood	Children under two years of age, possibly because they sit in 'a soup of urine and feces'
Diabetes mellitus	Glycosuria favors bacterial growth and there may be underlying renal disease
Structural abnormalities	Any structural abnormality to the urinary tract increases the risk of infection. For example, patients with polycystic renal disease are prone to infections
Spinal injuries	A neurogenic bladder may lead to incomplete emptying and stasis of urine
Analgesic nephropathy	Damage to the renal papillae. Dead tissue separates from the medulla and the resultant cavities are prone to bacterial infection
Renal stones	Stones can diminish urine flow and bacteria invade the crevices of stones
Instrumentation	Pathogenic organisms can be introduced during catheterization and cystoscopy. Indwelling catheters frequently predispose to bacterial and fungal infection

Fig. 10.12 Predisposing factors for urinary tract infections.

Urinary tract infections during pregnancy may be asymptomatic, but analysis of urine frequently reveals the presence of protein and possibly blood.

The majority of urinary tract infections are caused by organisms that originate from the patient's own intestinal flora, and the pathogen is frequently a Gram-negative bacillus such as *Escherichia coli*, which accounts for most cases of infection. However, some infections are caused by Gram-positive cocci such as *Streptococcus faecalis* and *Staphylococcus saprophyticus* (Fig. 10.14).

Trimethoprim is a first-line drug for acute uncomplicated lower and upper infections except in pregnancy

Trimethoprim is a first-line drug for preventing and treating acute uncomplicated lower and upper urinary tract infections (see Chapter 23). It can be used alone or in conjunction with sulfamethoxazole (i.e. co-trimoxazole). Amoxicillin, fluoroquinolones, such as ciprofloxacin and norfloxacin, and nitrofurantoin are suitable alternatives. Trimethoprim or co-trimoxazole (folate antagonists or sulfonamides) is contraindicated in pregnancy, and there is a risk of hemolysis in patients with glucose-6-phosphate dehydrogenase deficiency if given fluoroquinolones or nitrofurantoin.

Urinary tract infection

- The most common pathogen is *Escherichia coli*
- The main drug for the treatment of acute infections is trimethoprim
- Co-trimoxazole, fluoroquinolones (norfloxacin, ciprofloxacin), amoxicillin, and nitrofurantoin are also useful for treating acute infections
- Trimethoprim and co-trimoxazole are contraindicated in pregnancy, but amoxicillin and nitrofurantoin are considered to be safe

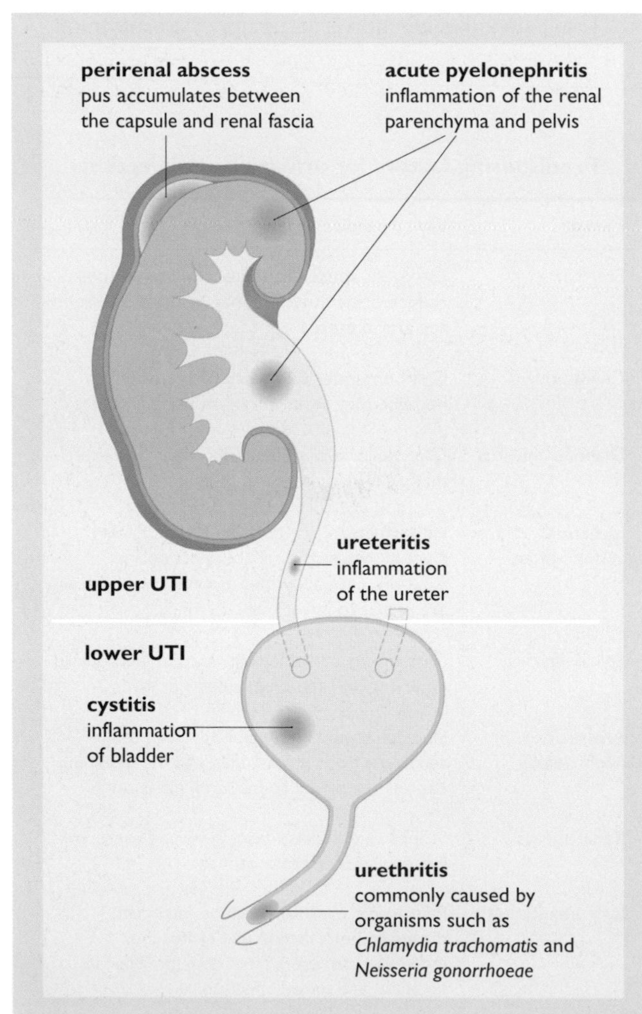

Fig. 10.13 Common sites of urinary tract infection (UTI).

The antibiotic of choice for chronic or recurrent infections depends on the microbiology

For chronic or recurrent urinary tract infections, the choice of drug should be made according to the microbiologic results.

The primary focus of some urinary tract infections can lie elsewhere (see Fig. 10.14). For example, the urinary tract is involved in about 5% of patients with pulmonary tuberculosis. The principal chemotherapy for renal tuberculosis is a combination of rifampicin, isoniazid, and pyrazinamide (see Chapter 9).

Parasitic diseases that commonly involve the urinary tract include schistosomiasis, which is the most common helminthic infection in man (see Fig. 10.14). Treatment is with praziquantel or metrifonate (see Chapter 25).

Some pathogens causing urinary tract infections

Primary infection	Secondary infection (primary source non-renal)
Bacteria	**Bacteria**
Gram-negative bacilli	*Mycobacterium tuberculosis*
Escherichia coli	*Salmonella* species
Klebsiella species	*Staphylococcus aureus*
Proteus species	
Pseudomonas species	**Fungi**
	Histoplasma duboisii
Gram-positive bacilli	
Streptococcus faecalis	**Parasites**
Staphylococcus aureus	*Schistosoma* species
Staphylococcus epidermidis	*Echinococcus* species
Staphylococcus saprophyticus	
Fungi	
Candida species	

Fig. 10.14 Some pathogens causing urinary tract infections.

Drugs used to treat nonrenal diseases that act on the kidney

Drugs used to treat nonrenal diseases that act on the kidney include:

- Diuretics, which are used in the treatment of edema arising from diseases of other systems such as congestive heart failure and hepatic cirrhosis.
- Drugs used in the prophylaxis of gout that facilitate the excretion of uric acid in the urine (uricosuric drugs).

Uricosuric drugs

Uric acid is cleared from the blood mainly by glomerular filtration with some secretion into the proximal tubule. However, the bulk of uric acid in tubule fluid is reabsorbed by countertransport systems in both the luminal and basolateral membranes of tubule cells. These exchange urate for either organic or inorganic anions. Uricosuric drugs inhibit the transport of urate across the luminal membrane (see Chapter 17).

The principal uricosuric drugs are probenecid and sulfinpyrazone, and these are useful in patients who have a low urine clearance of uric acid. To prevent urate crystallization in the early stage of uricosuric therapy, patients need to maintain a high fluid intake (2 liters/day) and to take sodium bicarbonate or potassium citrate to produce an alkaline urine (pH $\geq$ 6.0) .

Adverse effects Uricosuric drugs should be avoided in patients who overproduce uric acid. Paradoxically, uricosuric drugs can cause gout in some patients and they should not be given during an acute attack.

Probenecid and sulfinpyrazone cause gastrointestinal disturbances and are contraindicated in patients with peptic ulceration. Probenecid blocks the renal tubule secretion of organic acid drugs, such as benzylpenicillin, which may prolong their effects and increase the risk of toxicity.

NEPHROTOXIC DRUGS

The kidney is vulnerable to drug-induced injury because of its central role in the removal of foreign compounds and their metabolites from the body. Furthermore, the reabsorption of filtered solutes is energy dependent, and these processes are susceptible to substances that interfere with cellular functions such as energy production. Many nephrotoxic drugs have their primary effects on discrete parts of the nephron. This may result from regional differences in transport characteristics, cellular energetics, repair mechanisms, and capacity to bioactivate or detoxify potential toxins. The sites of action of some nephrotoxic drugs are shown in Fig. 10.15.

Antimicrobial drugs

Aminoglycosides, amphotericin B, and some first-generation cephalosporins are nephrotoxic

Aminoglycosides play an important role in the treatment of severe Gram-negative infections, but 10–15% of patients who receive these drugs develop acute renal failure. The primary

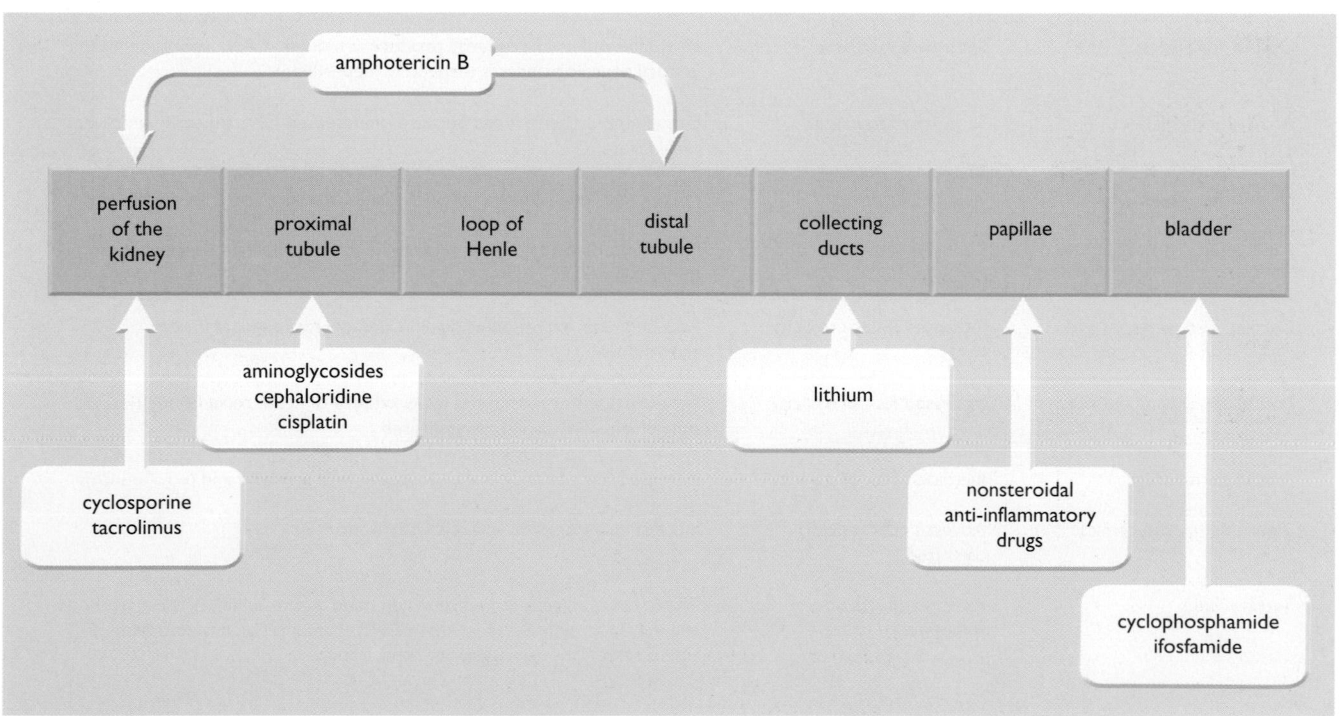

Fig. 10.15 Primary renal sites of action of some nephrotoxic drugs.

focus of injury is the proximal tubule and the order of these drugs in terms of their toxicity with the most toxic first is gentamicin, tobramycin, amikacin, and netilmicin.

The systemic antifungal drug amphotericin B is also nephrotoxic and it has been estimated that about 80% of patients given amphotericin B develop impaired renal function. This agent causes renal vasoconstriction, and although several regions of the nephron are affected by amphotericin B, the primary target is the distal tubule. A significant renal loss of Mg^{2+} and K^{+} can develop which, if uncorrected, will result in hypomagnesemia and hypokalemia. Recently, amphotericin B has been encapsulated in liposomes to produce a formulation that is less nephrotoxic than the parent drug.

Some first-generation cephalosporins (cephaloridine and cephalothin) are potential nephrotoxins, but are not as toxic to the kidney as aminoglycosides and amphotericin B.

Antineoplastic drugs

Alkylating agents, platinum derivatives, and increased urate excretion due to cell destruction can cause renal damage

Nephrotoxicity is a prominent feature of many alkylating agents. Cyclophosphamide and ifosfamide are metabolized to products that release acrolein, a nephrotoxic compound that induces hemorrhagic cystitis. This adverse effect can be prevented by the simultaneous administration of mesna (2-mercaptoethane sulfonate), which reacts with acrolein in the urinary tract and prevents toxicity.

The platinum derivatives, cisplatin and to a lesser degree carboplatin, are also nephrotoxic. Cisplatin-induced injury mainly affects the straight portion of the proximal tubule. To minimize the renal damage, it is routine to hydrate the patient with an infusion of 1–2 liters of saline before drug administration. Electrolyte disturbances such as hypocalcemia and hypomagnesemia are a common complication of therapy with cisplatin, but are rarely symptomatic.

The destruction of cells by antineoplastic drugs results in the release of purines from the breakdown of nucleic acids. Further catabolism of purines leads to excessive urate formation and excretion, the latter leading to increased risk of renal stone formation.

Analgesics

Acetaminophen and nonsteroidal anti-inflammatory drugs can damage the kidney

Acute renal failure develops as a result of acute tubular necrosis in about 2% of patients who have taken an overdose of acetaminophen (paracetamol). Renal dysfunction is usually accompanied by severe hepatic failure, but in a few cases there is acute renal failure in the absence of hepatic damage. Acute renal

Key classes of drugs to be avoided or used with caution in renal failure

Class of drug	Type of reaction	Comment
Opioid analgesics	Sensitivity increases	Morphine and its analogs may produce prolonged CNS depression and unusual neurologic effects (especially meperidine)
Anxiolytics/sedatives	Sensitivity increases	Dosage should be reduced because of increased CNS sensitivity in severe renal failure
Uricosuric agents	Reduced activity	Probenecid and sulfinpyrazone are ineffective
Antibacterial drugs	Reduced activity	Nitrofurantoin and nalidixic acid fail to achieve effective concentrations in the urine
Cardiac glycosides	Increased risk of toxicity	Reduced renal excretion of digoxin and increased risk of cardiac arrhythmias
Potassium-sparing diuretics	Increased risk of toxicity	Such drugs will aggravate the hyperkalemia of acute renal failure. Potassium supplements are also contraindicated
Antibacterial drugs	Increased risk of toxicity	Increased risk of peripheral neuropathy with isoniazid and nitrofurantoin.
Biguanide hypoglycemics	Adverse effects poorly tolerated	Increased risk of lactic acidosis with metformin
Tetracyclines	Adverse effects poorly tolerated	Tetracyclines, except doxycycline and minocycline, inhibit protein synthesis and induce a catabolic effect that results from increased metabolism of amino acids. This may aggravate renal failure

Fig. 10.16 Key classes of drugs to be avoided or used with caution in renal failure.

failure arises several days after ingestion and is mainly oliguric in type.

Chronic nonsteroidal anti-inflammatory drug (NSAID)-induced nephropathy is characterized by interstitial nephritis and renal papillary necrosis, and results from long-term ingestion of NSAIDs. It is unusual in patients under 30 years of age and occurs mainly in women aged 40–60 years. The loss of papillary tissue may lead to secondary nephron damage and eventually to impaired renal function.

Immunosuppressant drugs

Cyclosporine and tacrolimus are markedly nephrotoxic

The structural basis for the nephropathy caused by cyclosporine and tacrolimus is unique as both drugs adversely affect the renal vasculature. Most patients who receive cyclosporine develop an acute reversible impairment of renal function during early treatment. This is associated with afferent arteriolar vasoconstriction, which can be reversed by dopamine and nifedipine. Chronic nephrotoxicity is also common among patients given cyclosporine and may result from arteriolopathy (loss of myocytes and mural hyalinosis) with sclerosis of downstream glomeruli.

Lithium

A minority of patients who are treated with lithium for affective disorders develop nephrogenic diabetes insipidus, which is usually reversible on stopping the drug. The mechanism for this effect is a reduction in V_2 receptor-mediated stimulation of adenyl cyclase by vasopressin.

Amiloride can be used to reverse lithium-induced diabetes insipidus by inhibiting reabsorption of lithium through Na^+ channels in the collecting ducts.

Drugs causing acute interstitial nephritis

Many drugs can lead to an acute deterioration of renal function by causing an inflammation of the renal interstitium (acute interstitial nephritis), which may be due to a hypersensitivity reaction. These drugs include:

- Penicillins.
- Sulfonamides (including co-trimoxazole).
- NSAIDs.
- Diuretics (thiazides and furosemide).
- Allopurinol.
- Cimetidine.

Patients often have a fever, skin rash, and hematuria.

DRUGS TO AVOID IN RENAL FAILURE

Drugs should be prescribed with care for patients with impaired renal function because:

- There may be increased sensitivity to the drug.
- Some drugs are not effective when renal function deteriorates.
- Failure to excrete the drug or its metabolites leads to accumulation and toxicity.
- Adverse effects may be poorly tolerated.

Examples of drugs that fall into these categories are given in Fig. 10.16. Nephrotoxic drugs should not be used in patients with renal disease, if possible, because the consequences of nephrotoxicity are likely to be more severe if the functional capacity of the kidney is already limited.

FURTHER READING

Brenner BM (ed.) *Brenner and Rector's The Kidney (Vols 1 & 2) 5th edition*. Philadelphia: WB Saunders; 1996. [A comprehensive reference text on renal physiology, pathophysiology, and the treatment of renal diseases.]

Greger RF, Knauf H, Mutschler E (eds) *Diuretics: Handbook of Experimental Pharmacology, Vol 117*. Berlin: Springer-Verlag; 1995. [A review of renal physiology coupled with a detailed analysis of the development, pharmacodynamics, pharmacokinetics, and clinical use of each class of diuretic agent.]

Hook JB, Goldstein RS (eds) *Toxicology of the Kidney, 2nd edition*. New York: Raven Press; 1993. [A detailed review of the adverse effects of chemicals on the kidney.]

Lote CJ. *Principles of Renal Physiology, 3rd edition*. London: Chapman & Hall; 1994. [A clear and concise introduction to renal physiology.]

Stamm WE, Hooton TM. Management of urinary tract infections in adults. *N Engl J Med* 1993; **329**: 1328–1334. [An excellent guide to the treatment of urinary tract infections.]

Make a provisional diagnosis and determine a rational pharmacologic treatment for the following hypothetical case.

A 25-year-old woman who is 26 weeks pregnant attends a routine antenatal check. Her blood pressure is normal and she has no edema. However, her urine test reveals proteinuria, but no other abnormalities. She has no pain on micturition and her body temperature is normal.

1. What test would you do?
2. Would you delay treatment until you received the result of the test?
3. What drug treatment would you choose and for how long?
4. What are the endpoints for therapy?
5. What adverse effects can be anticipated with this drug treatment?

?

Indicate whether the following answers are true or false.

1. Furosemide
- a) is a loop diuretic
- b) is a high-ceiling diuretic
- c) produces hypokalemia
- d) is sometimes administered with triamterene
- e) can produce ototoxicity

2. Thiazide diuretics
- a) are aldosterone antagonists
- b) act on the proximal tubule
- c) decrease calcium excretion
- d) inhibit Na^+/Cl^- cotransport
- e) produce hyperkalemia

3. Spironolactone
- a) is a potassium-sparing diuretic
- b) binds to intracellular receptors
- c) acts on the thick ascending loop of Henle
- d) increases proton secretion
- e) is used in the treatment of primary aldosteronism

4. Osmotic diuretics
- a) have a direct action on renal tubule cells
- b) inhibit Na^+ reabsorption in the distal convoluted tubule
- c) increase medullary blood flow
- d) are used to relieve oliguria
- e) are used in the treatment of pulmonary edema

5. The following drugs are useful in the treatment of diabetes insipidus
- a) insulin
- b) desmopressin
- c) chlorothiazide
- d) mannitol
- e) chlorpropamide

6. The following statements are correct
- a) uricosuric drugs increase the secretion of uric acid in urine
- b) the primary drug treatment of gout is either probenecid or sulfinpyrazone
- c) patients treated with uricosuric drugs should maintain an alkaline diuresis
- d) probenecid and sulfinpyrazone should not be given during an acute attack of gout

7. In the treatment of urinary tract infection
- a) the most likely pathogens are Gram-positive cocci such as *Streptococcus faecalis*
- b) trimethoprim is usually effective
- c) fluoroquinolones should not be given to patients with glucose-6-phosphate dehydrogenase deficiency
- d) amoxicillin is contraindicated in pregnancy

8. Nephrotoxicity may be anticipated following administration of
- a) gentamicin
- b) amphotericin B
- c) cisplatin
- d) cephradine
- e) amoxicillin

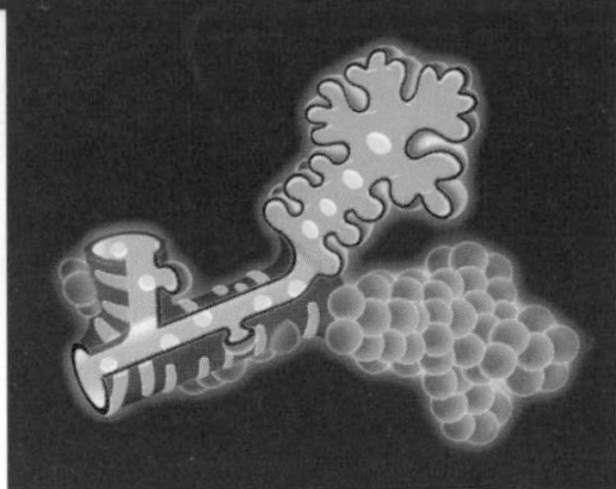

11. Drugs and the Respiratory System

PHYSIOLOGY OF THE RESPIRATORY SYSTEM

Blood is oxygenated and carbon dioxide is removed by the respiratory system

The body's metabolic processes use large quantities of oxygen and produce large amounts of carbon dioxide. The oxygen-absorbing surface of the lung (the gas-exchange surface) is therefore large (80 m^2). It can fit into the body because it is folded and shaped into a branching tree-like system of air-conducting tubes (bronchi and bronchioles), which end in millions of tiny sacs called alveoli (Fig. 11.1).

Respiration is controlled by spontaneous rhythmic discharges from the respiratory center in the medulla of the brain, which is regulated by higher centers in the brain and vagal afferents from the lungs (Fig. 11.2) and influenced by:

- Changes in blood pCO_2, which activate chemoreceptors in the medulla.
- Changes in blood pO_2, which activate chemoreceptors in the aortic arch and carotid bodies.

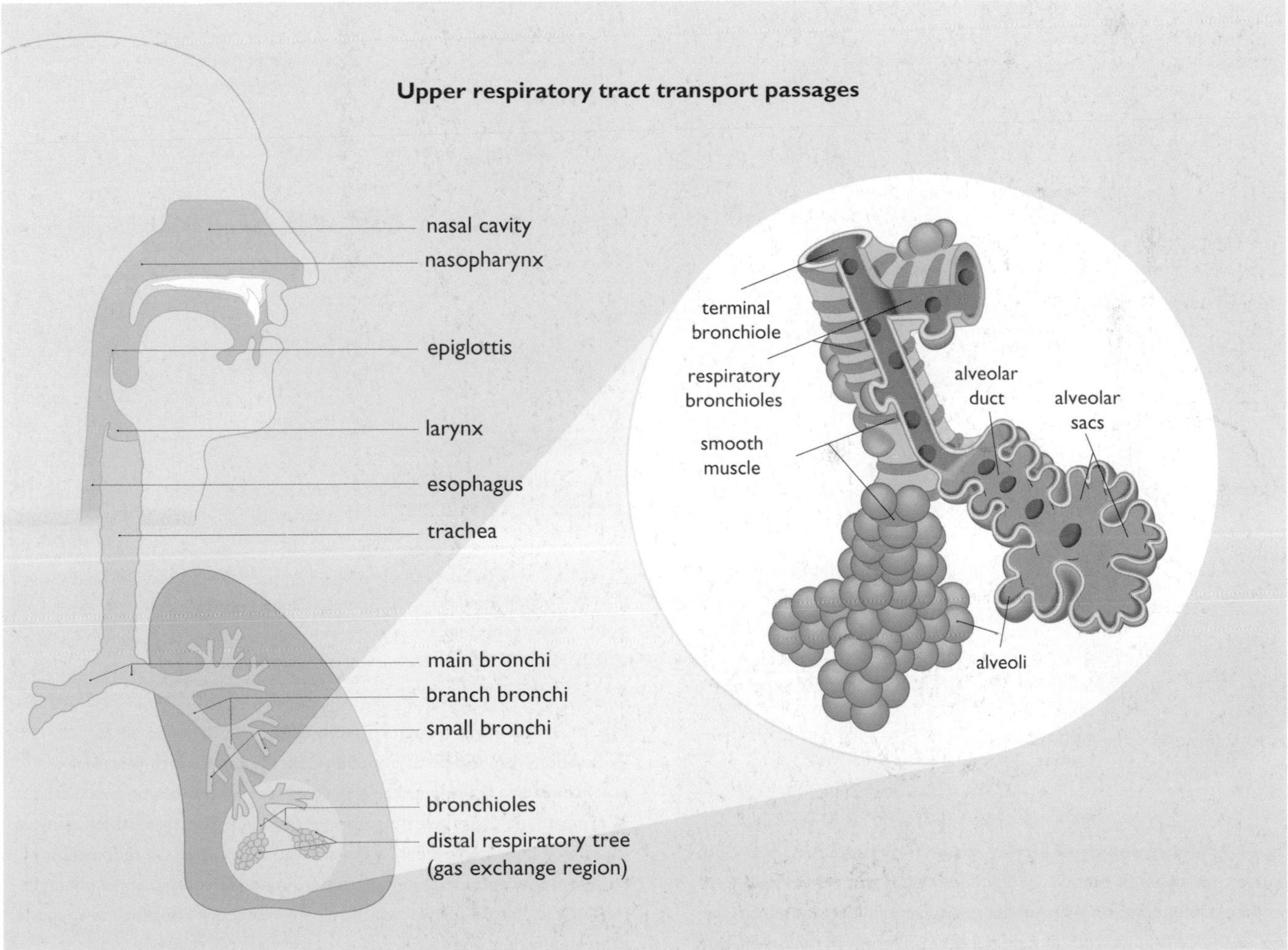

Fig. 11.1 Structure of the respiratory tract.

Drugs that alter respiration

- Narcotic analgesics, barbiturates, certain H_1 receptor antagonists, and ethanol cause respiratory depression
- Doxapram is a respiratory stimulant and is used for patients in ventilatory failure
- Respiratory stimulants are believed to stimulate both carotid chemoreceptors and the respiratory center
- They should be used with caution as they may have unwanted effects on the CNS such as convulsions, and their efficacy is uncertain

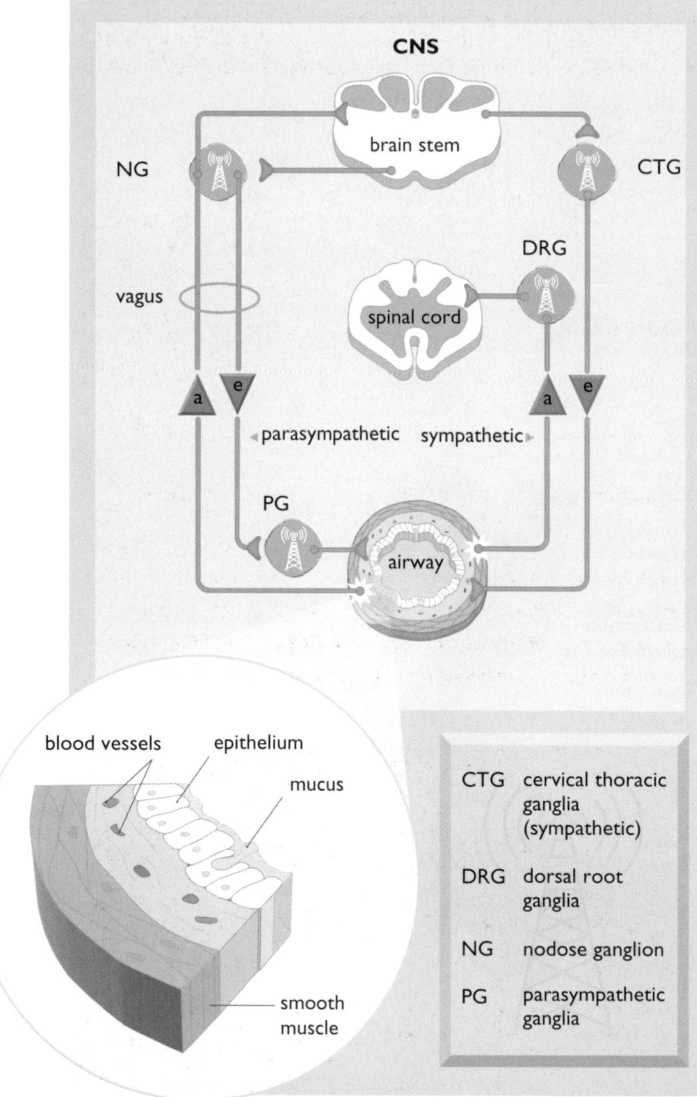

Fig. 11.2 Nerve supply of airway smooth muscle. Airway smooth muscle tone depends on both parasympathetic (vagus nerve) and sympathetic innervation. Afferent fibers also send information from the lung to the central nervous system (CNS). (a, afferent nerves; e, efferent nerves)

Airway smooth muscle tone is produced by parasympathetic, sympathetic, and nonadrenergic noncholinergic nerves and circulating epinephrine

Airway smooth muscle is innervated by:

- The parasympathetic nervous system via the vagus nerve (cranial nerve X), and airway smooth muscle tone is generated by acetylcholine acting on muscarinic receptors (Figs 11.2 and 11.3).
- The so-called 'third nervous pathway,' with the neurotransmitters (nitric oxide and vasoactive intestinal polypeptide [VIP]) used by the nonadrenergic noncholinergic (NANC) nerves of this system (see Fig. 11.3) producing muscle relaxation and bronchodilation.

Bronchial smooth muscle relaxation (bronchodilation) is also produced by circulating epinephrine (adrenaline) interacting with β_2 adrenoceptors on the muscle. Although the bronchial smooth muscle has little or no direct sympathetic innervation, there is a sympathetic supply to the parasympathetic ganglia (see Fig. 11.3).

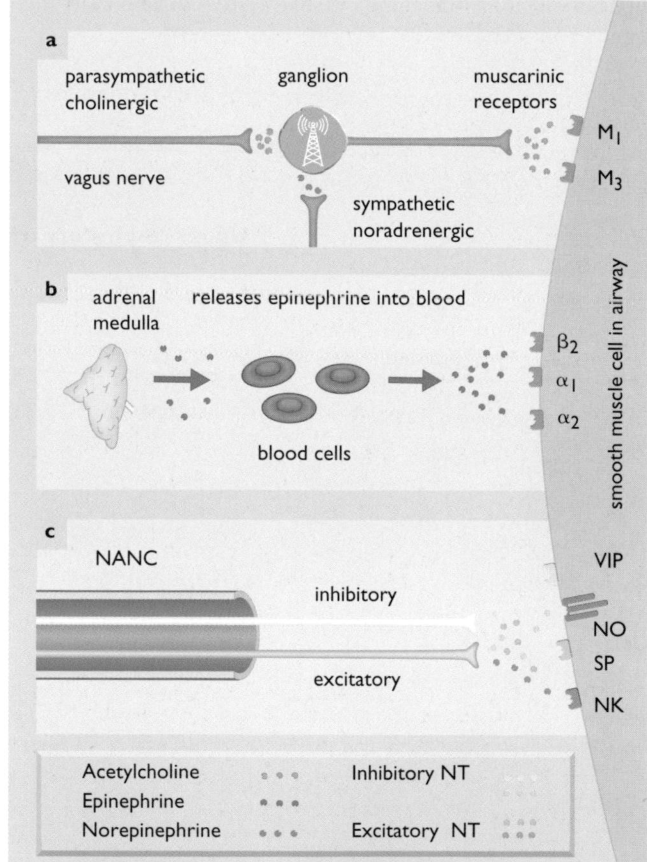

Fig. 11.3 Airway smooth muscle tone. This depends on: (a) innervation from the parasympathetic vagus nerve, which releases acetylcholine to act on muscarinic receptors, and this can be modulated by sympathetic fibers releasing norepinephrine at parasympathetic ganglia; (b) release of epinephrine into the circulation, which acts predominantly on β_2 adrenoceptors; (c) innervation from nonadrenergic noncholinergic (NANC) inhibitory nerves, which release vasoactive intestinal polypeptide (VIP) and nitric oxide (NO), and excitatory nerves releasing substance P (SP) and neurokinin A (NK). (NT, neurotransmitter)

Airway smooth muscle tone therefore depends on the balance between:

- The parasympathetic input.
- The inhibitory influence of circulating epinephrine.
- The NANC inhibitory nerves.
- The sympathetic innervation of the parasympathetic ganglia (Figs 11.3, 11.4).

Noninfectious diseases of the respiratory tract

- The most common diseases are asthma, allergic rhinitis, chronic bronchitis and cystic fibrosis
- Asthma is an inflammatory disease
- Cystic fibrosis is a genetic disease
- Cough is usually a symptom of an underlying disease

PATHOPHYSIOLOGY AND DISEASES OF THE RESPIRATORY SYSTEM

Respiratory disease can cause coughing, wheezing, shortness of breath, and abnormal gas exchange

Coughing, wheezing, shortness of breath, and abnormal gas exchange can result from:

- Changes in airway smooth muscle tone (e.g. bronchial asthma).
- Vascular congestion of the upper respiratory tract (e.g. rhinitis).
- Mucous plugging (e.g. chronic bronchitis).

BRONCHIAL ASTHMA

Bronchial asthma is a chronic inflammatory disease of the airways that causes acute bronchospasm and dyspnea

Bronchial asthma is a common disease, affecting up to 20% of the population in some countries. Its associated morbidity and mortality are increasing in most countries despite increasing use of anti-asthma drugs.

The characteristic clinical features of bronchial asthma are believed to result from a chronic inflammatory response in the airways involving local eosinophil accumulation, which is evident following bronchoalveolar lavage (BAL) and on biopsy and at autopsy (Fig. 11.5). It is thought that the granules of infiltrating eosinophils release cytotoxic mediators (Fig. 11.6), which damage the respiratory ciliated epithelial layer. The tissue damage contributes to increased airway irritability (bronchial hyperresponsiveness), which causes coughing and wheezing in response to stimuli that do not normally provoke such responses (Fig. 11.7).

Bronchial hyperresponsiveness may result from exposure of sensory nerves beneath the damaged epithelium (Fig. 11.8). Activation of these nerves on exertion or exposure to environmental irritants results in local axon and vagal reflexes, which can produce bronchoconstriction, mucus secretion, and airway vasodilation (Fig. 11.8).

Bronchodilators and anti-inflammatory drugs are used to treat asthma

Bronchodilators

Acute reversible bronchospasm contributes to the characteristic wheezing of asthma. It is readily treated by three different classes of bronchodilator drugs: β_2 adrenoceptor agonists, anticholinergics, and xanthines.

Clinical features of bronchial asthma

- Acute attacks of dyspnea associated with acute airway obstruction due to contraction of airway smooth muscle
- Mucus hypersecretion, which may lead to mucus plugging
- Airway inflammation
- Bronchial hyperresponsiveness

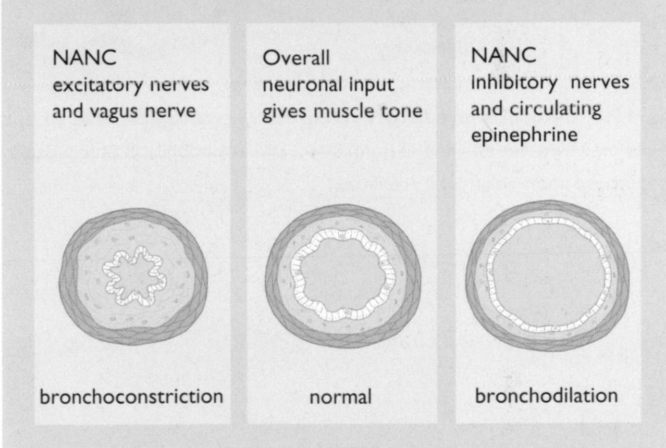

Fig. 11.4 Bronchial smooth muscle tone. Bronchial smooth muscle tone depends upon the balance between the parasympathetic input, circulating epinephrine, nonadrenergic, noncholinergic (NANC) inhibitory nerves, and sympathetic innervation of the parasympathetic ganglia.

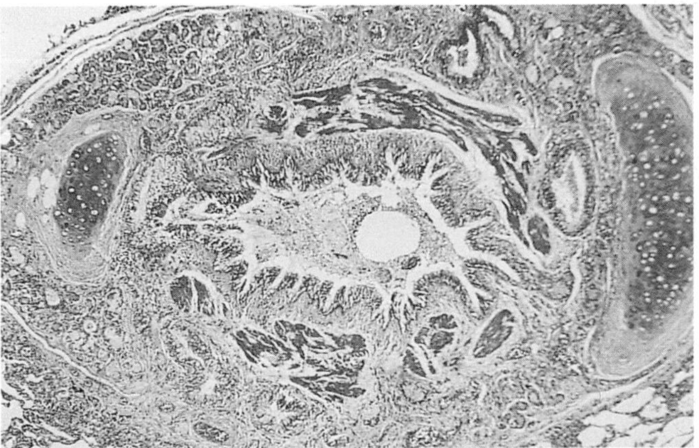

Fig. 11.5 Asthmatic airway. A section of asthmatic airway showing the pathophysiologic changes. (Courtesy of Dr Alan Stevens and Professor James Lowe.)

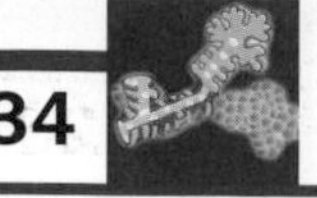

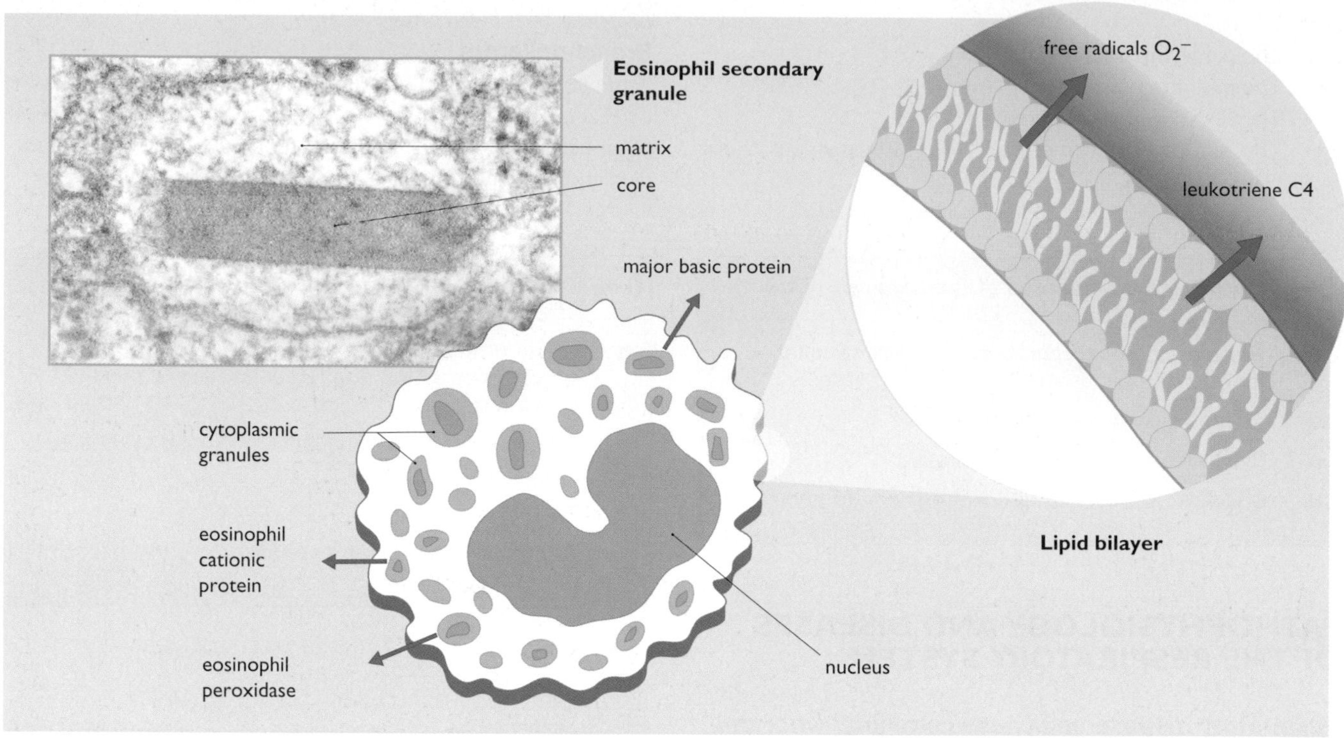

Fig. 11.6 Cytotoxic mediators released by eosinophils lead to epithelial damage. Infiltrating eosinophils release cytotoxic mediators, including major basic protein, eosinophil peroxidase, and eosinophil cationic protein from their granules. Certain inflammatory mediators can be released from the lipid bilayer upon eosinophil activation.

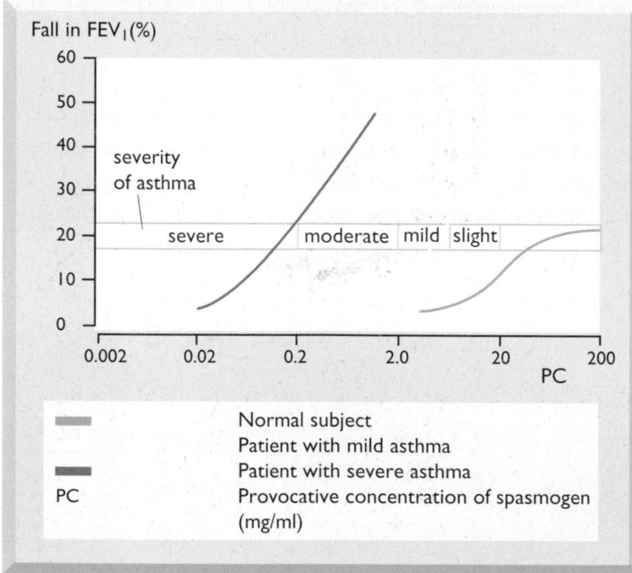

Fig. 11.7 Bronchial hyperresponsiveness. People with bronchial asthma have bronchial hyperresponsiveness, which causes them to cough and wheeze in response to stimuli that would not provoke such responses in normal subjects. Clinically, this hyperresponsiveness can be demonstrated by measuring the change in lung function, which is shown by a reduction in FEV_1 (forced expiratory volume in one second) in response to an inhaled spasmogen such as histamine or methacholine. Increased irritability is observed with increasing disease severity.

β_2 Adrenoceptor agonists are the most widely prescribed drugs for the treatment of the bronchoconstriction in asthma and are available by inhalation from a metered-dose inhaler or nebulizer as well as orally. Short-acting β_2 adrenoceptor agonists for the acute relief of bronchospasm include albuterol, terbutaline, and fenoterol*.

β_2 Adrenoceptor agonists relax airway smooth muscle through the activation of adenylyl cyclase (Fig. 11.9). They are excellent functional antagonists of the bronchoconstriction caused by a wide range of stimuli. One of their drawbacks, however, has been their short biologic half-life (2–3 hours), but a variety of long-acting β_2 adrenoceptor agonists have now been introduced that produce effective bronchodilation for up to 15 hours. The long-acting β_2 adrenoceptor agonists include salmeterol, aformoterol, and bambuterol*. The prolonged action of salmeterol is believed to be due to the presence of a long lipophilic tail, which binds to an 'exoreceptor' in the vicinity of the β_2 adrenoceptor on airway smooth muscle (see Fig. 11.9). These long-acting drugs are intended for long-term prevention of asthma attacks, but are not recommended for acute relief. particularly salmeterol, which has a delayed onset of action. They are particularly useful for treating nocturnal asthma.

The adverse effects of β_2 adrenoceptor agonists include tremor and hypokalemia, and, when given in excessive amounts, tachycardia.

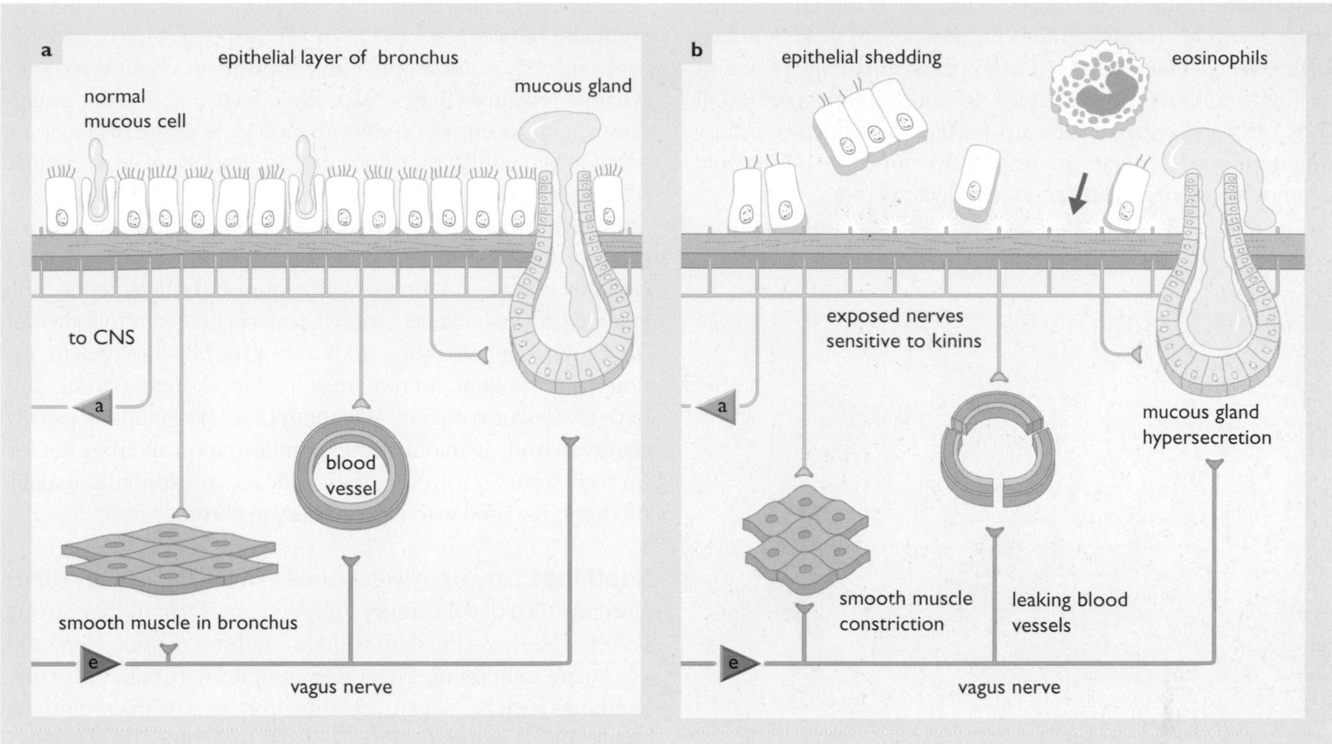

Fig. 11.8 Mechanism of bronchial hyperresponsiveness. This may result from exposure of sensory airway nerves following damage to the ciliated epithelial layer by cytotoxic mediators released by infiltrating eosinophils, which may then become hypersensitive as a result of exposure to inflammatory mediators such as prostaglandins and cytokines. (a) Normal lung; (b) asthmatic lung.

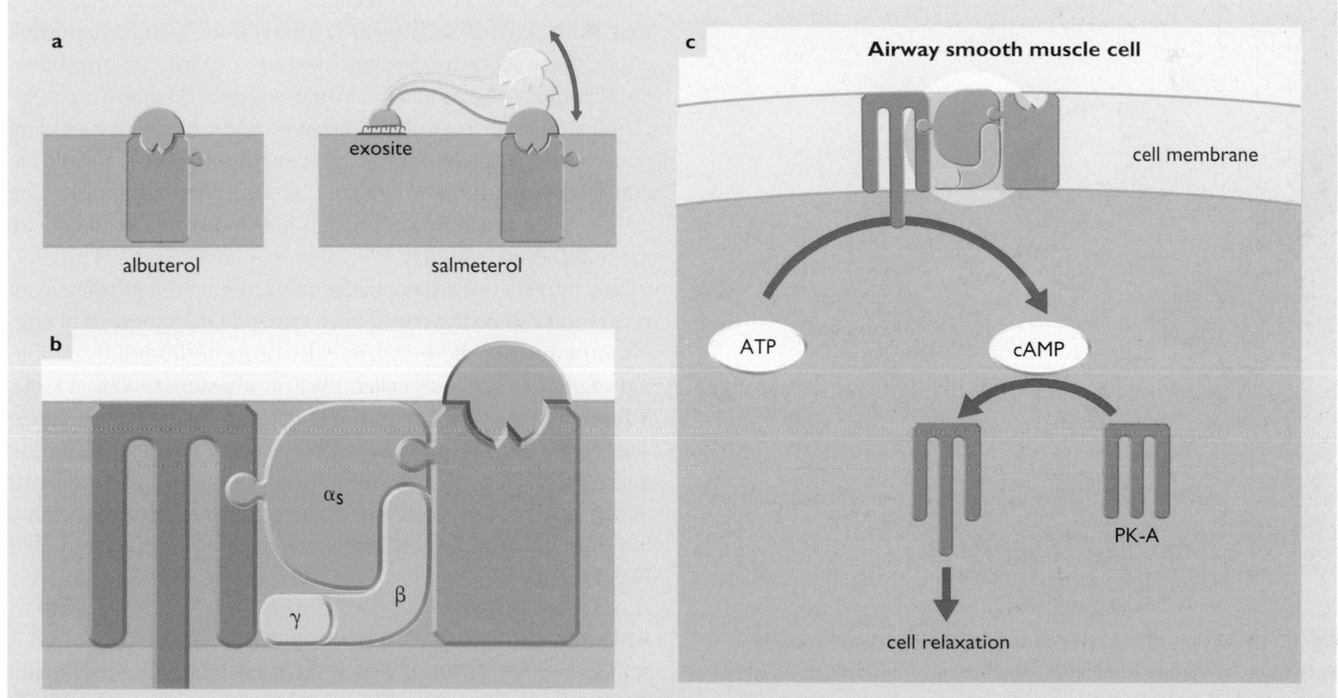

Fig. 11.9 Action of β_2 adrenoceptor agonists on airway smooth muscle. (a,b) β_2 Adrenoceptor agonists (e.g. short-acting albuterol or long-acting salmeterol) relax airway smooth muscle via the activation of G protein-coupled receptors. (c) This leads to the activation of adenylyl cyclase and generation of cAMP. Theophylline may relax airway smooth muscle by inhibiting cAMP phosphodiesterase in the cell, thereby increasing the intracellular concentrations of this second messenger. (PK-A, protein kinase A)

Anticholinergics cause bronchodilation by binding to muscarinic receptors on airway smooth muscle and thereby antagonizing acetylcholine released from parasympathetic nerves in the vagus nerve. Anticholinergics do not therefore prevent all types of bronchospasm, but are particularly effective against irritant-induced changes in respiratory function. Muscarinic receptor antagonists also decrease mucus secretion.

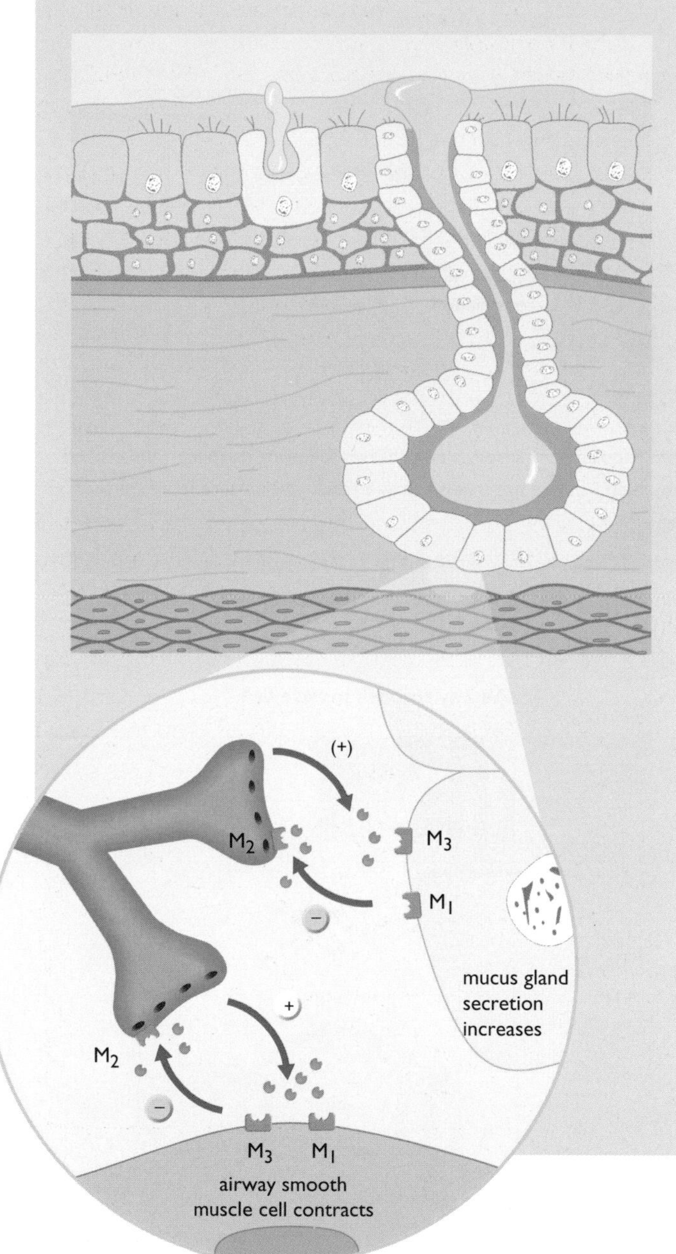

Fig. 11.10 Action of acetylcholine (ACh) on airway smooth muscle. ACh released from parasympathetic neurons acts on M_1 and M_3 muscarinic receptors on airway smooth muscle and submucosal glands to bring about muscle constriction and mucus secretion. In addition, some of the released ACh acts on presynaptic M_2 muscarinic receptors on the nerve terminal to reduce further release of ACh. These M_2 receptors are known as 'autoreceptors.'

Currently available muscarinic receptor antagonists do not discriminate between M_2 and M_3 receptors (Fig. 11.10), and it is likely that M_2 autoreceptor antagonism on cholinergic presynaptic terminals may reduce the effectiveness of the antagonism at M_3 receptors on smooth muscle. Selective M_3 receptor antagonists could therefore be an important therapeutic advance.

Muscarinic antagonists include ipratropium bromide, oxitropium bromide*, and atropine. The first two drugs are used clinically in many countries by the inhaled route to reduce the systemic adverse effects otherwise associated with this class of drugs. When inhaled they are poorly absorbed into the circulation from the lung, do not cross the blood–brain barrier, and have few adverse effects. Maximum bronchodilation is usually observed from 30 minutes after administration and they last for up to 5 hours. However, their efficacy in asthma is usually modest compared with their efficacy in chronic bronchitis.

Xanthines have been widely used in the treatment of asthma since the turn of the century following observations that 'strong coffee' relieved the symptoms of asthma. Coffee, tea, and chocolate-containing beverages contain naturally occurring xanthines such as caffeine and theobromine. The main xanthine used clinically is theophylline, which is sometimes used as theophylline ethylenediamine (aminophylline). Both drugs are usually given orally.

Xanthines are rapidly metabolized and have a short biologic half-life. However, this limitation is overcome by using a 'slow-release' preparation, which will maintain effective plasma concentrations over 16–18 hours.

The major problem with using xanthines as bronchodilators is that they have a very narrow therapeutic window: plasma concentrations over 10 μg/ml are required for effective bronchodilation, but plasma concentrations over 20 μg/ml are associated with an increased likelihood of adverse effects, including nausea, cardiac arrhythmias, and convulsions. Plasma xanthine concentrations should therefore be measured. Aminophylline can be given as a slow intravenous infusion with a loading dose for acute severe asthma.

Drug interactions are important as the serum theophylline concentration can be increased or decreased by a variety of drugs.

Xanthines are believed to produce bronchodilation by inhibiting a family of enzymes called phosphodiesterases (Fig. 11.11). These enzymes take part in the metabolism of the second messengers involved in relaxing airway smooth muscle (i.e. cAMP and cGMP). In particular, inhibition of phosphodiesterase III and IV in airway smooth muscle leads to intracellular accumulation of cAMP and therefore smooth muscle relaxation (see Figs 11.9, 11.12).

Anti-inflammatory and prophylactic drugs

Anti-inflammatory drugs may resolve existing bronchial inflammation and/or prevent subsequent inflammation in asthma. Most anti-inflammatory drugs prevent subsequent inflammation and are therefore classed as prophylactic drugs. As anti-inflammatory drugs are unable to cause bronchodilation, they are not recommended for acute asthma attacks.

Glucocorticosteroids are the best established anti-inflammatory drugs for the treatment of the chronic inflammatory process underlying asthma. They inhibit inflammatory cell infiltration into the airways and reduce edema formation by acting on the vascular endothelium. Glucocorticosteroids:

- Induce synthesis of the polypeptide lipocortin-1, which inhibits phospholipase A_2, a key enzyme in the production of inflammatory mediators, including prostaglandins, leukotrienes, and platelet activating factor (PAF) (Fig. 11.13). It is thought that this is why they are effective in asthma.
- Interact with 'glucocorticosteroid response elements' in inflammatory cells, which are believed to neutralize the transcription factors for the synthesis of cytokines such as interleukin (IL)-5 and tumor necrosis factor (TNF)-α (Fig. 11.14).
- Are unique in having the ability to resolve established inflammatory responses in the airways, though the mechanism responsible for this is not clear.

Drugs for asthma

- All β adrenoceptor agonists promote bronchodilation
- The principal action of glucocorticosteroids is suppression of the inflammatory response
- Xanthines combine bronchodilator and anti-inflammatory properties
- Muscarinic receptor antagonist-induced bronchodilation is occasionally useful

Glucocorticosteroids can be given prophylactically by inhalation to achieve a local anti-inflammatory effect without causing systemic adverse effects. Inhaled glucocorticosteroids used for bronchial asthma include beclomethasone, budesonide, and fluticasone. Oral glucocorticosteroids may be required for severe asthma unresponsive to inhaled glucocorticosteroids, and usually prednisone, methylprednisolone, or prednisolone is prescribed.

Both oral and intravenous glucocorticosteroids are useful in the treatment of acute severe asthma. However, oral glucocorticosteroids have systemic adverse effects suppression of the hypothalamus–pituitary axis. Chronic use can lead to a variety of serious adverse effects, including stunting of growth in children.

Classification of phosphodiesterase isozymes

Family	Isozyme	Tissue	Inhibitors
I	Ca^{2+}/calmodulin dependent	Brain, airway smooth muscle	Vinpocetine Theophylline
II	cGMP stimulated	Heart, vascular smooth muscle, platelets, airway smooth muscle	Theophylline
III	cGMP inhibited	Lymphocyte, platelets, heart, vascular smooth muscle, airway smooth muscle	Milrinone Theophylline
IV	cAMP selective	Inflammatory cells (neutrophil, macrophage, mast cell, eosinophil, lymphocyte) airway smooth muscle, heart, brain, striated muscle	Rolipram Theophylline
V	cGMP selective	Trachea, platelets, vascular smooth muscle	Zaprinast Theophylline

Fig. 11.11 Classification of phosphodiesterase isozymes.

Xanthines not only produce bronchodilation, as described above, but also inhibit inflammatory cell activation and infiltration in the airways of asthmatics. Furthermore, xanthine withdrawal from some asthmatics leads to a worsening of asthma,

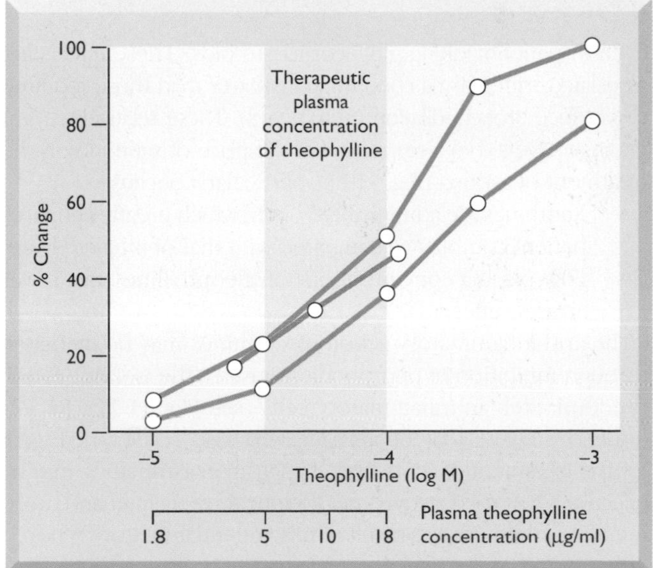

Fig. 11.12 Effects of theophylline at therapeutic concentrations. Percentage change in FEV_1 (red), percentage inhibition of airway smooth muscle relaxation (green), or percentage inhibition of phosphodiesterase activity in airway smooth muscle (purple) in relation to plasma concentrations of theophylline (μg/ml) or theophylline concentration (logM in an isolated tissue experiment). (Adapted with permission from Rabe et al. *Eur Resp J* 1995; 289: 600–603.)

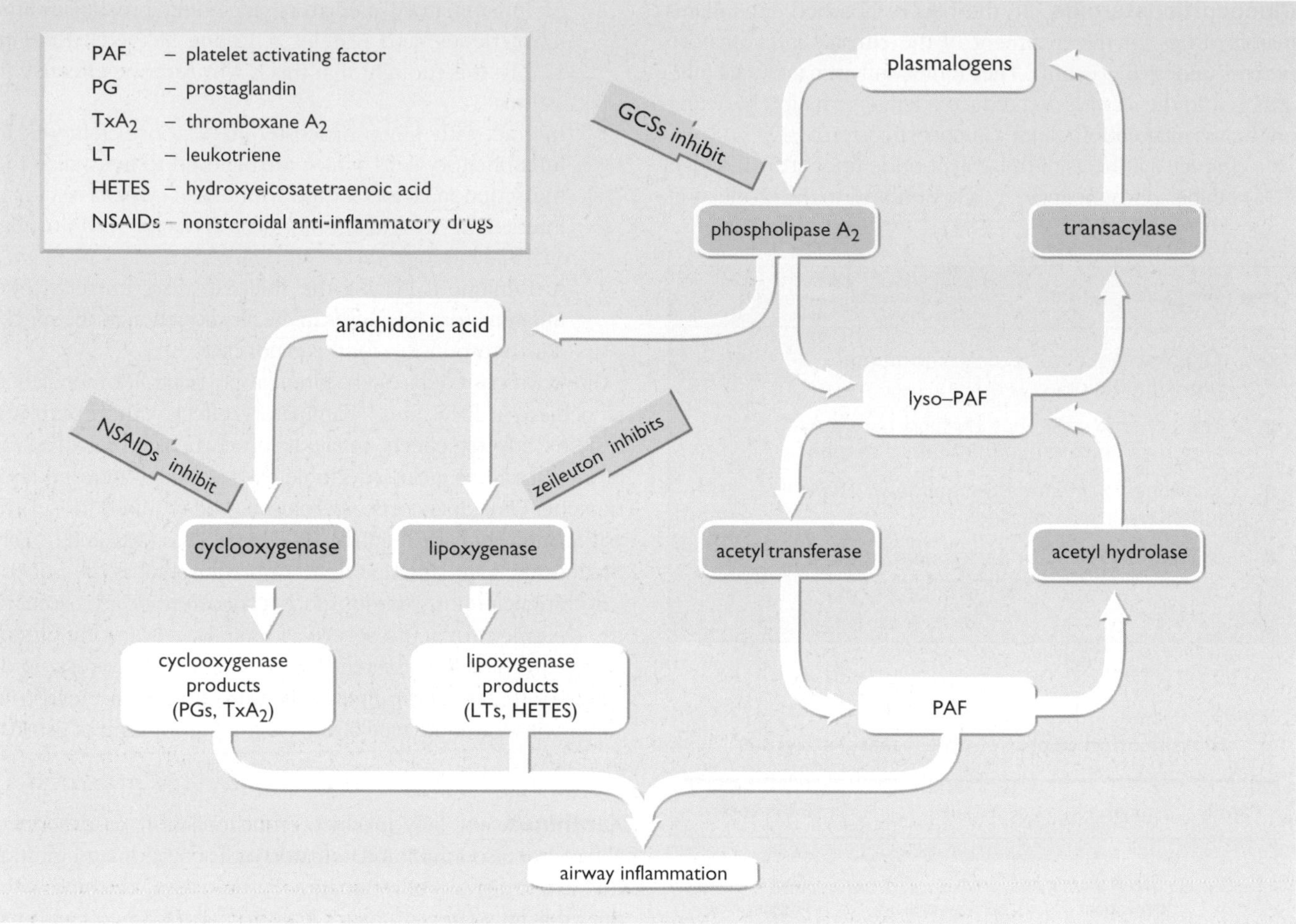

PAF – platelet activating factor
PG – prostaglandin
TxA_2 – thromboxane A_2
LT – leukotriene
HETES – hydroxyeicosatetraenoic acid
NSAIDs – nonsteroidal anti-inflammatory drugs

plasmalogens
GCSs inhibit
phospholipase A_2
transacylase
arachidonic acid
lyso–PAF
NSAIDs inhibit
zeileuton inhibits
cyclooxygenase
lipoxygenase
acetyl transferase
acetyl hydrolase
cyclooxygenase products (PGs, TxA_2)
lipoxygenase products (LTs, HETES)
PAF
airway inflammation

Fig. 11.13 Glucocorticosteroids (GCSs) reduce the production of a variety of lipid inflammatory mediators.

even in patients taking glucocorticosteroids. These effects are associated with plasma concentrations lower than those required to produce bronchodilation (5–10 μg/ml). These relatively recent findings have led to a reappraisal of the place of xanthines in the treatment of asthma (Fig. 11.15), particularly because:

- Xanthines are administered orally, which greatly enhances patient compliance compared with that of inhaled drugs.
- Low plasma concentrations of theophylline have fewer adverse effects.

The anti-inflammatory action of xanthines may be mediated through inhibition of phosphodiesterase IV, the isozyme found predominately in inflammatory cells (see Fig. 11.11). Recent evidence suggests that theophylline, which is an established agent for the treatment of acute bronchospasm in asthmatics, may be effective when used at low doses for long-term maintenance treatment in asthmatics as a result of this anti-inflammatory action.

Cromolyn sodium, ketotifen, and nedocromil sodium are anti-inflammatory drugs used prophylactically in the treatment of bronchial asthma. Cromolyn and nedocromil sodium are active by inhalation. Ketotifen is orally active and is used worldwide except in the US. The mechanisms of action of these prophylactic drugs are not clearly understood, but cromolyn sodium was originally thought to be a 'mast cell stabilizer,' preventing the release of histamine and other inflammatory mediators. It is now clear that this action is not the only effect of these prophylactic drugs. They are capable of affecting many inflammatory cell types including alveolar macrophages, thereby preventing inflammatory cell recruitment into the airway wall. In addition, cromolyn

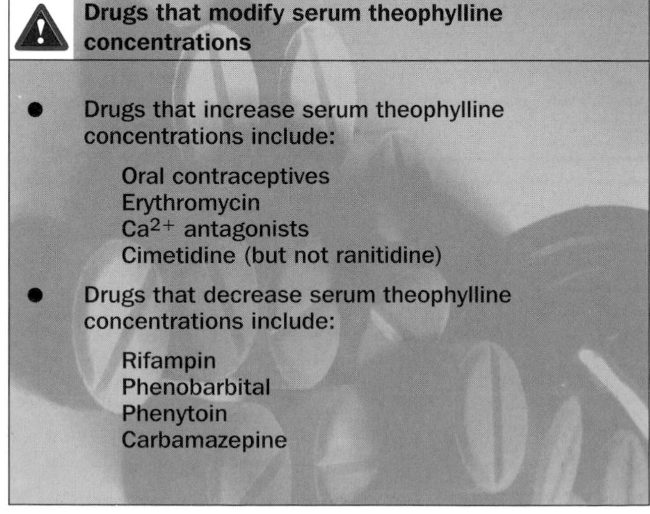

Drugs that modify serum theophylline concentrations

- **Drugs that increase serum theophylline concentrations include:**

  Oral contraceptives
  Erythromycin
  Ca^{2+} antagonists
  Cimetidine (but not ranitidine)

- **Drugs that decrease serum theophylline concentrations include:**

  Rifampin
  Phenobarbital
  Phenytoin
  Carbamazepine

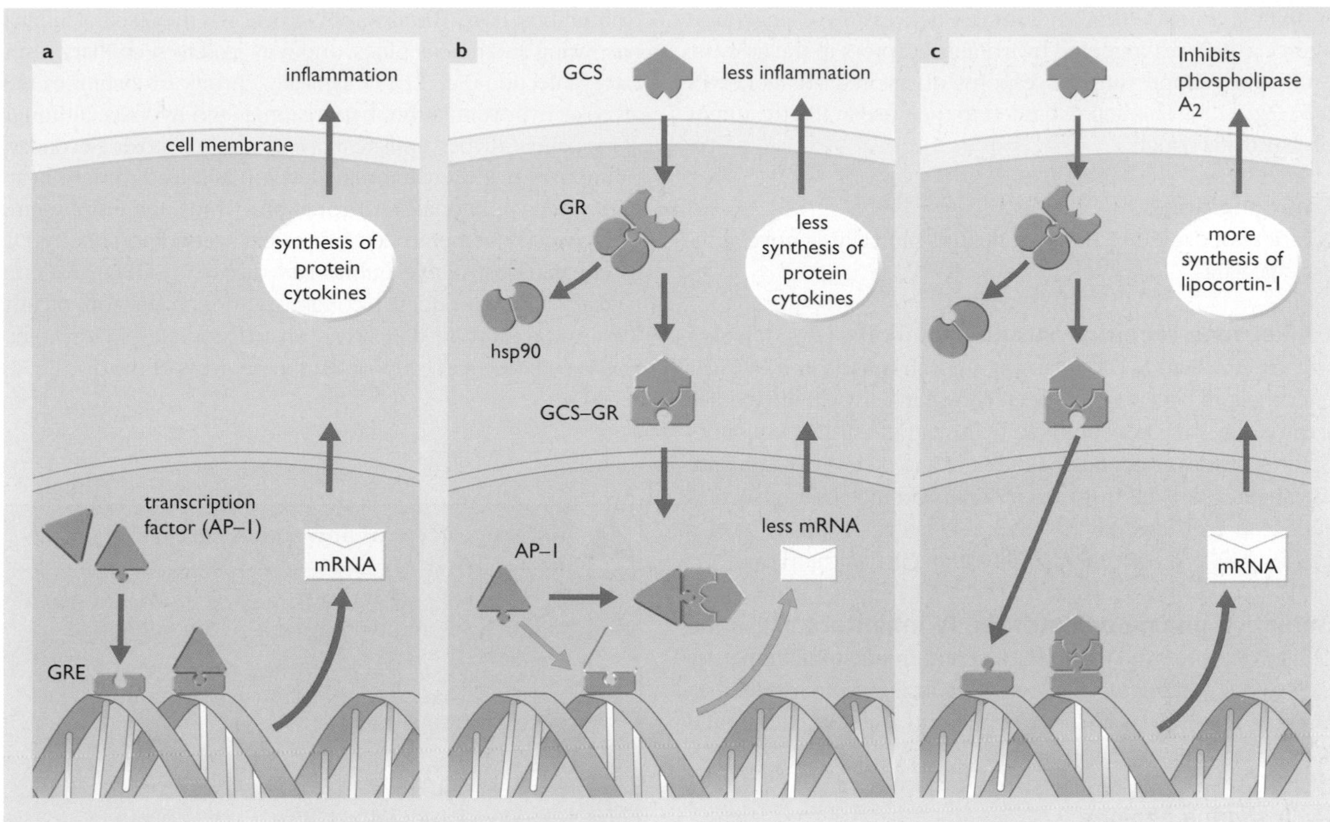

Fig. 11.14 Effect of glucocorticosteroids on gene transcription. (a) Transcription factors (e.g. AP-1) bind to receptors on DNA to bring about mRNA synthesis. This then leads to the synthesis of new proteins (e.g. cytokines), which are released by the cell to cause inflammation. (b) Glucocorticosteroids (GCS) bind to cytosolic glucocorticosteroid receptors (GR), which are normally associated with two molecules of a 90 kD heat shock protein (Hsp90). The GCS–GR complex translocates to the nucleus and binds to glucocorticosteroid response elements (GRE) in the promoter sequences of target genes. (c) This leads to increased transcription of new proteins (e.g. lipocortin-1), or decreased transcription of proteins via binding to transcription factors (e.g. AP-1) resulting in reduced synthesis of inflammatory products (i.e. cytokines, neurokinin 1 [NK1] receptors, inducible nitric oxide synthase [NOS], cyclooxygenase-2, endothelin-1, phospholipase A_2 [PLA_2]).

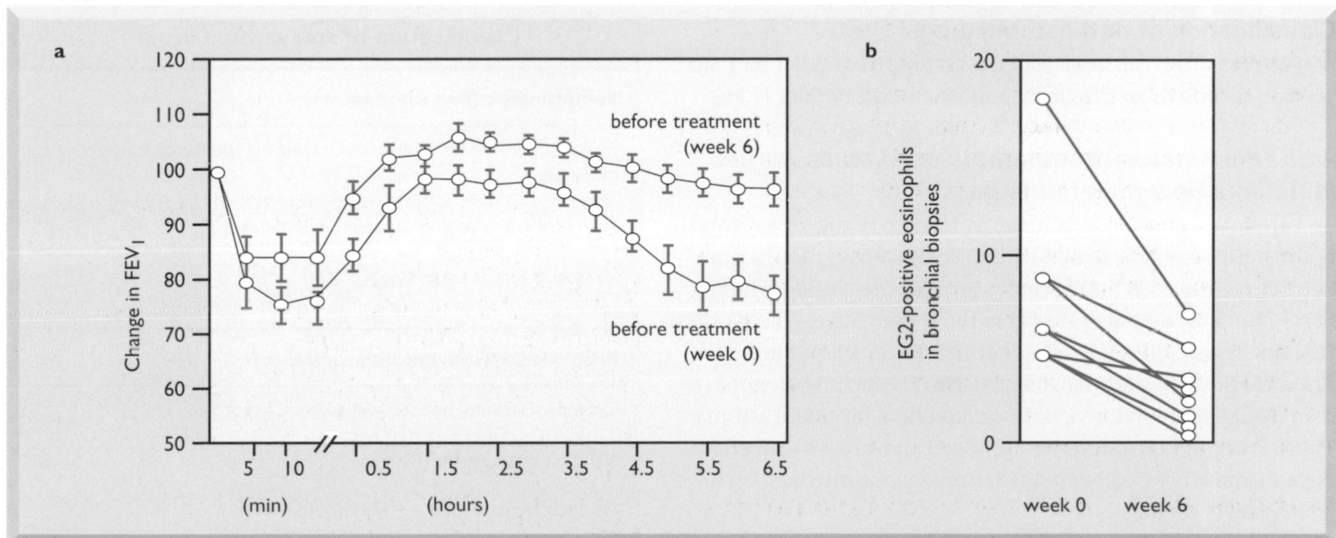

Fig. 11.15 Effect of exposure to allergen in asthma. (a) Exposure to allergen induces immediate bronchoconstriction (shown as a fall in FEV_1 in the first 15 minutes) followed by a later fall in lung function (shown as a fall in FEV_1 from 3.5 to 6.5 hours. (b) The allergic response is associated with recruitment of activated eosinophils into bronchial tissue, which is assessed by the number of eosinophils staining positively with the antibody EG2. EG2 recognizes eosinophils actively secreting the eosinophil derived protein, eosinophil cationic protein (ECP). After 6 weeks of treatment with low-dose theophylline (200 mg twice daily), the magnitude of the late response (a) and the number of infiltrating EG2-positive cells (b) are reduced.

sodium and nedocromil sodium can depress the exaggerated neuronal reflexes triggered by irritant receptors in the airways, probably by suppressing the response of exposed irritant nerves (see Fig. 11.8). This action has led to their use in the treatment of 'asthmatic cough.'

Emerging drugs

A variety of drugs are being evaluated clinically as novel anti-asthma drugs.

Leukotriene receptor antagonists for the peptidoleukotrienes LTC4 and LTD4 on airway smooth muscle and vascular endothelium have recently been shown in early clinical studies to produce some benefit in the treatment of asthma. Inhibitors of the synthesis of peptidoleukotrienes and other 5-lipoxygenase metabolites derived from arachidonic acid metabolism such as zeileuton (see Fig. 11.13) have also been shown to have a modest effect in the treatment of asthma in clinical trials.

Selective phosphodiesterase IV inhibitors inhibit the phosphodiesterase IV isozyme present in most inflammatory cells and are being investigated in clinical trials in asthmatics. Many of these drugs are active orally and are being developed as novel anti-inflammatory agents.

Cyclosporine analogs

Lymphocytes play an important role in regulating eosinophil infiltration into the lungs of asthmatics. Cyclosporine has been successfully used in the treatment of immune disorders involving lymphocytes and has recently been shown to have some clinical benefit in asthmatics resistant to therapy with glucocorticosteroids. However, it has considerable adverse effects and so there is a growing interest in finding safer analogs of this drug to use in the treatment of asthma and other diseases.

Classification of anti-asthma drugs

Anti-asthma drugs can be classified according to whether they are bronchodilator, prophylactic, or anti-inflammatory (Fig. 11.16).

Anti-inflammatory treatment is used much earlier in asthma now than in the past

As asthma is a chronic inflammatory disease of the airways and not just a disease associated with bronchoconstriction, a number of organizations and societies around the world including the National Institutes of Health in the United States, the World Health Organization, the Canadian Thoracic Society, the British Thoracic Society, and the Australasian Thoracic Society have issued guidelines on the optimal treatment of bronchial asthma. These are based on a stepwise approach, but stress the need for anti-inflammatory treatment much earlier in the disease than has been used in the past.

CHRONIC BRONCHITIS

Chronic bronchitis is caused by airway luminal narrowing and mucus plugs

Chronic bronchitis is defined in functional terms as a disorder associated with the excessive production of sputum and cough daily or most days. The airway obstruction is the result of luminal narrowing and mucus plugs, and may lead to secondary respiratory infection (Fig. 11.17). Typically, chronic bronchitis causes alveolar hypoventilation, hypercapnia, and hypoxia, although some patients hyperventilate to avoid severe hypoxia. Secondary pulmonary hypertension may develop and lead to right heart failure (cor pulmonale). Chronic bronchitis and emphysema often occur together in heavy smokers, a condition referred to as chronic obstructive pulmonary disease (COPD). Patients typically have a productive cough, sputum production, breathlessness on exertion, and airway obstruction. Respiratory infection is common and can worsen the progress of the disease.

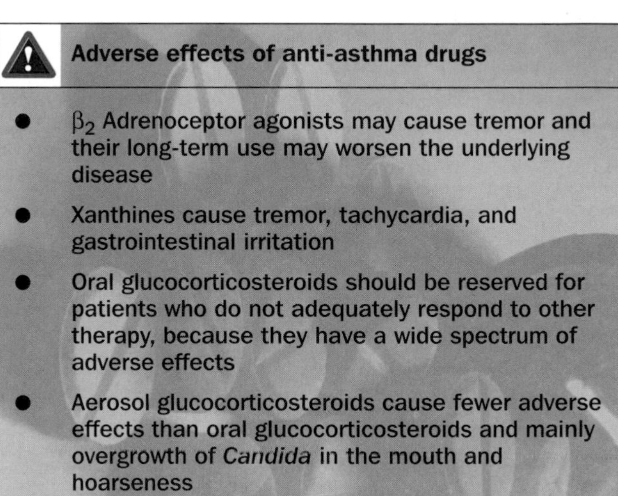

Adverse effects of anti-asthma drugs

- β_2 Adrenoceptor agonists may cause tremor and their long-term use may worsen the underlying disease
- Xanthines cause tremor, tachycardia, and gastrointestinal irritation
- Oral glucocorticosteroids should be reserved for patients who do not adequately respond to other therapy, because they have a wide spectrum of adverse effects
- Aerosol glucocorticosteroids cause fewer adverse effects than oral glucocorticosteroids and mainly overgrowth of *Candida* in the mouth and hoarseness

Classification of anti-asthma drugs
Symptomatic (bronchodilators)
β_2 Adrenoceptor agonists (short-acting e.g. albuterol; long-acting e.g. salmeterol)
Anticholinergics (e.g. ipratropium bromide)
Xanthines (e.g. theophylline)
Prophylactic (prevent inflammation)
Cromolyn sodium, nedocromil sodium, ketotifen
Xanthines (e.g. theophylline)
Glucocorticosteroids (e.g. budesonide)
Anti-inflammatory (resolve inflammation)
Glucocorticosteroids (e.g. budesonide)

Fig. 11.16 Classification of anti-asthma drugs.

Bronchodilators, mucolytics, and antibiotics are used to treat chronic bronchitis

Bronchodilators

β_2 Adrenoceptor agonists (short- and long-acting) are used to treat breathlessness on exertion in chronic bronchitis, but are generally less effective than in the treatment of bronchial asthma because less of the airways obstruction is due to abnormal airway smooth muscle contraction.

Xanthines are used in the treatment of chronic bronchitis, particularly for their effects on airway smooth muscle. They also have central nervous system (CNS) effects, leading to increased alertness, which may be important in chronic bronchitis, and can increase diaphragm contractility.

Mucolytic drugs

***N*-Acetylcysteine** breaks the disulfide bonds that hold mucus glycocoproteins together and thereby reduce the viscosity of mucus. *N*-Acetylcysteine and a related drug ambroxil have been shown to have some clinical benefit in the treatment of COPD.

Anticholinergics are the mainstay of therapy for chronic bronchitis because they can reduce much of the bronchospasm associated with smoking and the subsequent inhalation of irritants. Their ability to reduce mucus secretion in the airway by antagonizing acetylcholine acting on muscarinic receptors in mucus glands is also very beneficial (see Fig. 11.9).

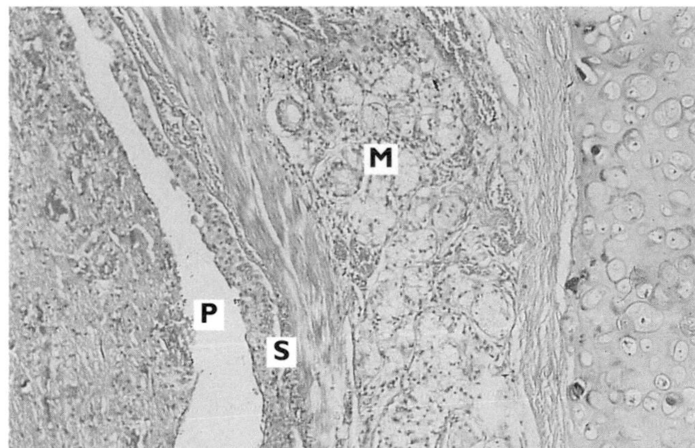

Fig. 11.17 Chronic bronchitis. The main abnormality is hypersecretion of mucus, which plugs the airway (P). Hypersecretion is associated with hypertrophy and hyperplasia of bronchial mucus-secreting glands (M). The Reid index, which is the ratio of gland:wall thickness in the bronchus, is increased in chronic bronchitis. Inflammation is typically absent, although excessive mucus production is frequently associated with the development of coincidental respiratory tract infections, leading to secondary inflammation. Squamous metaplasia (S) is common in patients who have persistent or recurrent superimposed infections. (Courtesy of Dr Alan Stevens and Professor James Lowe.)

Antibiotics

Patients with chronic bronchitis commonly get secondary bacterial infections colonizing the sputum. Antibiotics are therefore often prescribed for these patients and are discussed in more detail on p. 247.

ADULT RESPIRATORY DISTRESS SYNDROME

Adult respiratory distress syndrome (ARDS) is an acute life-threatening condition. It results from increased leakiness of the pulmonary capillary network leading to hypoxia, reduced lung compliance, alveolar infiltrates, and noncardiogenic pulmonary edema. It is common in patients with sepsis, which accounts for 50% of ARDS cases. The mortality rate of ARDS is approximately 60–70%.

Current therapy for ARDS is inadequate

No widely available drug prevents the onset of ARDS or lessens its lethality. However, there are promising studies in animals and case reports of emerging therapies for the future including monoclonal antibodies directed against cytokines, PAF, TNF, and IL-1 receptor antagonists.

CYSTIC FIBROSIS

Cystic fibrosis is usually associated with a mutation in a specific protein essential for apical Cl^- clearance

Cystic fibrosis is an inherited disease that starts early in childhood and affects the airways and ducts in various organs, principally the lungs, pancreas, and sweat glands.

Most patients with cystic fibrosis have a mutation in a specific protein that is essential for apical Cl^- clearance (Fig. 11.18). This results in defective Cl^- clearance and excessive Na^+ reabsorption and, as a consequence of osmotic changes, excessive water reabsorption. The defect results in thick and viscous secretion in ducted organs, typically in the airways of the lung, and ducts of the pancreas and sweat glands in homozygotes. In the lungs this gives rise to areas in which inspired air is poorly circulated, and subsequent bacterial infection (involving *Staphylococcus aureus, Pseudomonas aeruginosa*, or other organisms) results in irreversible lung damage (bronchiectasis). Analogous processes involving retained secretions occur in the other organs.

Mucolytics, antisecretory agents, antibiotics, and physiotherapy are used to treat cystic fibrosis

The recent discovery of the nature of the genetic defect underlying cystic fibrosis has increased the chance of developing effective therapies, including gene therapy, to produce a true cure. At present, gene therapy is not available.

People with cystic fibrosis have a markedly reduced life expectancy, but it can be significantly extended by aggressive therapy with drugs and physiotherapy. Current therapy of the pulmonary effects centers on:

- Thinning secretions and thereby keeping airways and organ ducts patent.
- Combating opportunistic infections (Fig. 11.19).

The purulent mucus secreted by people with cystic fibrosis is characteristically yellow and rich in DNA tangles (from killed

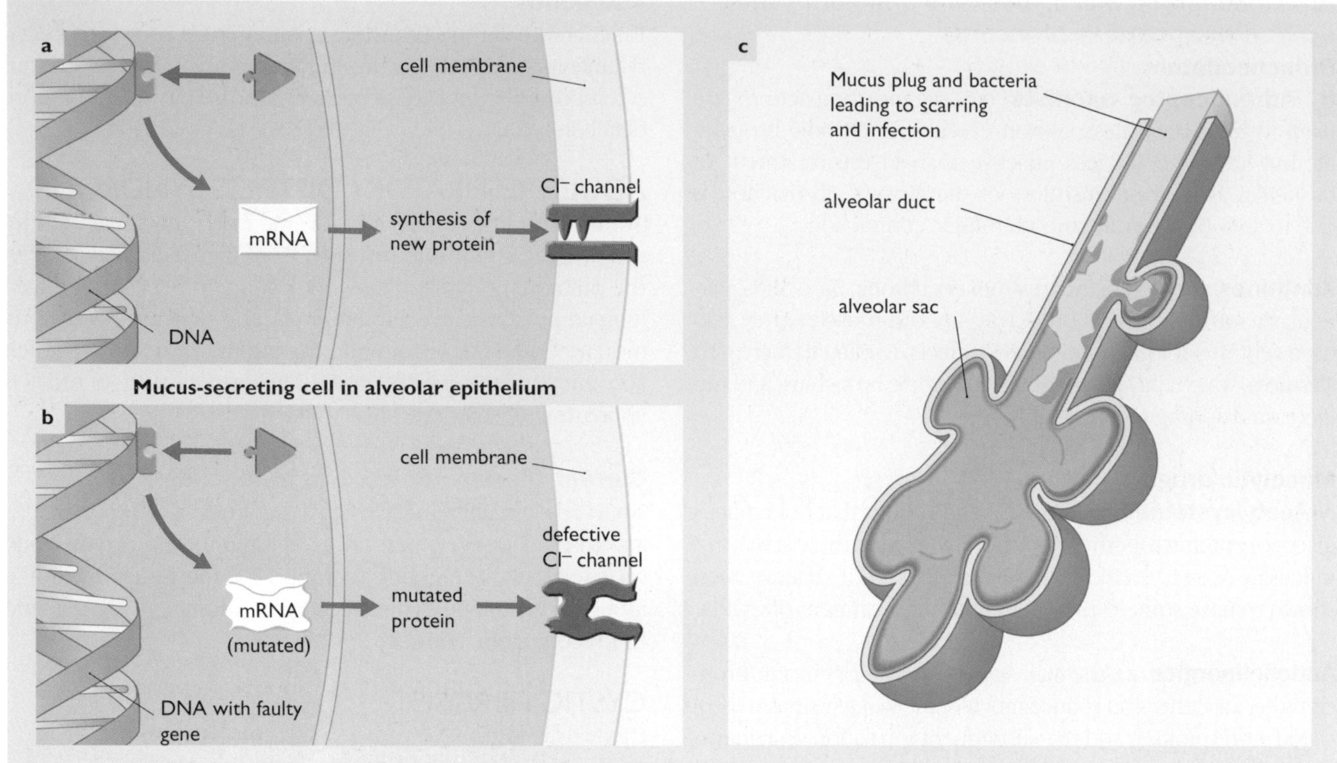

Fig. 11.18 Pathophysiologic elements of cystic fibrosis. Mutations in a specific protein essential for the Cl^- channel result in defective Cl^- clearance and water resorption. This results in thick and viscous secretions in ducted organs.

cells), which has led to the use of DNAases to loosen secretions further (see below).

Mucolytics and antisecretory agents

Respiratory tract fluid secretion is reduced by anticholinergic drugs (muscarinic receptor antagonists). A variety of other drugs will increase the movement of fluid and reduce its viscosity.

- Expectorants increase the fluidity of the secretions and thereby improve the productivity of coughing. Typical expectorants include glyceryl guaiacolate, which can be given orally, and menthol* and camphor, which are given as a vapor, but the effectiveness of these agents is limited. Potassium iodide may have better expectorant properties.
- Mucolytic agents decrease the viscosity of secretions. *N*-Acetylcysteine breaks the disulfide bonds that help pack the mucin molecule and thereby make it more viscous. However, it has many adverse effects including nausea, vomiting, stomatitis, and rhinorrhea.
- Agents that break down DNA tangles (e.g. recombinant DNAases given by aerosol) have recently been shown to be effective in the treatment of cystic fibrosis.

Therapeutic approaches to cystic fibrosis

Problem	Approach
Defective gene	Replace
Defective gene product	Add
Increased Na^+ reabsorption	Increase Na^+ excretion (amiloride)
Thick stagnant mucus	Expectorants, mucolytics, DNAases, physical therapy
Bacterial infection (*Staphylococcus aureus, Pseudomonas aeruginosa*)	Antibiotics
Irreversible lung damage	Lung transplant

Fig. 11.19 Therapeutic approaches to cystic fibrosis.

Antibiotics

The typical bacteria found in the lungs of patients with cystic fibrosis are *S. aureus* (early in the disease) and *P. aeruginosa*. Pneumonia is therefore particularly common. The first-line antibiotics used to treat this are gentamicin, tobramycin, or amikacin together with one of the following: ciprofloxacin, ticarcillin, imipenen, ceftazidime, and piperacillin. Tobramycin is often given as an aerosol. If there is excessive lung damage the patient may require a lung transplant.

NONSPECIFIC COUGH

Coughing is a valuable reflex, but may require treatment if it becomes distressing and exhausting

Cough is a reflex triggered by mechanical or chemical stimulation of the upper respiratory tract, or by central stimuli

(Fig. 11.20). It is a protective mechanism that serves to expel foreign bodies and unwanted material from the airways (Fig. 11.21). However, coughing is sometimes both useless and distressing and can psychologically and physically exhaust the patient. Cough suppression is then indicated.

As a reflex mechanism, a cough involves an arc (see Fig. 11.20) with sensor, central, and efferent components. The exact nature of the sensory receptors for cough are unknown. However, anatomically, cough-sensitive nerves extend from the larynx to the division of the segmental bronchi. The exact pathway of afferent fibres involved in cough and the exact location of the CNS relay (cough center) are also unknown. The efferent pathway for cough involves the intercostal and phrenic nerves. Abrupt contraction of the respiratory muscles leads to an explosive rise in intrathoracic pressure, which forces air out of the alveoli and through the airways.

The sensor and central components of the reflex arc are targets for drugs used to suppress cough

Drugs to suppress cough reduce either:

- Receptor activation and therefore the activity in afferent nerves.
- The sensitivity of the 'cough center.'

Drugs that reduce receptor activation

A variety of agents act at peripheral sites. These drugs act directly in some way to reduce the sensitivity of 'cough receptors' to substances such as irritant chemicals and autacoids, which activate the receptors.

Menthol* vapor inhalation reduces the sensitivity of peripheral cough receptors in animals. This probably also occurs in humans. Sucking lozenges impregnated with menthol* or eucalyptus oil will also reduce the tendency to cough.

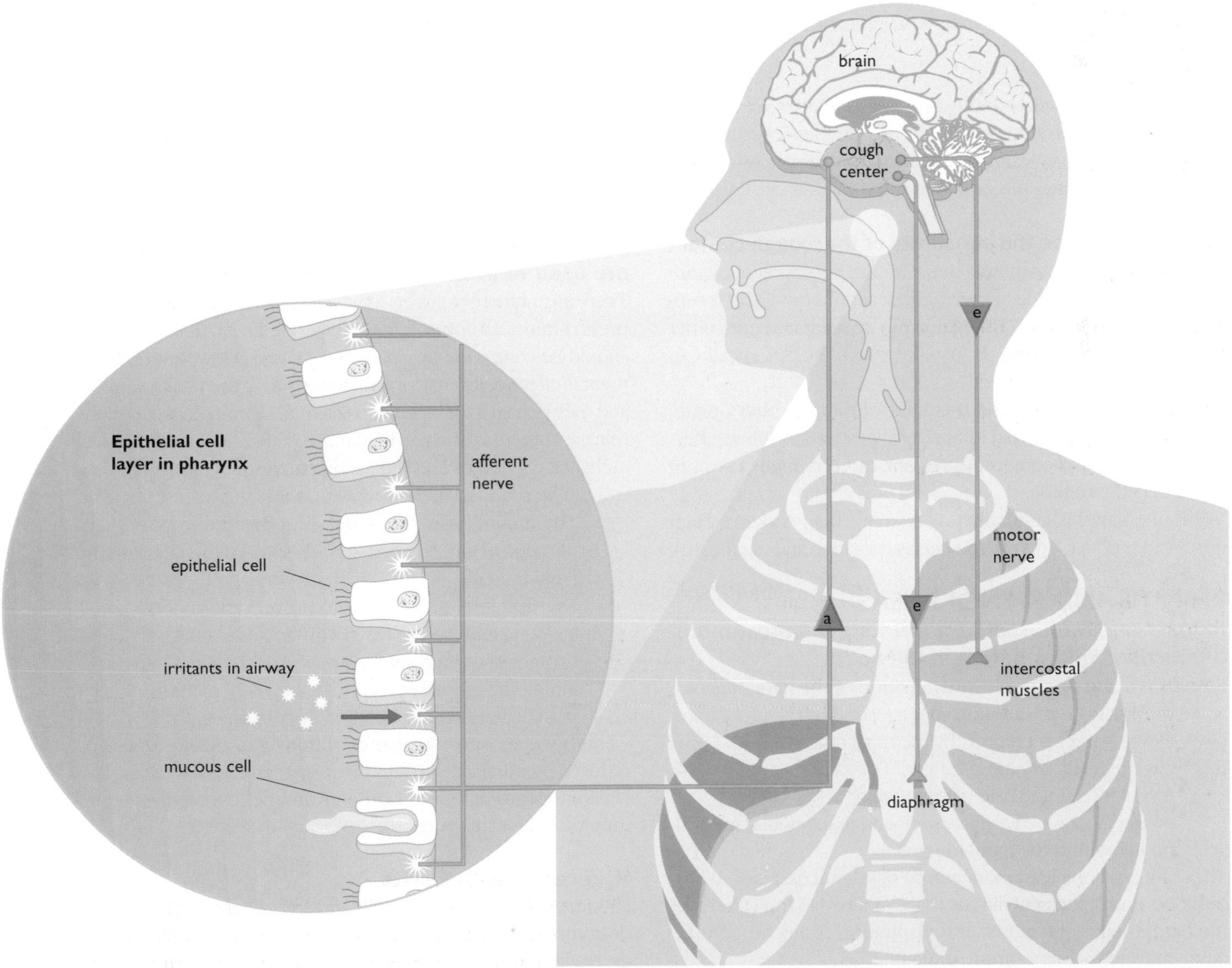

Fig. 11.20 Cough reflex arc. Coughing may be triggered by mechanical, chemical, or central stimuli. (a, afferent nerves; e, efferent nerves)

Causes of cough				
Mechanical	**Inflammatory**	**Extrathoracic**	**Abnormal cough reflex**	**Central**
Bronchitis	Asthma	Postnasal drip	Viral infection	Psychogenic
Pneumonia	Viral infection	Esophageal reflux	Asthma	
Cystic fibrosis and asthma	Pollutants	Middle ear disease	ACEI	
Tumor, granuloma, blood, edema	ACEI		Idiopathic	
Foreign body	Interstitial disease			

Fig. 11.21 Causes of cough. (ACEI, angiotensin-converting enzyme inhibitor) (Adapted with permission from *Cough* by Fuller, in *The Lung* by Crystal and West, Raven Press, New York, 1991.)

Topical local anesthetics such as benzocaine applied to the pharynx and larynx, can reduce the sensitivity of the 'cough receptors' in these areas to irritant chemical or physical stimuli.

Benzonatate is taken orally and is thought to act on both peripheral and central receptors. It is probably less effective than codeine (see below) and is chemically related to the local anesthetic tetracaine. It is available in the US, but not Canada.

Drugs that reduce the sensitivity of the 'cough center'

Opioids Heroin, morphine, and codeine possess central antitussive actions by virtue of their agonist actions on opiate receptors in the cough center. This action can be separated from other opioid effects. Codeine is usually used therapeutically in proprietary 'cough mixtures.'

Dextromethorphan is the *d*-isomer of methyl ether opiate, levorphanol, and is devoid of analgesic properties. It is as effective as codeine as a cough suppressant, but very high doses can cause CNS depression.

Chlophedianol is generally less effective than codeine. High doses can produce CNS effects such as excitation and nightmares.

RHINITIS AND RHINORRHEA

Rhinitis and rhinorrhea are irritating manifestations of mucosal inflammation in the nose

Rhinitis is acute or chronic inflammation of the nasal mucosa, while rhinorrhea is a condition characterized by the production of excessive watery secretions by the nasal mucosa. Both occur mainly as the result of either:

- A viral infection of the nasal mucosa.
- An interaction between antigens and tissue-bound IgE antibodies within the nasal mucosa.

These interactions lead to increased nasal mucosal blood flow, or blood vessel permeability, or both. As a result, the volume of the nasal mucosa increases and inspiration of air through the nasal passages becomes more difficult.

The blood supply to the nasal mucosa includes extensive collaterals and venous sinuses to provide sufficient blood flow to keep the nasal mucosa warm and moist. The most important physiologic controlling mechanism for nasal blood flow is sympathetic neural tone, though autacoids also play a role (Fig. 11.22). Sympathetic activity reduces rhinitis and rhinorrhea, clears the nasal passages, and facilitates breathing. Sympatholytic drugs (adrenergic neuron blockers and α adrenoceptor antagonists) can cause nasal congestion.

H_1 receptor antagonists (antihistamines), anti-inflammatory drugs, and nasal vasoconstrictors are used to treat rhinitis and rhinorrhea

There are a variety of targets at which drugs can be aimed to suppress rhinitis and control rhinorrhea (Fig 11.23). Ideally, rhinitis should be controlled by targeting its cause. However, no treatment is effective against viral infections (e.g. the common cold) and they remain a therapeutic challenge. Immunologic reactions release autocoids such as histamine, which is one of the final mediators of rhinitis and the accompanying sneezing, and control can be achieved in the following ways:

- The immune reaction can be moderated by a local application of glucocorticosteroids sprayed directly onto the nasal mucosa.
- The next level of control is to prevent the antibody interaction resulting in release of autocoids.
- Cromolyn sodium can be applied to the nasal mucosa to inhibit the release of histamine and other autacoids from mast cells and other inflammatory cells.

The hypersecretory phase of rhinitis can be prevented or reduced by using a drug to vasoconstrict the nasal mucosa, and α adrenoceptor agonists (sympathomimetics) are most commonly used for this purpose.

H_1 receptor antagonists

Histamine is stored in mast cells and can be released by physical or chemical stimuli. The major autacoid released during an allergic reaction in the nasal mucosa is histamine, which acts on the nasal mucosa, predominantly via H_1 receptors. H_1 receptor

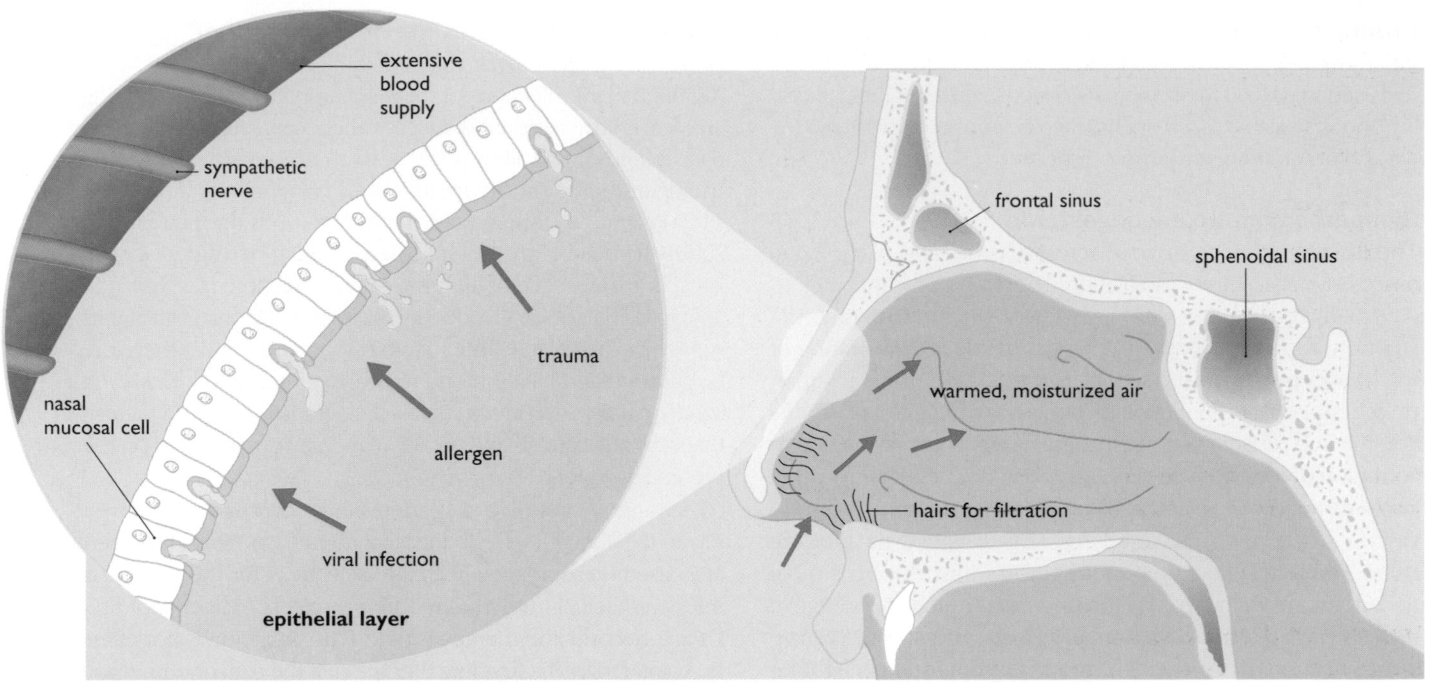

Fig. 11.22 Mechanisms of rhinitis and rhinorrhea. Sympathetic input is the most important physiologic controlling system regulating the extensive blood supply to the nasal mucosa. Fluid hypersecretion occurs in response to a variety of stimuli.

Targets in the treatment of rhinitis and rhinorrhea

Target	Treatment
Nasal blood flow	Vasoconstrictors
Anti-inflammatory	Glucocorticosteroids
Suppression of mediator release	Cromolyn sodium
Mediator receptor blockade	H_1 receptor antagonists Leukotriene antagonists

Fig. 11.23 Targets in the treatment of rhinitis and rhinorrhea.

antagonists (antihistamines) are therefore useful in the treatment of allergic rhinitis. It cannot be assumed that there is no H_2 receptor involvement, but there have been no reports that H_2 antihistamines are effective against allergic rhinitis, even though the vasodilation associated with rhinitis may have an H_2 mediated component.

Newer H_1 receptor antagonists with longer half-lives produce less sedation

There are various different chemical types of H_1 receptor antagonist (antihistamines). H_1 receptor antagonists can also be divided into two groups:

- One group with a relatively short metabolic half-life (less than 12 hours) (e.g. mepyramine* and chlorpheniramine).
- The other group has a longer half-life (over 12 hours) (e.g. cetirizine, astemizole, and terfenadine).

The H_1 receptor antagonists with a longer half-life are a more recent development and have been developed to overcome the major incapacitating adverse effect of sedation produced by the older H_1 receptor antagonists. The sedation produced by H_1 receptor antagonists may involve both specific and nonspecific effects. The effect of the newer agents with longer half-lives to produce less sedation may be partly explained by their different pharmacokinetic characteristics: they may take longer to accumulate in the CNS and so sedation develops more slowly.

The degree of sedation produced by the older H_1 receptor antagonists varies according to the chemical type of the drug, the dose, and the patient. Although not all patients develop the same degree of sedation, it is sufficiently common to warn the patient against taking other CNS depressants (e.g. alcohol). The sedation produced by these older H_1 receptor antagonists is unsurprising since they have chemical structures similar to those of other CNS depressants.

Anti-inflammatory drugs

Glucocorticosteroids have marked anti-inflammatory actions. They also produce many adverse effects, including excessive suppression of the immune system, exacerbation of infections, and suppression of the adrenocortical axis, which are mainly seen following oral administration (see Chapter 17). Most of these adverse effects can be avoided if smaller doses are applied regionally or topically, although this can be associated with a local suppression of the immune reaction, giving rise to the possibility of subsequent local infection.

The most widely used glucocorticosteroids applied topically to the nasal mucosa are beclomethasone, budesonide, and fluticasone, which are regularly sprayed as an aerosol into the nostril. The use of beclomethasone in this way is not associated with major systemic adverse effects.

Cromolyn sodium suppresses the release of autacoids from inflammatory cells involved in an allergic reaction (see p. 240). It is used to reduce the itching associated with rhinitis and sneezing and is available as a suspension to be applied topically to the nasal mucosa using an aerosol dispenser.

Sympathomimetic decongestants

The inflammatory and hypersecretory processes of the nasal mucosa involve active vasodilation. Therefore, one approach to control hypersecretion is to oppose vasodilation with vasoconstriction, which is effectively achieved by the administration of α adrenoceptor agonists (see Chapter 8). These drugs act upon α_1 adrenoceptors in the nasal mucosa which decreases its volume and resistance to movement of air. This may be due to activation of receptors on venous capacitance vessels. Activation of α adrenoceptors, possibly α_2, in nutrient arteries may lead to vasoconstriction of these vessels, possibly damaging the mucosal layer. The α adrenoceptor agonists were introduced as nasal decongestants many years before there was much knowledge of the subtypes of α adrenoceptors. Systematic attempts to evaluate selective agonists for their efficacy as decongestants might be useful.

α Adrenoceptor agonists will produce a degree of nasal vasoconstriction and decongestion when taken orally, but commonly cause generalized vasoconstriction and a tendency to elevate blood pressure. Nevertheless, drugs such as phenylephrine are included in proprietary (over-the-counter) oral mixtures for the treatment of rhinitis and rhinorrhea.

Emerging drugs

Leukotriene antagonists have been shown to be effective against allergic rhinitis in clinical trials.

RESPIRATORY INFECTIONS

The respiratory tract is a warm, moist environment lined with epithelial tissue that encounters inspired air laden with pathogens (see Fig. 11.1). Invading organisms include viruses, bacteria, fungi, and parasites.

Most common infections of the respiratory tract are due to viruses and bacteria. Some are relatively innocuous (e.g. the common cold), while others can be life-threatening (e.g. viral or bacterial pneumonia). The ease with which infection occurs in the respiratory tract varies according to the health of the individual. For example lung infection with *Pneumocystis carinii* is common in patients with the acquired immunodeficiency syndrome (AIDS). Furthermore, certain organisms invade only certain parts of the tract.

The oropharyngeal cavity is liable to infection by bacteria, viruses, and fungi. Viral infection is usually self-limiting, although it leaves the tissue susceptible to secondary infection by bacteria and fungi. *Candida albicans* is the most common fungal infection and follows a disturbance of immune status (e.g. systemic immunosuppression therapy or aerosol treatment of asthma with glucocorticosteroids).

The trachea and bronchi can be infected by viruses and bacteria. Viral infection often leaves the respiratory tract liable to superinfection with bacteria.

Antibiotics can lead to the development of resistant organisms

Although many infections of the respiratory tract are self-limiting and leave little residual damage, others can cause permanent damage and chronically reduce the total capacity of the lungs. The use of antibiotics in the treatment of bacterial infections (Fig. 11.24) carries a unique potential risk to both the patient and society because of the possible development of resistant organisms. In the absence of life-threatening infection, the choice of antibiotic is based on the identity of the invading organism and its sensitivity to available antibiotics. The organism must therefore be cultured and its antibiotic sensitivity determined. However, some organisms produce such a characteristic infection pattern that clinical diagnosis and choice of therapy can be based on the presentation alone.

The range of antibiotics sharing similar properties has given rise to the concept of first-line, second-line, and third-line therapy based on their specificity and selectivity for the particular infective bacterium. First-line therapy refers to agents of first choice. Second-line therapy is used if the infection is not effectively treated by the first-line therapy, or if the patient cannot tolerate the first-line therapy.

Antibiotics used for specific respiratory tract infections

Epiglottitis The cephalosporin derivatives cefuroxime, cefotaxime, and ceftriaxone are used to treat life-threatening epiglottitis due to *Haemophilus influenzae* (type B), with chloramphenicol as a second-line drug. Chloramphenicol is effective, but can cause a lethal aplastic anemia (incidence approximately 1/30,000).

Pharyngitis There are no effective drugs to treat infectious inflammation of the pharynx caused by viruses. Streptococcal group A bacteria produce the most troublesome infection and penicillins (V initially) are first-line antibiotics. Erythromycin is second-line therapy and cephalexin third line (Fig. 11.25).

Laryngitis and acute rhinitis of the common cold are viral infections. They are usually not treated, although the secondary bacterial infection that may occur can be treated with antibiotics. It is generally accepted that prescribing antibiotics specifically for viral infections of the upper respiratory tract is poor medical practice because of the risk of encouraging the development of resistant organisms.

Factors determining the use of antibiotics

- Clinical presentation of infection
- Identity of the infecting organism and its risk to the patient
- Sensitivity of the organism to individual antibiotics
- Likelihood of emergence of resistance
- Accessibility of drugs to the organism
- Availability of an effective antibiotic
- Adverse effects of effective antibiotics
- Pharmacodynamics and pharmacokinetics
- Pharmacoeconomics

Fig. 11.24 Factors determining the use of antibiotics.

Sinusitis A variety of organisms are responsible for sinusitis in adults including *Streptococcus pneumoniae, H. influenzae, Micrococcus catarrhalis*, streptococci, Gram-negative bacilli, anaerobes, and respiratory viruses. Amoxicillin is generally the first-line antibiotic, while trimethoprim/sulfamethoxazole, rifampin, cefuroxime axetil, cefaclor, cefixime, amoxicillin/clavulanate are second line. Trimethoprim, doxycycline, and clarithromycin are third line.

In children with acute sinusitis, with or without perforation and infection with bacteria such as *S. pneumonia, H. influenzae, M. catarrhalis*, group A streptococci, *Staphylococcus aureus*, Gram-negative bacilli or anaerobes, then amoxicillin and pivampicillin are first-line, while trimethoprim/sulfamethoxazole and cefuroxime axetil are second line. Trimethoprim and clarithromycin are third line.

Bronchitis There are no effective therapies for viral infections of the bronchi.

- If the bronchitis is mild to severe and bacterial in origin (i.e. due to *Mycoplasma pneumoniae, S. pneumoniae, Chlamydia pneumoniae*) the first-line antibiotics are tetracycline and erythromycin. The second-line antibiotics are doxycycline and clarithromycin.
- If an adult presents with a mild to moderate acute exacerbation of chronic bronchitis following infection with organisms such as *S. pneumoniae, H. influenzae, M. catarrhalis* or *M. pneumoniae*, the first-line antibiotics are tetracycline, trimethoprim/sulfamethoxazole and amoxicillin. The second-line antibiotics are doxycycline, cefuroxime axetil, cefaclor, amoxicillin/clavulanate, and clarithromycin.
- If the bronchitis is accompanied by moderate to extensive underlying lung disease due to *S. pneumoniae, H. influenzae, M. catarrhalis* or *M. pneumoniae*, the first-line antibiotics are trimethoprim/sulfamethoxazole, cefaclor, cefuroxime axetil, amoxicillin/clavulanate, and any one of the above. The second-line antibiotics are floxacin and ciprofloxacin.
- If there is an acute infective exacerbation of chronic bronchitis in the presence of bronchiectasis and infection due to *H. influenzae, S. pneumoniae, M. catarrhalis* or *Pseudomonas aeruginosa*, the first-line antibiotics are tetracycline, trimethoprim/sulfamethoxazole and ciprafloxin. The second-line antibiotics are floxacin, ciprofloxacin, cefaclor, cefuroxime axetil, amoxicillin/clavulanate, and any one of the above with erythromycin or clarithromycin.

Pneumonia is an infection of the alveoli and small bronchioles that can involve the pleura (pleurisy) (Fig. 11.26). It can occur in a variety of situations and treatment varies according to the situation (Fig. 11.27).

In bronchopneumonia the primary infection is centered on the bronchi and spreads to involve adjacent alveoli, which become filled with an acute inflammatory exudate. Affected areas of lung become consolidated, at first in a patchy distribution involving only the lobules but, if untreated, the consolidation becomes confluent and involves one or both lobes. This pattern of disease is most common in infancy and old age, and predisposing factors include debility and immobility. Immobility leads to retention of secretions, which gravitate to the dependent parts of the lungs and become infected; bronchopneumonia, therefore, most commonly involves the lower lobes. The causative organisms depend upon the circumstances predisposing to infection.

Macroscopically, affected areas of the lung are firm and airless, and have a dark red or grey appearance in bronchopneumonia. There may be pus in the peripheral bronchi. Histologically, there is acute inflammation of the bronchi and the alveoli contain acute inflammatory exudate (see Fig. 11.26). The pleura is commonly involved, leading to pleurisy.

If the pneumonia is treated, recovery usually involves focal organization of the lung by fibrosis. Common complications include lung abscess, pleural infection, and septicaemia.

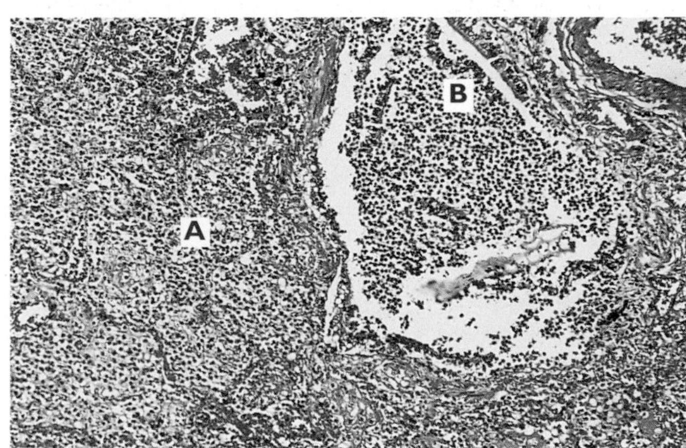

Fig. 11.26 Bronchopneumonia. Inflammation centered on bronchi (B) spreads out to cause inflammation in the alveoli (A), which contain acute inflammatory infiltrate. Consolidation occurs in the dependent part of the lung. (Courtesy of Dr Alan Stevens and Professor James Lowe.)

Treatment of bacterial pharyngitis

Type of infection	*Group A streptococci*		
In adults	**First-line**	**Second-line**	**Third-line**
	Penicillin V	Erythromycin	Cephalexin, clarithromycin
In children	Penicillin V, amoxicillin, pivampicillin	Erythromycin estolate	Cephalexin

Fig. 11.25 Drug treatment of bacterial pharyngitis.

Treatment of bacterial pneumonia

Type of infection		
Adults	**First-line**	**Second-line**
When community acquired and mild to moderate disease. No comorbidity *S. pneumoniae, M. pneumoniae, C. pneumoniae, H. influenzae*	Tetracyline, erythromycin	Doxycycline, clarithromycin
With comorbidity. Mixed infections with *S. pneumoniae, H. influenzae, H. influenzae,* oral anaerobes, Gram-negative bacilli, *S. aureus, Legionella* sp.	Cefaclor, cefuroxime axetil, amoxicillin/clavulanate or any of these *plus* erythromycin or clarithromycin	
When community acquired severe disease in hospital, with or without comorbidity *S. pneumoniae, H. influenzae, Legionella* sp., *M. pneumoniae, S. aureus, C. pneumoniae.* Comorbidity pathogens: anaerobes, Gram-negative bacilli	Cefuroxime axetil, cefuroxime, cefotaxime, ceftiaxone, or any of these *plus* erythromycin or clarithromycin ± rifampin	Trimethoprim/sulfamethoxazole *plus* erythromycin
With severe disease in intensive care environment *S. pneumoniae, H. influenzae, Legionella* sp., Gram-negative bacilli, *P. aeruginosa, S. aureus, M. pneumoniae, C. pneumoniae*	Erythromycin ± rifampin plus one of ciprofloxacin, imipenem, or ceftazidime	
In institutionalized elderly patients with mild to moderate disease *S. pneumoniae, H. influenzae,* oral anaerobes, Gram-negative bacilli, *S. aureus, Legionella* sp.	Trimethoprim/sulfmethoxazole, cefaclor, cefuroxime axetil, amoxicillin/clavulanate, or any one of the above ± erythromycin or clarithromycin	
With severe disease *S. pneumoniae, H. influenzae,* oral anaerobes, Gram-negative bacilli, *S. aureus, Legionella* sp.	Cefaclor or cefuroxime axetil or amoxicillin/clavulanate or ceftriaxone or combinations, penicillin or amoxicillin *plus* ciproxfloxacin	Ciprofloxacin plus clindamycin
Children		
With mild disease *S. pneumoniae, S. aureus,* streptococci Group A, *M. pneumoniae, H. influenzae*	Amoxicillin, pivampicillin, erythromycin estolate	Trimethoprim/sulfamethoxazole, clarithromycin, erythromycin/ sulfisoxazole, amoxicillin/clavulanate, cefixime, cefaclor, cefuroxime axetil chloramphenicol ± erythromycin or clarithromycin
With severe disease *S. pneumoniae, S. aureus* streptococci Group A, *M. pneumoniae, H. influenzae*	Cefuroxime ± erythromycin estolate or clarithromycin	Trimethoprim/sulfamethoxazole, clarithromycin, erythromycin/ sulfisoxazole, amoxicillin clavulanate, cefixime, cefaclor, cefuroxime axetil, chloramphenicol ± erythromycin or clarithromycin

Fig. 11.27 Treatment of bacterial pneumonia.

Whooping cough is a potentially debilitating condition resulting from infection with *Bordetella pertussis*, and children can be vaccinated against it. Erythromycin (the estolate is preferred for children) is the first-line antibiotic, while trimethoprim/sulfamethoxazole is second line and tetracycline, amoxicillin, and ampicillin are third line.

> **Antibiotics**
>
> - Antibiotics should not be used to treat viral respiratory infections
> - Different antibiotics act at different stages in bacterial growth and development
> - Combinations of antibiotics may be synergistic and prevent the occurrence of resistant bacteria
> - The full course of any antibiotic treatment must be completed or resistance is likely to develop

Tuberculosis

Tuberculosis is a bacterial infection with unique characteristics that make it difficult to treat. Infections with the mycobacteria (*Mycobacterium tuberculosis*) responsible for tuberculosis have occurred in man throughout recorded history and are more common where there is crowding and poverty. With the general improvement in world economies, housing, and hygiene, the incidence of tuberculosis, particularly in the wealthier countries, decreased remarkably in the latter half of this century, but has recently begun to increase in incidence and importance. Much of the increase in wealthier countries is associated with AIDS, and strains of tubercle bacillus resistant to conventional or previously effective therapy continue to emerge.

M. tuberculosis can infect tissue other than respiratory tissue (e.g. brain and intestine), and the mycobacteria can be found in both closed and caseous cavity lesions and in macrophages. Often the disease is self-limiting and the body seals the mycobacteria in a calcified lesion, where they remain dormant. This prevents spread of the infection, but prevents drugs from readily penetrating the lesion. Therefore, there is a risk of subsequent rupture of the lesion and renewed infection. An additional complication of this dormant phase is that antimycobacterial drugs exert their lethal actions only on actively growing organisms. These features mean that, in order to kill all organisms, therapy must be continued for 9–18 months and combinations of drugs are used. Prophylactic therapy is required for the contacts of people with active disease. The main therapeutic aim is to achieve the lowest relapse rate possible, which is ideally less than 5%.

> **Antitubercular drugs**
>
> - Mycobacteria readily develop drug resistance
> - The main antitubercular drugs are isoniazid, rifampin, streptomycin, ethambutol, and pyrazinamide
> - Drug combinations are always required in the treatment of tuberculosis

Isoniazid is a derivative of isonicotinic acid and was first introduced in 1952. It is a very effective first-line antitubercular drug for those who can tolerate it, and in whom infection is due to isoniazid-susceptible mycobacteria. The mechanism of action of isoniazid is not clear. At low concentrations, it is bactericidal against actively growing organisms. It is less effective against atypical strains of the mycobacterium. Resistance is encountered in approximately 1 in 10^7 organisms, which accounts for the growth of resistant strains if isoniazid is given alone. Fortunately there is no crossresistance between isoniazid and other effective agents, namely rifampin and ethambutol.

Isoniazid is usually given in combination therapy: adult doses are 300 mg (5 mg/kg daily) with children receiving twice the dose. Isoniazid is readily absorbed and distributes freely into the intra- and extracellular space although its distribution into the cerebrospinal fluid (CSF) is limited. Its hepatic metabolism (acetylation) is genetically determined, with a 1.5-hour half-life in fast acetylators, and a 3-hour half-life in slow acetylators.

The adverse effects of isoniazid depend on the dose and route of administration and include peripheral neuritis, insomnia, restlessness, convulsions, and psychosis. Isoniazid-induced neuritis appears to result from a relative pyridoxine deficiency due to substrate competition between pyridoxine and isoniazid. It is prevented by pyridoxine administration. Although isoniazid is a pyridoxine analog, this does not interfere with the antibacterial actions of isoniazid. Hepatotoxicity can occur, is age related, and is more common if there is pre-existing liver damage. Allergic reactions such as fever and skin rashes are other adverse effects of isoniazid treatment.

Rifampin is a first-line drug. It is one of the semisynthetic derivatives of the antibiotic rifampicin B and has activity against some Gram-negative and Gram-positive cocci, chlamydiae, and poxviruses, as well as against mycobacteria. The mechanism of rifampin's antibacterial action is inhibition of RNA synthesis in bacteria as a result of binding to bacterial RNA polymerase. Rifampin is able to penetrate mammalian cells and kill mycobacteria within them. Selectivity for bacterial RNA polymerase versus mammalian RNA polymerase is complete, and rifampin does not therefore inhibit human cell division.

Resistance is encountered in approximately 1 in 10^7 organisms and is not associated with crossresistance to other drugs. The mechanism of resistance remains unclear, but the indiscriminate use of rifampin for minor infections undoubtedly facilitates its development.

Rifampin is well absorbed when administered orally, undergoes enterohepatic recirculation, and distributes widely throughout the body. The concentration within the CNS may reach approximately 25% of that in the serum. It is primarily excreted in the feces.

Rifampin is usually administered with isoniazid, ethambutol or other antitubercular drugs at an adult dose of 600 mg/day. It is used with dapsone for the treatment of atypical mycobacteria, as well as for prophylaxis against *H. influenzae* type B in children. It can be used to eradicate staphylococci in the nasopharynx when combined with trimethoprim and sulfamethoxazole.

Treatment of tuberculosis

- The first-line treatment of tuberculosis is a combination of rifampin, isoniazid, and pyrazinamide
- Treatment is usually for 6 months and the pyrazinamide may be discontinued after 2 months

Adverse effects reported with rifampin include rashes, thrombocytopenia, nephritis, and a flu-like syndrome. It colors body secretions orange and although this may cause concern to patients, there is no associated morbidity.

Rifampin induces microsomal enzymes in the liver and therefore increases the elimination of drugs metabolized by these enzymes (e.g. anticoagulants, oral contraceptives, cortisol, and antibiotics such as ketoconazole, cyclosporine, and chloramphenicol).

Ethambutol is a first-line antitubercular drug that inhibits many strains of mycobacteria. The mechanism of action is, however, not known, but it is believed to be bacteriostatic. Resistance develops rapidly, so it is always given in combination with other drugs. Usually 15 mg/kg is given once daily in combination with isoniazid or rifampin.

The most common adverse effect is a visual disturbance with a loss of color vision and, in the most severe cases, retinal damage. Such changes are usually reversible and regress after discontinuing the drug.

Pyrazinamide is an analog of nicotinamide and strongly inhibits the growth of mycobacteria. It is a first-line drug, is well absorbed, and is widely distributed in the body. Tolerance develops fairly readily, but does not cross with isoniazid or other antitubercular drugs. The main adverse effect occurs in 1–5% of patients and involves the liver. Other adverse effects include nausea, vomiting, and hyperuricemia. Drug-induced fever has also been reported.

Streptomycin was one of the first aminoglycoside antibiotics discovered and was found to be effective against tuberculosis. In common with other aminoglycoside antibiotics it causes eighth cranial nerve damage, resulting in disturbances of balance and deafness. Such damage may be permanent. Streptomycin resistance is encountered in $1/10^8$–10^{10} organisms. It is therefore never given alone, but always in combination with other antitubercular drugs. Streptomycin penetration into cells is poor, and poor absorption characteristics mean that it must be given intramuscularly. Streptomycin is used chiefly in patients with severe tuberculosis and when the infection is life threatening.

Capreomycin is a polypeptide antibiotic that is effective against many mycobacteria, but it shows crossresistance with related antibiotics. It is highly toxic, damaging the kidney and the eighth nerve, and because of this it is a second-line drug. Toxicity is dose related.

Cycloserine, an analog of D-alanine, inhibits the enzyme alanine racemase and thereby inhibits many strains of *M. tuberculosis*. Its adverse effects involve the CNS, can be severe, and include CNS dysfunction and psychotic reactions. It is a second-line drug.

Ethionamide is chemically similar to isoniazid and also blocks mycolic acid synthesis. However, there is no crossresistance with isoniazid. It is a second-line drug because resistance develops quickly and it is poorly tolerated because it causes gastric irritation and neurologic symptoms.

***para*-Aminosalicylic acid** (PAS) is similar to *para*-aminobenzoic acid (PAB) and sulfonamides. It is not generally antibacterial, but is effective against mycobacteria. Its close similarity to PAB probably means that it competes with PAB to prevent the formation of dihydropteroic acid in a manner that is specific to typical mycobacteria. It is a second-line drug.

Viomycin is another polypeptide antibiotic derived from *Streptomyces*. It is given twice weekly as a 2 g injection. However, resistance develops quite readily and this crosses with streptomycin, kanamycin, and capreomycin; in addition, viomycin is more toxic than streptomycin in terms of eighth nerve-related damage. For these reasons it is a second-line drug.

Other drugs are either less effective than the drugs discussed above or have not been extensively evaluated. They include rifabutin (ansamycin), tetracyclines, fluoroquinolones, and amikacin.

DRUGS WITH ADVERSE EFFECTS IN PATIENTS WITH RESPIRATORY DISEASE

β Adrenoceptor antagonists

β_2 Adrenoceptor antagonists such as propranolol, with its potent capacity to block β_2 adrenoceptors, are strictly contraindicated in patients who have bronchial asthma because they precipitate severe bronchoconstriction, which may be lethal. This adverse effect results from the dependence of asthmatics on circulating epinephrine and/or the innervations of parasympathetic ganglia by sympathetic nerves as inhibitory mechanisms to offset vagal tone, which tends to reduce airway diameter. β Adrenoceptor antagonist eyedrops can also induce life-threatening asthma attacks in asthmatic subjects.

Adverse effects of drugs used for respiratory diseases other than asthma and infection

- Mucolytic agents have relatively few adverse effects
- The opioids are the only cough suppressant with a major adverse effect (i.e. the potential for drug abuse and social withdrawal)

Angiotensin-converting enzyme inhibitors

Angiotensin-converting enzyme (ACE) inhibitors such as captopril and enalapril are used increasingly in the treatment of hypertension and congestive heart failure. However, ACE inhibitors such as captopril can induce coughing in some patients with concomitant allergic airway diseases. The mechanism is believed to be local generation of bradykinin because ACE inhibitors inhibit peptidyl peptidase enzymes involved in the metabolism of bradykinin in addition to inhibiting the conversion of angiotensin I to angiotensin II. The concentration of bradykinin in the lung can then become elevated and stimulate the afferent receptors, initiating cough. ACE-induced coughing is effectively treated with cromolyn sodium.

Nonsteroidal anti-inflammatory drugs

Approximately 20% of people with asthma can develop severe bronchoconstriction following ingestion of nonsteroidal anti-inflammatory drugs (NSAIDs). The mechanism is not fully understood, but may relate to the generation of lipoxygenase metabolites of arachidonic acid because it can be inhibited by 5-lipoxygenase inhibitors. NSAIDs, including aspirin, must therefore be used with caution in patients with asthma.

Adverse effects of antibiotics

- The principal adverse effect of penicillin and cephalosporins is allergy
- The principal adverse effect of aminoglycosides is renal toxicity
- The principal adverse effects of sulfonamides are allergy and skin photosensitivity
- The principal adverse effect of antitubercular drugs vary with the drug

FURTHER READING

Barnes PJ. Neural control of the lung. *Am Rev Resp Dis* 1993; **134**: 1289–1314. [A detailed review of the biology of the neural mechanisms involved in regulating the biology of the lung.]

Barnes PJ. Anti-inflammatory therapy for asthma. *Ann Rev Resp Med* 1993; **44**: 229–249. [This review provides an in-depth discussion of recent advances in the treatment of bronchial asthma.]

Holgate, S (ed.) *Immunopharmacology of the Respiratory System*. London: Academic Press; 1995. [An up-to-date review of the immunologic mechanisms contributing to lung disease.]

Karlsson JA. A role for capsaiscin-sensitive tachykinin-containing nerves in chronic coughing and sneezing but not in asthma. *Thorax* 1993; **48**: 396–400. [A review of the pathogenesis and treatment of coughs and sneezes.]

Nadel JA, Murray J (eds) *Textbook of Respiratory Medicine 2e*. London: WB Saunders; 1994. [An excellent textbook written by two distinguished American authors covering the clinical aspects of respiratory medicine.]

Make a provisional diagnosis and determine a rational pharmacologic treatment for the following hypothetical case.

A mother reports that her 6-year-old son had a fever the previous night of 38°C and had woken periodically with coughing and wheezing. She also reported that he had been ill for 3 days with an unproductive cough. His symptoms are less severe during the day, although he has been physically less active than usual. On examination, her son has a runny nose and slightly red eardrums and throat. His respiration is not labored and his general appearance is normal. The only other signs are audible wheezing and rhonchi on auscultation that do not clear upon coughing.

1. Would you reassure the mother that all is well, and that the disease will resolve quickly without drug treatment?
2. If you decided to prescribe an antibiotic, which antibiotic would you use?
3. If you decided to prescribe an antibiotic plus a bronchodilator, which bronchodilator would you use?
4. Would you order further tests (total and differential white cell count, throat swab for bacterial culture and sensitivity)?
5. Would you prescribe anti-inflammatory drugs?
6. What is the probable diagnosis? How should this be treated?

?

Indicate which is the correct answer for each question.

1. One of the effects of theophylline in biologic tissues is
   a) stimulation of Na^+K^+ ATPase
   b) inhibition of Na^+K^+ ATPase
   c) inhibition of cyclic nucleotide phosphodiesterase
   d) stimulation of cyclic nucleotide phosphodiesterase
   e) stimulation of adenylyl cyclase

2. Cough suppression is indicated
   a) if phlegm production is excessive
   b) if there is severe rhinitis
   c) if there is bronchiectasis
   d) if the cough is induced by extrabronchial irritation

3. Prominent antitussive activity produced by therapeutic doses is characteristic of
   a) morphine
   b) theophylline
   c) albuterol
   d) dexamethasone

4. In the treatment of tuberculosis
   a) up to 30% of the *Mycobacterium* cultures isolated from cases in New York City are resistant to multiple anti-microbial agents
   b) oral streptomycin is effective
   c) compliance in drug taking is a major problem
   d) the molecular mechanisms of antibacterial resistance are well characterized

5. In treatment and prophylaxis
   a) isoniazid (INH) is useful on its own for treatment of tuberculosis
   b) INH is useful on its own for prophylaxis of tuberculosis
   c) rifampin is useful on its own for treatment of tuberculosis
   d) rifampin is useful on its own for prophylaxis of meningitis

6. Erythromycin
   a) is a macrolide antibiotic
   b) binds to motilin receptors
   c) is useful for treating *Mycoplasma pneumoniae* infections
   d) is an agent of choice for the treatment of infections due to β lactamase-producing Gram-positive staphylococci
   e) first line treatment of tuberculosis is with a combination of rifampin, INH, and pyrazamide

7. When applied to the airways of an asthmatic individual, drug X causes bronchodilation. The effect is not blocked by propanolol. Drug X does not normally have any central nervous system effect and, if it is given by mouth, has a bioavailability of less than 40%. Drug X is most likely
   a) atropine
   b) scopolamine
   c) terbutaline
   d) ipratropium
   e) salbutamol

8. Acute administration of the following drugs induces bronchodilation except
   a) metaproterenol
   b) aminophylline
   c) cromolyn sodium
   d) epinephrine
   e) theophylline

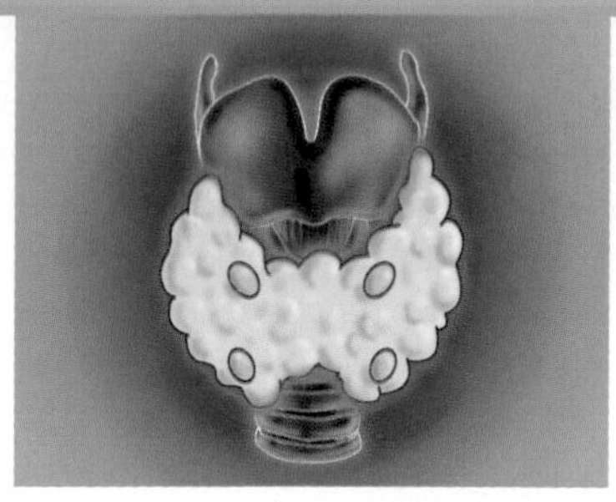

12. Drugs and the Endocrine and Metabolic Systems

GENERAL PHYSIOLOGY OF THE ENDOCRINE AND METABOLIC SYSTEMS

The endocrine system regulates many of the body's activities. It consists of a variety of organs that secrete substances into the blood which affect the function of target tissues elsewhere in the body. The organs of the endocrine and metabolic system include the hypothalamus, pituitary, thyroid, adrenals, gonads, pancreatic islets of Langerhans, and the parathyroids. The endocrine organs and hormones regulate seven major physiologic parameters (Fig. 12.1), each of which requires an endocrine organ, regulatory inputs, and target tissue responses. Despite this diversity, endocrine organs share common features in the mechanisms of hormone action and the patterns of hormonal regulation. A cardinal feature of the drug therapy of endocrine diseases is the interaction between exogenously

Functional anatomy of the endocrine and metabolic systems

Endocrine function	Regulatory factors	Endocrine organ/hormone	Target tissues
Availability of fuel	Serum glucose, amino acids, enteric hormones (somatostatin, cholecystokinin, gastrin, secretin), vagal reflex, sympathetic nervous system	Pancreatic islets of Langerhans/insulin, glucagon	All tissues, especially liver, skeletal muscle, adipose tissue, indirect effects on brain and red blood cells
Metabolic rate	Hypothalamic thyrotropin releasing hormone (TRH), pituitary thyrotropin (TSH)	Thyroid gland/ triiodothyronine (T_3)	All tissues
Circulatory volume	Renin, angiotensin II, hypothalamic osmoreceptor	Adrenals/aldosterone Pituitary/vasopressin	Kidney, blood vessels, CNS
Somatic growth	Hypothalamic growth hormone releasing hormone (GHRH), somatostatin, sleep, exercise, stress, hypoglycemia	Pituitary/growth hormone Liver/insulin-like growth factors (IGFs)	All tissues
Calcium homeostasis	Serum Ca^{2+} and Mg^{2+} concentration	Parathyroid glands/parathyroid hormone, calcitonin, vitamin D	Kidney, intestines, bone
Reproductive function	Hypothalamic gonadotropin releasing hormone (GnRH), pituitary follicle stimulating hormone (FSH) and luteinizing hormone (LH), inhibins	Gonads/sex steroids Adrenals/androgens	Reproductive organs, CNS, various tissues
Adaptation to stress	Hypothalamic corticotropin releasing hormone (CRH), pituitary adrenocorticotropic hormone (ACTH), hypoglycemia, stress	Adrenals/glucocorticosteroids, epinephrine	Many tissues: CNS, liver, skeletal muscle, adipose tissue, lymphocytes, fibroblasts, cardiovascular system

Fig. 12.1 Functional anatomy of the endocrine and metabolic systems. The endocrine and metabolic systems regulate seven major bodily functions. For each target tissue effect, endocrine glands release hormones in response to regulating factors, which include physiologic (e.g. sleep and stress), biochemical (e.g. glucose and Ca^{2+}), and hormonal (e.g. hypothalamic and enteric hormones) stimuli.

administered drugs and the 'endogenous pharmacology' of endocrine hormones.

The endocrine regulation of Ca^{2+} homeostasis is discussed in Chapter 17 and disorders of circulatory volume in Chapter 10. Additional information on disorders of reproductive function is presented in Chapter 13.

THE HYPOTHALAMIC–PITUITARY AXIS

The hypothalamus and pituitary integrate physiologic signals and release hormones that regulate the function of other endocrine glands

With the exception of fuel metabolism and electrolyte homeostasis, pituitary hormones regulate most endocrine systems. The pituitary regulates thyroid, glucocorticosteroid, sex steroid, and growth factor secretion by synthesizing and secreting specific hormones which regulate other endocrine organs. The pituitary also secretes two hormones that act directly on target tissues (prolactin and vasopressin). It consists of anterior and posterior divisions (Fig. 12.2). The anterior pituitary (or adenohypophysis) is derived from Rathke's pouch in the embryonic oropharynx, whereas the posterior pituitary (or neurohypophysis) is an extracranial extension of neuronal tissue from the diencephalon. A portal venous system from the hypothalamus supplies blood to the anterior pituitary and provides a direct conduit for hypothalamic hormones, which regulate anterior pituitary function. Because of the low perfusion pressure of portal venous systems, the anterior pituitary is vulnerable to ischemic damage, particularly during postpartum hemorrhage (Sheehan's syndrome). The cells of the anterior pituitary are a mixed population of cell types that secrete different peptide hormones.

Regulation of thyroid hormone secretion is typical of a hypothalamic–pituitary–endocrine axis (Fig. 12.3). A lowered concentration of circulating thyroid hormone is detected by hypothalamic thyroid hormone receptors. This results in the release of thyrotropin releasing hormone (TRH) from the hypothalamus (tertiary level of regulation) into portal veins supplying the anterior pituitary. Stimulation of TRH receptors on pituitary thyrotroph cells leads to the release of thyroid stimulating hormone (TSH, thyrotropin) into the systemic venous system (secondary level of regulation). TSH stimulates thyroid hormone release from the thyroid gland (primary level of hormone production). Thyroid

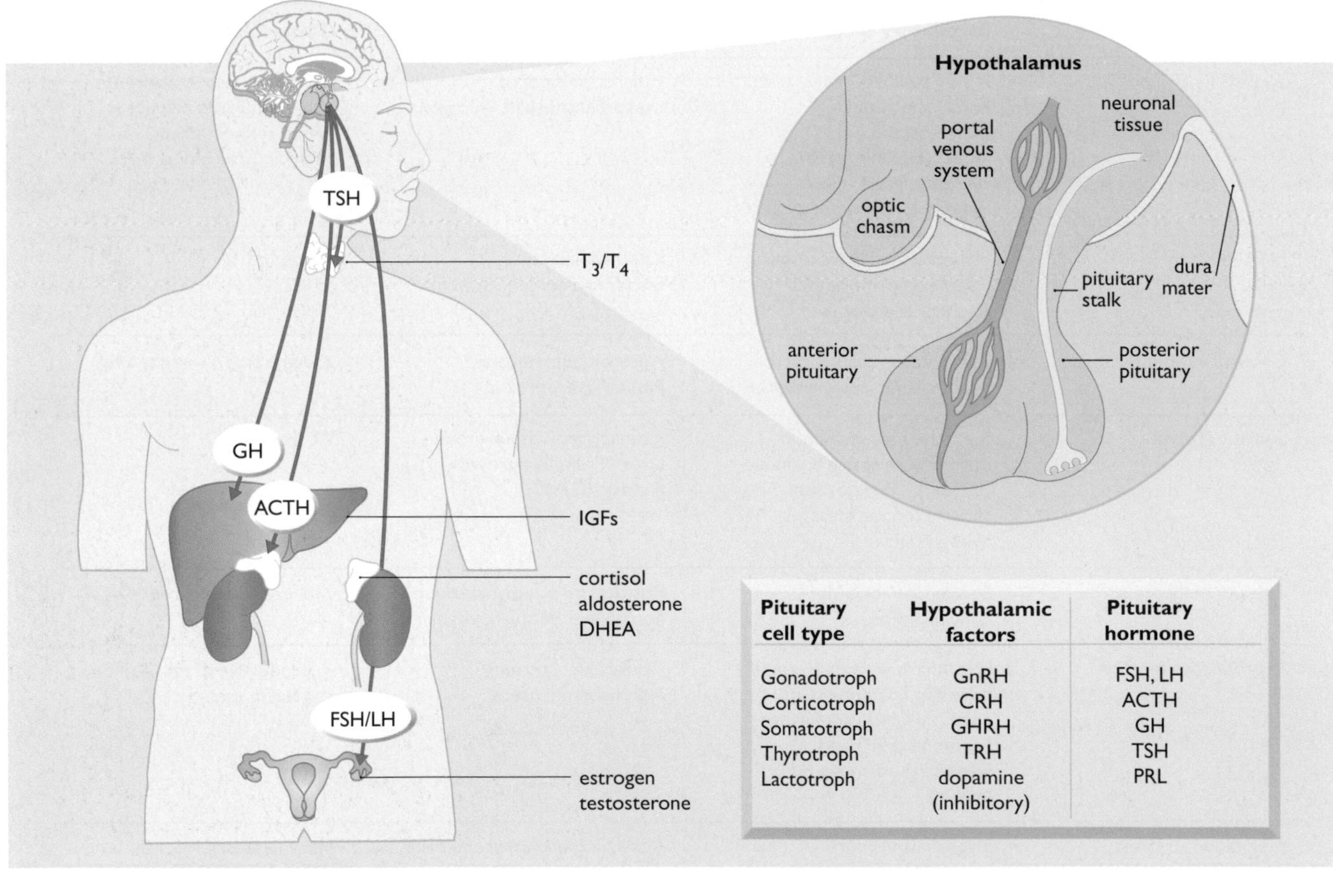

Pituitary cell type	Hypothalamic factors	Pituitary hormone
Gonadotroph	GnRH	FSH, LH
Corticotroph	CRH	ACTH
Somatotroph	GHRH	GH
Thyrotroph	TRH	TSH
Lactotroph	dopamine (inhibitory)	PRL

Fig. 12.2 The hypothalamic–pituitary axis. The cells of the anterior pituitary are regulated by hypothalamic hormones, which are released into the portal veins leading from the hypothalamus to the anterior pituitary via the pituitary stalk. Anterior pituitary hormones are released into the inferior petrosal veins for delivery to endocrine organs elsewhere in the body. The posterior pituitary consists of specialized neurons that synthesize the peptide hormones, vasopressin and oxytocin, for release into the systemic circulation. (ACTH, adrenocorticotropic hormone; CRH, corticotropin releasing hormone; DHEA, dehydroepiandrosterone; FSH, follicle stimulating hormone; GH, growth hormone; GHRH, growth hormone releasing hormone; GnRH, gonadotropin releasing hormone; IGFs, insulin-like growth factors; LH, luteinizing hormone; T_3, triiodothyronine; T_4, tetraiodothyronine; TRH, thyrotropin releasing hormone; TSH, thyroid stimulating hormone; PRL, prolactin)

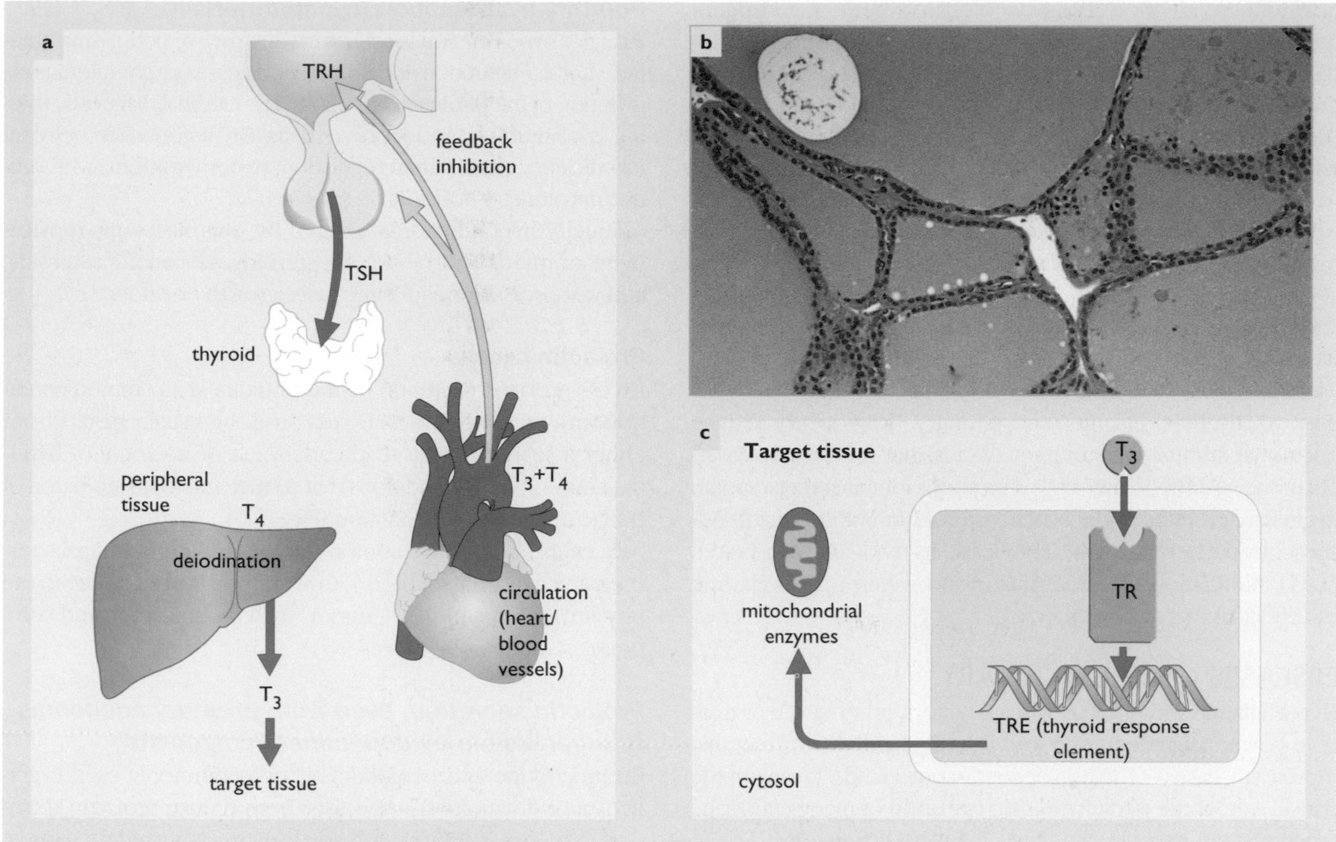

Fig. 12.3 The hypothalamic–pituitary–thyroid axis. (a) Thyroid hormone regulation illustrates the features of endocrine systems regulated by the hypothalamus and pituitary. Hypothalamic thyrotropin releasing hormone (TRH) is released into the portal circulation and stimulates pituitary thyroid stimulating hormone (TSH) release. Circulating TSH stimulates the thyroid gland to release thyroxine (tetraiodothyronine or T_4) and triiodothyronine (T_3) from stores in the thyroid follicles (b). Thyroid hormones are largely bound to the proteins thyroid binding globulin (TBG) and prealbumin in the circulation. The major circulating hormone (T_4) is metabolized in the peripheral tissues to the more active hormone T_3, which enters cells and binds thyroid hormone receptors in the nucleus (c). Bound thyroid hormone receptors (TR) interact with specific thyroid response elements (TREs) of thyroid hormone responsive genes. The hypothalamus and pituitary also contain thyroid hormone receptors, which mediate feedback inhibition by circulating thyroid hormone. Thyroid hormone is stored in the follicles of the thyroid gland. TSH stimulates endocytosis of thyroglobulin stores and release of thyroid hormone into the circulation. The scalloped margins of the thyroglobulin stores result from resorption by the cells lining the thyroid follicle. (b, Courtesy of Dr Thomas Ulbright.)

hormone acts on target tissues and also has negative feedback effects on the hypothalamus and pituitary. The endocrine systems regulating the sex steroids and the adrenal response to stress share this four-tiered pattern of hypothalamic, pituitary, primary endocrine gland, and target tissue response.

Many endocrine systems share a common pattern of diseases

Endocrine systems regulating metabolic rate (thyroid hormone), reproductive function (sex steroids), adaptation to stress (glucocorticosteroids) and somatic growth (growth hormone–IGF axis) share a common pattern of diseases affecting each level of endocrine regulation. While disease at any level in the regulatory system may produce a similar effect (i.e. hypo- or hyperstimulation of end-organ effects), different approaches to drug therapy may be preferred depending on the site of pathology. For example, hypogonadism due to failure of pituitary gonadotrophs may respond to therapy with exogenous gonadotropins, but gonadal failure will not. Diagnostic strategies in endocrine disease attempt to identify the site of pathology by identifying the pattern of hormonal responses, which is characteristic for different diseases (Fig. 12.4). The primary alterations and compensatory responses of regulatory hormones accompanying the different patterns of endocrine disease must be understood to allow both diagnosis and treatment.

PATHOPHYSIOLOGY AND DISEASES OF THE ENDOCRINE AND METABOLIC SYSTEMS

PHARMACOLOGIC PRINCIPLES

Drugs affecting the endocrine and metabolic systems act at a variety of steps in the process of hormonal signaling where they promote or inhibit target tissue effects. This allows for different pharmacotherapeutic approaches to achieve the same pharmacologic effect by either modifying hormone action or altering hormone production. For example, treatment of androgen-dependent prostate cancer may involve either an androgen receptor antagonist (flutamide) or an inhibitor of androgen production (finasteride).

Another key point in the interaction of drugs with hormonal systems is that a partial agonist at a receptor may act as as an agonist when the endogenous hormone is absent, but as an antagonist when it is present (see Chapter 4). For example, tamoxifen is a mixed agonist/antagonist of estrogen receptors and produces some estrogen effects in postmenopausal women who lack endogenous estrogen, but has an antagonist effect in premenopausal women by blocking the action of endogenous estrogen.

In endocrine systems that are regulated by hormonal feedback to the hypothalamus and pituitary, drugs which reduce hormonal stimulation of target tissues may lead to increased hormone secretion. The cortisol synthesis inhibitor metyrapone, for instance, reduces glucocorticosteroid inhibition of adrenocorticotropic hormone (ACTH) release. Its use leads to increased ACTH stimulation of the adrenal gland which may overcome the effect of metyrapone therapy.

DISEASES OF THE PITUITARY

Hypothalamic and pituitary diseases affect either single or multiple hormonal systems and lead to symptoms which resemble those of diseases of the primary endocrine glands. Owing to the critical role of the pituitary in the regulation of many endocrine functions, pituitary disease affects many body functions.

Common patterns of endocrine disease

	Primary hormone	Regulatory hormones	Target tissue effects
Primary hormone deficiency	Decreased	Increased	Decreased
Secondary hormone deficiency	Decreased	Decreased	Decreased
Primary hormone excess	Increased	Decreased	Increased
Secondary hormone excess	Increased	Increased	Increased
Target tissue resistance	Increased	Increased	Decreased

Fig.12.4 Common patterns of endocrine disease. Hyperfunction and hypofunction of an endocrine system may result from disease of the primary endocrine organ, at the secondary regulatory level, or at the target tissues. Diagnosis and treatment must consider patterns of adaptation to disease at these different levels. For example, symptoms of adrenal insufficiency associated with a low cortisol and high adrenocorticotropic hormone (ACTH) concentrations suggest a diagnosis of primary adrenal failure (Addison's disease), whereas similar symptoms associated with a low ACTH concentration suggest pituitary disease.

Pituitary hypofunction (hypopituitarism)

Pituitary hypofunction is caused by destructive neoplasms, trauma, vascular infarction, inflammatory diseases or granulomatous infection of the pituitary (Fig. 12.5). The cardinal diagnostic finding is of multiple endocrine deficits (hypogonadism, adrenal insufficiency, altered fluid regulation, hypothyroidism) with subnormal pituitary hormonal responses.

Pituitary hypofunction is treated by pharmacologic replacement of thyroid hormone, sex steroids, glucocorticosteroids, and vasopressin, and in some cases growth hormone.

Prolactin excess

Excess prolactin secretion by the pituitary is a common condition with multiple causes. Excess prolactin usually results from either a secretory lactotroph adenoma or a variety of hypothalamic–pituitary conditions that reduce the tonic inhibition of prolactin release by dopamine (Fig. 12.6).

Excess prolactin is a common cause of infertility and galactorrhea, and may be associated with symptoms and signs due to the physical size of a pituitary tumor, such as headaches and compression of the optic nerves.

Prolactin secretion, even from pituitary adenomas, is suppressible by dopaminergic agonists

Bromocriptine and pergolide are two commonly used ergot-derivative dopaminergic agonists. Both reduce prolactin secretion, but are associated with adverse effects including nausea. Tolerance develops to these adverse effects, but the therapeutic effect on pituitary lactotrophs is maintained. Dopaminergic agonist therapy also leads to prompt shrinkage of pituitary lactotroph adenomas, even those compressing the optic chiasm. These agents have therefore now replaced surgery as the primary treatment for this type of pituitary tumor.

Causes of hypopituitarism

Mass lesions	Pituitary tumors Craniopharyngioma Meningioma
Infarction	Postpartum pituitary necrosis (Sheehan's syndrome)
Inflammatory/infiltrative diseases	Sarcoidosis Histiocytosis X Hemochromatosis Lymphocytic hypophysitis
Infectious diseases	Tuberculosis Syphilis
Physical insults	Trauma Surgery Radiation
Isolated hypothalamic/pituitary hormone deficiencies	

Fig 12.5 Causes of hypopituitarism.

Prolactin-lowering dopaminergic agonists

- Nausea and vomiting
- Orthostatic hypotension
- Nasal congestion
- Exacerbation of psychosis
- Digital vasospasm

GROWTH HORMONE–INSULIN-LIKE GROWTH FACTOR AXIS

Growth hormone excess (acromegaly)

The growth hormone–IGF axis is another endocrine system for which the pathology lies largely within the pituitary and hypothalamus. Growth hormone is a peptide hormone which promotes protein synthesis and tissue growth. Many of the effects are mediated by the release of insulin-like growth factors from the liver. These are peptide hormones which produce anabolic effects by stimulating receptors that contain tyrosine kinase activity. Growth hormone excess is rare and is usually due to an adenoma of pituitary somatotrophs. Growth hormone excess in adulthood after closure of the epiphyseal plates does not usually increase stature. The main signs are coarse facial features, enlargement of hands and feet, thickening of soft tissues, and enlargement of organs such as the heart (cardiomegaly) (Figs 12.7, 12.8). In children, growth hormone excess may lead to giantism.

Treatment of growth hormone-secreting tumors with a dopaminergic agonist or octreotide may be indicated

Treatment of growth hormone-secreting tumors usually involves surgery and radiation therapy. If appropriate, two types of drug can be used:

- A dopaminergic agonist (e.g. bromocriptine, pergolide), which suppresses growth hormone secretion from some somatotroph adenomas.
- Octreotide, a synthetic somatostatin analog and agonist that is useful in the treatment of acromegaly, carcinoid tumors, and gastrointestinal diseases.

Octreotide is an octapeptide that shares the physiologic effects of the native hormone somatostatin. Somatostatin is produced at many sites in the body, including the central nervous system (CNS), the digestive tract, and pancreatic δ cells, where it inhibits the release of a variety of hormones (Fig. 12.9). Somatostatin receptors are G protein-coupled receptors that inhibit hormone release by reducing cAMP formation.

Octreotide has a longer half-life than somatostatin and is therefore a more practical therapeutic agent. As a peptide, octreotide requires parenteral administration by subcutaneous injection. Owing to its inhibitory effects on a wide variety of endocrine tissues, it is also used to treat endocrine tumors in the pancreas and gastrointestinal tract (carcinoid tumors) and hormonally responsive diarrheal conditions.

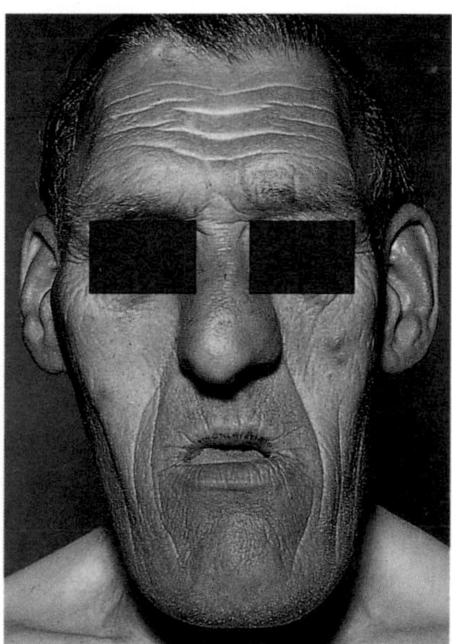

Fig. 12.7 Characteristic facial features of acromegaly. (Courtesy of Dr CD Forbes and Dr WF Jackson.)

Causes of hyperprolactinemia

Compression of pituitary stalk by mass lesions	
Pituitary lactotroph adenoma	
Physiologic stimuli	Suckling Chest wall trauma
Hormonal effects	Pregnancy Estrogen therapy Hypothyroidism
Drugs	Antipsychotic drugs (dopamine antagonists) Cimetidine Verapamil Opiates
Renal failure and hepatic cirrhosis	

Fig. 12.6 Causes of hyperprolactinemia.

Symptoms and signs of acromegaly

- Coarse facial features
- Enlargement of hands and feet
- Thickening of soft tissues
- Dental misalignment
- Arthralgias
- Excessive sweating
- Glucose intolerance
- Enlargement of organs (e.g. heart)
- Hypertension
- Skin tags

Fig. 12.8 Signs and symptoms of acromegaly.

Growth hormone deficiency

Short stature is a common clinical disorder and is only rarely caused by deficiency in growth hormone (Figs 12.10, 12.11). Growth hormone deficiency may result from panhypopituitarism, selective impairment of pituitary somatotrophs, or deficient hypothalamic GHRH release.

Pituitary extracts have been used pharmacotherapeutically in the past, but have been replaced by recombinant human growth hormone, somatropin, and a closely related recombinant protein, somatrem. Since endogenous growth hormone release occurs in an irregular pattern of periodic brief elevations that elicit sustained IGF secretion, continuous plasma levels of exogenous growth hormone are not necessary for therapeutic efficacy. Recombinant growth hormone can be given daily or even several times weekly. Although growth hormone therapy has been studied in other conditions of short stature such as constitutional short stature and Turner's syndrome, there is no consensus that adult height is favorably influenced by growth hormone therapy of these conditions. The use of growth hormone is being investigated as a therapy for frail elderly patients in view of its anabolic effects on muscle and bone.

THE THYROID AND DISORDERS OF METABOLIC RATE

Thyroid hormone controls the metabolic activity of all tissues by regulating genes whose protein products are critical in cellular respiration

Many tissues respond to hormonal and paracrine stimuli by increasing cellular respiration. Skeletal muscle, for example, responds to nicotinic receptor stimulation by activating myosin–ATPase and subsequently increasing glycolysis to sustain muscle contraction. Independent of this type of tissue and function-specific regulation of cell metabolism, thyroid hormone exerts a broad regulation of cell respiration and protein synthesis, which is loosely referred to as 'metabolic rate.' The effects of thyroid hormone are varied (Fig. 12.12), but are best understood as regulating the body's overall level of cellular metabolic activity and energy expenditure.

Conditions such as starvation or severe illness reduce thyroid hormone activity and conserve energy expenditure by many tissues. Conversely, the hypothalamic–pituitary–thyroid axis is stimulated under conditions of CNS arousal such as fear and anxiety. Although thyroid hormone is not considered to be part of the hormonal 'fight or flight' response because of its slow time course of effect, it has a complementary function in modulating the body's response to more prolonged periods of stress.

The synthesis, release and end-organ effects of thyroid hormones involve numerous steps, several of which are sites of drug action

Active thyroid hormone (triiodothyronine or T_3) and its precursor (thyroxine, tetraiodothyronine, or T_4) are formed by the addition of I^- anions to two sites on the aromatic rings of tyrosine residues on a large peptide (thyroglobulin) stored in the thyroid gland. The iodination of tyrosine molecules, and the linkage of two iodotyrosine molecules together to form thyronine requires three key features of the thyroid epithelial cell:

- The ability to accumulate high intracellular concentrations of I^- by active transport from the blood (I^- transport).

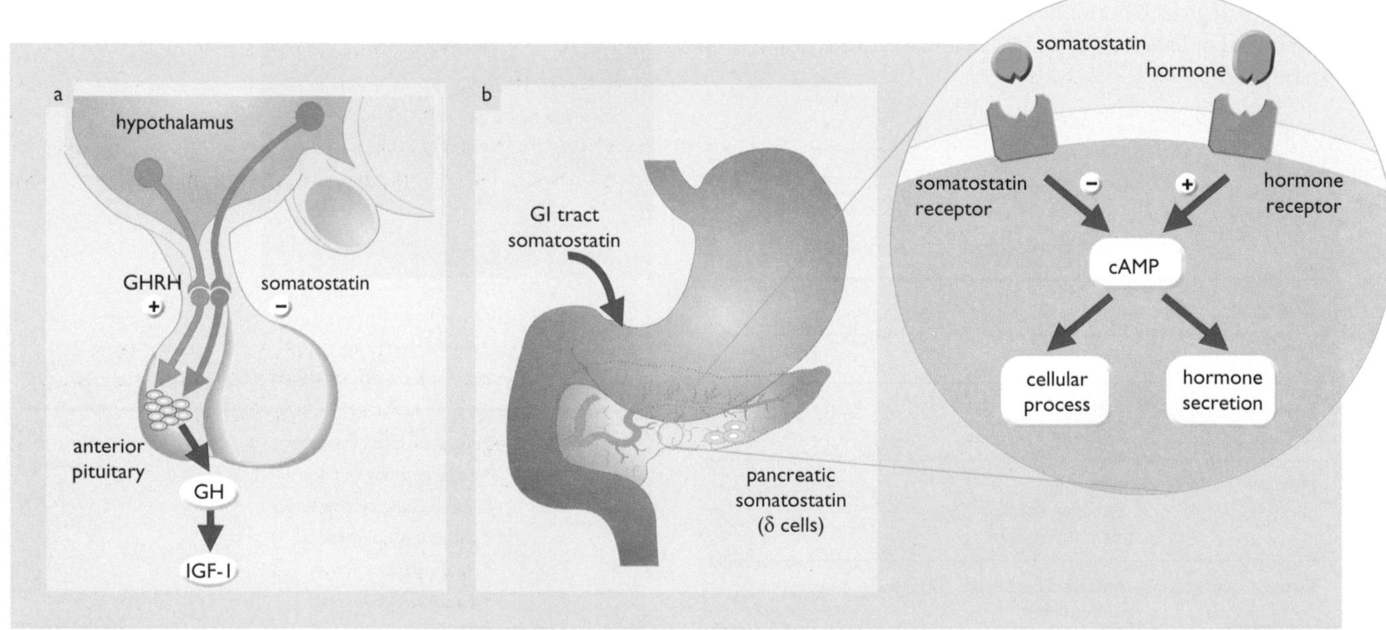

Fig. 12.9 Somatostatin physiology. Somatostatin is synthesized and released locally in the hypothalamus, pancreatic δ cells (a) and gastrointestinal (GI) tract (b). Stomatostatin inhibits cellular processes related to growth hormone (GH), insulin, glucagon, and enteric hormone secretion by reducing cAMP accumulation and inhibiting cellular depolarization (inset). Octreotide is a synthetic peptide analog of somatostatin used in the treatment of GI carcinoid tumors, hormone-mediated bowel disease, and occasionally, acromegaly. (GHRH, growth hormone releasing hormone; IGF-1, insulin-like growth factor-1)

- The action of an oxidizing enzyme, thyroid peroxidase, to catalyze the binding of hypoiodate (IO^-) to the tyrosine ring and the coupling of two iodinated tyrosines.
- The large polypeptide, thyroglobulin, with numerous tyrosine residues suitable for iodination and coupling (Fig. 12.13).

Thyroglobulin in the extracellular thyroid follicles stores iodinated thyronine, which is released as thyroid hormone into the blood after endocytosis and cleavage by thyroid follicular cells. The thyroid follicles store preformed thyroid hormone, usually in sufficient amounts to sustain T_4 release for approximately 6 weeks. T_3 has a tenfold greater binding affinity for the thyroid receptor than T_4, and is therefore considered to be the active form of the hormone. Although some T_3 is released from the thyroid gland, most is formed by deiodination of T_4 by deiodinase enzymes distributed throughout the body (peripheral conversion).

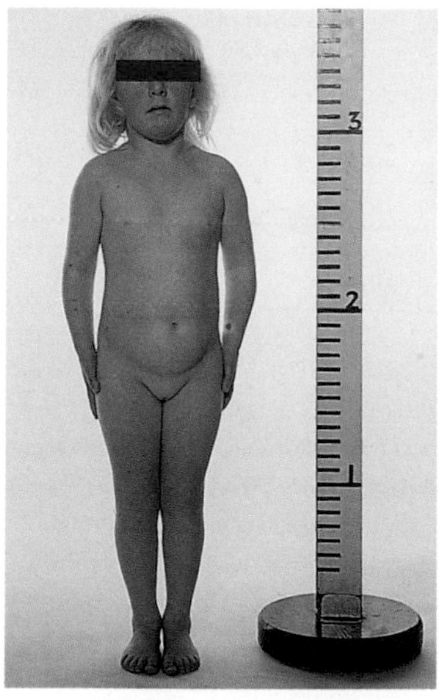

Fig. 12.10 Growth hormone deficiency in a 10-year-old girl. (Courtesy of Dr WF Jackson.)

Causes of short stature	
Constitutional short stature	
Familial (genetic) short stature	
Chronic illness	
Intrauterine growth retardation	
Psychosocial dwarfism	
Endocrine conditions	Hypopituitarism Growth hormone (GH) deficiency GH resistance (dwarfism) Hypothyroidism Glucocorticosteroid excess Vitamin D disorders
Genetic syndromes	Achondroplasia Turner's syndrome Noonan's syndrome Genetic obesity syndromes

Fig. 12.11 Causes of short stature.

Hypothyroidism

Thyroid hormone deficiency is a common disorder and is usually caused by autoimmune destruction of the thyroid gland. It produces the symptoms of lethargy, weight gain, cold intolerance, dry skin, and mental sluggishness. In its most severe form (myxedema), it may cause coma, while in neonates, hypothyroidism is an important cause of lifelong cognitive impairment and abnormal skeletal development (cretinism).

Primary failure of the thyroid gland due to autoimmune disease (Hashimoto's thyroiditis) is the most common cause of hypothyroidism, although other inflammatory conditions and physical damage may also impair thyroid gland activity (Fig. 12.14). Autoimmune thyroid disease, like many autoimmune diseases, is more prevalent in women, and in rare cases may be associated with other autoimmune endocrine deficiencies, such as adrenal failure, insulin-dependent diabetes mellitus, or hypogonadism. Impaired thyroid hormone action may also be due to reduced pituitary TSH secretion (secondary) or the rare condition of cellular resistance (thyroid hormone resistance).

Synthetic thyroid hormones are widely used to treat hypothyroidism

Synthetic levothyroxine is a convenient, orally active hormone replacement therapy. Although it requires metabolic activation to form active T_3, it is commonly used because of its long elimination half-life of 6 days. This prolonged action is largely due to its high degree of binding to plasma thyroid binding globulin and to prealbumin, which reduces clearance and provides a large store of circulating drug. Drugs with long elimination half-lives are useful in the treatment of chronic diseases as the impact of a single missed dose on the steady-state plasma concentration is small. The disadvantage of levothyroxine therapy is its slow rate of achieving steady-state effects: dose adjustments can be evaluated only after treatment for 5 weeks.

Physiologic effects of thyroid hormone

- Fetal development (physical and cognitive)
- Metabolic rate
- Body temperature
- Cardiac rate and contractility
- Peripheral vasodilation
- Red cell mass and circulatory volume
- Respiratory drive
- Peripheral nerves (reflexes)
- Hepatic metabolic enzymes
- Bone turnover
- Skin and soft tissue effects

Fig. 12.12 Physiologic effects of thyroid hormone.

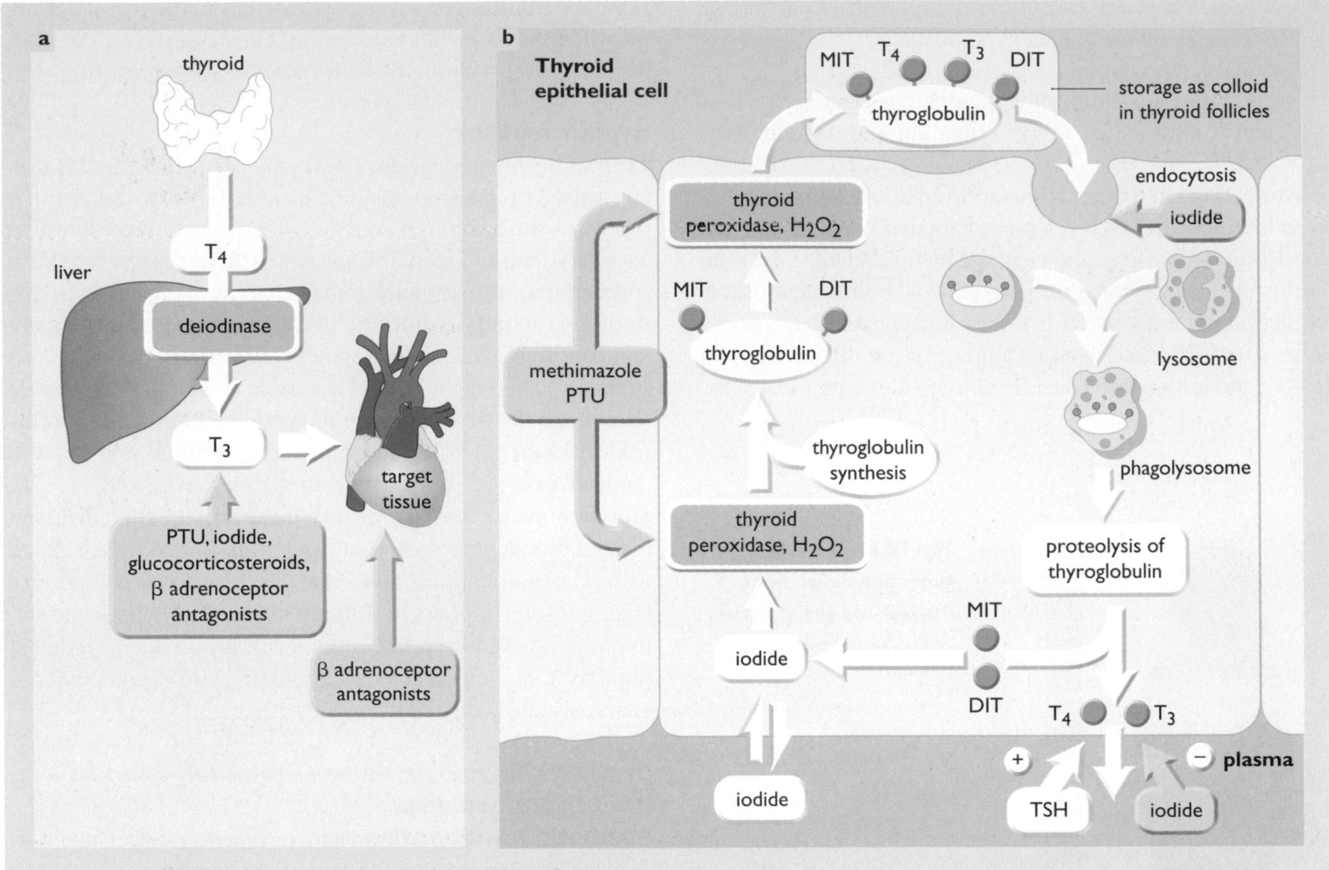

Fig. 12.13 Thyroid hormone pharmacology. (a) Thyroxine (tetraiodothyronine or T_4) undergoes deiodination to triiodothyronine (T_3) by diodinase at peripheral sites such as the liver. The sites of action of antithyroid drugs are also shown. (b) Iodide is actively transported into thyroid epithelial cells. Thyroid peroxidase, a microsomal enzyme, catalyzes the iodination of the aromatic rings of tyrosine at the 3 and 5 positions, creating monoiodotyrosine (MIT) and diiodotyrosine (DIT). Thyroid peroxidase also couples iodotyrosines to form thyronine residues in thyroglobulin. Thyroglobulin is secreted and stored in the thyroid follicles. Thyroid stimulating hormone (TSH) causes stored thyroglobulin to undergo endocytosis and lysosomal proteolysis to release thyroid hormone. (PTU, propylthiouracil)

Causes of hypothyroidism	
Primary	Chronic lymphocytic thyroiditis (Hashimoto's disease)
	Subacute thyroiditis
	Painless thyroiditis (postpartum thyroiditis)
	Radioactive iodine ingestion
	Iodine deficiency or excess
	Inborn errors of thyroid hormone synthesis
Secondary	Pituitary disease
Target tissues	Thyroid hormone resistance

Fig. 12.14 Causes of hypothyroidism.

Liothyronine (L-triiodothyronine sodium) is poorly bound to thyroid binding globulin and therefore achieves biologic effects more rapidly than levothyroxine, but there are wide fluctuations in plasma concentrations between doses.

Other forms of thyroid hormone replacement include dessicated thyroid gland preparations from beef or pork and pork thyroglobulin preparations, but their usage is declining.

Hyperthyroidism

Hyperthyroidism is a syndrome of excessive tissue metabolism due to excessive thyroid hormone action resulting from either:

- Overproduction of endogenous hormone.
- Ingestion of exogenous hormone.

Thyroid hormone excess is usually due to immunologically stimulated thyroid hormone release or a hormone-producing thyroid

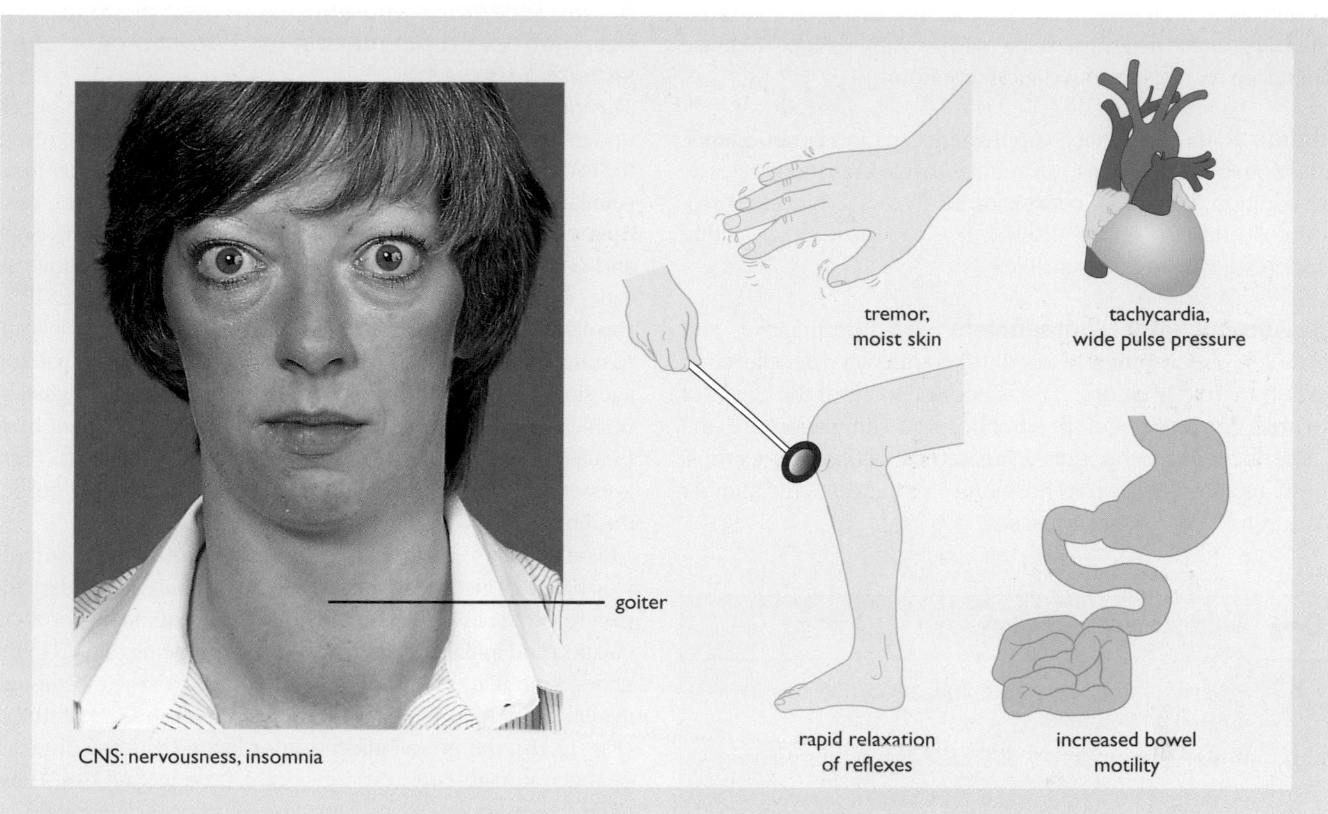

Fig. 12.15 Signs, symptoms, and causes of hyperthyroidism. Hyperthyroidism leads to characteristic symptoms of nervousness, weight loss, heat intolerance, and fatigue. Signs such as tachycardia, tremor, accelerated reflexes, smooth skin, hyperhidrosis, and ocular stare are common to hyperthyroidism of any cause. Proptosis, diplopia, and corneal inflammation are specific findings in Graves' disease. (Photograph courtesy of Dr CD Forbes and Dr WF Jackson.)

adenoma. Autoimmune disease (Graves' disease) is the most common cause. In Graves' disease antibodies activate TSH receptors, leading to diffuse enlargement of the thyroid gland, excess hormone, and the classic stigmata of hyperthyoidism (i.e. nervousness, weight loss, tremor, eyelid retraction, sweating, and heat intolerance) (Figs 12.15, 12.16). Other forms of hyperthyroidism share these features, but Graves' disease is the only form of hyperthyroidism in which there is an immunologic attack on the extraocular muscles, which causes protrusion of the globe (proptosis, exophthalmos). Other immunologic forms of thyroiditis may also result in excess thyroid hormone production by allowing preformed thyroid hormone to leak from an inflamed thyroid gland.

The major types of nonimmunologically mediated hyperthyroidism are adenomas, either single (hyperfunctioning adenoma) or multiple (multinodular goiter). Multinodular goiter is common in the elderly and is usually clinically insignificant. Occasionally, thyroid hormone production by an adenoma exceeds daily requirements and leads to hyperthyroidism.

Causes of hyperthyroidism

- Thyroid hormone ingestion
- Diffuse toxic goiter (Graves' disease)
- Hyperfunctioning adenoma (toxic nodule)
- Toxic multinodular goiter
- Painless thyroiditis
- Subacute thyroiditis
- Thyroid stimulating hormone (TSH)-secreting adenoma
- Human chorionic gonadotropin (HCG)-secreting tumors

Fig. 12.16 Causes of hyperthyroidism.

Antithyroid drugs inhibit thyroid hormone synthesis, release, peripheral conversion, and target tissue effects

The agents used to treat hyperthyoidism can act at almost every step of thyroid hormone synthesis and release (see Fig. 12.13).

Methimazole and propylthiouracil inhibit the thyroid peroxidase enzyme leading to reduced thyroid hormone formation and storage in the thyroid follicles. However, the effect of these drugs may not be detectable for several weeks if there are stores of previously synthesized hormone. Propylthiouracil also inhibits the deiodination reaction that produces active T_3 from T_4. This may be desirable if the hyperthyroidism is life-threatening. Methimazole, however, has a longer elimination half-life allowing once- or twice-daily doses and so improving compliance. Both drugs can cause allergic reactions and rarely are hepatotoxic and cause bone marrow suppression. Their use therefore requires careful clinical monitoring.

Iodide found in dietary supplements, radiocontrast agents, and some cough syrups can reduce thyroid hormone release. In addition, I^- reduces conversion of T_4 to T_3. In acute thyrotoxicosis due to Graves' disease, I^- is the most rapidly acting suppressive treatment available.

β Adrenoceptor antagonists (e.g. propranolol and esmolol) are commonly used to counteract the effects of excess thyroid hormone. This is because many of the effects of thyroid hormone and β adrenoceptor stimulation are the same, including tachycardia, increased metabolic rate, nervousness, and tremor. Thyroid hormone also increases the number of adrenoceptors in many tissues.

Antithyroid drug therapy

- Propylthiouracil and methimazole inhibit thyroid hormone synthesis
- I^- blocks the release of stored thyroid hormone
- I^-, propylthiouracil, and β adrenoceptor antagonists inhibit conversion of thyroxine (tetraiodothyronine or T_4) to triiodothyronine (T_3)
- β Adrenoceptor antagonists functionally antagonize the target organ effects of thyroid hormone

DISORDERS OF CARBOHYDRATE METABOLISM

Although thyroid hormone regulates the basal metabolic rate of tissues, its effect on the delivery of fuel precursors to cells is minor. Instead this critical endocrine function is performed mainly by the endocrine pancreas. Unlike most other endocrine systems, regulation of the endocrine pancreas does not occur through a hypothalamic–pituitary axis. Instead, carbohydrate and lipid metabolism is regulated by:

- Signals from the gut (released by gastric distension and food content).
- Signals from the blood stream (circulating glucose levels).
- Intracellular signals (intracellular energy stores).

The overall homeostatic function of both carbohydrate and lipid metabolism is to deliver fuel substrates for use and storage after eating, and to mobilize fuel stores during the fasting (postabsorptive) state.

The regulation of carbohydrate and fatty acid metabolism is the key function of insulin and associated counterregulatory hormones. The maintenance of adequate levels of circulating glucose is essential for brain tissue and red blood cells since these tissues lack insulin-dependent glucose transporters and depend on circulating glucose concentration for their energy supply.

Insulin receptor stimulation activates glucose transporters on the plasma membranes of insulin-sensitive tissues

The intracellular mechanism of insulin action is not completely understood. The insulin receptor is a membrane-bound receptor with tyrosine kinase activity (Fig. 12.17). As with other intracellular kinases, phosphorylation of intracellular proteins alters their enzymatic activity resulting in sequential phosphorylating and dephosphorylating steps in an intracellular signaling cascade. One important substrate for the insulin receptor is IRS-1 (insulin receptor substrate-1). Insulin receptor stimulation leads to translocation of glucose transporters from an endosomal storage site to the plasma membrane, leading to increased glucose uptake. The regulation of glucose transporters on peripheral tissues is essential to fuel delivery, while on pancreatic β cells it is essential to the glucose sensing mechanism, which regulates insulin release.

Insulin release occurs in response to food-related stimuli, which reflect increasing fuel availability. Insulin released by the pancreatic β cells in the islets of Langerhans enters the portal circulation and initially acts on the liver before being diluted in the general circulation and delivered to other tissues. Although insulin has numerous effects on fuel metabolism in these tissues (Fig. 12.18), the overall effect is coordinated glucose disposal, glycogen storage, fatty acid storage, and protein synthesis. These different metabolic effects of insulin can occur at different doses. Inhibition of ketone body formation in the liver occurs at lower doses of insulin than those required to stimulate glucose uptake in skeletal muscle.

Counterregulatory hormones from the pancreas, pituitary, adrenal cortex, and adrenal medulla protect against hypoglycemia

In the fasting state, glucose concentrations decline and insulin release is suppressed. Multiple neurohormonal responses occur if the plasma glucose falls below a critical concentration. These include:

- Pancreatic glucagon release.
- Sympathetic nervous system activation.
- Hypothalamic–pituitary–adrenal release of growth hormone, cortisol, and epinephrine.

These counterregulatory hormones increase glycogenolysis and inhibit insulin release. The prodromal symptoms of hypoglycemia (nervousness, tachycardia, tremor, sweating) result from sympathetic nervous system activity. Failure of the counterregulatory response, as seen in extreme insulin excess and panhypopituitarism, leads to an insufficient supply of glucose to the brain and coma.

Somatostatin, which is synthesized in pancreatic δ cells and elsewhere, inhibits the release of both insulin and counterregulatory hormones, providing a mechanism to dampen the escalating insulin and counterregulatory hormone release.

Diabetes mellitus

Two types of diabetes mellitus share the features of hyperglycemia and vascular pathology. They differ in their pathogenesis and in the ability of residual insulin to suppress ketone formation from fatty acids (Fig. 12.19).

Deficient insulin action is a feature of several syndromes.

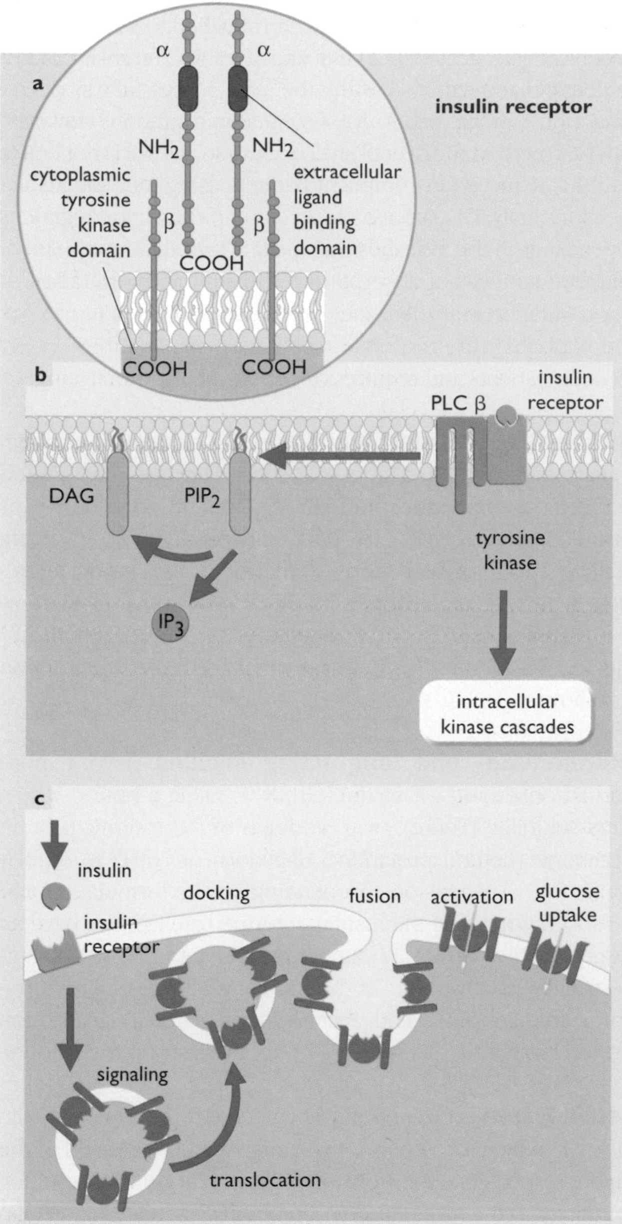

Fig. 12.17 Insulin action. (a) The insulin receptor is a heterodimeric transmembrane receptor consisting of two α and two β subunits. The intracellular portions of the β subunits contain tyrosine kinase activity (see Chapter 3). (b) Insulin receptor stimulation leads to phosphorylation of multiple intracellular signaling molecules. Phosphorylation of tyrosine kinase residues on intracellular kinases leads to activation of serine/threonine kinase cascades. Phosphorylation of phospholipase C (PLC) leads to intracellular Ca^{2+}-mediated signaling events. (c) Intracellular signals cause translocation of glucose transporters from an endosomal compartment to the plasma membrane where they increase glucose uptake. (DAG, diacylglycerol; IP_3, inositol-1,4,5-triphosphate; PIP_2, phosphoinositol)

Insulin-dependent diabetes mellitus (IDDM or Type 1 diabetes mellitus) results from autoimmune destruction of pancreatic β cells. The autoimmune attack begins years before insulin secretion fails and by the time diabetes mellitus is diagnosed the β cells are irreversibly damaged. This usually occurs at less than 30 years of age, hence the former description as 'juvenile onset' diabetes mellitus. The cardinal finding in this diabetic syndrome is an inability to secrete even the modest amounts of insulin needed to suppress ketone formation, resulting in recurrent episodes of diabetic ketoacidosis.

Effects of insulin on fuel homeostasis

Carbohydrates	Increases glucose transport Increases glycogen synthesis Increases glycolysis Inhibits gluconeogenesis
Fats	Increases lipoprotein lipase activity Increases fat storage in adipocytes Inhibits lipolysis (hormone sensitive lipase) Increases hepatic lipoprotein synthesis Inhibits fatty acid oxidation
Proteins	Increases protein synthesis Increases amino acid transport

Fig. 12.18 Effects of insulin on fuel homeostasis.

Features of insulin-dependent (IDDM) and non-insulin-dependent (NIDDM) diabetes mellitus

	IDDM	**NIDDM**
Age at onset	< 30 yrs	> 30 yrs
Family history of diabetes mellitus	Uncommon	Common
Body weight	Not obese	Obese
Ketoacidosis	Common	Rare
Insulin treatment	All patients	Some patients
Other autoimmune endocrine deficiencies	Yes (rare)	No
Prevalence in adult population	0.5%	5%
HLA association	Yes	No

Fig. 12.19 Features of insulin-dependent (IDDM) and non-insulin-dependent (NIDDM) diabetes mellitus.

Noninsulin dependent diabetes mellitus (NIDDM or Type 2 diabetes mellitus) is the other major form of diabetes mellitus. Insulin is secreted, but is ineffective in normalizing plasma glucose. However, the circulating insulin concentrations are adequate to suppress ketone formation under most circumstances, so patients do not have repeated bouts of diabetic ketoacidosis. Although insulin may be used therapeutically, NIDDM patients are not dependent on insulin therapy to prevent ketoacidosis. The cardinal finding is that increments in plasma insulin do not lead to the expected increases in glucose disposal. This phenomenon is termed 'insulin resistance.' Resistance syndromes in other endocrine systems are caused by receptor mutations, but NIDDM is not usually due to a mutated insulin receptor. The term NIDDM defines a syndrome that may include several different disease processes including:

- Glucose transporter defects.
- Desensitization of insulin receptors.
- Toxic effects of hyperglycemia.
- The metabolic demands of obesity.
- Conditions associated with excessive counterregulatory hormones (e.g. pheochromocytoma, Cushing's syndrome, and acromegaly).
- Conditions associated with a loss of pancreatic function (e.g. pancreatic cancer surgery and pancreatitis).

Insulin resistance can occur in the absence of hyperglycemia

Severe insulin resistance leads to impaired glucose regulation and the development of clinical diabetes mellitus, but many patients with hypertension and hypercholesterolemia demonstrate insulin resistance without abnormal glucose regulation. This observation has led to the term 'syndrome X' to describe patients with hypertension, hypercholesterolemia, and insulin resistance. Such patients constitute a large fraction of the population at risk of premature arteriosclerosis. The pathogenetic mechanism underlying this syndrome is not known, but impaired insulin action is associated with increased hepatic very low density lipoprotein (VLDL) production and lower circulating high density lipoprotein (HDL) concentrations (see below), which increase the risk of arteriosclerosis.

Both types of diabetes mellitus lead to microvascular and neuronal dysfunction which contribute to the 'end organ complications'

Although IDDM and NIDDM differ in disease etiology, the prevalence of ketoacidosis, and the role of insulin resistance, they both produce the same pathologic sequelae. The so-called 'end-organ complications' include retinal disease, renal failure, peripheral nerve dysfunction, peripheral vascular disease, and arteriosclerosis.

Owing to the prevalence of obesity in affluent societies, NIDDM is nine times more common in the adult population of such societies than IDDM. Diabetes is a leading cause of blindness and renal failure, and a major cause of morbidity and mortality due to arteriosclerosis resulting in cerebrovascular thrombosis, myocardial infarction, and amputations of the extremities.

Different insulin preparations with different patterns of absorption are used to match insulin delivery to caloric intake

Before the isolation of insulin for therapeutic use in the 1930s, IDDM was fatal in childhood. A variety of insulin preparations have since been developed to provide a 'physiologic' pattern of insulin replacement. An insulin pump attached to a small subcutaneous needle, delivering a basal rate of insulin and small boluses on demand at mealtimes, is the the most successful way of creating a physiologic pattern of insulin administration. However, with this method the overall level of glucose control is not better than that achieved in compliant patients using multiple insulin injections daily. The success of such multiple injection regimens depends upon the availability of insulins with different pharmacokinetic patterns of absorption. Estimates of the duration of action of different insulins (see below) are, however, imprecise. The hypoglycemic response to a given insulin varies widely between patients and requires close therapeutic monitoring.

Short-acting regular insulins most resemble endogenous insulin in their duration of action. They are precipitated with Zn^{2+} to maintain solubility, but contain no additives or formulation strategies to delay absorption. Short-acting insulins spontaneously form dimeric or hexameric aggregates which retard absorption. Since subcutaneous absorption is slower than pancreatic release, such preparations are injected 30–45 minutes before a meal and exert their action for 6 hours.

Intermediate- and long-acting insulins have a more gradual onset and offset due either to using a buffer, which alters solubility (Lente), or to addition of the cationic protein protamine (neutral protamine Hagedorn or NPH) to regular insulin Zn^{2+} suspensions. Depending on the formulation and the species origin of the insulin, intermediate insulins have an onset of action within 2 hours, a peak effect at 10 hours, and are usually inactive after 20 hours. Long-acting insulin (Ultralente) contains Zn^{2+} and acetate buffer to delay absorption further. It begins to act within 4 hours and lasts up to 36 hours.

Insulin lyspro is a genetically engineered recombinant insulin analog in which the order of two amino acids is reversed in the region responsible for hormone dimerization. The resulting homology to the monomeric hormone IGF-1 creates an insulin that is absorbed rapidly as a monomer. This analog has a onset and duration of action shorter than that of regular insulin and is therefore given immediately before meals.

Insulin regimens generally include an intermediate insulin given to provide a maximal effect during meal ingestion and a minimal effect during fasting periods such as sleep. Treatment of IDDM requires a close matching of insulin administration with caloric intake and therefore a combination of regular and intermediate insulin is usually necessary. Many NIDDM patients, who have residual β cell function, only need intermediate or long-acting insulin to improve glycemic control. Insulin administration is guided by the timing and pattern of food intake, but the early morning increase in activity of the hypothalamic–pituitary–adrenal (HPA) hormones such as cortisol and epinephrine may increase blood sugar even without food intake. The slow rate of absorption of intermediate insulin and the 'dawn phenomenon' of the HPA axis allows intermediate insulin to be taken at bedtime with minimal nocturnal hypoglycemia. Typical insulin replacement schedules are depicted in Figs 12.20 and 20.21.

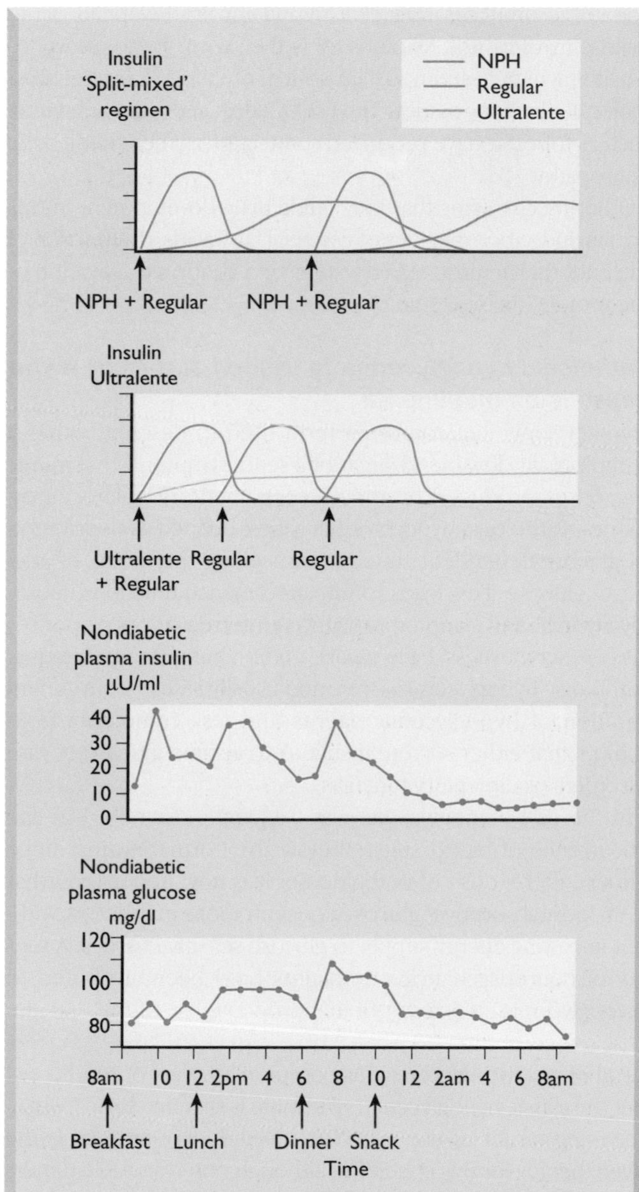

Fig. 12.20 Insulin therapy. Exogenously administered insulin does not mirror the rapid meal-related increases of pancreatic insulin secretion owing to delayed absorption from the site of injection. The goal of insulin dosing regimens is to coordinate peaks in insulin delivery with the times of calorie ingestion. Systemic insulin levels are higher during insulin therapy of IDDM than with endogenous pancreatic regulation. Pancreatic insulin release into the portal venous system may suppress hepatic gluconeogenesis at lower doses than those needed with systemic insulin administration.

Oral hypoglycemic agents increase insulin secretion or increase the sensitivity of tissues to endogenous insulin

Oral hypoglycemic agents are used to treat patients with diabetes mellitus who do not require insulin to prevent ketoacidosis. These drugs can be categorized according to whether they increase insulin release, increase sensitivity to insulin, or block glucose uptake.

Sulfonylurea drugs are the mainstay of oral hypoglycemic therapy. They:

- Block K^+/ATP channels in pancreatic β cells.
- Cause depolarization and subsequent activation of voltage-sensitive Ca^{2+} channels and increased insulin release.

The sulfonylurea hypoglycemics used clinically differ in their potency, duration of effect, and adverse effects profile (Fig. 12.22).

Insulin preparations

Insulin preparation	Action	Peak activity (h)	Duration (h)
Regular	Rapid	1–3	5–7
Semilente	Rapid	3–4	10–16
Neutral protamine Hagedorn (NPH)	Intermediate	6–14	18–28
Lente	Intermediate	6–14	18–28
Ultralente	Prolonged	18–24	30–40

Fig. 12.21 Insulin preparations.

Oral hypoglycemic agents

	Major mechanism	Typical daily dose (mg)	Duration of action (h)
Second-generation sulfonylureas	Insulin release		
Glyburide		5–20	10–24
Glipizide		5–40	10–16
First-generation sulfonylureas	Insulin release		
Tolbutamide		500–2000	6–12
Chlorpropamide		100–500	60
Tolazamide		200–1000	12–24
Acetohexamide		250–1500	12–24
Biguanides			
Metformin	Insulin sensitivity	500–2500	6–12

Fig. 12.22 Oral hypoglycemic agents.

Biguanides (metformin, phenformin) are another class of hypoglycemic agents. Their predominant effect is to increase tissue sensitivity to insulin. Clinical use of phenformin may lead to lactic acidosis, but this adverse effect is less common with the newer generation biguanide, metformin. Combined use of biguanides with sulfonylureas produces additive hypoglycemic effects, which may reduce the need for insulin therapy in some Type II diabetics. Troglidazone is a new hypoglycemic agent which is chemically distinct from the biguanides which has similar effects on tissue sensitivity to insulin.

Acarbose provides an alternative strategy for increasing insulin action. It reduces glucose absorption by inhibiting polysaccharide hydrolysis by α-glucosidase in the intestine.

Agents that target the pathophysiology of end-organ complications may reduce the morbidity of diabetes mellitus

The large-scale prospective Diabetes Control and Complications Trial (DCCT) has demonstrated that maintenance of near normoglycemia using fastidious dietary control and insulin reduces the rate of development of retinal disease, nephropathy, and peripheral neuropathy in IDDM. Indirect evidence suggests that these benefits may extend to atherosclerotic complications in IDDM, as well as to the same spectrum of complications in NIDDM. Despite these benefits, such control is difficult to achieve clinically and therefore other therapies that can reduce the severity of diabetic complications are needed. Drug development in this area is based on animal studies and the clinical observations of diabetic pathophysiology. Streptozotocin and alloxan are β cell toxins used to produce IDDM in animals. Based on data from such animal models, a number of hypotheses have emerged to explain the mechanism of diabetic end-organ complications (Fig. 12.23).

One hypothesis focuses on the effect of chronic hyperglycemia on extracellular proteins such as the renal basement membrane. Chronic hyperglycemia leads to nonenzymatic glycation of proteins. Glycated proteins spontaneously form abnormal cross-linkages, which resist normal mechanisms for protein turnover and thereby produce a dysfunctional extracellular matrix. These advanced glycosylation end products (AGEs) may also lead to the release of cytokines from activated macrophages with growth-promoting effects on renal mesangial and vascular smooth muscle cells. Agents that reduce the formation of AGEs, such as aminoguanidine, are under investigation for clinical use.

Another therapeutic strategy for reducing the complications of diabetes mellitus is based on the observation that the 6-carbon polyol, sorbitol, accumulates in tissues that develop end-organ complications, such as the optic lens, retina, endothelium, and Schwann cells of peripheral nerves. Sorbitol is produced from glucose by the enzyme aldose reductase and is metabolized by conversion to fructose, but this path cannot eliminate the large amounts of sorbitol produced by chronic hyperglycemia. Sorbitol accumulates intracellularly and impairs the uptake of the hexose myoinositol. Myoinositol is the precursor to phosphoinositol, which is an important source of intracellular signaling molecules in many tissues. The use of aldose reductase inhibitors such as tolrestat have produced some improvement in diabetic neuropathy.

Other mechanisms that may guide drug development in this area include abnormalities of essential fatty acids, dysfunction of the endothelial nitric oxide system, and abnormal activation of the protein kinase C signaling pathway.

> **Oral agents for noninsulin-dependent diabetes mellitus (NIDDM)**
>
> - **Sulfonylureas stimulate insulin release by inhibiting K^+ channels on pancreatic β cells**
> - **Biguanides and troglidazole enhance the insulin sensitivity of target tissues**
> - **All hypoglycemic therapies improve insulin release and action by reducing hyperglycemic β cell dysfunction (glucose toxicity)**

Pathologic hypoglycemia is treated surgically if the cause is an insulinoma

Hypoglycemia is a confusing term used to describe either a pathologically low blood sugar or a set of symptoms that mimic responses produced by the glucose counterregulatory hormones. Pathologic hypoglycemia is best defined as deprivation of glucose-dependent tissues (particularly the brain) of adequate glucose. This leads to impaired mental function (neuroglycopenia) and symptoms of the counterregulatory responses such as nervousness, tachycardia, tremor, hunger, and sweating. Pathologic hypoglycemia is rare and usually results from administration of hypoglycemic agents and less commonly from tumors that either secrete insulin or consume glucose or rare disorders of alimentary function.

In the past, hypoglycemia was frequently diagnosed by the occurrence of blood sugars below the normal fasting range 3hours after a dose of oral glucose. It is now understood that such 'post-absorptive' glucose concentrations may be low without impairing energy supply to glucose-sensitive tissues. A variety of neuropsychiatric complaints have been attributed to 'hypoglycemia' as a result of inappropriate use of the oral glucose tolerance test.

Pathologic hypoglycemia may occur in a variety of conditions, but the classic hypoglycemic syndrome is that due to an insulin-secreting tumor of the pancreas (insulinoma). Surgery is the main therapy for this condition, although non-resectable tumors are occasionally treated pharmacologically with octreotide or diazoxide.

Diazoxide is a drug that reduces insulin secretion by activating K^+/ATP channels in β cells. This contrasts with the opposite effects of sulfonylurea hypoglycemic agents.

Glucagon The natural counterregulatory hormone, glucagon, is available as a therapeutic agent for parenteral administration, but its short half-life limits its use to the short-term correction of hypoglycemia resulting from the treatment of diabetes mellitus. However, glucose is usually preferred.

DISORDERS OF LIPID METABOLISM

Ingested fats are the body's main source of stored fuel. These fats, and those that are synthesized endogenously, form a variety of functionally important compounds such as cell membrane components, bile, steroid hormones, and intercellular signaling molecules (e.g. prostaglandins and leukotrienes).

The processes of dietary fat intake, hepatic synthesis of fat molecules, and delivery to target tissues is known collectively as lipoprotein metabolism (Fig. 12.24).

The lipoprotein system shuttles triglycerides to the peripheral tissues and orchestrates the movement of cholesterol

At the point of origin, the lipoprotein aggregate (intestinal chylomicron or hepatic VLDL particle) has its highest triglyceride

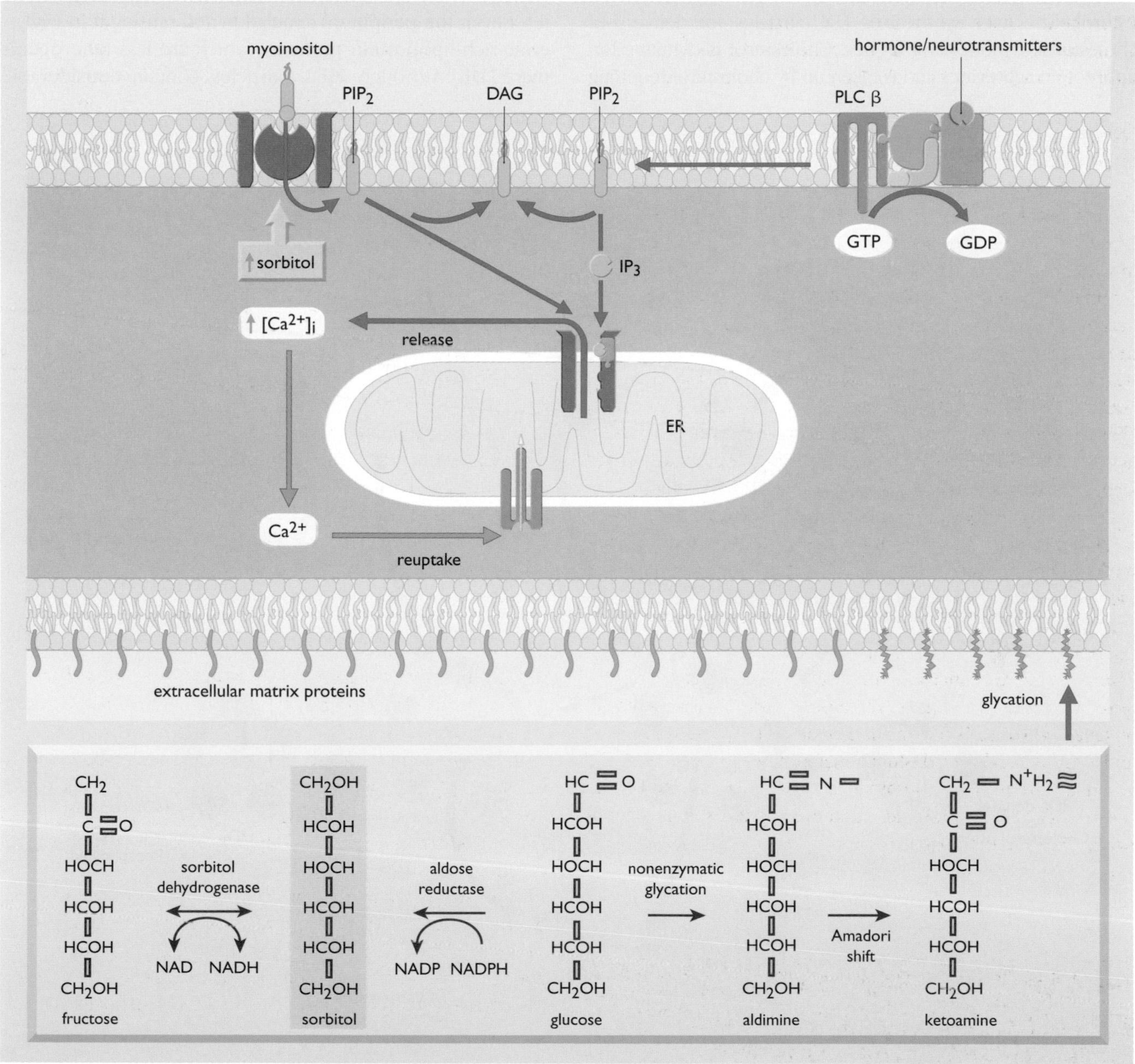

Fig. 12.23 Mechanisms of diabetic end-organ complications. High intracellular sorbitol concentrations accumulate owing to the action of aldose reductase on glucose. Intracellular sorbitol inhibits the cellular uptake of myoinositol which is a precursor for phosphatidylinositol (PIP_2) in the cell membrane. PIP_2 is the substrate for phospholipase C (PLC β), which is activated by G protein-coupled hormone or neurotransmitter stimulation in many tissues. Diacylglycerol (DAG) and inositol-1,4,5-triphosphate (IP_3) lead to protein kinase C activation and Ca^{2+}-mediated cellular responses. Hyperglycemia also impairs other functions by nonenzymatic glycation of extracellular proteins. The glycated amino acid residues undergo rearrangements that lead to abnormal covalent crosslinks. The function of these proteins may be impaired and they may resist normal turnover in the renal glomerulus and in the vasculature. (ER, endoplasmic reticulum)

content and therefore its lowest density. While circulating through peripheral vascular beds, lipoprotein lipase removes triglycerides from these aggregates for uptake by the tissues. Apoproteins of the C class act as cofactors for lipase activity and are exchanged between triglyceride-rich particles and circulating HDL. As the triglyceride content is progressively lost and the density increases, intermediate-density lipoprotein (IDL) particles and chylomicron remnants are eventually taken up by a hepatic uptake mechanism that recognizes B and E class apolipoproteins.

In addition to shuttling triglycerides to peripheral tissues, the lipoprotein system also orchestrates the movement of cholesterol. The liver synthesizes LDL particles for delivery of cholesterol to peripheral tissues. Cholesterol is contained in lipoprotein aggregates and is taken up by cholesterol-requiring tissues via the LDL receptor, the LDL receptor-related protein, and nonreceptor-mediated pathways. Defects of the LDL receptor lead to familial hypercholesterolemia, a lipoprotein disorder characterized by premature arteriosclerosis.

The liver also synthesizes components of the HDL particle that contain apolipoproteins which facilitate cholesterol esterification and transfer of cholesterol esters to triglyceride-rich particles. HDL also recovers non-esterified cholesterol and Apo C components from chylomicrons and VLDL remnants for reuse by new triglyceride-rich particles. This 'centripetal' cholesterol transport is one mechanism for removing cholesterol from the peripheral circulation and reusing it in triglyceride-rich lipoprotein particles, which are less atherogenic than LDL. Although HDL particles contain considerable

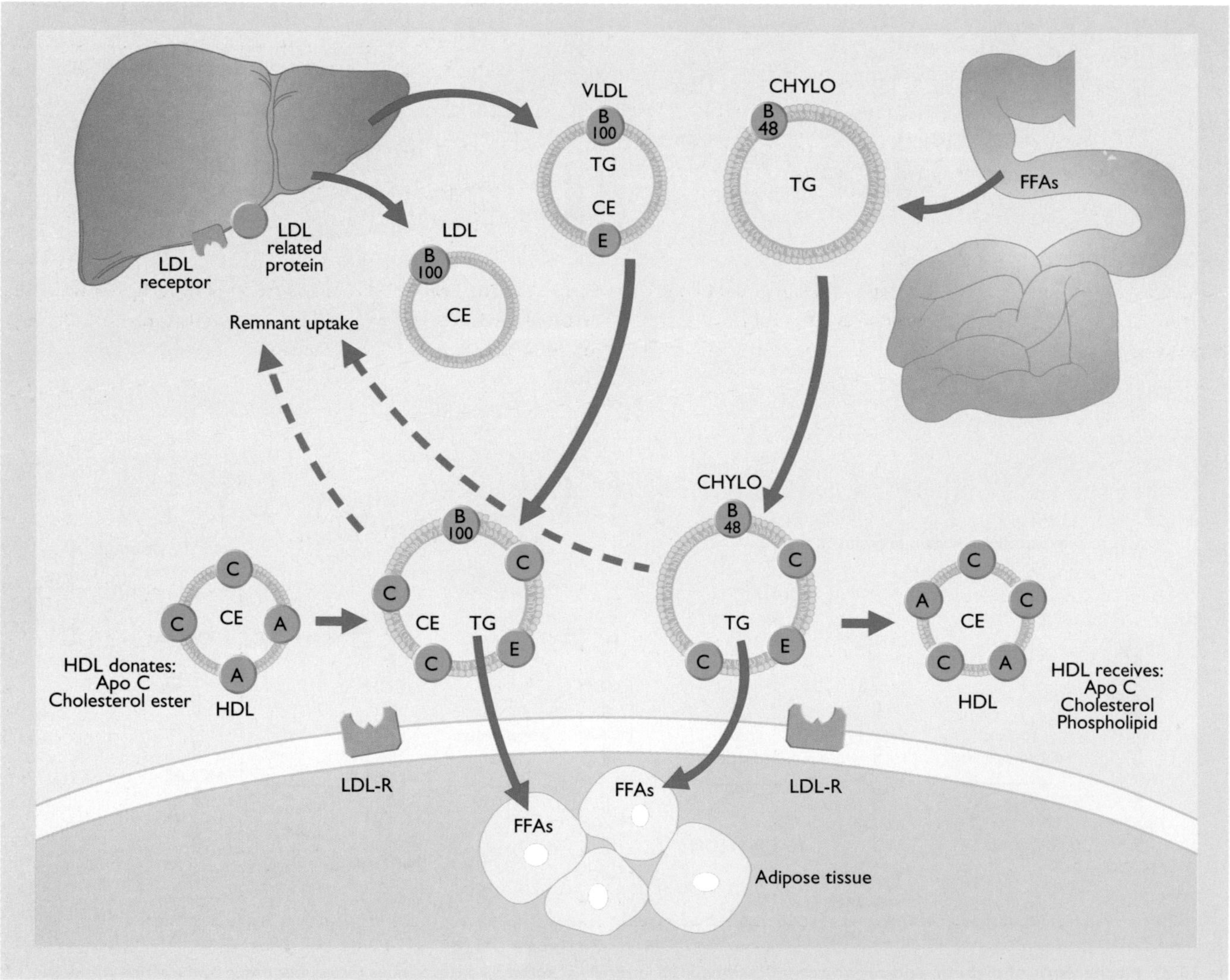

Fig. 12.24 Lipoprotein metabolism. Ingested fatty acids (FFAs) are converted to triglycerides (TG), combined with apoprotein (Apo) B-48, and covered by a phospholipid monolayer to form chylomicrons (CHYLO) in the intestinal lymph. Similarly, triglycerides synthesized in the liver are combined with Apo B-100 to form very low density lipoprotein (VLDL) in the liver. These triglyceride-rich lipoproteins acquire Apo C proteins from high density lipoprotein (HDL). Apo C is a cofactor for lipoprotein lipase (LPL) in the vascular endothelium, which delivers fatty acids to target tissues. As triglyceride-rich particles are metabolized, HDL recovers Apo C and phospholipids for reuse by other nascent particles. Remnant particles are taken up by the liver and secreted by the liver in LDL particles, which contain cholesterol ester (CE) as their predominant core constituent.

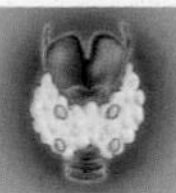

amounts of cholesterol, they do not contain the B and E class lipoproteins needed for receptor-mediated uptake of LDL and IDL particles.

Lipid-lowering drugs act at multiple steps in the lipoprotein metabolic pathway

Hyperlipidemias are common disorders in many countries. The most commonly encountered conditions are elevations of LDL, VLDL, or both lipoproteins produced by a combination of familial tendencies and dietary excess. Several hyperlipidemic syndromes have specific pathogenetic mechanisms, but these account for a minority of hypercholesterolemic patients. The specific mechanisms include:

- Defective LDL receptors (familial hypercholesterolemia).
- Deficiency of lipoprotein lipase (Type I hyperlipidemia, primary hypertriglyceridemia).
- Deficient remnant particle clearance (Type III hyperlipidemia, familial dysbetalipoproteinemia).

The Fredrickson classification of hyperlipidemias is commonly used for these disorders (Figs 12.25, 12.26).

Drug treatment of hyperlipidemia includes a variety of agents that affect cholesterol synthesis, cholesterol losses in bile, and LDL and VLDL metabolism. The steps involved in cholesterol and lipoprotein metabolism affected by such drugs are shown in Fig. 12.27.

HMG CoA reductase inhibitors

Cholesterol is synthesized in a variety of tissues from acetyl CoA. The rate-limiting step is the enzyme hydroxymethylglutaryl (HMG) CoA reductase, which releases the cholesterol precursor mevalonic acid from coenzyme A. Competitive inhibition of this enzyme by drugs such as lovastatin, pravastatin, simvastatin, and fluvastatin leads to compensatory cellular responses such as increased expression of HMG CoA enzyme and LDL receptors. Owing to the compensatory increase in HMG CoA, cellular cholesterol synthesis is only slightly reduced, but clearance of

The Fredrickson classification of hyperlipidemias

Type	Serum cholesterol and TG concentrations	Specific lipoproteins
I	TG very elevated Cholesterol mildly elevated	Chylomicrons increased VLDL normal
IIa	Cholesterol increased TG normal	LDL increased
IIb	Cholesterol increased TG increased	LDL and VLDL increased
III	Cholesterol increased TG increased	Excess IDL remnant particles
IV	TG increased Cholesterol normal	VLDL increased LDL normal
V	TG very elevated Cholesterol mildly elevated	Chylomicrons increased VLDL increased

Fig. 12.25 The Fredrickson classification of hyperlipidemias. (IDL, intermediate density lipoprotein; LDL, low density lipoprotein; VLDL, very low density lipoprotein; TG, triglyceride)

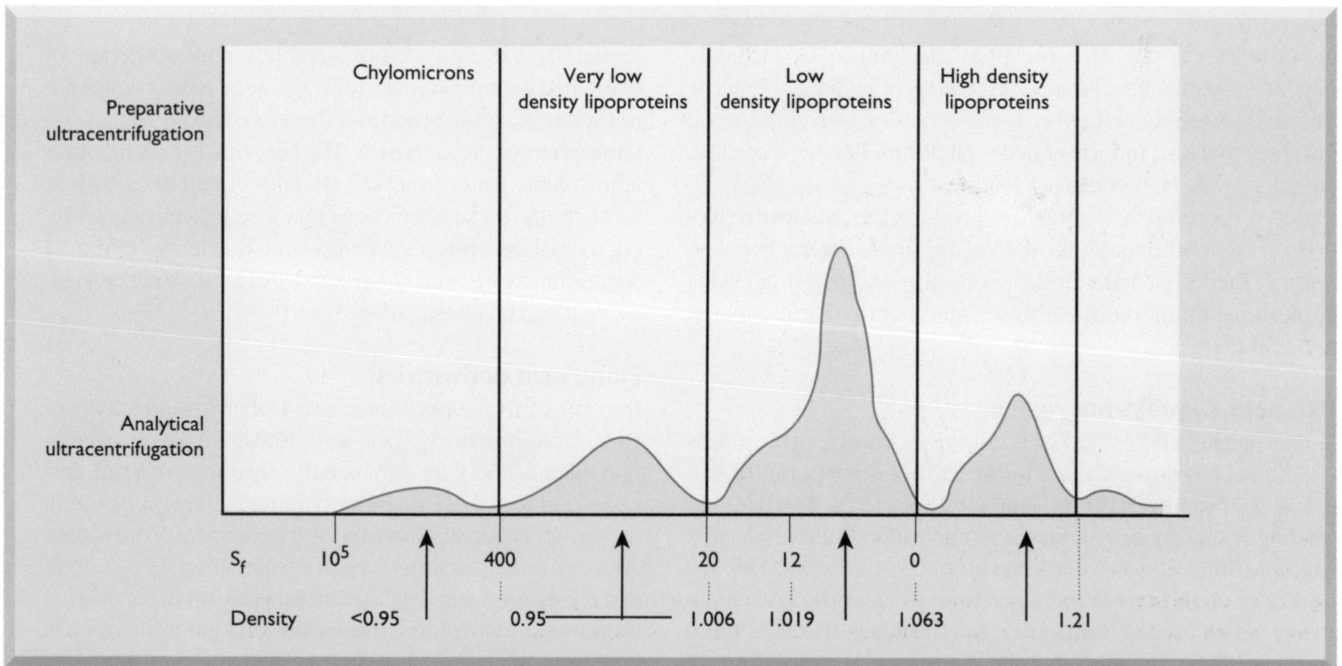

Fig. 12.26 Lipoprotein fractions. Ultracentrifugation of plasma reveals lipoprotein fractions of differing densities. The low density fraction contains both low (LDL) and intermediate-density lipoproteins (very low density lipoprotein remnants). The most commonly used cholesterol assays do not use ultracentrifugation, but instead estimate the concentration of LDL after measuring triglycerides and high density lipoproteins.

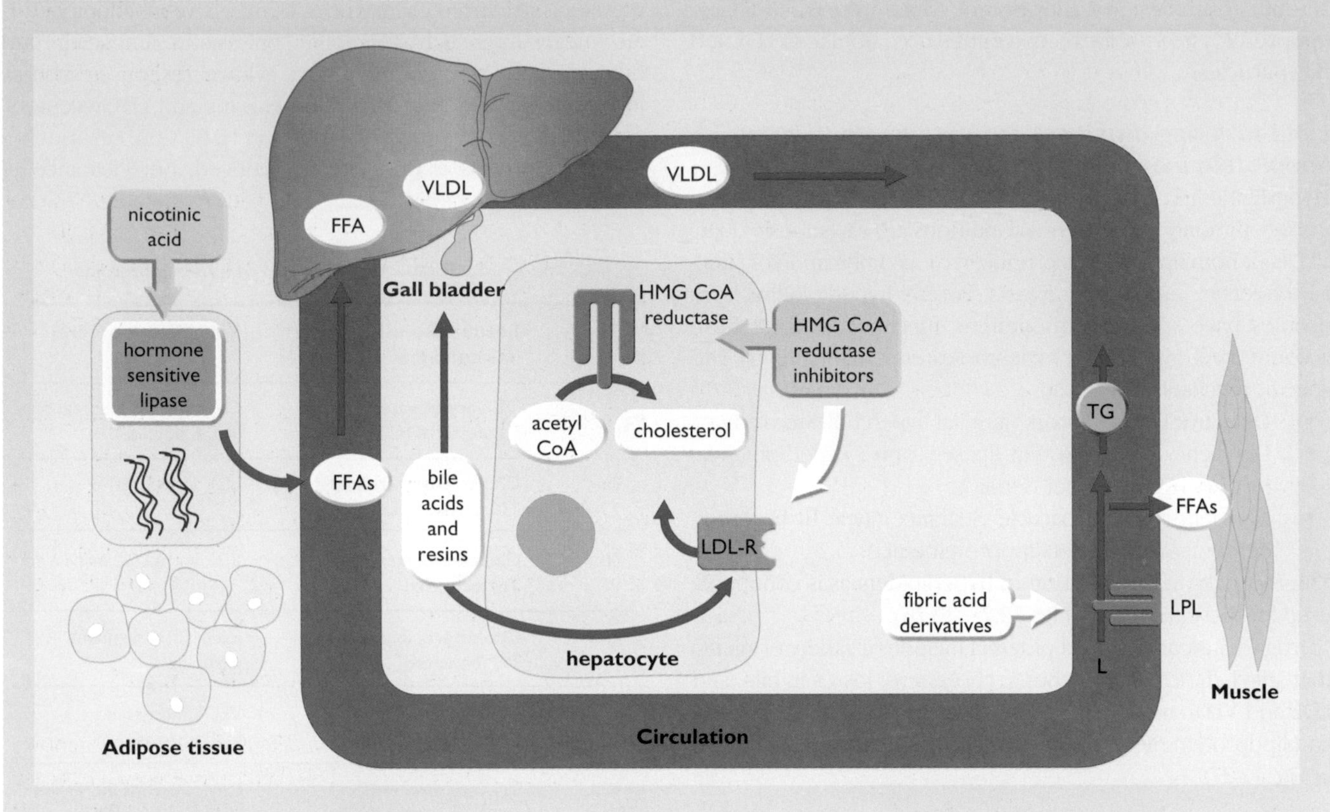

Fig. 12.27 Sites of action of hypolipidemic agents. HMG CoA reductase inhibitors lead to increased low density lipoprotein (LDL) receptor expression on hepatocytes and improved clearance of LDL from the plasma. Bile acid resins similarly lead to an increased LDL clearance as well as increased cholesterol losses in bile. Fibric acid derivatives enhance lipoprotein lipase (LPL) action in peripheral tissues, which leads to improved clearance of triglyceride-rich particles. Nicotinic acid limits the flux of free fatty acids (FFAs) from adipose tissue, which reduces the stimulus for hepatic very low density lipoprotein (VLDL) production. By reducing VLDL production, fewer remnant particles are available for LDL synthesis.

cholesterol via the LDL receptor mechanism is markedly enhanced, leading to sustained reductions in serum cholesterol. The most pronounced effect is reduction of LDL cholesterol, but there is also a reduction in the cholesterol content of VLDL particles, while HDL cholesterol increases.

HMG CoA reductase inhibitors produce the greatest reductions in LDL cholesterol (30–40%) of any single class of hypolipidemic agents. Their modest efficacy at lowering VLDL cholesterol limits their use as a monotherapy for combined hyperlipidemias.

Bile acid sequestrant resins

Lower plasma cholesterol concentrations can be achieved by combining a reduced dietary intake of cholesterol with the use of bile acid sequestrants to eliminate cholesterol. The bile acid binding resins cholestyramine and cholestipol inhibit bile acid reabsorption, allowing cholesterol loss in the feces. Hepatic uptake of cholesterol is then increased to meet the body's ongoing needs for bile synthesis, and this leads to more rapid clearance of circulating LDL and IDL particles. Maximal doses of resin lead to reductions of LDL cholesterol of approximately 20%, but HDL cholesterol concentrations are not affected. VLDL cholesterol usually increases during the initial period of therapy; hence these agents are not suitable for monotherapy of combined hyperlipidemias. Bile acid sequestrant resins are not systemically absorbed and therefore have no direct systemic pharmacologic activity. They do, however, bind other lipid-soluble factors such as vitamins A and D as well as some drugs. These interactions may lead to symptoms related to malabsorption of drugs and nutrients. Bile acid sequestrants cause mild gastrointestinal adverse effects such as bloating and constipation.

Fibric acid derivatives

In contrast to the predominantly LDL-lowering effects of HMG CoA inhibitors, fibric acid derivatives such as gemfibrozil and clofibrate enhance the clearance of VLDL particles. They increase the activity of peripheral lipoprotein lipase, which facilitates entry of triglycerides from VLDLs and chylomicrons into target tissues. Transfer of cholesterol esters from HDL to triglyceride-rich particles is therefore reduced and the cholesterol content of HDL increases, while less cholesterol circulates in atherogenic remnant particles. With maximal doses of gemfibrozil, HDL cholesterol increases by approximately 20% while circulating triglyceride concentrations are reduced by approximately 50%. Through poorly understood mechanisms, LDL cholesterol is reduced by approximately 10%.

Fibric acid derivatives are most appropriate for the clinical disorders associated with increased circulating triglycerides (Type IIb and Type IV hyperlipidemias), and are particularly effective for familial dysbetalipoproteinemia (Type III hyperlipidemia), which results from impaired remnant clearance due to Apo E abnormalities. A genetic deficiency of lipoprotein lipase (Type I hyperlipidemia) is characterized by markedly elevated triglycerides, but is not responsive to fibric acid derivatives. One of the most common causes of hypertriglyceridemia and low levels of HDL is diabetes mellitus, in which enhanced lipolysis in peripheral tissues increases hepatic VLDL production and reduces HDL cholesterol levels.

Nicotinic acid

Nicotinic acid (niacin) is a vitamin precursor of the nicotine adenine dinucleotides (NAD and NADP), which are important enzymatic cofactors. In pharmacologic doses the effects of nicotinic acid on lipoprotein metabolism are independent of its role as a precursor for nicotinamide. However, although nicotinic acid has been used to treat hyperlipidemia for many years, its mechanism of action is poorly understood. Its major effect is to decrease production of VLDLs by reducing the flux of fatty acids from adipose tissue to the liver. Lower VLDL concentrations lead to a reduced exchange of cholesterol with HDL (and therefore higher HDL cholesterol concentrations) as well as reduced delivery of IDL to the liver for LDL formation. Because of these compensatory changes in lipoprotein metabolism, nicotinic acid therapy produces the optimal therapeutic effect of increasing HDL while lowering LDL cholesterol and triglycerides. For these reasons, it is useful in the treatment of combined hyperlipidemias.

The adverse effects of nicotinic acid include acute dose-related effects such as flushing and pruritus, which are the most common. These are prostaglandin mediated and may be prevented by concurrent aspirin administration. Patients become tolerant to such adverse effects, but not to the therapeutic effect on lipoproteins with gradual increases in dose and prolonged exposure. Other adverse effects, such as an aggravation of peptic ulcer disease, hyperuricemia, glucose intolerance, and hepatic and skeletal muscle toxicities may, however, limit the use of this inexpensive and effective agent.

Lipid-lowering agents

- HMG CoA reductase inhibitors: elevation of liver enzymes and creatine phosphokinase (myositis)
- Bile acid sequestrant resins: gastrointestinal bloating, constipation, impaired drug absorption
- Fibric acid derivatives: cholelithiasis, elevation of creatine phosphokinase (myositis)
- Niacin: vasomotor flushing, pruritus, hyperuricemia, glucose intolerance, peptic ulcer, cholestatic jaundice, hyperpigmentation
- Sustained-release niacin preparations and combined use of HMG CoA reductase inhibitors and fibric acid derivatives lead to an increased risk of myositis

Other hypolipidemic agents

Probucol is a hypolipidemic agent with minimal cholesterol lowering effects, but may act by reducing the oxidation of LDLs. Oxidized LDL is taken up more avidly by macrophages to produce foam cells and atherosclerotic plaques. However, probucol is not commonly used because it reduces HDL to a greater degree than LDL cholesterol.

Fish oils contain ω_3 fatty acids such as eicosapentaenoic acid, which is an essential fatty acid constituent of biologic membranes. Ingestion of fish oils results in decreased VLDL synthesis and improved clearance of remnant particles. The hypolipidemic effect of this dietary constituent is thought to contribute to the low prevalence of coronary artery disease in many maritime cultures.

Secondary causes and combined therapy of hyperlipidemia

Dietary reduction of cholesterol intake and treatment of cholesterol-elevating conditions such as diabetes mellitus, renal disease, cholestatic disorders, hypothyroidism, and hypogonadism are recommended before starting drug therapy for hyperlipidemia. Weight loss is associated with the combined health benefits of improved lipoprotein metabolism, reduced blood pressure, and improved insulin sensitivity. In postmenopausal women, estrogen replacement leads to modest reductions in cholesterol as well as additional cardiovascular benefits. If lifestyle modification is inadequate and complicating medical conditions have been appropriately managed, cholesterol-lowering therapy can be initiated according to the predominantly elevated component, for example:

- Nicotinic acid or fibric acid derivatives for triglycerides.
- Bile acid sequestrants or HMG CoA reductase inhibitors for LDL cholesterol.

Combined therapy with bile acid sequestrants and other agents is safe and usually produces additive cholesterol-lowering effects. Combinations of nicotinic acid, HMG CoA reductase inhibitors, and fibric acid derivatives are effective, but may cause either hepatic or skeletal muscle toxicity.

DISORDERS OF GLUCOCORTICOSTEROIDS AND THE STRESS RESPONSE HORMONES

The hypothalamic–pituitary–adrenal (HPA) axis releases adrenal hormones such as glucocorticosteroids and epinephrine. These mediate a complex set of physiologic effects best characterized by the term 'general adaptation syndrome.' In the 1940s Hans Selye coined this term to describe the adrenal response to 'fight or flight' situations. This concept of hormonally regulated adaptation to acute stress provides a general framework for understanding the varied actions of glucocorticosteroids and catecholamines, and for recognizing the patterns of disturbance in this system (Fig. 12.28). Under conditions of stress, the hypothalamic hormone corticotropin releasing hormone (CRH)

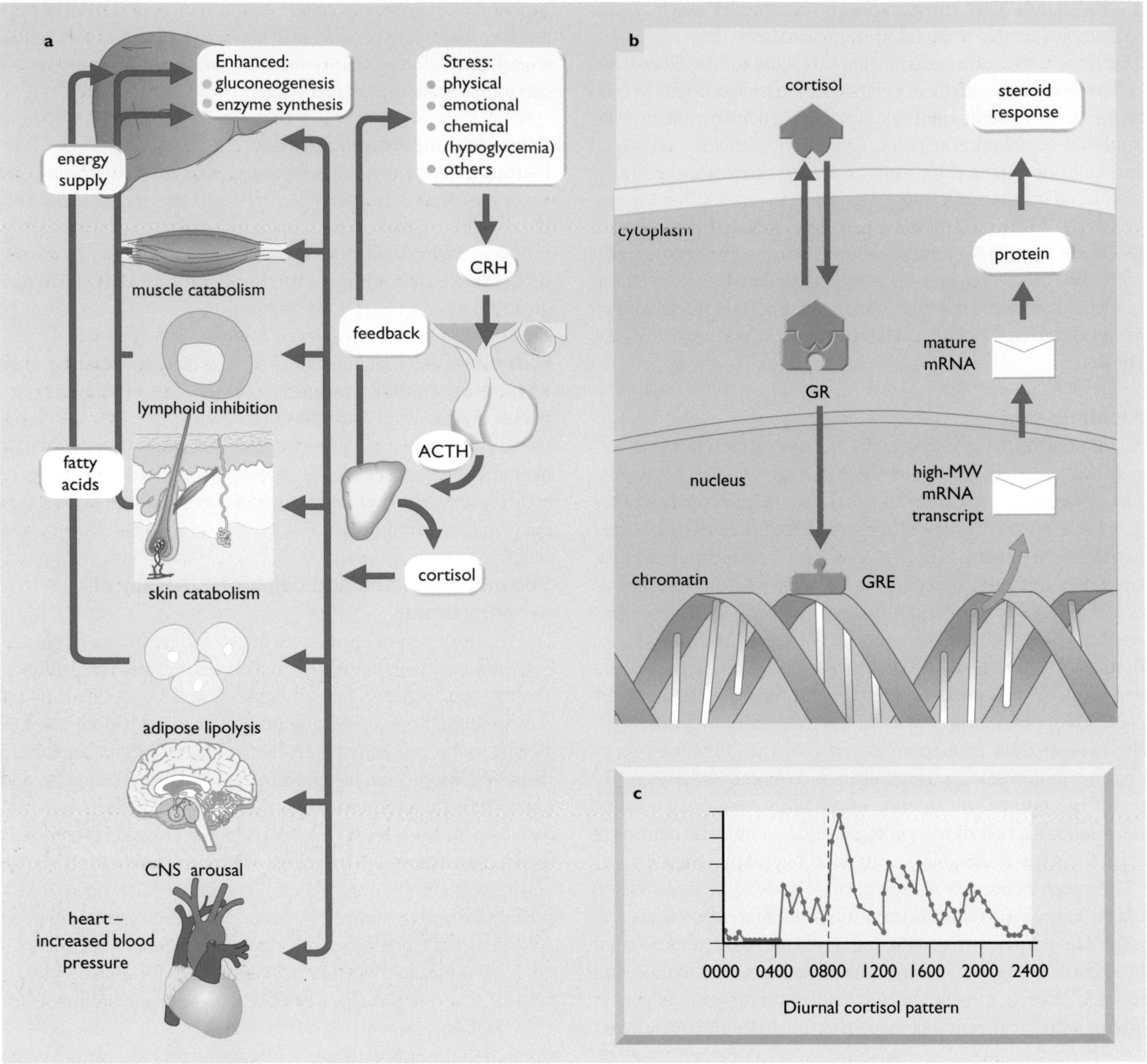

Fig. 12.28 Glucocorticosteroids and adaptation to stress. (a) A variety of sensorineural inputs regulate the pattern of corticotropin releasing hormone (CRH) release in the hypothalamus. CRH releases adrenocorticotropic hormone (ACTH). ACTH leads to cortisol production in the adrenal zona fasciculata. Cortisol circulates to peripheral tissues where it binds cytosolic glucocorticosteroid receptors (GR) (b). After hormone binding, these receptors are translocated to the nucleus where they lead to transcription of glucocorticosteroid-responsive genes. The products of these genes lead to diverse target tissue effects such as enhanced gluconeogenesis, lipolysis, tissue catabolism, inhibition of lymphocyte function, pressor effects in the vasculature, and CNS behavioral effects. (c) The diurnal cortisol pattern reflects peak activity of the hypothalamic–pituitary–adrenal axis in the early morning.

causes pituitary ACTH release, resulting in increased production of cortisol in the zona fasciculata of the adrenals. The sympathetic nervous system, activated under similar conditions, releases neuronal norepinephrine and secretes epinephrine from the adrenal medulla. Among its varied effects, cortisol enhances epinephrine synthesis and sensitizes the peripheral tissues to the effects of catecholamines. The net effect of glucocorticosteroid and catecholamine action is to prepare the body for short periods of high performance. In this light, the varied effects of glucocorticosteroids—to increase gluconeogenesis and lipolysis, mobilize fuel substrates from muscle, increase CNS arousal, increase blood pressure, suppress inflammation, and delay wound healing—seem to serve a common purpose. The sympathetic nervous system reinforces these effects by increasing blood pressure, cardiac output, blood glucose, lipolysis, CNS arousal, skeletal muscle blood flow, and platelet coagulability.

Sustained increases of stress hormones lead to widespread physiologic derangements

While short-term activation of the stress responses may have been useful during evolution, major disorders can result from prolonged excess of the hormones that mediate the general adaptation syndrome:

- Chronic suppression of lymphocyte function by glucocorticosteroids predisposes to a variety of infections, including opportunistic parasitic and fungal diseases.
- Similarly, chronic glucose counterregulation may lead to diabetes mellitus.
- Chronic cardiovascular effects may result in hypertension.

Glucocorticosteroids also have other poorly understood effects. These include:

- Stimulation of bone resorption.
- Inhibition of intestinal Ca^{2+} absorption.
- Inhibition of gonadotropin release.
- An increase in abdominal adipose tissue.
- Permissive effects on vasopressin action in the kidney.

As sex steroids are important anabolic agents for bone, the combined effects of glucocorticosteroid therapy on gonadotropins, Ca^{2+} balance, and bone physiology mean that it is an important risk factor for osteoporosis in both men and women.

Glucocorticosteroid deficiency

Glucocorticosteroid deficiency leads to profound symptoms even under nonstressed conditions. Glucocorticosteroid deficiency results from either:

- Hypothalamic–pituitary disease leading to reduced ACTH secretion.
- Destruction of the adrenal cortex by autoimmunity (Addison's disease), destructive tumors, infarction, or infection.
- Suppression of HPA function following treatment with exogenous glucocorticosteroids for inflammatory, autoimmune, or allergic diseases (iatrogenic adrenal insufficiency).

All these syndromes share the hallmark clinical features of glucocorticosteroid deficiency: poor appetite, weight loss, fatigue, myalgia, arthralgia, and impaired cardiovascular reserve.

Patients with glucocorticosteroid deficiency due to deficient pituitary function, do not demonstrate:

- Deficiency of the salt-retaining hormone aldosterone, which is maintained by the renin–angiotensin system.
- Compensatory rises in ACTH and POMC-derivative hormones such as melanocyte stimulating hormone (MSH), which leads to increased skin pigmentation.

Patients with primary adrenal deficiency (Addison's disease) demonstrate the additional features of low blood pressure and hyperkalemia, owing to loss of aldosterone.

Synthetic glucocorticosteroids differ in potency, duration of effect, and concurrent mineralocorticosteroid actions

Glucocorticosteroids are used to correct adrenal insufficiency, to suppress an overactive HPA axis, to suppress autoimmune diseases, to prevent organ transplant rejection, and to treat lymphocyte-derived tumors. As a result, glucocorticosteroids are among the most commonly prescribed drugs in clinical use. In the treatment of adrenal insufficiency, the goal is to mimic the physiologic patterns of cortisol action. In the treatment of other diseases, glucocorticosteroids are given in supraphysiologic doses, the therapeutic goal being to maximize the therapeutic benefit while minimizing dose-related adverse effects such as iatrogenic adrenal insufficiency, osteoporosis, arteriosclerosis, infections, and neuropsychiatric disorders.

Dosing and drug-delivery strategies are used to reduce the adverse effects of glucocorticosteroid therapy

One strategy to minimize the adverse effects of glucocorticosteroid therapy is that of intermittent dosing, for example the alternate-day therapy of allergic diseases. This strategy exploits the differences in pharmacodynamic half-life of different glucocorticosteroid effects. It has been demonstrated that glucocorticosteroids may suppress allergic phenomena when given every 48 hours, whereas pituitary suppression is shorter lived. Even with the same average dose, glucocorticosteroid administration every 2 days may achieve the desired therapeutic effect with less iatrogenic adrenal insufficiency than more frequent dosing.

Glucocorticosteroid therapy

- Osteoporosis
- Glucose intolerance
- Increased risk of atherosclerotic disease
- Myopathy
- Immune suppression
- Cataracts
- Avascular necrosis of bones (e.g. hip)
- Neuropsychiatric disorders

Another strategy for optimizing therapy is local administration. Topical glucocorticosteroids used for psoriasis and contact dermatitis (see Chapter 18) and inhaled glucocorticosteroids used for asthma and chronic lung disease may achieve high local concentrations, but produce only a modest elevation of systemic glucocorticosteroid (see Chapter 11). Such relative localization depends on dose, however, since topical glucocorticosteroids can be systemically absorbed in sufficient quantities to suppress pituitary function. Therapy is further enhanced using topical glucocorticosteroids with high rates of drug metabolism, leading to rapid elimination of any systemically absorbed drug (e.g. triamcinolone acetonide).

The potencies and durations of effect of different glucocorticosteroids must be compared before any therapeutic substitution between them

The therapeutic effect of glucocorticosteroid therapy is determined by four factors:

- Drug concentration at the effector tissue.
- Potency.
- Elimination half-life.
- Half-life of biologic responses.

Comparisons of potency between glucocorticosteroids provide a general guideline for therapeutic substitution (Fig. 12.29). However, estimates of relative potency are imprecise because they do not fully reflect the duration of effect. For example, dexamethasone has sevenfold greater binding affinity for the glucocorticosteroid receptor than hydrocortisone, but is 150-fold more potent in suppressing adrenal function on the day after a single dose. In general, long-acting synthetic glucocorticosteroids such as dexamethasone and betamethasone are more likely to produce pituitary suppression than short-acting agents.

When hydrocortisone therapy is used for adrenal insufficiency in an attempt to mimic physiologic release of cortisol, unequally divided doses are given in the early morning and afternoon (Fig. 12.30). Endogenous cortisol production is approximately 10 mg/day (28 μmol/day), and although hydrocortisone is highly bioavailable, greater daily exposure to glucocorticosteroid is often needed in replacement therapy.

Although synthetic glucocorticosteroids also have mineralocorticosteroid activity to varying degrees, a synthetic mineralocorticoid (e.g. fludrocortisone) is also administered in the treatment of adrenal insufficiency.

Glucocorticosteroid excess

The physiologic role of glucocorticosteroids is best seen in periods of acute stress, but cortisol is secreted in biologically active amounts under nonstressed conditions. Cortisol synthesis and release follows a diurnal pattern, with increased activity in the pre-dawn hours due to the activation of the HPA axis. Cortisol secretion is highest in the early morning, and may wane to very low levels at night.

Excess glucocorticosteroid action leads to Cushing's syndrome, which is characterized by muscle weakness, central fat deposition, 'moon' facies, purple abdominal striae, atrophic skin, capillary fragility, hypertension, glucose intolerance, and neuropsychiatric disorders. Cushing's syndrome results from a variety of causes (Fig. 12.31, 12.32), but is usually due to an ACTH-secreting pituitary adenoma (Cushing's disease), a cortisol-secreting adrenal tumor, or ectopic ACTH production from other neoplasms (e.g. neuroendocrine tumors of the lung and gut).

Inhibitors of cytochrome P-450 steroidogenic enzymes have different effects on glucocorticosteroid, mineralocorticosteroid, and androgen production

The mainstay of treatment for Cushing's syndrome is surgical removal of the hormone-secreting tumor from the pituitary, adrenal gland, or elsewhere. When surgery is not successful, pharmacologic therapy is used to counteract the glucocorticosteroid excess. The most useful drugs are inhibitors of adrenal glucocorticosteroid synthesis such as ketoconazole, metyrapone, aminoglutethimide, and mitotane. There are no drugs that reduce ACTH secretion from pituitary adenomas, and the glucocorticosteroid receptor antagonist mifepristone (RU-486) has not proved practical for treating chronic hypercortisolism.

Inhibitors of steroid biosynthesis have characteristic activity at different steps in cortisol synthesis, and lead to predictable effects on other adrenal steroids (Fig. 12.33).

Metyrapone predominantly inhibits the terminal step in cortisol synthesis, 11-β-hydroxylation, leading to an increase in the precursor 11-deoxycortisol. An accumulation of precursors such as 17-hydroxyprogesterone may lead to increased adrenal androgen formation and hirsutism in women. Although metyrapone has no effect on aldosterone synthesis, the

Some characteristics of synthetic glucocorticosteroids

	Equipotent dose (mg)	Relative glucocorticosteroid potency	Relative mineralocorticosteroid potency	Elimination half-life (h)	Duration of effect (h)
Hydrocortisone (cortisol)	20	1	1	1.5–2	8–12
Prednisone	5	4	0.8	3.5	18–36
Prednisolone	5	4	0.8	3.5	18–36
Methylprednisolone	4	5	0.5	2–3	18–36
Triamcinolone	4	5	0	3	18–36
Dexamethasone	0.75	20–50	0	3.5	18–36
Betamethasone	0.6	20–50	0	4.0	18–36

Fig. 12.29 Some characteristics of synthetic glucocorticosteroids.

precursor, 11-deoxycortisol, has mineralocorticosteroid activity, which may result in salt retention and hypertension.

Ketoconazole and aminoglutethimide Ketoconazole, an imidazole antifungal agent, and aminoglutethimide, an antiseizure medicine, inhibit multiple sites in steroidogenesis, including the entry point of cholesterol side-chain cleavage as well as important steps in androgen and cortisol biosynthesis. Ketoconazole's effectiveness as an antifungal agent is due to inhibition of a cytochrome P-450 enzyme involved in fungal ergosterol biosynthesis (see Chapter 26).

Adverse effects of ketoconazole, aminoglutethimide and metyrapone All the steroidogenic enzymes inhibited by ketoconazole, aminoglutethimide, and metyrapone are part of the large family of cytochrome P-450 enzymes, which catalyze monooxygenation reactions. Cytochrome P-450 enzymes are involved in many biosynthetic and drug metabolism reactions, which may be the basis of the adverse drug interactions that occur with these types of agents. Since input into the steroidogenic pathway is reduced and multiple enzyme sites are inhibited, biologically active steroid precursor molecules do not accumulate. However, these drugs do inhibit sex steroid production and this may lead to hypogonadism in men.

Mitotane inhibits steroidogenesis at the ACTH-regulated step of cholesterol side-chain cleavage and also causes atrophy of the adrenal cortex. Its only use is in the treatment of adrenal cancer because of its gastrointestinal toxicity.

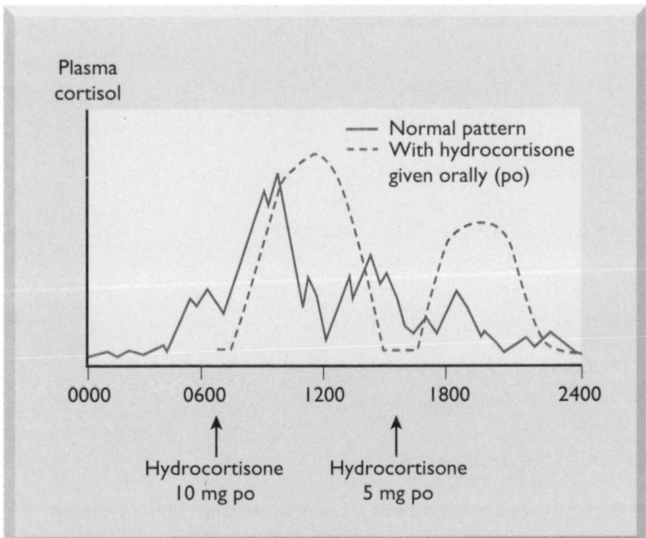

Fig. 12.30 Glucocorticosteroid replacement therapy. An average adult produces approximately 10 mg/day of cortisol. Cortisol production shows marked diurnal variation, with an initial elevation in the pre-waking hours. Physiologic replacement with oral hydrocortisone attempts to mimic this endogenous pattern.

MINERALOCORTICOSTEROIDS, VASOPRESSIN, AND DISORDERS OF CIRCULATORY VOLUME

The hypothalamus, pituitary, and the adrenal glands are also involved in the hormonal regulation of extracellular fluid volume (Fig. 12.34). The pituitary and adrenal glands regulate

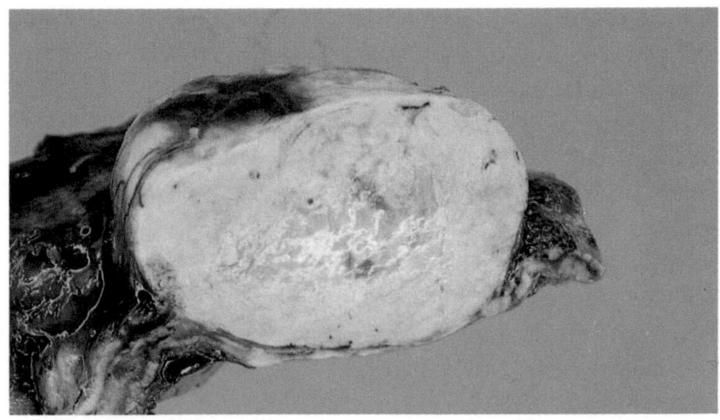

Fig. 12.31 An adrenocortical adenoma, a cause of Cushing's syndrome. (Courtesy of Dr Thomas Ulbright.)

Signs and symptoms of Cushing's syndrome

- Myopathy
- Peripheral muscle wasting
- Central obesity
- 'Moon' facies
- Supraclavicular and dorsocervical fat pads
- Pigmented abdominal striae
- Acne
- Hirsutism
- Plethora
- Bruising and capillary fragility
- Hypertension
- Glucose intolerance
- Hypokalemia
- Arteriosclerosis
- Infections
- Neuropsychiatric disorders
- Osteoporosis
- Hypogonadism

Fig. 12.32 Signs and symptoms of Cushing's syndrome. Causes of pathologic hypercortisolism are adrenocorticotropic hormone (ACTH)-secreting pituitary adenomas (Cushing's disease), ectopic ACTH production from other neoplasms (ectopic ACTH syndrome), and adrenocortical adenomas. Cushing's syndrome, unlike mild hypercortisolism seen in obesity, acute psychiatric disease, and alcoholism, leads to progressive physiologic derangements.

circulatory volume by two interdependent mechanisms regulating Na^+ balance (adrenal mineralocorticosteroids) and free water balance (pituitary vasopressin).

Since Na^+ and its accompanying anions (Cl^- and HCO_3^-) are the main osmotic constituents of extracellular fluid, regulation of Na^+ loss through the kidney, gut, and skin is critical in determining extracellular fluid volume. Extracellular fluid is partitioned between the vascular and interstitial compartments and therefore extracellular volume is a major determinant of circulatory blood volume and blood pressure homeostasis. The osmotic content of extracellular water drives free water from the large intracellular reservoir to the extracellular fluid compartments.

Sodium retention in the distal renal tubule is modulated by aldosterone via genes responsible for the synthesis of Na^+/K^+ and Na^+/H^+ exchangers

Body Na^+ is regulated in the kidney by the mineralocorticosteroid hormone aldosterone, angiotensin II, the sympathetic nervous sysyem, atrial natriuretic peptides, and intrinsic renal mechanisms.

The renal sensing mechanism for circulatory volume as well as its effector limb, the renin–angiotensin–aldosterone (RAA) axis, are described in Chapter 10. Afferent inputs such as renal afferent arteriole baroreceptors, the renal tubular Na^+ sensor, and volume receptors in the central veins, stimulate renin release in response to decreased blood volume or reduced renal perfusion. Renin's actions lead to the synthesis of the peptides angiotensin II and angiotensin III, which act on the adrenal zona glomerulosa to increase the synthesis of aldosterone (Fig. 12.35). Aldosterone synthesis is similar to cortisol synthesis except for the two-step formation of the 18-aldehyde group by the angiotensin II-sensitive enzyme, corticosterone methyloxidase I and II. This enzyme is present only in the zona glomerulosa.

Like other steroid hormones, aldosterone induces genes found in the tissues expressing the mineralocorticosteroid receptor (i.e. kidney, brain, vasculature). Although the mineralocorticosteroid receptor can bind both aldosterone and cortisol, it is protected from stimulation by glucocorticosteroids by a unique enzyme, 11β-hydroxysteroid dehydrogenase. This enzyme is expressed in mineralocorticosteroid target tissues and selectively inactivates any cortisol in the proximity of mineralocorticosteroid receptors.

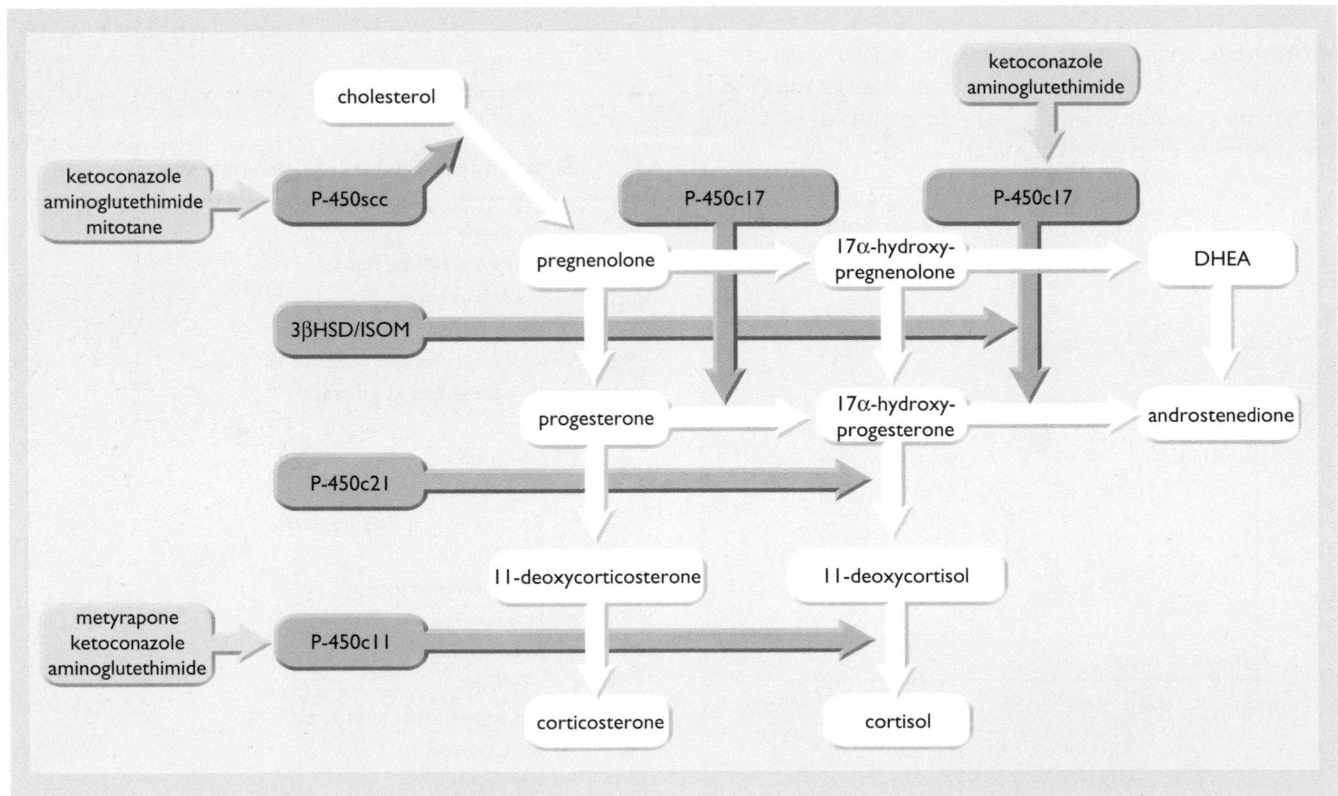

Fig. 12.33 Inhibitors of glucocorticosteroid synthesis. Inhibitors of adrenal glucocorticosteroid synthesis act at different steps of the synthetic pathway. Ketoconazole, aminoglutethimide, and mitotane act at the initial step of cholesterol side-chain cleavage (P-450scc), which delivers steroidogenic substrate into the pathway. Ketoconazole and aminoglutethimide are competitive inhibitors of cytochrome P-450 enzymes, and have other sites of action in the synthetic pathway. These agents reduce the production of adrenal androgen (DHEA and androsteredione) by inhibition of 17α-hydroxylase (P-450c17) and may lead to androgen deficiency in males. Metyrapone inhibits the terminal step in cortisol synthesis, 11β-hydroxylase (P-450c11), leading to a build-up of precursors with androgenic and mineralocorticosteroid potency. (DHEA, dehydroepiandrosterone; 3βHSD/ISOM, 3β-hydroxysteroid isomerase, P-450c21, 21α-hydroxylase)

The classic target tissue for mineralocorticosteroids is the renal distal convoluted tubule epithelial cell where mineralocorticosteroid stimulation induces genes for the Na^+/K^+ ATPase transporter, ion channels, and mitochondrial enzymes critical to Na^+ recovery and K^+ or H^+ excretion. Outside the kidney, mineralocorticosteroids conserve Na^+ in the gastrointestinal tract and skin, and increase blood pressure by effects on the brain and the vasculature.

Aldosterone secretion is also stimulated by high serum K^+, and is the major mechanism of protection against life-threatening hyperkalemia.

Excess mineralocorticosteroid action leads to a renal loss of K^+ and H^+ (i.e. hypokalemia and alkalosis) and increased extracellular fluid volume, while a lack of mineralocorticosteroid leads to hyperkalemia and volume depletion.

Free water balance is coupled to Na^+ balance by the hypothalamic osmoreceptor and release of vasopressin from the posterior pituitary

While the RAA axis and the sympathetic nervous system regulate the Na^+ content of extracellular water, such control extends to extracellular volume only if the free water balance is regulated to maintain osmotic equilibrium. Marked Na^+ retention by aldosterone leads to both an increased Na^+ content and an increased osmolality of the extracellular water. As a result, water shifts from the intracellular to the extracellular space, and a hyperosmotic stimulus is received by the osmoreceptor cells in the hypothalamus. The osmotic sensing mechanism in the brain causes vasopressin (antidiuretic hormone, ADH) release from the posterior pituitary (Fig. 12.36).

Vasopressin is a nine amino acid peptide hormone. Circulating vasopressin stimulates V_2 receptors, which increase the permeability of the renal collecting tubules by a cAMP-mediated mechanism. This allows water in the tubule to move into the extracellular space of the renal interstitium. As a result, free water is recovered into the circulatory compartment, and then provides negative feedback to the osmoreceptor in the brain. Thirst is also activated and suppressed by similar circumstances. In addition to free water regulation, vasopressin stimulates V_1 receptors on the vasculature to cause vasoconstriction via a Ca^{2+}-dependent intracellular signaling pathway.

Vasopressin release is suppressed by reduced osmolality, resulting in increased free water losses in response to excess fluid intake. If there is a severe reduction in blood pressure

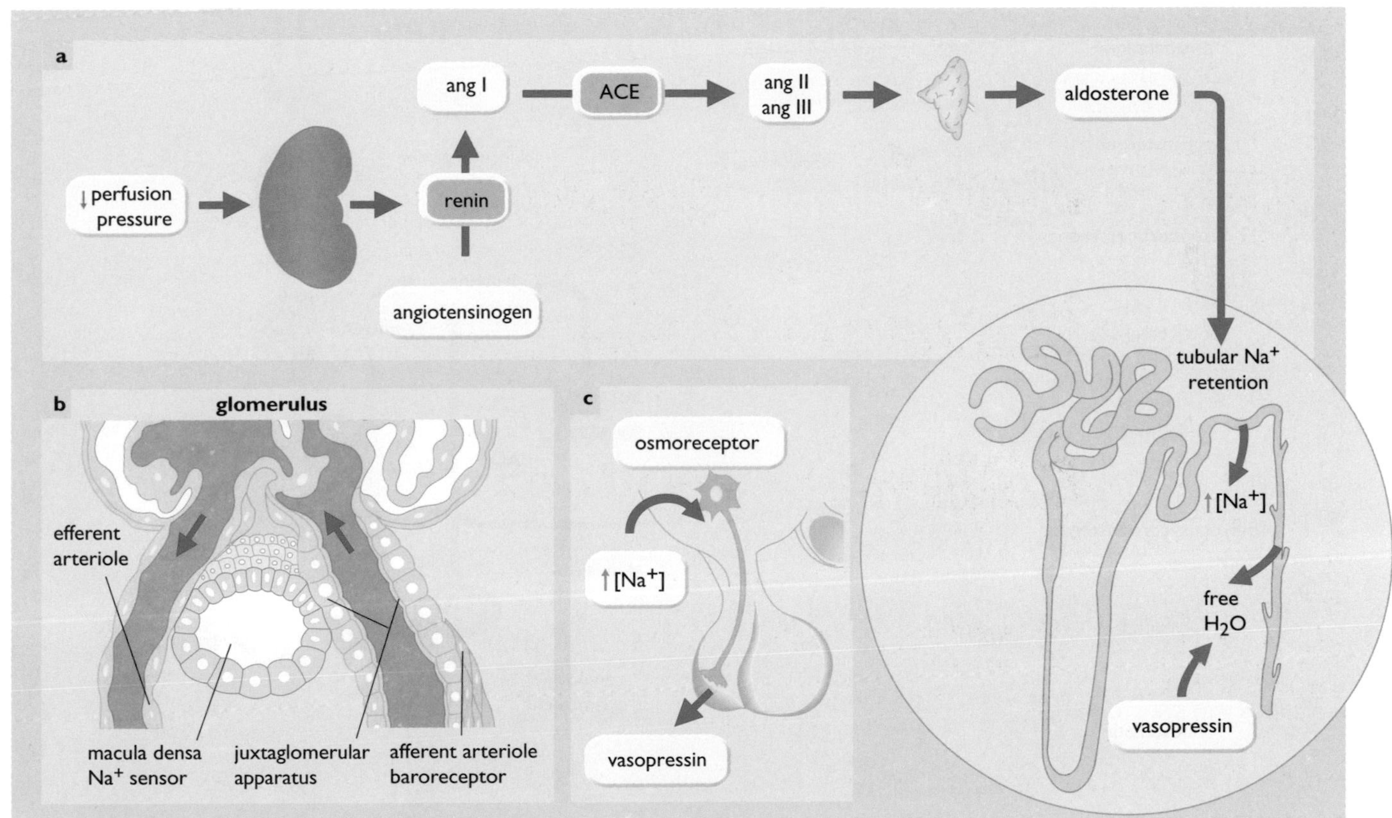

Fig. 12.34 Hormonal regulation of circulatory volume. Central cardiovascular reflexes, renal baroreceptors, and the distal tubular Na^+ sensor provide physiologic input about circulatory volume (a, b). In response to decreased renal perfusion, the juxtaglomerular cells of the afferent glomerular arteriole release renin. Renin converts circulating angiotensinogen to angiotensin (ang) I, which is then converted to ang II by the converting enzyme (ACE) in the vascular endothelium (a). Ang II and ang III stimulate aldosterone production, which leads to Na^+ reabsorption in the distal convoluted tubule. Na^+ reabsorption increases the osmolality of extracellular fluids. This stimulates the hypothalamic osmoreceptor to release vasopressin from the posterior pituitary. Vasopressin leads to enhanced free water reabsorption in the collecting duct, which expands extracellular volume and reduces plasma osmolality (c).

(shock), vasopressin is released regardless of osmolality in an attempt to maintain circulatory volume at the expense of osmolality.

Mineralocorticosteroid deficiency

Mineralocorticosteroid deficiency is usually caused by destruction of the adrenal cortices (Addison's disease), in which there are symptoms of such deficiency (hyperkalemia, acidosis, hypovolemia) as well as symptoms of glucocorticosteroid deficiency (anorexia, weakness, weight loss). The hallmark of mineralocorticosteroid deficiency is reduced extracellular volume and resulting postural hypotension, poor skin turgor, and reduced urine output. Since intracellular water passively follows its osmotic gradient, serum Na^+ concentration may be normal despite reductions in total body Na^+.

Mineralocorticosteroid deficiency may also result from secondary deficiency of renin and/or angiotensin release in chronic renal disease (hyporeninemic hypoaldosteronism).

Sodium supplements and mineralocorticosteroid replacement are used to treat mineralocorticosteroid deficiency whatever the cause. Synthetic mineralocorticosteroids include 9α-fludrocortisone, which is a potent mineralocorticosteroid agonist with minimal glucocorticosteroid activity (see Fig. 12.35b).

Vasopressin deficiency (diabetes insipidus)

A deficiency of action of vasopressin results from either impaired release or impaired action on the kidney:

- Impaired vasopressin release is usually due to destructive lesions (neoplasms, granulomatous inflammation or trauma) of the posterior pituitary.
- An impaired renal response to vasopressin is caused by renal disease and certain drugs (Fig. 12.37).

Vasopressin deficiency is diagnosed by an inability to concentrate urine when the extracellular fluid osmolality increases (hypernatremia). In contrast to the normal serum Na^+

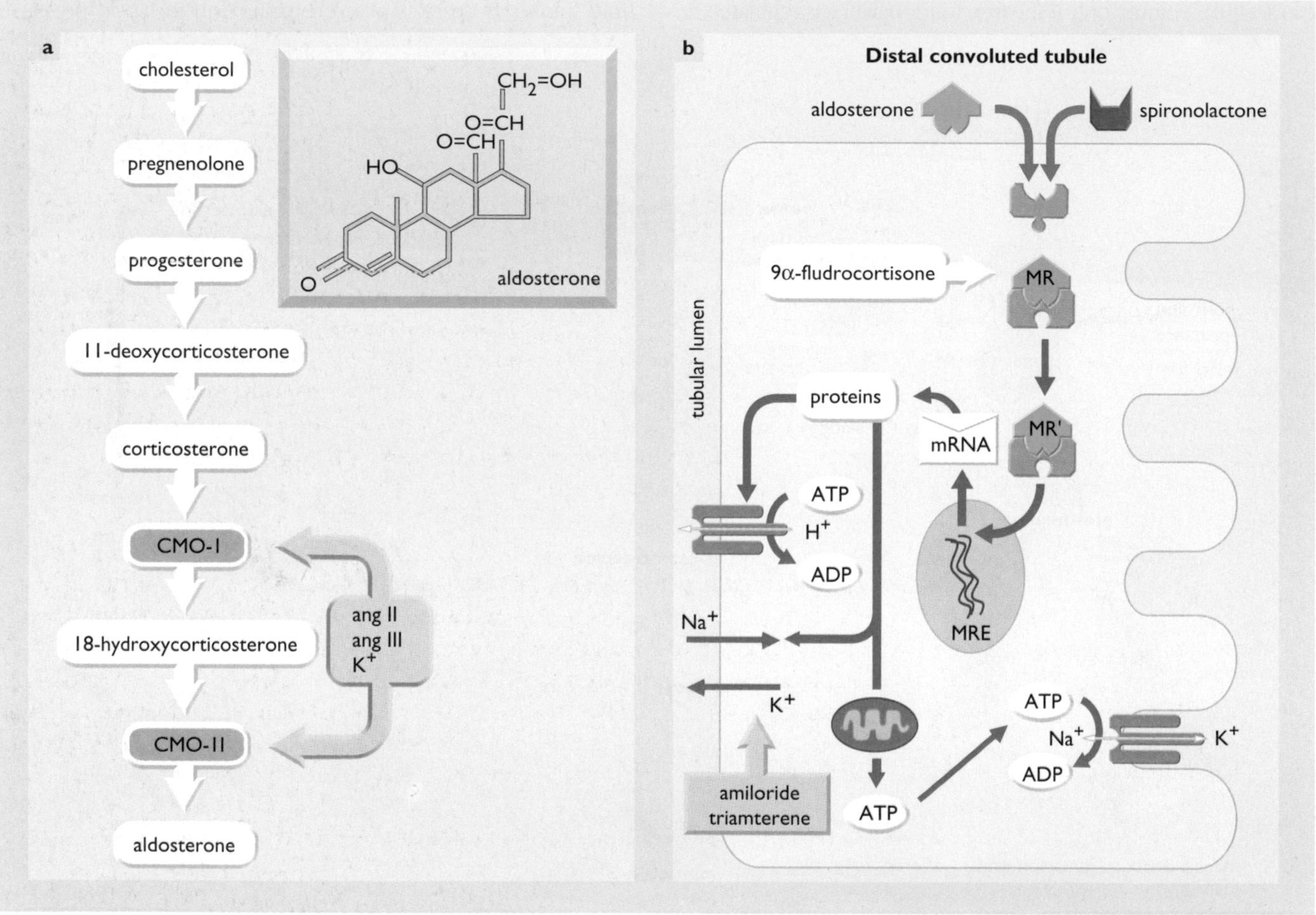

Fig. 12.35 Mineralocorticosteroids and regulation of Na^+ balance. Angiotensins (ang II and III) regulate the corticosterone methyloxidase (CMO) I and II enzymes, which catalyze the hydroxylation and aldehyde formation at 18-C of corticosterone (a). Circulating aldosterone binds to cytosolic mineralocorticosteroid receptors (MR), which then translocate to the nucleus to regulate the expression of genes containing a mineralocorticosteroid response element (MRE) In the renal tubular epithelial cell, the Na^+/K^+ ATPase, the luminal Na^+ permease, the luminal proton pump, and mitochondrial enzymes necessary for the production of ATP. The net effect of aldosterone stimulation in the distal convoluted tubule is to reabsorb Na^+ while excreting K^+ and H^+ (b). Spironolactone is a competitive antagonist at mineralocorticosteroid receptors, while diuretics such as amiloride and triamterene functionally antagonize Na^+/K^+ ATPase.

concentration found with mineralocorticosteroid deficiency, serum Na^+ concentration is increased in free water deficiency states.

Treatment of diabetes insipidus requires differentiation between pituitary and renal causes

Nephrogenic diabetes insipidus is treated by removal of any causative drugs and treatment of the intrinsic renal disease.

Pituitary disease leading to vasopressin deficiency is not usually reversed by treatment of the underlying tumor or inflammation.

Vasopressin replacement therapy involves administration of synthetic vasopressin analogs (desmopressin or lypressin). These compounds differ from native vasopressin by either a lysine substitution at the eighth amino acid position (lypressin) or deamination of the first-position cysteine residue (desmopressin). They can be administered by nasal spray (currently the preferred route of administration) or subcutaneous or intramuscular injection. Twice-daily treatment is usually required, with at least one dose in the evening to allow uninterrupted sleep. Desmopressin is also used intravenously in the management of hemophilia owing to its unexplained ability to increase the activity of von Willebrand's factor.

Mineralocorticosteroid excess

Mineralocorticosteroid excess is an important, but uncommon, cause of hypertension. Like other hormonal excess syndromes, it is caused by either:

- A primary excess of adrenal mineralocorticosteroid production.
- A secondary excess of the mineralocorticosteroid-regulating hormone angiotensin II.

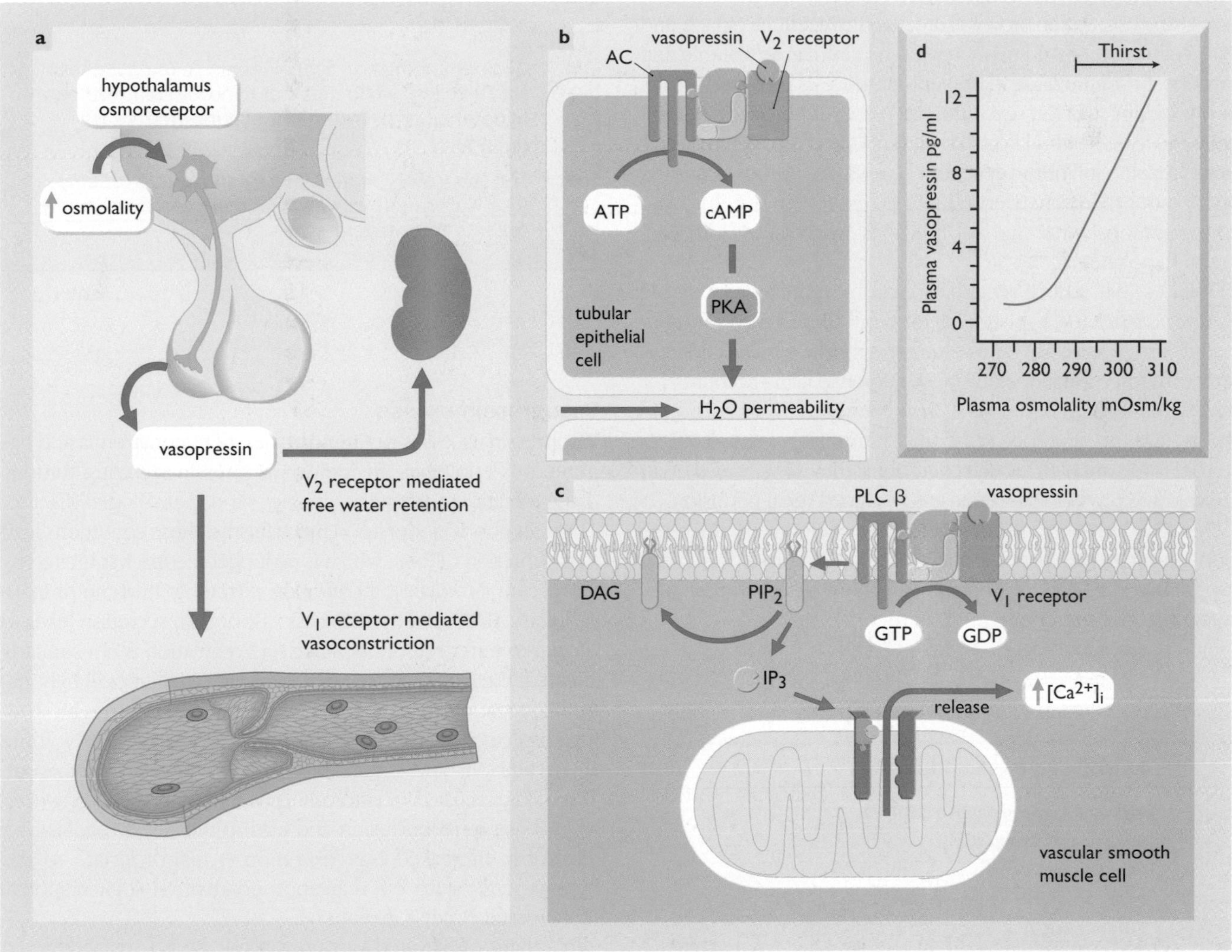

Fig. 12.36 Vasopressin and regulation of free water balance. Osmotic stimulation leads to vasopressin release from the posterior pituitary (a), and vasopressin then stimulates V_2 receptors on distal tubular epithelial cells. V_2 receptors are G protein-coupled receptors that stimulate adenylyl cyclase (AC) to increase intracellular cAMP and activate protein kinase A (PKA). This leads to enhanced permeability of the tubular epithelium (b). Increase in permeability of the collecting duct results in free water movement into the hypertonic renal medullary interstitium. Vasopressin also acts on other tissues. In the vasculature, via V_1 receptors that are linked to a phospholipase C (PLC β) signaling pathway. Release of inositol-1,4,5-triphosphate (IP_3) and diacylglycerol (DAG) from phosphoinositol (PIP_2) increases intracellular Ca^{2+} and potentiates vasopressor responses (c). As plasma osmolality increases with an increase in plasma vasopressin levels, so thirst mechanisms are activated (d).

Secondary mineralocorticosteroid excess due to excessive production of renin and angiotensin is usually caused by renal diseases such as renal artery stenosis, which impair the kidney's ability to sense systemic arterial pressure. The mineralocorticosteroid excess is mild and the pressor effects of angiotensin II dominate.

Primary mineralocorticosteroidism usually results from either single functioning adenomas of the zona glomerulosa (aldosterone-producing adenoma), or angiotensin II hypersensitivity leading to bilateral hypertrophy of the zona glomerulosa (idiopathic hyperaldosteronism). Surgical resection of an aldosterone-producing adenoma often reverses the hypertension, but bilateral adrenalectomy will not correct the hypertension in idiopathic hyperaldosteronism.

Mineralocorticosteroid excess increases extracellular Na^+

As a result of the increased extracellular Na^+ and indirect stimulation of vasopressin release produced by mineralocorticosteroid excess, water moves from the intracellular space and extracellular fluid volume increases. As circulatory volume and renal perfusion increase a pressure–natriuresis response occurs in the kidney and Na^+ excretion increases. The effects of mineralocorticosteroid-related Na^+ retention and pressure–natriuresis reach equilibrium at a modest level of volume expansion, but do not progress to overt volume excess (edema). Serum Na^+ concentrations remain normal, but K^+ is progressively lost, leading to hypokalemia.

Diseases that reduce renal perfusion by reducing circulatory volume as a result of hypoalbuminemia or reduced cardiac output lead to progressive Na^+ and volume retention, which is not corrected by the pressure–natriuresis response. This accounts for the edema seen in conditions such as congestive heart failure, cirrhosis, and the nephrotic syndrome. Although mineraolcorticosteroid levels are high in such conditions, they are elevated by an appropriate physiologic response to reduced renal perfusion.

There are no therapeutic agents that selectively decrease aldosterone production. The major therapy for an aldosterone-producing adenoma is surgery, but many cases of mineralocorticosteroidism require medical therapy.

Causes of diabetes insipidus
Neurogenic (vasopressin deficiency)
Hypothalamic and pituitary tumors
Lymphocytic hypophysitis
Sarcoidosis
Infections (tuberculosis, syphilis)
Histiocytosis X
Nephrogenic (renal vasopressin resistance)
Chronic renal disease
Hypokalemia
Drugs (lithium, demeclocycline, anesthetics)

Fig. 12.37 Causes of diabetes insipidus.

Spironolactone is a selective mineralocorticosteroid receptor antagonist in the kidney, and this accounts for its natriuretic and potassium-sparing effect. Spironolactone also antagonizes androgen receptors, leading to gynecomastia and hypogonadism in some males, and such actions have led to its use to treat hirsutism in women.

Diuretics that functionally antagonize the mineralocorticosteroid effects on renal tubules provide another common pharmacologic strategem for treating mineralocorticosteroidism. The potassium-sparing diuretics amiloride and triamterene reduce tubular sodium reabsorption but do not interact with androgen receptors to cause hypogonadal symptoms in male patients. However, they may cause hyperkalemia and their use requires close monitoring.

Clinical and laboratory diagnosis of volume disorders

- **Clinical findings of hypervolemia (edema) reflect Na^+ excess, while signs of hypovolemia (orthostatic hypotension, dehydration, oliguria) reflect Na^+ deficiency**
- **The laboratory finding of hypernatremia reflects free water deficiency, while hyponatremia usually reflects free water excess**

Vasopressin excess

Vasopressin excess is a common cause of hyponatremia and has numerous etiologies, including vasopressin-secreting tumors, drug effects, pulmonary disease, and neurologic disease. Through poorly understood mechanisms, these conditions lead to vasopressin release, which is no longer feedback inhibited by low serum osmolality, a condition termed 'syndrome of inappropriate ADH secretion.' Excess vasopressin secretion leads to renal free water retention. Since Na^+ regulation is not similarly affected, the excess water retention leads to dilutional hyponatremia. Most of the excess free water diffuses into the intracellular space, and therefore increases in circulatory volume (hypertension) and extracellular water (edema) do not occur. The mild expansion of extracellular water is sufficient, however, to increase renal perfusion and lead to increased tubular Na^+ excretion. Increased Na^+ excretion is inappropriate to the hyponatremic state, but is an appropriate physiologic response to increased circulatory volume.

Treatment of elevated vasopressin release is usually directed toward correcting its underlying cause. In some cases, vasopressin secretion by tumors or neurologic disease requires medical therapy, including restriction of free water intake.

Pharmacologic therapy Antibiotic tetracyclines such as demeclocycline antagonize the action of vasopressin on the kidney, but can cause renal toxicity. Paradoxically, diuretics improve the hyponatremia, probably by reducing the renal medullary osmotic gradient for free water reabsorption.

DISEASES OF THE TESTIS AND OVARY

Unlike other endocrine systems, which regulate important physiologic functions on a short-term basis, the hypothalamic–pituitary–gonadal (HPG) axis regulates the differential expression of secondary sexual characteristics that take place over a lifetime. Functions such as sustaining spermatogenesis, follicular development, and the menstrual cycle require short-term regulation, while others such as puberty and menopause take place over long periods. Hypothalamic gonadotropin hormone releasing hormone (GnRH) and pituitary gonadotropin release are coordinated by complex neuroendocrine mechanisms. The major regulator of sex steroid production is luteinizing hormone (LH), while that for gamete development is follicle stimulating hormone (FSH). These hormones are secreted in an episodic or 'spiking' pattern with lower basal levels during much of the day. Androgens and estrogens exert feedback inhibition on gonadotropin secretion, but these effects vary during the menstrual cycle.

Androgens are produced in the gonads and the adrenals, while estrogens are produced from androgen precursors in the gonads and adipose tissue

LH and FSH stimulate both gonadal steroidogenesis and conversion of adrenal androgens to testosterone and estrogens in the gonads (Fig. 12.38, see Chapter 13, Fig. 13.4). The syntheses of estrogens and androgens share biosynthetic steps with other adrenocortical steroids, but glucocorticosteroids and mineralocorticosteroids are not synthesized because the gonads do not express key enzymes in cortisol and aldosterone production. Under normal conditions, most sex steroids are produced in the gonads. With adrenal disease, however, production of the steroid dehydroepiandrosterone in large quantities in the zona reticularis can lead to the production of substantial amounts of sex steroids. Dehydroepiandrosterone has only slight androgenic activity but is readily converted to other sex steroids in the gonads, leading to the production of potent androgens. Estrogens are also produced as a result of aromatase activity in the gonads and adipocytes. The aromatase enzyme converts androgens to estrogens and is expressed in adipose tissue where it is responsible for most postmenopausal estrogen production and higher estrogen levels in obese men and women.

Estrogen-responsive diseases

In women, many disorders are influenced by estrogens, but few are directly caused by altered estrogen production. Common conditions such as menstrual abnormalities, uterine neoplasms, breast cancer, and the predisposition to autoimmune diseases are influenced by estrogen levels, but are not caused by an estrogen excess or deficit. Excess estrogen production in women, like excess testosterone production in men, does not produce readily noticeable signs or symptoms.

Estrogen therapy is used:

- To replace normal hormone production in deficiency states.
- To suppress endogenous hormone production (contraceptives).
- To treat other hormone-responsive conditions.

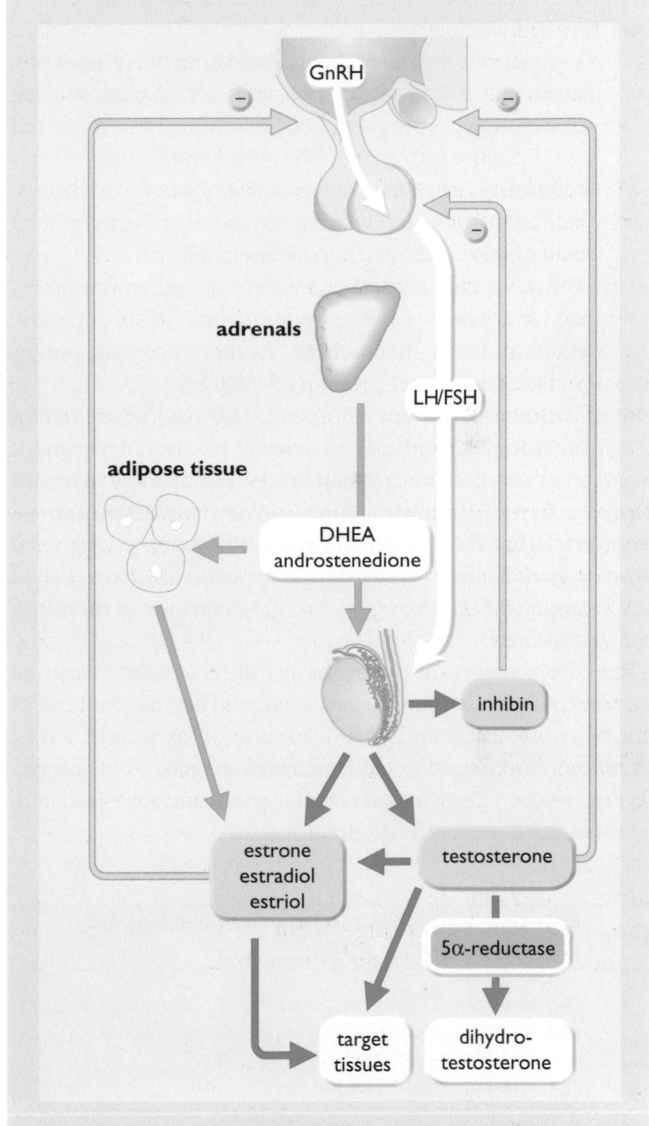

Fig. 12.38 Regulation of sex steroids. Hypothalamic gonadotropin releasing hormone (GnRH) stimulates the release of luteinizing hormone (LH) and follicle stimulating hormone (FSH) from the gonadotrophs of the anterior pituitary. LH and FSH stimulate sex steroid production in the gonads. Adrenal androgens are further metabolized to more potent androgens in the gonads. The aromatase enzyme in both the gonads and adipose tissue converts androgens to estrogens. In certain target tissues, the enzyme 5α-reductase converts testosterone to the more potent androgen dihydrotestosterone. In postpubertal males, sex steroid production is constant. In females, gonadotropins and sex steroids are released in a complex pattern during the menstrual cycle (see Fig. 13.4). (ACTH, adrenocorticotropic hormone; DHEA, dehydroepiandrosterone)

Estrogens and estrogen agonists Normal daily production of estrogen (largely estradiol and estrone) in premenopausal women varies during the menstrual cycle from 20 to 100 μg/day (69.4–347 nmol/day). Estrogens are readily conjugated in the liver by sulfation and subsequently excreted in bile and urine. This first-pass hepatic metabolism limits oral estrogen therapy and daily doses of 1–2 mg synthetic estradiol are needed to achieve adequate hormone replacement. Most estrogen therapies use drugs that are less susceptible to first-pass hepatic metabolism:

- Conjugated estrogens, either isolated from the urine of preganant mares or synthetic, contain predominantly estrone sulfates, which are subsequently hydrolyzed and converted to more active estrogens in the peripheral tissues.
- Transdermal estrogen patches deliver estradiol to the systemic circulation and increase exposure of the peripheral tissues before eventual hepatic metabolism.
- Ethinylestradiol is used in a variety of oral contraceptive pills. It contains a substitution at the C-17 of estradiol, which reduces metabolism. It therefore has potent estrogenic effects at doses of 20–50 μg/day.

One of the oldest synthetic estrogens, diethylstilbestrol (DES), is a nonsteroidal synthetic estrogen. Its use in pregnant women to prevent miscarriage in the 1970s was found to cause reproductive tract abnormalities in the daughters of these women and has led to a greater recognition of the long-term developmental effects of sex steroid exposure *in utero*. Use of any estrogen or antiestrogen during pregnancy is therefore contraindicated.

The adverse effects of estrogens include abnormal menstrual bleeding, water retention, nausea, increased hepatic synthesis of hormone binding globulins, an elevation of triglyceride levels, increased blood clotting, and an increased risk of breast and uterine cancer. The increased risk of uterine cancer is eliminated by concurrent progesterone therapy.

Estrogen and progesterone replacement in the menopause

- **Benefits are lower overall mortality rates, decreased risk of arteriosclerotic disease, prevention of osteoporosis, atrophic vaginitis, and neuropsychiatric effects**
- **Risks are menstrual bleeding, venous thromboembolism, cholestatic disease, breast tenderness, fluid retention, migraine headaches, and a slightly increased risk of breast cancer**

Antiestrogen therapy The role of estrogen in promoting the growth of breast and uterine neoplasms has led to the use of estrogen receptor antagonists for these conditions and other indications.

Tamoxifen is a partial agonist of the estrogen receptor, with weak intrinsic potency. Tamoxifen behaves as an estrogen antagonist in breast tissue but has weak agonist effects on the endometrium, the genitourinary epithelium, bone remodeling, and cholesterol metabolism. Not all responses are equally sensitive to tamoxifen's partial agonist actions. Much of tamoxifen's antagonist activity results from its metabolism to 4-hydroxy-tamoxifen, an active metabolite with greater antagonist potency. Some patients with breast cancer respond to the weak agonist effects of tamoxifen with an initial increase in tumor mass, a phenomenon termed 'tamoxifen flare,' but this is usually short-lived since antagonist effects soon predominate.

Clomiphene is another mixed estrogen agonist/antagonist and is commonly used to stimulate ovarian follicle development in the treatment of infertility (see Chapter 13). Clomiphene antagonizes estrogen-mediated negative feedback on pituitary gonadotropin release. This leads to increased FSH secretion and stimulation of folliculogenesis. Clomiphene has not been used as an antiestrogen in breast cancer.

Newer agents currently in clinical trials, such as raloxifene*, show greater tissue selectivity, producing agonist effects on the bone and liver, but not on the breast and reproductive tissues.

Progesterone pharmacology

Progesterone is produced in large quantities (10–20 mg/day) by the ovary during the luteal phase of the menstrual cycle, and by both ovaries and the placenta during pregnancy. Acting with estrogen, progesterone modulates the phenotype of endometrial and breast tissues, producing secretory endometrium and mammary duct maturation in preparation for pregnancy and parturition. The decline in progesterone secretion that regularly follows 14 days after the mid-cycle LH surge is the primary signal for the onset of menses.

Progestational agents are used therapeutically for:

- Contraception.
- Menstrual irregularities.
- Endometriosis.
- Postpartum suppression of lactation.

Progestins share binding affinity for the androgen receptor, and many progestational agents show androgenic adverse effects. Progestins also have limited binding affinity for mineralocorticosteroid and glucocorticosteroid receptors. Many synthetic progestins are in clinical use (see Chapter 13).

The progesterone receptor antagonist mifepristone (RU-486) is a potent antagonist at both progesterone and glucocorticosteroid receptors. It is used as an abortifacient.

Androgen excess and deficiency

The adrenals and the testes produce a variety of compounds capable of stimulating androgen receptors. Dihydrotestosterone and testosterone are the most potent, but androgenic precursors such as dehydroepiandrosterone and androstenedione also exert androgenic effects. 17-Carbon androgenic precursors from either the adrenals or the gonads can be converted to testosterone by 17-hydroxysteroid dehydrogenase in the testis or in the ovary. The enzyme 5α-reductase produces the more potent androgen dihydrotestosterone.

Androgens are important therapeutic factors in the treatment of disorders of puberty, prostatic disease, and hirsutism

Certain androgenic effects such as male pattern baldness, facial hair, and prostatic hypertrophy appear to depend on stimulation by dihydrotestosterone, whereas other effects are fully agonized by the less potent androgen testosterone.

Androgen excess in prepubertal boys due to unregulated testicular testosterone production ('testotoxicosis') leads to premature puberty, short adult stature, and behavioral problems. Conversely, constitutional pubertal delay can be treated with short courses of androgen therapy. After puberty, androgen excess is clinically silent in men, but leads to androgenic responses ranging from hirsutism to virilization in women. Androgen deficiency in adult males is an important cause of male osteoporosis.

Androgen replacement Like the estrogens, testosterone has poor bioavailability owing to hepatic metabolism and as a result synthetic analogs, transdermal delivery systems, and intramuscular formulations are used clinically. Commonly used intramuscular testosterone preparations (testosterone enanthate, testosterone cypionate, testosterone propionate) use an oil-based vehicle to slow absorption from the site of injection. This leads to dosing intervals of 2–4 weeks, in contrast to the 3-day dosing interval with aqueous testosterone injections. Transdermal testosterone delivery systems provide another mechanism of bypassing first-pass hepatic metabolism of exogenous testosterone.

The orally active androgens, methyltestosterone and fluoxymesterone, are not commonly used for androgen replacement, but are commonly abused by body builders. Other orally active androgenic steroids (testolactone, oxandrolone, stanozolol, oxymetholone) and intramuscular preparations (nandrolone) have weak androgenic effects and are used clinically for their anabolic actions in cancer and refractory anemia. Close monitoring for hepatic dysfunction is needed during oral androgen therapy, and for a variety of androgen-related adverse effects during all androgen therapies (Fig. 12.39).

Antiandrogens are commonly used to treat hirsutism in women and prostatic disease in men:

- Cyproterone acetate*, a progesterone derivative, is an androgen receptor antagonist. It is also a partial agonist at progesterone receptors, and this effect may reduce LH secretion even when its antiandrogen effect reduces the androgenic inhibition of gonadotropin secretion.
- Flutamide is a nonsteroidal androgen antagonist devoid of effects on other steroid receptors. Its use leads to increased LH secretion and testosterone synthesis, which may result in therapeutic failure.
- Spironolactone, the mineralocorticosteroid antagonist, is also an androgen agonist and is a common used therapy for female hirsutism.

In men, the observation that androgen effects such as prostatic growth and male pattern baldness depend on androgen receptor stimulation by dihydrotestosterone has led to the therapeutic use of the 5α-reductase inhibitor finasteride. Testosterone is converted to the more potent dihydrotestosterone by the enzyme 5α-reductase, which is expressed in the skin, liver, and genital tissues. Finasteride therapy improves the symptoms of prostatic hypertrophy and leads to a reduction in prostatic volume.

Gonadotropin axis modulators

A variety of disorders in women respond to a reduction in estrogen action. These include breast and uterine neoplasms, endometriosis, dysfunctional uterine bleeding, and estrogen-responsive immunologic syndromes. Estrogen receptor antagonism is one therapeutic option, but modulators of pituitary FSH and LH secretion also reduce estrogen production (Fig. 12.40).

Danazol is weak androgen that inhibits gonadotropin secretion resulting in a subsequent reduction in estrogen synthesis. More recently, leuprolide, nafarelin, and histrelin, which are potent agonists of GnRH, have proven useful. These agents have greater potency for the GnRH receptor on the pituitary than the endogenous agonist GnRH. After a brief period of stimulation they

Androgen replacement therapy

- **Intramuscular preparations (testosterone enanthate, or cypionate) are inexpensive and can be given at 2–4-week intervals**
- **Transdermal testosterone delivery systems are effective, but more expensive**
- **Oral androgens are associated with a high risk of hepatic disease**

The effects of androgen therapy

Central nervous system	Gonadotropin suppression Behavioral effects
Body habitus	Hirsutism Virilization Acne Baldness Gynecomastia
Hematologic	Erythrocytosis
Metabolic	Dyslipidemia
Hepatic	Cholestatic jaundice Peliosis hepatis Hepatocellular carcinoma
Genitourinary	Priapism Prostatic hypertrophy Prostatic cancer

Fig. 12.39 The effects of androgen therapy.

desensitize the GnRH receptor and so reduce gonadotropin secretion. However, these agents require parenteral administration and lead to menopausal adverse effects such as vasomotor symptoms, bone loss, and genitourinary atrophy.

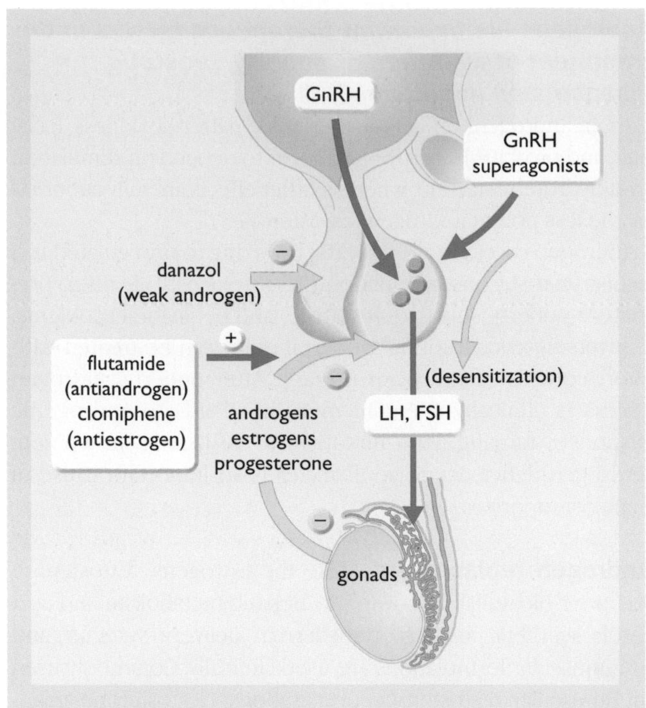

Fig. 12.40 Modulators of the gonadotropin axis. Several commonly used drugs act by altering the function of the hypothalamic–pituitary–gonadal axis. Agonists of the gonadotropin receptor (leuprolide, nafarelin, histrelin) produce desensitization of gonadotroph responses, leading to reduced concentrations of luteinizing hormone (LH) and follicle stimulating hormone (FSH). The weak synthetic androgen, danazol, mimics the feedback inhibition of endogenous androgens and reduces gonadotropin secretion without marked peripheral androgenic adverse effects. Androgen and estrogen receptor antagonists interrupt feedback inhibition of gonadotropin secretion by sex steroids. The resultant rise in gonadotropins that occurs with the estrogen antagonist, clomiphene, promotes ovarian folliculogenesis in the treatment of infertility, whereas the reflex LH increase that occurs with the androgen receptor antagonist, flutamide, may stimulate testosterone synthesis and lead to failure of the antiandrogen effect. Flutamide may therefore be combined with a gonadotropin releasing hormone (GnRH) agonist in the treatment of prostatic cancer.

FURTHER READING

Klibanski A, Zervas NT. Diagnosis and management of hormone-secreting pituitary adenomas. *N Engl J Med* 1991; **324**: 822–831. [A review of diagnostic and treatment issues in acromegaly, hyperprolactinemia, Cushing's disease, and other pituitary tumors.]

Oppenheimer JH, Braverman LE, Toft A, Jackson IM, Ladenson PW. A therapeutic controversy. Thyroid hormone treatment: when and what. *J Clin Endocrinol Metab* 1995; **80**: 2873–2883. [A discussion of clinical controversies in thyroid hormone therapy for treatment of hypothyroidism and thyroid cancer.]

Strobl JS, Thomas MJ. Human growth hormone. *Pharmacol Rev* 1994; **46**: 1–34. [A thorough review of the pharmacology and clinical use of growth hormone in the treatment of short stature.]

Summary of the second report of the National Cholesterol Education Program (NCEP) expert panel on detection, evaluation, and treatment of high blood cholesterol in adults. *JAMA* 1993; **269**: 3015–3023. [Current recommendations from an expert panel on the evaluation of arteriosclerotic risk factors and the integration of pharmacologic and nonpharmacologic approaches to hyperlipidemia.]

Tyrrell JB. Glucocorticoid therapy. In *Endocrinology and Metabolism 3e*. New York: McGraw-Hill; 1995. [A thorough review of pharmacologic issues in the use of glucocorticosteroids.]

Zinman B. The physiologic replacement of insulin. An elusive goal. *N Engl J Med* 1989; **321**: 363–370. [A detailed review of therapeutic issues in the treatment of diabetes mellitus with insulin.]

Make a provisional diagnosis and determine a rational pharmacologic treatment for the following hypothetical case.

A 32-year-old Caucasian woman has been fatigued and anorexic for several months. She lives in the tropics, spends a lot of time in the sun, and eats mainly tropical fruits. She reports feeling faint on standing upright over the past three weeks, has lost 5 kg in weight, and frequently feels nauseated. She has no other medical problems. Her family history includes a sister and mother with hypothyroidism. On examination she is tanned and excessively thin. Lying blood pressure is 100/77 mmHg with a pulse of 86 bpm. Standing blood pressure is 88/– mm Hg with a pulse higher than 100 bpm. Her skin is darkest over the extensor surfaces of her elbows, knees, and wrists. Her oral mucosa is hyperpigmented. Serum Na^+ is slightly low (132 mmol/liter), serum K^+ is elevated (5.6 mmol/liter), urinary Na^+ concentration is high (100 mmol/liter), and urinary K^+ concentration is low (<10 mmol/liter).

1. What would your initial approach be?
2. The patient is clinically stable. Which medications would you prescribe her?
3. What guidance do you give the patient about monitoring therapy and dose adjustment?
4. What are the adverse effects of overtreatment?

Indicate which is the correct answer for each question.

1. Which of the following is the agent of choice for combined hyperlipidemia with significant elevations of both low density lipoprotein (LDL) cholesterol and triglycerides?
a) an HMG CoA reductase inhibitor
b) a bile acid sequestrant resin
c) a fibric acid derivative
d) niacin
e) levothyroxine

2. A patient with diabetes mellitus who takes a single injection of intermediate insulin each morning experiences elevated blood sugars at 7 a.m., but near-normal blood sugars at 6 p.m. Which change in therapeutic regimen would you recommend?
a) add intermediate insulin at bedtime
b) increase the dose of intermediate insulin each morning
c) add short-acting insulin each morning on waking up
d) reduce food intake in the evening
e) add an oral hypoglycemic drug

3. A 30-year-old woman experiences cessation of previously normal menses. An evaluation of hormone concentrations reveals low estradiol, low gonadotropins, elevated prolactin, normal cortisol, normal growth hormone, and normal thyroid hormone. Pituitary imaging reveals a small adenoma in the anterior pituitary. Which treatment would you recommend?
a) estrogen replacement therapy
b) a long-acting dopaminergic agonist
c) gonadotropin replacement therapy
d) octreotide therapy
e) surgery

4. A 30-year-old woman develops secondary amenorrhea. An evaluation of hormone concentrations reveals low gonadotropins, low estradiol, mildly elevated prolactin, normal growth hormone, low thyroid hormone, normal thyroid stimulating hormone, and normal cortisol. Pituitary imaging reveals a large pituitary tumor with deviation of the pituitary stalk. Which treatment would you recommend?
a) a long-acting dopaminergic agonist alone
b) a dopaminergic agonist in addition to estrogen and thyroid hormone replacement therapy
c) surgery followed by hormone replacement therapy
d) octreotide therapy
e) estrogen replacement therapy

5. Which drug treatment for diabetes mellitus improves sensitivity to the action of insulin?
a) sulfonylureas
b) biguanides
c) long-acting insulin
d) intermediate-acting insulin
e) short-acting insulin

6. Which medication is likely to cause gynecomastia in men treated for excess mineralocorticosteroid secretion?
a) amiloride
b) spironolactone
c) triamterene
d) fludrocortisone
e) cortisol

7. A 57-year-old woman presents with rapid atrial fibrillation, a low blood pressure, exophthalmos, tremor, hyperreflexia, and a goiter. After a blood sample for thyroid hormone has been sent to the laboratory which of the following would you recommend?
a) a radioiodine uptake and scan of the thyroid to determine the etiology of the hyperthyroidism while awaiting the results of the hormone concentrations
b) antithyroid therapy (propylthiouracil)
c) a short-acting β adrenoceptor antagonist (e.g. esmolol) and antithyroid therapy
d) I^-, a short-acting β adrenoceptor antagonist, and antithyroid therapy
e) I^- alone

8. A 60-year-old woman presents with a moon face, supraclavicular fat pads, central obesity, recent onset of noninsulin-dependent diabetes mellitus (NIDDM), and myopathy. She takes no medications other than a skin cream for psoriasis. An evaluation of hormone concentrations reveals low cortisol and adrenocorticotropic hormone (ACTH) levels.
Administration of ACTH produces a normal rise in cortisol. What is your diagnosis?
a) glucocorticosteroid deficiency (secondary)
b) Cushing's syndrome due to adrenal tumor
c) iatrogenic Cushing's syndrome
d) Cushing's disease due to a pituitary tumor
e) mineralocorticosteroid deficiency

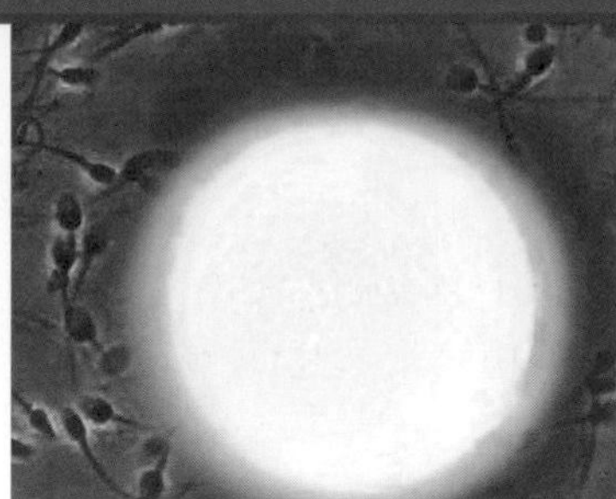

13. Drugs and the Reproductive System

PHYSIOLOGY OF THE FEMALE REPRODUCTIVE TRACT

The ovary provides the gametes for fertilization and synthesizes hormones to maintain the secondary female sex characteristics and the rest of the reproductive tract

The ovary consists of spherical follicles embedded in a stroma, which is surrounded by a membrane (the tunica albuginea, Fig 13.1). Each follicle contains a gamete (oocyte, ovum, egg). All the ova are laid down in early fetal life and start to undergo meiosis. This, however, is arrested at the prophase of the first meiotic division. There are about 7 million initially, but a large proportion die before birth and during childhood. By puberty there are about 400,000 ova left, and of these 0.1% (i.e. 400) will ovulate. The rest die within the ovary by approximately 50 years of age.

The most important hormones produced by the ovary are the sex steroids estrogen (mainly estradiol, but also estrone and estriol) and progesterone, and their production is controlled by the hypothalamic–pituitary axis (Fig. 13.2) (see also Chapter 12). Other ovarian peptide hormones also influence gonadotropin release, and some of those acting only on the pituitary are:

- Inhibin, which selectively inhibits FSH release.
- Activin, which selectively stimulates FSH release.
- Gonadotropin-surge-attenuating-factor, which selectively prevents the release of the LH.

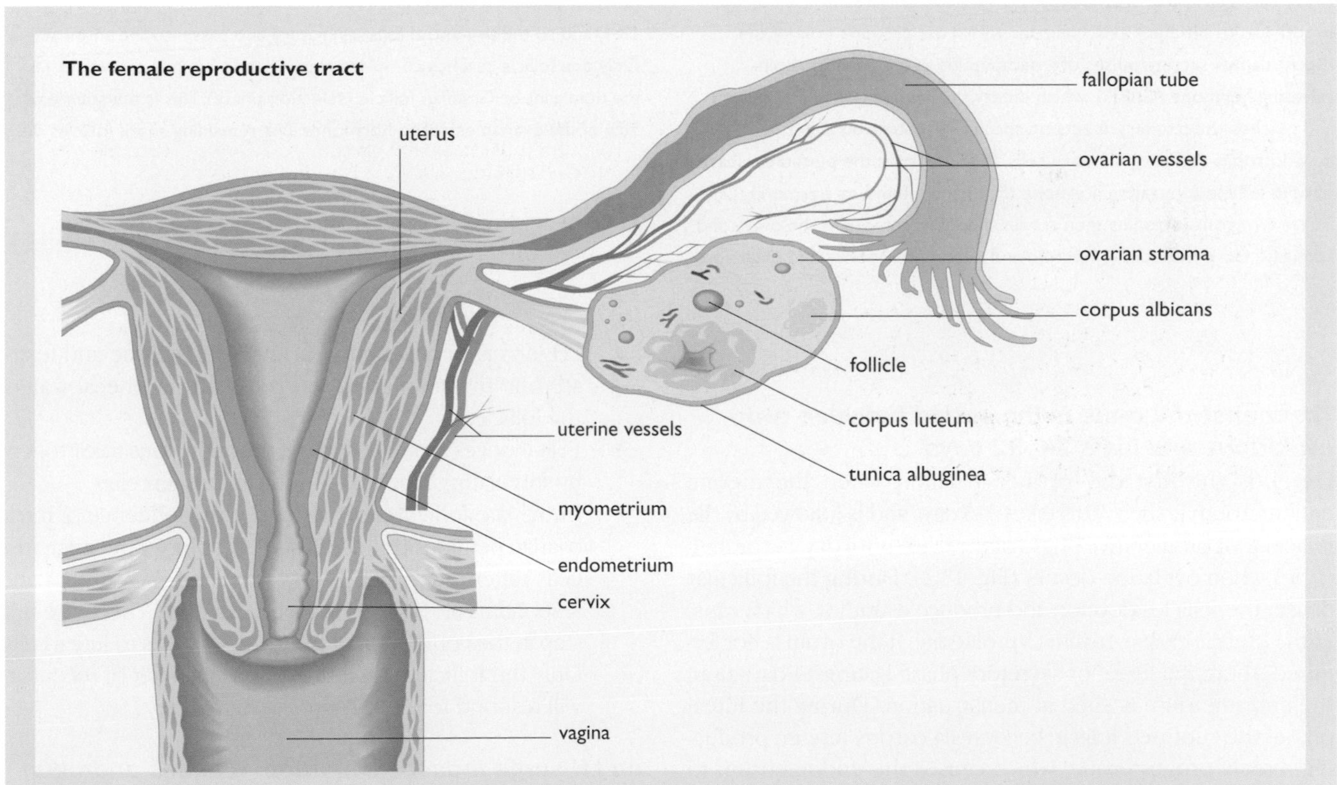

Fig. 13.1 Structure of the female reproductive tract. This consists of two ovaries, each surrounded by a fallopian tube that is approximately 10 cm long and joins a short muscular organ, the uterus. The lower end of the uterus narrows to form the cervix, which is a muscular structure containing many secretory glands and protruding into the vagina. The cervix produces mucus to act as a barrier to infection between the vagina and uterus. The vagina is a thick-walled muscular tube lined by stratified nonkeratinized squamous epithelium. The outer layers of epithelium are constantly shed and these cells form the bulk of the cells seen in vaginal smears, which are taken to determine whether the vaginal mucosa is atrophic or being stimulated by estrogen, and to reveal the presence of infection.

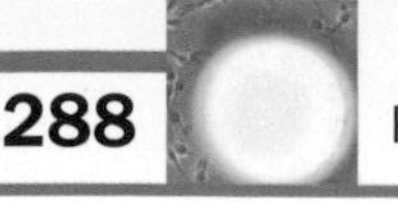

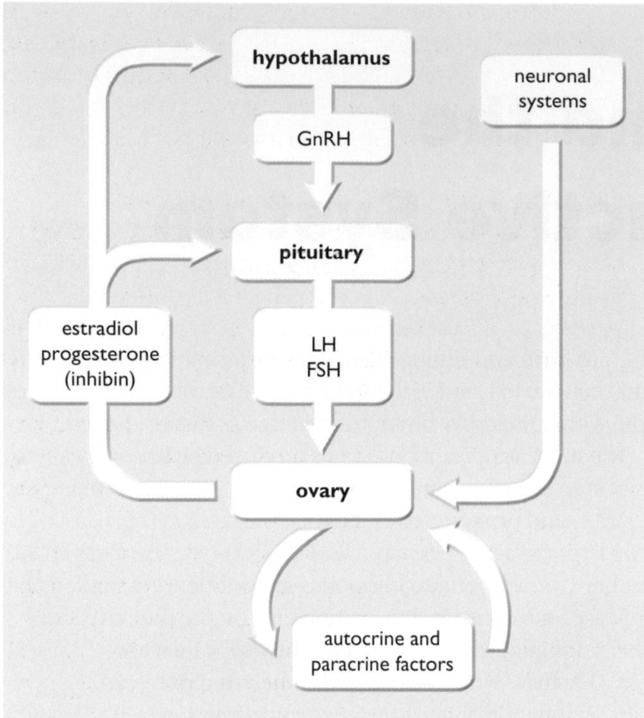

Fig. 13.2 The hypothalamic–pituitary–ovarian axis. Endocrine control of ovarian function is exerted by hormones, the most important being estrogen and progesterone. Their production is controlled by the hypothalamic–pituitary axis. Neurons within the preoptic area of the hypothalamus secrete pulses of a decapeptide called gonadotropin-releasing hormone (GnRH), which enters the hypophysial portal system and reaches the pituitary. It acts on specific receptors on the gonadotropin-secreting pituitary cells, and stimulates the pulsatile release of both follicle stimulating hormone (FSH) and luteinizing hormone (LH). These two gonadotropins then act on specific receptors in the ovary and stimulate the production of steroid and peptide hormones and ovulation.

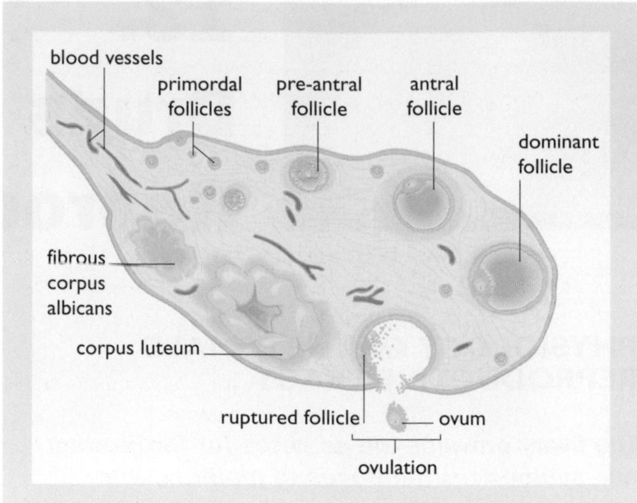

Fig. 13.3 The life cycle of the follicle. The follicles formed in fetal life consist of the ovum surrounded by two or three layers of granulosa cells and are called primordial follicles. Each day, some of these primordial follicles start maturation and begin to form a wall (theca) which becomes vascularized. This is the pre-antral stage and any further maturation is under the control of follicle stimulating hormone (FSH) and luteinizing hormone (LH). If the FSH levels are below a critical concentration, the pre-antral follicles die (hence the huge losses over a lifetime). In the early follicular phase, FSH levels are above a critical concentration (see Fig. 13.4) and so the pre-antral follicles mature and pass into the antral stage. Only one follicle reaches complete maturity and is ready to ovulate, i.e. the dominant or Graafian follicle (selection phase). This is the source of 90% of the ovarian estrogen hormones. The remaining antral follicles die.

The menstrual cycle is the period between two ovulations and lasts 24–32 days

Day 1 is the first day of menstruation when the uterine endometrium is shed. This takes 3–5 days and is followed by the follicular or proliferative phase of the cycle until day 14 (or mid-cycle) when ovulation occurs (Fig. 13.3). During the follicular phase, the follicles develop and produce estradiol, which causes the uterine endometrium to proliferate. If the ovum is not fertilized, there is a luteal or secretory phase lasting 14 days until the endometrium is shed at menstruation. During the luteal phase, the ruptured follicle becomes a corpus luteum producing mainly progesterone, which causes the endometrium to become secretory.

LH increases androgen and progesterone production, while FSH increases estrogen production from androgens

The production of estrogen and progesterone is controlled by the hypothalamic–pituitary axis (see Fig. 13.2):

- LH increases production of androstenedione and testosterone by stimulating receptors on the thecal wall of the follicle.
- FSH induces aromatization of the androgens to estrogens by stimulating receptors on the granulosa cells.
- In the late follicular phase, under the influence of intra-ovarian peptides (induced by FSH), some of the granulosa cells differentiate. They now possess LH receptors and respond to LH by secreting progesterone. This is the first step in the conversion of the granulosa cells to luteal cells. Only the follicle possessing this second set of receptors will respond to the LH surge and ovulate.

An LH surge induces ovulation, reduces androgen and estrogen synthesis, and increases progesterone production

The maturation of growing follicles is controlled by the gonadotropin hormones follicle stimulating hormone (FSH) and luteinizing hormone (LH), while a variety of intrafollicular regulators exert autocrine and paracrine effects, especially on the proliferation of the granulosa cells.

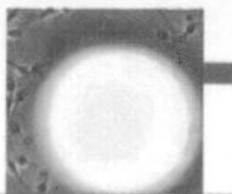

Estrogen concentrations rise as the follicles mature. Normally the sex steroids control the rate of their own secretion by negative feedback, but this becomes positive at both the hypothalamic and pituitary level when the estradiol concentration reaches a critical concentration (> 200 pg/ml) for a critical length of time (2 days), resulting in an enhanced release of LH (the LH surge, Fig. 13.4) and, to a lesser extent, FSH.

The LH surge:

- Appears to desensitize the LH receptors on the theca, thereby terminating androgen and therefore estrogen synthesis, resulting in a rapid decline of the circulating estrogen concentration.
- Stimulates LH receptors on the differentiated granulosa cells, which start to secrete progesterone.
- Stimulates the resumption of meiosis in the ovum. The second meiotic division then starts, but is arrested in the metaphase and is completed only at fertilization. Thus, the ovum is never 'foreign' and need not be protected from the immune system.
- Induces the release of ovarian cytokines, plasminogen activators, prostaglandins, and histamine, causing the first dissolution of the thecal wall and then contraction of the weakening structure resulting in its rupture (ovulation). This occurs approximately 36 hours after the surge.

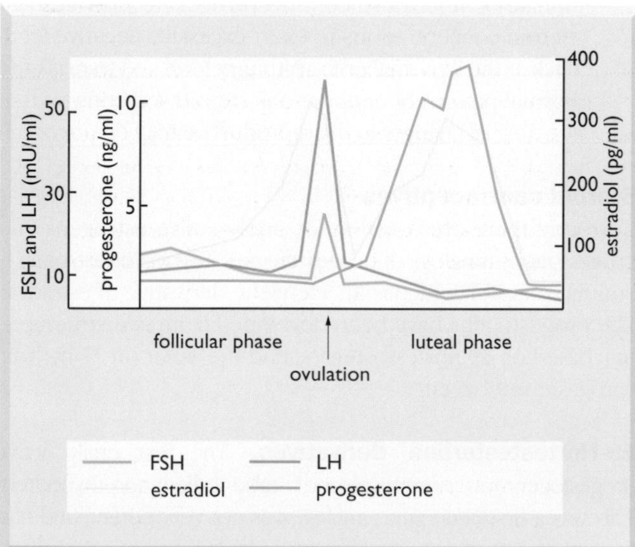

Fig. 13.4 Changes in the concentrations of circulating hormones during the menstrual cycle. Note that the hormone concentrations are drawn to different scales. During menstruation and in the early follicular phase, the steroid concentrations are low and as there is little steroid negative feedback gonadotropin secretion (especially FSH) is slightly elevated. FSH stimulate the follicles in the ovary to grow, mature, and secrete estrogen. The increasing estrogen concentration then exerts negative feedback, reducing gonadotropin concentrations. However, when the estrogen concentration reaches a critical concentration (> 200 pg/ml) for a critical length of time (2 days), the negative feedback switches to a positive feedback, stimulating a dramatic transient release of LH (the LH surge) and to a lesser extent FSH from the pituitary. The increased concentration of LH appears to desensitize the LH receptors on the theca, thereby terminating androgen and therefore estrogen synthesis, resulting in a rapid decline of the circulating estrogen concentration. However, LH receptors on the differentiated granulosa cells continue to respond to LH and start to secrete progesterone.

A corpus luteum forms after ovulation and produces large quantities of progesterone, which maintains the uterine endometrium

After ovulation the granulosa cells all become differentiated, all possess LH receptors (luteinization). They hypertrophy and fill the ruptured structure which becomes a solid body called the corpus luteum (see Fig. 13.3).

The main function of the corpus luteum is steroidogenic, and it produces large quantities of 17-hydroxyprogesterone and progesterone as well as estrogen. Progesterone is needed to prepare the uterine endometrium for the fertilized egg.

The LH concentration at this time is low under the influence of progesterone, but is sufficient to maintain the corpus luteum. If fertilization does not take place the corpus luteum becomes senescent and starts to regress in the mid-luteal phase (day 21 onward of the cycle). At this point there is a rise in $PGF_{2\alpha}$ synthesis within the corpus luteum resulting in local vasoconstriction, hypoxia, and death of the tissue with a consequent fall in hormone production. As the progesterone concentrations decline in the second half of the luteal phase the endometrial cells die and are eventually shed at menstruation.

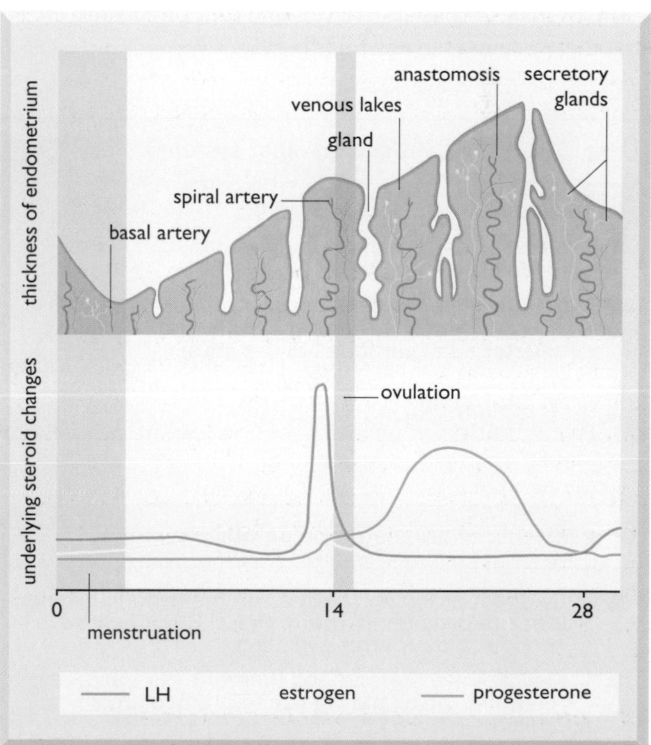

Fig. 13.5 Changes in human endometrium during human menstrual cycle. Underlying steroid changes are indicated (LH, luteinizing hormone.).

The uterine endometrium and myometrium, cervix, and vagina undergo characteristic changes during the menstrual cycle

The uterus is a muscular organ consisting of an endometrium and myometrium. At the beginning of the menstrual cycle during menstruation the endometrium is shed down to the basal laminalis (Fig. 13.5). The increasing estrogen concentration that follows leads to reconstruction of the endometrium, while under the influence of progesterone:

- The myometrial cells enlarge and their excitability and movement is depressed.
- The stroma becomes edematous and the glands become convoluted and distended and start to secrete a viscous fluid rich in glycoproteins, sugars, and amino acids.

Menstruation occurs when the steroid levels fall at the end of the luteal or secretory phase (see Fig. 13.5). The endometrial lining regresses and is discarded, and this is facilitated by an increased $PGF_{2\alpha}$ production by the endometrium as $PGF_{2\alpha}$ stimulates uterine myometrial contractions.

The characteristics of cervical mucus also vary during the menstrual cycle:

- Under the influence of estrogen it is a watery secretion containing glycoprotein structures that sperm can penetrate easily.
- Under the influence of progesterone the mucus is reduced in quantity and thickens, with the glycoproteins forming a mesh-like micelle structure that restricts penetration by sperm. This is the basis of the contraceptive action of the progesterone-only pill.

The vaginal epithelium is stimulated by estrogen.

The ovarian steroids also have significant physiologic effects on other systems (see Key Facts boxes).

Effects of estrogen on other systems

- Increases tendency to clotting
- Increases high density lipoproteins (HDL), which reduce the risk of arteriosclerosis
- Increases concentrations of binding protein in plasma for steroids and therefore can reduce effector concentrations of the latter
- Decreases osteoclast activity and therefore bone resorption

Effects of progesterone on other systems

- By direct or indirect actions on the hypothalamous, it raises body temperature 0.2–0.6°C. This rise is seen for 4 days after ovulation
- Elevates aldosterone and therefore Na^+ and water retention, which may relate to premenstrual edema
- Decreases the ratio of high density lipoproteins (HDL) to low density lipoproteins (LDL), which is associated with increased myocardial infarctions

PHARMACOLOGY OF THE FEMALE REPRODUCTIVE SYSTEM

Drugs can be used to:

- Inhibit normal functioning and prevent fertility (i.e. contraception).
- Replace missing hormones or correct patterns of hormone secretion and either induce full fertility with ovulation and maintenance of the reproductive tract or prevent amenorrhea (absence of menstruation) without inducing fertility.

CONTRACEPTION

Contraceptive agents prevent fertility by acting at a variety of sites along the reproductive tract:

- The condom (male or female) prevents access of the sperm to the ovum.
- The intrauterine device makes the uterine endometrium unsuitable for implantation of the fertilized ovum.
- Female steroid hormone contraceptives prevent ovum release from the ovary and/or make the reproductive tract inhospitable should fertilization take place. The main rationale behind these contraceptives is to provide high steroid concentrations to exert excessive negative feedback at the hypothalamic—pituitary level and to mask the normal pattern of endogenous steroid secretion so that the normal changes in the reproductive tract do not occur.

Steroid contraceptives

Currently there are a variety of orally active estrogens and progestogens (analogs of progesterone). The major estrogen is ethinyl estradiol, which is an acetylene derivative of estradiol. The progestogens have been developed from two structures, one based on 19-nortestosterone and the other on 17-hydroxyprogesterone acetate.

19-Nortestosterone derivatives. The first orally active progestogen was norethisterone* (also called norethynodrel). This was a first generation analog, was not very potent, and had the extreme disadvantage of having androgenic activity that affected women and if the contraception failed, caused virilization of a female fetus. Levonorgestrel (the *d*-isomer of norethisterone) is an example of the second generation analogs and is more potent. Both first and second generations of progesterone analogs reduce the ratio of high density lipoprotein (HDL) to low density lipoprotein (LDH) and therefore increase the risk of cardiovascular disease. The third generation progestogens include desogestrel, gestodene, and norgestimate, and tend to increase the HDL:LDL ratio, possibly owinge to some inherent estrogenic activity.

17-Hydroxyprogesterone acetate derivatives. These analogs have no androgenic or estrogenic activity and are used only as injectable or depot preparations. The most commonly used is Depo-Provera, which is medroxyprogesterone acetate.

Combined oral contraceptives

Combined oral contraceptives (COCs) include any of the 19-nortestosterone derivatives combined with ethinyl estradiol. In the 1960s the daily dose of ethinyl estradiol was 150 µg, but the currently recommended doses of 20–35 µg greatly reduce cardiovascular risks. The combination is usually taken for 21 days and then stopped for 7 days to allow withdrawal bleeding (monophasic preparation). Triphasic preparations consist of pills containing a three stepwise increase in steroids in an attempt to mimic the natural pattern of cyclic steroid release and allows better menses control. It is possible to take the monophasic preparation daily for 12 weeks (i.e. four packets) before having a 7-day break, particularly if there are adverse effects during the pill-free week.

Advantages of combined steroid contraceptives result from their ability to suppress the menstrual cycle and establish an endocrine condition similar to that of pregnancy or lactation and include:

- Highly effective contraception (i.e. 0.5 pregnancies/100 woman-years).
- A reduction in the incidence and/or severity of premenstrual tension, dysmenorrhea, and menstrual loss, and therefore a lower incidence of anemia.
- Improved acne (some preparations).
- Suppression of benign breast disease.
- Suppression of ovarian cysts.
- Possible suppression of endometriosis.
- Suppression of uterine fibroids.
- Reduced risk of pelvic inflammatory disease, possibly by thickening the cervical mucus so that bacteria cannot penetrate into the reproductive tract.

Fertility and pregnancy in ex-pill and pill users

- The incidence of spontaneous abortion and abnormalities among ex-pill users is not increased, and there is a decreased incidence of stillbirths
- Most women experience a rapid return to fertility on stopping 'the pill' and conception can occur after only a 1- or 2-day delay in starting a new packet

Disadvantages of combined steroid contraceptives Figure 13.6 shows that the relative risk of taking steroid contraceptives compared with that of other voluntary and involuntary risks such as cigarette smoking is small, and less than the risk of childbirth. However, adverse effects include:

- Vascular diseases, as estrogen doses over 50 µg may be associated with an increased risk of cardiovascular disease, and this risk is magnified in cigarette smokers. Most preparations now contain 35 µg or less, which greatly reduces the risk. The main causes of death are ischemic heart disease and cerebrovascular disease. Estrogen is primarily the cause of thrombotic disorders as it affects clotting factors. Progesterone may induce alterations in the long-term and this is in part due to reduction in the ratio of the HDL:LDL cholesterol complexes. Although these risks are increased in COC users, the risks of dying from them is nearly always confined to those who also smoke; there is a small increased risk with age, which is enhanced in smokers.
- Breast cancer. Although oral contraceptives reduce the incidence of ovarian and endometrial cancer, some data suggest that they may increase the risk of breast cancer but the causes are multifactorial and further investigation is required.
- Impaired glucose tolerance, especially if the patient is predisposed to diabetes mellitus, but this usually returns to normal within six months of stopping treatment. The combined pill is therefore relatively contraindicated for women with diabetes mellitus who also have a higher risk of a cardiovascular disorder. They are usually given the progestogen-only pill to avoid estrogen treatment.

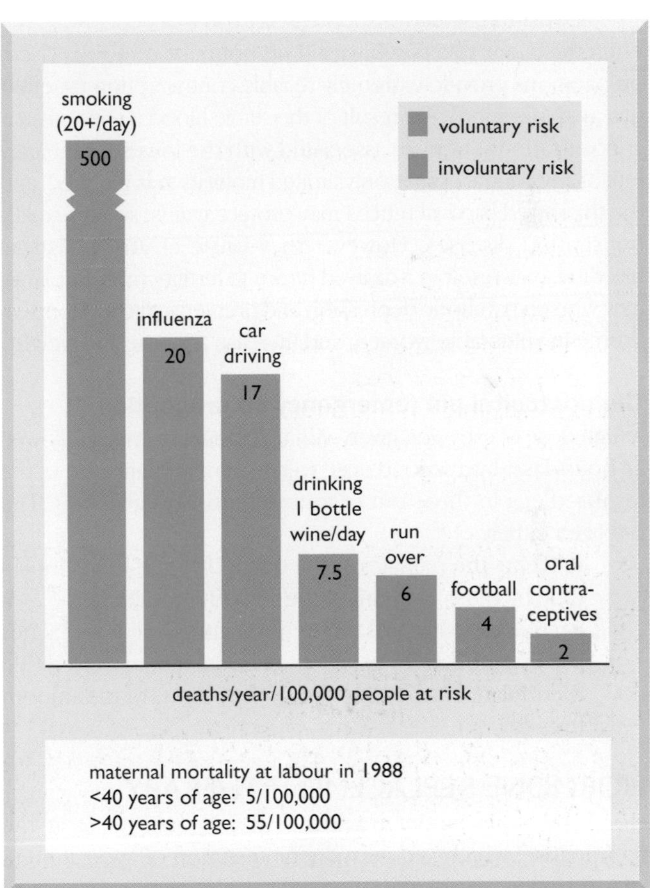

Fig. 13.6 The risk of taking the pill compared with other voluntary and involuntary risks.

Progestogen-only pill (minipill)

The progestogen-only pill (POP) consists of a low dose of progestogen given alone. It is taken continuously and, since ovulation still takes place in many women, menstruation is normal, although its timing can be irregular. The steroid acts on all the other sites listed above for the combined pill, but particularly induces a thick viscous cervical mucus for approximately 18–20 hours after taking the pill. The pill is therefore best taken in the middle of the day so that the mucus will be thick in the evening and early morning.

Depot progestogen preparations

These include:

- A short-term treatment, lasting 12 weeks, of depot medroxyprogesterone acetate 150 mg given intramuscularly.
- Netta Noristerat (norethisterone) 200 mg given intramuscularly at 8-week intervals.
- Subdermal implants of either ethinyl estradiol combined with a progestogen or progestogen only. There is a 5-year progestogen-only type (Norplant), which consists of 30 mg levonorgestrel releasing a constant and continuous amount of hormone.

The two main sites of action of depot preparations are:

- Cervical mucus, which is thickened and therefore prevents sperm penetration.
- Ovulation, which is suppressed in 50% of cycles.

The effects are reversible within 48 hours of removal. These preparations provide extremely reliable contraception (as effective as sterilization) as a result of the stable blood levonorgestrel concentration. They are associated with the lowest pregnancy rate of any contraceptive, only limited motivation is required, and the thickened cervical mucus may protect against some sexually transmitted diseases. However they cause erratic menstrual bleeding, may result in a delayed return to fertility (not Norplant), may worsen psychotic depression and premenstrual tension/syndrome in vulnerable women, and increase appetite and weight.

The postcoital pill (emergency contraception)

A high dose of estrogen given within 72 hours of coitus followed 12 hours later by a second dose will prevent implantation of the fertilized egg in three out of four potential pregnancies. The estrogen either:

- Prevents the passage of the ovum through the fallopian tube by causing spasm of the smooth muscle wall.
- Accelerates the passage of the ovum so that it reaches the uterine lumen before the endometrium is prepared for implantation by inducing contractions of the smooth muscle.

HORMONE REPLACEMENT THERAPY

Hormone replacement therapy (HRT) is used to treat the menopause, which is a permanent cessation of cyclical menstruation due to loss of ovarian follicular activity and is judged to have occurred retrospectively after 12 months of amenorrhea. In developed countries it occurs at a mean age of 51 years, while premature menopause occurs before 40 years of age.

All the unwanted symptoms of menopause are due to estrogen deficiency affecting estrogen-sensitive tissues

Estrogen-sensitive tissues include the urogenital tract, the cardiovascular system, and the skeletal system. Early-onset menopausal symptoms involve urogenital tissue and include vaginal dryness, dyspareunia (painful intercourse), recurrent urinary tract infections, urinary incontinence, and atrophy of the urethral mucosa. Other early symptoms are hot flushes, sweats, and palpitations. These latter symptoms cease spontaneously after some years or even months, but can recur. The mechanisms underlying menopausal vasomotor problems (e.g. hot flashes) are not clearly understood.

Osteoporosis is associated with any estrogen deficiency

More serious menopausal symptoms result from progressive loss of bone mineral mass and collagen over several years, leading to osteoporosis (a systemic skeletal disease characterized by a low bone mass and deterioration of the bone microarchitecture with an increased susceptibility to fracture, see Chapter 17). Estrogen usually reduces bone resorption by inhibiting gene expression of interleukin-6, which is known to activate osteoclasts. Causes of osteoporosis therefore include any state that involves estrogen deficiency, i.e. the menopause, amenorrhea (either congenital or due to anorexia nervosa), excessive exercise, and certain drug treatments. Alcohol and smoking not only inhibit Ca^{2+} absorption, but also are toxic to osteoblasts and therefore inhibit bone formation.

The rate of myocardial infarction increases after the menopause

There is evidence indicating that estrogen replacement therapy after the menopause may substantially decrease the greater risk of myocardial infarction and hypertension. The longer-term effects of estrogen deficiency are related to the tendency for atheroma formation leading to myocardial infarctions. This is due to reduced HDL, which normally carries cholesterol away from the circulation to the liver. More recently, it has been established that there are estrogen receptors on the vascular endometrium and estrogen can stimulate the synthesis of nitric oxide, a potent vasodilator of endometrial origin. Nitric oxide normally exerts a tonic inhibitory efffect on vascular tone, modulating the tonic vasoconstrictor effect of the sympathetic nervous sytem. Reduced nitric oxide production therefore leads to hypertension and hence the ensuing dangers to the cardiac system.

Drug treatment of menopausal symptoms

Hormonal treatments. Estrogen replacement therapy relieves the early-onset symptoms and reduces the risk of osteoporosis and cardiovascular disease. In contrast to the synthetic estrogen used for contraception, menopausal hormone replacement conventionally uses natural estrogens. These include microionized estradiol or estriol, estradiol valerate, and most commonly, conjugated equine estrogens extracted from pregnant mare's urine (Premarin) and containing 17β-estradiol, sodium estrone sulfate, and equilin (an estrogen not produced in the human).

When estrogen replacement is administered alone it:

- Induces endometrial hyperplasia, which may become neoplastic.
- Stimulates uterine fibroids to grow, which may lead to heavy irregular break-through bleeding.

The estrogens are therefore usually given with a progestogen to inhibit endometrial growth. If the progestogen is given over the last 10 days of a 28-day cycle, it induces a withdrawal break-through bleeding. If this is unacceptable the two steroids can be given together continuously. Progestogen does not reduce the benefits provided by the estrogen to the cardiovascular and skeletal systems. The steroids are usually given orally but can be applied in transdermal patches, gels or subcutaneous implants which can reduce the minor adverse effects (nausea, vomiting, migraine and weight gain).

Nonhormonal treatments can be provided as a second-line treatment for menopausal symptoms if estrogenic compounds are contraindicated (usually in women who have, or have had, breast or uterine carcinoma). They do not, however, relieve the urogenital symptoms, or prevent cardiovascular disease.

Clonidine (an α_2 adrenoceptor agonist) and veralipride (a dopamine antagonist) can prevent hot flashes. Propranolol (a β adrenoceptor antagonist) is useful for palpitations. The treatment of osteoporosis is discussed in Chapter 17.

PATHOPHYSIOLOGY AND DISEASES OF THE FEMALE REPRODUCTIVE SYSTEM

The common disorders of the female reproductive tract are shown in Fig. 13.7.

HYPOTHALAMIC AND PITUITARY DISORDERS

Primary disorders (hypogonadotropic hypogonadism)

Isolated gonadotropin deficiency is a congenital deficiency of gonadotropin releasing hormone (GnRH) leading to hypogonadotropic hypogonadism, which is characterized by eunuchoid features, incomplete development of secondary sex characteristics, and absence of menarche (onset of menstrual cycles).

Secondary disorders

Hypothalamic function is closely controlled by peripheral systems, steroid feedback being an obvious example, but body composition and diet are also important controlling influences. For instance, the onset of puberty (menarche) occurs at a critical body weight and fat:lean ratio. More than a 20% loss in body weight or strenuous physical exercise causing a specific reduction in fat can cause both amenorrhea and oligomenorrhoea (infrequent menstrual cycles) and is associated with low stroid levels and anovulation (infertility). These changes may lead in turn to a diminished bone mass.

Gonadotropin therapy

Exogenous gonadotropins are indicated for congenital or acquired gonadotropin deficiency and when clomiphene fails (see below). An FSH preparation is given to stimulate follicular growth, and when this is optimal an LH preparation is given to induce follicular rupture 24–36 hours later. As the normal feedback mechanisms are bypassed, this treatment can result in multiple ovulations and multiple pregnancy.

Gonadotropin preparations include:

- Human menopausal gonadotropin (HMG), which is extracted from postmenopausal urine and has equal FSH and LH bioactivity. (After the menopause, when steroidogenesis ceases, gonadotropin release and excretion is greatly enhanced and it can be extracted from urine in high concentrations.) As HMG is a biologic extract it is difficult to standardize and only 1% of the protein in the preparation is actually gonadotropin.
- Metrodin*, which is a purified preparation also obtained from postmenopausal urine, contains 94% FSH and no LH activity.
- Recombinant FSH and LH, which are currently under clinical development.
- Human chorionic gonadotropin (HCG), which is produced by the blastocyst in very early pregnancy and eventually by the syncytiotrophoblast of the placenta. Structurally it is similar to LH and acts on LH receptors. It therefore has similar biologic actions, but a much longer half-life (20 hours compared with 12 minutes).

To avoid multiple pregnancies, low doses of an FSH preparation are injected for 14 days and daily ultrasound is used to observe follicular growth. The dose is increased only if maturation fails. Alternatively, a higher dose of FSH can be given at

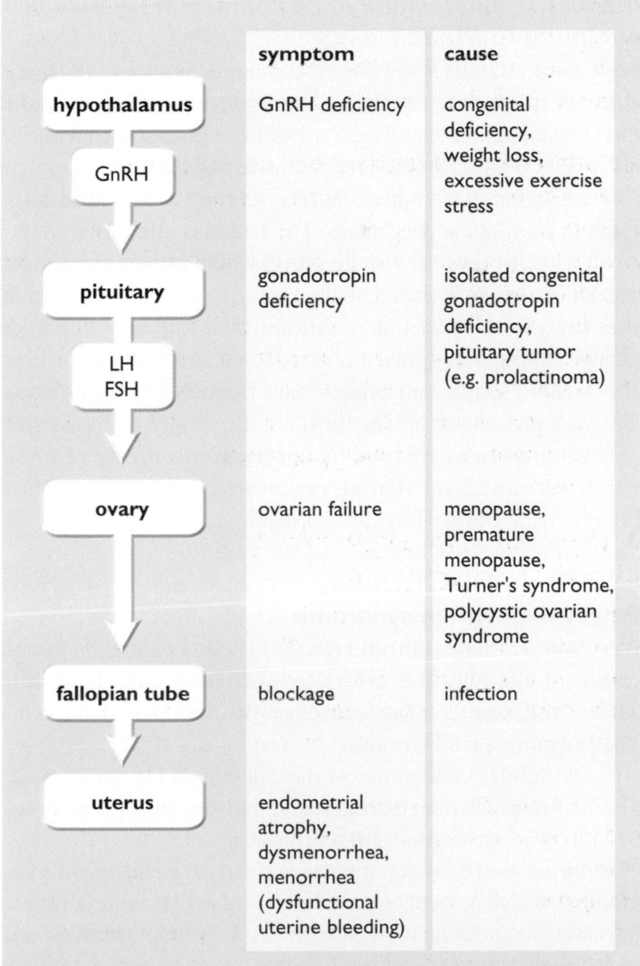

Fig. 13.7 Causes and symptoms of common reproductive disorders. (FSH, follicle stimulating hormone; GnRH, gonadotropin releasing hormone; LH, luteinizing hormone)

the start of treatment with stepwise decrements thereafter mimicking the natural cyclic pattern of FSH secretion. Another regime is to obliterate all endogenous gonadotropin secretion by suppressing GnRH release with a GnRH analog. This allows for more precise monitoring of the gonadotropin dosage and timing, and it has been reported that this method reduces miscarriage rates

Gonadotropin releasing hormone and its agonist analogs

GnRH is a decapeptide and analogs are obtained by substitution of the amino acids in the 6 and 10 position to increase potency and the duration of action. Currently used preparations are gonadorelin (GnRH itself), buserelin, goserelin, and leuprorelin*.

Chronic administration of GnRH agonists can ultimately inhibit the release of pituitary gonadotropins after a period of the expected stimulation. The continuous high levels desensitize the GnRH receptors on the gonadotrophs, resulting in a hypogonadal hypopituitary state. Attempts have been made to use this effect for contraception by administering the analogs as a nasal spray. However, they can induce marked estrogenic deficiency, leading to menopausal symptoms.

Administering exogenous GnRH in a pulsatile manner is most useful in patients with relative or complete GnRH deficiency

Endogenous GnRH is released in a pulsatile manner, which presumably avoids desensitization. Administering exogenous GnRH in a similar manner stimulates endogenous gonadotropin release and preserves the feedback mechanisms that allow development of a single dominant follicle, thereby tending to avoid the development of multiple pregancies. The GnRH is administered by a small battery-powered syringe pump leading to an intravenous or subcutaneous cannula. Usually a pulse is applied every 90 minutes for a few minutes, and although the rate and amplitude change during the normal menstrual cycle, good ovulation rates (i.e. > 90%) result from a fixed pulse frequency and amplitude, although pregnancy rates are lower. If the patient has no interest in fertility, replacement therapy can be given with the COC pill, which will provide the steroids necessary for the maintenance of bone density and healthy vasculature.

OVARIAN DISORDERS

Polycystic ovarian syndrome

Polycystic ovarian syndrome (PCOS) is one of the commonest causes of infertility. It is associated with infertility, obesity, hirsutism, and many cyst-like follicles on the periphery of the ovary. The hormone profile reveals:

- A high LH concentration (i.e. a low FSH:LH ratio).
- Chronically high estrogen and androgen concentrations.
- Low progesterone concentration.

The unopposed estrogen increases the risk of endometrial carcinoma, while the high concentrations of active androgens lead to hirsutism and acne in most patients. Treatment varies according to the symptoms and can involve:

- Prevention of amenorrhea or oligomenorrhoea and unopposed estrogen effects.
- Induction of ovulation and fertility.
- Prevention and removal of the virilizing effects of the androgens.

Amenorrhea, oligomenorrhea, and dysfunctional uterine bleeding are treated with progestogens, which overcome the unopposed estrogen, while ovulation is induced with clomiphene or other anti-estrogens (sse below). If clomiphene fails to induce ovulation, gonadotropin preparations or pulsatile administration of GnRH analogs can be tried (see above).

Clomiphene is usually the first-choice treatment for PCOS patients who are infertile

Clomiphene citrate is an anti-estrogen that antagonizes the normal negative feedback of endogenous estrogen at the hypothalamic and pituitary level resulting in an increased endogenous FSH release, which induces follicular growth. Although the ovulation rate after clomiphene is 70%, the pregnancy rate is only 30% and this was thought to be due to the anti-estrogenic effect of clomiphene preventing normal uterine endometrial growth or inducing impenetrable cervical mucus. However, uterine biopsies do not show any abnormalities and possibly more precise timing of intercourse by carefully monitoring follicular maturation and ovulation using currently available techniques will improve pregnancy rates.

Clomiphene is well tolerated and adverse effects are seen only with higher doses or prolonged treatment and include ovarian enlargement and vasomotor symptoms (i.e. flashing and palpitations).

Antiandrogens, combined oral contraception, or GnRH analogs can be used to treat hirsutism and virilization associated with PCOS

Androgens act on the pilosebaceous unit, which consists of the sebaceous gland and hair follicle, inducing conversion of vellus to terminal hair and increasing growth rate. Removal of the androgenic stimulation cannot reverse the conversion, but prevents further conversion and growth.

Steroidal antiandrogens block testosterone receptors and include:

- Cyproterone acetate* (CPA), which is also progestogenic, so treatment should be interrupted to allow breakthrough bleeding. Alternatively, it can be given with ethinyl estradiol and so provide contraceptive protection.
- Spironolactone, which is an aldosterone antagonist as well as a potent antiandrogen with a higher affinity for androgen receptors than CPA. It also interferes with the cytochrome P-450 monooxygenases and alters steroidogenesis, reducing testosterone synthesis and increasing its metabolism. Potassium retention is a potentially serious adverse effect (see Chapter 10).

Nonsteroidal antiandrogens include:

- Flutamide, which blocks androgen receptors.
- Finasteride, which inhibits 5α-reductase, preventing the formation of dihydrotestosterone from testosterone (see Chapter 12).

Combined oral contraception is a widely used treatment; the gonadal steroid activity suppresses endogenous gonadotropin release and so reduces endogenous androgen production.

GnRH agonist analogs administered chronically suppress gonadotropin release and ovarian steroidogenesis. However, postmenopausal symptoms can result from the absence of estrogen and so these drugs should be given in conjunction with an oral contraceptive or an HRT preparation.

Prolactinemia

Prolactin is a hormone of the anterior pituitary and is tonically inhibited by hypothalamic dopamine. Like GnRH, dopamine enters the blood supply to the pituitary, where it acts on D_2 receptors on pituitary lactotrophs to inhibit the synthesis and release of prolactin. The symptoms of hyperprolactinaemia are amenorrhea, infertility, postmenopausal symptoms (e.g. a reduction in bone mineral density and adverse vascular effects due to estrogen deficiency), and galactorrhea. Drug therapy is discussed in Chapter 12.

UTERINE DISORDERS

Dysmenorrhea

Dysmenorrhea is characterized by cramps of the lower abdomen, gastrointestinal and neurologic disturbances, and general malaise, associated with an increased frequency and amplitude of uterine contractions and increased resting tone. It is probable that excess prostaglandin (PG) production, especially of $PGF_{2\alpha}$ and PGE_2 (with an increased ratio of $PGF_{2\alpha}$ to PGE_2), as well as an excess production of leukotrienes and vasopressin are involved in the pathogenesis.

Menorrhea or dysfunctional uterine bleeding

Menorrhea is a frequent, prolonged, heavy and unpredictable menstruation. The causes are not known, as steroid levels and uterine endometrial changes are normal. There are higher than normal levels of PGs and plasminogen activation which would enhance uterine contractions and bleeding.

Endometriosis

Endometriosis is characterized by the presence of functioning endometrial cells outside the uterine cavity. It can be the cause of secondary menorrhea, with menstrual periods lasting longer than 8 days. The symptoms are severe cyclical abdominal pain and backache, dyspareunia, and infertility. It results from retrograde menstruation leading to the deposition of normal endometrial tissue in the peritoneum.

Uterine fibroids

Uterine fibroids are benign tumors of the myometrium consisting of smooth muscle surrounded by a capsule of connective tissue. They occur in 25–30% of women of reproductive age and can distort the uterine cavity. They can cause menorrhea, irregular bleeding, iron deficiency, and spontaneous abortions.

All these uterine disorders are treated somewhat empirically by a similar set of preparations, the choice depending on the predominant symptoms

Steroid contraceptive preparations are used to reduce endometrial thickness. The progesterone-only contraceptive preparations are less effective than the combined pill, but are similarly effective if given at a higher dose. In addition to the usual norethinderone or medroxyprogesterone acetate preparations, gestrinone* (an androgenic progestogen) has also been used. The progestogens prolong shortened cycles and induce a secretory endometrium, thereby preventing hyperplasia.

Danazol is a weak nonselective steroid that reduces gonadotropin release and estrogen levels, resulting in amenorrhoea and therefore relieving most symptoms. However, it has many unwanted adverse effects including menopausal symptoms (this limits its use to six months), virilization, weight gain, depression, and irregular breakthrough bleeding.

GnRH agonists given daily cause amenorrhea and are given as a nasal spray, but for no longer than 6 months to avoid menopausal complications. They can be given with 'addback therapy' (i.e. an HRT preparation is provided as a supplement).

Nonsteroidal anti-inflammatory drugs (NSAIDs) are analgesic and anti-inflammatory and can reduce blood loss by 20–40%, presumably by reducing PG production. Their advantage is that they are taken cyclically for only a few days each month.

Ethamsylate* is a hemostatic drug that increases capillary resistance and platelet adhesion and leads to a modest reduction in blood loss.

Tranexamic acid is an antifibrinolytic agent and can be used only if there is a low risk of thrombosis and bleeding is heavy.

INFECTIONS IN THE FEMALE REPRODUCTIVE TRACT

Infections of the female reproductive tract can be classified as either vulvovaginal infections (e.g. candidiasis, bacterial vaginosis, endocervicitis) or pelvic inflammatory disease (PID).

The presence of microorganisms in the vagina is common and not necessarily associated with disease. Under certain predisposing conditions the normal vaginal flora can produce an infection (e.g. *Candida albicans* infections). Other infections are caused by nonresident organisms.

Candidiasis

Candidiasis, caused by the fungus *Candida albicans*, inflames the ectocervix, vaginal walls, and vulva resulting in itching, irritation, dyspareunia, dysuria, and a white cheese-like discharge. Predisposing factors include high estrogen concentrations (as in late pregnancy or when using high-dose oral contraceptives), uncontrolled diabetes mellitus, immunosuppressive or broad-spectum antibiotic therapy, and local factors such as tight clothing, douching, and cosmetics.

Treatment involves the use of topically applied antifungal agents such as nystatin

Other antifungals can be taken orally such as azole compounds (e.g. clotrimazole), imidazole compounds (e.g. ketoconazole), and bistriazole compounds (e.g. fluconazole). Intravaginal boric acid capsules, or locally applied 1% gentian violet, can be used for those cases that are resistant to the antifungals.

Bacterial vaginosis

Bacterial vaginosis is typically due to a disturbance of the vaginal ecology rather than an infection by a particular organism. There appears to be a loss of normal flora, especially Gram-positive lactobacilli, and an unusual predominance of anaerobic bacteria. There is an increased number of squamous epithelial cells coated with anaerobic coccobacilli, mycoplasma, and *Gardnerella vaginalis*. As the latter is generally found in this disease, it can be used as a marker. There is also an overgrowth of several other organisms including *Prevotella melaninogenica*, *P. bivia*, and peptostreptococci.

Bacterial vaginosis is a noninflammatory nonirritative condition associated with an excessive grey discharge that has a low viscosity and a distinctive fishy odor. The odor results from the products of the anaerobic bacteria, including putrescine and cadaverine.

Oral metronidazole is the treatment of choice of bacterial vaginosis

Metronidazole, given orally over 7 days, is very effective against anaerobic bacteria. Metronidazole resistance can occur and treatment is then difficult as there are few alternatives. Clindamycin, given topically, is one alternative and is used in pregnancy as it is less toxic to the fetus. Another approach is to attempt to return the pH of the discharge to normal with acetic or lactic acid, or even yoghurt. The recurrence rate is relatively high at 40%.

Trichomonas vaginalis infection

Trichomonas vaginalis is an anaerobic flagellated protozoan that is sexually transmitted. It produces ectocervical and vaginal inflammation, and approximately 50% of patients have a profuse malodorous yellow-green frothy discharge.

Treatment involves the use of trichomonacidal imidazole derivatives, particularly metronidazole or tinidazole, given orally as a single dose.

Endocervicitis

Infection with the bacteria *Neisseria gonorrhoeae* and/or *Chlamydia trachomatis*, which are both sexually transmitted organisms, produces cervical inflammation. The lumen of the cervix is lined by columnar cells, which are preferred by *N. gonorrhoeae* and *C. trachomatis*. The major problem is that such infection of the lower reproductive tract is asymptomatic in 50% of cases and can therefore spread. This can lead to pelvic inflammatory disease (see below) and even extrapelvic complications such as endocarditis, septic arthritis, and perihepatitis.

The symptom of either *N. gonorrhoeae* or *C. trachomatis* infection is a non-irritating vaginal discharge containing polymorphonuclear leukocytes:

- The discharge due to *N. gonorrhoeae* is green–yellow and pus-like.
- The discharge due to *C. trachomatis* is less severe and milky white.

In asymptomatic patients, a gonorrheal infection is often recognized only via the infected partner in whom the symptoms are more obvious; however, *C. trachomatis* infection can go unrecognized in many women as the symptoms are also mild in men.

N. gonorrhoeae *infection is treated with penicillin, a quinolone, or a third generation cephalosporin*

N. gonorrhoeae can be treated with penicillin (amoxicillin), but owing to the increased resistance to this antibiotic, one of the newer quinolones (e.g. ciprofloxacin) or a third generation cephalosporin (e.g. cefoxitin or ceftriaxone) are often used instead. Erythromycin is preferred during pregnancy (Fig. 13.8).

Treatment of endocervicitis

Drug	Chemical group	Administration	Action	Other features
Amoxicillin, imipenem, carbapenem	β Lactam	Oral as single dose	Predominantly anti-*Neisseria gonorrhoeae*	Resistance common
Ciprofloxacin	Quinolone derivative	Oral as single dose	Predominantly anti-*N. gonorrhoeae*	
Ceftriaxone	Cephalosporin derivative	Intramuscular	Predominantly anti-*N. gonorrhoeae*	
Erythromycin, clindamycin, azithromycin	Macrolides	Oral for 7 days (azithromycin single dose)	Anti-*N. gonorrhoeae*, but more potent against *Chlamydia trachomatis*. Erythromycin is the drug of choice in pregnancy	
Doxycycline	Tetracycline derivative	Oral for 7 days	Predominantly anti-*C. trachomatis*	

Fig. 13.8 Treatment of endocervicitis.

C. trachomatis *responds to tetracyclines and macrolides*

C. trachomatis is a highly specialized intracellular bacterium that has a preference for the columnar epithelial cells of the female reproductive tract. It cannot produce ATP and so enters cells and uses the ATP produced by cell mitochondria. It responds to tetracyclines (e.g. doxycycline) and the macrolides such as azithromycin and erythromycin (see Fig. 13.8).

Treatment of endocervicitis is often aimed at both N. gonorrhoeae *and* C. trachomatis

A typical antibiotic combination to treat both *N. gonorrhoeae* and *C. trachomatis* infection is amoxicillin plus ciprofloxacin given as a single dose, followed up by doxycycline for 5–7 days.

Herpes vulvovaginitis

The treatment of herpes vulvovaginitis due to infection with herpes simplex virus (HSV) is discussed in Chapter 24.

Pelvic inflammatory disease

Pelvic infections are usually polymicrobial involving two to four organisms, which can be a mixture of aerobic and anaerobic bacteria. They are often caused by vaginal flora ascending to the upper genital tract, and the organisms can be either components of the normal vaginal flora or exogenous infections such as *C. trachomatis*. PID can also be associated with bacterial vaginosis, endometriosis, and pelvic peritonitis.

The clinical features include acute and severe abdominal pain, a palpable adnexal mass, a vaginal discharge, fever, and abnormal menstrual bleeding.

Salpingitis (inflammation of the fallopian tube) is a serious and important component of PID as PID is the major cause of tubal occlusion leading to infertility or ectopic pregnancy.

In developed countries, PID is usually treated with a combination of antibiotics

In developed countries, *C. trachomatis* are the major cause of PID. Combined antibiotic treatment is therefore usual to cover such a wide variety of organisms. A typical treatment would include:

- Clindamycin or metronidazole, which are highly effective against anaerobic organisms.
- Gentamicin or aztreonam, which are effective against aerobic Gram-negative bacilli.

Doxycycline may be given as a follow-up to cover *C. trachomatis*. Another combination includes:

- Cefoxitin, which is effective against *N. gonorrhoeae,* group B streptocci, anaerobic streptococci, and most aerobic and anaerobic Gram-negative bacilli.
- Doxycycline, which is effective against *C. trachomatis*, but this needs to be continued for longer than cefoxitin if the infection is in the uterine endometrium and fallopian tube.

N. gonorrhoeae is the major cause of PID in in Africa and the first-line treatment in Africa is usually a penicillin or a cephalosporin (Fig. 13.9).

Treatment of pelvic inflammatory disease

Drug	Chemical group	Action
Ampicillin	β Lactam antibiotic	Anti-Group B streptococci, anaerobic streptococci, enterococci, *N. gonorrhoeae*
Cefoxitin, ceftriaxone	Cephalosporin derivative	Anti-Group B streptococci, *N. gonorrhoeae*, anaerobic Gram-negative bacilli
Clindamycin, erythromycin	Macrolides	Anti-Group B streptococci, anaerobic streptococci, *C. trachomatis*
Metronidazole	Imidazole derivative	Anti-anaerobic organisms, *Trichomonas*, amebic infections
Doxycycline	Oxytetracycline derivative	Anti-*C. trachomatis*
Gentamicin, tobramycin	Aminoglycoside derivatives	Anti-aerobic gram-negative bacilli (e.g. *N. gonorrhoeae*) and staphylococci (used with clindamycin, metronidazole or ampicillin)
Aztreonam	Monobactam antibiotic	Anti-aerobic Gram-negative bacilli
Ciprofloxacin	Quinolone derivative	Anti-aerobic Gram-negative bacilli

Fig. 13.9 Treatment of pelvic inflammatory disease. Aerobic pathogens include group B streptococci, enterococci, *Escherichia coli, pneumoniae, proteus* spp. Anaerobic pathogens include *peptococci, peptostreptococci, Bacteroides, Neisseria gonorrhoeae, Chlamydia trachomatis.*

PHYSIOLOGY OF THE MALE REPRODUCTIVE TRACT

The male reproductive system includes the external genitalia, testes, epididymis, vas deferens, prostate gland, and associated tissues such as the urethra (Fig. 13.10). Endocrinologic aspects are discussed in Chapter 12. The testes produce spermatozoa, which are stored in the epididymis, from where they are propelled to the vas deferens, the prostate, and posterior urethra before ejaculation.

The hormonal control of testicular function begins in the hypothalamus

The hypothalamus secretes GnRH (Fig. 13.11), which stimulates the synthesis and secretion of FSH and LH:

- FSH acts upon Sertoli cells in the testicular tubules to increase synthesis of the intracellular receptor for testosterone.
- LH acts on Leydig cells to induce testosterone synthesis.

Testosterone acts on the surrounding testicular tubules at high

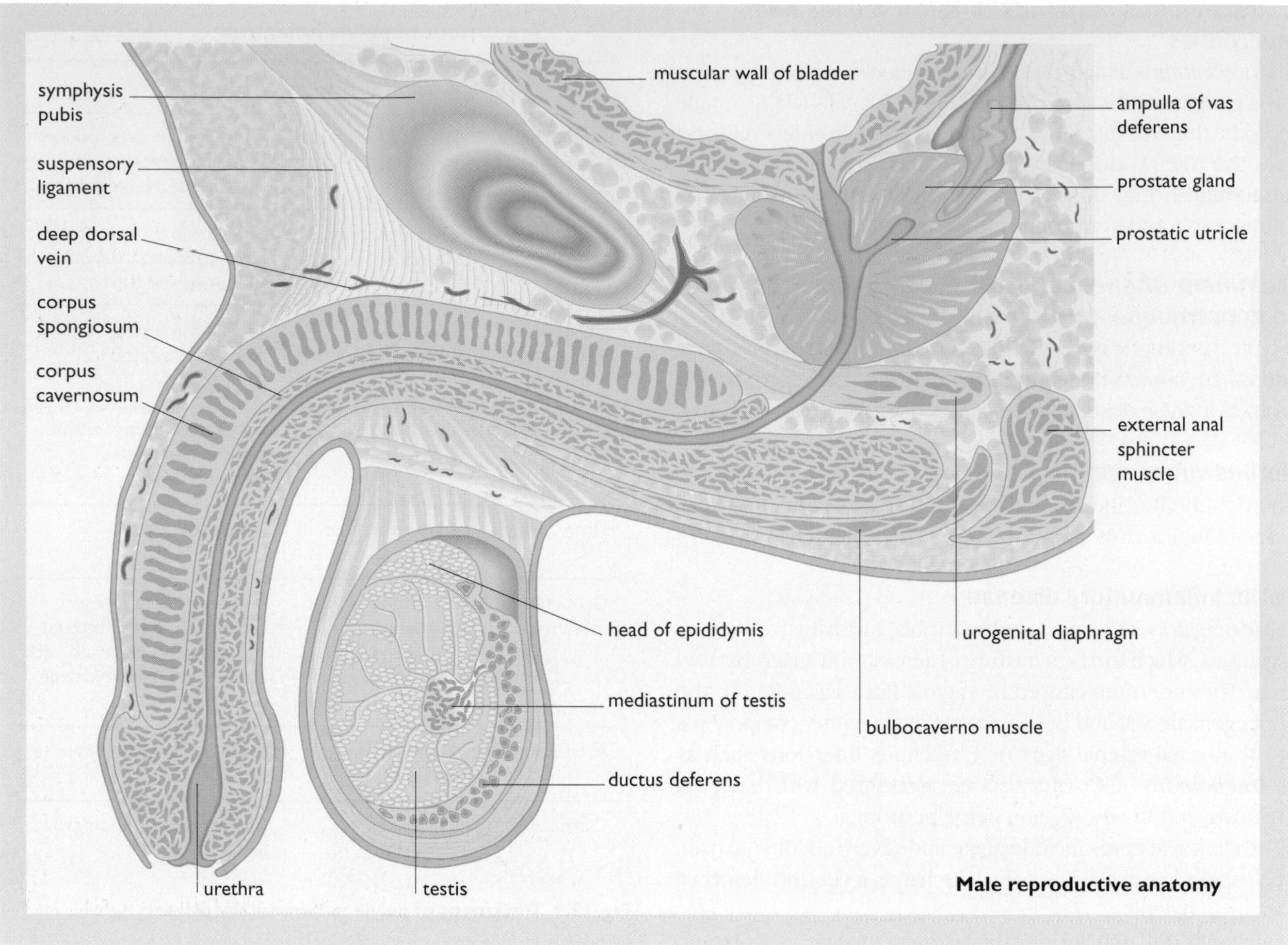

Fig. 13.10 Structure of the male reproductive tract. This shows the gross anatomy of the male reproductive tract, particularly the testes (the site of sperm production) and the duct (vas deferens), which transfers sperm from their storage site to the prostate. From the prostate the ejaculate is presented to the posterior portion of the urethra and subsequent ejaculation from the penis is due in part to contractions of the bulbus cavernosa.

concentrations to increase sperm production and on other testosterone-sensitive tissue throughout the body. In some tissues the active form of testosterone is dihydrotestosterone, which is produced by the action of 5α-reductases.

Testicular function is regulated by two feedback loops (see Fig. 13.11):

- Testosterone acts on the anterior pituitary to reduce LH secretion.
- Inhibin, produced by Sertoli cells, limits FSH secretion.

Various agonists, antagonists, and enzyme inhibitors act at different points in this system.

The ejaculate is a mixture of sperm and secretions from the prostate, epididymis, and urethra

Spermatogenesis is the production of sperm, which accumulates in the seminiferous tubules and the epididymal tract, where they mature and are stored. The vas deferens contains large smooth muscle cells and is innervated by sympathetic nerves. Norepinephrine, an α adrenoceptor agonist, produces coordinated contractions of the vas deferens, and as a result sperm and secretions move toward the prostate.

Transport of sperm and its expulsion from the penis involves erection, emission, and ejaculation

Emission is the movement of semen into an already dilated posterior urethra, and this is followed by the forceful ejection (i.e. ejaculation) of sperm. Sperm does not usually pass into the bladder as a result of the increased tone in the trigone muscle and closure of the internal urethral sphincter. Failure of these mechanisms (e.g. in autonomic neuropathy) may cause retrograde ejaculation. The pressure for ejaculation is derived from coordinated squeezing of the urethra by surrounding smooth muscle, especially the bulbocavernosus. The ejaculate contains spermatozoa and secretions from all parts of the tract, but most of its volume is provided by seminal vesicle fluid.

An erect penis is needed for ejaculation and is produced by a variety of neuronal reflexes and coordinated vascular events in the penis

Stimuli for erection are both psychologic and tactile. Sensory nerves run in the pudendal branch of the dorsal nerve of the penis, and the efferent nerves are both sympathetic (in the hypogastric nerve from the twelfth thoracic and upper lumbar segments) and parasympathetic (from the second to fourth segments of the sacral cord). The different innervations have either an erectile or anti-erectile effect:

- Sympathetic activation of the penis is anti-erectile.
- Parasympathetic activation is erectile.
- Nonadrenergic noncholinergic (i.e. NANC) and probably nitrergic (i.e. nitric oxide) nerve activation is erectile.

These basic anti-erectile and erectile functions are modulated by substances such as PGE_1 and vasoactive intestinal polypeptide (VIP) acting on persistent adrenergic tone to unmask the erectile effect. PGs may play a role in erection, but this erection is unaffected by NSAIDs, which block PG production.

Detumescence results from contraction of the smooth muscle of the corpora cavernosa, while relaxation promotes tumescence and erection. Continuous adrenergic activity maintains the flaccid state and has to be removed or opposed before erection can occur. The physiology of ercetion is also modulated by autacoids, for example:

- Histamine, which acts on H_1 receptors to cause contraction of the corpora nervosa and on H_2 receptors to cause relaxation.
- 5-hydroxytryptamine (5-HT), which activates various types of 5-HT receptors to cause contraction of the corpora cavernosa smooth muscle.

An erection can occur only when the smooth muscles of the arteries and sinusoids in the penis (Fig. 13.12) have relaxed. The erectile tissue can then fill with blood at arterial pressure. The swelling that results from the inflow of blood is limited by the nondistensible nature of the tunica albuginea. As the pressure rises, venous drainage is impaired by physical compression and venoconstriction. The reduction of penile blood flow maintains the high pressure, but limits the share of the cardiac output demanded by an erect penis. An erection can therefore occur only if there is:

- Adequate neurologic control.
- Adequate arterial flow.
- Appropriate venous drainage and blocking mechanism.

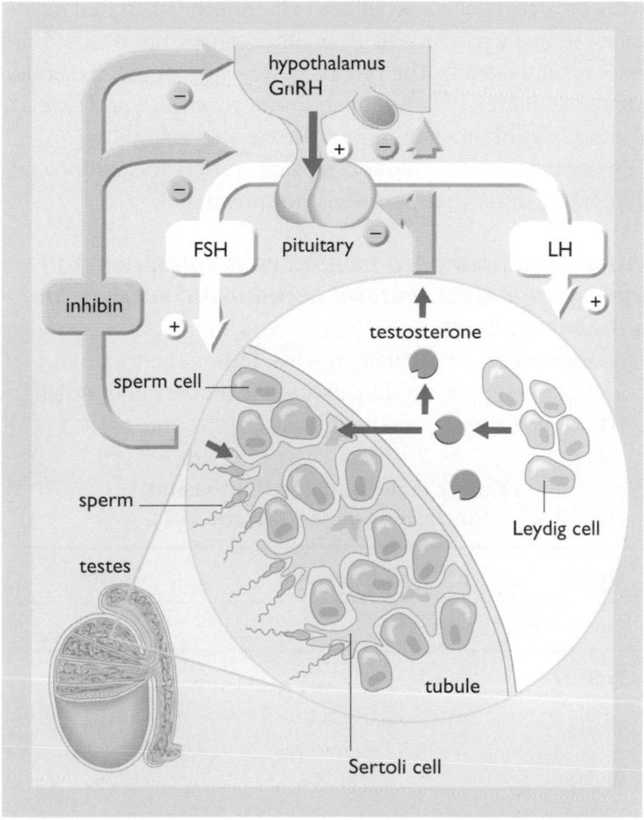

Fig. 13.11 Hormonal control of Sertoli, Leydig, and sperm cell function. Testicular development and function is critically dependent upon the production of testosterone. This is achieved by a system of positive and negative feedback involving hypothalamic gonadotropin releasing hormone (GnRH), anterior pituitary luteinizing hormone (LH) and follicle stimulating hormone (FSH), and proteins such as inhibin from the Sertoli cells. Testosterone acts on the anterior pituitary to reduce LH secretion, while inhibin limits FSH secretion.

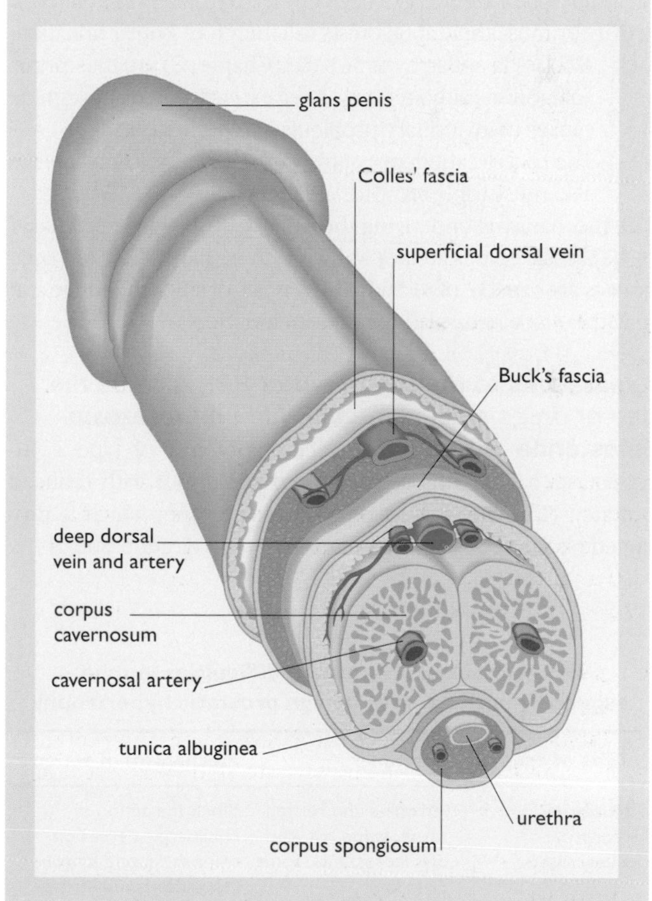

Fig. 13.12 Structure of the penis. The procreative function of the penis depends upon erection, which results from dilation of the cavernosal artery and filling of the corpora cavernosa and corpus spongiosum with arterial blood. The various fascia, particularly the tunica albuginea, prevent excessive dilation of the penis and limit venous drainage. Both arterial dilation, increasing flow, and reduction of venous outflow are important for maintaining erection.

PATHOPHYSIOLOGY AND DISEASES OF THE MALE REPRODUCTIVE SYSTEM

BENIGN PROSTATIC HYPERPLASIA

Growth of the prostate is increasingly common with increasing age, and by 70 years of age most men have benign prostatic hyperplasia (BPH).

The symptoms of BPH result from urinary obstruction

Pathologically, BPH is characterized by an increased number of stromal and epithelial cells. The resulting prostatic enlargement causes difficulties with urination such as frequency, urgency, and retention. There are two components to these symptoms:

- Continuous static obstruction as a result of the enlargement of the gland.
- Dynamic obstruction due to the activation of bladder smooth muscles.

A variety of drugs can increase the symptoms of BPH and even cause acute urinary retention (Fig.13.13). Urination depends upon cholinergic (and NANC) activation and, to a lesser extent, on inhibition of adrenergic mechanisms. Blockade of cholinergic activity by muscarinic antagonists will therefore impair urination:

- All class Ia antiarrhythmics (see Chapter 8) are muscarinic antagonists, although to varying extents, and disopyramide causes many urinary problems in elderly males.
- The tricyclic antidepressants, particularly amitriptyline, are also muscarinic receptor antagonists.

The mechanisms underlying the urinary obstruction produced by benzodiazepines are not known with certainty. Calcium antagonists are capable of relaxing many types of smooth muscle and may therefore relax bladder smooth muscle.

Approaches to the treatment of BPH include the use of drugs such as finasteride and terazosin

Finasteride is a partially selective inhibitor of type 2 5α-reductase. It also inhibits type 1 reductase, but with reduced potency. (In many tissues dihydrotestosterone, which is produced by the action of 5α-reductases in the target tissue, is the active form of testosterone.) Selective inhibitors of tissue-specific reductases are being developed to treat androgen-dependent conditions (e.g. baldness). When used by patients with BPH, finasteride slowly reduces the size of the prostate and, as a result, improves urinary symptoms, but such an improvement is relatively slow and often only modest.

Terazosin is a reversible α_1 adrenoceptor antagonist that improves the dynamic components of urination and reduces the symptoms of BPH. Adrenoceptor activation of the trigone muscle and urethra increases the resistance to urine flow. α_1 Adrenoceptor antagonists remove such activation and acutely lower the resistance to urine flow, thereby quickly relieving symptoms. Other drugs of this class, such as prazosin and doxazosin, appear to have similar beneficial actions. Terazosin has a long half-life of 12 hours, so it can be given as a single daily dose. It is usually given at bedtime to decrease the need for nocturnal urination.

PROSTATE CANCER

Prostate cancer is a common cancer (Fig. 13.14), accounting for 28% of all male cancers, and its incidence is almost equal to that of gastrointestinal cancer, although its associated mortality is less. Many prostate cancers occur late in life and are of limited malignancy, so many patients die from other causes, but over 10% of cases result in death. The prognosis depends on the size of the tumor, its degree of differentiation (invasiveness), and spread. The majority of prostate cancers are carcinomas.

Prostate cancers produce a wide variety of symptoms, depending upon their location and spread.

Prostate cancers are treated with hormones and their antagonists and are cured using surgery and anticancer drugs

Prostate cancers are usually testosterone dependent and so hormone therapy is used in addition to surgery and radiation

Drugs that worsen urinary difficulties in men, especially in those with benign prostatic hypertrophy

Type of drug	Examples	Mechanism of action
Muscarinic receptor antagonists	Atropine and related drugs, some tricyclic antidepressants, some class Ia antiarrhythmics (e.g. disopyramide)	Block the action of cholinergic nerves on smooth muscle (trigone relaxation and detrusor contraction) involved in urination
Benzodiazepines	–	
Ca^{2+} antagonists	–	Smooth muscle relaxants

Fig. 13.13 Drugs that worsen urinary difficulties in men, especially in those with benign prostatic hypertrophy.

Yearly incidence and death rates for various cancers in the US

Origin	Incidence	Deaths
Urinary tract		
Prostate	200,000	38,000
Testes	6800	325
Bladder	51,200	10,500
Kidney	27,600	11,300
Others		
Gastrointestinal	220,000	120,000
Lung	172,000	153,000

Fig. 13.14 Yearly incidence and death rates for various cancers in the US.

therapy. Testosterone, FSH, and LH are vital in regulating and controlling male sexuality, and hypogonadism is an important cause of lack of libido. However, testosterone concentrations do not correlate directly with either libido or erectile function. It is generally believed that androgen therapy improves sexual thoughts and arousal. Treatment of hyperprolactinemia, which is associated with erectile dysfunction and lack of libido, with the agonist bromocriptine restores normal sexual function.

Drugs that alter the actions and concentrations of testosterone are useful in the treatment of BPH and prostate cancer.

The action of testosterone on prostate cells can be controlled at a number of levels

FSH and LH release from the pituitary can be blocked in at least two ways (Fig. 13.15):

- Estrogens (diethylstilbestrol) inhibit the release of GnRH from the hypothalamus, thereby reducing LH and FSH release and decreasing testosterone production.
- GnRH analogs such as leuprolide act as partial agonists, stimulating and then reducing FSH and LH release from the pituitary.

Other methods of control include:

- Removing the testes (bilateral orchidectomy), leaving only the adrenal cortex as a source of androgens.
- Using ketoconazole (a fungicide) or aminoglutethimide, which inhibit various enzymes, including those responsible for the synthesis of testosterone, and reduce the adrenal production of androgens.
- Using 5α-reductase inhibitors such as finasteride to inhibit the conversion of testosterone to the active hormone dihydrotestosterone.
- Using drugs that block intracellular receptors for dihydrotestosterone, such as flutamide, cyproterone*, and certain progestin analogs.

TESTICULAR TUMORS

Testicular tumors are uncommon, the incidence being 2–3/100,000 men aged 18–44 years. Men with undescended testes and those who have had mumps-induced orchitis have an increased risk of developing testicular cancer, most (95%) of which are germ cell in origin. Nonseminomas are embryonal cancers, teratomas, and choriocarcinomas. Less than 10% of

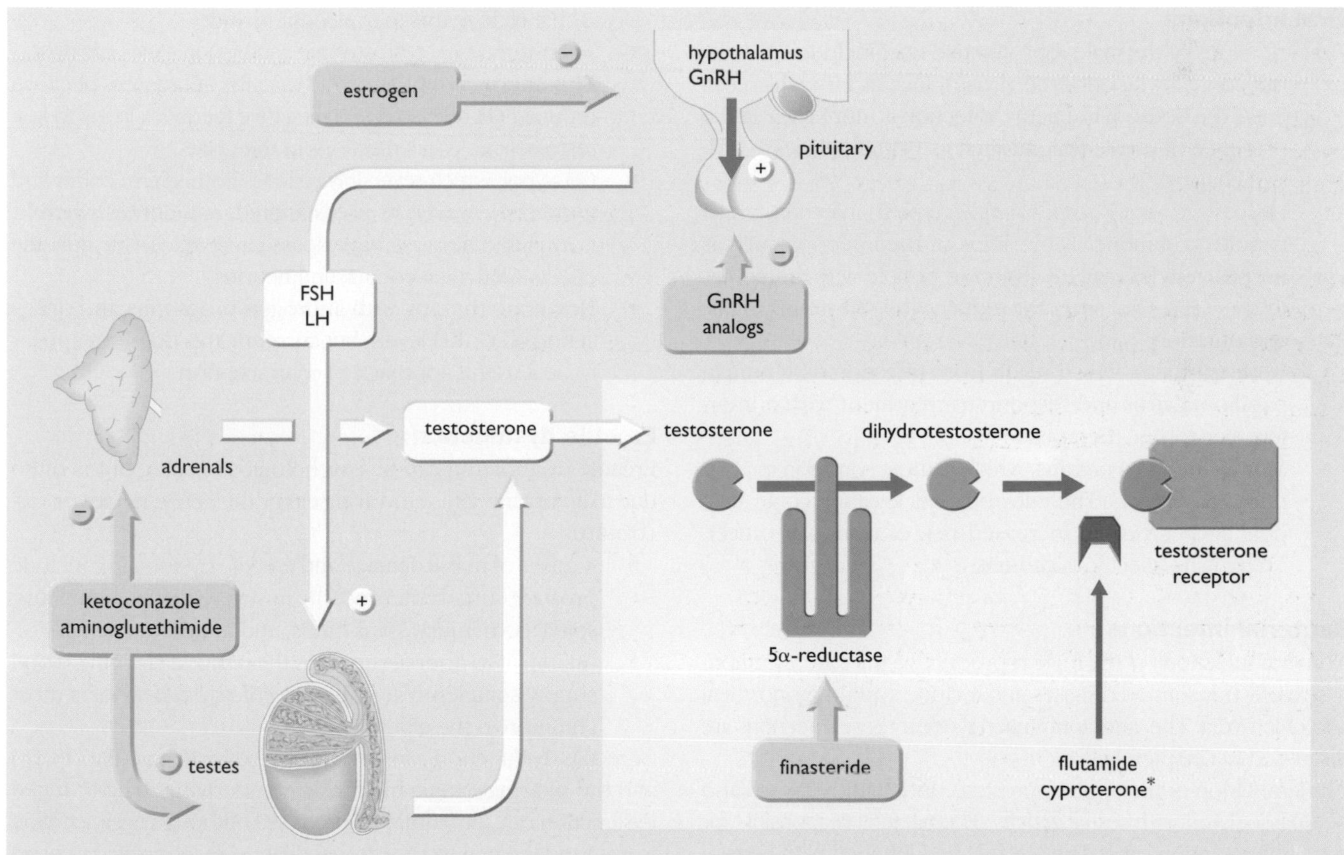

Fig. 13.15 Prostate cancer can be controlled by reducing the action of testosterone on the prostate. This can be achieved using a variety of methods. Release of the gonadotropin releasing hormone (GnRH) from the hypothalamus can be inhibited by estrogens, while the effects of luteinizing hormone releasing hormone (LHRH) to release FSH and LH can be blocked by LHRH analogs. Alternatively, testosterone synthesis can be inhibited by ketoconazole and aminoglutethimide, while the conversion of testosterone to its prostate-activating derivative, dihydrotestosterone, can be prevented by 5α-reductase inhibitors such as finasteride. Another approach is to block the testosterone receptor with flutamide or cyproterone*.

testicular tumors arise from the specialized gonadal stroma (e.g. interstitial cells) and most of these are benign. Testicular cancers in men over 50 years of age are generally lymphomas.

Tumors are not common in other parts of the male reproductive tract.

The cure rate of testicular cancer is 85–95% with appropriate surgery, radiation, and chemotherapy

Combination therapy is used, usually cisplatin, etoposide, and bleomycin. Other drugs include vinblastine, ifosfamide, dactinomycin, doxorubicin, and cyclophosphamide. The same chemotherapeutic regimens are used for seminomas and nonseminomas.

INFECTIONS OF THE MALE REPRODUCTIVE TRACT

The male reproductive tract can be infected by viruses, bacteria, and parasites, and many infections occur as a result of sexual activity. All parts of the male reproductive tract can become infected, but the main sites are the urethra, prostate, and epididymis.

Urinary tract infections are much less common in men than in women, presumably because the penis and urethral secretions confer protection against infection (see Chapter 10).

Viral infections

Viral infections of the male reproductive tract include:

- Infections by bloodborne viruses such as HIV, which can enter the body via the penis. Infection is more likely in the presence of penile lesions such as genital herpes, warts, and chancre.
- Herpes (generally herpes simplex type II) infection, which is quite common. Visible signs of the infection such as herpes vesicles may be absent in people with antibodies to the virus. Oral acyclovir reduces the symptoms, signs, and duration.
- Venereal warts, which result from infection with human papilloma virus and respond to treatment with α interferon or topical therapy.
- Mumps-induced orchitis, which is most common in postpubertal patients. The infected testicle can become atrophic and carries an increased risk of testicular cancer. There is no specific treatment.

Bacterial infections

Nonviral infections of the male reproductive tract are commonly sexually transmitted diseases and include syphilis, gonorrhea, and chlamydia. The antibiotics used to treat these infections are discussed in Chapter 24.

Inflammation of the urethra, prostate, and epididymis can also be unassociated with sexual activity. The bacteria responsible for such inflammation cannot necessarily be identified with certainty and therefore the choice of appropriate antibiotic can be uncertain. Adequate treatment of prostatitis with antibiotics is complicated by the poor penetration of antibiotics into all parts of the gland. Infectious foci in the prostate are hard to eradicate and may require long-term treatment (i.e. 4–6 weeks or longer) with trimethoprim–sulfamethoxazole or fluoroquinolone*.

MALE INFERTILITY

Male infertility may result from:

- A failure of the testes to produce sperm in adequate quantities and of sufficient vitality.
- Failure of emission if the contractile activity of the vas deferens is impaired (e.g. by agents that block sympathetic nerves and α adrenoceptors).
- Reflux emission into the bladder so that sperm fail to reach the anterior urethra.
- Erectile dysfunction.

Some drugs induce sterility, but most cannot be used as contraceptives

An adequate sperm count is needed for fertilization, but fertilization has occurred when the sperm count is only 15% of normal. It has proved difficult to reduce the sperm count as a useful stratagem for male contraception since:

- Drugs and chemicals that irreversibly impair sperm production (e.g. antineoplastics, cadmium, nitrofuranes, dinitropyrrole) are toxic.
- The induction of irreversible sterility for contraception is not usually acceptable.

Drugs that reduce the sperm count include:

- Testosterone (or testosterone analogs) in excessive doses. The sperm count is paradoxically decreased because reduced LH release due to negative feedback leads to low testosterone concentrations in the testes.
- Gossypol, which reversibly reduces both sperm count and motility. However, its use is limited in countries where it is available because high doses cause excessive adverse effects (diarrhea, edema, and neuritis).
- Hormone therapy with androgen/progestins and drugs acting on GnRH levels, but currently this does not appear to be a useful approach to contraception.

Erectile dysfunction

Erectile dysfunction can be psychologic in origin, but is often due to an organic cause involving either the penile nerves or vasculature:

- Causes of nerve damage and erectile dysfunction include prostate surgery, neuropathy in severe diabetes mellitus, spinal cord injury, spina bifida, and multiple sclerosis.
- An impaired arterial supply to the penis, disrupting blood supply sufficiently to cause erectile dysfunction, is most common in the elderly.

Erectile dysfunction can also be caused by drugs (Fig. 13.16) and the pharmacologic mechanism underlying drug-induced dysfunction can sometimes be predicted. Although acetylcholine is not fundamental to the arterial dilation responsible for erection, muscarinic antagonists prevent any involvement of muscarinic receptor activation. Drugs that affect central aspects of the autonomic system, such as some antihypertensives and central nervous system (CNS) depressants, can therefore be

Drugs that can cause erectile dysfunction

Class of drug	Specific drugs
Antihypertensives	Clonidine, methyldopa, hydrochlorothiazide, β adrenoceptor antagonists
Psychotropics	Monoamine oxidase inhibitors, tricyclic antidepressants, phenothiazines, benzodiazepines
CNS depressants	Sedatives, narcotics, ethanol, anxiolytics
Miscellaneous	Atropinics, estrogens, cimetidine, anticancer drugs

Fig. 13.16 Drugs that can cause erectile dysfunction. These drugs cause erectile dysfunction either indirectly by actions within the central nervous system or directly by actions on the smooth muscle of the penis or on penile innervation.

expected to disturb erectile reflexes. CNS sedatives such as narcotics and ethanol can also be expected to affect either libido or integration of the cortical and subcortical systems involved in generating libido and integrating it with the central autonomic nervous systems controlling erection. However, the mechanisms underlying erectile dysfunction induced by other drugs (e.g. diuretics) are not clear

Diagnosis of erectile dysfunction can involve a full investigation of:

- The psychologic status of the patient.
- Nerve and blood supplies of the penis.
- Endocrinologic function, especially in relation to testosterone, LH, and prolactin.

The functional integrity of erectile mechanisms is determined objectively by measuring nocturnal penile tumescence. However, this is not an infallible test, since nocturnal tumescence may be inhibited by depression, drugs, and disorders of rapid eye movement (REM) sleep.

Treatment of erectile dysfunction can involve psychotherapy, surgery, or regional drug administration

Some of the psychologic factors responsible for erectile dysfunction, such as a lack of libido, respond to appropriate psychotherapy, whereas surgery (e.g. changing venous drainage and implanting externally controllable penile prostheses) is needed to cure other cases. Physical measures such as vacuum devices and constricting bands are commonly used before resorting to surgery or implantable inflatable prostheses.

Erection can be induced by the intracavernosal injection of a variety of drugs. These include papaverine, α adrenoceptor antagonists, PGE_1, Ca^{2+} agonists, VIP, ketanserin, histamine, and β adrenoceptor antagonists. Mixtures of such drugs have also been used when a single agent is ineffective. Intraurethral pellets of PGE_1 provide a less invasive method of application.

The three drugs most commonly given by intracavernosal injection are papaverine, α adrenoceptor antagonists and PGE_1

These are effective for psychogenic, neurogenic, and even vasculogenic erectile dysfunction. PGE_1 may be the best drug to use because its use is associated with a lower incidence of priapism and cavernosal fibrosis. The corpora cavernosa contain enzymes (i.e. PG dehydrogenases) responsible for metabolizing PGE_1, which is a constituent of semen. This metabolic breakdown of PGE_1 in the cavernosum may account for its superiority in the treatment of erectile dysfunction. Swift degradation of PGE_1 minimizes the possible adverse effect of priapism.

Adverse effects of intracavernosal injections of papaverine, α adrenoceptor antagonists and PGE_1

The injection may cause a painful sensation (especially for PGE_1) and, rarely, long-term fibrosis. Papaverine and α adrenoceptor antagonists produce prolonged erection (priapism) lasting 4–6 hours in 5–10% of patients. More prolonged priapism is treated with α agonists, general anesthesia, and aspiration of blood from the corpus.

FURTHER READING

Gilbert GL. Infectious diseases: challenge for the 1990s. *Baillière's Clin Obstet Gynaecol* 1993; **7**: 1. [A detailed account of the treatment of infections in the female reproductive system, including treatments used in pregnanacy.]

Ginsberg J (ed.) *Drug Therapy in Reproductive Endocrinology*. London: Arnold and New York: Oxford University Press; 1996. [Up-to-date and comprehensive series of reviews.]

Pollard I. *A Guide to Reproduction*. Cambridge: Cambridge University Press; 1994. [Provides details fo the physiology and endocrinology of the female reproductive system.]

Zuspan F, Raeburn W. *Drug Therapy in Obstetrics and Gynaecology*. London: Mosby London; 1992. [A detailed account of the treatment of infections in the female reproductive system, including treatments used in pregnanacy.]

Make a provisional diagnosis and determine a rational pharmacologic treatment for the following hypothetical case.

A couple has been referred to a fertility clinic because of a failure of the female partner to conceive. Neither partner has a history of sexually transmitted disease. The female partner complains of hirsutism and a tendency to obesity, whereas both partners complain of the male partner's failure to achieve an erection at appropriate times.

1. What examination and tests should the female be subjected to?
2. What is the likely diagnosis, what treatment would you suggest, and why?
3. What investigations would you perform on the male?
4. What treatment would you suggest, and why?

Indicate which is the correct answer for each question.

1. All the following are correct about the combined oral contraceptive, except
- a) is a mixture of a steroid and a peptide hormone
- b) inhibits gonadotropin release
- c) produces changes in the fallopian tube, uterus, and cervix
- d) often contains ethinyl estradiol

2. The following statements about hormone replacement therapy are all correct, except
- a) should consist of both estrogen and progestogen components
- b) protects against cardiovascular disease
- c) protects against osteoporosis
- d) often contains ethinyl estradiol

3. Polycystic ovarian syndrome
- a) is always associated with infertility
- b) is always associated with a large number of cyst-like ovarian follicles
- c) can be treated by enhancing estrogen levels using clomiphene
- d) can be treated with a combined oral contraceptive

4. Disorders of the uterus (dysmenorrhea, menorrhea, endometriosis, fibroids) can be treated with all of the following, except
- a) oral progestogens
- b) combined oral contraceptives
- c) gonadotropin preparations
- d) nonsteroidal anti-inflammatory drugs

5. Metronidazole can be used in the treatment of all of the following, except
- a) trichomoniasis
- b) candidiasis
- c) bacterial vaginosis
- d) *Chlamydia trachomatis*

6. The symptoms of benign prostatic hypertrophy are rapidly alleviated with
- a) finasteride
- b) terazosin
- c) flutamide
- d) atropine

7. All of the following can be expected to reduce the severity of prostate cancer, except
- a) estrogen
- b) finastride
- c) testosterone
- d) aminoglutethimide

8. All of the following drugs are capable of causing erectile dysfunction, except
- a) atropine
- b) PGE_2
- c) clonidine
- d) ethanol

9. All of the following drugs can produce urinary difficulties in elderly males, except
- a) atropine
- b) Ca^{2+} antagonist
- c) antiarrhymics
- d) finasteride

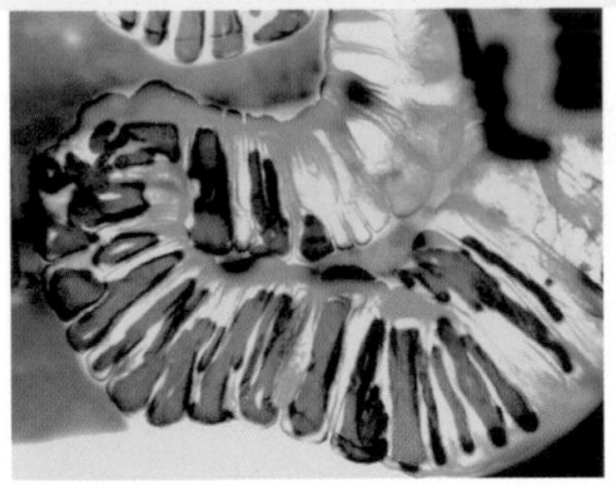

14. Drugs and the Gastrointestinal System

PHYSIOLOGY OF THE GASTROINTESTINAL SYSTEM

The alimentary tract is a muscular tube lined internally by an epithelium that varies in structure depending on its functions (Fig. 14.1). Functions of the alimentary tract include:

- Food ingestion.
- Breaking food up into small portions.
- Converting large food molecules into smaller molecules (amino acids, small peptides, carbohydrates, sugars, and lipids) by enzymes and other secretions so that they can be absorbed into the blood and lymph circulation. Most of the small molecules are then transported to the liver where they are used as building blocks for essential proteins, carbohydrates, and lipids.
- Excretion of undigested and previously digested matter as waste products.
- Water and electrolyte balance.
- Regulation of hormone secretion in various segments of the alimentary tract to enable controlled digestion and excretion.

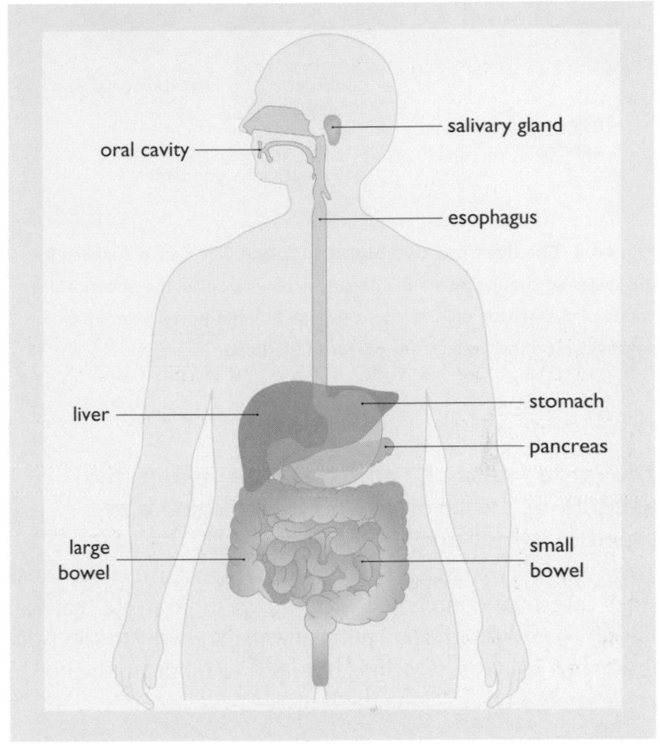

Fig.14.1 Structure of the alimentary tract.

The esophagus transports food in an undigested fragmented form from the pharynx to the stomach where digestion begins

The esophagus is about 25 cm long and opens into the stomach at the esophagogastric junction. The stomach is a dilated portion of the digestive tract where the fragmented food is retained while it is macerated and partially digested.

The gastric epithelium secretes hydrochloric acid, digestive enzymes, and mucus. It also contains hormone-secreting cells. The acid and digestive enzymes convert food into a thick semi-liquid paste (chyme), while mucus lubricates ingested food and protects the stomach from the corrosive effects of the acid and enzymes.

The liver is a metabolic, secretory, and immunologic organ

The liver's metabolic role includes:

- Anabolism and catabolism of many endogenous substances, including glycogen and hemoglobin.
- Metabolism of many drugs and foods.

The metabolic and secretory systems metabolize, transport, or secrete endogenous and exogenous chemicals, and can be modified by chemicals, including drugs. The Kupffer cells of the liver play an important role in immune responses.

The liver is also part of the biliary tract. It manufactures and secretes bile, which is collected by the bile ducts and stored in the gall bladder, from where it is discharged into the duodenum to aid fat digestion.

The liver has two blood supplies (Fig. 14.2). Blood from these supplies then flows into the hepatic venous system and hepatic vein.

The liver is exposed to drugs that enter the circulation from any site of administration

All substances, including drugs, absorbed from the upper intestine are carried immediately to the liver by the portal vein, while substances in the systemic circulation can reach the liver through the hepatic artery. Oral drugs can lead to a double exposure via the portal vein and then the systemic circulation. Drugs can also be secreted into the bile, which is excreted via the bile duct into the lumen of the duodenum. The drug can then be reabsorbed and reach the liver again via the portal vein. This phenomenon is called enterohepatic circulation of drugs.

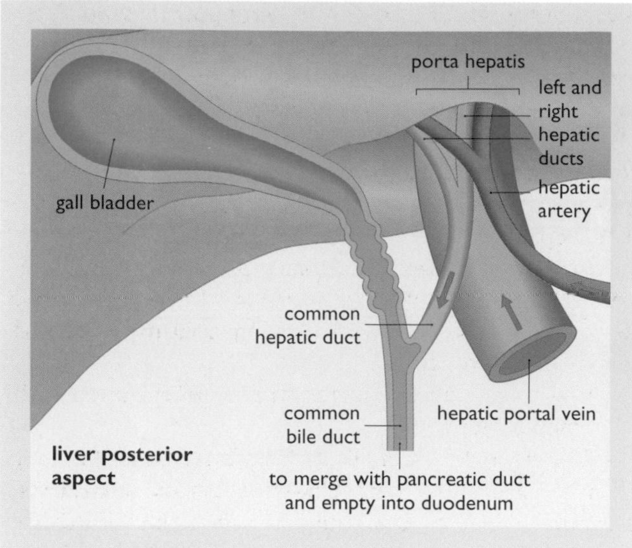

Fig. 14.2 The liver has two blood supplies. The liver is supplied by the systemic circulation via the hepatic artery to serve the nutritional needs of the hepatic cells. It is also supplied by the portal vein, which delivers blood that has already perfused the upper intestine.

The large intestine comprises the cecum, the ascending, transverse, and descending and sigmoid colon, and the rectum

The main function of the large intestine is to convert the liquid small intestinal contents to solid indigestible waste material (feces) by extensive reabsorption of water and soluble salts from the bowel contents. Mucin is required to lubricate the bowel contents as it passes along the bowel.

PATHOPHYSIOLOGY AND DISEASES OF THE GASTROINTESTINAL SYSTEM

PEPTIC ULCER DISEASE

Helicobacter pylori *plays a significant role in the pathogenesis of gastritis, peptic ulcer disease, and gastric cancer*

Peptic ulcer disease is chronic, recurs, and affects at least 10% of the population in developed countries. Although 50–80% of the adult population worldwide is infected with *H. pylori*, which if untreated can persist for decades, no more than 10–20% of infected people develop peptic ulcer disease or neoplasia, although many more may have low-grade gastritis. However, almost all patients with gastritis and duodenal ulceration and 80–90% of patients with gastric ulcers have an *H. pylori* infection in their gastric antrum.

Risk factors for acquiring *H. pylori* infection are under investigation. There appears to be a positive relationship with better economic conditions in childhood, but others report a positive relationship with crowded living conditions and growing up in rural areas. The methods of transmission are uncertain: contact with animals and contaminated sewage are possibilities.

The additional factors that cause infected individuals to develop clinical disease may involve the different virulences of strains of *H. pylori*, genetic differences in the host, age at which the host acquired the infection, and compounding environmental factors. The importance of each of these factors is poorly understood. The virulent strains of *H. pylori* causing cytotoxicity and peptic ulcer are associated with the gene termed *vacA*, but this relationship is far from absolute.

Treatment of peptic ulcer disease should include eradication of H. pylori

To reduce the incidence of recurrence of peptic ulcer associated with *H. pylori* infection, treatment regimens must include eradication of the *H. pylori*, and many practitioners argue that this should be included for all cases of peptic ulcer disease. Recurrence of duodenal ulceration after healing can be as high as 80% within 1 year when *H. pylori* eradication is not part of the treatment, but less than 5% when *H. pylori* is eradicated. If *H. pylori* eradication is not part of the treatment, recurrence can be reduced by maintenance doses of acid secretion inhibitors. At present there are two main types of eradication regimen and peptic ulcers associated with *H. pylori* infection are treated with either:

- Antibiotics and bismuth ('classic' triple therapy).
- Antibiotics combined with an acid secretion inhibitor—either a proton pump inhibitor (PPI) or an H_2 receptor antagonist.

The optimum drug combinations, duration of therapy, and doses are an evolving issue.

The 'classic' triple therapy includes about 2 weeks' treatment with bismuth, metronidazole, and tetracycline or amoxicillin. This eliminates *H. pylori* in 90% of patients and heals the ulcers in virtually all patients. Drawbacks are:

- Problems with compliance because approximately 30% of patients have adverse effects leading to treatment withdrawal in about 20%.
- The rapid development of resistance, particularly to metronidazole.
- An adverse response to alcohol with metronidazole.

Dual therapy comprises omeprazole (a PPI) given with a single antibiotic, usually either amoxicillin or clarithromycin. However, omeprazole has also been used with both antibiotics or as quadruple therapy with both antibiotics plus metronidazole. Some studies report that omeprazole plus a single antibiotic treatment is as effective as classic triple therapy, but others are less encouraging. One study has indicated that omeprazole given for a total of 7 days with the addition of metronidazole, bismuth, and tetracycline for the last 4 days resulted in eradication in 91% of patients. There is little doubt that omeprazole improves the ability of antibiotics to eradicate *H. pylori*, perhaps by increasing gastric pH, but the optimum treatment regimen has not yet been decided.

Combinations of ranitidine with bismuth are also available and there have been reports of good success rates when this formulation is given with clarithromycin.

Gastric acid secretion inhibitors

Gastric acid secretion depends on the activation of gastrin, histamine type 2, and muscarinic type 3 receptors

Parietal cells (Fig. 14.3) are located in the oxyntic glands of the gastric mucosa. Their unique acid pump is contained within vesicles in the cytosol, and cell stimulation leads to insertion of the vesicle membranes into the canalicular membranes, thereby enabling acid secretion. During stimulation, vesicles are depleted, but their number is restored when there is no acid secretion. Acid secretion depends on the activation of three main receptors on the basolateral membrane of the parietal cell:

- Gastrin receptors, which respond to gastrin secreted from the G cells in the antrum.
- Histamine type 2 receptors (H_2), which respond to histamine secreted from the enterochromaffin-like (ECL) cells that lie close to the parietal cell.
- Muscarinic type 3 receptors (M_3) on the parietal cell, which respond to acetylcholine released from neurons innervating the parietal cell. These enteric neurons also synapse at interneurons in which the muscarinic receptor appears to be an M_1 subtype.

Muscarinic and gastrin receptors are found on ECL cells as well as on parietal cells and ECL receptor stimulation leads to increased histamine release. Stimulation of the different parietal cell receptors acts through various signal transduction mechanisms to stimulate acid secretion. Histamine stimulates the adenylyl cyclase system, while gastrin and acetylcholine both increase intracellular Ca^{2+}, but by different mechanisms.

Proton pump inhibitors and H_2 receptor antagonists inhibit acid secretion by the parietal cell

Peptic ulcers treated with gastric acid inhibitors heal rapidly, but recurrence is common unless *H. pylori* is eliminated.

Proton pump inhibitors include omeprazole and its fluorinated counterpart lanzoprazole, which irreversibly inhibit the H^+/K^+-dependent ATPase proton pump that controls H^+ secretion from the parietal cell into the secretory canaliculi (see Fig. 14.3). They inhibit acid secretion by more than 90% and frequently produce achlorhydria. Amoxicillin is combined with omeprazole because:

- It is more effective at the higher pH achieved with omeprazole.
- PPIs alone do not eradicate *H. pylori*, indeed they may increase the risk of worsening gastritis in infected patients.

Omeprazole is better at eradicating *H. pylori* as part of a 12-day classic triple therapy than the H_2 receptor antagonist famotidine, which inhibits acid secretion by about 60%.

PPIs are inactive prodrugs and are converted at acid pH in the canaliculi to sulfenamide, which combines covalently with SH groups on the H^+/K^+ ATPase. They are given as enteric-coated formulations to prevent sulfenamide formation in the stomach lumen. Sulfenamide, unlike omeprazole, does not readily cross biologic membranes, and therefore it accumulates in the canaliculi of parietal cells; because of this and the unique nature of the pump, PPIs have little action on ion pumps elsewhere in the body. PPIs have a considerably longer duration of action than H_2 antagonists and are given once daily.

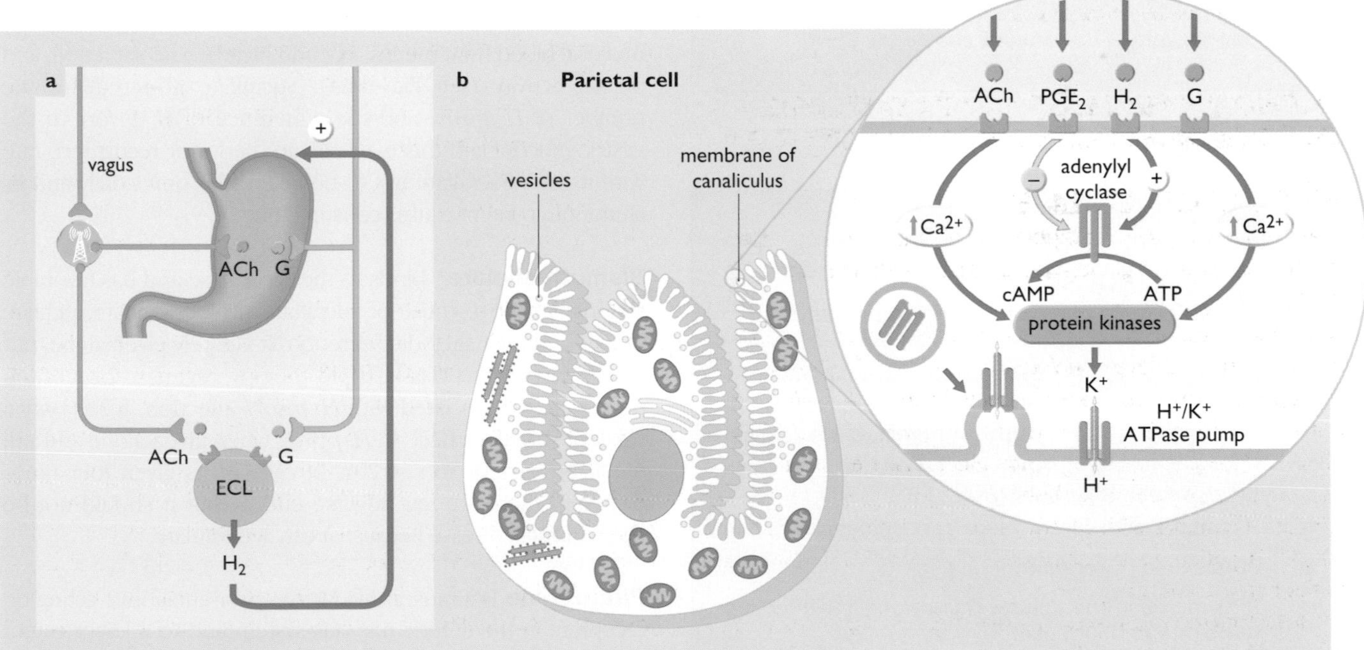

Fig. 14.3 Acid secretion from the parietal cell. (a) Gastrin (G) and acetylcholine (ACh) stimulate the parietal cell directly to increase acid secretion, and also stimulate the enterochromaffin-like (ECL) cells to secrete histamine, which then acts upon the H_2 receptors of the parietal cell (b). The H^+/K^+ ATPase pump is in tuberovesicles, which fuse with the canalicular membrane upon stimulation and release H^+ into the lumen; Cl^- is transported into the lumen by a separate carrier system. The parietal cell also has receptors for prostaglandin (PG) E_2 and their stimulation inhibits acid secretion.

It is debatable whether long-term acid suppression with a PPI is completely safe. Atrophic changes have been reported in the gastric corpus after 36 months of treatment in patients with gastroesophageal reflux disease (GERD), especially if there was gastritis before PPI administration. These changes may be due to untreated *H. pylori* in many patients already infected with this organism. There was also a marked increase in ECL cell hyperplasia.

H_2 receptor antagonists including cimetidine, ranitidine, famotidine, and nizatidine, competitively block histamine-induced acid release by the parietal cell. Acid secretion suppression is less than with a PPI because only the histamine component is inhibited, but is sufficient to result in ulcer healing in a high percentage of patients. Night time administration is particularly important for ulcer healing because acid buffering is less at night. The dosage is either twice daily or a single dose at night for 4–8 weeks.

Drugs for peptic ulcer and gastroesophageal reflux disease (GERD)

- Acid suppression enhances *Helicobacter pylori* eradication by antibiotics
- *H. pylori* eradication reduces ulcer recurrence rates
- Proton pump inhibitors (PPIs) suppress acid secretion more than H_2 antagonists
- Sucralfate and bismuth can increase prostaglandin, mucus, and bicarbonate secretion, and reduce the number of *H. pylori*
- Omeprazole is the drug of choice for GERD

Anti-ulcer drugs

- Overall proton pump inhibitors (PPIs) and H_2 antagonists have a low incidence of adverse effects
- Cimetidine and omeprazole, but not ranitidine, nizatidine, or famotidine, inhibit cytochrome P-450 liver enzymes. Cimetidine and omeprazole reduce the metabolism of drugs such as warfarin, theophylline, phenytoin, and 'ecstasy'
- H_2 antagonists rarely cause gynecomastia
- PPIs cause hypergastrinemia
- PPIs increase the risk for *Campylobacter* infection tenfold in patients over 45 years of age
- Sucralfate interacts with tetracyclines, cimetidine, digoxin, and phenytoin
- Bismuth produces a black tongue and stools

Cimetidine and famotidine are now available without prescription in some countries in packs containing only 2 weeks' supply for the treatment of dyspepsia. The unrestricted use of cimetidine and omeprazole needs careful consideration because their inhibition of cytochrome P-450 hepatic enzymes can lead to reduced metabolism of drugs that are detoxified by this enzyme system.

Other drugs used in peptic ulcer disease

Misoprostol is an analog of prostaglandin (PG) E_1. Endogenous PGE_2 and PGI_2 are important for maintaining the integrity of the gastroduodenal mucosal barrier (Fig. 14.4) and synthesis of the endogenous concentrations of PG required for mucosal barrier integrity is thought to be via pathways involving the cyclooxygenase type 1 (COX-1) enzyme. Nonsteroidal anti-inflammatory and antipyretic drugs (NSAIDs) such as aspirin inhibit COX-1 (see Chapter 7) and thereby reduce mucosal, and possibly parietal cell, PG synthesis, resulting in erosions and reduced healing of peptic ulcers and increased acid secretion. Misoprostol can be used to heal and prevent NSAID-induced damage when co-prescribed with the NSAID. Also, if appropriate, the type of NSAID should be changed to one having less effect upon COX-1 (e.g. ibuprofen). Although misoprostol replaces the prostaglandins that have been depleted by NSAIDs, some reports suggest that its effectiveness is no better than H_2 antagonists for treating or preventing NSAID-induced erosions.

Sucralfate is a polymer of aluminum and sucrose. Its structure results in minimal systemic absorption in healthy individuals, but it can accumulate in renal impairment. Sucralfate binds to the ulcer base, has antacid activity, and provides a mucosal barrier against acid, allowing healing. It has favorable effects on mucosal blood flow, mucus, PG, and bicarbonate secretion, and pepsin activity (see Fig. 14.4). Sucralfate also reduces the number of *H. pylori* and the adherence of *H. pylori* to the gastric mucosa and this may explain the lower recurrence rate with its use. Sucralfate has to be taken four times daily and its aluminum content causes constipation.

Bismuth chelate* binds to the ulcer base and has favorable actions similar to those of sucralfate on bicarbonate, pepsin, mucus and prostaglandin secretion. It is rarely given alone, but forms part of the classic triple therapy regimen for treating peptic ulcers associated with *H. pylori* infection. It has only a weak destructive effect on *H. pylori* when given alone and will eradicate bacteria in just 20% of cases. It is given four times daily and there are few adverse effects, but it should not be given in renal disease because it can accumulate.

Pirenzepine is a muscarinic M_1 receptor antagonist acting on receptors in the enteric nervous system and to a lesser extent on M_3 receptors on the parietal cell. The type of muscarinic receptor present on the ECL cell is uncertain. Pirenzepine inhibits acid and pepsin secretion, but this class of drug is relatively unpopular as a first choice because there is a high incidence of anticholinergic effects (dry mouth and blurred vision).

Antacids consist of Al^{3+} and Mg^{2+} salts, and less commonly Na^{+} and Ca^{2+} salts and are used for nonulcer dyspepsia and GERD (see p. 310). They neutralize acid and increase gastric pH and as a result may reduce the damaging effect of pepsin, which is pH dependent; additionally, Al^{3+} and Mg^{2+} salts bind and inactivate pepsin. Many different formulations are available. They have been shown to facilitate ulcer healing but few controlled studies have been performed. Healing takes longer than with H_2 receptor antagonists. A maintenance regimen of antacid can reduce the recurrence rate of duodenal ulcers over 1 year when compared with a placebo, and in one study was as effective as a maintenance regimen of H_2 receptor antagonists.

Both Al^{3+} and Mg^{2+} salts are poorly absorbed from the stomach. Doses are given 1–3 hours after meals and will keep the pH elevated until the next meal, though their duration of action is less than that of H_2 receptor antagonists. Mg^{2+} salts can cause diarrhea, whereas Al^{3+} salts can cause constipation. Both can bind many drugs, including a variety of antibiotics and phenytoin, and can increase the urinary excretion of weak acid drugs such as aspirin by increasing renal tubular pH.

GASTROESOPHAGEAL REFLUX DISEASE

One in ten people have GERD in which stomach and duodenal contents reflux into the esophagus. This can lead to an inflamed esophageal mucosa (esophagitis). Chronically this can progress to erosive esophagitis and transformation of the esophageal mucosa into a columnar gastric-type mucosa (Barrett's metaplasia), which is a significant premalignant condition for esophageal adenocarcinoma. GERD reflux is often associated with gastric distension, a transiently reduced lower esophageal sphincter pressure, and diminished esophageal peristalsis, although reflux may occur in the absence of reduced lower esophageal sphincter pressure in severe erosive esophagitis. As a result of these associations the injurious low pH gastroduodenal contents reside in the esophagus for damaging lengths of time because of the tendency for the reflux to move upwards. This upward movement in people with GERD is in contrast to events in people without GERD, in whom reflux results in increased esophageal peristalsis and rapid emptying of the esophagus. Neutralization of the esophageal contents by esophageal and salivary secretions is an important protective factor. In addition, nonadrenergic noncholinergic (NANC) control may also be important, partly through the involvement of nitric oxide and cholecystokinin, which induce relaxation of the lower esophageal sphincter.

In achalasia, there is a significant reduction in nitrergic neurons in the sphincter and lower esophageal sphincter pressure is increased. This raised pressure can be reduced by local administration of botulinum toxin.

Drugs used to treat gastroesophageal reflux disease increase gastrointestinal motility and sphincter pressure and reduce acid and bile secretion

Treatment regimens depend on the severity of the disease (Fig. 14.5). Occasional uncomplicated GERD (heartburn) is most often treated by self-medication, frequently with H_2 receptor antagonists or antacids.

Causes of damage to the gastrointestinal mucosal barrier and treatment

Cause of damage	Treatment
Helicobacter pylori infection	Antibiotics plus PPI or H_2 antagonists
Increased acid	Reduced by PPI, H_2 antagonists, or prostaglandins
Reduced thickness of mucus layer	Heal ulcer, prostaglandins and sucralfate stimulate mucus secretion
Reduced bicarbonate	Prostaglandins and sucralfate stimulate
Increase in type I pepsin	Increase stomach pH, bind to Al^{3+} salts or sucralfate
Decreased mucosal blood flow	Increase prostaglandins, sucralfate increases blood flow
NSAID-induced ulcer erosion potential	NSAID withdrawal, substitute with an NSAID with a low erosion potential combined with a prostaglandin analog

Fig. 14.4 Causes of damage to the gastrointestinal mucosal barrier and treatment. (NSAID, nonsteroidal anti-inflammatory drug; PPI, proton pump inhibitor)

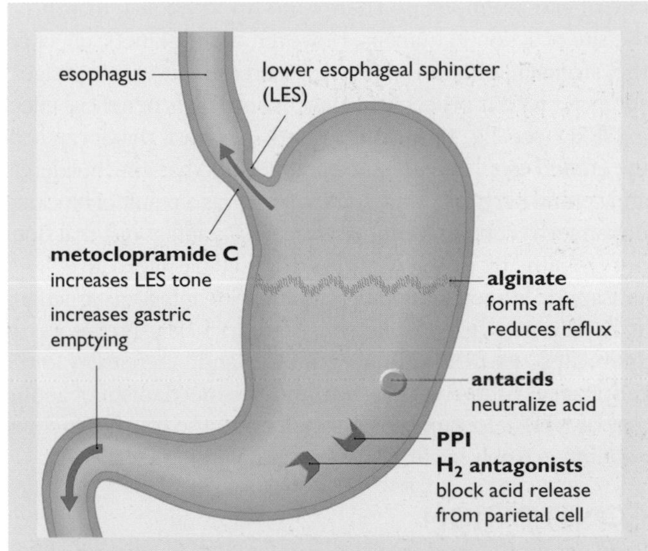

Fig. 14.5 The sites of action of drugs used to treat gastroesophageal reflux disease (GERD). (PPI, proton pump inhibitors)

Antacids and alginic acid Mg^{2+} and Al^{3+} antacids are often given in combination with alginic acid, an inert substance that foams in acid and forms a raft on the stomach contents, thereby reducing reflux. The foaming raft has a high pH, but much of the benefit of these preparations may be derived from the antacid constituents. Alginates are also available in combination with cimetidine.

H_2 antagonists If there is no response to simple measures, one study has found that a 12-week course of H_2 antagonists produced healing in up to 75% of patients with erosive esophagitis. This rate was not improved with 24 weeks of treatment. However, other studies contend that H_2 antagonists are purely symptomatic and do not produce healing.

Proton pump inhibitors Long-term maintenance of erosive oesophagitis with a PPI has been shown to be associated with fewer relapses than long-term maintenance with H_2 antagonists. Omeprazole produced healing in 95% of patients. It was then followed by 12 months of maintenance with 20 mg omeprazole once daily or 150 mg ranitidine twice daily, which resulted in 77% and 46% remission rates, respectively. However, in another study 47% of patients with GERD resistant to healing with H_2 antagonist treatment and treated for 36 months with 20 mg omeprazole daily relapsed after initial healing. There is some evidence that Barrett's metaplasia regresses with omeprazole treatment.

Prokinetic (motility-promoting) drugs In GERD, prokinetic drugs are best used as adjuncts to PPI and H_2 antagonist drug therapy.

Metoclopramide is a dopamine type 2 (D_2) receptor antagonist (see Chapter 7) and a 5-hydroxytryptamine (5-HT) receptor stimulant. From animal studies it is said to act on 5-HT_4 interneurons in the stomach enteric nervous system, resulting in acetylcholine release, increased gastric motility, and an increased rate of gastric emptying. There is no firm evidence that this is the site of action in humans. However, the prokinetic effect on the stomach plus an ability to increase lower esophageal sphincter tone is probably the mechanism of its beneficial effect in GERD (see Fig. 14.5). There is little evidence that it can heal the eroded esophagus. Metoclopramide also has anticholinergic and central nervous system (CNS) effects as a result of blocking dopamine receptors. Domperidone*, a D_2 antagonist that does not cross the blood–brain barrier, is a suitable alternative.

Cisapride is a substituted benzamide with antagonistic actions at 5-HT_3 receptors while stimulating 5-HT_4 receptors. It stimulates gastrointestinal motility and increases lower esophageal sphincter pressure, and the mechanism of action may be 5-HT_4 receptor stimulation. It can cause diarrhea in some patients, possibly by an action on the colon.

CONSTIPATION

Regulation of normal gastrocolonic motility involves the CNS, the enteric nervous system, and gastrointestinal hormones. There are many causes of constipation, but ultimately it results from an absence of propagating contractions in the colon, which may be associated with either decreased or increased segmenting contractions. In some patients there may be abnormalities of propulsion affecting just the proximal or distal parts of the colon. Normal defecation of formed stools can vary from three times a day to only once every 3 days.

The incidence of severe chronic constipation, excluding that due to organic disease or an iatrogenic cause, is not known, but it is significantly greater in women than in men. The definition of constipation is also clouded, sometimes being described as an altered frequency of defecation and sometimes as difficult defecation.

Constipation is managed by dietary improvement, eliminating any drugs that can cause constipation, excluding the presence of underlying pathology, and laxatives

Laxatives

The mechanisms of action of laxatives are illustrated in Fig. 14.6. Laxatives are widely misused in some societies for many reasons, including eating disorders when they are used to reduce calorie intake. Sometimes laxative use may disguise the presence of underlying disease (e.g. obstruction).

Bulk laxatives Constipation and diarrhea can be treated with fiber bulking. Unprocessed fiber (e.g. bran from unprocessed wheat or citrus sources) forms a readily available nondigestible source of bulk-forming laxative that can be recommended if sufficient fiber cannot be obtained from a normal balanced diet. It may take several days for full effectiveness and sometimes causes flatulence. It works by absorbing water and promoting

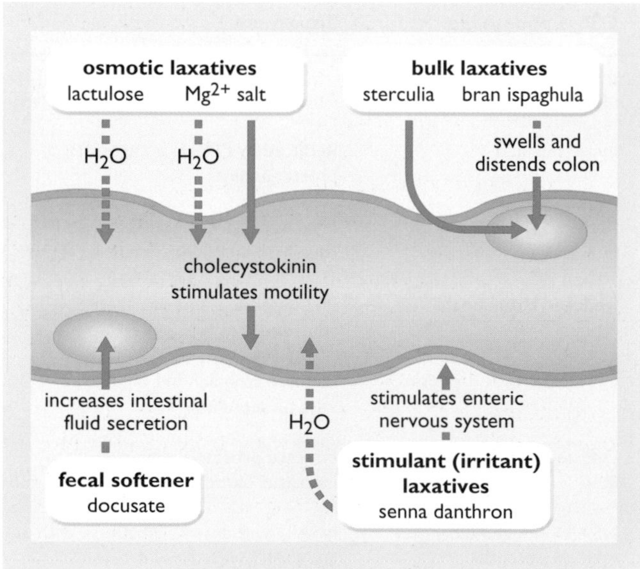

Fig. 14.6 Mechanism of action of laxatives. Bulk laxatives absorb water and on swelling slowly distend the colon and increase peristaltic motility; osmotic laxatives enhance peristalsis by osmotically increasing the bowel fluid volume; stimulant (irritant) laxatives stimulate the enteric nervous system; fecal softeners increase intestinal fluid secretion.

bacterial growth; on swelling, it distends the colon and increases peristaltic motility. Other bulk laxatives include preparations of ispaghula* husk, sterculia* gum, and methylcellulose, which are available in more palatable forms than unprocessed fiber and are gluten free; some preparations are also sugar free. They have essentially the same action as bran, but sterculia contains polysaccharides, which are broken down by bacteria, and the resulting fatty acids can have an additional osmotic effect. Fiber is thought to normalize stool texture and is also used to treat patients with loose stools (see p. 313).

Osmotic laxatives are widely prescribed. They are poorly absorbed and increase the small and large bowel fluid volume by osmosis and as a result increase peristaltic motility.

Lactulose is widely used and is a semisynthetic disaccharide of galactose and fructose. It passes unchanged to the colon and is then broken down by bacteria to lactic and acetic acids, which act osmotically to increase fluid volume and lower pH. It is effective within 2–3 days. Mg^{2+} salts and Na^{+} acid phosphate are used less often than lactulose; they are poorly absorbed and are osmotically active. Mg^{2+} also increases the synthesis of cholecystokinin, which increases colon motility and fluid secretion into the lumen.

Stimulant contact or irritant laxatives should not be given long-term. They have limited or restricted uses and can cause long-term pathologic problems. They act within hours and include:

- Senna, which is obtained from plantains. The constituent anthroquinones are hydrolyzed by gut bacteria to yield glycosides and subsequently anthracenes. These stimulate the enteric nervous system and alter fluid balance across the gut wall to promote propulsive motility.
- Bisacodyl, which is a diphenolic compound similar to phenolphthalein that can be given rectally for a rapid response.
- Danthron, which has similar properties to senna, but is carcinogenic in animal studies.
- Sodium picosulfate*, which is frequently used for bowel preparation before endoscopy or surgery.

The mechanisms of action of this group of drugs are poorly understood, but it has been suggested that they damage enterocytes and weaken intercellular junctions. They also stimulate PG, cAMP, and possibly cholecystokinin, and vasoactive intestinal polypeptide (VIP) synthesis. These changes can all affect fluid balance and motility.

Chronic use of the anthroquinone laxatives can lead to melanosis coli, a black discoloration of the colonic mucosa, which can persist for years. Chronic administration of stimulant laxatives can also lead to the development of a 'cathartic colon,' which is a progressive deterioration of colon function that can exacerbate an existing bowel dysfunction.

Fecal softeners Docusate is dioctyl sodium sulfosuccinate. It has detergent properties, increases intestinal fluid secretion, and has weak stimulatory activity on intestinal motility. It relieves constipation within 1–2 days.

Prokinetic drugs Bethanechol, metoclopramide, cisapride, and naloxone can stimulate colon motility, but reports of their use in the treatment of severe chronic constipation are insubstantial and require further clarification.

Chronic laxative use

- Chronic use of stimulant (irritant) laxatives can lead to the development of a 'cathartic colon' with reduced propagative motility, dilatation, and exacerbation of any underlying disease
- Can damage the enteric nervous system
- Can lead to electrolyte imbalance

DIARRHEA

There are many causes of diarrhea including:

- An existing chronic disease (e.g. loss of functioning mucosa in inflammatory bowel diseases and gut resections, the motor abnormalities of irritable bowel syndrome, malabsorption diseases, endocrine abnormalities such as thyrotoxicosis).
- Infectious agents.
- Drugs.
- Psychologic factors.

Acute secretory diarrhea usually results from an infection.

Acute infectious diarrhea is extremely common and usually lasts just a few days. A common cause is acute viral gastroenteritis, and in children it is a rotavirus that is usually identifiable. In many cases, particularly adults, viral causes are often not identified, but bacterial pathogens such as *Campylobacter* are commonly cultured (Fig. 14.7).

Causes of acute diarrhea in developed countries

Cause	Proportion of cases (%)	
	In children under 2 years of age	Adult
Identified viruses	22 (predominantly rotavirus)	–
Bacteria	14	33[1]
Protozoa	2	2

[1] Approximately 50% are due to *Campylobacter*; the rest are largely undiagnosed, but are likely to be viral gastroenteritis

Fig. 14.7 Causes of acute diarrhea in developed countries.

Worldwide, acute diarrhea (mainly of infectious origin) causes up to five million deaths every year as a result of dehydration. Approximately 85% of these deaths are in children less than 2 years of age and many could be prevented by simple measures. In Britain about 12 children younger than 1 year of age die each year from infectious diarrhea, while 20% of all health service consultations in the UK are for children less than 2 years of age with acute diarrhea.

The vigor of treatment for acute diarrhea depends upon the differential diagnosis and the patient's age. Young children are particularly prone to dehydration as 15% of the body weight turns over each day as water. Classifying enteropathogenic bacteria according to whether or not they invade the intestine is also important when deciding upon treatment (Fig. 14.8):

- Generally invasive bacteria cause bloody, relatively small volume, diarrhea.
- Adhesive but noninvasive enterotoxigenic bacteria produce toxins, which can increase cyclic AMP and result in a massive secretion of Cl^- followed by water and Na^+ secretion. More than 1 liter of fluid can be lost every hour, but with effective rehydration the infection tends to be short lived.

It needs to be borne in mind that diarrhea is the body's defense mechanism for ridding itself of the invading organisms.

Approximately 20% of travellers abroad suffer an acute episode of diarrhea. It is estimated that the predominant infectious causes are noninvasive *Escherichia coli* (40%), *Shigella* (10%), *Campylobacter jejuni* (3%), protozoa (5%), and viruses (10%), while no pathogen is isolated in about 22%. This pattern is quite different from that of home-acquired pathogens.

Rotavirus is the most important pathogen causing dehydrating diarrhea in infants in both developed and developing countries. In the USA there are an estimated 3.5 million cases of rotavirus diarrhea every year among infants and up to 125 related deaths. Worldwide there are an estimated 800,000 deaths from rotavirus-related gastroenteritis. Successful vaccines against some strains are being evaluated.

The mainstay of treatment of acute diarrhea is the correction of dehydration and not the reduction of stool fluid output

Rehydration therapy

Oral rehydration therapy (ORT) is the first priority in the treatment of acute diarrhea of all causes and promptly administered oral formulations save many lives. In many cases, particularly those of viral origin, oral rehydration is the only therapy needed, but intravenous therapy is needed if there is a severe electrolyte imbalance. ORT will not immediately reduce the volume of diarrhea, but absorption of the administered electrolytes leads to correction of the electrolyte imbalance, fluid balance and acidosis, while the body systems eliminate the pathogens. The success of this will depend upon the nutritional and physical status of the patient. There are several oral formulations (in powder form).

The World Health Organization (WHO) oral rehydration therapy (ORT) recommended formulation contains:

- NaCl 3.5 g/liter (Na^+ 90 mmol/liter).
- KCl 1.5 g/liter (K^+ 20 mmol/liter).
- NaCitrate 2.9 g/liter (citrate 30 mmol/liter).
- Chloride (80 mmol/liter).
- Glucose 20 g/liter (111 mmol/liter).

Pathologic features of some enteroinfective organisms that cause diarrhea

Infective organism	Mechanism	Volume of diarrhea
Rotavirus	Damages small bowel villi	+ (watery stools)
Adhesive enterotoxigenic bacteria *Escherichia coli* *Salmonella enteritidis*[1] *Cholera*	Noninvasive. Adhere to brush borders of intestinal absorptive cells. Secrete enterotoxins that alter fluid electrolyte transport and increase prostaglandin activity. Stimulate enteric nervous system	 ++ (watery stools) ++ (watery stools) +++ (watery stools)
Invasive bacteria *Shigella*[1] *E. coli*[1,2] *Salmonella typhimurium* *Campylobacter jejuni*[1]	Invade epithelium. Secrete enterotoxins. Cause inflammation and tissue destruction. Some move between epithelial cells	Bloody stools

[1]Sometimes causes vomiting
[2]Some strains

Fig. 14.8 Pathologic features of some enteroinfective organisms that cause diarrhea. (The mechanisms stated are a generalization. Each bacterium uses distinct mechanisms to penetrate the epithelium and produce damage and diarrhea.)

Other formulations contain considerably less Na^+ than this WHO formula, which can sometimes produce hypernatremia, and formulations containing less Na^+ (approximately 50 mmol/liter) should probably be used in developed countries. Clearly, a source of uninfected drinkable water is required for reconstituting the solutions. The correct amount of water must be added to avoid worsening the dehydration if the solutes are too concentrated. In fact, the WHO formulation is slightly hypertonic. Some formulations contain HCO_3^- rather than citrate, but these tend to deteriorate in hot conditions. More recently, formulations that produce a hypotonic solution, containing a glucose polymer have been tested; this reduces volume loss by about 30% when compared with no treatment. Glucose is necessary because it facilitates Na^+ absorption via the Na^+/glucose cotransporter, and this also increases water absorption. Other formulations that replace glucose with amino acids or even cooked cereal have also been used with similar results to the WHO formulation.

Drugs used to treat diarrhea

Many drugs have an antidiarrheal action because they alter intestinal propulsive motility and increase the time for fluid absorption; however, only a small number are commonly used for acute infective diarrhea. Not only do these drugs enhance absorption by slowing transit time, but some also accelerate absorption as a separate action.

Opiate-like antidiarrheal agents include:

- Diphenoxylate* and loperamide, which are congeners of meperidine.
- Codeine, which is a congener of morphine.

They act on μ opiate receptors in the myenteric plexus and possibly on 5-HT receptors, and by modulating acetylcholine release reduce peristaltic activity, but enhance segmental activity and tone and increase transit time. They may also enhance absorption by acting on opiate receptors.

Although these drugs have been available for many years, it is difficult to gain a consensus about their use, which has been largely based on individual preference and divergent advice.

Patients with viral gastroenteritis or traveller's diarrhea generally require no antidiarrheal treatment, but opiates can reduce the duration of diarrhea by about 12 hours. Some reports suggest that these drugs should not be given for infections caused by enteroinvasive bacteria such as *Shigella* (Fig. 14.8) because they delay clearance of the organism, prolonging the diarrhea and accompanying fever, but other reports state that this is of little clinical consequence.

Co-phenotrope* is a combination of diphenoxylate* and atropine. It can produce the typical antimuscarinic adverse effects of blurred vision and dry mouth and there is little evidence to suggest that the combination has advantages.

Loperamide has relatively selective actions on the gut and undergoes enterohepatic recycling, extending the drug concentration in the gut.

Stool modifiers such as the absorbent clay, kaolin, are given in combination with morphine. Kaolin has a bulking action, improving stool consistency. Other bulking agents, such as wheat bran, increase stool viscosity. It is critical that fluid and electrolyte balance is maintained when bulking agents are used. Kaolin may also absorb toxins, although this effect is largely anecdotal.

Antibiotic treatment of diarrhea should be undertaken sparingly. It is rarely required for the treatment of communally acquired infectious diarrhea in developed communities because this is likely to be self-limiting and viral in origin. Tetracycline can be given for severe cholera and *Salmonella typhimurium*, although substantial outbreaks of infections can be resistant, as happened with a cholera outbreak in the Ruandan refugee camps in Tanzania in 1994. *Shigella* can be treated with ampicillin, although again there are marked individual variations, with a high level of resistance in some strains, and alternative antibiotics may be necessary. *Campylobacter jejuni* is sensitive to erythromycin or ciprofloxacin. (Antibiotics are discussed in detail in Chapter 23.)

The indiscriminate use of broad-spectrum antibiotics has led to a high level of resistance in many enteropathogenic bacteria. The use of antibiotics that destroy the normal flora as well as the pathogen may allow overgrowth of organisms such as *Clostridium difficile,* which can cause serious pseudomembranous colitis requiring treatment with either metronidazole or vancomycin. Commonly used drugs that can cause diarrhea or constipation are shown in Fig. 14.9.

Opiate antidiarrheals

- **Codeine and diphenoxylate, but not loperamide, cross the blood–brain barrier and produce euphoria and respiratory depression, particularly in children**
- **Can delay clearance of enteroinvasive bacteria such as *Shigella*, but some investigators suggest that this is of little clinical consequence**
- **Chronic use of opiates can cause paralytic ileus and toxic megacolon**

Drugs that can cause diarrhea or constipation

Constipation	Diarrhea
Al^{3+} salts	Mg^{2+} salts
Anticholinergics	Erythromycin
Antidepressants	Ampicillin
Fe^{3+} preparations	Prokinetics
Antispasmodics	Theophylline
Opiates	Indomethacin
Ca^{2+} antagonists	Fe^{3+} preparations
Sympathomimetics	Levodopa
	Propranolol
	Parasympathomimetics

Fig. 14.9 Drugs that can cause diarrhea or constipation.

Drugs for diarrhea and constipation

- Rehydration is of prime importance in diarrhea
- Opiates decrease peristalsis and increase overall gut tone
- Antibiotics should be necessary only for specific infectious diarrheas such as cholera
- Mechanisms of action of laxatives include an osmotic effect, bulking, irritation, stimulation of the enteric nervous system, and fecal softening
- Bulk laxatives and osmotic laxatives act within days, but irritant laxatives act within hours

INFLAMMATORY BOWEL DISEASE

The incidence of inflammatory bowel disease (IBD), which includes ulcerative colitis (UC) and Crohn's disease (CD), is about 1/10,000/year. The etiologies of UC and CD are unknown, but there is considerable overlap between the two conditions. Multifocal infarction and infection with *Mycobacterium* and other pathogens have been implicated, but their relevance is far from clear. Products of nonpathogenic intestinal flora may also play a role. Genetic factors, environmental conditions, and alterations in the mucosal immune system are also thought to be involved.

IBD follows a course of flare-ups (with chronic intestinal inflammation, which may be accompanied by fever and anemia) and periods of remission. Frequent, bloody, loose stools and abdominal pain are common, and patients are prone to infection.

Aminosalicylates, glucocorticosteroids, and immunosuppressants are used to treat inflammatory bowel disease

Aminosalicylates such as sulfasalazine are widely used in the treatment of CD and UC to maintain remission. They have only limited use for treating acute relapses. Sulfasalazine is broken down by gut flora, mainly in the cecum and colon, to the active component 5-aminosalicylate (5-ASA) and sulfapyridine, which appears to cause the adverse effects of nausea, toxic effects on red cells, and oligospermia. The mechanism of action of 5-ASA is unknown. The use of sulfasalazine to treat CD is largely limited to where 5-ASA is released (i.e. colonic involvement).

Mesalazine* is 5-ASA and olsalazine is two molecules of 5-ASA linked by a diazo bond, which is cleaved in the colon. They have a lower incidence of adverse effects than sulfasalazine, but olsalazine tends to cause diarrhea in some patients.

Aspirin worsens IBD and should be avoided.

Glucocorticosteroids are widely used to treat relapses of IBD. They are of limited use in maintaining remission. Their adverse effects (see Chapter 12) have led to the development of local acting, poorly absorbed glucocorticosteroids such as budesonide.

Immunosuppressants can be useful in the treatment of IBD:

- Azathioprine and 6-mercaptopurine reduce the need for glucocorticosteroids and are particularly useful for glucocorticosteroid-refractory and glucocorticosteroid-dependent patients, but it takes several months before their effect becomes evident.
- Cyclosporine produces improvement in symptoms within 2 weeks, but has to be given as a high-dosage intravenous administration because oral therapy is ineffective.
- Methotrexate appears to be beneficial in some patients, but its usage and benefits require further evaluation.

New therapies under consideration include antitumor necrosis factor antibody, interferon-γ and anti-CD4 antibody. Treatment with 5-lipoxygenase inhibitors, nicotine, and short-chain fatty acids has also been reported.

Drugs and inflammatory bowel disease

- Aminosalicylates such as mesalazine and olsalazine maintain remission
- Glucocorticosteroids are effective for acute relapses of the disease
- Poorly absorbed glucocorticosteroids (e.g. budesonide) have little effect on the hypothalamic–pituitary–adrenal axis
- Nonsteroidal anti-inflammatory drugs exacerbate inflammatory bowel disease

PATHOPHYSIOLOGY AND DISEASES OF THE LIVER

JAUNDICE

Jaundice is a yellowing of the skin and conjunctiva. It is produced by increased serum concentrations of bilirubin, which result in the deposition of bilirubin and its metabolic products in the skin and other organs. Causes of increased serum bilirubin concentrations include:

- Increased formation of bilirubin due to increased breakdown (hemolysis) of red blood cells so that bilirubin production exceeds the capacity of the liver to metabolize it.
- Inadequate bilirubin metabolism in the liver due to congenital abnormalities or disease of the liver parenchyma.
- Obstruction to bile outflow from the liver so that bilirubin 'spills' into the blood.

Many drugs can cause jaundice by one or more of these mechanisms (Fig. 14.10).

There is no specific drug treatment for jaundice.

CONGENITAL LIVER DISEASE

The three congenital diseases of the liver of particular note in pharmacology are Wilson's disease and hemochromatosis, because drug treatment is useful, and Dubin–Johnson syndrome, which can alter liver metabolism of drugs.

Wilson's disease (hepatolenticular degeneration) is a rare (1/million population) autosomal recessive trait in which there is defective copper excretion into the bile. This leads to an accumulation of copper in the tissues, including the brain, resulting in neurologic and hepatic dysfunction.

Treatment involves the use of drugs that chelate copper (usually penicillamine, see Chapter 29) and promote its removal from the body.

Dubin–Johnson syndrome is characterized by hyperbilirubinemia and jaundice because the liver is unable to secrete conjugated bilirubin efficiently. This results from a congenital impairment of an ATP-dependent transport system that is specific for a variety of multivalent organic anions, including conjugated bilirubin. Drugs such as oral contraceptives are also metabolized by this method and should be avoided by individuals with Dubin–Johnson syndrome.

ACQUIRED LIVER DISEASE

Chemical-induced liver disease Many chemicals are toxic to the liver (e.g. halogenated hydrocarbons such as carbon tetrachloride). Ethanol is the most commonly ingested hepatotoxic substance and chronic excess intake produces a fatty liver and cirrhosis (see Chapter 30).

Liver infections Hepatitis A, B, and C, are among the most common infectious diseases, and their consequences can include cirrhosis and possibly carcinoma of the liver. They are best controlled by the prophylactic use of specific vaccines.

Parasitic infections such as *Schistosoma mansoni*, *Echinococcus*, *Ameba histolytica*, and *Chlonorchis sinesis* occur in the liver, and can be treated with the appropriate antiparasitic agents (see Chapter 25).

Mechanism of action of some drugs that cause jaundice

Mechanism	Drug	Comment
Hemolysis (increased bilirubin production)	Antimalarials Sulfonamides Aspirin Phenacetin	Occurs in people with glucose-6-phosphate dehydrogenase (G6PD) deficiency
	Cephalosporins Methyldopa	Immunologic basis
Altered hepatic bilirubin uptake	Rifampin	
Hepatotoxicity	Carbon tetrachloride	
	Acetaminophen overdose	Treat with *N*-acetylcysteine
	Tetracycline	Avoid in pregnancy
Diffuse hepatocellular damage	Tricyclic antidepressants	Uncommon
	Isoniazid	Related to dose and patient's age
Intrahepatic cholestasis	Anabolic steroids Phenothiazines	
	Erythromycin	Incidence probably not related to type of salt used (e.g. estolate)

Fig. 14.10 Mechanism of action of some drugs that cause jaundice.

PATHOPHYSIOLOGY AND DISEASES OF THE BILIARY TRACT

Bile consists of approximately:

- 65–90% bile salts (e.g. cholic acid, deoxycholic acid, chenodeoxycholic acid, and lithocholic acid, coupled to glycine or taurine).
- 5–25% cholesterol.
- 2–25% phospholipids.
- Bilirubin, fatty acids, electrolytes, and water.

There is a tendency for stones to form in the bile (cholelithiasis) and this is frequently accompanied by inflammation of the gall bladder (cholecystitis).

Cholelithiasis The chemical nature of gall bladder stones varies widely and only stones formed from cholesterol can be dissolved by drugs. Such stones are particularly common when there has been rapid weight loss (e.g. during treatment of morbid obesity).

The naturally occurring bile acid ursodiol (ursodeoxycholic acid) is the oral agent of choice for dissolving cholesterol stones. It has largely superseded chenodiol (chenodeoxycholic acid), which is associated with liver toxicity and diarrhea. Ursodiol:

- Decreases cholesterol secretion into the bile.
- May decrease cholesterol absorption from the intestine.
- May increase bile flow.

The net effect is a reduced cholesterol concentration in the bile and a tendency for dissolution of existing cholesterol stones. Cholesterol synthesis is not decreased.

Cholecystitis Since the inflammation of cholecystitis is caused by stones and bacterial infection, the definitive treatment is an appropriate antibiotic followed by surgery. Pain associated with cholycystitis can be severe, and morphine is usually required to control it. Patients with cholecystitis also need adequate intravenous fluids, as nausea and vomiting are common and can be severe.

PATHOPHYSIOLOGY AND DISEASES OF THE PANCREAS

The pancreas is an endocrine and exocrine organ that secretes insulin and glucagon into the blood and digestive enzymes into the dudodenum.

Pancreatic inflammation can be acute or chronic.

- Acute pancreatitis is a medical emergency and treatment is supportive (i.e. parenteral fluids and relief of pain and nausea).
- Chronic pancreatitis is associated with ethanol ingestion and ethanol should therefore be avoided. There can be a lack of pancreatic digestive enzymes (see cystic fibrosis below for treatment).

Diabetes mellitus is characterized by a relative lack of the endocrine secretion of insulin and/or resistance to insulin (see Chapter 12).

Cystic fibrosis There can be a lack of pancreatic digestive enzymes in cystic fibrosis (see Chapter 12), in which secretory mechanisms are impaired, and in chronic pancreatitis. Pancreatic enzymes (lipase, amylase, and protease) can then be given orally to aid fat, starch, and protein digestion. The formulations are acid resistant so that the enzymes reach the duodenum intact.

FURTHER READING

Millward-Sadler GH, Wright R Arthur MJP (eds) *Liver and Biliary Disease (I and II)*. London: WB Saunders; 1992. [These are a classic pair of books for understanding the basic sciences and clinical correlates in liver disease.]

Walsh JH, Peterson WL The treatment of *Helicobacter pylori* infection in the management of peptic ulcer disease. *N Engl J Med* 1995; **333:** 984. [This article outlines the current thinking in the treatments of ulcer disease.]

Make a provisional diagnosis and determine a rational pharmacologic treatment for the following hypothetical case.

A 40-year-old man was seen by his physician 12 months ago because of dyspepsia, which occurred some time after eating. The discomfort was relieved by eating a meal or taking antacids. The physician diagnosed a peptic ulcer and prescribed an expensive drug, which provided rapid (within 2 days) relief. The patient continued to take the drug for 1 month and had no further dyspepsia for another 6 months. However, over the next few months his symptoms grew progressively worse. Now, on a return visit to the same physician, further investigations have demonstrated the presence of a duodenal ulcer, while a culture from the ulcer shows the presence of *Helicobacter pylori*. This time the physician prescribes different drugs.

1. What drugs can be prescribed to relieve the symptoms of peptic ulcer?
2. What was the drug prescribed on the first visit?
3. Why did the ulcer relapse?
4. What drugs would probably be prescribed on the second visit?
5. If the most appropriate drugs are prescribed, what are the chances of a cure?

?

Indicate which is the correct answer for each question.

1. Metoclopramide is thought to act as a prokinetic drug as a result of
a) its action as an H_2 antagonist of histamine
b) its action as an inhibitor of gastrin
c) a vagolytic action caused by muscarinic blockade
d) its action as an antagonist at dopamine receptors
e) its action as an antagonist at opiate receptors

2. The drug to treat ulcerative colitis is
a) loperamide
b) sulfasalazine
c) diphenoxylate
d) carboxymethylcellulose
e) paregoric

3. An example of a drug used in the treatment of peptic ulcer disease that acts by enhancing mucosal defense mechanisms is
a) cimetidine
b) atropine
c) doxepin
d) sucralfate
e) aminosalicylate (ASA)

4. Which of the following cathartics does not itself act as a laxative?
a) mineral oil
b) phenolphthalein
c) castor oil
d) diphenyl isatin
e) bisacodyl

5. To which class do dioctyl sodium sulfosuccinate and mineral oil belong?
a) saline cathartic
b) stimulant cathartic
c) stool-softening laxative
d) bulk-forming laxative
e) stimulant laxative

6. The most rational of the following drug combinations for treating mild diarrhea is
a) kaolin, pectin, and atropine
b) atropine and tincture of opium
c) kaolin and pectin
d) kaolin and pectin with phenobarbital
e) tincture of opium with neomycin

7. The saline cathartics such as magnesium sulfate owe much of their cathartic effect to
a) increased peristalsis due to interaction with emodin receptors of the intestinal mucosa
b) decreased reabsorption of water due to the formation of an insoluble barrier
c) a lowering of surface tension allowing water to penetrate the fecal mass
d) osmotic forces, which retain water in the digestive tract
e) formation of an emollient gel that maintains soft stools

8. All of the following statements are correct, except
a) antacids containing Mg^{2+} should be given with caution to patients with impaired renal function
b) aluminum hydroxide can decrease phosphate absorption from the gastrointestinal tract
c) stimulant (contact) cathartics (e.g. phenolphthalein) are believed to stimulate peristalsis by increasing the mucosal content of prostaglandins and 3'5'-cAMP
d) antacid mixtures are preferred to proton pump inhibitors for treating gastroesophageal reflux
e) excessive use of cathartics and laxatives may lead to functional bowel disturbances

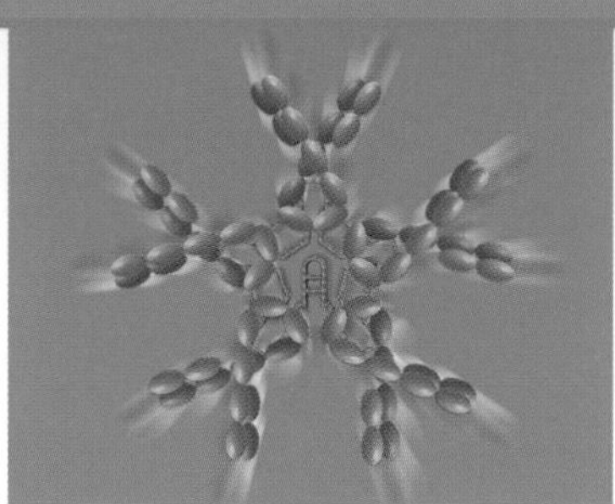

15. Drugs and the Immune System

PHYSIOLOGY OF THE IMMUNE SYSTEM

Lymphocytes are wholly responsible for the specific immune recognition of antigens or pathogens, which is a key feature of the immune response. They are derived from bone marrow stem cells. T lymphocytes then develop in the thymus, while B lymphocytes develop in the bone marrow (Fig. 15.1).

T cells have T cell antigen receptors (TCRs) on their cell surfaces

T cells specifically recognize antigens in association with the major histocompatibility complexes (MHC) (HLA antigens) on antigen-presenting cells (APCs) such as macrophages. When T cells are activated by an antigen through a TCR, they produce soluble proteins, called cytokines, which signal to T cells, B cells, monocytes/macrophages, and other cells (Fig.15.2).

T cells are classified in two subsets:

- CD4-positive ($CD4^+$) T cells, which interact with B cells and help them to proliferate, differentiate, and produce antibody. They are therefore called helper T (TH) cells.
- CD8-positive ($CD8^+$) T cells, which destroy host cells that have become infected by viruses or other intracellular pathogens. This kind of action is called cytotoxicity and these T cells are therefore called cytotoxic T (Tc) cells.

B cells use surface immunoglobulins as their antigen receptors.

B cells specifically recognize a particular antigen. They are stimulated when their surface immunoglobulin interacts with its specific antigen. They then proliferate and differentiate into plasma cells, which produce large amounts of the receptor immunoglobulin in a soluble form. This is known as an antibody, which is present in the blood and tissue fluids and can bind to the antigen that initially activated the B cells. The presence of antibodies activates other parts of the immune system, which then eliminate the pathogen carrying that antigen.

Cytokines are a large group of molecules that signal between cells during immune responses

A variety of cytokines and growth factors are produced by various cell populations involved in the immune response (Fig. 15.3) and have a vital role in the initiation and regulation of these immune responses. All are proteins or peptides, and some contain sugar molecules (glycopeptides). In general, cytokines:

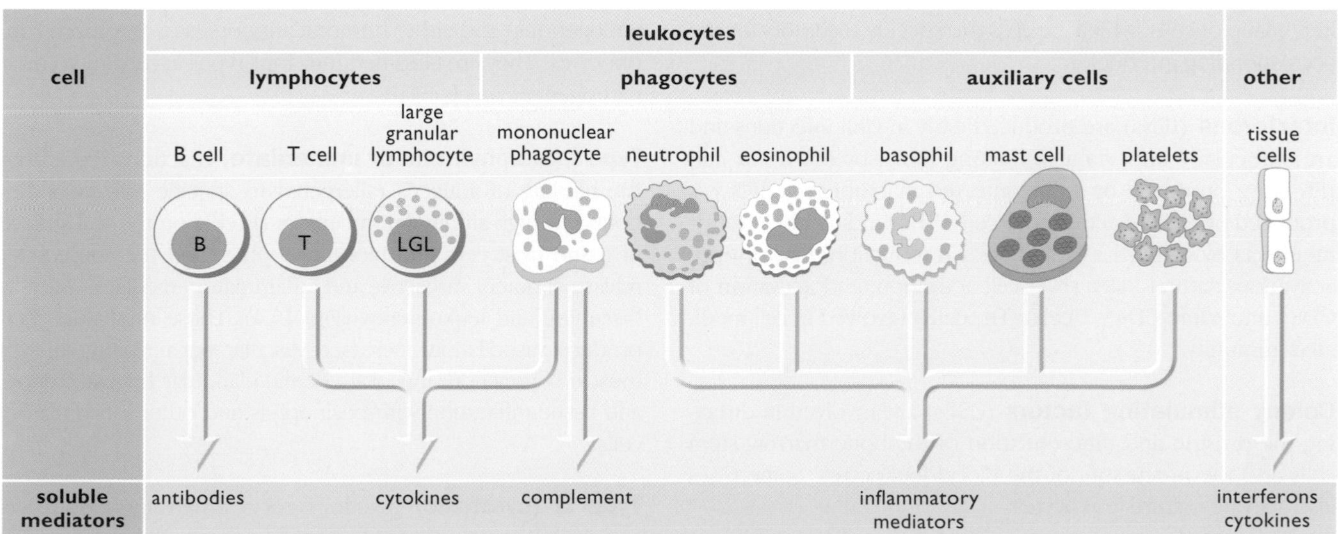

Fig. 15.1 The principal components of the immune system. Complement is made primarily by the liver, although there is some synthesis by mononuclear phagocytes. Each cell produces and secretes only a particular set of cytokines or inflammatory mediators.

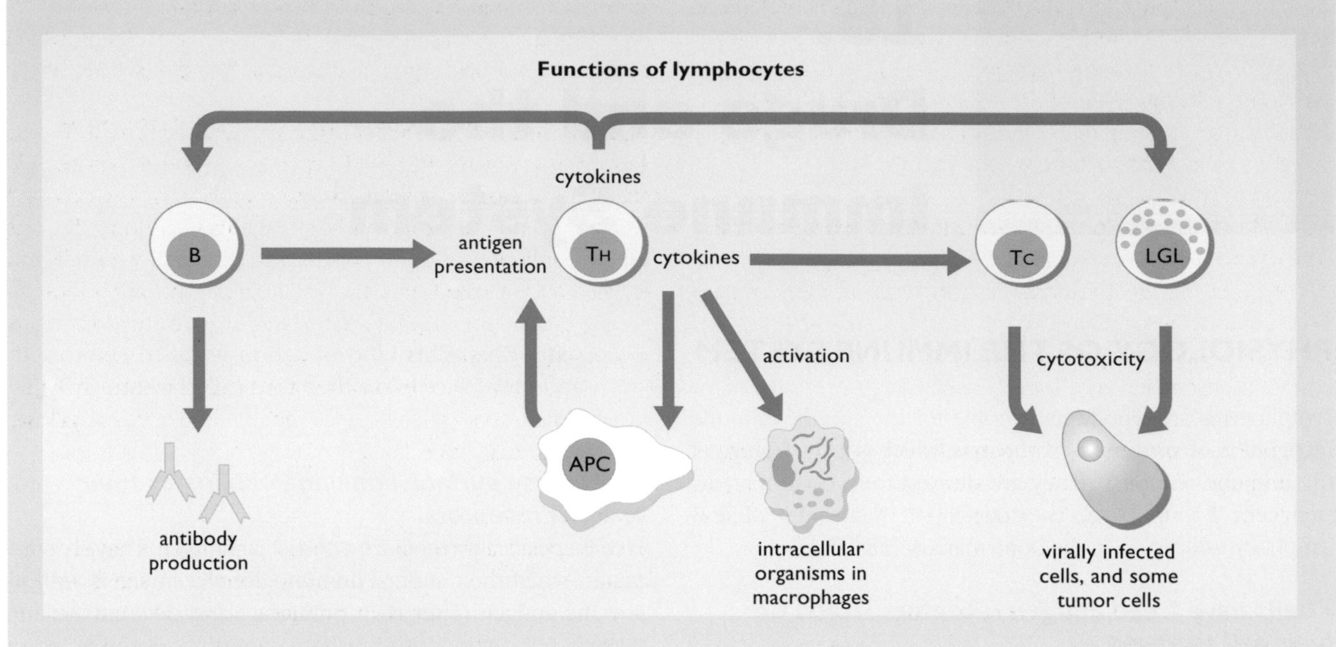

Fig. 15.2 Functions of B cells and T cells. B cells produce antibodies, while T helper (TH) cells are stimulated by antigen-presenting cells (APCs) and B cells to produce cytokines, which control immune responses. Macrophages are activated to kill intracellular microorganisms. Cytotoxic T (Tc) cells and large granular lymphocytes (LGL) recognize and kill target host cells.

- Have multiple effects on different cell types.
- Often share similar or synergistic effects.
- Presumably act in the immune response as an array of molecular messages that orchestrate the interplay and control of individual component cells.

Interleukins are a large group of cytokines (IL-1 to IL-12) produced mainly by T cells, but some are also produced by macrophages and other cells. Those produced by lymphocytes (T cells) are often called lymphokines. They have a variety of functions but most are involved in directing other cells to divide and differentiate. Each interleukin acts on a specific limited group of cells, which express the specific receptors for the corresponding interleukin.

Interferons (IFNs) are produced early in viral infections and are particularly important in limiting their spread. IFN-α and IFN-β are produced by virally infected macrophages; IFN-γ is produced by certain activated T cells. They induce their antiviral effects by MHC class I and class II induction, macrophage activation, natural killer (NK) cell activation, and activation of $CD8^+$ and some $CD4^+$ T cells (TH_1 cells) involved in cell-mediated immunity.

Colony stimulating factors (CSFs) are involved in directing the division and differentiation of the bone marrow stem cells and the precursors of the blood leukocytes. Some CSFs also activate mature leukocytes.

Other cytokines include tumor necrosis factors (TNF-α and TNF-β) and transforming growth factor-β (TGF-β), which have a variety of functions, but are particularly important in mediating inflammation and cytotoxic reactions.

PATHOPHYSIOLOGY AND DISEASES OF THE IMMUNE SYSTEM

HYPERSENSITIVITY REACTIONS AND IMMUNOLOGIC DISEASES

Hypersensitivity reactions

Hypersensitivity reactions are pathologic processes resulting from specific interactions between antigens (exogenous or endogenous) and either humoral antibodies or sensitized lymphocytes. They are classified into four types according to their pathogenetic mechanisms.

Type I (anaphylactic or immediate) reactions result from the binding of antigens (allergens) to specific IgE antibodies bound to high-affinity IgE receptors (FcεRI) on the cell surface of tissue mast cells and blood basophils, and the subsequent release of potent vasoactive and inflammatory mediators such as histamine and leukotrienes (Fig. 15.4). These mediators then produce vasodilation, increased vascular permeability, smooth muscle contraction, mucosal edema, glandular hypersecretion, and tissue infiltration with eosinophils and other inflammatory cells.

Type II (cytotoxic) reactions occur when antibody reacts with antigenic components of a cell or tissue. This leads to cell lysis or tissue damage as a result of antibody-dependent cell-mediated cytotoxicity (ADCC) by NK cells and macrophages through Fc receptors or by activation of the full complement system (Fig. 15.5). Such reactions often form the basis of adverse reactions to drugs, particularly when the drug binds to red blood cells. Ingestion of the offending drug leads to a type II cytotoxic reaction on the surface of red blood cells, leading to lysis of red blood cells and hemolytic anemia.

Type III (immune complex-mediated) reactions result from deposition of soluble antigen–antibody complexes in vessels or other tissues. The immune complexes activate complement components and thereby initiate a sequence of events that results in polymorphonuclear leukocyte chemotaxis, tissue injury, and vasculitis (Fig. 15.6).

Type IV (cell-mediated or delayed) reactions are mediated by sensitized CD4+ T cells following contact with antigen. Circulating antibodies are not involved and are not needed to produce tissue injury. The activation of sensitized CD4+ T cells results in their proliferation and the release of cytokines, which activate macrophages, granulocytes, and NK cells (see Fig. 15.3).

Cytokine effects in the immune response

Cytokines	Cell sources	Target cells and functions
IL-1	Macrophages	T and B cell activation
IL-2	T cells	T cell activation and proliferation
IL-3	T cells	Stem cell proliferation and differentiation
IL-4	T cells	B cell differentiation and IgE class switch TH_2 cell differentiation
IL-5	T cells	Eosinophil differentiation and activation
IL-6	T cells	B cell differentiation
IL-7	Stromal cells	B cell proliferation and differentiation
IL-8	Macrophages	Neutrophil chemotaxis
IL-10	T cells	Inhibition of TH_1 cells
IL-12	Macrophages	TH_1 cell differentiation
GM-CSF	T cells	Eosinophil activation
IFN-γ	T cells, NK cells	Inhibition of TH_2 cells, macrophage activation MHC class I and II induction
IFN-α	Macrophages	NK cell activation, MHC class I induction
TNF-α	Macrophages	Activation of macrophages, granulocytes, and TC cells

Fig. 15.3 Cytokine effects in the immune response. (GM-CSF, granulocyte–monocyte colony stimulating factor; IFN, interferon; IL, interleukin; MHC, major histocompatibility complex; NK cells, natural killer cells; TC cells, cytotoxic T cells; TH cells, helper T cells; TNF, tumor necrosis factor)

ALLERGIC DISEASES AND DRUG THERAPY

Disorders involving the type I hypersensitivity reaction include the atopic diseases (asthma, allergic rhinitis, conjunctivitis, and urticaria) and systemic anaphylaxis. Patients with atopic diseases have an inherited predisposition to develop IgE antibodies to inhaled and ingested substances (allergens) that are not usually antigenic to people who are not atopic. (Bronchial asthma is discussed in Chapter 11.)

Type III and IV hypersensitivity reactions are involved in hypersensitivity pneumonitis, allergic bronchopulmonary aspergillosis, and eosinophilic pneumonias.

Anaphylaxis

Anaphylaxis is a systemic, life-threatening, IgE-mediated type I hypersensitivity reaction that occurs in a previously sensitized person exposed to the sensitizing antigen. It occurs when antigen (proteins and haptens) reaches the circulation. The most common causative antigens are foreign serum, parenteral hormones and enzymes, blood products, penicillins, cephalosporins, allergen extracts, and insect stings.

Histamine, leukotrienes, prostaglandins, and other mediators are generated or released when the antigen binds to IgE on basophils and mast cells. These mediators induce the features that characterize anaphylaxis—smooth muscle contraction (bronchial and gastrointestinal), vasodilation, and an increase in vascular permeability (see Fig. 15.4). Airway obstruction due to laryngeal edema and bronchospasm causes asphyxia and hypoxia, while vasodilation and plasma extravasation into the tissues cause hypovolemic shock, urticaria, and angioedema. Urticaria and angioedema are customarily attributed to histamine. The vascular collapse is probably due to the release of histamine and the generation of prostaglandin D_2, while leukotrienes are the most likely mediators of the marked peripheral airway obstruction. In humans the potency of leukotrienes C_4 and D_4 is 3000 times that of histamine in terms of inducing airflow limitation.

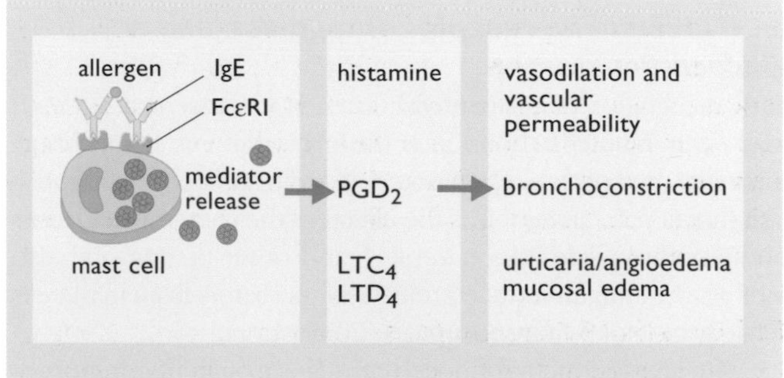

Fig. 15.4 Mechanism of type I hypersensitivity reaction. The binding of allergens to specific IgE antibodies bound to the cell surface IgE receptors (FcεRI) induces degranulation and release of mediators such as histamine and leukotrienes (LT) from mast cells and basophils. (PG, prostaglandin)

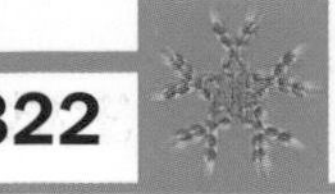

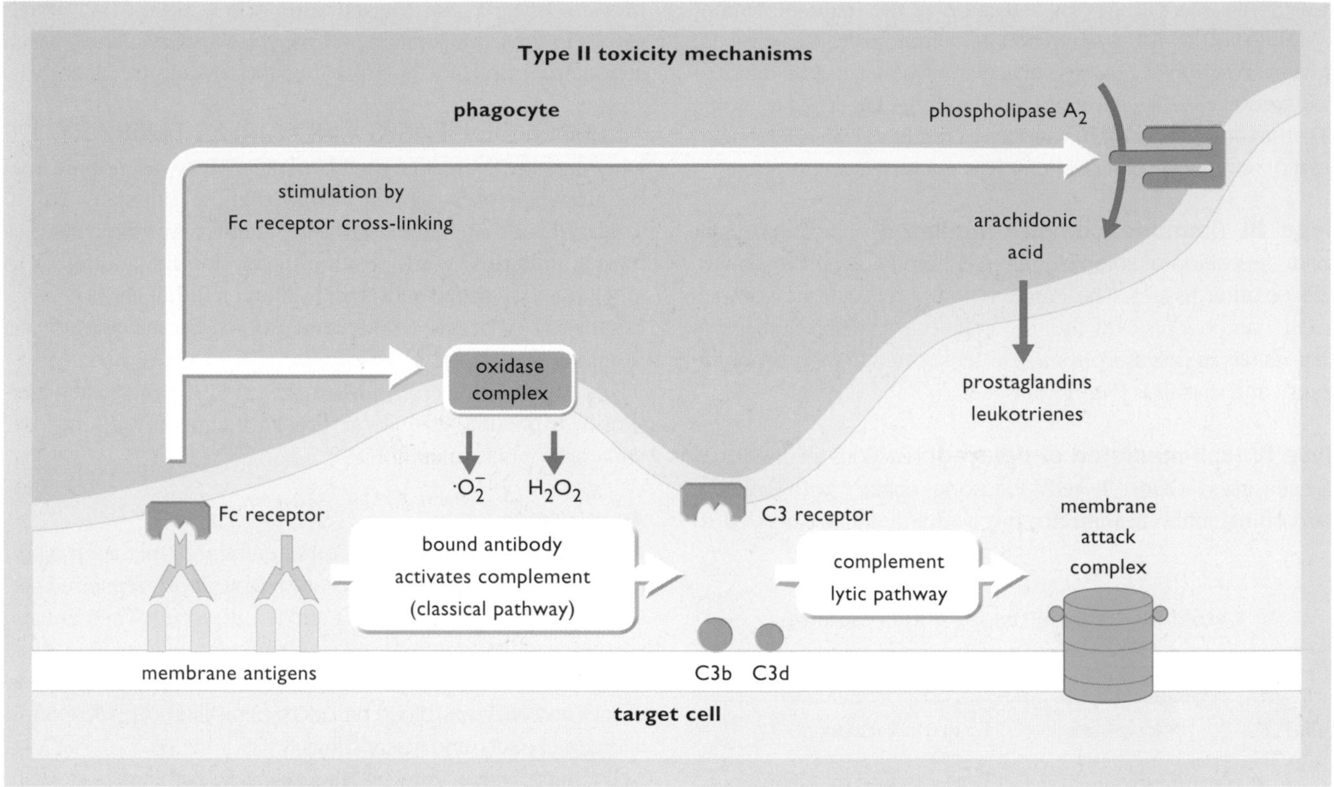

Fig. 15.5 Mechanism of type II hypersensitivity reaction. Antibody bound to membrane antigens on target cells opsonizes them for phagocytes. Cross-linking of the Fc receptors on the phagocyte activates a membrane oxidase complex to secrete oxygen radicals and increases arachidonic acid release from membrane phospholipids (effected by phospholipase A_2). Immune complexes induce complement C3b deposition, and this can also interact with receptors on phagocytes. Activation of the lytic pathway results in the assembly of the membrane attack complex by components C5–C9 of the complement cascade.

Typically, within 1–15 minutes after exposure to the antigen, the patient feels uneasy and complains of nausea, abdominal distress, palpitation, pruritus, urticaria, and difficulty in breathing due to laryngeal edema or bronchospasm. The manifestations of shock may develop within another 1–2 minutes, and primary cardiovascular collapse can occur without respiratory symptoms.

Drug treatment includes immediate epinephrine, an H_1 histamine receptor antagonist, and a glucocorticosteroid

Early recognition of an anaphylactic reaction is essential, as death may occur minutes to hours after the first symptoms. Epinephrine, the initial drug of choice, is a potent α and β adrenoceptor agonist that functionally antagonizes the effects of the chemical mediators on smooth muscle, blood vessels, and other tissues, and also inhibits the antigen-induced release of mediators from mast cells via activation of β_2 adrenoceptors. Epinephrine:

- Relaxes bronchial smooth muscle through β_2 adrenoceptors.
- Constricts arterioles through α_2 adrenoceptors (Fig. 15.7).

Epinephrine should be given immediately subcutaneously. If the antigenic material has been injected into an extremity, the rate of absorption may be reduced by prompt application of a tourniquet proximal to the injection site, and epinephrine administration into the site. An intravenous infusion is needed to maintain intravascular volume and allow additional medication.

When the above measures have been instituted, an H_1 histamine receptor antagonist should be given intravenously to forestall laryngeal edema and block the effect of further histamine release. The additional use of an H_2 histamine receptor antagonist may provide additional benefit.

Glucocorticosteroids (40 mg methylprednisolone or equivalent) have no effect on the acute event, but should be given intravenously to suppress slow-onset urticaria, angioedema, bronchospasm, laryngeal edema, or hypotension.

Intravenous aminophylline to maintain a plasma theophylline level of 10–20 μg/ml is indicated for bronchospasm that does not respond to epinephrine.

Anaphylactoid reactions are clinically similar to anaphylaxis, but the mechanism is quite different. They occur after the first injection of certain drugs (aspirin, polymyxin, pentamidine, opioids, and radiographic contrast agents) in susceptible patients and are due to a dose-related, pharmacologically induced mediator release from basophils and mast cells rather than an immunologically mediated mechanism. Treatment is as for anaphylactic reactions.

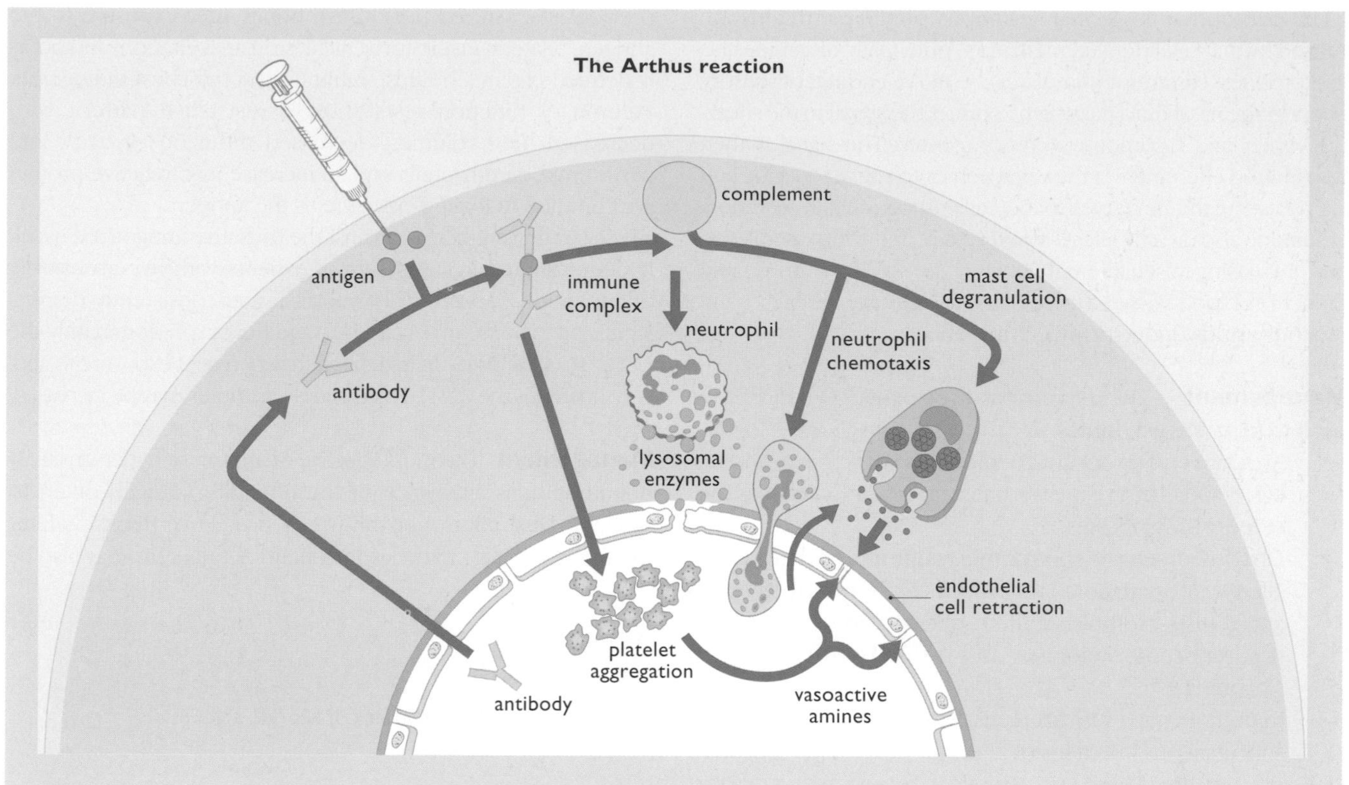

Fig. 15.6 Mechanism of type III hypersensitivity reactions. Antigen injected intradermally combines with specific antibody from the blood to form immune complexes. The complexes activate complement and act on platelets, which release vasoactive amines. Immune complexes also induce macrophages to release tumor necrosis factor (TNF) and interleukin-1 (IL-1) (not shown). Complement C3a and C5a fragments cause mast cell degranulation and attract neutrophils into the tissue. Mast cell products, including histamine and leukotrienes, increase blood flow and capillary permeability. The inflammatory reaction is potentiated by lysosomal enzymes released from the polymorphs. Furthermore, C3b deposited on the complexes opsonizes them for phagocytosis. The Arthus reaction can be seen in patients with precipitating antibodies (e.g. those with extrinsic allergic alveolitis associated with farmer's lung disease).

Causes of anaphylaxis and anaphylactoid reactions

- Anaphylaxis is IgE-mediated hypersensitivity that occurs in a previously sensitized person and penicillins, cephalosporins, many other drugs, and insect stings are the most common causes
- Anaphylactoid reactions are due to a dose-related pharmacologically induced mediator release and aspirin, other non-steroidal anti-inflammatory drugs, and radiographic contrast media are the most common causes

Allergic rhinitis

Allergic rhinitis is an IgE-mediated disorder and results from the deposition of airborne allergens (e.g. pollens, molds, animal danders, and house dust mites) on the nasal mucosa. It is characterized by sneezing, watery rhinorrhea, and nasal congestion, and generally presents in atopic individuals (i.e. those with a family history of a similar or related symptom complex and a personal history of other allergy such as eczematous dermatitis, urticaria, and asthma).

Actions of epinephrine

Target	Receptor	Function
Mast cell	β_2	Inhibition of secretion
Bronchial smooth muscle	β_2	Relaxation
Heart	β_1	Increased rate and force
GI tract	α/β_2	Decreased motility
Liver	α/β_2	Glycogenolysis
Kidney	β_2	Increased renin secretion
Piloerector muscle	α_1	Contraction
Eye	α_1	Mydriasis
Blood vessels of skeletal muscle	β_2	Dilation
Blood vessels of skin and gut	α_1	Constriction

Fig. 15.7 Actions of epinephrine. (GI, gastrointestinal)

The pathophysiologic manifestations of allergic rhinitis are caused by mast cell-derived mediators, principally histamine and leukotrienes. Histamine stimulates the nerve endings of sensory fibers in the nasal mucosa, which conduct the signal to the sneezing center and vasomotor/secretion center. The signal is then transmitted efferently via the vagal nerves to cause sneezing and via parasympathetic nerves to increase mucous gland secretion. Histamine also directly affects blood vessels, inducing vasodilation and increasing vascular permeability. The leukotrienes C_4 and D_4 act on blood vessels (increasing vascular permeability) and mucous glands (inducing mucus secretion).

Management Three principal therapeutic measures are used to treat allergic rhinitis:

- Avoidance of exposure to allergens, which is a simple, basic, and effective measure that significantly reduces the severity of symptoms.
- Drug treatment to control the symptoms of rhinitis and allergic inflammation. This includes histamine H_1 receptor antagonists, cromolyn sodium, glucocorticosteroids, and α adrenoceptor agonists, and is discussed in detail in Chapter 11.
- Immunotherapy with allergens, which consists of repeated subcutaneous injections of gradually increasing concentrations of the allergen, is used if drug treatment is poorly tolerated, if systemic glucocorticosteroids are needed during the season, or if the patient has perennial allergic rhinitis.

Urticaria

Urticaria and angioedema are essentially anaphylaxis limited to the skin and are manifested by wheals and erythema in the dermis and a diffuse swelling of subcutaneous tissues, respectively. Causes of urticaria include drug allergy, insect stings or bites, injections of allergen extracts, or ingestion of certain foods (particularly eggs, shellfish, nuts, or fruits).

Acute urticaria is a self-limiting condition that generally subsides within one to a few days. The symptoms are usually relieved with oral H_1 antagonists (e.g. diphenhydramine, chlorpheniramine, or terfenadine). Parenteral administration of an H_1 antagonist (e.g. diphenhydramine) and/or a glucocorticosteroid (e.g. prednisone) may be necessary for more severe reactions, particularly when associated with angioedema. Topical glucocorticosteroids are of no value. Epinephrine is the first treatment to use for acute pharyngeal or laryngeal angioedema.

Hypersensitivity pneumonitis

Hypersensitivity pneumonitis (allergic alveolitis) is a lymphocytic and granulomatous interstitial pneumonitis caused by type III and IV hypersensitivity reactions to repeated inhalation of a variety of antigens. Farmer's lung, caused by repeated inhalation of dusts in hay containing thermophilic actinomycetes, is the prototype of this disorder. The etiologic agents are most commonly thermophilic actinomycetes, fungi, or animal proteins inhaled in large quantities (Fig. 15.8).

Hypersensitivity pneumonitis is characterized by the development of a cough, fever, chills, malaise, and dyspnea in a previously sensitized person 6–8 hours after exposure to the antigen, bilateral inspiratory crackles on auscultation, and poorly defined patchy or diffuse infiltrates on the chest radiograph. Pulmonary function tests show a restrictive pattern with decreased lung volumes, decreased diffusion capacity, and hypoxemia. Neutrophilia and an increase in C-reactive protein are common following exposure to the antigen.

Precipitating antibodies against the causative antigen are usually demonstrated in the serum of patients with hypersensitivity pneumonitis, and bronchoalveolar lavage consistently demonstrates an increase in T cells in lavage fluids (predominantly the $CD8^+$ Tc cell subset). In patients with very recent exposure to antigen, however, the $CD4^+$ TH cells in lavage fluids may be increased.

Management The most effective treatment of hypersensitivity pneumonitis is avoidance of the offending antigen or environment. Dust control or the use of protective masks to filter the offending dust particles in contaminated areas may also be

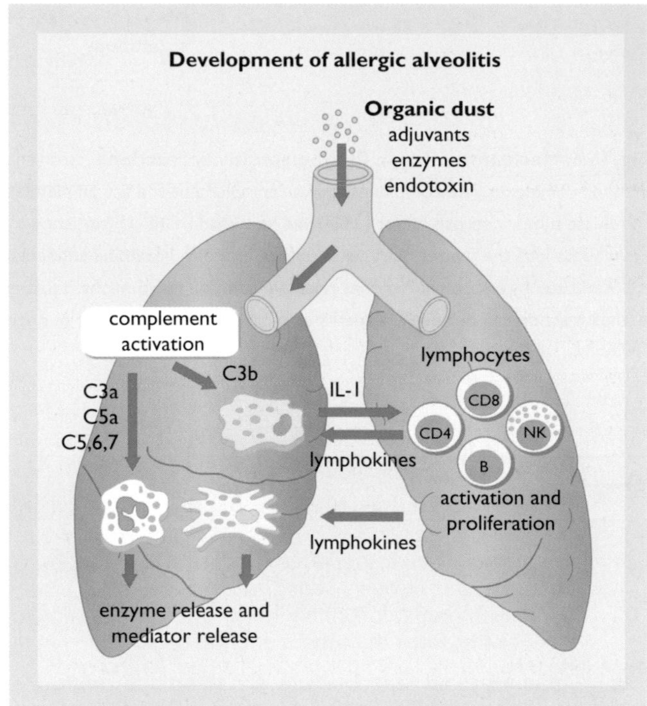

Fig. 15.8 Development of allergic alveolitis. In this simplified scheme, organic dust antigens, which contain large amounts of enzymes, endotoxin, and immunologic adjuvant activity are inhaled, resulting in an initial nonspecific activation of the complement system in resident alveolar macrophages. This leads to early chemoattraction of neutrophils and further recruitment of macrophages into the lesions. Antigen is appropriately presented to resident bronchoalveolar T and B cells by dendritic cells or macrophages, and macrophage-derived interleukin-1 (IL-1) and other cytokines are released. These mediators lead to clonal expansion of T helper/suppressor ($CD4^+$TH/$CD8^+$Tc) cells, natural killer (NK) cells, and B cells in the lung. B cells subsequently produce antibody and a wide array of cytokines. Macrophage- and T cell-derived suppressor factors are also produced and ultimately modulate or dampen the granulomatous response.

effective. Glucocorticosteroids are the drug treatment of choice and markedly reduce the pulmonary inflammatory process.

Allergic bronchopulmonary aspergillosis

Allergic bronchopulmonary aspergillosis (ABPA) occurs in asthmatic patients and is an eosinophilic pneumonia resulting from an allergic reaction to *Aspergillus fumigatus*. The presence of *A. fumigatus* growing in the bronchial lumen provokes an allergic response in the airways and parenchyma. Type I and III (and possibly type IV) hypersensitivity reactions are involved in the pathogenesis. Histopathologic studies reveal eosinophilic infiltrations of the pulmonary parenchyma with a bronchiocentric infiltration of lymphocytes, plasma cells, and monocytes. ABPA is clinically characterized by bronchial asthma, which is usually long standing, pulmonary infiltrates, sputum production, blood eosinophilia, an immediate wheal and flare skin test, precipitating antibody in the serum to *A. fumigatus*, and high levels of total (and specific) IgE.

Management Treatment with glucocorticosteroids and other antiasthmatic drugs (theophylline, sympathomimetics) usually controls the asthma attacks, resolving the inflammatory process and allowing expectoration of the mucus plugs and *A. fumigatus*. Glucocorticosteroid therapy leads to decreased serum IgE levels and the pulmonary infiltrates disappear. A long-term maintenance dose of prednisone (7.5–15 mg/day) may be needed to prevent the development of progressive irreversible disease. Inhaled beclomethasone dipropionate is also useful. Antifungal agents are not effective in resolving the inflammatory process. Immunotherapy with extracts of *A. fumigatus* is contraindicated because it produces bothersome local reactions and may cause exacerbation of symptoms.

MECHANISM OF ACTIONS OF DRUGS USED FOR AUTOIMMUNE DISEASES

Systemic lupus erythematosus

Systemic lupus erythematosus (SLE) is an autoimmune disease that occurs predominantly in young women and is characterized by the production of autoantibodies, especially anti-DNA antibodies. It is discussed in more detail in Chapter 17.

Glucocorticosteroids have a profound inhibitory effect on many cells in the immune system

The immunosuppressive effects of glucocorticosteroids in relation to the treatment of autoimmune diseases such as SLE are summarized in Fig. 15.9. They suppress the proliferative responses of T cells to antigens and mitogens by inhibiting the synthesis of IL-2, and *in vivo* delayed-type hypersensitivity reactions with antigens are suppressed after 2 weeks of glucocorticosteroid therapy. Glucocorticosteroids also suppress the early stages of B cell activation and proliferation but, once activation and proliferation have occurred, B cells are resistant to glucocorticosteroid-mediated suppression of immunoglobulin (antibody) production. After several weeks of glucocorticosteroid therapy, the serum levels of IgG and IgA, and to a lesser degree IgM, are lowered, probably as a result of decreased production.

Glucocorticosteroids also modulate monocyte activity. They reduce the production of monocyte-derived cytokines such as IL-1, markedly inhibit the expression of Fc and C3 receptors and monocyte chemotaxis *in vitro* and *in vivo*, and suppress the bactericidal capacity of monocytes.

Glucocorticosteroids improve immune complex-mediated diseases by inhibiting the clearance of immune (antigen–antibody) complexes by the reticuloendothelial system, perhaps by downregulating Fc receptors and thereby interfering with antibody–Fc receptor interaction.

Glucocorticosteroids also:

- Downregulate endothelial cell functions such as vascular permeability and the expression of adhesion molecules, which probably have an inhibitory effect on leukocyte migration into inflammatory sites.
- Block prostaglandin synthesis by inhibiting the release of arachidonic acid from the phospholipid of cell membranes, which may be mediated by the inhibition of cyclooxygenase transcription. This decrease in prostaglandin production probably accounts for the favorable effects of glucocorticosteroids in inflammatory states (see Chapters 11, 17).

Adverse effects of long-term glucocorticosteroid treatment include the development of a cushingoid habitus, weight gain, hypertension, opportunistic infections, capillary fragility, acne, hirsutism, osteoporosis, ischemic necrosis of bone, cataracts, glaucoma, diabetes mellitus, hyperlipidemia, myopathy, ulcers, hypokalemia, irregular menses, irritability, insomnia, and psychosis.

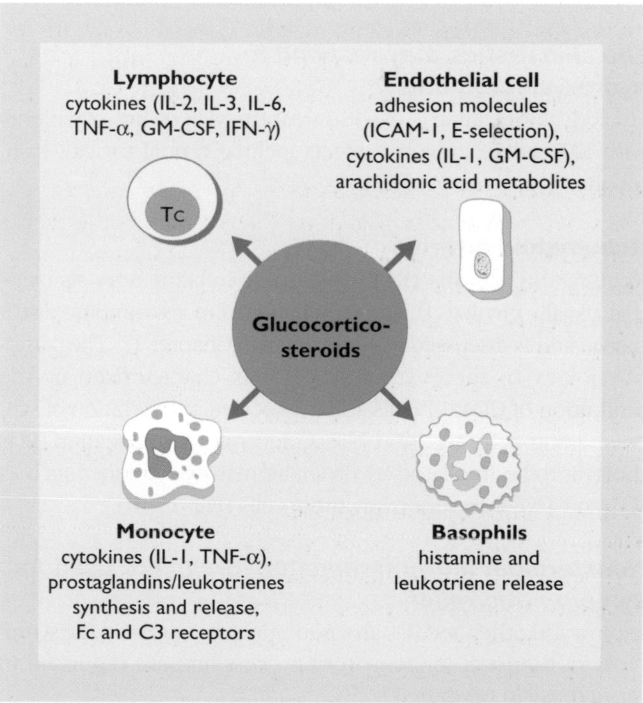

Fig. 15.9 Suppressive effects of glucocorticosteroids on immune and inflammatory responses. (GM-CSF, granulocyte–monocyte colony stimulating factor; ICAM, intercellular adhesion molecule; IFN, interferon; IL, interleukin; TNF, tumor necrosis factor)

Cytotoxic drugs such as cyclophosphamide are used in combination with glucocorticosteroids in the treatment of SLE

Cyclophosphamide acts as an immunosuppressive agent by alkylating DNA and thereby interfering with DNA synthesis and cell division. It is active during all phases of the cell cycle including the resting (G0) stage, but is most active during the S phase of DNA synthesis.

Cyclophosphamide prevents the clonal expansion of both B and T cells and induces lymphocytopenia by depleting these cells. B cells are more sensitive than T cells. Cyclophosphamide:

- Inhibits B cell antibody production and serum immunoglobulin levels *in vitro*.
- Suppresses the antigen-induced proliferative response and cytokine production of T cells.
- Inhibits T cell-mediated activities such as delayed-type hypersensitivity reactions.
- Inhibits many of the inflammatory and immune activities of monocytes.

Adverse effects of cyclophosphamide include bone marrow suppression, hemorrhagic cystitis, permanent amenorrhea and azoospermia, and an increased risk of malignancy. The bone marrow suppression is dose dependent and leukopenia is usually self-limiting and reversible once the drug therapy has ceased.

Nonsteroidal anti-inflammatory drugs (NSAIDs) including salicylates can improve arthralgia

Although NSAIDs can improve arthralgia in SLE, some adverse effects of NSAIDs such as hepatitis, aseptic meningitis, and renal impairment are particularly common in patients with SLE.

The skin rashes may respond to hydroxychloroquine

Hydroxychloroquine is used to treat the skin rashes of patients with SLE, but its adverse effects include retinal toxicity, rash, myopathy, and neuropathy.

Rheumatoid arthritis

Rheumatoid arthritis (RA) is a chronic inflammatory synovitis that usually involves the peripheral joints in a symmetric distribution and is discussed in more detail in Chapter 17. The pathophysiology of rheumatoid synovitis is characterized by the infiltration of CD4+ T cells and monocytes, proliferation of synovial lining cells and fibroblasts, and neovascularization. It is thought to be mediated by proinflammatory cytokines such as IL-1 and TNF-α produced by these cells (Fig. 15.10).

Nonsteroidal anti-inflammatory drugs are used for symptomatic relief

Aspirin and other NSAIDs are used primarily to relieve the symptoms of the local inflammatory process and are discussed in more detail in Chapter 17.

Disease-modifying drugs may alter the course of rheumatoid arthritis

A heterogeneous group of agents has been classified as disease-modifying drugs and may have the capacity to alter the course of RA. They include:

- Gold salts.
- D-Penicillamine.
- The antimalarials.
- Sulfasalazine.

These agents have minimal direct nonspecific anti-inflammatory or analgesic effects, usually have a slow onset of efficacy, reduce clinical symptoms over 1–3 months, and induce remissions in a few patients. As many as two-thirds of patients show some clinical improvement as a result of therapy with any of these agents, but the induction of true remissions is unusual. In addition to clinical improvement, there is frequently an improvement in the serologic parameters of disease activity such as C-reactive protein concentration, titers of rheumatoid factor, and the erythrocyte sedimentation rate. Despite this, there is minimal evidence that disease-modifying drugs actually retard the development of bone erosions in the joints.

Gold salts are used in the treatment of RA, but have limited efficacy as single agents. Approximately 20–35% of patients treated with the intramuscular preparation show a significant response, which is maximal at 6–12 months. This remission is sustained in about 50% of the responders. A 5-year follow-up

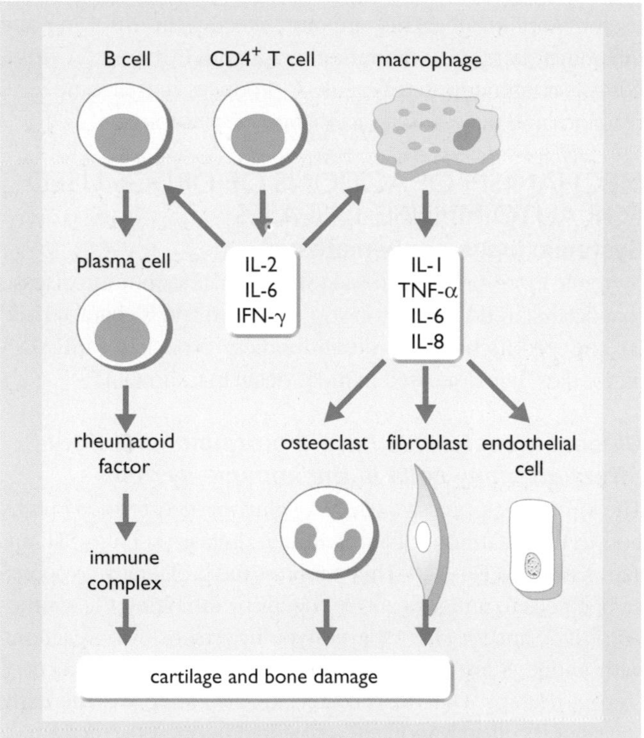

Fig. 15.10 Cytokine network in the pathogenesis of rheumatoid arthritis. Activation of CD4+ T cells, B cells, and macrophages is involved in the initiation of rheumatoid synovitis. These cells release proinflammatory cytokines such as interleukin-1 (IL-1) and tumor necrosis factor (TNF)-α, resulting in proliferation of synovial lining cells and fibroblasts, neovascularization, and cartilage and bone injury.

revealed no difference between treated and untreated patients when gold salt therapy was used alone.

Gold salts act mainly on monocytes and macrophages, inhibiting their functions. They reduce the migration, phagocytosis, and expression of Fc and CR3 receptors of macrophages as well as accessory cell function, as indicated by the suppression of lymphocyte blastogenesis. They may also inhibit aggregation of γ globulin and induce complement C1 inactivation.

The adverse effects of gold salts include rashes, leukocytopenias, and proteinuria. Oral gold salt therapy is less effective when used as a single agent, but is easier to administer than the parenteral courses of gold salt therapy and has fewer adverse effects.

D-Penicillamine has been used in the treatment of RA. Although its mechanism of action remains unknown, it has immunomodulatory effects *in vitro*, the most important of which may be inhibition of TH cell function. Its adverse effects include gastrointestinal intolerance, skin rash, nephrotoxicity, and elicitation of autoantibodies with associated autoimmune diseases.

Hydroxychloroquine can also control the symptoms of RA, but its mechanism of action in the therapy of RA is unknown. It may inhibit the release of prostaglandins or lysosomal enzymes, inhibit lymphocyte proliferation and immunoglobulin production by interfering with IL-1 production by macrophages, or alter the processing and presentation of peptide antigen in the macrophage. Hydroxychloroquine is principally used as the basal agent for attenuating a mild inflammatory process or stabilizing a remission. It should be discontinued if the patient fails to show any improvement after 6 months.

The adverse effects of hydroxychloroquine include dermatitis, myopathy, and corneal opacity, which is usually reversible. Irreversible retinal degeneration can occur and is a cause for concern, but is not common at the doses currently used. Ophthalmologic examination is required every 6 months during treatment.

Sulfasalazine may reduce the rate of progression of erosions in RA. Its adverse effects include gastric symptoms, neutropenia, hemolysis, hepatitis, and rash.

Glucocorticosteroids can be used in the treatment of RA and this is discussed in more detail in Chapter 17.

Methotrexate is another immunosuppressive drug that is useful in the treatment of RA. It is a folic acid antagonist and is given in a single oral low dose (7.5–15 mg) once a week. This treatment of RA is discussed in more detail in Chapter 17. Methotrexate inhibits cell division by competitively binding dihydrofolate reductase, resulting in decreased thymidine and purine nucleotide synthesis. Its action is therefore cell cycle specific, destroying cells during the S phase of DNA synthesis but having little to no effect on resting cells. Methotrexate suppresses primary and secondary antibody responses *in vivo*, but few effects have been observed on pre-existing delayed-type hypersensitivity reactions.

The effect of weekly low-dose methotrexate may be anti-inflammatory and not immunosuppressive. Methotrexate significantly reduces the generation of the 5-lipoxygenase pathway products by leukocytes, and may also decrease IL-1 production by macrophages.

The major adverse effects of methotrexate include bone marrow suppression (leukopenia and thrombocytopenia), opportunistic infections, and hepatotoxicity with fibrosis. Liver fibrosis is most common in those who have a cumulative dosage of 1.5 g, in those receiving the drug daily, and in those with preexisting liver disease, alcoholism, or diabetes mellitus. Other adverse effects include interstitial pneumonitis, gastrointestinal upset, stomatitis with oral ulcerations, dermatitis, osteoporotic fractures, and fetal malformation. Unlike other cytotoxic drugs, methotrexate is not associated with an increased risk of malignancy.

Cyclosporine and T cell suppression Cyclosporine has a selective inhibitory effect on T cells by inhibiting the TCR-mediated signal transduction pathway. It specifically binds to its cytoplasmic binding protein, cyclophilin, and this complex then binds to calcineurin, inhibiting phosphatase activity and therefore the nuclear translocation of the nuclear factor of activated T cells (NF-AT) (Fig. 15.11). Cyclosporine inhibits IL-2 production, T cell proliferation, TH cell activity for antibody production, and TC cell generation, and so could have a beneficial effect on autoantibody production and immune complex-mediated diseases. Cyclosporine has therefore been used to treat autoimmune diseases, though most available data are for RA. A clinical improvement is generally observed, but the adverse effects of cyclosporine as well as the flares that occur after cyclosporine is discontinued may limit its use. Cyclosporine is also an effective therapy for ocular Behçet's disease, psoriasis, atopic dermatitis, aplastic anemia, and nephrotic syndrome, and may have therapeutic activity in polymyositis, dermatomyositis, and severe glucocorticosteroid-dependent asthma.

The major adverse effect of cyclosporine is renal toxicity (primarily proximal renal tubular changes), which is usually dose related and reversible. Other adverse effects include hypertension, hepatotoxicity, tremor, hirsutism, and gingival hyperplasia. Bone marrow suppression is unusual. Lymphomas have been reported in some cyclosporine-treated renal transplant recipients.

Immunosuppressive drugs

- The major adverse effects of cytotoxic drugs are bone marrow suppression and opportunistic infections
- Cyclophosphamide causes hemorrhagic cystitis, amenorrhea and azoospermia, and an increased risk of malignancies
- Methotrexate causes hepatotoxicity and interstitial pneumonitis
- Cyclosporine causes renal toxicity

Polymyositis and dermatomyositis

Polymyositis and dermatomyositis are immunologically mediated inflammatory muscle diseases characterized by lymphocyte infiltration in the skeletal muscle. Patients with polymyositis have symmetric proximal muscle weakness, elevated serum levels of muscle-associated enzymes such as creatine kinase (CK), electromyographic abnormalities characteristic of inflammatory myopathy, and histologic evidence of muscle damage and lymphocyte infiltration in a muscle biopsy. These features are also seen in patients with dermatomyositis in addition to a characteristic heliotrope skin rash and Gottron's erythema.

The pathogenetic mechanisms of polymyositis and dermatomyositis may differ. Interstitial infiltration of $CD8^+$ T cells surrounding and invading otherwise normal-appearing myocytes is a prominent feature in polymyositis. In contrast, perivascular infiltration of $CD4^+$ T cells and B cells and perifascicular muscle fiber atrophy are prominent in dermatomyositis. The myositis-specific autoantibodies may also play a pathogenetic role: for example, anti-Jo-1 autoantibody is directed against histidyl-tRNA synthetase and is found in 20–30% of patients with myositis.

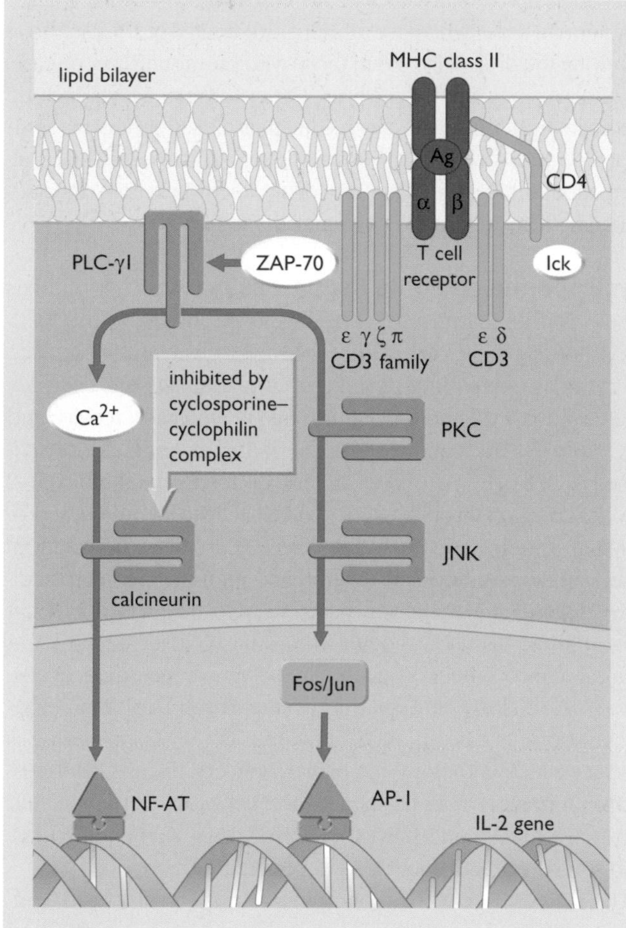

Fig. 15.11 Cyclosporine and T cell suppression. Stimulation of T cells through the T cell receptor (TCR) phosphorylates the CD3ζ chain of the TCR–CD3 complex. Phosphorylated CD3ζ then binds and activates ZAP-70, a tyrosine kinase. Subsequently, phospholipase C (PLC)-γ1 is activated by tyrosine phosphorylation and cleaves phosphatidylinositol bisphosphate to the second messengers inositol 1,4,5-triphosphate and diacylglycerol. The former produces a sustained rise in intracellular calcium ($[Ca^{2+}]_i$), while the latter activates protein kinase C (PKC). These two signals then synergize to induce and activate transcription factors required for interleukin-2 (IL-2) gene transcription. The rise in $[Ca^{2+}]_i$ activates the calmodulin-dependent phosphatase calcineurin, which leads to alteration of the preformed cytoplasmic component of the nuclear factor of activated T cells (NF-AT), allowing it to move into the nucleus. There it combines with newly formed Fos and Jun proteins induced by the PKC pathway to create NF-AT, which binds to a response element in the IL-2 enhancer. Fos and Jun also bind as an AP-1 complex to a separate enhancer site (TRE; TPA responsive element). Other transcription factors NF-kB and NF-IL-2A are also involved in IL-2 gene transcription. Cyclosporine specifically binds to its cytoplasmic binding protein (cyclophilin) and thereby inhibits IL-2 production by T cells. (lck, a tyrosine kinase)

Glucocorticosteroids are the mainstay of therapy for polymyositis and dermatomyositis

Polymyositis and dermatomyositis are treated with high doses of glucocorticosteroids (prednisone or prednisolone 1–2 mg/kg/day). The glucocorticosteroid is continued in a high dose until the serum CK level returns to normal. The dose is then tapered very slowly. The condition may improve within 1–4 weeks, but in some patients treatment may be needed for 3 months before there is an improvement. Muscle strength may not improve for weeks to months after the serum concentrations of muscle-derived enzymes have normalized. Patients who have a poor prognosis (i.e. patients with acute severe myositis who have bedridden muscle weakness, dysphagia or respiratory muscle weakness, and patients with interstitial pneumonitis) are treated with intravenous 'pulses' of 1000 mg methylprednisolone for 3 days, followed by maintenance with daily glucocorticosteroids. Sometimes it is difficult to distinguish glucocorticosteroid-induced myopathy (increasing muscle weakness during glucocorticosteroid therapy) from a relapse of the myositis.

Other immunosuppressive drugs are sometimes used

Immunosuppressive drugs are used:

- For severe polymyositis or dermatomyositis.
- If the response to glucocorticosteroids is inadequate after 1–3 months of treatment.
- If there are frequent relapses.

 **Long-term administration of glucocorticosteroids**

- The major adverse effects of high-dose glucocorticosteroids are opportunistic infections and psychosis
- Other major adverse effects of long-term glucocorticosteroids are ischemic necrosis of bone, osteoporosis, diabetes mellitus, hyperlipidemia, cataracts, and glaucoma

Oral methotrexate is a major therapeutic option for glucocorticosteroid-resistant patients. Cyclosporine may be beneficial for conditions such as interstitial pneumonitis.

Systemic sclerosis

Systemic sclerosis (SSc) is a multisystem disorder of unknown etiology characterized by fibrosis of the skin, lungs, and gastrointestinal tract, Raynaud's phenomenon, and microvascular abnormalities of the skin and visceral organs. Its characteristic immunologic and microvascular abnormalities include:

- Antinuclear antibodies, particularly anti-Scl-70 autoantibody found in 30–70% of patients and directed against the nuclear enzyme DNA topoisomerase I.
- Hypergammaglobulinemia.
- Perivascular infiltration of $CD4^+$ T cells and macrophages in the dermis.
- Intimal thickening with narrowing of the vascular lumen in the skin and kidneys.

Management D-Penicillamine has been used to reduce fibrosis and prevent the development of skin thickening and significant organ involvement. This drug interferes with inter- and intramolecular cross-linking of collagen and is also immunosuppressive, including the inhibitory effect on TH cell function. Its immunosuppressive activity may also lead to decreased collagen production.

Glucocorticosteroids are indicated for inflammatory myositis in SSc. They also reduce edema associated with the edematous phase of early skin involvement, but are not indicated in the long-term treatment of SSc. High doses of glucocorticosteroids may cause acute renal failure.

Polyarteritis nodosa

Polyarteritis nodosa (PN) is an immune complex-mediated necrotizing vasculitis that characteristically affects small- and medium-sized muscular arteries, especially at their bifurcations. Most lesions occur in the kidney, heart, liver, gastrointestinal tract, musculoskeletal system, testes, peripheral nervous system, and skin. The symptoms and signs depend on the severity and location of vessel involvement and the resulting ischemic changes. Nonspecific features include fever, weight loss, malaise, neutrophilia, increased C-reactive protein, and increased erythrocyte sedimentation rate. Circulating immune complexes have also been detected. The lesions contain immunoglobulins and complement components, and in some cases hepatitis B antigen is detected. The deposited immune complexes produce lesions by activating complement components and attracting and activating inflammatory cells.

Management Glucocorticosteroids are the mainstay of therapy, but the addition of cyclophosphamide nearly doubles the 5-year survival rate to 90%.

Characteristic features of autoimmune diseases

- Autoimmune diseases are characterized by the presence of autoantibodies and autoreactive T cells against self-antigens
- Disease-specific autoantibodies are frequently detected: anti-DNA antibody in systemic lupus erythematosus, rheumatoid factor (autoantibody to IgG) in rheumatoid arthritis, anti-Jo-1 antibody in polymyositis, and anti-Scl-70 antibody in systemic sclerosis
- Glucocorticosteroids and immunosuppressive drugs are effective treatments

FURTHER READING

Frank MM, Austen KF, Calman HN, Unanue ER (eds) *Samter's Immunologic Diseases 5e*. Boston: Little, Brown and Company; 1995. [This book describes, in depth, the mechanism and therapy of immunologic diseases, including hypersensitivity and autoimmune diseases.]

Holgate ST, Church MK (eds) *Allergy*. London: Gower; 1993.

Roitt IM, Brostoff J, Male DK (eds) *Immunology 4e*. London: Mosby; 1993. [These two books are updated standard textbooks, with well-drawn illustrations, for understanding the basics of clinical allergy and immunology.]

Make a provisional diagnosis and determine a rational pharmacologic treatment for the following hypothetical case.

A 23-year-old female presents with a history of facial rash, low-grade fever (up to 37.2°C), and general fatigue. On examination, the patient has facial erythema and pretibial pitting edema but is otherwise normal. Laboratory examination reveals a decreased white blood cell count, an increased serum creatinine, and massive proteinuria.

1. Which of the following serologic tests—antinuclear antibody, anti-DNA antibody, serum complement, anti-streptolysin O titer, rheumatoid factor—would you order to determine the diagnosis of this autoimmune disease? Explain your answer.
2. Which of the following examinations—chest radiograph, renal function tests, renal angiography, renal biopsy, muscle biopsy—would you order to determine the severity of the disease?
3. If you decided to treat this patient with drugs, what would you use? For each drug list its class, for how long it should be used, what the end points of therapy are, and what its adverse effects are.

Indicate whether the following answers are true or false.

1. The following cytokines are produced by T cells
   a) interleukin (IL)-1
   b) IL-2
   c) IL-3
   d) IL-4
   e) interferon (IFN)-γ
2. The first choice of drug for anaphylaxis is
   a) diphenhydramine
   b) cromolyn sodium
   c) aminophylline
   d) hydrocortisone
   e) epinephrine
3. Mediators responsible for anaphylaxis is/are
   a) major basic protein
   b) histamine
   c) tumor necrosis factor (TNF)-α
   d) leukotriene C4
4. The following diseases is/are mediated by IgE antibodies
   a) hypersensitivity pneumonitis
   b) allergic rhinitis
   c) contact dermatitis
   d) anaphylaxis
5. Systemic lupus erythematosus
   a) is characterized by the presence of anti-DNA antibodies
   b) anti-DNA antibody titer is decreased by glucocorticosteroid therapy
   c) is treated with intravenous 'pulse' cyclophosphamide for lupus nephritis
   d) is treated with intravenous 'pulse' cyclophosphamide because it has less urinary bladder toxicity
6. Methotrexate is used for
   a) systemic lupus erythematosus
   b) polymyositis
   c) rheumatoid arthritis
   d) polyarteritis nodosa
7. Drugs specific for T cells include
   a) cyclophosphamide
   b) gold salts
   c) cyclosporine
   d) sulfasalazine
   e) methotrexate
8. Bone marrow suppression is a major adverse effect of which of the following immunosuppressive drugs?
   a) cyclosporine
   b) cyclophosphamide
   c) methotrexate
   d) prednisone

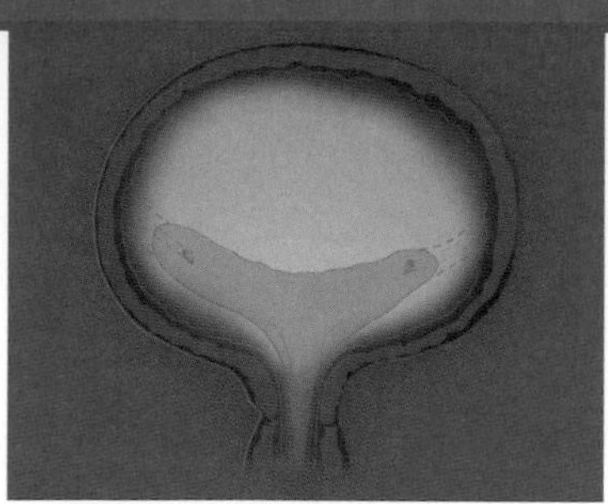

16. Drugs and the Bladder

PHYSIOLOGY OF THE BLADDER

The bladder stores urine, emptying itself at appropriate intervals

The lower urinary tract includes the detrusor muscle, the trigone, and the urethra (Fig. 16.1). These are mainly smooth muscle structures that differ in morphology and innervation, but form a functional unit controlled by complex central and peripheral nervous mechanisms.

The lower urinary tract is innervated by the parasympathetic, sympathetic, and somatic nervous systems (Figs 16.2, 16.3). The detrusor smooth muscle receives a dominating cholinergic innervation and in humans the main excitatory transmitter is acetylcholine, which stimulates muscarinic (M_1, M_2, and M_3) receptors to produce bladder contraction and emptying. The M_3 receptor is probably the most important for contraction. The detrusor also receives a relatively sparse adrenergic innervation: β adrenoceptors (β_2 subtype) dominate over α adrenoceptors and the response to norepinephrine is relaxation. It has been assumed that sympathetic activity during bladder filling facilitates urine storage by relaxing the detrusor. The importance of such a mechanism is uncertain.

The trigone and the urethra (the outflow region) receive a rich adrenergic innervation: α adrenoceptors (α_1 subtype) dominate over β adrenoceptors and the response to norepinephrine is contraction. During bladder filling ongoing sympathetic activity keeps the urethra closed. The outflow region also has a noncholinergic nonadrenergic (NANC) innervation. These nerves contain various peptides including vasoactive intestinal polypeptide, neuropeptide Y, and nitric oxide synthase (the nitric oxide-forming enzyme). Nitric oxide relaxes the outflow region, but its functional importance is unknown. It should be noted that both adrenergic and cholinergic nerves contain transmitters other than norepinephrine and acetylcholine, respectively. The urethra also contains a striated muscle component, the external urethral sphincter (rhabdosphincter), which together with the pelvic floor muscles plays an important role in maintaining continence.

Distension of the detrusor initiates the micturition reflex (Fig. 16.4).

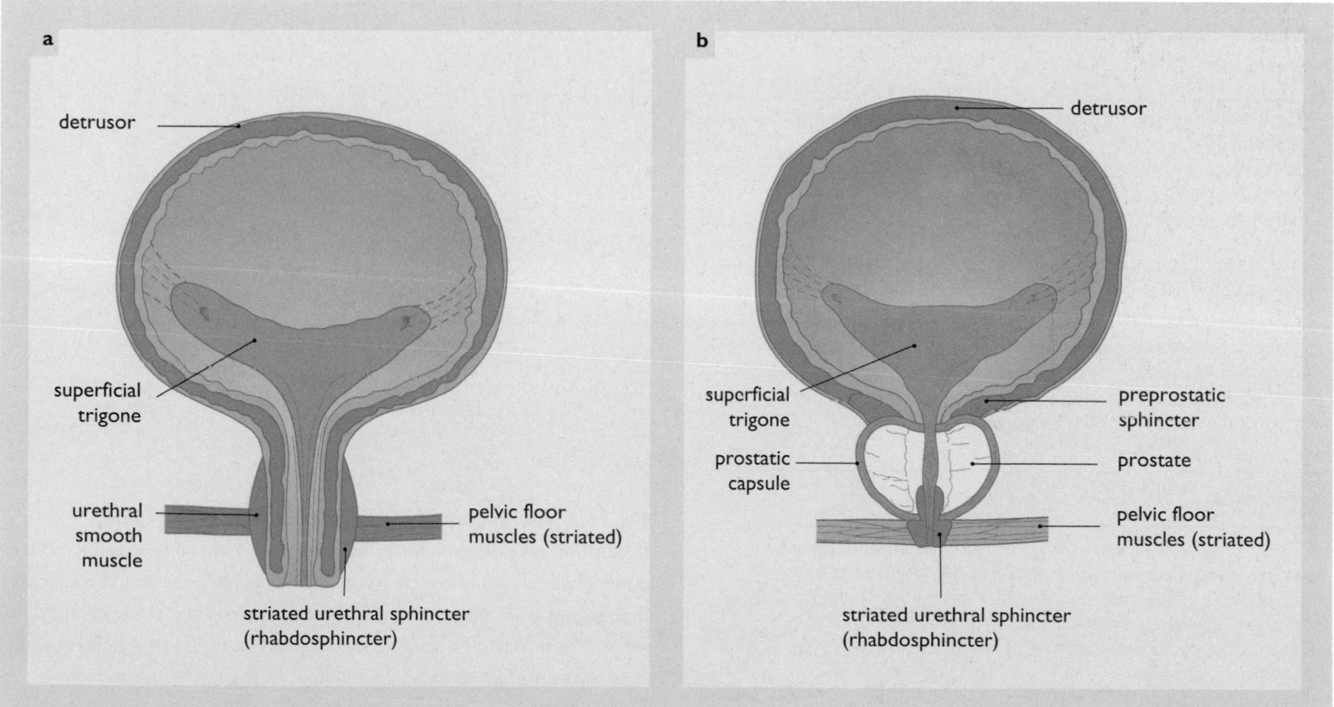

Fig. 16.1 Structure of the lower urinary tract in women (a) and in men (b).

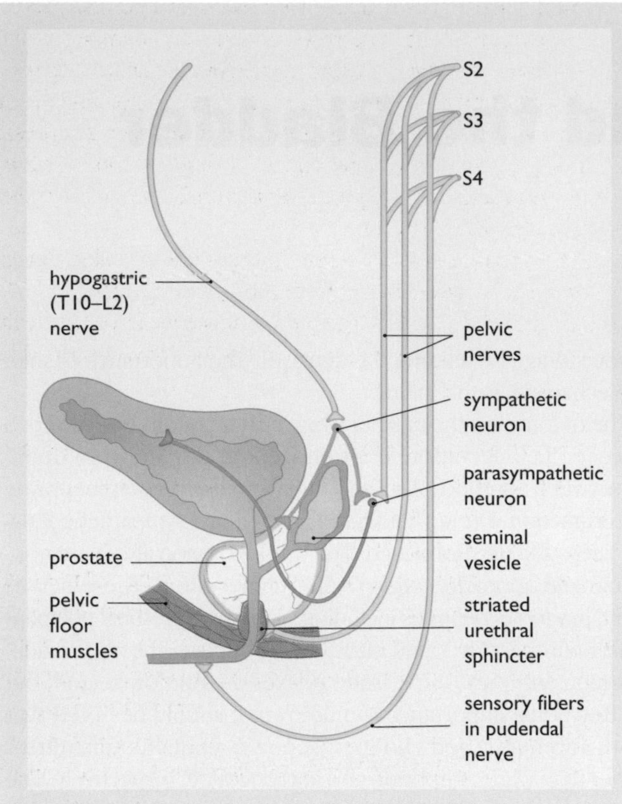

Fig. 16.2 Innervation of the lower urinary tract. The parasympathetic, sympathetic, and somatic nervous systems supply the lower urinary tract through the pelvic, hypogastric, and pudenal nerves.

Receptor functions in the lower urinary tract
Detrusor
• Contraction-mediating muscarinic (M_3) receptors dominate functionally • Relaxation-mediating β adrenoceptors (β_2 adrenoceptors) dominate over contraction-mediating α adrenoceptors (α_1 adrenoceptors)
Urethra
• Contraction-mediating α adrenoceptors (α_1 adrenoceptors) dominate functionally over relaxation-mediating β adrenoceptors (β_2 adrenoceptors) • Muscarinic receptors, but function is unknown
Prostate
• Contraction-mediating α adrenoceptors (α_1 adrenoceptors) dominate in the prostatic stroma, and may contribute to the increased outflow resistance found in benign prostatic hyperplasia (i.e. the 'dynamic' component of obstruction) • Muscarinic receptors localized to the epithelium may have a secretory function

Fig. 16.3 Receptor functions in the lower urinary tract.

PATHOPHYSIOLOGY AND DISEASES OF THE BLADDER

Urinary incontinence results from a failure to store urine, while urinary retention results from a failure to empty

Micturition disorders can be roughly classified into disturbances of storage or of emptying.

URINARY INCONTINENCE

Urinary incontinence is common, occurring in 10% of the population. It is defined as an objectively demonstrable

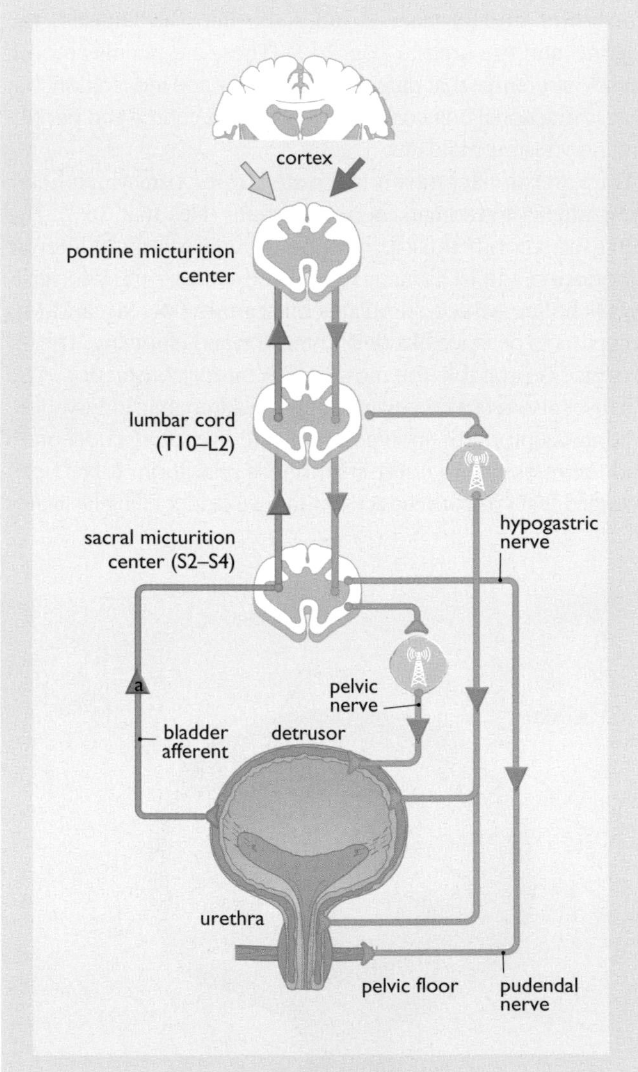

Fig. 16.4 The micturition reflex. The afferent branch of the micturition reflex runs in the spinal cord via the dorsal root ganglia to the pontine micturition center, which is under voluntary control. The efferent branch runs from the pontine micturition center to the sacral micturition center, from which the preganglionic nerves run to the pelvic plexus and then to the bladder to cause contraction. At the same time, the efferent branch inhibits the hypogastric and pudendal nerves, leading to relaxation of the outflow region and the pelvic floor.

involuntary loss of urine. It may be a symptom, a sign, or a condition (Fig. 16.5).

Stress incontinence is involuntary loss of urine in the absence of detrusor contraction and occurs when the intravesical pressure exceeds the urethral pressure. A primary cause is defective transmission of the intra-abdominal pressure to the proximal urethra owing to a change in position of the urethra from being a mainly intra-abdominal to a partly extra-abdominal structure (Fig. 16.6). This, in turn, may be a consequence of trauma of the outflow region (e.g. following parturition or as a result of aging). A contributing factor may be deficient mucosal function due to lack of estrogen.

Urge incontinence is involuntary loss of urine accompanied by a strong desire to void (urgency) and can be subdivided into motor urge incontinence and sensory urge incontinence. Motor urge incontinence is associated with detrusor overactivity and/or decreased detrusor compliance. Detrusor activity is interpreted from the measurement of detrusor pressure and may be normal or overactive. Overactivity is characterized by involuntary detrusor contractions during the filling phase that may be spontaneous or provoked and which the patient cannot completely suppress. Detrusor overactivity can be found in outflow obstruction, inflammation, and irritative processes in the bladder, or the cause may be unknown (idiopathic).

Hyperreflexia describes the condition of uncontrolled detrusor contractions associated with neurologic disorders.

The drugs used to treat urge incontinence and hyperreflexia and stress incontinence are shown in Fig. 16.7 and described in detail below.

Types of urinary incontinence

Urge incontinence
- Motor urge incontinence (involuntary detrusor contractions)
- Sensory urge incontinence

Hyperreflexia: involuntary detrusor contractions associated with neurologic disorders (e.g. multiple sclerosis, trauma)

Stress incontinence: defective urethral closure mechanism
- Defective transmission of intra-abdominal pressure to the proximal urethra
- Lack of estrogen

Fig. 16.5 Types of urinary incontinence.

Treatment of urge incontinence and hyperreflexia is aimed at decreasing detrusor activity and increasing bladder capacity

Antimuscarinic agents

Muscarinic receptors probably mediate the main part of the contraction in the overactive detrusor in addition to their role in normal bladder contraction. However, although atropine and other antimuscarinic drugs produce almost complete paralysis of the normal bladder when injected parenterally, the efficacy of antimuscarinic drugs given orally for overactive detrusor contractions can be inadequate. It is not clear whether this can be attributed to low bioavailability, adverse effects limiting the dose that can be given, or atropine resistance. Atropine resistance has been attributed to the occurrence of NANC transmitters which, even when the muscarinic receptors are blocked, may mediate contraction of the bladder.

Atropine and related antimuscarinic drugs are tertiary amines. They are well absorbed from the gastrointestinal tract and enter

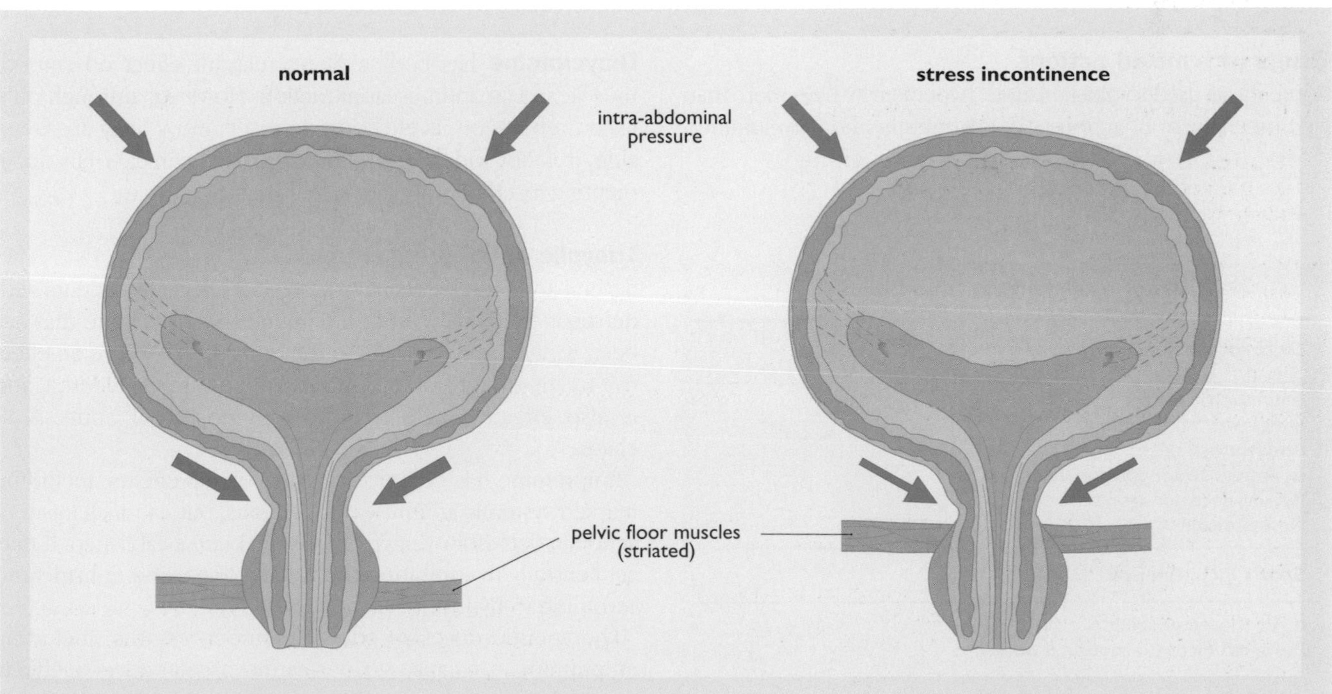

Fig. 16.6 Stress incontinence. There is defective transmission of intra-abdominal pressure (arrows) to the proximal urethra.

the central nervous system (CNS). CNS adverse effects may therefore limit their use. Quaternary ammonium compounds (e.g. emepronium and propantheline) are not well absorbed and their entry into the CNS is limited. They therefore have a lower incidence of CNS adverse effects, but still produce peripheral antimuscarinic adverse effects such as accommodation paralysis, constipation, tachycardia, and a dry mouth. None of the currently available antagonists can discriminate between the muscarinic receptor subtypes, and systemic adverse effects often limit their clinical use.

Atropine is generally not used to treat detrusor instability because of its systemic adverse effects. However, intravesical atropine administered via a catheter can increase bladder capacity without causing any systemic adverse effects in patients with detrusor hyperreflexia.

Emepronium and propantheline have pronounced effects on bladder function when given parenterally. They are quaternary ammonium compounds with a low oral bioavailability of 5–10%, which varies markedly between individuals. To obtain an optimal effect, the drug dose should be titrated: the oral dose is increased until there is no incontinence or until adverse effects preclude any further increase. Both drugs reduce detrusor overactivity and can be clinically useful.

New drugs

Antimuscarinic drugs with selectivity for the urinary bladder have been developed to improve treatment of bladder overactivity. One such a drug is darifenacin, which has a selective effect on the muscarinic M_3 receptor. Another drug, tolterodine, has no selectivity for muscarinic receptor subtypes, but is selective for the bladder over the salivary glands in an animal model and is currently in phase III clinical trials.

Drugs with mixed actions

Some drugs used to block bladder hyperactivity have more than one mechanism of action (e.g. oxybutynin and dicyclomine). They all have a fairly pronounced antimuscarinic effect in addition to a 'direct' action on the detrusor muscle, which is often poorly defined.

Drugs used to treat incontinence
Urge incontinence and hyperreflexia
Antimuscarinic drugs Drugs with mixed actions Antidepressants α_1 Adrenoceptor antagonists β_2 Adrenoceptor agonists Desmopressin
Stress incontinence
α Adrenoceptor agonists Estrogens (in postmenopausal women)

Fig. 16.7 Drugs used to treat incontinence.

Oxybutynin has a well-documented efficacy in the treatment of detrusor overactivity and is probably the drug of first choice for this disorder, despite its adverse effect profile (see below). It has both an antimuscarinic and a direct muscle relaxant effect, in addition to local anesthetic actions. The latter effect may be important when the drug is administered intravesically, but probably plays no role when it is given orally. *In vitro*, oxybutynin is 500 times weaker as a smooth muscle relaxant than as an antimuscarinic agent and, when given systemically, it probably acts mainly as a muscarinic antagonist. Oxybutynin has a high affinity for muscarinic receptors in both the bladder and salivary glands, and a higher affinity for M_1 and M_3 receptors than for M_2 receptors.

Oxybutynin is a tertiary amine and is well absorbed, but undergoes an extensive first-pass metabolism. Its bioavailability is 6% in healthy volunteers and its plasma half-life is approximately 2 hours, but shows wide interindividual variation. An active metabolite of oxybutynin, *N*-desethyl oxybutynin, has pharmacologic properties similar to those of the parent compound, but occurs in much higher concentrations. It therefore appears that the effect of oral oxybutynin is largely exerted by the metabolite. The presence of an active metabolite may also explain the lack of correlation between plasma oxybutynin concentration and adverse effects.

The therapeutic effect of oral oxybutynin is associated with a high incidence (up to 80%) of adverse effects. These are typically antimuscarinic (i.e. dry mouth, constipation, drowsiness, blurred vision) and are often dose limiting. However, when administered intravesically, oxybutynin increases bladder capacity and produces clinical improvement with few adverse effects.

Dicyclomine has both a direct relaxant effect on smooth muscle and an antimuscarinic action. However, although published reports on its effect on detrusor overactivity are favorable, it is not widely used, and controlled clinical trials documenting its efficacy and adverse effects are scarce.

Tricyclic antidepressants

Several antidepressants have beneficial effects in patients with detrusor overactivity, but imipramine is the only one that has been widely used clinically to treat this disorder. It is an effective treatment for bladder overactivity (e.g. in the elderly), and is also effective as a treatment of nocturnal enuresis in children.

Imipramine has complex pharmacologic effects, including marked systemic antimuscarinic actions, but its mechanism of action in detrusor overactivity has not been established. It may act centrally by inhibiting the uptake of norepinephrine and serotonin (5-hydroxytryptamine).

Therapeutic doses of tricyclic antidepressants, including imipramine, can cause serious cardiovascular adverse effects (e.g. orthostatic hypotension, ventricular arrhythmias), and children seem to be particularly sensitive. The risks and benefits of imipramine in the treatment of voiding disorders, particularly children with enuresis, are not clearly defined.

α Adrenoceptor antagonists

Detrusor overactivity and symptoms related to a disturbed detrusor function (e.g. urgency and nocturia) can be improved in patients with benign prostatic hyperplasia treated with α adrenoceptor antagonists such as prazosin, terazosin, and doxazosin. Prazosin can also decrease detrusor overactivity and increase bladder capacity in patients with detrusor hyperreflexia (clinical observations suggest that neurologic damage may be associated with a change in α adrenoceptor function with an effect on detrusor activation). α Adrenoceptor antagonists may provide a therapeutic alternative in the treatment of detrusor overactivity in some patient groups, but their value has not yet been established.

β Adrenoceptor agonists

β_2 Adrenoceptor agonists can increase bladder capacity, but few investigations have been performed in patients with detrusor overactivity. Favorable effects have been reported in studies with terbutaline, albuterol, and clenbuterol*, but the therapeutic efficacy and value of β_2 adrenoceptor agonists in the treatment of detrusor overactivity have not been established.

Desmopressin

Desmopressin is a synthetic vasopressin analog acting on V_2 receptors to produce a pronounced antidiuretic effect. It has practically no vasopressor actions (V_1 receptors). It decreases the nocturnal production of urine and is an effective short-term treatment for enuresis in children. Desmopressin reduces the frequency of nocturia in men with benign prostatic hyperplasia and in patients with multiple sclerosis, and may be of value in some adults with detrusor overactivity, particularly with nocturia.

Treatment of stress incontinence is aimed at increasing outlet resistance

Pharmacologic treatment of stress incontinence aims at increasing outlet resistance. This can be obtained by increasing a low intraurethral pressure or by improving the function of the urethral mucosa.

α Adrenoceptor agonists

α Adrenoceptor agonists increase intraurethral pressure and the most widely used is ephedrine. Ephedrine directly stimulates both α and β adrenoceptors and, in addition, releases norepinephrine from nerve terminals and inhibits catecholamine reuptake. It produces systemic adverse effects including increasing blood pressure, sleep disturbances, headache, tremor, and palpitations. Ephedrine may be effective when used prophylactically in certain stress situations, but the results with long-term therapy can be disappointing.

Estrogens

The beneficial effects of estrogen include proliferation of the urethral mucosa with a consequent improvement of the mucosal ability to increase outflow resistance. Estrogens may also increase the effect of α adrenoceptor stimulation on the urethral smooth muscle. Estrogen treatment, particularly in combination with an α adrenoceptor agonist, may be effective in women who lack estrogen.

URINARY RETENTION

The primary cause of a failure of bladder emptying may be:

- In the bladder: the detrusor contraction is insufficient.
- In the urethra: the outflow resistance is too high and cannot be overcome by detrusor activity.

Treatment of urinary retention aims to increase detrusor activity or decrease outlet resistance

Parasympathomimetic drugs

Detrusor contraction is mediated mainly through stimulation of muscarinic receptors. However, muscarinic receptor agonists (e.g. bethanechol and carbachol) or anticholinesterase agents (e.g. neostigmine) do increase bladder tone, but do not improve bladder emptying, since they do not change outflow resistance. These drugs are rarely used because of their predictable adverse effects, including perspiration and gastrointestinal discomfort.

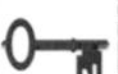

Treatment of urinary incontinence and urinary retention

- **Treatment of a failure to store urine (urinary incontinence) is aimed at decreasing detrusor activity, increasing bladder capacity, or increasing outlet resistance**
- **Treatment of a failure to empty urine (urinary retention) is aimed at increasing detrusor activity or decreasing outlet resistance**

α Adrenoceptor antagonists

Prazosin blocks urethral α adrenoceptors. It can be an effective treatment in patients with parasympathetic decentralization of the bladder (autonomous bladder) who are unable to empty the bladder voluntarily because the outflow resistance is too high to be overcome by detrusor activity.

INFECTIONS OF THE URINARY TRACT

Approximately 35% of all women will have a symptomatic urinary tract infection, most often cystitis, at some time in their life

Urinary tract infections are among the most common bacterial infections, and the most common manifestations are cystitis and pyelonephritis. Pyelonephritis is usually preceded by cystitis. The risk of developing an acute pyelonephritis before puberty is approximately 3% for girls and 1–2% for boys. In the latter part of childhood and in adults, cystitis is the most common infection, with peak frequencies in young and postmenopausal women. In men, urinary tract infections are uncommon, but increase in frequency with prostatic hypertrophy and other types of outflow obstruction. Urinary tract infections are the most common nosocomial infections and are seen in 3–4% of acute hospital patients.

Escherichia coli is the most common urinary tract pathogen and is responsible for 80% of all urinary tract infections acquired outside hospital. However, only a small fraction of the many existing clones cause urinary tract infections. Other Enterobacteriaceae (e.g. *Proteus*) can cause infection in boys and men, and in women with complicating disorders. *Staphylococcus saprophyticus* is common in young women.

Urinary tract pathogens

- *Escherichia coli*
- *Staphylococcus saprophyticus*
- *Klebsiella/Enterobacter*
- *Proteus*
- *Pseudomonas*
- Enterocci
- *Staphylococcus epidermidis*

The significance of a urinary tract infection differs in small children and adults and therefore the treatment approaches can differ. The treatment approaches can also differ between men and women. The drugs most commonly used for treating urinary tract infections are listed in Fig. 16.8.

Lower urinary tract infections in women

The cardinal symptoms of acute cystitis are pain during micturition, urgency, and frequency, and bacteriuria can be demonstrated in up to 75% of patients with these symptoms.

*The first-line treatment of acute sporadic cystitis in nonpregnant women is trimethoprim, pivmecillinam, or pivampicillin**

Acute sporadic cystitis in a healthy young women is not a serious condition and the first-line treatment in nonpregnant women (Fig. 16.9) is either trimethoprim, which is effective against both Gram-negative (*E. coli*) and Gram-positive bacteria (*S. saprophyticus*), or pivmecillinam, which is effective against Gram-negative bacteria and *S. saprophyticus*, but has no effect against *Enterococcus faecalis*. Pivampicillin* may also be used. If these drugs cannot be used (e.g. because of allergy or other adverse effects, alternatives include:

- Cephalosporins (e.g. cefadroxil, which has appropriate pharmacokinetic properties for the treatment of urinary tract infections), which are effective against most Gram-negative and Gram-positive urinary tract pathogens, including *Proteus* and *S. saprophyticus*, though *E. faecalis* is resistant.
- Fluoroquinolones (e.g. norfloxacin, ciprofloxacin, and ofloxacin). These have few adverse effects and are effective against most urinary tract pathogens, including *Pseudomonas aeruginosa*, which can be found in patients with an in-dwelling catheter.
- Nitrofurantoin, which has an antibacterial effect only in the urinary tract. Antibacterial concentrations are not achieved in the plasma after recommended doses because it is rapidly eliminated. Rarely, nitrofurantoin causes serious pulmonary adverse effects and neuropathy.

In pregnant women with acute cystitis, other treatment alternatives are needed (see Fig. 16.9).

Pregnant women with asymptomatic bacterimia, of whom 20–40% may develop an acute pyelonephritis later in pregnancy, also require treatment. In these cases the treatment alternatives are:

- Nitrofurantoin.
- Cephalosporins (e.g. cefadroxil).
- Pivmecillinam.
- Pivampicillin*/pivmecillinam.

Lower urinary tract infections in men

Symptomatic urinary tract infections are unusual in men, and should always be investigated. *E. coli* is less frequently the cause than in women, and infections by *Proteus, Klebsiella, Enterobacter,* enterococci, and coagulase-negative staphylococci are relatively common.

Infections of the lower urinary tract in men often involve the prostate. The first-line antibiotics are therefore drugs that can penetrate the prostate and are trimethoprim and quinolones (e.g. norfloxacin) (see Fig. 16.9). Tetracyclines (e.g. doxycycline, which has a high lipid solubility and reaches therapeutic tissue concentrations in most organs) are a second-line alternative. The recommended treatment time is usually 10 days, but may be extended to 3 weeks if there are clinical signs of prostatitis.

Lower urinary tract infections in children

The symptoms of urinary tract infections in children are variable: the younger the child, the more nonspecific the symptoms. Urgency, pain during micturition, and bladder pain, together with a temperature higher than 38°C, generally lead to a diagnosis of cystitis. The first-line treatment (see Fig. 16.9) is trimethoprim for boys, and trimethoprim or

Drugs used to treat urinary tract infections

- Trimethoprim
- Trimethoprim/sulfonamides
- Penicillins (broad-spectrum)
- Cephalosporins
- Fluoroquinolones
- Nitrofurantoin
- Tetracyclines

Fig. 16.8 Drugs used to treat urinary tract infections.

nitrofurantoin for girls (there is a high frequency of nitrofurantoin-resistant *Proteus* infection in boys). The second-line treament is pivmecillinam.

Upper urinary tract infections

Treatment of acute pyelonephritis should be started before a bacteriologic diagnosis has been established

Acute pyelonephritis is a potentially life-threatening infection, characterized by a high fever, chills, flank pain, malaise, and vomiting. The antibiotics used to treat it are those that achieve high concentrations in both blood and renal tissue. Oral treatment is often sufficient (see Fig. 16.9). Parenteral treatment is indicated if the general condition of the patient is impaired and in pregnancy (pregnant women should be treated in hospital and cephalosporins are the first-line drugs).

The first-line antibiotic both in nonpregnant women and men is a quinolone (e.g. norfloxacin) or trimethoprim/sulfamethoxazole. The second-line alternatives are cephalosporins (e.g. cefadroxil) and pivmecillinam/pivampicillin*.

A urinary tract infection with a high fever in a child is often considered to be pyelonephritis, and the first-line treatment is trimethoprim/sulfamethoxazole. Alternative treatment is a cephalosporin (e.g. cefadroxil) or pivmecillinam.

First-line oral treatment of uncomplicated urinary tract infection

	Cystitis	Acute pyelonephritis
Women (nonpregnant)	Trimethoprim Pivmecillinam	Norfloxacin Trimethoprim/sulfamethoxazole
Treatment time	7 days	10–14 days
Women (pregnant)	Nitrofurantoin Cefadroxil Pivmecillinam Pivampicillin*/pivmecillinam	Hospitilization
Treatment time	7 days	
Men	Trimethoprim Norfloxacin	Norfloxacin Trimethoprim/sulfamethoxazole
Treatment time	10–14 days	
Children	Trimethoprim (boys) Trimethoprim or nitrofurantoin (girls)	Trimethoprim/sulphamethoxazole
Treatment time	3–5 days	10 days

Fig. 16.9 First-line treatment of uncomplicated urinary tract infections.

FURTHER READING

Anderson RU. Treatment of complicated and uncomplicated urinary tract infections. In: Mulholland SG (ed) *Antibiotic Therapy in Urology*. Philadelphia: Lippincott-Raven Publishers; 1996: pp. 23–37. [Aspects of modern treatment of lower urinary tract infections.]

Andersson K-E. The pharmacology of lower urinary tract smooth muscles and penile erectile tissues. *Pharmacol Rev* 1993; **45**: 253–308. [Overview of the peripheral regulation of the lower urinary tract.]

de Groat WC, Booth AM, Yoshimura N. Neurophysiology of micturition and its modification in animal models of human disease. In: Maggi CA (ed) *The Autonomic Nervous System*. Vol. 6, Chapter 8, Nervous Control of the Urogenital System. London; Harwood Academic Publishers; 1993: pp. 227–289. [Overview of the central nervous regulation of the lower urinary tract.]

Hooton TM, Stamm WE. Management of acute uncomplicated urinary tract infection in adults. *Med Clin North Am* 1991; **75**: 339–357. [Principles for treatment of lower urinary tract infections.]

Wein AJ. Pharmacology of incontinence. *Urol Clin North Am* 1995; **22**: 557–577. [Detailed review of the principles and drugs used for the treatment of different forms of urinary incontinence.]

Make a provisional diagnosis and determine a rational pharmacologic treatment for the following hypothetical case.

A 72-year-old man developed burning on urination and urgency, and urinalysis demonstrated many white blood cells and bacteria in his urine. On physical examination he had an enlarged nontender prostate, and additional history revealed that he had longstanding prostatism. He did not have features suggestive of an upper urinary tract infection. A urine culture was obtained and he was started on antibiotic treatment. He was also noted to have hypertension, which had not been treated for several years, and he was therefore prescribed diltiazem. The burning on urination improved over the next 2 days. However, 4 days later the patient developed acute urinary retention requiring catheterization.

1. What would be appropriate choices for antibiotics before knowing the results of the urine culture?
2. How might the results of the culture modify the treatment?
3. How long should a course of antibiotics be continued for this indication?
4. What are the possible explanations for the development of acute urinary retention?
5. By what mechanism could diltiazem impair bladder emptying?
6. Which classes of drugs are associated with urinary retention?
7. What measures can be taken to improve bladder emptying?

Indicate which is the correct answer for each question.

1. Which is the most commonly used drug for treatment of motor urge incontinence?
- a) atropine
- b) prazosin
- c) phenylpropanolamine
- d) terbutaline
- e) oxybutynin

2. Which is the most common urinary tract pathogen outside hospitals?
- a) *Proteus*
- b) *S. saprophyticus*
- c) *E.coli*
- d) *Pseudomonas*
- e) *Enterococci*

3. Which of the following statements is correct?
- a) the main excitatory transmitter of the human detrusor is norepinephrine
- b) the main excitatory transmitter of the human urethra is acetylcholine
- c) the main excitatory transmitter of the human detrusor is acetylcholine
- d) the normal detrusor response to norepinephrine is contraction
- e) the normal urethral response to norepinephrine is relation

4. Which of the following statements is correct?
- a) the main contraction-mediating receptor of the human detrusor the α_1 adrenoceptor
- b) the main contraction-mediating of the human urethral smooth muscle is the muscarinic M_3 receptor
- c) the main relaxation-mediating receptor of the human detrusor is the muscarinic M_3 receptor
- d) the normal detrusor contains more α adrenoceptors than muscarinic receptors
- e) the main contraction-mediating of the human urethral smooth muscle is the α_1 adrenceptor

5. α_1 Adrenoceptor antagonists can be useful for treatment of
- a) acute cystitis
- b) acute pyelonephritis
- c) benign prostatic hyperplasia
- d) stress incontinence
- e) acute prostatitis

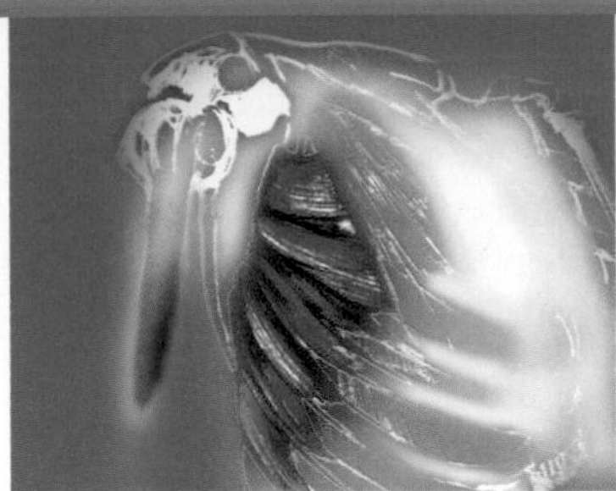

17. Drugs and the Musculoskeletal System

PHYSIOLOGY OF THE MUSCULOSKELETAL SYSTEM

The musculoskeletal system protects vital structures and is responsible for a variety of mobility-related functions

The integrity of the musculoskeletal system depends on interactions between skeletal muscles, which usually cross joints and move the bones to which they are attached. Joints link two or more bones and provide a low-friction surface on which bones can move. Muscle function is controlled by voluntary and involuntary discharges from the motor cortex in the central nervous system (CNS). Muscle tone is modulated by spinal reflexes at the level of the spinal cord where the motor nerve exits.

The skeleton is made up of a series of bones and joints that maximize range while maintaining stability. The two types of bone are:

- Cortical compact bone, which provides strength when torsion is the dominant force, is dense, and is the main component of long bones.
- Trabecular bone, which resists compressive forces, is found at the end of long bones, and makes up the major component of the vertebral body.

There are also two types of joint:

- A synovial (true) joint (e.g. the knee joint) allows extensive movement. Its stability is maintained by ligaments as well as muscles that pass across it.
- A fibrocartilaginous joint (e.g. the sacroiliac joint) maximizes joint stability, but limits movement of the skeleton.

PATHOPHYSIOLOGY AND DISEASES OF THE MUSCULOSKELETAL SYSTEM

Bone diseases

- Can cause fractures and pain
- Osteoporosis is characterized by a reduced quantity of bone
- Osteomalacia is characterized by a lack of mineralization
- Paget's disease is characterized by the production of abnormal bone

OSTEOPOROSIS

Osteoporosis is a thinning of normal bone with aging, but may be accelerated by a premature natural or surgical loss of ovarian function, medications (e.g. glucocorticosteroids), or lifestyle factors (e.g. alcohol, smoking). It is a common disorder in women and may result in forearm, hip, and spinal fractures. The increasing morbidity and mortality due to osteoporosis in Europe and North America reflect the increasingly aging population.

An assessment of bone density using imaging studies provides the best estimate of fracture risk

Bone quality is normal in osteoporosis, but its quantity is reduced (Fig. 17.1). The balance between formation (a function of osteoblasts) and bone resorption (a function of osteoclasts) determines whether the amount of bone increases or decreases over time. Bone mass is determined by the net effect of these two active ongoing processes. It increases from birth to about 30 years of age in both men and women (Fig. 17.2), and then slowly declines, with a more rapid decline in women in the early postmenopausal years.

Bone formation and resorption can be semiquantified by histomorphologic analysis on bone biopsy or indirectly assessed using markers of bone formation and resorption. Serum Ca^{2+} concentrations and Ca^{2+}-regulating hormones are normal.

Drugs used to treat osteoporosis in postmenopausal women include estrogen replacement therapy, progesterone, calcitonin, bisphosphonates, and calcium

Hormone replacement therapy Estrogen replacement therapy (ERT) at the time of the menopause inhibits the effect of osteoclasts on bone resorption (see Chapters 12 and 13). It therefore slows bone loss and may actually increase bone quantity in the first few years following cessation of normal ovarian function. It can be provided orally, by injection, or transdermally, as estrogens and their esters are easily absorbed through the skin, mucous membranes, and gastrointestinal tract. The different routes of administration have different pharmacokinetics and other properties. Oral estrogen (e.g. conjugated equine estrogen, estrone sulfate, and micronized estradiol-17β) is the most widely prescribed drug to treat postmenopausal osteoporosis.

Estrogens circulate in the blood with sex hormone binding globulin and albumin and, like other steroid hormones, act in the cell nucleus. They diffuse passively through cell membranes and bind to the nuclear estrogen receptor found in estrogen-responsive tissues. Following activation, the estrogen receptor

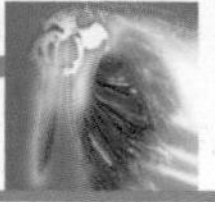

binds to specific DNA sequences that result in transcription of adjacent genes.

The decision to start ERT and compliance depend not only on its effect on bone but also on its other clinical effects.

ERT will relieve vasomotor symptoms if given in the first few years of the menopause. Usually treatment can be tapered, but occasionally long-term treatment is required. ERT inhibits bone loss and may initially increase bone density. In addition, it influences lipoprotein metabolism (Fig. 17.3), resulting in decreased low density lipoprotein (LDL) cholesterol and increased high density lipoprotein (HDL) concentrations, thereby protecting against cardiovascular disease. Clinical studies have shown a reduced rate of myocardial infarction, decreased mortality from cardiovascular disease, and an overall reduction in total mortality in postmenopausal women who receive ERT. Transdermal estrogen usually controls postmenopausal symptoms and osteoporosis, but has little effect on lipoproteins.

Progesterone should be considered for all patients started on ERT who have not had a hysterectomy, because it will reduce the significantly increased risk of endometrial cancer associated with ERT to below the native risk. Unopposed estrogens should only be given to women who have had a hysterectomy and therefore have no risk of developing endometrial hyperplasia. The addition of cyclic progesterone therapy usually results in the continuation of monthly menstruation, but menstrual bleeding can be reduced by using lower doses or continuous progesterone. Continuous use of progesterone inhibits endometrial proliferation and reduces the risk of endometrial cancer, but can cause 'breakthrough bleeding.' There is some evidence that progesterone diminishes the favorable effect of estrogens on the lipoprotein profile. Progesterone can be given orally, transdermally, or by injection. Common oral progesterones used include medroxyprogesterone, norethindrone, and micronized progesterone.

Calcitonin, a 32-amino acid peptide that directly inhibits osteoclasts, can slow bone loss (Fig. 17.4). It acts on a well-defined receptor that is seen in a variety of cells, but most

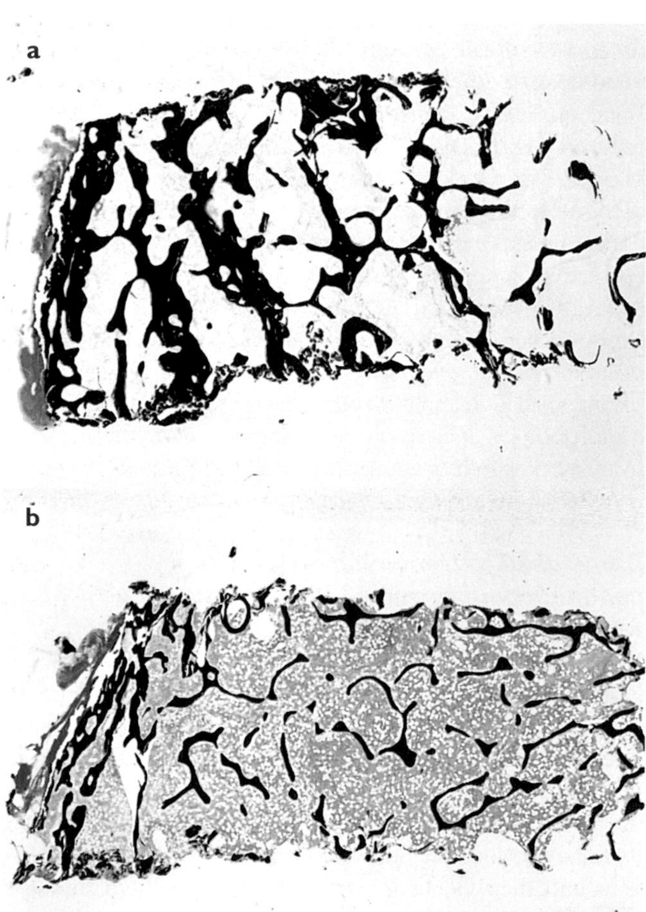

Fig. 17.1 Osteoporosis. (a) Micrograph of a resin section of a bone biopsy from the iliac crest showing normal cortical and trabecular bone stained with a silver method, which makes calcified bone show up as black. (b) Micrograph of bone from a patient with osteoporosis. When compared with (a), which shows the bone mass of a healthy patient of the same age, it is clear that the cortical zone is narrower and that the trabeculae are thinner and less numerous. (Courtesy of Dr Alan Stevens and Professor Jim Lowe.)

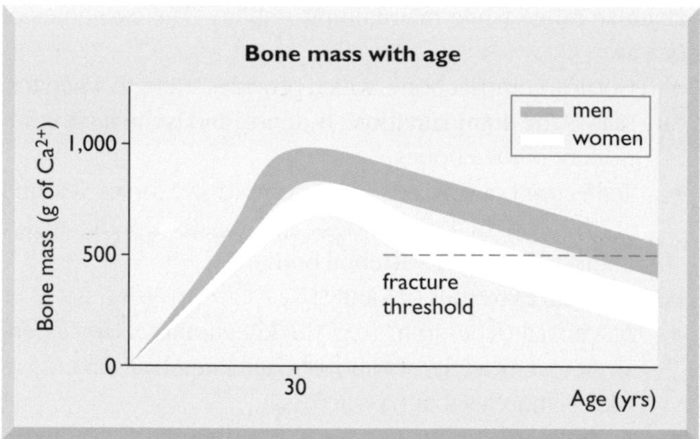

Fig. 17.2 Bone mass with age.

Advantages and disadvantages of estrogen

Advantages	Disadvantages
Reduced menopausal symptoms	Cost
Decreased bone loss	Breast symptoms
Decreased risk of fracture	Possibly associated with breast malignancy
Improved lipid profile	Return of menstrual flow (if cycled with progesterone)
Reduced cardiovascular disease	Increased risk of endometrial malignancy (unless used with progesterone)

Fig. 17.3 Advantages and disadvantages of estrogen.

importantly osteoclasts. There is homology between this receptor on osteoclasts and the parathyroid hormone (PTH) receptor on osteoblasts. The membrane receptor is coupled to adenylyl cyclase so that its activation increases the intracellular concentration of cAMP, resulting in an inhibitory effect on the osteoclasts. Calcitonin may exert an effect on the osteoblasts, but this is less clear.

Oral calcitonins are ineffective because they are broken down by aminopeptidases and proteases in the gastrointestinal tract. Parenteral calcitonin is well absorbed, but this inconvenient route of administration limits its widespread use. Intranasal calcitonin is therefore used instead, although it is not well absorbed, with low peak plasma concentrations, but it is more practical and has wider patient acceptance. Recent randomized controlled trials of nasal calcitonin have demonstrated an improved bone density of 2–3% over 2 years. Further studies are needed to confirm that it leads to a significant reduction of fractures in the long term. Injected calcitonin at higher doses (50–100 IU/day) has analgesic properties and is frequently used in patients with severe pain due to recent vertebral compression fractures.

Intranasal or subcutaneous calcitonin can be given to produce beneficial effects on the bone without causing serious systemic adverse effects. Marine (salmon or eel) calcitonins are usually used because they are many times more potent than human calcitonin. Minor adverse effects include flushing and gastrointestinal symptoms (nausea, vomiting, or diarrhea).

Bisphosphonates are analogues of pyrophosphate, but have a carbon rather than an oxygen atom. The P–C–P structure allows for many variations by changing the side chains on the carbon atom. Small changes in the side chain structure can result in significant physicochemical, biologic, and therapeutic differences, and every phosphonate needs to be considered individually.

Bisphosphonates have a strong affinity for calcium phosphate and act exclusively in calcified tissues. The mechanism of bisphosphonate inhibition of bone resorption is unclear. It was postulated that it was physicochemical, but a direct cellular effect may be more important. Unlike calcitonin, which has an immediate effect on resorption, bisphosphonates take about 48 hours to block resorption.

Different bisphosphonates have significantly different antiresorptive potency, the potencies of etidronate, clodronate*, tiludronate*, pamidronate, alendronate*, and risedronate* being 1, 10, 10, 100, 1000, and 5000, respectively.

Oral absorption of most bisphosphonates is 1–10% of a given dose. They should never be given with milk products, food, or at the same time as Ca^{2+} supplements, as this inhibits absorption.

Recent large prospective studies in osteoporosis have shown that at least two bisphosphonates (etidronate and alendronate*) increase bone density 4–8% over the first 3 years of treatment and reduce vertebral and nonvertebral fractures by at least 50%. If given continuously, etidronate can cause osteomalacia. This can be avoided by intermittent administration with periods of several weeks to 3 months off the drug. Bone biopsy studies up to 7 years after cyclic etidronate have not shown mineralization defects. Bisphosphonates such as alendronate* do not have this effect and can be given continuously.

Bisphosphonates are slowly released from the skeleton and may have actions on bone tissue for years. There is some concern that this prolonged action may have an undetermined accumulative effect 10–20 years later.

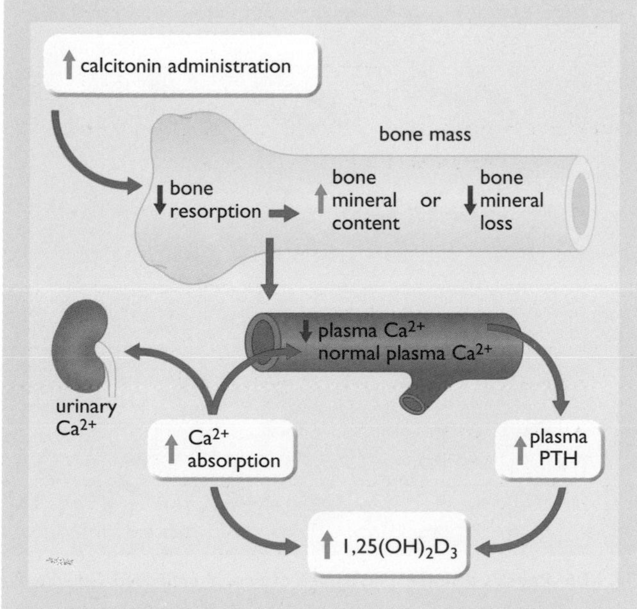

Fig. 17.4 The effect of calcitonin on bone and calcium homeostasis. (PTH, parathyroid hormone; $1,25(OH)_2D_3$, 1,25-dihydroxyvitamin D_3)

Calcium supplements have a small beneficial effect on preventing bone loss. Calcium in the form of either dietary Ca^{2+} or oral Ca^{2+} supplements is inexpensive and safe and should be recommended to all patients to slow bone loss. It is recommended that postmenopausal women have a Ca^{2+} intake of more than 1500 mg daily.

Emerging drugs A variety of drugs are being assessed for treating osteoporosis.

Vitamin D analogs facilitate Ca^{2+} absorption and may have an undetermined effect on both bone resorption and formation.

PTH hormone analogs used in cyclic doses are being evaluated in clinical trials. They stimulate osteoblasts and thereby result in increased bone formation. Although they can only be given by injection, they may be a highly effective treatment for increasing bone in the first few years after menopause.

Selective estrogen receptor modulators are being evaluated in clinical trials. These drugs have been developed since the observation that tamoxifen used to treat breast cancer increased bone density. This occurred despite tamoxifen being an estrogen partial agonist and therefore acting as an estrogen antagonist. It is possible that newer analogs of tamoxifen may have an action on bone that is beneficial without the potential risk of breast cancer associated with estrogen.

Tamoxifen-like drugs may have a differential effect in tissues possessing estrogen receptors, resulting in beneficial effects in endometrial, bone, and breast tissues.

OSTEOMALACIA AND RICKETS

Osteomalacia is a relatively uncommon condition of bone in which there is decreased mineralization of new bone matrix (Fig. 17.5). In children this lack of calcification may result in growth failure and deformity and is called rickets. Adults may present with bone pain, proximal myopathy, or fractures with minor trauma.

Osteomalacia is most commonly due to acquired vitamin D deficiency. Biochemical markers include hypocalcemia, a secondary elevation of PTH concentration, and a low plasma 25-hydroxyvitamin D concentration. Other less common hereditary types of osteomalacia also occur.

The major source of vitamin D is the skin, where it is produced by a photochemical reaction. Individuals who lack exposure to sunlight because of climate, type of clothing, or institutionalization (such as long-term geriatric care) are at risk of vitamin D deficiency (see Chapter27).

Vitamin D is used to treat and prevent osteomalacia

Vitamin D-deficient osteomalacia responds well to vitamin D, 25-hydroxyvitamin D, 1α-hydroxyvitamin D, or 1,25-dihydroxyvitamin D. It may also respond to sun exposure. In the US, dairy products are fortified with vitamin D and osteomalacia is relatively rare.

PAGET'S DISEASE OF BONE

Paget's disease is a bone condition that presents with bone pain, skeletal deformity, neurologic complications, or fractures. The incidence is highly variable: it is common in central Europe, the UK, Australia, New Zealand, and the US, and rare in Africa, the Middle and Far East, and Scandinavia.

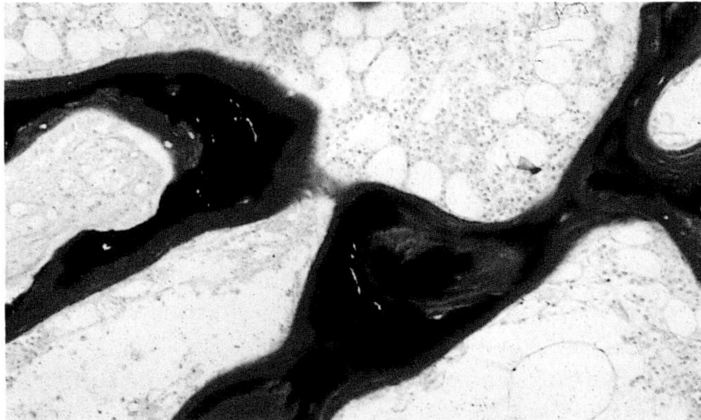

Fig. 17.5 Osteomalacia. Micrograph of iliac crest bone embedded in acrylic resin without previous decalcification from a patient with osteomalacia. There is a broad zone of unmineralized osteoid (red) and a central zone of mineralized bone (black) in this section stained by the von Kossa's silver technique. (Courtesy of Dr Alan Stevens and Professor Jim Lowe.)

The pathology reveals excessive bone resorption and formation (Fig. 17.6) and there are three phases: osteolytic, osteoblastic, and quiescent. All three patterns may be present in one patient at the same time. The presence of inclusion bodies has led to the suggestion that the disease may have a viral origin.

Drugs used to treat Paget's disease of bone include analgesics, calcitonin, and bisphosphonates

Analgesics Simple analgesics (aspirin, acetaminophen) are often used for pain due to Paget's disease. Nonsteroidal anti-inflammatory drugs (NSAIDs) also reduce the pain, but do not reduce the long-term complications.

Calcitonin inhibits resorption and can reduce pain by a variety of potential mechanisms (see p. 341). Marine (salmon and eel) calcitonins are more potent than human calcitonin, but can be associated with the development of antibodies, resulting in

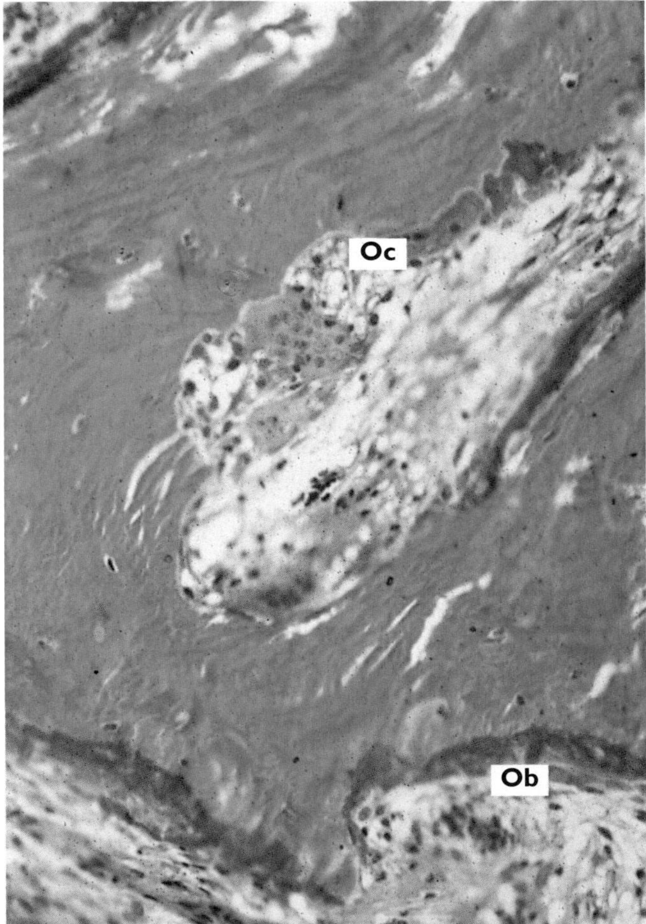

Fig. 17.6 Paget's disease. Micrograph of a resin-embedded, Gouldner-stained section from a patient with active Paget's disease. There is uncontrolled osteoclast (Oc) resorption of a bone, and osteoblasts (Ob) are attempting to fill in sites of recent osteoclast erosion in an adjacent site. (Courtesy of Dr Alan Stevens and Professor Jim Lowe.)

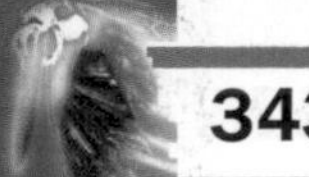

resistance to treatment. The treatment needs to be given subcutaneously to achieve adequate blood concentrations to be effective in reducing bone pain. These high doses (50–100 IU/day) are commonly associated with adverse effects including cutaneous flushing and gastrointestinal effects.

Bisphosphonates are an effective treatment of Paget's disease. They reduce the turnover of both 'pagetic' and normal bone (see p. 341). Gastrointestinal intolerance is the main adverse effect.

OSTEOARTHRITIS

Osteoarthritis is the most common joint disease. It is characterized pathologically by a loss of articular cartilage, bone remodelling and hypertrophy, subchondral bone sclerosis, and bone cysts. It may be the result of either:

- Excessive loads on the joint.
- The presence of abnormal cartilage or bone.

The most characteristic feature of osteoarthritis is gradual progressive cartilage loss. However, the rate of glycosaminoglycan hyaluronic acid, collagen, and proteoglycan synthesis is increased. Local factors, including lysosomal proteases and neutral metalloproteinases, and cytokines, including interleukin-1 (IL-1), are involved in the cartilage destruction.

The pathophysiologic changes cause the localized pain that initially occurs with use and is relieved with rest, but which later occurs with minimal activity or movement. Joint stiffness, which is characteristic of inflammatory arthritis, is minimal or short lived.

Drug treatment of osteoarthritis includes analgesics and nonsteroidal anti-inflammatory drugs

Treatments for osteoarthritis

- Mechanical devices to relieve stress in the joint
- Analgesics
- Anti-inflammatory drugs
- Surgical intervention

Analgesics, including acetaminophen, often relieve the pain of osteoarthritis and are the preferred drug therapy. Data from large clinical studies show the effectiveness of analgesics in comparison to NSAIDs in osteoarthritis, showing they are as effective. Narcotic analgesics should only be used for short periods, intermittently, or for acute flares.

NSAIDs are frequently used to treat patients with osteoarthritis. They are effective analgesics and can also treat any associated inflammation, but have no major effect on the underlying process. NSAIDs inhibit cyclooxygenase, the enzyme that converts arachidonic acid to prostaglandins (Fig. 17.7). However, currently available NSAIDs have minimal effect on lipooxygenase, the enzyme that plays an important role in transforming arachidonic acid to to leukotrienes. NSAIDs also have other immunoregulatory effects, but these are not thought to be clinically significant.

Highly selective inhibitors of cyclooxygenase 2 (COX-2) could be important therapeutically

There are two forms of the enzyme cyclooxygenase: cyclooxygenase 1 (COX-1) and cyclooxygenase 2 (COX-2) (Fig. 17.8). COX-1 is an enzyme linked to the production of physiologic prostaglandins in the kidney and stomach, whereas COX-2 is linked to proinflammatory prostaglandin production. Current NSAIDs preferably inhibit COX-1 or are nonselective, but NSAIDs that are 200–300 times more selective for COX-2 might have improved gastrointestinal and kidney safety profiles.

NSAID use is limited by their significant adverse effects, which particularly affect the gastrointestinal tract, the kidney, the CNS, and the hematopoietic system.

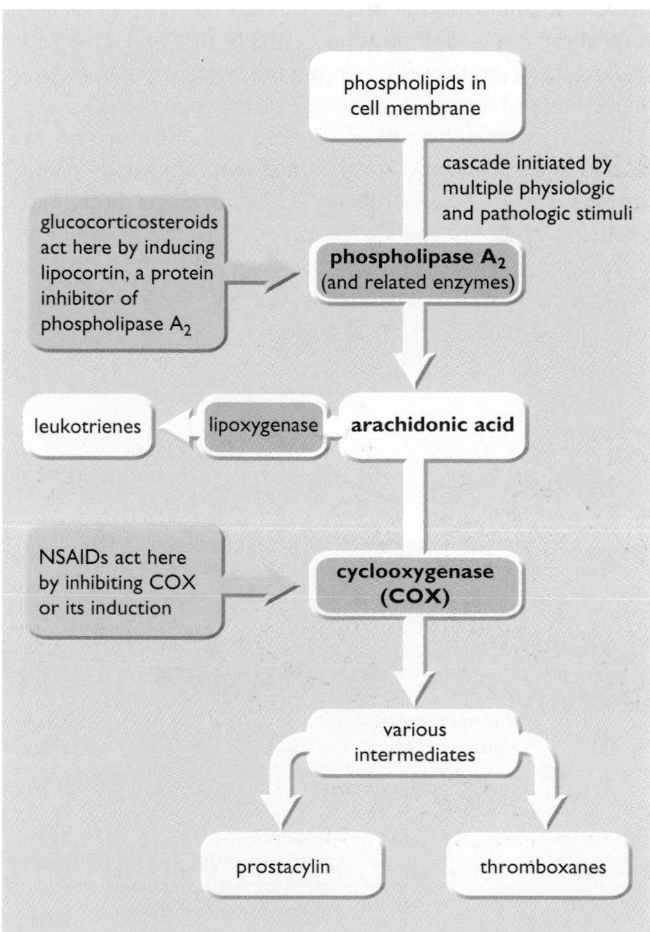

Fig. 17.7 Arachidonic acid and its metabolites. (NSAIDs, nonsteroidal anti-inflammatory drugs)

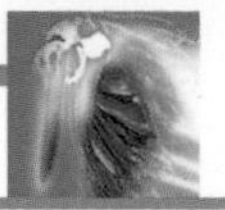

Adverse effects of nonsteroidal anti-inflammatory drugs

- Gastrointestinal tract: gastric irritation, peptic ulcers, bleeding, perforation
- Kidney: decreased renal blood flow, decreased creatinine clearance, rarely interstitial nephritis or nephrotic syndrome
- CNS: headaches, confusion, tinnitus, aseptic meningitis (rare)
- Hematopoietic system: bleeding, inhibited platelet adhesion (irreversible effect with aspirin persisting 10–12 days)

RHEUMATOID ARTHRITIS

Rheumatoid arthritis is a chronic inflammatory disease of joints that results in joint pain, swelling, and destruction. It affects an estimated 1% of the adult population throughout the world. Progression of the disease results in joint destruction, deformity, and significant disability.

Rheumatoid arthritis is characterized by chronic inflammation in the synovium, which lines the joint. The synovium is inflamed, with an accumulation of polymorphonuclear leukocytes in the superficial layers and mononuclear cells (CD4-positive T lymphocytes and plasma cells) beneath the lining cell layer and deep in the synovial tissues. With disease progression there is massive synovial hypertrophy, with invasion by both inflammatory cells and fibroblast-like cells. Fibrovascular tissue known as 'pannus' invades and destroys both bone and cartilage. Proteinases, prostaglandins, leukotrienes, and reactive oxidants have all been implicated as mediators in the inflammatory changes and tissue destruction in the synovial lining.

Rheumatoid arthritis is associated with a variety of nonarticular clinical syndromes including vasculitis, subcutaneous nodules, interstitial pulmonary fibrosis, pericarditis, mononeuritis multiplex (vasculitis of peripheral nerves), Sjögren's syndrome (inflammation of the salivary glands), Felty's syndrome (splenomegaly and leukopenia), and ocular inflammation.

Early diagnosis and intervention with disease-modifying agents may reduce the significant associated morbidity of rheumatoid arthritis

The treatment of rheumatoid arthritis involves the use of anti-inflammatory drugs and other disease-modifying agents.

NSAIDs inhibit the cyclooxygenase enzyme, resulting in decreased prostaglandin synthesis (see Figs 17.7, 17.8). The two main classes are:

- Aspirin.
- Non-aspirin NSAIDs.

Aspirin is an effective, inexpensive anti-inflammatory if used in therapeutic doses. It is distinct from other NSAIDs because it is an irreversible cyclooxygenase inhibitor and acetylates the active site in the cyclooxygenase enzyme.

Other NSAIDs may be better tolerated than aspirin, but significant gastrointestinal adverse effects (bleeding or perforation) occur with all NSAIDs. Other NSAIDs have no proven increased efficacy over aspirin, and specific NSAIDs may have certain reactions that are more commonly associated with that particular drug. Significant adverse effects other than those affecting the gastrointestinal system include an elevated serum creatinine,

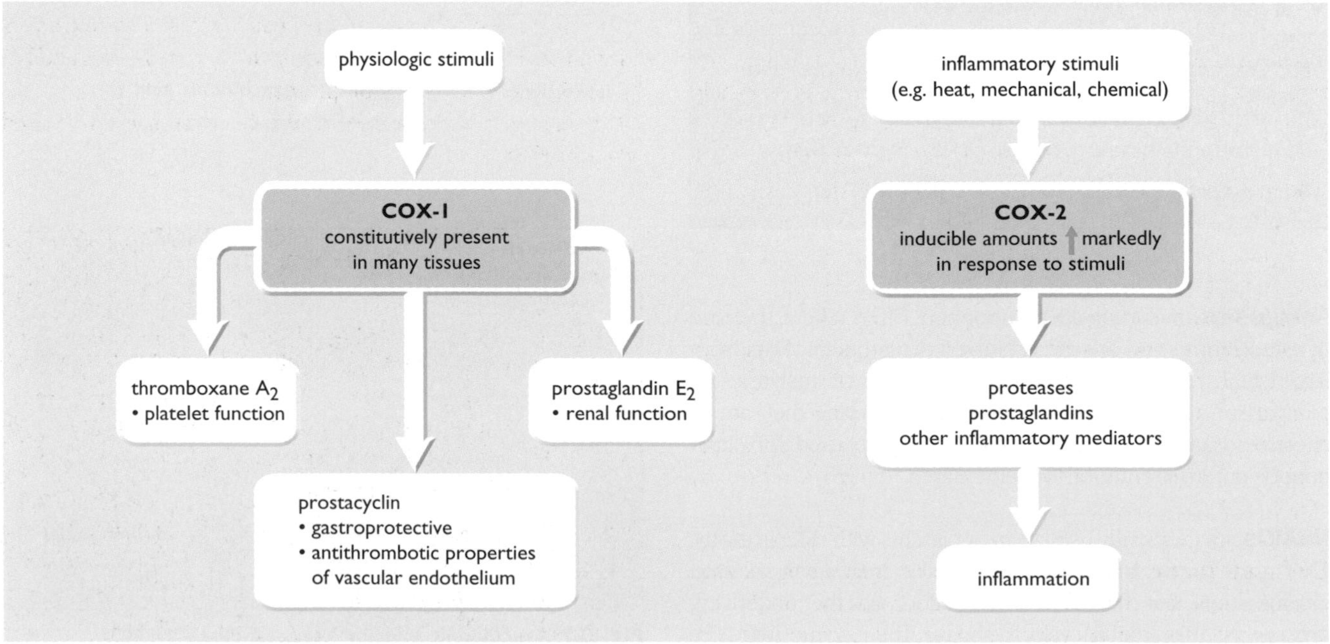

Fig. 17.8 The two cyclooxygenase isoforms COX-1 and COX-2.

fluid retention (especially in congestive heart failure), headaches, and confusion. Both aspirin and other NSAIDs can cause hypersensitivity reactions. Regimens with a once- or twice-daily dose may be more convenient and increase compliance, but do not improve effectiveness or reduce adverse effects of drugs.

Low-dose glucocorticosteroids probably do not have a long-term effect on rheumatoid arthritis

Glucocorticosteroids are not the first-choice treatment of rheumatoid arthritis and should be avoided if possible. Low-dose glucocorticosteroids (less than or equal to prednisone 7.5 mg/day) are effective anti-inflammatory and immunosuppressive drugs, but probably do not have a long-term effect on the disease. They can be added to NSAID therapy to control symptoms in severe disease until other agents become effective. They are an option if NSAIDs are not tolerated or in individuals who are unable to work.

The common adverse effects of glucocorticosteroids depend on the dose and duration of treatment. In addition to bruising and skin thinning, the major long-term concern is bone loss. The need to use the minimum dose of glucocorticosteroids should be emphasized to the patient.

Intra-articular glucocorticosteroids are highly effective, have fewer systemic adverse effects than oral treatment, and are only used if one or two joints are affected. The major risk is the potential to introduce joint infection and the possible risk of accelerating joint cartilage destruction.

If active rheumatoid arthritis is not controlled with nonsteroidal anti-inflammatory drugs or glucocorticosteroids, other antirheumatic drugs should be considered

Clinically useful agents include antimalarials, sulfasalazine, injectable gold salts or oral gold, penicillamine, methotrexate, azathioprine, and cyclosporine. Severe active rheumatoid arthritis is usually treated with one of these disease-modifying drugs in addition to an NSAID and/or low-dose prednisone.

Antimalarials Hydroxychloroquine and chloroquine are examples of antimalarials used to induce a remission or help reduce inflammation in rheumatoid arthritis. However, although antimalarials are thought to be the least effective disease-modifying agent, they have the lowest toxicity. The dose should be maintained for a trial of six months to determine their effectiveness. Color and peripheral vision should be monitored from 6–12 months, depending on the dose.

The anti-inflammatory mechanism of action of chloroquine and hydroxychloroquine is unclear. There is some evidence that they interfere with a wide variety of leukocyte functions. They may inhibit IL-1 production by macrophages, lymphoproliferative responses, and cytotoxic responses of T lymphocytes. At high doses (which are now rarely used) they also have an inhibitory effect on DNA synthesis.

Sulfasalazine is frequently used in the UK as the first-choice disease-modifying agent, but is used less commonly in the US. It is thought to be as effective as gold, but probably has fewer adverse effects. Sulfasalazine is a combination of 5-aminosalicylic acid linked covalently to sulfapyridine*. It is poorly absorbed orally, but is cleaved to its active components by colonic bacteria. It is believed that sulfapyridine* is absorbed systemically and is possibly responsible for its therapeutic effect. Sulfapyridine* is eventually excreted in the urine. The mechanism of action is unclear, but there is some evidence that it reduces natural killer cell activity and alters other lymphocyte functions.

The adverse effects are primarily caused by sulfapyridine*. Severe reactions include acute hemolysis in individuals with glucose-6-phosphate dehydrogenase deficiency, and rarely agranulocytosis. Rashes occur in 20–40% of patients. Other adverse effects include nausea, fever, and arthralgias.

Gold Intramuscular gold salts have historically been the formulation for rheumatoid arthritis in the US. Adverse effects include dermatitis, proteinuria, and bone marrow suppression. Monitoring should include a complete blood count and urinalysis before each injection. Oral gold preparations have become available in recent years; although they appear to be as effective as injectable gold, oral gold is used less frequently. There are two parenteral gold salts (gold sodium thiomalate and aurothioglucose) and one oral form (auranofin).

Gold salts are taken up by reticuloendothelial cells (i.e. in the bone marrow, lymph nodes, liver, and spleen), and in these tissues they impair macrophage function and cytokine activity. Other possible mechanisms of action include inhibition of prostaglandin synthesis, interference with complement activation, cross-linking of collagen, and inhibition of lysosomal activity.

Penicillamine Oral penicillamine, which is a chelator of heavy metals, is a useful agent in the treatment of rheumatoid arthritis and its effectiveness is comparable to that of injectable gold. It is well absorbed orally (40–70%), although food will decrease its absorption. It is metabolized in the liver and is excreted in the urine and feces.

The mechanism of action of penicillamine in rheumatoid arthritis is unclear. It suppresses antibodies to IgM antibodies and has other effects on immune complexes.

The main disadvantage of penicillamine is its many and varied adverse effects.

Adverse effects of penicillamine

- Cutaneous: macular or papular rashes, urticaria, pemphigoid, lupus erythematosus, dermatomyositis
- Hematologic: fatal hematologic reactions are rare, but include thrombocytopenia, leukopenia, agranulocytosis, aplastic anemia
- Renal: reversible proteinuria in the nephrotic range
- Unusual adverse effects: acute pneumonitis, myasthenia gravis (with long-term treatment)
- Less serious effects: nausea, other gastrointestinal effects, transient anosmia

Methotrexate is a folic acid antagonist that is effective in the treatment of rheumatoid arthritis if given orally or parenterally in weekly doses of 5–20 mg/week (see Chapter 28) The mechanism of action is not clearly understood. However, it decreases inflammatory cells in the synovium, and this may prevent erosions and joint damage. There is concern that methotrexate is associated with liver damage with cumulative doses over 1.5 g. In patients with certain coexisting diseases, including alcoholic liver disease, obesity, and diabetes mellitus, the risk of liver toxicity may warrant avoidance of the drug. Monthly complete blood counts and measurement of liver enzyme and serum albumin concentrations are recommended. If there are persistent elevations of liver enzyme concentrations, or hypoalbuminemia, methotrexate should be discontinued and appropriate investigations done to determine the cause of the liver disease. Investigations might include a liver biopsy to look for evidence of early fibrosis or cirrhosis, which warrants permanent discontinuation of methotrexate. The significant risks of liver biopsy need to be explained to the patient before recommending this procedure. Other common adverse effects of methotrexate include nausea, oral ulcers, hair loss, acute pneumonitis, and bone marrow suppression.

Azathioprine is an orally active purine analog that is cytotoxic to inflammatory cells (see Chapter 15). Treatment may be necessary for 3–6 months to be clinically effective. As azathioprine can cause serious adverse effects, including bone marrow suppression and liver toxicity, close monitoring is necessary (see Chapter 28).

Cyclosporine The importance of the lymphocyte in the inflammatory response in rheumatoid arthritis provides a theoretic basis for trials of cyclosporine and its analogs in the treatment of this disease, as cyclosporine is known to influence lymphocyte function (Fig. 17.9, see Chapter 15). There is recent evidence that, despite potential toxicity, cyclosporine may control resistant synovitis in selected patients.

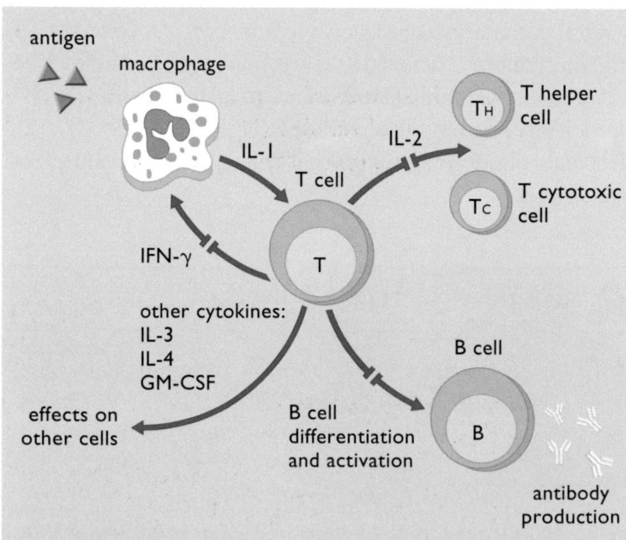

Fig. 17.9 Effects of cyclosporine on the immune system. Cyclosporine acts at a number of levels, denoted by breaks in arrows. (GM-CSF, granulocyte/macrophage colony stimulating factor; IFN-γ, interferon-γ; IL-1, interleukin-1) (Adapted with permission from *Sandorama Special 2* by Dr Gino Maulucci, Sandoz Medical Publications, 1993.)

GOUT AND OTHER TYPES OF CRYSTAL ARTHRITIS

Gout is a common disease characterized by the precipitation of monosodium urate crystals in tissues

Gout predominantly affects men in their thirties and forties, but also occurs in postmenopausal women. The clinical manifestations include acute inflammatory arthritis (acute gout), chronic articular and periarticular inflammation, uric acid, kidney stones (urolithiasis), and gouty nephropathy, which is rare. Hyperuricemia is common, but unless associated with symptoms and signs should not be treated.

Uric acid production and secretion is usually balanced to keep the tissue uric acid concentration below levels at which urates precipitate and crystals form (Fig. 17.10). Genetic and environmental factors may affect both the production and renal secretion of uric acid. Hyperuricemia is associated with obesity,

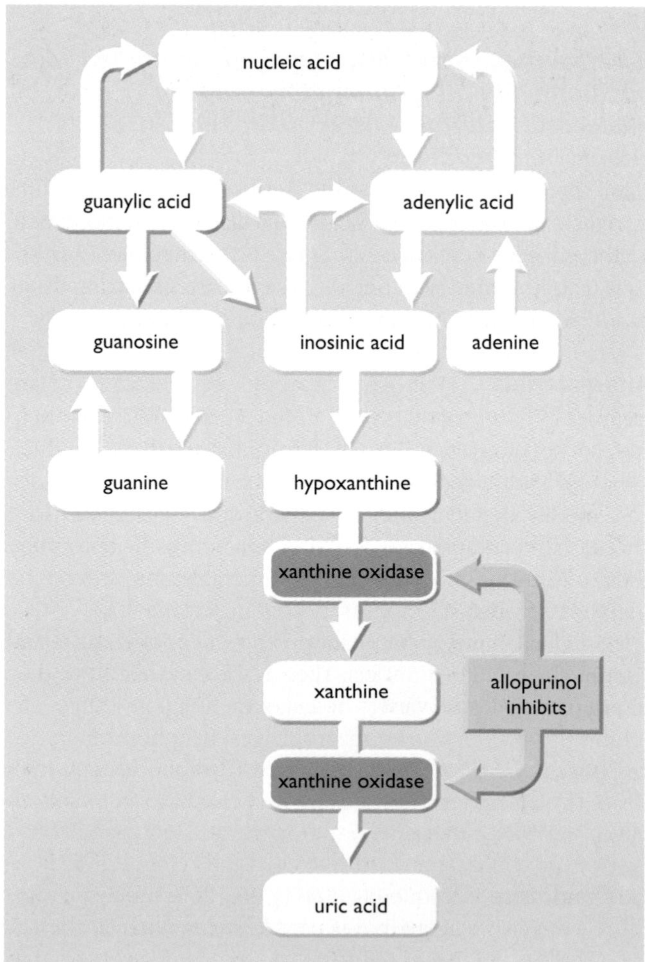

Fig. 17.10 Simplified outline of purine metabolism.

diabetes mellitus, hypertension, and renal insufficiency, and treatment with thiazide diuretics and low-dose salicylates.

Uric acid overproduction, which is seen in 10% of individuals with gout, can be associated with inherited enzyme deficiencies or myeloproliferative disorders. A reduced renal clearance of uric acid is responsible for the remaining 90% of cases.

Calcium pyrophosphate dihydrate (CPPD) deposition disease and hydroxyapatite deposition

Calcium pyrophosphate dihydrate (CPPD) deposition disease has been reported in association with a variety of conditions and may result in acute inflammation (pseudogout) or joint degeneration. Pseudogout is a relatively common disease with clinical features indistinguishable from those of acute gout. The characteristic acute inflammatory response involves neutrophils reacting to calcium pyrophosphate crystals. The tissue inflammation responds to the same medical treatment as gout.

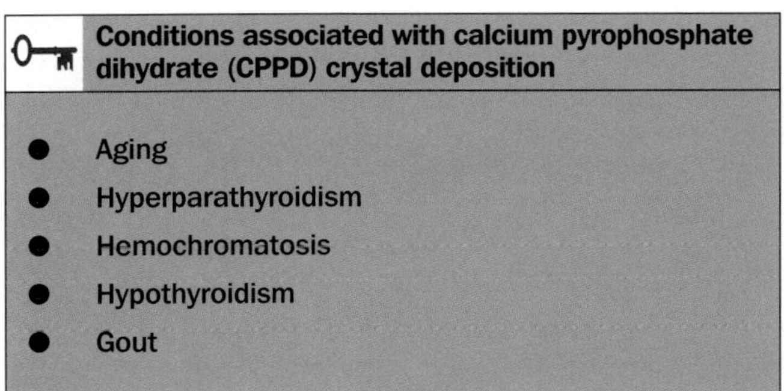

Conditions associated with calcium pyrophosphate dihydrate (CPPD) crystal deposition

- Aging
- Hyperparathyroidism
- Hemochromatosis
- Hypothyroidism
- Gout

Hydroxyapatite deposition may result in acute joint inflammation, periarticular inflammation, and subcutaneous tissue deposition. It is frequently associated with osteoarthritis, but the importance of apatite crystals in the pathogenesis of osteoarthritis is not clear.

Drugs used to treat acute crystal arthritis include nonsteroidal anti-inflammatory drugs, colchicine, and glucocorticosteroids

NSAIDs are usually started at the first sign of an acute attack of crystal arthritis and continued until the signs of inflammation resolve. Most commonly indomethacin is started in a dose of 50 mg three times a day and then slowly tapered over 10–14 days. Other NSAIDs that may be effective include diclofenac, ketoprofen, tolmetin, and naproxen. The adverse effects of NSAIDs are discussed on p. 344.

Colchicine is effective in acute gout and other types of crystal arthritis. It penetrates inflammatory cells and migrates into the microtubular system where it has a direct inhibitory action on the microtubules so the inflammatory cells lose their ability to respond. The maximal dose of 6 mg (10 tablets) over 24 hours should not be exceeded and then no further colchicine should be given for the next 7 days. Intravenous colchicine should be used rarely, if at all.

Adverse effects include gastrointestinal toxicity, with nausea, vomiting, and diarrhea in up to 80% of individuals at higher doses. Colchicine has also been associated with bone marrow suppression, renal failure, disseminated intravascular coagulation, hypocalcemia, seizures, and death. Rarely, chronic use is associated with a neuromuscular disorder resembling polymyositis.

Glucocorticosteroids may be an effective treatment in acute crystal arthritis when alternatives, including NSAIDs or colchicine, are not tolerated or are contraindicated. Options include oral prednisone or intravenous or intraarticular glucocorticosteroids. Intramuscular adrenocorticotropin hormone (ACTH, corticotropin) offers no advantage over glucocorticosteroids.

Symptomatic treatment Acute gout and pseudogout can be precipitated by major illnesses. These patients frequently cannot tolerate the above medical treatments and, as crystal arthritis is commonly a self-limited acute process, symptomatic treatment with ice, rest (splints), and simple analgesics, although less effective, is often sufficient.

Regulating serum uric acid concentrations provides an effective method of preventing recurrent episodes of gout

Initial preventive management of gout should include weight and blood pressure control, a low purine diet, and avoidance of medications that can contribute to hyperuricemia. Blood uric acid concentration can be reduced by uricosuric agents or a xanthine oxidase inhibitor.

Uricosuric agents are the treatment of choice for individuals who:

- Have diminished renal clearance of uric acid (i.e. do not overproduce uric acid).
- Do not have renal stones or renal dysfunction.
- Have had a previous reaction to a xanthine oxidase inhibitor.

Uricosuric agents block the reabsorption of filtered and secreted uric acid in the renal tubules (Fig. 17.11). They include probenecid, sulfinpyrazone, and high-dose aspirin.

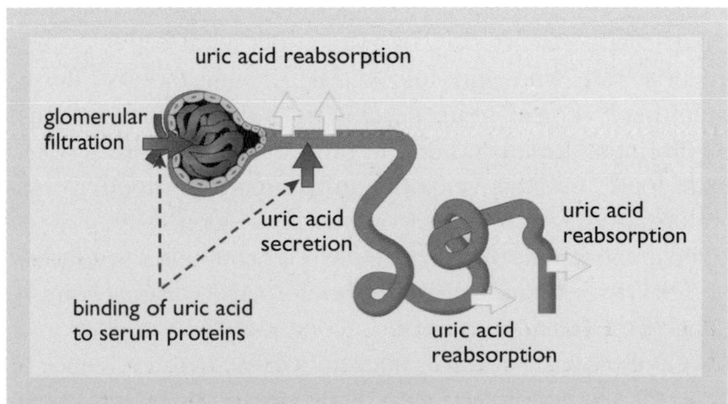

Fig. 17.11 Uric acid secretion and reabsorption in kidney. Uricosuric agents block uric acid reabsorption in the proximal tubules.

Allopurinol is a xanthine oxidase inhibitor. It competitively binds to the enzyme xanthine oxidase, which controls the last two steps in purine metabolism of both adenine and guanine to uric acid, and is indicated for lowering uric acid in patients with:

- Uric acid overproduction.
- Nephrolithiasis.

Allopurinol is commonly preferred to a uricosuric agent by patients because of the ease of administration. The typical dose is 300 mg/day orally, but may need to be increased to 600–800 mg/day. The dose must be decreased if glomerular filtration is decreased, and should be less than 200 mg/day when the creatinine clearance is 10–20 ml/min (0.17–0.33 ml/s).

The adverse effects of allopurinol are independent of the dose, and are commonly headaches, dyspepsia, and diarrhea. A pruritic rash develops in 5% of patients. Rarely, a life-threatening syndrome of allopurinol hypersensitivity may occur with fever, renal failure, and toxic epidermal necrolysis.

Allopurinol is readily absorbed, with 80% being bioavailable within 2–6 hours. It is oxidized by xanthine oxidase to oxypurinol. Both allopurinol and oxypurinol inhibit xanthine oxidase, thereby decreasing the conversion of hypoxanthine and xanthine to uric acid. These precursors of uric acid are readily soluble and excreted in the urine (see Fig. 17.10).

Drug interactions with allopurinol are common. Allopurinol interferes with:

- The metabolism of other purine analogs such as azathioprine and 6-mercaptopurine and the doses of these drugs need to be reduced by 25–50% when allopurinol is given.
- Hepatic inactivation of other drugs, including that of oral anticoagulants. Prothrombin activity must be closely monitored if allopurinol is given, and the dose of oral anticoagulant may need adjusting.
- Treatment with theophylline, leading to increased accumulation of the active metabolite of theophylline. In addition, plasma theophylline concentration may be increased.

SYSTEMIC LUPUS ERYTHEMATOSUS

Systemic lupus erythematosus (SLE) is a relatively common autoimmune disease that affects approximately 1 in 1000 individuals. It is more prevalent in young females. Its associated morbidity and mortality are decreasing in most parts of the world as a result of early recognition and treatment. Its associated complications are higher in poorer socioeconomic groups, and the incidence of SLE is higher in black, Hispanic, and oriental individuals. SLE is characterized by a variety of clinical features, which include skin and musculoskeletal manifestations. Renal, pulmonary, serosal, neuropsychiatric and reticuloendothelial involvement are less common, but potentially more serious. Pathologic findings include inflammation, blood vessel abnormalities, and immune complex deposition.

The immunologic disturbance includes antibodies to a variety of 'self' tissues. Antinuclear antibodies (ANA) against components of the cell nucleus are most common. The contribution of ANA to the clinical events is unclear because of the presence of antibodies in nondisease states and because the target antigen in the nucleus would normally be protected from antibody binding. The immune disturbance promotes B cell hyperactivity to both self and foreign antigens. Activation of an antibody response to a foreign antigen such as a virus may be a triggering mechanism.

Treatment of systemic lupus erythematosus involves anti-inflammatory and immunosuppressive drugs

Glucocorticosteroids The symptoms and signs of acute inflammation in the skin and joints in SLE are readily treated with glucocorticosteroids (Fig. 17.12). Options include:

- Topical preparations for inflammatory rashes.
- Low-dose oral therapy for mild disease.
- Higher-dose oral or pulse intravenous infusions for severe and life-threatening disease.

The mechanism of action of glucocorticosteroids is unclear. They have a direct effect on the bone marrow cells, resulting in demargination of circulating neutrophils (neutrophilia) and at the same time, leukopenia, with fewer circulating eosinophils and monocytes. At high doses, glucocorticosteroids inhibit cytokine release and action. They have minimal effect on lymphokine production and cytotoxic, helper, and suppressor activity of T cells. High-dose glucocorticosteroids may act by inducing the synthesis of a peptide that inhibits phospholipase A_2, which controls both prostaglandin and leukotriene production (see Chapter 11).

The dose is chosen to minimize the risk of adverse effects yet provide adequate drug to suppress the inflammatory response. Oral prednisone or prednisolone is used in preference to other longer-acting oral drugs such as dexamethasone and is usually given in a single morning dose. Prednisone is available in convenient doses (5 mg tablets) to facilitate dose increases or reductions. Adverse effects of glucocorticosteroids include skin thinning and bruising, central obesity, muscle wasting, hypertension, glucose intolerance, and osteoporosis.

Antimalarials are particularly effective treatment for the manifestations of SLE, cutaneous lesions, and inflammatory arthritis. Once they have been started and have produced

Classification of drugs used for systemic lupus erythematosus

Mild disease	Nonsteroidal anti-inflammatory drugs Glucocorticosteroids (low-dose prednisone) Antimalarials Methotrexate
Severe disease	Glucocorticosteroids (high-dose prednisone, methylprednisolone) Azathioprine Alkylating agents (cyclophosphamide)
Investigational	Cyclosporine Immune globulin

Fig. 17.12 Classification of drugs used for systemic lupus erythematosus.

clinical benefit, their discontinuation may result in a recurrence of disease manifestations. Antimalarial drugs include hydroxychloroquine, quinacrine, and chloroquine. The first two drugs are used extensively in many countries, while chloroquine is a less expensive but less well tested alternative. The relative safety of antimalarials makes them attractive drugs for early intervention. Their mechanism of action is described on p. 345. Common adverse effects include nonspecific symptoms, cutaneous rashes, and gastrointestinal complaints. Less frequently there are CNS reactions. Retinal toxicity is the major clinical concern, but is rarely seen at low doses of antimalarials. Visual field and color vision should be tested at baseline and then every 6 months (see Chapter 19).

Azathioprine is widely used for many of the manifestations of SLE including renal disease to reduce requirements for glucocorticosteroids. Azathioprine reduces inflammation in lupus nephritis and improves renal function. However, it has significant adverse effects, including bone marrow suppression, so monthly blood counts should be obtained. Significant hepatic toxicity has been observed, but is usually reversible if the medication is discontinued. It is not clear whether azathioprine increases the risk of malignancy, particularly hematopoietic and lymphoreticular malignancy.

Azathioprine is a derivative of 6-mercaptopurine. It acts by inhibiting cellular replication by reducing purine synthesis. It is selective primarily for T cell responses and has little effect on antibody responses at doses of less than 4 mg/kg/day.

Alkylating agents are the most effective agents after glucocorticosteroids for treating life-threatening SLE (Fig. 17.13). They inhibit the activation and division of inflammatory cells (see Chapter 15). Cyclophosphamide is an alkylating agent that kills both T and B lymphocytes. It is commonly used with other agents for cancer chemotherapy. At lower daily doses or monthly pulse intravenous doses it preferentially inhibits B lymphocytes. Cyclophosphamide is the most studied alkylating agent and may be given as a daily oral dose or a monthly intravenous bolus.

Cyclophosphamide is usually added to high-dose glucocorticosteroids to treat severe SLE that is either life threatening or does not respond to glucocorticosteroids and azathioprine. The dose of glucocorticosteroid should be reduced slowly following clinical improvement. Cyclophosphamide is a more effective treatment of diffuse lupus nephritis than other treatments.

Cyclophosphamide has significant adverse effects. Common effects include nausea, alopecia, and bone marrow suppression. Monthly blood monitoring is recommended to detect drug-related leukopenia. Cyclophosphamide may also produce gonadal failure with decreased ovarian function and azoospermia. It is therefore not recommended for individuals who may want to have children in the future if other treatments are available. However, if cyclophosphamide is given to a young individual and time permits, sperm or embryo storage should be considered and discussed with the patient and family. Cyclophosphamide is also associated with an increased risk of malignancy, and has been associated with cutaneous, bladder, hematopoietic, and lymphoreticular malignancies. Furthermore, acrolein, a final metabolite of cyclophosphamide, may accumulate within the bladder and cause mucosal inflammation and bleeding. Such injury can be minimized by encouraging a high fluid intake to irrigate the bladder or giving acetylcysteine or other sulfhydryl compounds to bind acrolein.

SERONEGATIVE SPONDYLOARTHROPATHIES

Seronegative spondyloarthropathies are a group of inflammatory types of arthritis characterized by common clinical features and associated to a varying degree with the HLA-B27 gene. Sacroiliitis is the characteristic lesion and the disorders include

Drugs affecting inflammation and the immune system

	Disease indication	Adverse effects
Antimalarials	RA, SLE	Retinopathy
Gold salts	RA	Dermatitis GI symptoms Proteinuria
Penicillamine	RA, scleroderma	Dermatitis GI symptoms Proteinuria
Methotrexate	RA, psoriasis Polymyositis Dermatomyositis SLE	Myelosuppression Pneumonitis Ulcerations Hepatotoxicity
Sulfasalazine	RA Inflammatory bowel disease	Dermatitis GI symptoms Hepatitis
Azathioprine	RA, SLE Polymyositis Transplantation	Myelosuppression GI symptoms Hepatotoxicity
Cyclophosphamide	Vasculitis SLE	Myelosuppression Alopecia GI symptoms Infertility Hemorrhagic cystitis Malignancy
Cyclosporine	RA Transplantation SLE Psoriasis Uveitis	Hypertension Renal toxicity Neurotoxicity Hepatotoxicity
Glucocorticosteroids	RA SLE Transplantation Vasculitis Connective tissue disease	Cushing's syndrome Osteoporosis Cataracts Ulcers

Fig. 17.13 Drugs affecting inflammation and the immune system. (GI, gastrointestinal; RA, rheumatoid arthritis; SLE, systemic lupus erythematosus)

ankylosing spondylitis, psoriatic arthritis, reactive arthritis, and the arthritis associated with inflammatory bowel disease.

Pathologically, granulation tissue erodes the fibrocartilaginous joint, resulting eventually in ossification and possible bony fusion. Inflammation similar to the inflammatory process of rheumatoid arthritis may involve the peripheral synovial joints. Enthesitis (inflammation of tendinous insertions to bone) is another characteristic feature. Extra-articular features include ocular inflammation, cutaneous inflammation, and occasionally cardiac involvement.

Nonsteroidal anti-inflammatory drugs are the most widely used drugs for treating the inflammation of seronegative spondyloarthropathies.

The most effective NSAIDs, including indomethacin, diclofenac, naproxen, and tolmetin, are recommended first. Other NSAIDs may be effective and can be tried if the above are not effective or are associated with adverse effects. Although various clinical trials suggest that certain NSAIDs are more effective than others, clinical experience and familiarity with doses is probably more important than selecting any one NSAID.

Other agents Glucocorticosteroids do not affect the long-term outcome of seronegative spondyloarthropathies, but might be beneficial in low doses to control symptoms. Sulfasalazine, which is frequently used to treat rheumatoid arthritis, may control the peripheral arthritis (see p. 345). All agents used to treat rheumatoid arthritis can be used to treat psoriatic arthritis.

MUSCULOSKELETAL INFECTIONS

Septic arthritis

Septic arthritis is characterized by fever, pain, swelling, and a reduced joint range. In sexually active individuals there should be a high index of suspicion for *Neisseria gonorrhoeae*. Otherwise, most cases are caused by Gram-positive organisms (*Staphylococcus aureus* and streptococci, Fig. 17.14). Important host factors include:

- Underlying joint disease (rheumatoid arthritis, osteoarthritis).
- Chronic illnesses (diabetes mellitus, chronic renal failure).
- Alcohol abuse.
- Drugs (glucocorticosteroids, cytotoxics, intravenous drug abuse).
- Extra-articular infections (urinary tract, skin).

Most joint infections are single, but 20% are polyarticular.

Organisms causing septic arthritis

Non-gonococcal	Gram-positive (65–85%) Gram-negative bacilli (10–15%) Mixed aerobic and anaerobic (5%) Mycobacteria and fungi (<5%)
Neisseria gonorrhoeae	

Fig. 17.14 Organisms causing septic arthritis.

Early effective management is important to prevent muscle contractures and, more importantly, joint destruction

If infection is suspected, the joint should be aspirated early and the aspirated fluid sent for Gram stain, culture, and cell count. Treatment involves the use of appropriate antibiotics and an effective method of drainage (e.g. arthroscopy, arthrotomy, repeated needle aspiration). Antibiotics need to be started immediately after early joint aspiration. Initial selection should be based on the patient's age and any associated diseases, and the Gram stain. The regimen can be adjusted at 24–48 hours when the culture results are available, and later modified when the sensitivities are known. Suggested initial antibiotic regimens include:

- Intravenous methicillin or cloxacillin ± intravenous aminoglycoside.
- Intravenous imipenen.
- Intravenous ceftriaxone (see Chapter 23).

Parenteral antibiotics produce excellent synovial and intra-articular antibiotic levels. Intra-articular antibiotics are not needed.

The duration of therapy is determined by the clinical response, the effectiveness of drainage, and the organism. Streptococcal infection can usually be effectively treated with 2 weeks of intravenous therapy followed by 2–4 weeks of oral high-dose treatment. Staphylococcal infections may require longer treatment. Good clinical studies comparing short versus long (i.e. 2–6 weeks) of intravenous antibiotic therapy are not available.

Osteomyelitis

Bacteria can invade bone in a variety of ways: as a result of direct trauma, surgery, or extension from a soft tissue infection, and in the blood. The resulting osteomyelitis may present acutely, subacutely, or chronically with bone pain, fever, and leukocytosis. Patients with sickle cell disease are 100 times more likely to present with osteomyelitis than the general population. Bone destruction with periosteal elevation may be seen radiographically. Abscess and sinus formation may occur. A bone scan is the most commonly used primary diagnostic tool for evaluating osteomyelitis in both adults and children. The diagnosis is often made late clinically so it is important to recognize early imaging findings.

Treatment includes:

- Splinting to prevent fractures.
- Consideration of surgical drainage.
- Intravenous antibiotics.

Prosthetic joint infections

Prosthetic joint infections are increasingly common, but are difficult to diagnose and treat. Over 100,000 total hip replacements are carried out each year in the US and one of the main clinical concerns is the risk of bacterial infection of the prosthetic implant. Such an infection may occur early postoperatively (i.e. within a year) or be a late complication and result from a bacteremia. Skin contaminants are isolated from early postoperative infection (i.e. *Staphylococcus epidermidis*, *S. aureus*, anaerobes). Late infections are usually due to staphylococci, streptococci and Gram-negative bacilli. There is increasing concern about the emergence of methicillin-resistant *S. aureus* (MRSA).

All bacteriologically confirmed infections should be treated with high-dose intravenous antibiotics, appropriate surgical debridement, and reimplantation

Six weeks of high-dose intravenous antibiotics alone results in low rates of cure (i.e. less than 20%). Adding antibiotic to the cement at the time of revision surgery may be beneficial. Results are further improved by carrying out a two-stage revision procedure, with a temporary prosthesis for 6 weeks to several months and then permanent reimplantation.

Prophylactic perioperative antistaphylococcal antibiotics are believed to prevent infection if used in a short course starting immediately before surgery and continuing 24–72 hours after surgery. In addition, antibiotics are often used empirically in the first 3–6 months following joint replacement to prevent prosthetic joint infection with procedures such as dental surgery and genitourinary manipulation, but this topic needs further study.

FURTHER READING

Favus MJ (ed.) *Primer of Metabolic Bone Diseases and Disorders of Mineral Metabolism 2e*. New York: Raven Press; 1993. [A good review of current treatment of osteoporosis, which also reviews uncommon bone disorders.]

Schumacher Jr HR (ed.) *Primer on the Rheumatic Diseases 10e*. Atlanta, Georgia: Arthritis Foundation; 1993. [A comprehensive and practical reference for primary care physicians and specialists.]

Make a provisional diagnosis and determine a rational pharmacologic treatment for the following hypothetical case.

A 42-year-old single mother comes to you with a 6-month history of pain and swelling in her wrists, hands, and feet. Recently she has noticed nodules over both her elbows. She reports that she has ringing in her ears because she is taking so much aspirin. She is concerned that she will be unable to run her small store. On examination the patient has synovitis affecting her wrists, metacarpophalangeal, proximal interphalangeal, and metatarsophalangeal joints as well as subcutaneous nodules.

1. Discuss appropriate management regarding the aspirin she is taking and other NSAIDs you might consider.
2. Discuss the advantages/disadvantages of starting low-dose glucocorticosteroids.
3. After being on intramuscular gold injections for 20 weeks she has had no clinical response. Discuss the available options.
4. Finally, after starting 12 weeks of methotrexate (10 mg po) given weekly, she is starting to improve but her hepatocellular liver enzymes increase to twice their normal levels. Explain why.

Indicate which is the correct answer for each question.

1. The most effective treatment to prevent early severe post-menopausal osteoporosis is
a) Ca^{2+} alone
b) Ca^{2+} and hormone replacement therapy
c) Ca^{2+} and calcitonin
d) Ca^{2+} and bisphosphonates

2. Glucocorticosteroids have the following effects, except
a) cushingoid features
b) osteoporosis
c) inhibition of the inflammatory response
d) increased high density lipoprotein (HDL) cholesterol

3. Methotrexate has the following significant adverse effects, except
a) liver toxicity
b) bone marrow suppression
c) acute pneumonitis
d) deposition in the retina resulting in visual loss

4. Nonsteroidal anti-inflammatory drugs have the following effects, except
a) analgesia
b) antipyretic
c) anti-inflammatory
d) decrease erosions in rheumatoid arthritis

5. Appropriate treatment for acute gouty arthritis in a man with congestive heart failure and renal insufficiency might include
a) rest, ice, and simple analgesics
b) allopurinol
c) indomethacin
d) high-dose intravenous colchicine

6. A woman with longstanding well-controlled rheumatoid arthritis presents with an acute painful swollen knee and a high fever. Reasonable management would include
a) injecting the knee with intraarticular glucocorticosteroids
b) changing medication to a more effective nonsteroidal anti-inflammatory drug
c) aspirating fluid from the knee to look for crystals and for culture and starting oral colchicine
d) aspirating fluid from the knee to look for crystals and for culture and starting intravenous antibiotics

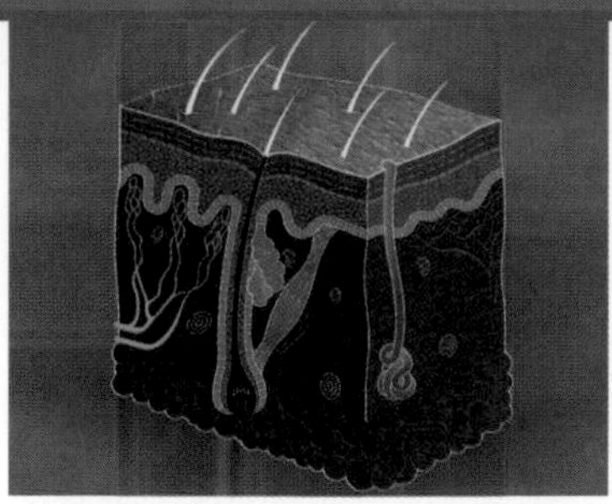

18. Drugs and the Skin

PHYSIOLOGY OF THE SKIN

Skin protects the body against the environment and prevents excessive loss of protein, electrolytes, water, and heat. It is one of the largest organs, with a surface area of approximately 1.8 m^2 and accounting for 16% of body weight. It is composed of epidermis, dermis, and subcutis (Fig. 18.1).

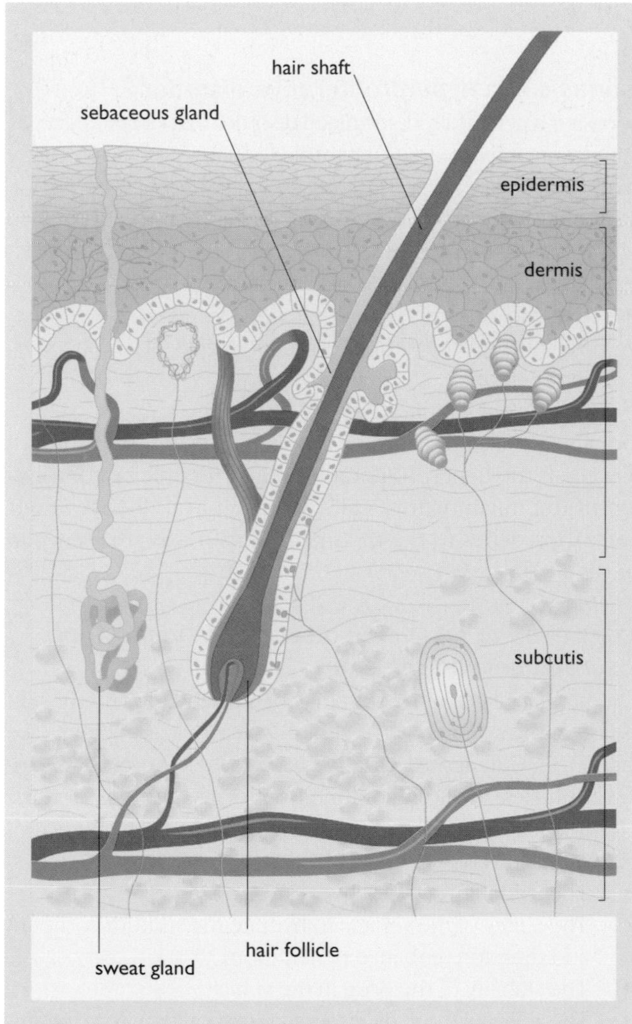

Fig. 18.1 Skin is composed of three layers. The most superficial layer of the skin is the epidermis, which varies in thickness from site to site. Beneath this lies the dermis composed of collagen and some elastic fibers. The subcutis is the deepest layer of the skin and consists mainly of adipose tissue intersected by fibrocollagenous septa.

PATHOPHYSIOLOGY AND DISEASES OF THE SKIN

The treatment of skin damage produced by trauma or disease is aimed at:

- Healing or eliminating the disease.
- Replacing or amplifying normal skin function.

Skin treatment preparations therefore include:

- Preparations aimed at the specific disease state.
- Preparations that increase protection from the environment and prevent loss of protein, electrolytes, water, and heat.

Although skin disease can be disfiguring and affect the quality of life, it is rarely life threatening. The risk–benefit ratio of any treatment must be considered when deciding on therapy. There are a number of skin disorders for which there is no safe and effective treatment, but under such circumstances the importance of camouflage creams and wigs must not be overlooked.

SKIN DISEASES

Skin disease is a common reason for seeking medical advice and accounts for 1–2% of all consultations in general practice. The most common skin complaints are dermatitis and eczema (5%), acne (1%), urticaria (1%), and psoriasis (0.5%). Viral warts account for over 1% and skin cancer for approximately 0.1% per year.

Eczema and dermatitis describe a pattern of inflammation in the skin

Eczema and dermatitis are interchangeable terms and describe a pattern of inflammation in the skin characterized by the presence of intercellular edema (spongiosis) in the epidermis rather than a single disease (Fig. 18.2). Many causes are recognized and include:

- Exogenous irritants and contact allergens.
- Infections.
- Atopy.
- Drugs.
- Environmental influences such as low humidity, friction, and ultraviolet light.
- Local factors such as venous stasis.

Approaches to the treatment of eczema are shown in Fig. 18.2.

Acne is a disease of the pilosebaceous unit

Acne is characterized by comedones (keratin plugs in the sebaceous duct opening), inflammatory papules, pustules, nodules, cysts, and scars. The rash occurs where there is a high density

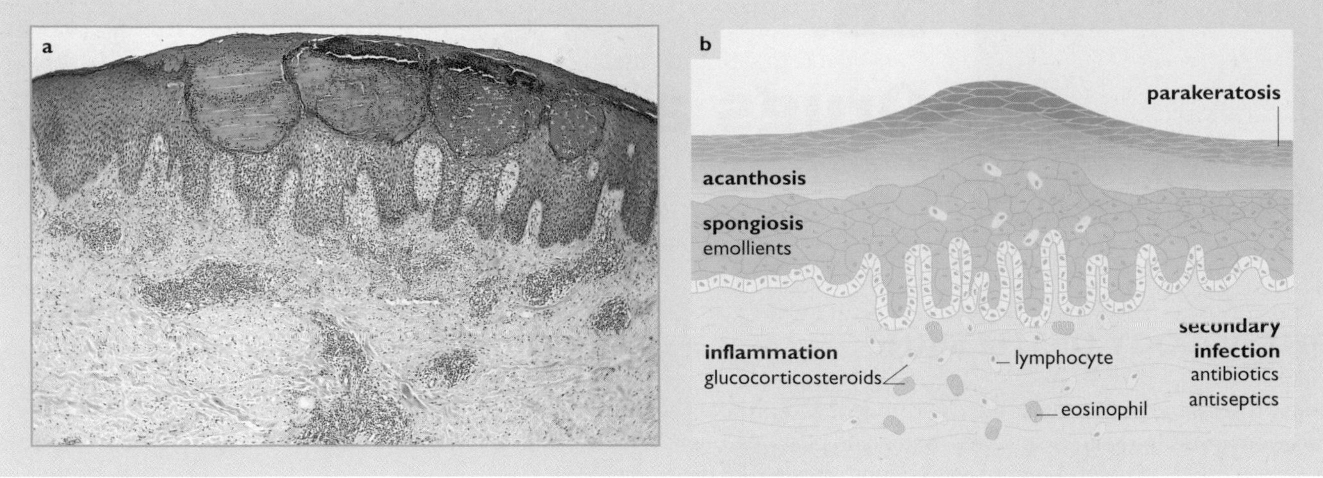

Fig. 18.2 Eczema. (a) Eczema is characterized histologically by epidermal spongiosis, permeated by an inflammatory infiltrate, predominantly of monocytes. (Courtesy of Dr P. McKee.) (b) Sites of drug action in eczema: Emollients help to reduce transepidermal water loss, which is increased as a result of spongiosis; glucocorticosteroids are anti-inflammatory and vasoconstricting and reduce keratinocyte cell division.

of pilosebaceous glands (e.g. on the face, back, and chest). Androgenic stimulation of the sebaceous glands at puberty accounts for the high prevalence of acne at puberty, and the active pilosebaceous follicles are heavily colonized by *Propionibacterium acnes*. The mechanism for keratin plug formation is poorly understood, but is thought to be pivotal. Continued gland secretion then results in swelling of the glands and ducts, with nodule and cyst formation and the induction of an inflammatory response, which produces inflammatory papules and pustules. Approaches to the treatment of acne are shown in Fig. 18.3.

Treatment of acne

- Keratolytics should be used as first-line therapy
- If a systemic antibiotic is needed, tetracyclines are indicated in children over 12 years of age, but should not be given to children under 12 because of their effects on maturing teeth
- Oxytetracycline should be given before minocycline because of the rare reaction to minocycline involving liver, joints, and fever
- In children under 12 years of age erythromycin is the systemic drug of choice
- In adults, tetracyclines should be given in preference to erythromycin as erythromycin is used for life-threatening infections such as *Mycoplasma pneumoniae*
- Antibiotic resistance to *Propionibacterium acnes* is as high as 40% in patients with acne referred to hospital

Psoriasis is a hyperproliferative disorder

Psoriasis is a genetically determined disorder that can be triggered by infection, trauma, drugs, ultraviolet light, and stress, and rarely by hypocalcemia.

Psoriatic skin turns over in 7 days rather than the normal 56 days. It is characterized by:

- Thickened skin plaques with superficial scales.
- Capillary dilatation in the papillary dermis.
- An inflammatory infiltrate, predominantly of lymphocytes, in the dermis.
- A neutrophil infiltrate in the epidermis.

The capillary dilatation may be an initiating event or an attempt to nourish the hyperproliferating skin. The precise contribution of the inflammatory cells to the clinical disease is not clear. Approaches to the treatment of psoriasis are shown in Fig. 18.4.

Drugs used to treat skin disease are ideally not absorbed beyond the skin

Treatment applied to the skin may be designed for use in skin disease or the skin may act as a transdermal delivery system (see Chapter 5). Cutaneously applied drugs are delivered by a variety of vehicles, including ointments, creams, pastes, powders, aerosols, gels, lotions, and tinctures (Fig. 18.5). The choice of vehicle depends on:

- The solubility of the active drug.
- The ability of the vehicle to hydrate the stratum corneum and therefore enhance penetration.
- The stability of the drug in the vehicle.
- The ability of the vehicle to retard evaporation from the surface of the skin. This is greatest for ointments, and least for tinctures.

However, absorption of the drug depends on:

- Body site (e.g. drug absorption is low from the palms and soles, higher from the scalp and face, and very high from the scrotum and vulva).
- Skin hydration (e.g. oil-in-water emulsions and occlusive dressings).
- Skin condition (e.g. damage due to inflammation or burns increases absorption).

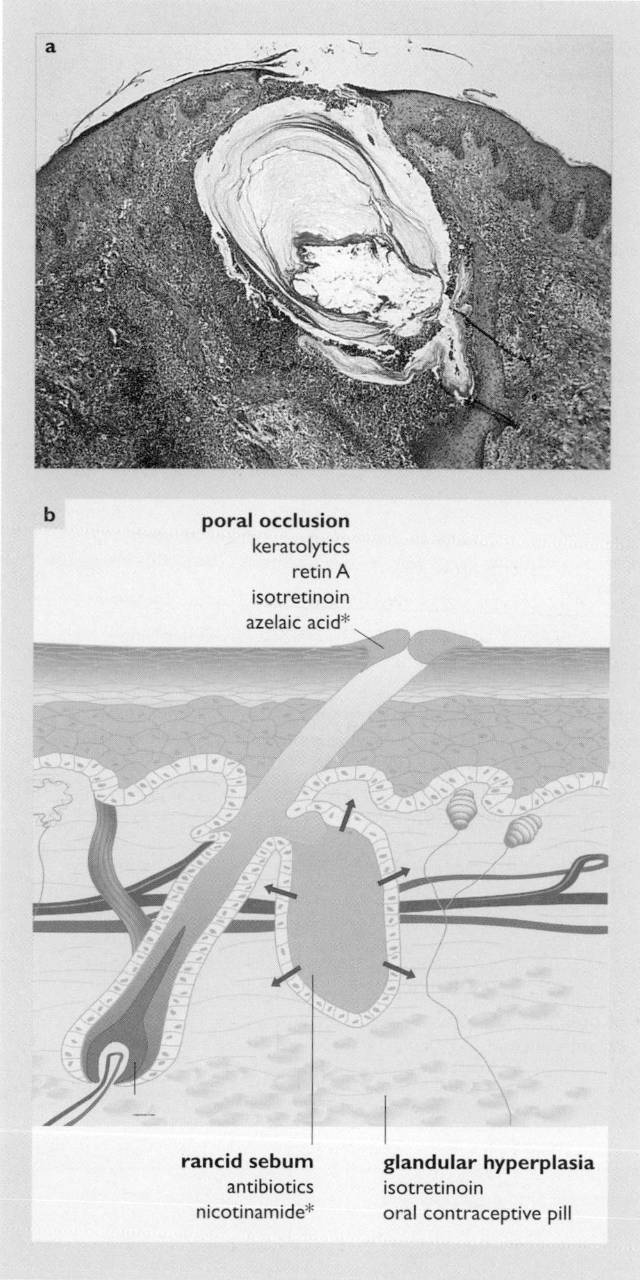

Fig. 18.3 Acne. (a) Histologically, acne is characterized by keratin plugs (comedones) which block the sebaceous follicle, so that sebum cannot escape. The sebaceous glands are often hyperplastic, and there can be an intense neutrophil influx. (Courtesy of Dr P. McKee.) (b) Sites of drug action in acne.

Increasing the concentration gradient across the skin, increases the mass of drug transferred per unit time. The ability of the skin to act as a reservoir for drugs must be considered when determining dosing schedules, as drugs with a short systemic half-life may have a longer local half-life in the skin.

Although topical treatment is attractive for treating skin disease, in terms of the risk–benefit ratio, many conditions require systemic therapy. The retinoids were specifically designed to treat skin diseases, but many other systemic agents used in the treatment of skin disease were originally developed for other conditions.

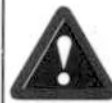 **Occlusive dressings and 'wet wraps'**

- An occlusive dressing can increase the absorption of a drug tenfold and can therefore lead to serious systemic toxicity
- The adverse effects of increased drug absorption must be considered when 'wet wraps' are used for eczema because the eroded stratum corneum is a further source of increased absorption

DRUGS THAT PROTECT THE SKIN FROM ENVIRONMENTAL DAMAGE

SUNSCREENS

The growing incidence of melanoma and nonmelanoma skin cancers and skin aging has been associated with exposure to ultraviolet light. Sunburn before 10 years of age is a major risk factor for malignant melanoma. Photosensitivity can be a manifestation of some diseases and the use of certain drugs. These conditions are best prevented by sun avoidance or using physical barriers to solar penetration, such as clothing. If exposure is unavoidable chemical sunscreens can be used to minimize exposure.

Sunscreens are classified as either absorbent or reflectant:

- Absorbent sunscreens are photo-absorbing chemicals and can be categorized according to their predominant active wavelength (Fig. 18.6).
- Reflectant suncreens are inert minerals such as titanium dioxide, zinc oxide, red petroleum, and calamine, which are cosmetically less attractive because they are greasy and sticky and do not vanish on the skin.

Commercial preparations contain these ingredients in various proportions.

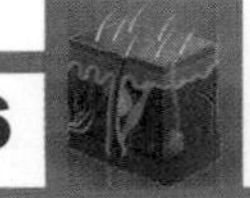

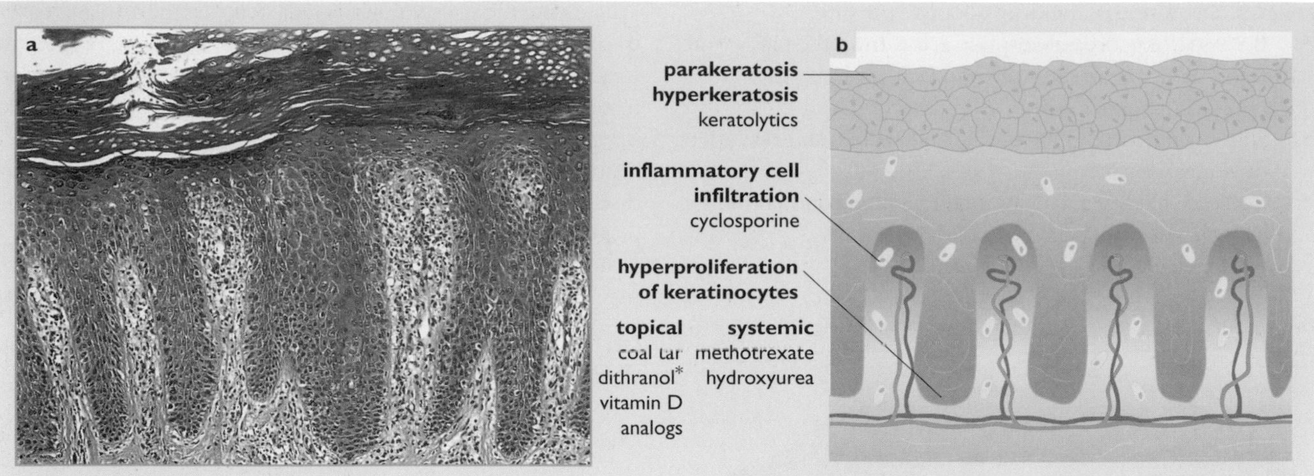

Fig. 18.4 Psoriasis. (a) Psoriasis is characterized by epidermal acanthosis, with clubbed papillae, suprapapillary thinning with dilatation of the capillaries, and hyper- and parakeratosis. Lymphocytes predominate in the dermis, whereas neutrophils may form microabscesses in the epidermis. (Courtesy of Dr P. McKee.) (b) Sites of drug action in psoriasis.

Vehicles used for topically applied skin preparations

Vehicle	Physical and chemical properties	Use	Commercial examples
Ointments	Thicker than creams		
Water-soluble	Mixtures of polyethylene glycols to form macrogels; consistency can be varied; easily washed off	Lubricants; burn dressings; to improve the penetration of active drugs (e.g. hydrocortisone) into the skin	Macrogels and polyethylene glycol mixtures
Emulsifying	Allow evaporation; mix with water and skin exudate		Emulsifying ointment
Nonemulsifying	Do not mix with water; act as occlusive dressings, therefore enhancing hydration and drug penetration, and softening crusts, but preventing evaporation and heat loss	Chronic dry skin conditions, but are difficult to remove except with oil or detergents, and are rather messy and inconvenient	Paraffin* ointment Simple ointment
Creams	Emulsion of oil in water or water in oil		
Oil in water	Vanish easily; washable; mix with serous discharge. Some contain a surface tension reducing agent	Cosmetically acceptable; a vehicle for water-soluble substances	Aqueous cream, cetomacroglycol
Water in oil	Act like oils (i.e. do not mix with serous discharge and aid skin hydration)	More cosmetically acceptable than ointments because they vanish easily, and are easy to apply; can be used on hairy areas; a vehicle for fat-soluble substances	Oily cream, zinc cream
Pastes	Thick, semi-occlusive ointment containing insoluble powders; very adhesive and can absorb some discharge		Zinc compound paste
Powders	Absorbent, but can cause crusting if applied to exudates; reduce friction between skin surfaces and have a cooling effect by increasing the effective surface area of the skin	A vehicle for antifungal powders	Zinc starch, talc
Gels	Semi-solid colloidal solutions or suspensions		
Lotions	Main component is water; evaporation of the water cools the skin and the subsequent vasoconstriction reduces inflammation	Can be used in hairy areas and in the presence of exudation	
Shake lotions	A means of applying powder to the skin, with additional cooling due to evaporation	Should not be used if there is much exudate	Calamine* lotion

Fig. 18.5 Vehicles used for topically applied skin preparations.

In practice, the sun protection of a sunscreen is about half that suggested by the skin protection factor (SPF)

The efficacy of a sunscreen is expressed as the skin protection factor (SPF), which is the ratio of the time required to produce minimal erythema with a sunscreen to the time required to produce minimal erythema without a sunscreen. However, the amount of drug applied in the laboratory to determine such protection is much greater per unit area than the same amount applied in practice; it is difficult to make allowances for loss of the sunscreen with sweating and swimming. The sun protection of a sunscreen is about half that suggested by the SPF in practise, therefore:

- If the SPF is less than 10, the sunscreen is only mild.
- If the SPF is 10–15, the sunscreen is moderate.
- If the SPF is higher than 15, the sunscreen will provide appreciable protection.
- If the SPF is higher than 25, the sunscreen will provide almost full protection, as required by patients with photosensitivity.

Sunscreen preparations have been refined to increase cosmetic acceptability, water resistance, durability, and effectiveness. However, the active ingredients, the base, the fragrances, and the stabilizers can all cause irritant, allergic, phototoxic, or photoallergic adverse reactions.

ANTIVIRAL AGENTS

Currently available antiviral agents are active against herpes viruses, but do not eliminate them, and must be given early (see Chapter 23).

Acyclovir

Acyclovir is a synthetic guanine analog. It is phosphorylated by viral thymidine kinase and in its triphosphate form interferes with herpesvirus DNA polymerase, leading to abnormal viral DNA replication (Fig. 18.7). It reduces viral shedding time and may aid healing. Acyclovir is available for topical use in the treatment of:

- Primary herpes simplex infections (e.g. cold sores, genital herpes).
- Limited mucocutaneous herpes in immunocompromised patients.

Absorbent sunscreens and the predominant wavelength screened

Sunscreen	Wavelength
Cinnamates	UVB
para-Aminobenzoic acid	UVB
Salicylates	UVB
Benzophenones	UVA
Camphor	UVA
Dibenzoylmethane	UVA
Aminobenzoates (padimate O)	UVB
Anthralin	UVA

Fig. 18.6 Absorbent sunscreens and the predominant wavelength screened. (Ultraviolet [UV] A, 320–360 nm; UVB, 290–320 nm)

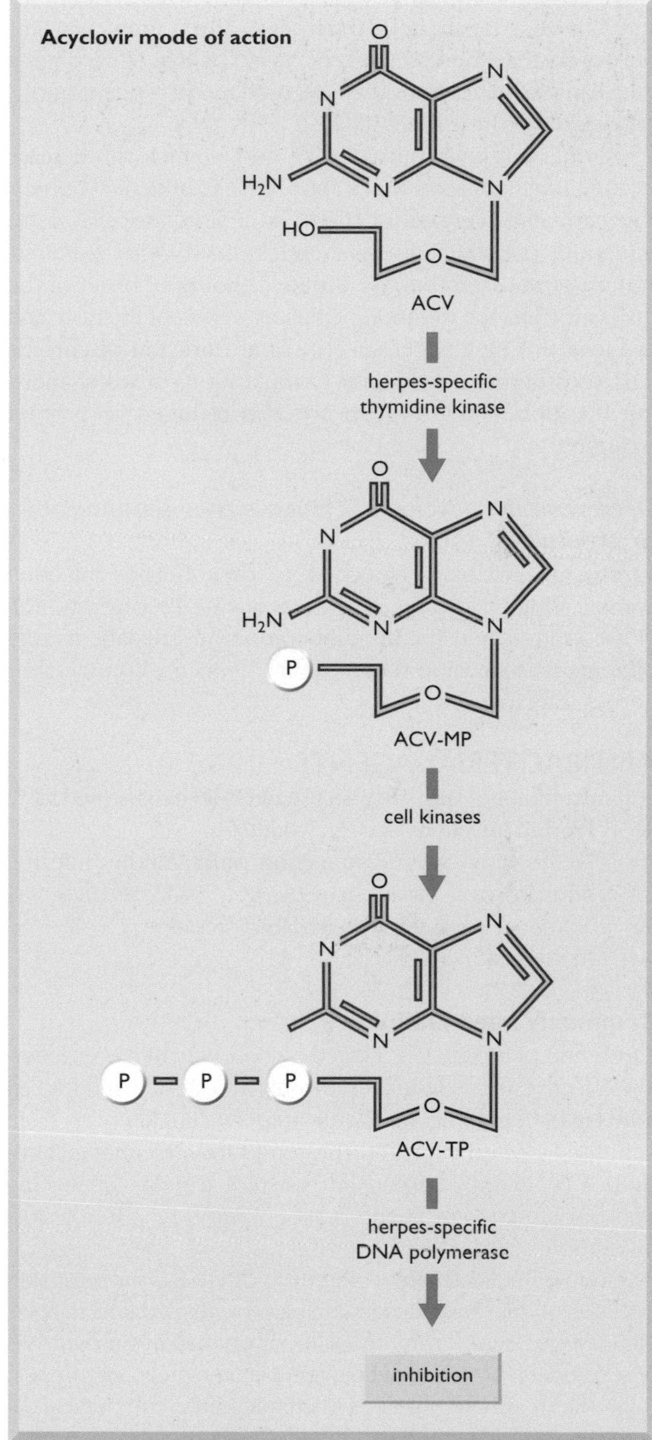

Fig. 18.7 Mechanism of action of acyclovir. Acyclovir is phosphorylated by the virus-specific thymidine kinase. Its triphosphate form interferes with herpesvirus DNA polymerase, inhibiting its replication.

Penciclovir is a more recent topical treatment for herpes labialis. There is no convincing evidence that topical acyclovir has a role in recurrent herpes simplex infections in immunocompetent patients.

The effectiveness of oral acyclovir is limited by its poor bioavailability

This has been partly overcome the use of a prodrug, valaciclovir*, which is metabolized in the liver to valine and acyclovir with a bioavailability of 54%. Valaciclovir* is administered twice a day for genital herpes or three times a day for herpes zoster, whereas acyclovir has to be taken five times a day. Famciclovir is another new oral antiviral agent and is administered three times a day.

Systemic acyclovir, valaciclovir*, and famciclovir decrease healing time and sometimes abort attacks of genital herpes. They are also licensed for the treatment of varicella zoster infections (i.e. chickenpox, shingles). In shingles, administration of antiviral therapy within 72 hours of onset of the rash, shortens the duration of pain as well as of the rash, and reduces the incidence, severity, and duration of chronic pain (postherpetic neuralgia). Complications of zoster affecting the ophthalmic branch are also reduced by prompt treatment.

Occasionally, acyclovir is given either parenterally or prophylactically

Parenteral acyclovir is needed to treat herpes infection complicating eczema (eczema herpeticum). Prophylactic acyclovir is indicated for immunocompromised patients and patients who develop recurrent erythema multiforme after herpes infections.

ANTIBACTERIAL AGENTS

Topical antibiotics (Fig. 18.8, see Chapter 24) can be used to:

- Prevent infections of clean wounds.
- Treat early wound infection and mildly infected dermatoses.
- To reduce nasal staphylococcal colonization.
- In the treatment of acne.

Commonly used antibiotics

Parenteral penicillin G followed by oral pencillin V is generally effective for cellulitis. Erythromycin can be used for cellulitis in patients who are allergic to penicillin. Recovery from cellulitis is often slow and the temptation to change antibiotics repeatedly should be resisted. A delay in starting appropriate therapy is the most common reason for slow resolution.

Systemic flucloxacillin* is the drug of choice for most skin infections, while systemic tetracyclines (oxytetracycline, minocycline, doxycycline), trimethoprim, or erythromycin (which is best reserved for women who might become pregnant) are useful in the treatment of acne. Oral tetracyclines and metronidazole are also used in the treatment of rosacea.

ANTIFUNGAL AGENTS

There are many topical and systemic antifungal agents for the treatment of skin, hair, and nail infections with fungi and yeasts (see Chapter 26).

ANTISEPTIC AGENTS

These may obviate the need for antibiotics.

- Chlorhexidine, benzalkonium chloride, triclosan*, and potassium permanganate solution (1 in 10,000 dilution) can be used as antiseptic skin cleansers.
- Cetrimide* has both disinfectant and detergent properties.
- Hydrogen peroxide can be used to disinfect deep wounds and ulcers.
- Streptokinase–streptodornase and dextranomer preparations aid ulcer desloughing, which helps eradicate local infection.
- Povidone-iodine is preferred to hexachlorophene because it is less irritant.

ANTIPARASITE PREPARATIONS

Lindane, malathion, and permethrin are indicated for scabies

Lindane should be avoided in pregnancy, breast-feeding mothers, patients with low body weight, young children, and those with a history of epilepsy. Malathion is an organophosphate cholinesterase inhibitor and kills both adult lice and ova *in vitro*. Permethrin is neurotoxic for scabies and lice, and there can be cross-sensitivity to pyrethrins or chrysanthemums. Aqueous preparations are preferred, as the alcoholic lotions are irritant. A hot bath is often recommended before treatment, but may increase absorption of the solutions and should be discouraged. One application is usually sufficient, but an application on two or three consecutive days is needed for hyperkeratotic scabies. All members of the household must be treated at the same time. Applications are usually applied from the neck down, but treatment of the scalp, face, and neck is recommended for children under 2 years of age, elderly patients, immunocompromised patients, and those for whom a previous treatment has failed.

Benzyl benzoate* is an older aracicide, but is irritant and should be avoided in children. Up to three applications on consecutive days may be needed.

A 5% precipitate of sulfur in petrolatum is also an effective treatment, but is rarely used because of its disagreeable odor and staining. However, it is a possible alternative for treating pregnant women and infants.

Patients must be told that the itch of scabies can persist for several weeks and that itching does not necessarily indicate treatment failure.

Malathion and carbaryl are recommended for head lice*

Both malathion and carbaryl* should be used as lotions rather than shampoos, and left in contact with the scalp for 12 hours. Aqueous formulations are preferred for asthmatic patients and small children to avoid alcoholic fumes. The treatment should be repeated after 7 days to kill lice emerging from any eggs that might have survived the first application.

Permethrin and phenothrin* are very effective against head lice, but resistance is emerging. Lindane is no longer recommended because of a high level of resistance.

Activities and uses of topical antibacterial drugs used in dermatology and their complications

Drug	Activity spectrum	Uses	Complications
Bacitracin	Gram-positive organisms. anaerobic cocci, *Neisseria*, tetanus bacilli, diphtheria bacilli	Nasal staphylococcal carriers	Resistance with long-term use Contact allergic dermatitis Rarely contact urticaria
Gramicidin (available only in combination with neomycin, polymixin, bacitracin, and nystatin)	As for bacitracin		Rarely contact allergic dermatitis
Mupirocin	Most Gram-positive aerobic bacteria including methicillin-resistant *Staphylococcus aureus* (MRSA)	Impetigo, nasal staphylococcal carriage	May cause irritation of nasal mucosa (contains propylene glycol)
Polymyxin B sulfate	Gram-negative organisms including *Psuedomonas, Escherichia coli, Enterobacter,* and *Klebsiella*	Used in compound antibiotic preparations	Neurotoxic and nephrotoxic if systemically absorbed, therefore to be avoided in open wounds or denuded skin Contact dermatitis uncommon
Neomycin	Gram-negative organisms including *E. coli, Proteus, Klebsiella,* and *Enterobacter*		Serum concentrations rarely detectable Contact dermatitis common with cross-sensitivity to streptomycin, kanamycin, paromomycin, gentamicin
Gentamicin	As for neomycin, but more effective against *Pseudomonas*, and active againststaphylococci and group A hemolytic streptococci		Use of topical gentamicin should be limited because of concerns about the emergence of resistance Neurotoxic, nephrotoxic, and ototoxic if absorbed Detected in plasma if applied to a large skin area, especially if denuded skin
Clindamycin	*Propionibacterium acnes*	Acne	10% absorption Rarely pseudomembranous colitis Skin irritation with alcohol vehicle, less with gel
Erythromycin Erythromycin in combination with benzoyl peroxide Erythromycin in combination with zinc acetate	*P. acnes*	Acne	Resistance increasing Combinations are claimed to reduce emergence of resistant strains
Metronidazole		Rosacea	Drying, burning, stinging
Tetracyclines (tetracycline, meclocycline)	*P. acnes*	Acne	Temporary yellow staining of skin Photosensitivity has not been a problem, but phototoxic Contraindicated in pregnancy, and in renal and hepatic disease

Fig. 18.8 Activities and uses of topical antibacterial drugs used in dermatology and their complications.

Malathion, lindane, and carbaryl* are effective for crab lice

Treatment should be applied to the whole body for 12 hours, and repeated 7 days later.

INSECT REPELLENTS

These agents repel insects primarily by vaporization of the active ingredients diethyltoluamide and dimethyl phthalate. The duration of action is limited by the rate of vaporization and washing and rubbing off. Few preparations currently available are effective for more than a few hours. Allergic reactions can develop, especially with prolonged use.

BARRIER PREPARATIONS

Barrier creams have been developed to protect the skin from irritants (e.g. in industry, for patients with dermatitis). They rely on:

- Water-repellent substances (e.g. silicones).
- Soaps.
- Impermeable deposits such as titanium, zinc, and calamine*.

Their efficacy is limited because they must be removable by washing and cannot be so occlusive that they block pores and follicles. They have a role in protecting skin from discharges and secretions and are used for diaper rash and colostomies.

BANDAGES AND DRESSINGS

A variety of bandages and dressings are prescribable and play an important role in the management of skin problems. Medicated bandages impregnated with zinc paste, with or without coal tar/ichthammol* are useful in the management of eczema, acting as an emollient, antipruritic, and barrier to scratching. Bandages containing calamine* and clioquinol and fabric dressings impregnated with povidone-iodine, chlorhexidine, framycetin*, sodium fusidate*, and paraffin* are also available.

Silicone gel sheets are clear, soft, and semi-occlusive, and conform well to awkward contours of the body. They have a role in the treatment of hypertrophic scars. Their mechanism of action is not fully understood: pressure, temperature of the scar, and oxygen tension within the scar are not involved, and it is currently believed that the gel may work by promoting scar hydration.

EMOLLIENTS

Emollients are used to reduce transepidermal water loss in patients with dry scaly skin. They are the mainstay of the long-term treatment of atopic dermatitis and ichthyoses, but are also useful in the treatment of other forms of eczema and in psoriasis.

There is a wide selection of commercially available emollients, containing a variety of ointments and creams (see Fig. 18.5), some of which are very greasy and can be too occlusive, while others are more water soluble and creamy, but less hydrating and need more frequent application. A mixture of soft white paraffin* and liquid paraffin* in equal parts is a thick emollient, whereas many of the cream formulations are thin emollients. Patient preference is an important consideration since these agents need to be used regularly and persistently. In practice this is influenced by stinging on application, ease of application, appearance on the skin (is it obviously greasy?), smell, duration of action, effect on clothing, and ease of removal.

DRUGS ACTING ON SKIN CONSTITUENTS

DRUGS ACTING ON KERATIN AND KERATINOCYTES

Keratolytics

Keratolytics are used to remove keratin. Mild keratolytics are used:

- To enhance the emollient effect of a cream of vehicle (e.g. urea).
- To reduce pore occlusion, which is characteristic of acne (e.g. salicylic acid, resorcinol, sulfur).

Methotrexate exerts a strong antimitotic effect on keratinocytes by inhibiting DNA synthesis by competitive inhibition of dihydrofolate reductase. At psoriatic doses methotrexate also inhibits neutrophil chemotaxis. It is administered once a week for the treatment of psoriasis. Renal, hepatic, and bone marrow function must be assessed prior to, and during, methotrexate treatment, and note should be taken of potential drug interactions (see Chapters 17 and 28).

Urea makes creams and lotions feel less greasy, increases the hydration of the stratum corneum (concentration, 2–20%), and is a keratolytic (20%). A concentration of 30–50% urea with occlusion can be used to soften the nail plate before nail avulsion.

Urea appears to act by modifying prekeratin and keratin, leading to increased solubilization. It may also cleave the hydrogen bonds that keep the stratum corneum intact. It is absorbed percutaneously, but is a natural product of metabolism, and is excreted in the urine without systemic toxicity.

Adverse effects include irritation and stinging, especially with occlusion and in the perineal area.

Salicylic acid is soluble in alcohol, but only slightly soluble in water. It is thought to act by solubilizing the cell surface proteins that keep the stratum corneum intact, resulting in desquamation. It is keratolytic at a concentration of 3–6%. Higher concentrations can destroy tissues. Low concentrations (up to 2%) of salicylic acid are used in the treatment of acne. Higher concentrations (up to 50%) can be used to eradicate warts and calluses, but are contraindicated in patients with diabetes mellitus or peripheral vascular disease because they can induce ulceration.

Salicylic acid is absorbed percutaneously, and 1 g of 6% salicylic acid results in plasma concentrations of approximately 0.5 mg/dl (0.04 mmol/liter). The drug is bound to albumin, but transiently increased levels of free salicylates can be detected in hypoalbuminemic patients. Salicylism and death have been recorded after topical application (the threshold for toxicity is 30–50 mg/dl [2.17–3.62 mmol/liter]). About 95% of a single dose of salicylate is excreted in the urine within 24 hours of absorption.

Adverse effects include urticarial and anaphylactic reactions in patients who are sensitive to salicylates.

Azelaic acid* is both keratolytic and mildly antibacterial, and is available as a topical cream for the treatment of acne.

Propylene glycol is keratolytic at a concentration of 40–70% and is useful in the treatment of hyperkeratotic conditions such as palmoplantar keratoderma, psoriasis, pityriasis rubra pilaris, and hypertrophic lichen planus.

Propylene glycol also increases the water content of the stratum corneum. This hygroscopic characteristic encourages the development of an osmotic gradient through the stratum corneum, increasing the hydration of the outermost layers and drawing water out of the inner layers of the skin.

Propylene glycol can be used alone or in a gel with 6% salicylic acid. It has the advantage of minimal absorption, and what is absorbed is oxidized in the liver to lactic acid and pyruvic acid, which are then used in general metabolism.

Its major adverse effect is irritancy, and it can cause contact allergic dermatitis.

Podophyllum resin is an alcoholic extract of *Podophyllum peltatum*, and is used in the treatment of condyloma acuminatum and plantar warts. Podophyllotoxin and its derivatives are cytotoxic agents that act on the microtubule proteins of the mitotic spindle, preventing normal assembly of the spindle and arresting epidermal mitoses in metaphase. The tincture needs to be applied accurately to the wart tissue to prevent severe erosion of the surrounding normal skin, and allowed a contact time of 2–3 hours (possibly increasing to 6–8 hours if tolerated) for 3–5 applications only. If this is not successful, alternative treatment modalities should be considered as the resin is absorbed and distributed in lipids, including those in the central nervous system. If extensive areas need treatment they should be treated in sections to minimize absorption, particularly from intertriginous areas and large moist warts.

Adverse effects include nausea, vomiting, muscle weakness, neuropathy, and even coma and death. Local irritation is common. Podophyllum resin is contraindicated during pregnancy because of its possible cytotoxic effects on the fetus.

Trichloracetic acid and silver nitrate are very strong keratolytics and are used to destroy tissues such as xanthelasma and excess granulation tissue.

Benzoyl peroxide penetrates the stratum corneum and follicular openings unchanged, but is converted to benzoic acid in the epidermis and dermis. It is keratolytic, and comedolytic, but is also thought to have some activity against *P. acnes*.

Adverse effects of benzoyl peroxide include irritancy with increasing concentrations, and sensitizing properties, with up to 1% of patients developing a contact allergic dermatitis. Its use in acne is therefore limited. Benzamycin* is a commercial preparation containing benzoyl peroxide (5%) and erythromycin (3%), which is said to be as effective as erythromycin, but reduces the emergence of erythromycin-resistant *P. acnes*.

Vitamin D analogs

Vitamin D analogs inhibit epidermal proliferation, induce terminal keratinocyte differentiation, and have anti-inflammatory properties *in vitro* and *in vivo*.

Vitamin D receptors (VDRs) are found in keratinocytes, melanocytes, Langerhans' cells, dermal fibroblasts, monocytes, and T lymphocytes in normal skin. They belong to the large family of structurally related ligand-inducible transcription factors, which includes the retinoid receptors and thyroid hormone receptors (see Chapter 3). In psoriasis, there is increased expression of VDRs in the basal and suprabasal layers of the epidermis, as well as a marked increase in the density of VDR positivity in intraepidermal and perivascular T cells and macrophages.

The effects of vitamin D analogs demonstrated to date include:

- Inhibition of T-cell proliferation by blocking the transition of T cells from the early to the late G1 phase of the cell cycle.
- Inhibition of the release of various cytokines, including interleukin (IL)-2, IL-6, IL-8, interferon (IFN)-γ, tumor necrosis factor (TNF)-β, and granulocyte–macrophage colony stimulating factor (GM-CSF).
- A reduction in the capacity of monocytes to stimulate T-cell proliferation and lymphokine release from T cells.
- Reduced neutrophil accumulation in psoriatic skin.

The mechanism of action of these analogs is not yet clearly elucidated. The goal is to develop analogs that induce the expression of the vitamin D-responding genes governing Ca^{2+} homeostasis and analogs that induce expression of the vitamin D-responding genes influencing the keratinocyte cell cycle. Clearly, for the treatment of skin disease, such analogs should optimally affect the cell cycle and have a minimal effect on Ca^{2+} homeostasis.

Calcipotriene is a vitamin D_3 analog (a side-chain modification of 1α 25-dihydroxyvitamin D_3). It is available for the topical treatment of psoriasis as a cream, ointment, and scalp solution. It is effective alone, and has been shown to have a sparing effect when used with ultraviolet light treatment, cyclosporine, methotrexate, and retinoids. Calcium metabolism is not affected at doses of less than 100 g/week.

Calcipotriene has become the drug of choice for mild to moderate psoriasis in primary care. Its nonstaining nonmessy formulation greatly improves patient compliance compared with that for coal tar and dithranol* preparations. It should not be applied to the face as it causes facial irritation in some patients. Calcipotriene has also been reported to be of benefit in the treatment of other dyskeratotic states and pityriasis rubra pilaris.

Tacalcitol* (1α 24-dihydroxyvitamin D_3) has recently become available in the UK for the topical treatment of psoriasis. It is applied once daily, and in clinical trials was tolerated on the face and in the flexures.

Anthralin

Anthralin has an antimitotic effect, but its mechanism of action remains unclear. Mitochondrial DNA production is reduced, glycolytic enzymes are inhibited (possibly as a result of lipid peroxidation leading to cross-linkage of enzyme proteins), and arachidonic acid levels are lowered. In human skin *in vitro* oxygen consumption is decreased and the pentose phosphate shunt is inhibited. Cyclic nucleotide levels are normalized (cGMP is increased in psoriasis).

Anthralin is the most potent topical treatment available for the treatment of psoriasis

Anthralin is unique because it can lead to remission. It must be kept in its reduced state until delivered to the skin. Oxidation then occurs on the skin, producing the therapeutic effect.

Anthralin is available as a cream (0.1–2%) and ointment (0.1–2%) for home use. The treatment is usually applied for 30–60 minutes (short-contact anthralin therapy) and then removed. Anthralin paste is largely confined to hospital use and can be applied for 24 hours or for shorter time periods (e.g. for Day Care patients). Anthralin must be applied to a test area first before treating the whole body, as patient tolerance varies. The strength of anthralin is gradually increased (e.g. doubling concentrations every 3–5 days). Therapy is discontinued when the plaques have flattened. Anthralin inevitably stains the skin and this stain can be removed with a keratolytic agent. It also stains clothing. Anthralin can be used in combination with light therapy, and coal tar baths (Ingram regimen).

No systemic toxicity has been reported with anthralin. However, it is irritant to normal skin and therefore must be applied accurately to the plaques of psoriasis.

Tar preparations

Therapeutic tars are products of the destructive distillation of wood, coal, or bitumen. They are highly complex mixtures with some 10,000 constituents. Petroleum tars have no therapeutic importance.

Wood tars (oil of cade, bee, birch, and pine) are available as ointments, pastes, and alcohol paints. They may sensitize, but do not photosensitize.

Bituminous tars were originally obtained from the distillation of shale deposits containing fossilized fish. Some have a high sulfur content. They are less effective than coal tars and do not photosensitize.

Coal tar is a black fluid with a characteristic smell. Different methods of distilling heated coal have been used to try to remove its color and odor. Coal tar modifies keratinization but its mechanism of action is poorly understood. The high boiling point tar acids (phenolics) may be responsible for its therapeutic effect, possibly by releasing lysosomes in the granular layer. Coal tars are also antipruritic (and are therefore used for eczema as well as psoriasis), mildly antiseptic, and photosensitizing. Refined tars are less phototoxic, but phototoxicity is directly related to therapeutic efficacy in psoriasis.

The carcinogenicity of pitch and heavy tar fractions is well established, but malignant tumors are extremely rare in relation to tar therapy. A few cases of genital cancer have been reported, but a recent study with a 25-year follow-up has shown that the incidence of skin tumors in patients using coal tar is not increased.

The photosensitizing potential of coal tars is exploited in the Goekerman regimen (i.e. combination therapy with ultraviolet light B) for psoriasis, which reduces epidermal DNA synthesis, possibly by forming cross-links between opposite strands on the DNA double helix.

The most common adverse effect is an irritant folliculitis. Phototoxicity and contact allergic dermatitis can also occur.

Retinoids

Retinoids include natural and synthetic derivatives of vitamin A and have potent effects on:

- Cell differentiation, which they reduce.
- Cell growth, inducing hyperplasia, hypergranulosis, and decreased numbers of tonofilaments and desmosomes in the epidermis. The latter effect is thought to account for the keratolytic effect.
- The immune response, stimulating cell-mediated cytotoxicity and acting as an adjuvant to stimulate antibody production to antigens that were not previously immunogenic.

They also reduce neutrophil migration, although the mechanism for this is not known.

At an intracellular level retinoids stabilize lysosomes, increase ribonucleic acid polymerase activity, increase incorporation of thymidine into DNA, and increase prostaglandin (PG) E_2, cAMP and cGMP concentrations. However, their mechanism of action is not yet clear. There are specific retinol and at least three retinoic acid receptors, which are all members of the family of glucocorticosteroid–thyroid VDRs (see Chapter 3).

Tretinoin is the acid form of vitamin A (i.e. retinoic acid). It is fomed by oxidation of the alcohol group in vitamin A alcohol, with all four double bonds in the side chain in the *trans* configuration. It is insoluble in water, but soluble in many organic solvents. It is available topically for use in acne, when its efficacy is attributed to decreased cohesion between epidermal cells and increased epidermal cell turnover. It is thought that this helps remove comedones, and convert closed comedones to open comedones.

The main adverse effect is irritation, but patients should be warned to avoid exposure to ultraviolet light while using tretinoin as it appears to increase the tumorigenic potential of ultraviolet light in animal studies.

A regular application of 0.05% tretinoin cream for a minimum of 4 months improves the appearance of photodamaged skin, and is licensed for the treatment of mottled hyperpigmentation and fine wrinkling caused by chronic sun exposure.

Isotretinoin is a synthetic retinoid that is now available for systemic and topical use. Its main effect seems to be to reduce the size and function of the sebaceous glands, and a 4–6-month course is highly effective in the treatment of acne in the majority of patients.

Isotretinoin is well absorbed, extensively bound to plasma proteins, and eliminated. It is given at a dose of 0.5–1 mg/kg.

The adverse effects of isotretinoin resemble the effects of hypervitaminosis A, producing dry skin and mucous membranes, and epidermal fragility. Rarely, visual disturbances, hair thining, myalgia and arthralgia, and raised liver enzymes have been reported. Cutaneous complications include allergic vasculitis, granulomatous lesions, and acne fulminans. Isotretinoin can cause benign intracranial hypertension (BIH), so frequent or unusual headaches are an indication to stop treatment and investigate as appropriate. As tetracyclines can also cause BIH, the two drugs should not be given together. Triglyceride concentrations increase during treatment, but with normal initial concentrations this increase is rarely sufficient to stop therapy and is reversible on stopping treatment.

Isotretinoin is teratogenic and should be given to women of child-bearing age only after appropriate counselling and with adequate contraception.

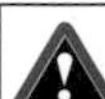 **Adverse effects of isotretinoin**

- Teratogenicity
- Dry skin and mucous membranes
- Epidermal fragility
- Rarely, visual disturbances, hair thinning, myalgia and arthralgia, and raised liver enzymes
- Allergic vasculitis
- Granulomatous lesions
- Acne fulminans
- Benign intracranial hypertension
- Increased triglyceride concentrations

Etretinate is an aromatic retinoid with a slow terminal elimination phase of several months. It is used in the treatment of psoriasis, particularly erythrodermic and generalized pustular psoriasis, at doses of 0.5–1 mg/kg. Higher doses are needed for chronic plaque psoriasis, but its use in combination therapy with psoralen* plus ultraviolet light A (PUVA) or ultraviolet light B is increasing because it has an ultraviolet light-sparing effect.

Adverse effects are similar to those of isotretinoin, but etretinate is more teratogenic. Particular caution is therefore needed when it is used in women of child-bearing age. Conception must also be avoided for 2 years after the drug is stopped in view of its long half-life. Skeletal hyperostosis is a recognized adverse effect of retinoid therapy, but is more common with etretinate than isotretinoin because etretinate is often used for longer periods of time in the treatment of psoriasis than isotretinoin is used for acne.

It has been claimed that tumors, including solar keratoses, kerato-acanthoma, epidermodysplasia verruciformis, basal cell epithelioma (BCE) and leukoplakia, sometimes clear following treatment with isotretinoin or etretinate. The use of retinoids in preventing skin tumors in high-risk patients, such as those with xeroderma pigmentosum, is currently being investigated in ongoing trials.

DRUGS ACTING ON MELANIN AND MELANOCYTES

Hydroxyquinone inhibits tyrosinase, thereby interfering with the synthesis of melanin. Topically, it causes temporary lightening of the skin. Monobenzone also affects tyrosinase, but may also be toxic to melanocytes, so producing permanent depigmentation.

Adverse effects of both drugs include irritant and allergic contact dermatitis. There is some absorption, since hypopigmentation may occur at sites other than that of monobenzone application.

Psoralens* are photoactivated chemicals that intercalate with DNA, forming cyclobutane adducts with pyrimidine in bases on subsequent exposure to ultraviolet light A. This forms the basis of PUVA photochemotherapy. This is an established treatment for psoriasis and mycosis fungoides, and clinical trials are being conducted to investigate its use in vitiligo.

DRUGS ACTING ON GLANDS

Isotretinoin reduces the size and sebum secretion of sebaceous glands (see above), while nicotinamide may act on the pilosebaceous unit (see below).

DRUGS ACTING ON NERVES

Topical nonsteroidal anti-inflammatory drugs and capsaicin can relieve pain*

Local pain can be transiently relieved by topical nonsteroidal anti-inflammatory drugs (NSAIDs) (see Chapter 7), while capsaicin* (0.075%) cream is licensed for the treatment of postherpetic neuralgia. Capsaicin* is a naturally occurring alkaloid found in fruits and capsicum. Crude extracts of capsicum or capsicum oleo-resin contain small amounts of capsaicin* and a number of co-capsaicinoids, which are thought to cause the counterirritant erythematous reaction that accompanies the application of these extracts. Capsaicin* itself acts by depleting sensory C fibers of neuropeptides, particularly substance P. It is not a traditional counterirritant and does not induce vasodilatation.

Topical applications relieve itch, partly by a cooling effect

Phenol, menthol*, and camphor are often added to topical applications to relieve itch and probably act as weak local anesthetics. Calamine*, astringents such as aluminum acetate and tannic acid, and coal tar also have some topical antipruritic effect.

Itch may be relieved systemically by histamine H_1 antagonists

There is a wide variety of histamine H_1 antagonists. They differ not only in their affinity for H_1 receptors, but also in their additional properties, which include sedation, anti-allergic effects, and actions at other receptors.

In the treatment of atopic eczema, most of the clinical trials suggest that their benefit is conferred by sedation rather than by histamine inhibition. Large clinical trials to test the hypothesis that anti-allergic antihistamines such as cetirizine and ketotifen might be beneficial are lacking.

In the treatment of urticaria, the choice of agent depends on the need for sedation, which is often desirable in acute urticaria but not in the chronic form.

For prolonged treatment, patients prefer longer-acting drugs. Astemizole is the longest -acting H_1 antagonist, but like terfenadine interacts with drugs commonly used in primary care (e.g. erythromycin) to produce prolongation of the QT interval, and this must be considered when using these agents. Loratadine is a long-acting antihistamine that appears not to produce these interactions.

Hypnotics, chlorpromazine, trimeprazine, and sedative antidepressants are sometimes helpful in the treatment of pruritus, possibly because they alter the perception of itch.

DRUGS ACTING ON HAIR

Topical minoxidil reverses androgenic alopecia in some patients. Its mechanism of action is unknown and its effect on androgenic alopecia is not permanent, with hair loss ocurrring within 4-6 months when it is stopped.

Cyproterone acetate*, in conjunction with ethinyl estradiol, is used to prevent the progression of androgenic alopecia in females.

Cyproterone acetate* is the treatment of choice for female hirsutism. It is an anti-androgen and:

- Decreases adrenal androgen secretion.
- Competes with both testosterone and dihydrotestosterone for the androgen receptor.
- Inhibits the 5α-reductase enzyme.
- Inhibits luteinizing hormone secretion by its progestational effects.

A dose of 2 mg daily is sufficient, and it is usually given in combination with an estrogen to ensure regular menstrual bleeding. An improvement may not be evident for 6–12 months. A male fetus will probably be feminized if a pregnancy occurs when cyproterone acetate* is used alone.

Luteinizing hormone releasing hormone analogs may improve hirsutism in patients with high androgen levels of ovarian origin. However, their use will be restricted by their propensity to reduce vertebral trabecular bone mass.

DRUGS THAT MODIFY INFLAMMATORY RESPONSES IN THE SKIN

GLUCOCORTICOSTEROIDS

Topical glucocorticosteroids are anti-inflammatory and vasoconstricting, and reduce keratinocyte cell division. They are classified into four groups (Fig. 18.9), according to their vasoconstricting potency, which correlates remarkably well with their clinical efficacy. Note that the different salts of hydrocortisone have very different potencies. Dermatologists therefore avoid generic prescribing of glucocorticosteroids. The fluorinated glucocorticosteroids are particularly potent and are absorbed systemically. It is claimed that the newer glucocorticosteroids fluticasone propionate and mometasone fumarate are potent topical glucocorticosteroids with less systemic absorption.

Glucocorticosteroids and their vasoconstricting potencies	
Mild potency	Hydrocortisone 0.1, 0.5, 1, 2.5% Hydrocortisone acetate 1% Fluocinolone acetonide 0.0025% Methylprednisolone acetate 0.25%
Moderate potency	Hydrocortisone with urea Alclometasone dipropionate 0.05% Betamethasone valerate 0.025% Clobetasone butyrate* 0.05% Deoxymethasone 0.05% Fluocinolone acetonide 0.00625% Fluocortolone hexanoate* 0.1%, 0.25% & fluocortolone pivalate* 0.1%, 0.25% Flurandrenolone* 0.0125%
Potent	Hydocortisone butyrate 0.1% Beclomethasone dipropionate 0.025%, 0.05% Betamethasone valerate 0.1% Budesonide 0.025% Deoxymethasole 0.25%, Diflucortolone valerate* 0.1% Fluclorone acetonide 0.025% Fluocinolone acetonide 0.025% Fluocinonide 0.05% Fluticasone propionate 0.05% Mometasone furoate 0.1% Triamcinolone acetonide 0.1%
Very potent	Clobetasol propionate 0.05% Diflucortolone valerate 0.3% Halcinonide 0.1%

Fig. 18.9 Glucocorticosteroids and their vasoconstricting potencies.

The potency of glucocorticosteroid required depends on:

- The skin disease (e.g. very potent for lichen planus).
- The site to be treated (e.g. mild to moderate only for facial application).
- The age of the patient (e.g. the indications for a potent glucocorticosteroid in a child are limited).

In general very potent glucocorticosteroids should be given to adults only under specialist supervision and should not be prescribed for children without consultation with a specialist.

Glucocorticosteroid penetration varies with:

- Body site. It is higher when applied to the genitals, face, and scalp than when applied to the trunk and limbs.
- State of the skin. It is enhanced by erythema or erosion.
- Occlusion, which increases penetration at least tenfold.
- The vehicle used. Ointments produce higher penetration than creams.
- Concentration of drug. A high concentration produces higher penetration than a low concentration, but penetration is not proportional to the concentration difference (e.g. increasing the concentration of hydrocortisone tenfold results in a fourfold increase in penetration).

Intralesional glucocorticosteroids are used for keloid and hypertrophic scars, chondrodermatitis nodularis helicis, and acne cysts

Intralesional administration of glucocorticosteroids overcomes the limited penetration of topical glucocorticosteroids and is used to provide a high local concentration of glucocorticosteroid. Relatively insoluble glucocorticosteroids (e.g. triamcinolone acetonide, triamcinolone diacetate, triamcinolone hexacetonide, betamethasone acetate–phosphate) are used to achieve high local doses, which are gradually released for 3–4 weeks. The injections must be limited to 1 mg per site to avoid local skin atrophy. Intralesional injections have a place in the management of keloid and hypertrophic scars, chondrodermatitis nodularis helicis, and acne cysts, for which the use of topical glucocorticosteroids is largely unsuccessful. Local injection is also sometimes helpful in alopecia areata and hypertrophic lichen planus that has not responded to topical glucocorticosteroids.

Topical glucocorticosteroids are used for eczema, vitiligo, and alopecia areata

Topical glucocorticosteroids are indicated in the treatment of inflammatory skin disorders and are a vital part of the acute treatment of most forms of dermatitis (eczema). The potency of topical glucocorticosteroid used must be titrated to the disease severity and the minimum effective strength determined for each patient. In seborrheic dermatitis, a combination of glucocorticosteroids and antipityrosporal agents is useful to calm the eczema, but antipityrosporal agents used early in relapse should be sufficient.

Topical glucocorticosteroids are useful in the treatment of flexural psoriasis, but should not be used as a first-line treatment elsewhere as a rebound exacerbation of the disease occurs on withdrawal. It is not uncommon for patients to require increasingly potent glucocorticosteroids to control the disease. If very potent glucocorticosteroids are then withdrawn, generalized pustular psoriasis can ensue, which is a medical emergency and often requires systemic treatment with agents such as methotrexate (see p. 360).

Potent topical glucocorticosteroids are used short-term in the treatment of vitiligo and alopecia areata, but should not be continued for more than 4 weeks.

A trial of topical glucocorticosteroids is worthwhile for sarcoidosis, discoid lupus erythematosus, and pemphigus, although systemic treatments are often necessary.

Systemic glucocorticosteroids are used for severe acute dermatoses, pemphigus, pemphigoid, and lichen planus

Systemic glucocorticosteroids are used only for severe dermatologic diseases because the treatment benefits must outweigh the risks of long-term use (see Chapter 12). They are indicated for:

- Severe acute dermatoses such as anaphylaxis, acute contact allergic dermatitis, acute autoimmune connective tissue diseases and generalized vasculitis, and generalized drug eruptions.
- Chronic disabling disorders such as pemphigus and pemphigoid.
- Severe lichen planus.
- Pyoderma gangrenosum.
- Sarcoidosis.
- Various other unusual dermatoses.

All the adverse effects of systemic glucocorticosteroids can be observed if there is significant systemic absorption of topical glucocorticosteroids

Local adverse reactions include worsening and spread of any infection (viral, bacterial, and fungal). Skin atrophy, striae, hirsutism, acne, and depigmentation may occur with long-term use, and the application of potent glucocorticosteroids on the face induces a 'perioral dermatitis.'

Significant systemic absorption has been documented with an application of a mildly potent agent under occlusion or with a very potent glucocorticosteroid without occlusion to 20% of the body area. Any of the adverse reactions of systemic glucocorticosteroids can then be observed. Plastic diapers act as an occlusive dressing so care is needed when prescribing for rashes in the diaper area. Rarely, suppression of the pituitary–adrenal axis results in iatrogenic Cushing's syndrome, but impaired stress responses are more common.

Contact dermatitis to the glucocorticosteroid molecules should be considered in any patient who fails to make the expected progress with appropriate-strength glucocorticosteroids.

CYCLOSPORINE

Cyclosporine acts mainly on T lymphocytes (see Chapter 15), but may also have a direct effect on DNA synthesis and proliferation in keratinocytes. A beneficial effect has been demonstrated in psoriasis and atopic dermatitis and its value in various more uncommon dermatoses is being evaluated.

Blood pressure and renal function must be monitored before and during treatment, and potential drug interactions must be considered (see Chapter 10).

GAMOLENIC ACID*

Patients with atopic dermatitis have elevated serum concentrations of linoleic acid and significantly reduced concentrations of γ linolenic acid and its metabolites. It has been postulated that this is due to a defect in δ6-desaturase activity in atopic individuals. Capsules of gamolenic acid* in evening primrose oil are therefore available for the treatment of atopic dermatitis. Individual patients mainly report an improvement in skin texture, which may take 8–12 weeks to become apparent, but the results of clinical trials are conflicting, and meta-analyses fail to show superiority over placebo.

NICOTINAMIDE*

Nicotinamide* is the amide of vitamin B_3. Physiologically, it is converted to nicotinamide adenine dinucleotide (NAD) or the dinucleotide phosphate (NADP), both of which function as coenzymes (see Chapter 27). Nicotinamide* is thought to act by electron scavenging, inhibition of phosphodiesterase, and/or increased tryptophan conversion to serotonin. It also has direct effects on inflammatory cells, inhibiting neutrophils, suppressing lymphocyte transformation, and inhibiting mast cell histamine release.

Nicotinamide may be a useful treatment for acne*

Clinical trials to date suggest that topical nicotinamide* gel is as effective as topical clindamycin for mild to moderate acne, and represents a nonantibiotic treatment that appears to be well tolerated. In acne its main effect seems to be inhibition of cyclic AMP phosphodiesterase and lymphocyte transformation, which may inhibit epithelial proliferation in the pilosebaceous unit.

Nicotinamide* has an established safety profile as it has been given systemically for schizophrenia and vitamin B deficiency states.

ANTIMALARIAL DRUGS

Hydroxychloroquine, chloroquine, and mepacrine* have a beneficial effect on discoid and systemic lupus erythematosus, polymorphic light eruption, and solar urticaria, and there is some evidence of a therapeutic response in sarcoidosis and porphyria cutanea tarda. Their mechanism of action in these disorders is unknown, but they have been shown to:

- Inhibit prostaglandin synthesis, chemotaxis, and hydrolytic enzymes.
- Stabilize membranes.
- Bind to DNA.

Alkylating agents and antimetabolites and their dermatologic disease indications

Drug	Uses
Cyclophosphamide	Pemphigus, pemphigoid Wegener's granulomatosis Lupus erythematosus Polymyositis Mycosis fungoides Histiocytosis X
Chlorambucil	Mycosis fungoides Behçet's disease Lupus erythematosus Wegener's granulomatosis Glucocorticosteroid-resistant sarcoidosis Sézary syndrome
Mustine* injection	Mycosis fungoides
Dacarbazine injection	Metastatic malignant melanoma
Methotrexate (given weekly; caution in the elderly and in renal impairment)	Psoriasis Reiter's syndrome Pityriasis rubra pilaris Ichthyosiform erythroderma Sarcoidosis Pemphigus/pemphigoid Glucocorticosteroid-resistant dermatomyositis
Hydroxyurea (less effective than methotrexate)	Psoriasis
Azathioprine (glucocorticosteroid-sparing agent)	Pemphigus/pemphigoid Lupus erythematosus Dermatomyositis Wegener's granulomatosis Actinic reticuloid Pityriasis rubra pilaris Intractable eczema in adults
Bleomycin	Squamous cell carcinoma Mycosis fungoides and other lymphomas Viral warts (intralesional)
Melphalan	Scleromyxedema
Cyclosporine	Psoriasis Atopic dermatitis Pemphigus/pemphigoid Mycosis fungoides/Sézary syndrome
5-Fluorouracil	Solar keratoses (topical) Keratoacanthoma (intralesional)

Fig. 18.10 Alkylating agents and antimetabolites and their dermatologic disease indications. Their use is justified only if the disease is sufficiently disabling.

SULFA DRUGS

Dapsone is the drug of choice for leprosy, and is also used in the treatment of dermatitis herpetiformis, immunobullous disorders, and numerous other rare dermatoses. Its mechanism of action is unclear, although neutrophils and immune complexes seem to play a part in the diseases influenced by the drug. Patients taking dapsone must be monitored for signs of hemolysis and methemoglobinemia because hemolytic anemia is a common adverse reaction and, although rare, methemoglobinemia can be a rapidly fatal complication.

Other sulfa drugs having some of the useful effects of dapsone are sulfapyridine* and sulfamethoxypyridazine.

OTHER DRUGS MODIFYING THE IMMUNE RESPONSE

Clofazimine is an antileprosy drug that has beneficial effects in inflammatory dermatoses such as pyoderma gangrenosum and lupus erythematosus.

Colchicine is an alkaloid derived from the autumn crocus that:

- Inhibits neutrophil and monocyte chemotaxis, collagen synthesis, and mast cell histamine release.
- Increases collagenolysis.
- Arrests mitosis in metaphase and is therefore antimitotic.

Colchicine has been used in the treatment of a variety of dermatologic diseases characterized by leukocyte infiltration of the skin, including Behçet's syndrome, psoriasis, palmoplantar pustulosis, dermatitis herpetifomis, Sweet's syndrome, necrotizing vasculitis, childhood dermatomyositis, and systemic sclerosis.

Adverse effects include gastrointestinal disturbances, which are almost universal as colchicine is usually administered at the maximum tolerated dose

Thalidomide is used, on a named-patient basis, for the treatment of recalcitrant aphthous ulceration, especially in patients with HIV, and has been beneficial in the treatment of pyoderma gangrenosum and Behçet's syndrome.

Adverse effects include teratogenicity and patients must be aware of this. They must also be monitored for subclinical neuropathy.

Fresh-frozen plasma is the treatment of choice for acute exacerbations of hereditary angioedema, as it replaces C1 esterase inhibitor that people with this condition lack.

Danazol stimulates the liver to produce more C1 esterase inhibitor and is therefore useful in the management of hereditary angioedema.

Stanozolol stimulates hepatic C1 esterase inhibitor production but, although it is less expensive than danazol, it can cause excess androgenization in women and should not be given during pregnancy. Stanozolol also increases fibrinolysis and may reduce the pain of liposclerosis of the legs.

Oral contraceptives Combination contraceptive pills containing cyproterone acetate*, ethinyl estradiol, and desogestrol are 'acne-friendly,' unlike most other contraceptive pills which tend to aggravate acne.

Alkylating agents and antimetabolites Drugs such as alkylating agents and antimetabolites (see Chapter 28) are used in dermatology only if the disease is sufficiently disabling to justify the risks of their use (Fig. 18.10).

CAMOUFLAGE CREAMS

Camouflage creams contain titanium dioxide in an ointment base with a variety of color shades that can be matched to the site and skin color of the patient. The best results are achieved by camouflage consultants.

FURTHER READING

Champion R, Burton J, Ebling F (eds) *Textbook of Dermatology 5 e.* Blackwell Science, Oxford; 1991. [Comprehensive textbook of dermatology in four volumes with excellent chapters on general aspects of treatment, systemic treatment, topical treatment and drug reactions, as well as detailed therapeutic suggestions for individual skin diseases.]

Leppard L, Ashton R. *Treatment in Dermatology.* Radcliffe Medical Press, Oxford; 1993. [Aimed at undergraduates and nonspecialists, explaining the rationale for treatment of skin diseases.]

Make a provisional diagnosis and determine a rational pharmacologic treatment for the following hypothetical case.

Carey is a 2-year-old girl with a red itchy rash in her elbow and knee flexures and on her neck. She continually scratches her skin until it bleeds, is losing a lot of sleep and is screaming at bathtime.

1. What is the likely diagnosis?
2. How often should Carey be bathed and what preparations should be used at bathtime?
3. Would you prescribe any topical treatment and if so what?
4. Would you prescribe any oral treatment and if so what?

Indicate whether the following answers are true or false.

1. The following vitamins or their analogs are indicated for use in dermatology
   a) vitamin A
   b) vitamin B
   c) vitamin C
   d) vitamin D
   e) vitamin E
2. The following drugs can be given orally for the treatment of chronic plaque psoriasis
   a) methotrexate
   b) acitretin
   c) cyclosporine
   d) glucocorticosteroids
   e) hydroxyurea
3. In the treatment of acne
   a) isotretinoin can be given topically or orally
   b) nicotinamide* is an anti-inflammatory non-antibiotic treatment
   c) minocycline is the antibiotic of choice for an 11-year-old girl
   d) *Propionibacterium acnes* resistance to antibiotics is not a problem
   e) benzoyl peroxide, azelaic acid*, and salicylic acid are all keratolytic
4. The following statements are correct
   a) valaciclovir is a prodrug
   b) oral acyclovir, valaciclovir, or famiciclovir should be prescribed for shingles.
   c) oral acyclovir is useful in the treatment of cold sores
   d) patients with eczema herpeticum should be hospitalized for intravenous acyclovir
   e) antiviral drugs are effective against cytomegalovirus
5. In the management of dermatitis
   a) ketoconazole cream can be used for seborrheic dermatitis
   b) systemic glucocorticosteroids may be needed to treat acute contact dermatitis
   c) lithium succinate can be used for seborrheic dermatitis
   d) allergy to the glucocorticosteroid molecule can be a problem
   e) diapers increase the potency of topical glucocorticosteroids

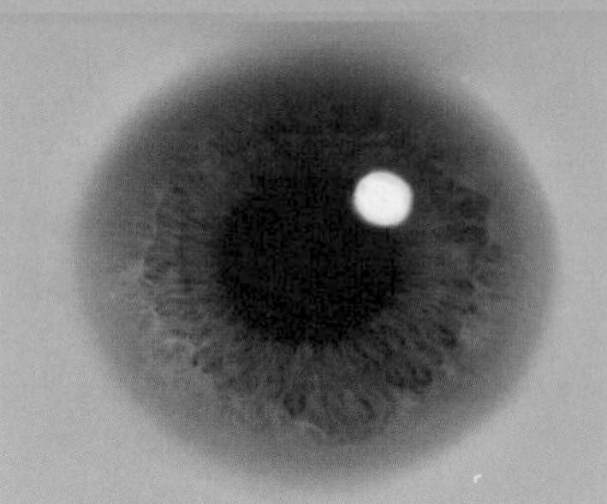

19. Drugs and the Eye

BIOLOGY OF THE EYE AND PRINCIPLES OF DRUG USE FOR THE EYE

STRUCTURE AND PHYSIOLOGY OF THE EYE

The eye focuses images from the external world onto the retina and converts them into electrical signals, which are then perceived by the brain. As vision is a major sense, a large area of the brain is used for processing this information, which is produced by two outposts of the central nervous system, the retinae. The retinae are contained within the eyeballs and are connected to the rest of the central nervous system by the optic nerves.

The eyeball is a spherical organ of about 25 mm in diameter. It contains a lens and two fluid-filled chambers, and is enclosed by the following four layers of specialized tissue:

- The cornea and sclera.
- The uveal tract (iris, ciliary body, and choroid).
- The pigment epithelium.
- The retina (Fig. 19.1).

The most anterior part of the eye around the eyeball is the

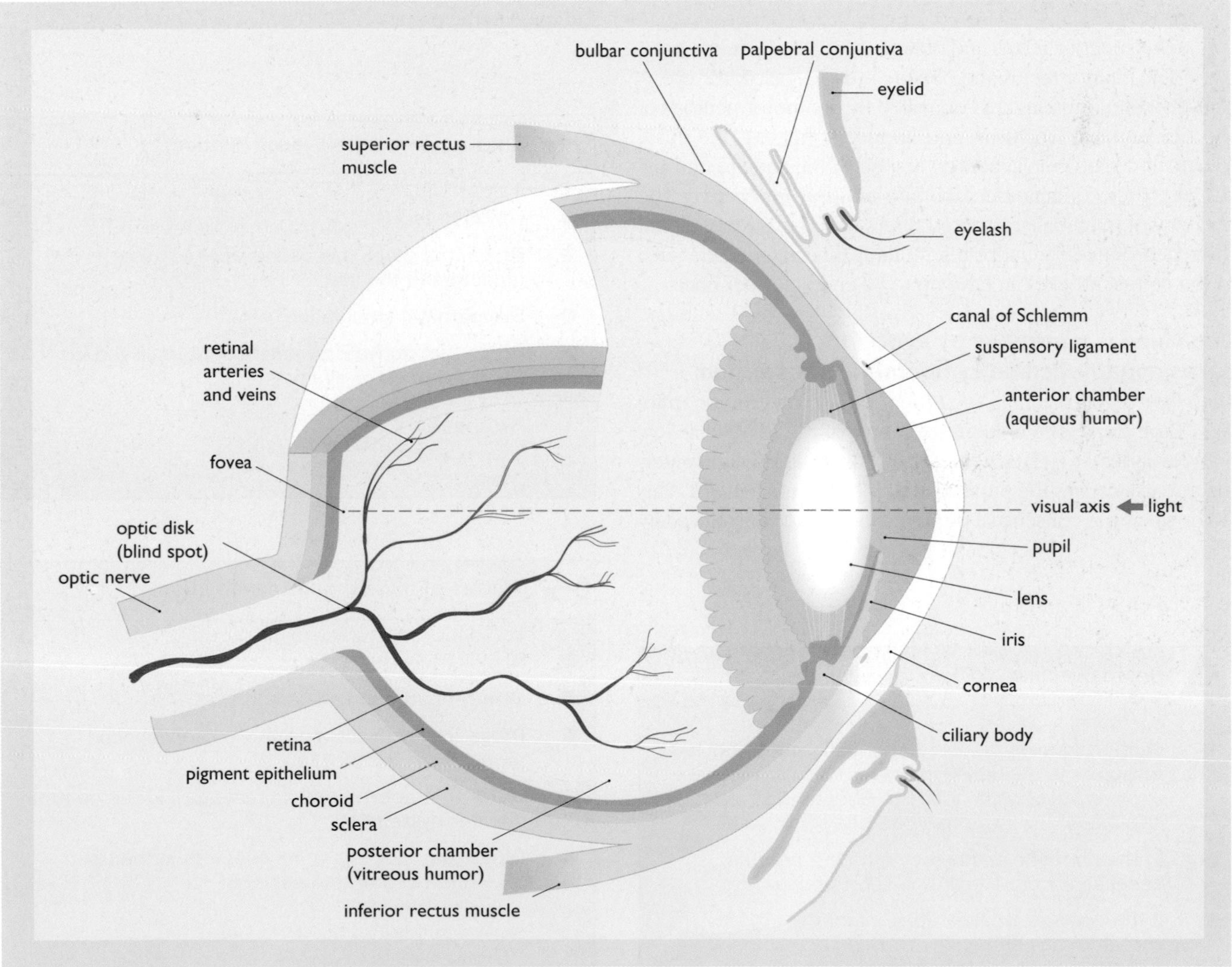

Fig. 19.1 Anatomy of the eye. A vertical cross-section through the eye ball.

bulbar conjunctiva, which also lines the inside of the eyelid where it becomes the palpebral conjunctiva.

The cornea is a transparent tissue at the front of the eye that allows light to enter the eyeball and contains fine sensory fibers. The majority of the eye's refractive power is at the air/corneal interface. The sclera is a continuation of the cornea and is the tough protective coat of the eye (the white of the eye), while the uveal tract is a layer of tissue beneath the sclera. From the front of the eye to the back, the uveal tract forms the iris (a pigmented smooth muscle), the ciliary body, and the choroid (a vascular bed beneath the retina). The retina is the neural tissue containing the eye's photoreceptor cells (rods and cones) and forms the innermost layer of the eyeball. To reach these photoreceptor cells, light must travel through the cornea, a fluid-filled anterior chamber, the lens, a fluid-filled posterior chamber, and the cellular layers of the retina. Obviously, all these tissues must be transparent to allow the light to pass through, and any condition that reduces the transparency of any of them will reduce visual capability.

The eye is moved within the orbit by six extraocular muscles

The six extraocular muscles are:

- The medial and lateral rectus muscles on either side of the eye.
- The superior rectus and oblique muscles above the eye.
- The inferior rectus and oblique muscles below the eye.

These striated muscles are controlled by the motor neurons of the oculomotor, trochlear, and abducens nerves (the third, fourth, and sixth cranial nerves, respectively), and are unusual because they contain fibers that are multiply innervated. The majority of mammalian striated fibers have between one and three neuromuscular endplates. Multiply innervated fibers, such as the rectus muscle, can have up to 80 endplates per fiber.

Pupil size is controlled by light and parasympathetic and sympathetic stimulation

High light levels reaching the retina lead to constriction (miosis) of the pupil (the hole in the center of the iris), while low light levels lead to dilation (mydriasis). In addition, light entering one eye causes the pupil of the other eye to constrict. This is known as the consensual pupil response and is produced by the brain. It only occurs if the brain is able to process the visual information it receives from the retina. This response is therefore a useful diagnostic tool for assessing brain damage in comatose or unconscious patients, and many doctors carry a small torch to test for it.

The parasympathetic nervous system maintains the tone of the iris and, when stimulated, causes miosis, while sympathetic stimulation (the 'fright, flight, and fight' response) causes mydriasis.

The dilator pupillae (the radial smooth muscle of the iris) is innervated by sympathetic fibers from the superior cervical ganglion. As elsewhere in the body, the sympathetic nervous system's neurotransmitter is norepinephrine, which acts on α_1 adrenoceptors resulting in pupil dilation. Drugs that are α_1 adrenoceptor agonists therefore contract the dilator pupillae and cause mydriasis (Fig. 19.2).

The constrictor pupillae (the sphincteric smooth muscle of the iris) is innervated by parasympathetic fibers from the ciliary ganglion. The parasympathetic nervous system's neurotransmitter acetylcholine acts on muscarinic receptors in the constrictor pupillae. Like adrenoceptor agonists, drugs that block muscarinic acetylcholine receptors are therefore also mydriatics (i.e. produce mydriasis).

Drugs that are clinically useful and cause miosis are confined to muscarinic agonists and are called miotics. Adrenoceptor antagonists such as phentolamine are miotics, but have little clinical value in the eye.

Neuromuscular blockers and the eye

- **Multiply innervated muscle tonically contracts in response to depolarizing neuromuscular blockers such as succinylcholine (see Chapter 21), and intraocular pressure may therefore increase**
- **In the normal eye this may not be a problem because succinylcholine is short acting**
- **If the eye has a penetrating injury the ocular contents may prolapse**

Causes of mydriasis (pupil dilation)

- **Low light levels****
- **Drugs that block muscarinic acetylcholine receptors in the iris****
- **Sympathetic stimulation***
- **Drugs that activate α_1 adrenoceptors in the iris (α_1 adrenoceptor agonists)***

*Weak dilation
**Strong dilation

Causes of miosis (pupil constriction)

- **High light levels****
- **Parasympathetic stimulation****
- **Drugs that activate muscarinic acetylcholine receptors in the iris****
- **Drugs that activate opioid receptors in the central nervous system****
- **Drugs that block α_1 adrenoceptors in the iris (α_1 adrenoceptor antagonists)***

*Weak constriction
**Strong constriction

Some drugs act at the level of the central nervous system to alter pupil size, for example an opioid receptor agonist, such as morphine, which produces the characteristic 'pinhole' pupil.

Accommodation is the mechanism that focuses the image on the retina

Accommodation is the ability of the eye to change its refractive power, which is a measure of how strongly it can bend a path of light. Refractive power is usually measured in units called diopters. The majority of the refractive power of the eye is located at the air/corneal interface and this is fixed. However, a small proportion of the refractive power is variable, owing to the ability of the lens to change its radius of curvature.

The lens is suspended in the eyeball from the ciliary muscle by suspensory ligaments. When the ciliary muscle relaxes, the suspensory ligaments are taut, stretching the lens into an ellipsoid shape (Fig. 19.3a). The low radius of curvature of the lens focuses distant objects onto the retina (far or distant vision). When the ciliary muscle contracts as a result of parasympathetic stimulation (i.e. acetylcholine acting on muscarinic receptors), the suspensory ligaments relax, and the lens takes up a more spherical shape (Fig. 19.3b). The curvature of the lens therefore increases and focuses near objects onto the retina (near vision). The contraction of the ciliary muscle for near vision explains why eyes get 'tired' after reading for long periods of time.

During accommodation for near vision, the pupil constricts, confining the light rays to the center of the lens to reduce spherical aberration and improve the quality of the image. This is the accommodation pupil reflex. Drugs that antagonize the accommodative event are often termed 'cycloplegics' and are exclusively muscarinic antagonists. There are no adrenoceptors in the ciliary muscle and accommodation is not therefore altered by sympatholytics or sympathomimetics.

The ability to accommodate (i.e. of the order of 12 diopters) in youth and young adulthood gradually decreases with age, because the lens becomes less flexible. By the age of 50 years, the accommodative power of the lens reduces to 1 or 2 diopters. This is why older people are generally 'long sighted' and need reading glasses. This natural condition of aging is termed 'presbyopia.'

Aqueous humor production is a continuous process

The anterior chamber of the eyeball is filled with a watery fluid called aqueous humor, which is continually produced by the blood vessels in the ciliary body at a rate of 3 ml/day. It flows first into the posterior chamber and then through the pupil into the anterior chamber (Fig. 19.4). The majority of the aqueous humor drains into the episcleral veins via the trabecular meshwork and

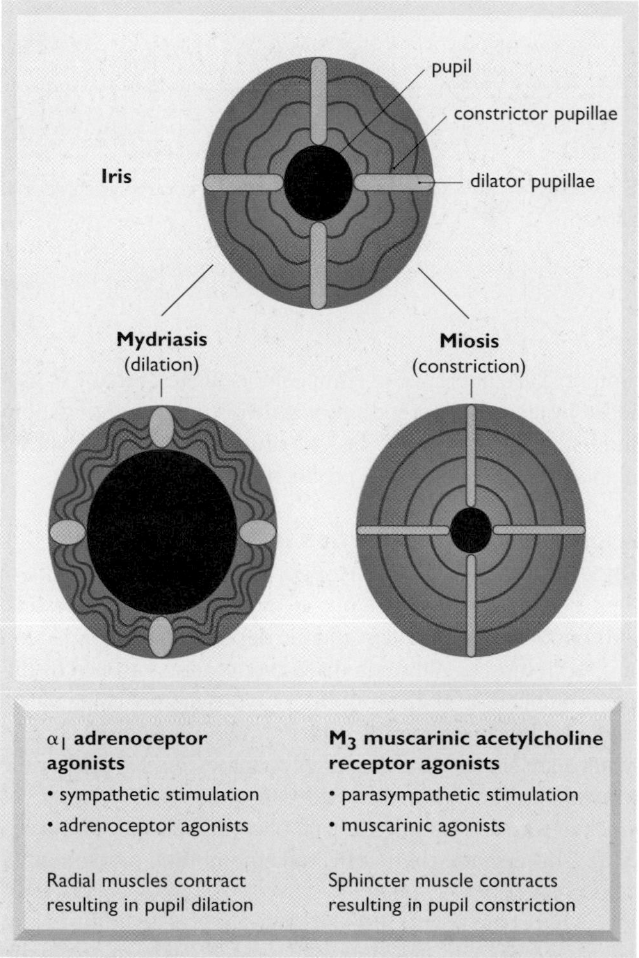

α_1 **adrenoceptor agonists**	M_3 **muscarinic acetylcholine receptor agonists**
• sympathetic stimulation	• parasympathetic stimulation
• adrenoceptor agonists	• muscarinic agonists
Radial muscles contract resulting in pupil dilation	Sphincter muscle contracts resulting in pupil constriction

Fig 19.2 Mechanisms involved in controlling pupil size.

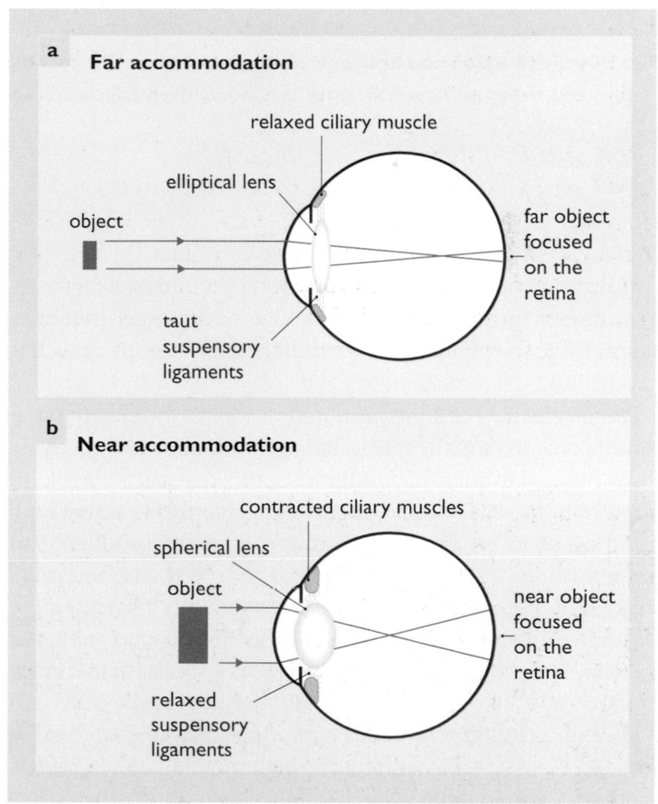

Fig. 19.3 Accommodation. The mechanisms of (a) far and (b) near accommodation to focus far and near objects onto the retina, respectively.

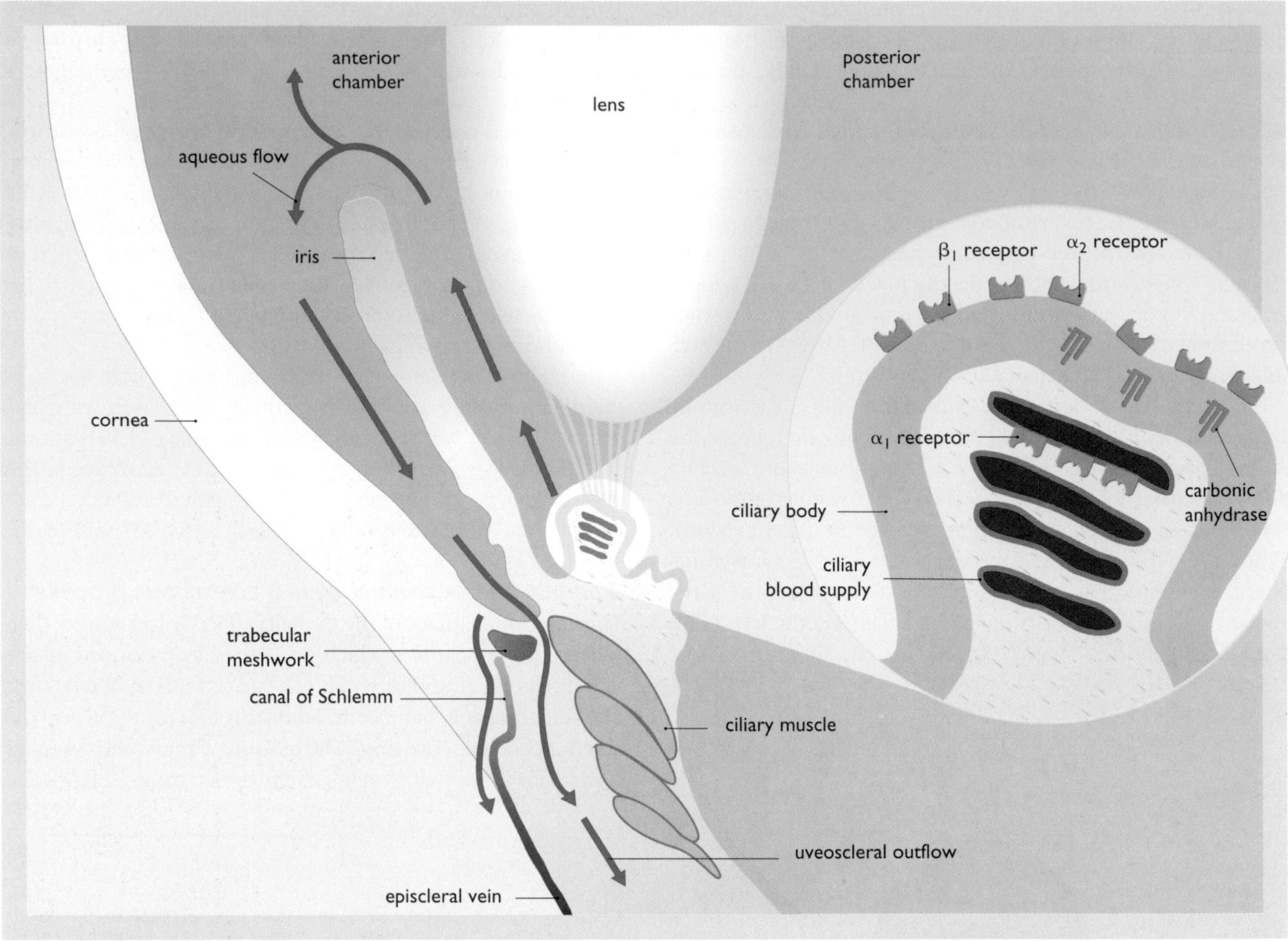

Fig. 19.4 Production and drainage of aqueous humor. The inset shows the location of α and β adrenoceptors and the enzyme carbonic anhydrase, which are all molecular targets for drugs that reduce the production of aqueous humor.

the canal of Schlemm, but some 10% drains through the uveoscleral outflow into the circulation by a trans-scleral route. The rate of production and drainage of aqueous humor is responsible for maintaining the intraocular pressure, which is normally 12–20 mmHg.

The production of aqueous humor is indirectly related to the blood pressure and the rate of blood flow in the ciliary body. As elsewhere, activation of α_1 adrenoceptors constricts the blood vessels in the ciliary body. Circulating epinephrine acting on β adrenoceptors on the ciliary body increases the production of aqueous humor. However, there may also be α adrenoceptors located on the ciliary body that reduce aqueous formation.

The enzyme carbonic anhydrase is important for aqueous humor formation (see Fig. 19.4). Its role in the eye is similar to that in the kidneys or other organs where fluid movement is involved.

The composition of aqueous humor is similar to that of blood plasma (Fig. 19.5), but without the high protein content, which, if present, would render the fluid translucent rather than transparent. However, aqueous humor is not purely an ultrafiltrate of plasma because it has a higher bicarbonate and ascorbic acid content. This difference in composition suggests that it is produced by an active secretion process. This point is important in understanding how one class of drugs (carbonic anhydrase inhibitors) acts to reduce its production (see p. 377).

Smooth muscle contraction is the key to many physiologic events in the eye

Pupil dilation and constriction, constriction of the blood vessels, and contraction of the ciliary muscle depend on the contraction of smooth muscle. Although these events are controlled by different branches of the autonomic nervous system using different neurotransmitters and receptors, their cellular transduction systems are similar. Both α_1 adrenoceptors and M_3 muscarinic acetylcholine receptors activate G proteins (see Chapter 3), which in turn activate the enzyme phospholipase C (PLC) (Fig. 19.6). This enzyme then converts a membrane phospholipid (phosphatidyl bisphosphate) into two second messengers, inositol-1,4,5-trisphosphate (IP_3) and diacylglycerol. IP_3 diffuses into the cytosol and activates intracellular receptors, resulting in the release of stored Ca^{2+}, which triggers muscle contraction.

Substance	Blood plasma mg/dl	Blood plasma (mmol/liter)	Aqueous humor mg/dl	Aqueous humor (mmol/liter)
Na^+	334	145	331	144
K^+	19.5	5.0	19.5	5.0
Ca^{2+}	10.4	2.6	6.8	1.7
Mg^{2+}	2.4	1.0	1.9	0.8
Cl^-	383	108	391	110
Protein	6000mg/100ml		10mg/100ml	
Ascorbic acid	0.35	0.02	17.6	1.0
HCO_3	165	27	207	34

Fig 19.5 Composition of aqueous humor.

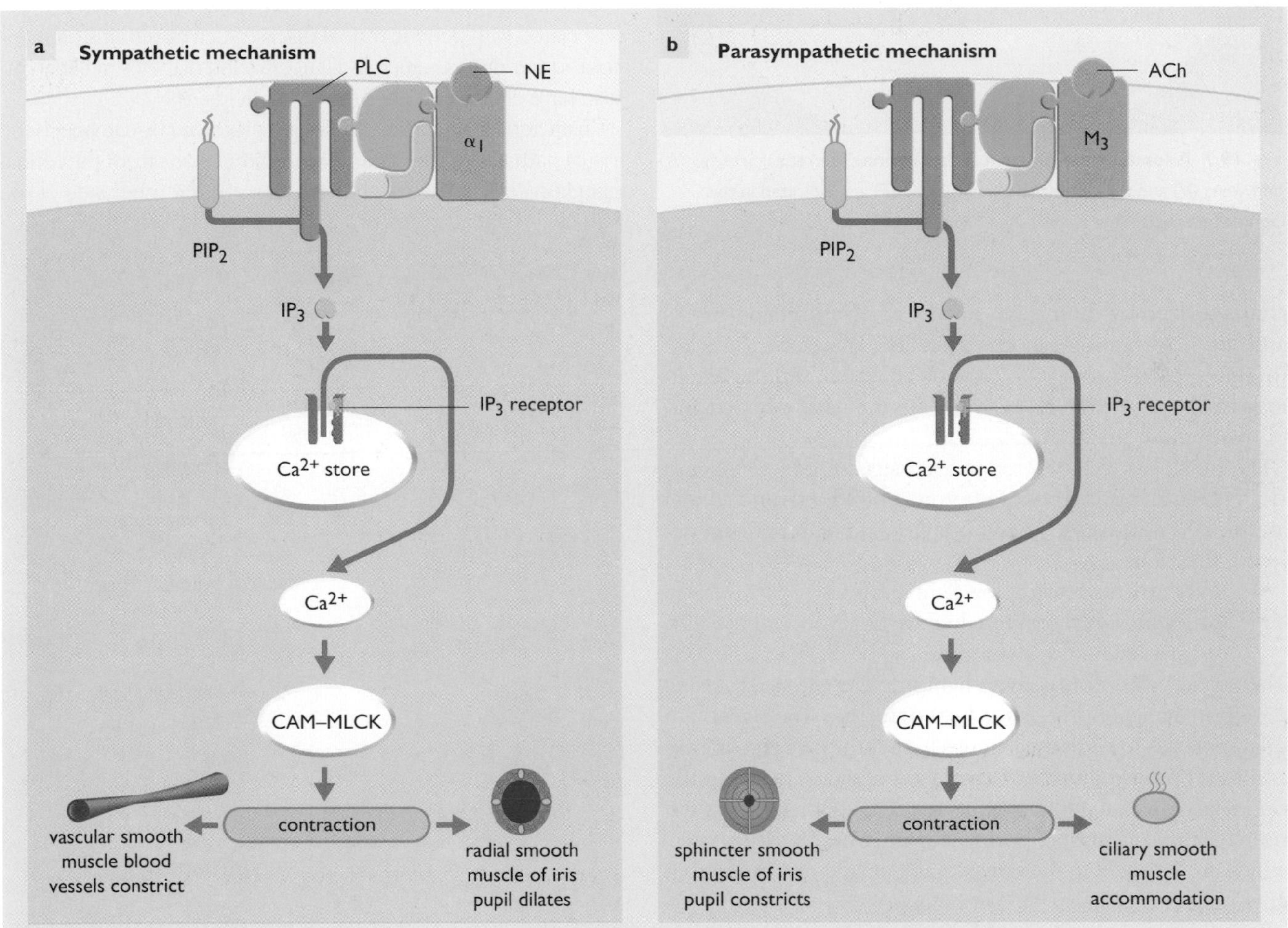

Fig.19.6 Cellular transduction pathway in smooth muscle. Activation of α_1 adrenoceptors (α_1) by norepinephrine (NE) or M_3 muscarinic receptors (M_3) by acetylcholine (ACh) leads to activation of G proteins, which stimulate inositol-1,4,5-trisphosphate (IP_3) production from phosphatidyl bisphosphate (PIP_2) by the enzyme phospholipase C (PLC). IP_3 releases Ca^{2+} from intracellular Ca^{2+} stores, and the Ca^{2+} then activates calmodulin–myosin light chain kinase (CAM–MLCK) and triggers contraction.

The retina converts light into electric signals

The retina is part of the central nervous system embryologically and can be considered as an extension of the brain. It receives oxygen and metabolic requirements from the choroid plexus behind and the retinal blood vessels in front, and is the only place where the circulatory system of the brain can be viewed directly. When viewed through the pupil with an ophthalmoscope, the image is called the fundus (Fig.19.7). The main features of this view are the retinal arteries and veins, and a pale moon-like disk, which is the end of the optic nerve. Other important areas include the macula lutea with the fovea at its center, both areas being

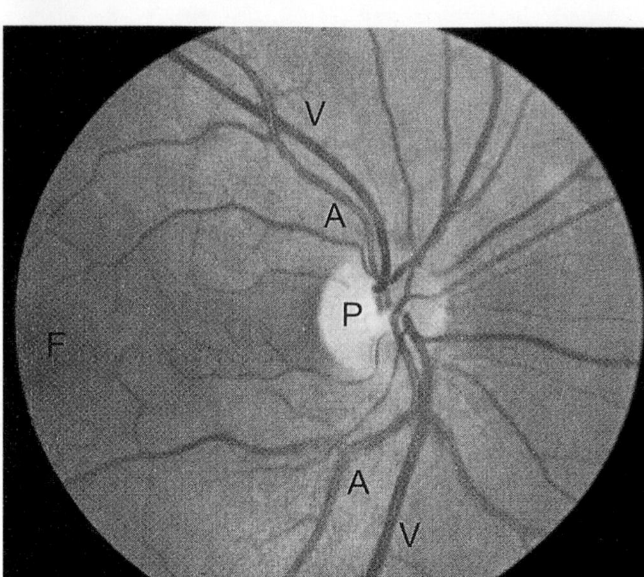

Fig. 19.7 A fundal view of the normal retina. The retinal arteries (A) and veins (V) and the optic disk (P) and fovea (F) are indicated in this ophthalmoscopic view.

characterized by their high density of photoreceptor cells and absence of retinal blood vessels. The sharpest images are therefore produced on this part of the retina, and the resulting visual images sent to the brain are the most detailed and of the highest quality.

The retina is a well-ordered layered structure of nerve cells (Fig. 19.8). The two types of photoreceptor (rods and cones) are located next to the pigment epithelium and perform different functions:

- Rods are only active at low light levels.
- Cones are only active at high light levels and are also responsible for color vision.

These photoreceptors convert light into electric signals using the opsin family of proteins as light detectors. The signals are then sent back towards the vitreous humor through bipolar cells and to retinal ganglion cells, the axons of which make up the optic nerve, which connects with the brain. Other cells in the retina include amacrine, horizontal, and interplexiform cells, which are involved in the considerable image processing that goes on in the retina.

Retinal function can be tested directly by recording the electric signal produced in response to a flash of light. This response is called the electroretinogram (ERG) (Fig. 19.9). The waveform is complex and different parts of it are generated by the different layers of the eye. The ERG is therefore a useful diagnostic tool for assessing both retinal and some systemic diseases.

Different areas of the visual field have different functions

Although the image produced by the central vision of the macula lutea and fovea is the most detailed, the visual field extends to some 200° binocularly. Most of the peripheral retina is concerned with detecting movement and triggers the eye to center on a new visual stimulus. For example, if someone walks into the peripheral visual field of someone who is reading, the reader will detect the movement, but will only identify who has entered their visual field when they look up and center their fovea on the person's face.

Peripheral vision is also responsible for low light vision as most of the rod photoreceptors, which are responsible for night vision, are located outside the fovea.

The visual fields are measured by a technique called perimetry, and small patches of lost vision in the visual field are called scotomas. Normally, each eye has one scotoma corresponding to the area of the optic disk (see Fig. 19.7) because it contains no photoreceptor cells and is therefore unable to perceive light: this scotoma is often called the blind spot.

Loss of peripheral vision is termed 'tunnel vision' and is often associated with genetic retinal disease such as retinitis pigmentosa. Other diseases such as glaucoma and diabetes mellitus can also have effects that alter the visual fields.

Characteristic visual field losses are produced by damage to the visual pathways in the brain because the axons from the retinal ganglion cells in the nasal retina cross to the other side of the

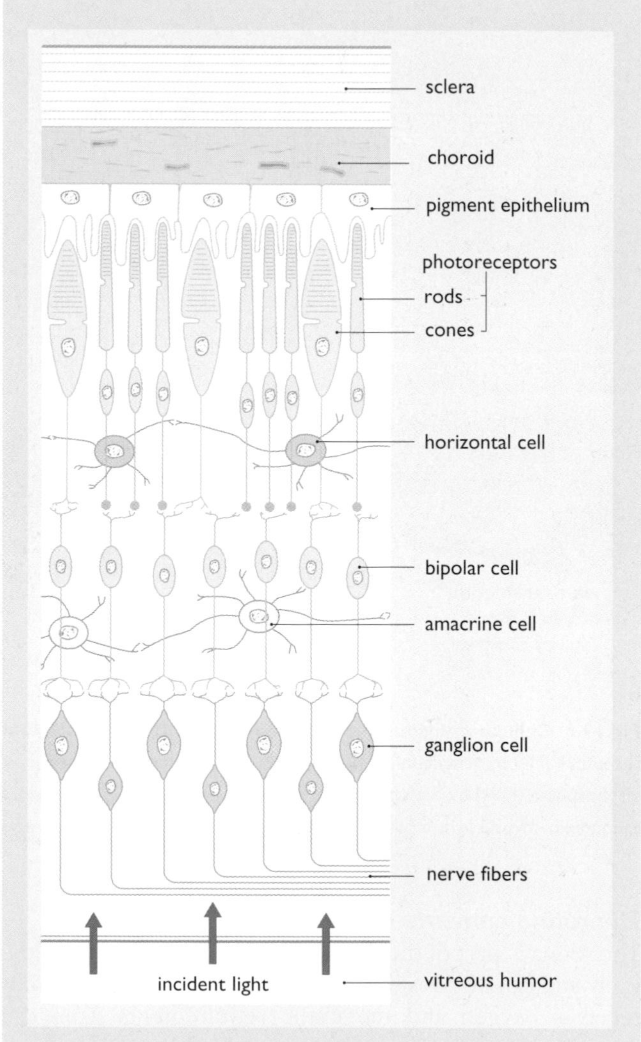

Fig. 19.8 Diagram of a cross-section through the retina.

brain at the optic chiasm. Damage to postchiasmal fibers on the right side of the brain therefore results in a loss of vision in the left half of the visual field of both eyes. Perimetry is a useful tool for investigating some retinal, pituitary, and neurologic diseases.

PROPERTIES OF DRUGS USED IN THE EYE

Drugs applied to the eye must be uncharged to cross the cornea

In order to act within the eye, all drugs applied topically to the eye must cross the cornea. They must therefore be lipophilic or uncharged. The ocular penetration of a weakly basic or acidic drug can be improved if the pH is appropriately adjusted to produce a larger proportion of uncharged drug (see Chapter 5). However, drug solutions do not need to be isotonic with lacrimal secretions (tears).

Most drugs for the eye are available as sterile eye drop preparations and care must be taken not to contaminate them or cause cross-contamination from one eye to the other. Single-use eye drops should be used, if possible.

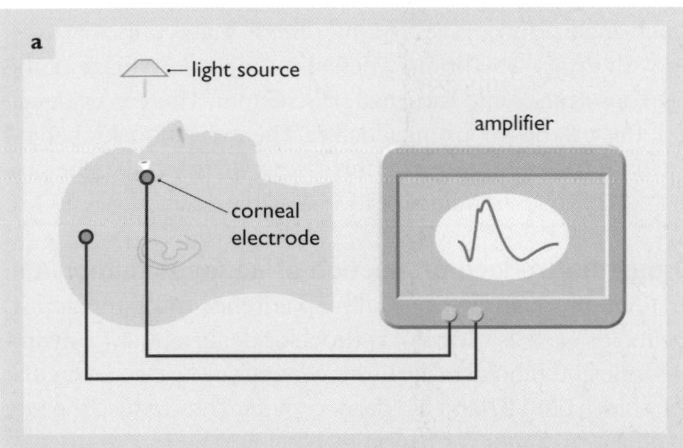

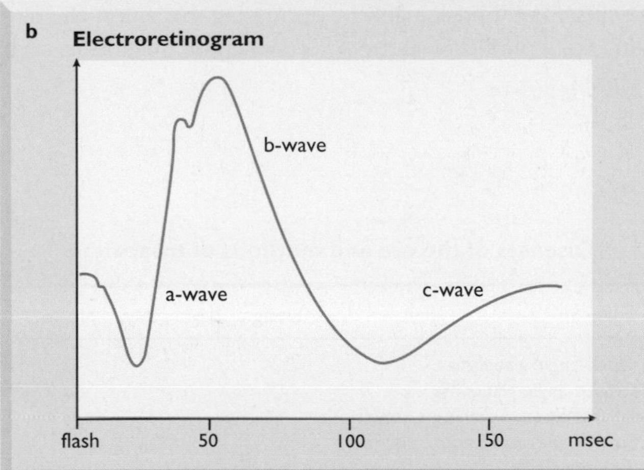

Fig. 19.9 The electroretinogram (ERG). (a) Electrodiagnostic recordings are performed by placing electrodes on the cornea and connecting them to an amplifier. A flash of light is used to produce a response called the ERG. (b) Components of the ERG are generated by different ocular layers: the a-wave from the photoreceptors; the b-wave from the bipolar cell layer; and the c-wave from the pigment epithelium (see Fig. 19.8).

Ophthalmic preparations

- Most drugs mentioned in this chapter are available as specific ophthalmic preparations (e.g. eye drops or creams)
- As the majority of eye drugs are applied locally, the risk of systemic adverse effects is minimized but not completely avoided
- Some locally applied drugs can cause systemic adverse effects
- Slow-release formulations may reduce the risk of adverse effects

Melanin in the iris binds some drugs and affects their action

The action of some drugs is related to eye color, which is produced by the content of the pigment melanin in the iris. Black or dark brown irises contain significantly more melanin than green, gray, or blue irises. Melanin binds a variety of drugs such as atropine and such drugs can therefore take longer to act and have longer-lasting effects if the patient has a dark iris. Care is needed to avoid overdosing patients with highly pigmented irises.

Eye color and drugs

- Iris pigmentation can affect the onset and duration of action of many drugs applied to the eye
- Black and brown irises contain more pigment (melanin) than green, gray, or blue irises
- The more pigment in the iris, the more drug can bind to it, resulting in a slower onset and longer duration of action

Preservatives in eye drops may cause allergic reactions

Many substances are used as preservatives in eye drops and may cause allergic responses in susceptible individuals. The preservative benzalkonium chloride should be avoided in patients using soft contact lenses as it can accumulate in the lens and may induce toxic reactions.

DRUGS USED IN OPHTHALMIC DIAGNOSIS

Muscarinic antagonists are used for mydriasis

Many systemic and retinal diseases can be diagnosed by looking at the fundus, and drugs that dilate the pupil (mydriatics) improve the view of the fundus. The most effective class of such drugs are the muscarinic antagonists (Fig. 19.10), and the particular drug used is chosen according to its duration of action and whether cycloplegia is required. They all act by blocking the muscarinic receptors in the iris and ciliary muscle, thereby antagonizing the parasympathetic control of these muscles. Cyclopentolate and atropine are the preferred drugs for producing cycloplegia in children.

Adrenoceptor agonists such as epinephrine and phenylephrine hydrochloride also dilate the pupil, but only to a small extent and they do not cause cycloplegia.

Muscarinic antagonists used as mydriatics

Drug	Duration of action (h)	Mydriatic effect	Cycloplegic effect
Tropicamide	1–3	++	+
Scopolamine	12–24	+++	+++
Homatropine	12–24	+++	+++
Cyclopentolate	12–24	+++	+++
Atropine	168–240	+++	+++

Fig. 19.10 Muscarinic antagonists used as mydriatics.

Local anesthetics are used to produce corneal anesthesia

The cornea is a particularly sensitive tissue and it is therefore commonly anesthetized in ophthalmic diagnosis because intraocular pressure measurement (tonometry) involves placing a device on the cornea for a short period of time. Such anesthesia is provided by a group of chemically related drugs, the local anesthetics (Fig. 19.11), which may also be used for minor eye operations. The mechanisms of action of these compounds are explained in Chapter 21.

Fluorescent dyes are used to detect foreign bodies

Fluorescent dyes such as fluorescein sodium and dichlorotetraiodofluorescein (rose bengal) are instilled into the eye to detect corneal lesions or foreign bodies. Rose bengal is only taken up by injured or infected cells, and is therefore useful for detecting corneal damage and viral infections.

Local anesthetics for corneal anesthesia

Drug	Uses
Oxybuprocaine hydrochloride*	Tonometry (short acting)
Proxymetacaine hydrochloride*	Children (less stinging)
Lidocaine hydrochloride	Tonometry and minor surgery
Amethocaine hydrochloride	Tonometry and minor surgery

Fig. 19.11 Local anesthetics used for corneal anesthesia.

PATHOPHYSIOLOGY AND DISEASES OF THE EYE

There are many eye diseases, some of which are listed in Fig. 19.12, but only those that can be treated by drugs are discussed in this chapter. Despite claims, there is no clear clinical evidence that any drug treatment or vitamin supplementation prevents or cures cataracts, age-related maculopathy or genetic retinal dystrophy.

GLAUCOMA

Glaucoma is caused by poor drainage of aqueous humor and can cause blindness

Glaucoma is characterized by:

- An increase in intraocular pressure to over 21 mmHg.
- Fundus changes, in particular optic disk 'cupping.'
- Visual field changes.

If untreated, it permanently damages the optic nerve and this can cause blindness. The two main types of glaucoma are open-angle (simple) and closed-angle glaucoma. The angle referred to is the filtration angle formed between the iris and the cornea.

Open-angle glaucoma

Open-angle glaucoma is a chronic disease that is primarily treated with drugs. The primary defect is reduced drainage of the aqueous humor into the canal of Schlemm. There is evidence that this can be a congenital defect. The two rationales behind the drug treatments used for this disease are to reduce the production of aqueous humor or to increase its drainage (Fig 19.13).

Drugs that reduce production of aqueous humor The first line of treatment is usually a β adrenoceptor antagonist. Examples such as carteolol hydrochloride, levobunolol hydrochloride and timolol maleate are generally nonselective in that they block both β_1 and β_2 adrenoceptors. They reduce the rate of aqueous humor formation by blocking these receptors on the ciliary body, presumably by decreasing the action of circulating epinephrine. Selective β adrenoceptor antagonists such

Diseases of the eye and methods of treatment

Disease	Drugs	Surgery	None
Open-angle glaucoma	✓	–	–
Closed-angle glaucoma	✓	✓	–
Inflammation and allergic conditions	✓	–	–
Squints and oculomotor disorders	✓	✓	–
Tear deficiency	✓	–	–
Infections	✓	–	–
Detached retina	–	✓	–
Cataracts	–	✓	–
Retinitis pigmentosa	–	–	✓
Amblyopia	–	–	✓
Retinopathy	–	–	✓

Fig. 19.12 Diseases of the eye and methods of treatment.

Drugs used to treat open-angle glaucoma

Type	Mechanism	Examples of drugs
Reduce aqueous humor formation		
β Adrenoceptor antagonists	Block β_1 receptors on the ciliary body	Timolol maleate Betaxolol hydrochloride Carteolol hydrochloride Levobunolol hydrochloride Metipranolol
α Adrenoceptor agonists	Agonism of α_2 receptors on the ciliary body and/or α_1 (vasoconstrictor) receptors on ciliary vessels	Epinephrine Dipivefrin hydrochloride Apraclonidine
Carbonic anhydrase inhibitors	Reduce bicarbonate formation	Acetazolamide Dichlorphenamide Dorzolamide
Increase drainage of aqueous humor		
Miotics	Activate muscarinic receptors on the iris and ciliary body causing pupil constriction and ciliary muscle contraction, which may improve uveoscleral outflow	Carbachol Pilocarpine

Fig. 19.13 Drugs used to treat open-angle glaucoma.

as betaxolol hydrochloride (β_1 selective) have also been shown to reduce intraocular pressure effectively. Metipranolol has been used in selected patients who are allergic to preservatives or who wear soft contact lens. However, its use (at least in the UK) is limited owing to reports of an associated granulomatous anterior uveitis.

Aqueous humor formation may also be reduced by α adrenoceptor agonists. Epinephrine is not very effective because it is poorly available at its site of action. This problem can be overcome by giving the prodrug dipivefrin hydrochloride. (A prodrug is a substance that is not itself biologically active, but is metabolized by the body into an active substance.) Dipivefrine hydrochloride is more highly lipophilic, and once in the eye it is converted to epinephrine, the active metabolite. The use of apraclonidine is confined to extreme or acute cases of raised intraocular pressure. It is a derivative of the α_2 adrenoceptor agonist, clonidine, but unlike clonidine it does not cross the blood–brain barrier and so has fewer unwanted systemic effects, but it is contra-indicated in patients with a history of cardiovascular disease. Apraclonidine is thought to act either on α_2 adrenoceptors on the ciliary body to reduce aqueous humor formation directly or via α_1 adrenoceptors to reduce ciliary blood flow in a manner similar to epinephrine. Its adverse effects include hyperemia, eyelid retraction, vasoconstriction of the conjunctiva (blanching), and mydriasis.

Carbonic anhydrase inhibitors are given systemically and work in the same way as when they are given as diuretics (see Chapter 10). The conversion of carbon dioxide and water to carbonic acid (and therefore bicarbonate) is catalyzed by the enzyme carbonic anhydrase. As the production of aqueous humor depends on the active transport of bicarbonate and Na^+ ions, reducing the activity of carbonic anhydrase ultimately reduces aqueous humor production. Adverse effects, particularly in the elderly, include paresthesia, hypokalemia, a lack of appetite, drowsiness, and depression. The recent introduction of slow-release carbonic anhydrase inhibitors has decreased the incidence of these adverse effects. Topical carbonic anhydrase inhibitors, such as dorzolamide, have been introduced recently to work synergistically with β adrenoceptor antagonists or miotics.

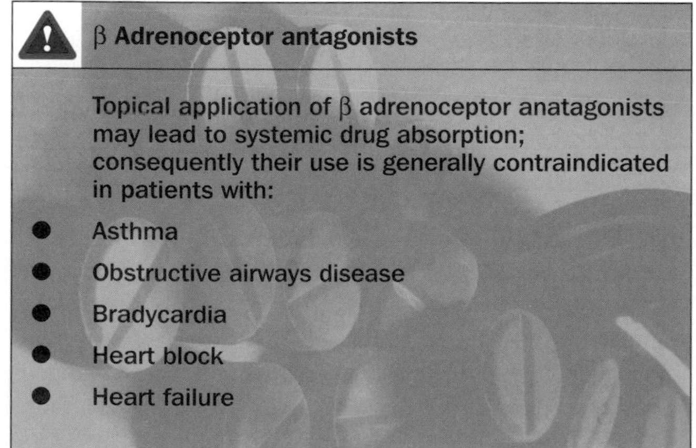

Drugs that increase the drainage of aqueous humor

Miotics may, to some degree, assist in the drainage of aqueous humor, possibly by increasing the uveoscleral outflow. Miotics have the obvious adverse effect of a permanently constricted pupil. Of more concern is the permanent accommodative spasm they produce which, over time, leads to blurred vision and headache. This occurs in all patients, but usually wears off with time in older patients. Slow-release formulations of miotics (e.g. modified-release pilocarpine) are available to minimize these adverse effects in younger patients.

Closed-angle glaucoma

Closed-angle glaucoma results from forward ballooning of the peripheral iris (iris bombé) so that it touches the back of the cornea, thereby reducing the flow of aqueous humor between the cornea and the iris.

In emergency situations, drug treatment is used to reduce the peripheral ballooning and so lower the acute rise in intraocular pressure. Drugs such as mannitol and glycerol given systemically increase the osmolarity of the blood and can reduce intraocular pressure, while topical miotics such as pilocarpine or carbachol can sometimes tauten the iris and temporarily relieve the problem.

A permanent cure is produced by laser surgery. An yttrium–aluminum–garnet (YAG) laser is used to form a hole in the iris (iridectomy) to increase the flow of aqueous humor.

 **Mydriatics and glaucoma**

- Mydriatics may be hazardous in patients suspected of closed-angle glaucoma as they may exacerbate the condition
- Pupil dilation and paralysis of the ciliary muscle reduce the drainage of aqueous humor

INFLAMMATION AND ALLERGY

Inflammation of the eye is treated with a short course of glucocorticosteroids

Local intraocular inflammation and uveitis (inflammation of the uveal tract) can be treated with a short course of glucocorticosteroids, which are are the first line of treatment for local inflammation. Their mechanism of action is explained in Chapter 11. However, these drugs are for short-term use only. With prolonged use they may cause 'steroid glaucoma' or cataracts. They should therefore only be given under ophthalmologic supervision. Examples of glucocorticosteroids in clinical use today are listed in Fig. 19.14. Systemic glucocorticosteroids may be appropriate for severe eye disease such as scleritis, episcleritis, and blinding uveitis.

A correct diagnosis is essential: glucocorticosteroids will worsen an inflamed eye produced by a dendritic ulcer resulting from a herpes simplex virus infection and may lead to blindness or even loss of the eye.

Allergic conditions such as allergic conjunctivitis can be treated with H_1 antihistamines such as antazoline or other drugs such as cromolyn sodium or nedocromil sodium. Topical glucocorticosteroids may also be needed for severe allergy.

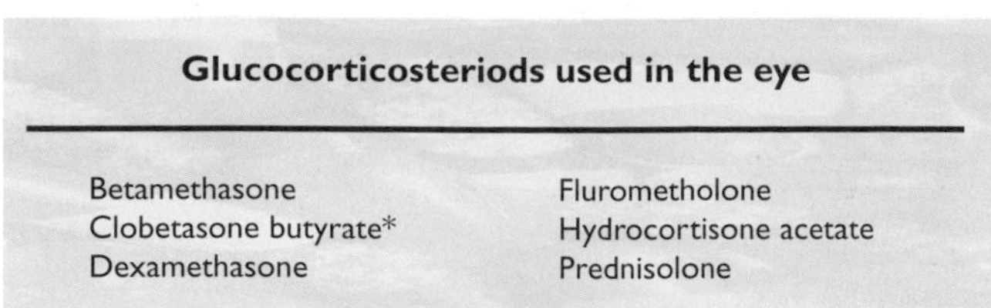

Glucocorticosteriods used in the eye	
Betamethasone	Flurometholone
Clobetasone butyrate*	Hydrocortisone acetate
Dexamethasone	Prednisolone

Fig. 19.14 Glucocorticosteroids used in the eye.

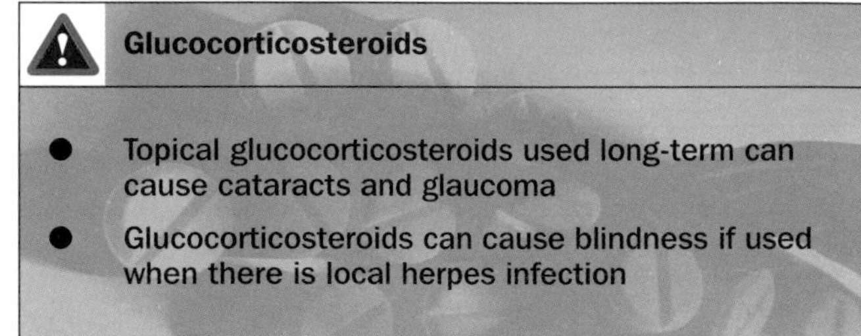

Glucocorticosteroids

- Topical glucocorticosteroids used long-term can cause cataracts and glaucoma
- Glucocorticosteroids can cause blindness if used when there is local herpes infection

TEAR DEFICIENCY

Tear deficiency is particularly associated with rheumatoid arthritis and is called Sjögren's syndrome. A variety of drugs can be used as artificial tears to prevent dry eyes becoming painful. Examples are listed in Fig. 19.15. Acetylcysteine is a mucolytic that can be used to break up mucoid secretions in the eye, which are often associated with a poor tear film over the eye.

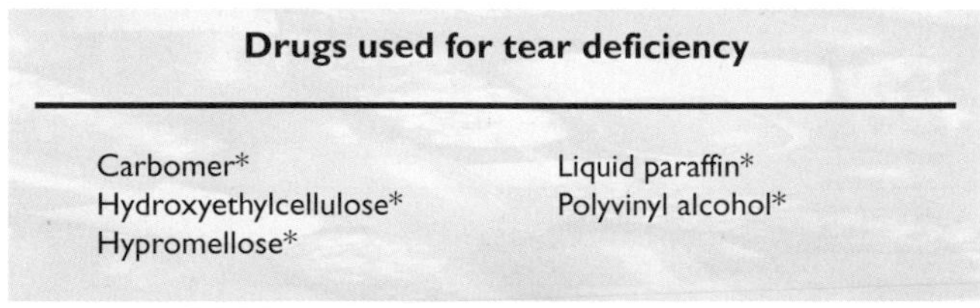

Drugs used for tear deficiency	
Carbomer*	Liquid paraffin*
Hydroxyethylcellulose*	Polyvinyl alcohol*
Hypromellose*	

Fig. 19.15 Drugs used as artificial tears.

SQUINT AND OCULOMOTOR DISORDERS

Some extraocular and eyelid muscle disorders can be treated with botulinum toxin

Some neuromuscular disorders of the extraocular muscles (squints) and eyelids (blepharospasms) can be treated with botulinum toxin A. This is one of the toxins produced by the bacteria *Clostridium botulinum*, which causes some forms of food poisoning. The skeletal muscles are injected with this toxin, and over a period of three days or so the muscle relaxes and stays relaxed for up to six weeks. Botulinum toxin A blocks acetylcholine release from the motor nerve terminals (Fig. 19.16). To ensure correct needle placement for the injection it is recommended that the procedure is performed with a special needle that allows recording of the electromyogram (EMG) at the same time.

The skeletal muscle autoimmune disease myasthenia gravis affects the muscles of the eyelids as well as the extraocular muscles. Systemic administration of anticholinesterase drugs such as neostigmine bromide and pyridostigmine bromide relieves the ocular and other symptoms (see Chapter 7).

DRUGS THAT HAVE ADVERSE EFFECTS ON THE EYE

Lacrimators

Lacrimators are drugs that are not used therapeutically. They cause intense irritation of the cornea and conjunctiva, for example tear gases such as orthochlorobenzylidenemalononitrite (CS gas) and Mace. CS gas is used as an harassing agent for controlling civil disorders, and in some countries these substances are legally available for use in personal protection.

These compounds activate capsaicin receptors, which are found on sensory nerves and are nonselective cation channels. Activation of the receptor opens the ion channel, allowing the flow of Na^+ and Ca^{2+} ions into the nerve; this depolarizes the nerve and can generate action potentials. The action potentials can then travel both orthodromically and antidromically along the fibers, depolarizing many nerve terminals (Fig. 19.17). A variety of mediators (neurokinins and tachykinins, which cause pain, inflammation, and lacrimal gland secretion) are then released from sensory nerve terminals in response to the stimulation. This sensation can be duplicated by touching the eyes after cutting up chilli peppers, and the sensory nerve receptors were therefore named after this 'lacrimator' in chilli peppers (i.e. capsaicin).

Cataractogenic drugs

When the lens becomes opaque it is called a cataract. Drugs that can cause cataracts include:

- Locally applied drugs such as glucocorticosteroids when given long term.
- Systemic drugs such as the phenothiazines (used to treat schizophrenia, see Chapter 7) (Fig. 19.18).

Retinopathic drugs

A number of systemically applied drugs can cause retinopathy. Ingestion of as little as 10 g of methanol, which is often found in illicit spirits such as moonshine and poteen, damages retinal ganglion cells. The axons of these cells form the

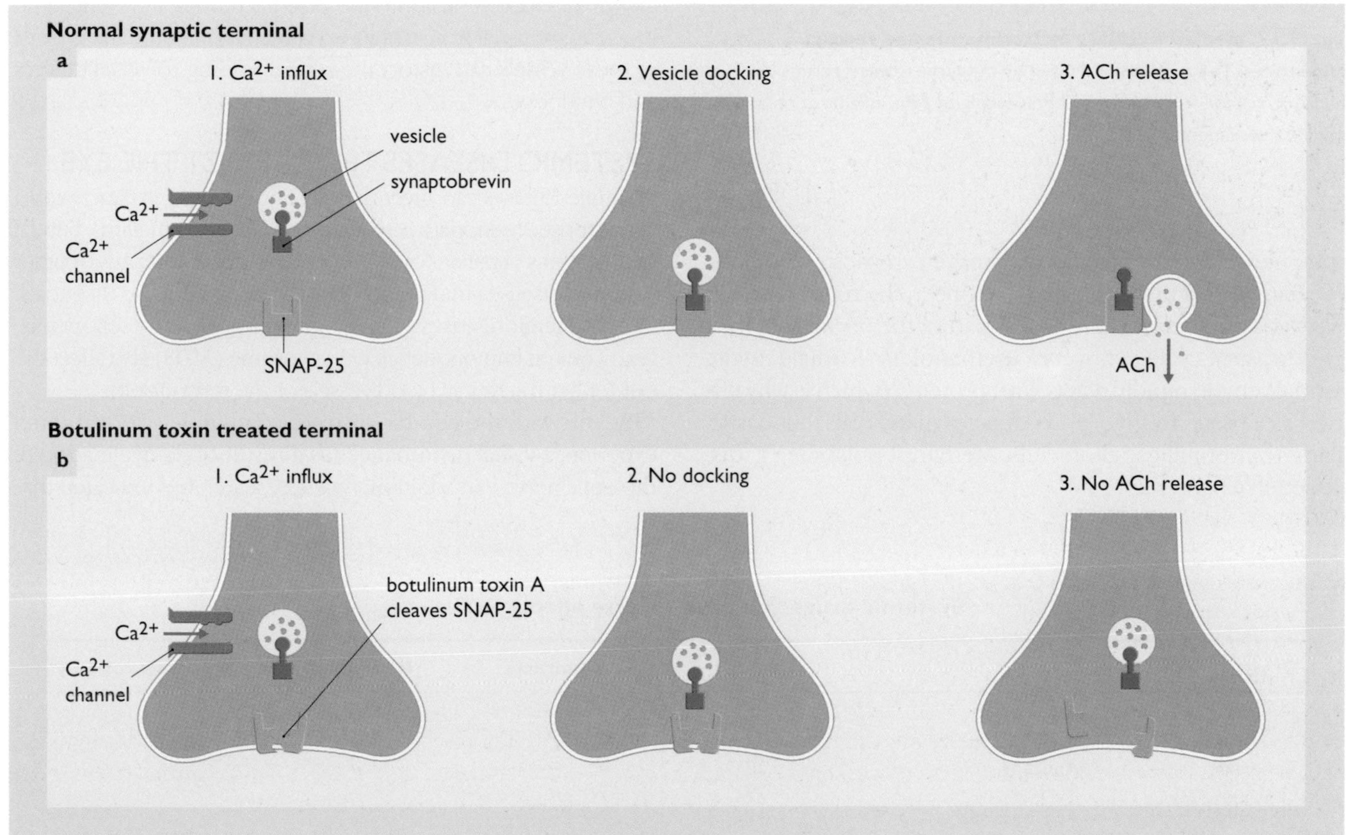

Fig. 19.16 The cellular mechanism of action of botulinum toxin. Botulinum toxin prevents vesicle docking and acetylcholine (ACh) release from motor nerves. It does this by cleaving synaptosomal-associated protein (SNAP-25), which is an important docking protein and has a molecular weight of 25 kD.

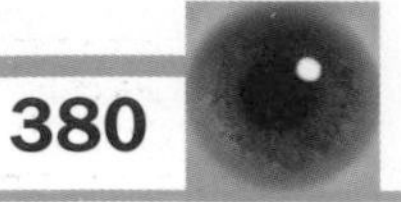

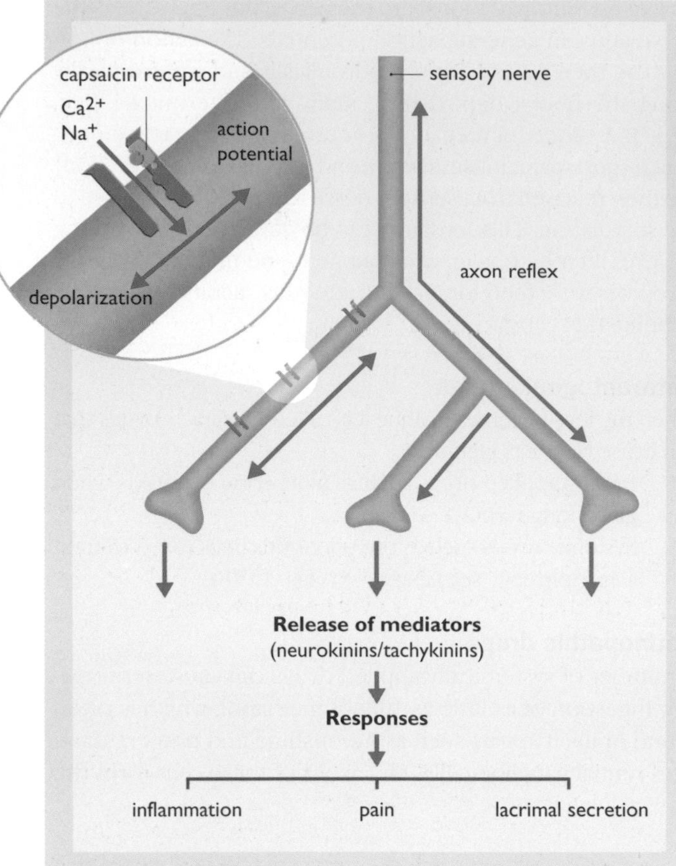

Fig. 19.17 Mediator release by lacrimators and related substances. The axon reflex caused by capsaicin agonists results in mediator release from sensory fibers leading to pain, inflammation, and glandular secretions.

optic nerves and the resulting damage can cause blindness. The damage occurs because an enzyme in the retina that normally converts retinol to retinal as part of the normal pigment (rhodopsin) cycle, converts methanol to formaldehyde. Formaldehyde rapidly reacts with proteins (which is why it is used as a tissue fixative) and damages many cells, but particularly the retinal ganglion cells. Methanol poisoning is discussed in Chapter 29.

Drugs that have adverse effects on the eye

- Cataracts can be caused by some locally applied drugs (e.g. ecothiopate)
- Cataracts can be caused by some systemically applied drugs (e.g. chloroquine)
- Retinopathies can be caused by some systemically applied drugs (e.g. tamoxifen)

Chloroquine, which was first used as an antimalarial drug and is now used for rheumatoid conditions, can cause reversible cataracts and also irreversible and very characteristic 'bull's eye' retinopathy. However, if the dose is kept below 250 mg/day this adverse effect is less common.

Indomethacin, ethambutol, tamoxifen, and phenothiazines are some of the other drugs that have adverse effects on the retina or the optic nerve. In some cases these retinal adverse effects are dose dependent. For example, retinal toxicity is rare if the dose of ethambutol is kept below 15 mg/kg/day. (It is prudent to arrange for ophthalmologic monitoring of patients taking these drugs.)

A specific problem of premature infants, who are often placed in a high-oxygen environment to aid their survival, is retrolental fibroplasia (Fig. 19.19). This is produced by the inappropriate growth of blood vessels into the vitreous humor and is triggered by abrupt removal from a high-oxygen environment. The growth of these vessels can distort the retina, leading to visual defects and blindness.

SYSTEMIC DISEASES THAT AFFECT THE EYE

Systemic diseases can affect the eye. For example, cataracts and a characteristic retinopathy are features of diabetes mellitus. Fundal examinations of patients with suspected diabetes mellitus or other systemic diseases may therefore help in making the diagnosis. Other systemic diseases such as hypertension, sickle cell anemia, and acquired immunodeficiency syndrome (AIDS) also affect the eye (either the retinal blood vessels or the retina itself).

Patients with the neurologic disease multiple sclerosis often experience visual disturbances as a result of demyelination of the optic nerves. In addition, recent research has indicated that

Systemic drugs that have adverse effects on the eye

Drug	Use	Chapter	Cataracts	Retinopathy	Optic neuropathy
Chloroquine	Antimalarial	25	✓	✓	–
Phenothiazines	Antipsychotic	7	✓	✓	–
Tamoxifen	Anticancer	28	–	✓	–
Methanol	Recreational	29	–	–	✓
Ethambutol	Antitubercular	11	–	–	✓
Indomethacin	Anti-inflammatory	17	–	✓	–
Oxygen	Neonatal care	–	–	✓	–

Fig. 19.18 Systemic drugs that have adverse effects on the eye.

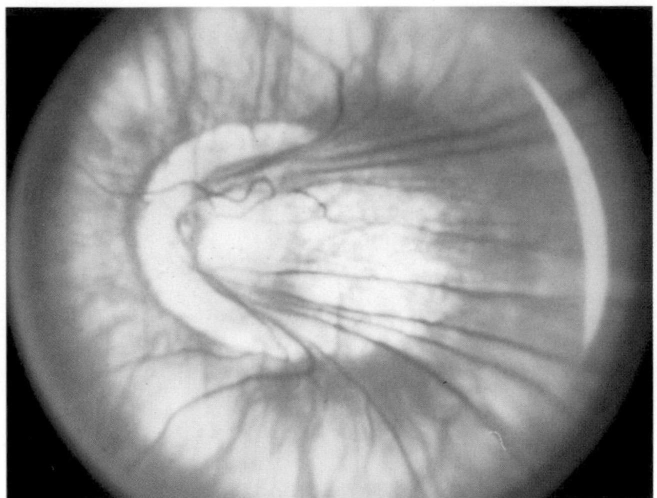

Fig. 19.19 Retrolental fibroplasia. A fundal photograph of a retina showing the characteristic retinal distortion caused by retrolental fibroplasia.

Antibacterial drugs used for eye infections

Use	Drugs
Broad-spectrum antibiotics	Chloramphenicol Ciprofloxacin Framycetin sulfate* Gentamicin Neomycin sulfate Ofloxacin
Pseudomonas aeruginosa infections	Gentamicin Tobramycin
Corneal ulcers	Ciprofloxacin
Chlamydial infections (trachoma)	Chlortetracycline
Staphylococcal infections	Fusidic acid
Acanthamoeba keratitis	Propamidine isethionate*

Fig. 19.20 Antibacterial drugs used for eye infections.

the retina itself may also be affected and contribute to these symptoms.

As the eye is controlled by the somatic motor system and both parasympathetic and sympathetic branches of the autonomic nervous system, and contains part of the central nervous system (retina), drugs that affect the function of any of these systems will in some way alter the function of the eye.

EYE INFECTIONS

Infections of the eye are commonly bacterial

Infections of the eye are commonly of bacterial or viral origin.

- Bacterial blepharitis and acute infective conjunctivitis are treated with topical antibacterial drops or creams.
- Gonococcal conjunctivitis requires both topical and systemic antibacterial therapy.
- Corneal ulcers and keratitis require specialist treatment involving the subconjunctival administration of antibiotics.
- Endophthalmitis is caused by infection and inflammation at the back of the eye and is a medical emergency. It may require intraocular injections of antibiotics.

Fungal eye infections are rare, but may occur in agricultural workers and require specialist treatment.

A wide range of antibacterial drugs are available (Fig. 19.20) for treating eye infections. Most can be used as broad-spectrum antibiotics, but some are reserved for specific infections.

Adverse effects associated with antibacterial drugs are minimal, and usually comprise transient stinging and itching. Chloramphenicol, the most widely used antibiotic, has been rarely associated with aplastic anemia, and ciprofloxacin is best avoided in children because it is particularly liable to cause local burning and itching sensations. The mechanisms of action of these drugs are discussed in Chapter 23.

There are fewer antiviral drugs available for ophthalmic use. Acyclovir is used to treat corneal ulcers caused by herpes simplex infection, and ganciclovir is used to treat cytomegalovirus infection of the eye, which occurs in patients with AIDS. The mechanisms of action of these drugs are discussed in Chapter 24.

FURTHER READING

Dowling JE. *The Retina: an Approachable Part of the Brain*. Cambridge USA: Harvard University Press; 1987. [An excellent book on the retina, written by a leading retinal scientist.]

Fraunfelder FT, Meyer SM. *Drug-induced Ocular Side Effects and Drug Interactions*. Philadephia USA: Lea & Febiger; 1989. [A major work for reference.]

Lee JP, Hogg C. Botulinum toxin therapy for squint and other ocular motility disorders. In: Easty DL (ed.) *Current Ophthalmology*. London: Baillière Tindal; 1990: 163–171. [A detailed description of BOTOX therapy in ophthalmology.]

Mauger TF, Craig EL. *Havner's Ocular Pharmacology 6e*. St Louis USA: Mosby-Year Book; 1994. [A major work for reference.]

Somlyo AP, Somlyo AV. Signal transduction and regulation in smooth muscle. *Nature* 1994; **372:** 231–236. [A recent review on cellular signalling in smooth muscle.]

Make a provisional diagnosis and determine a rational pharmacologic treatment for the following hypothetical case.

A 52-year-old woman visited an optician for a routine eye test. On learning of a family history of glaucoma, the optician examined her eyes thoroughly and noted a slight increase in intraocular pressure and mild cupping of the optic disk with some loss of visual acuity. He advised her to go to her family practitioner.

1. What two effects are needed from drug treatment in a patient with glaucoma?
2. What is the first-line group of drugs for treating this problem?
3. Give an example of one of the above drugs and explain how it works.
4. What coexisting conditions might preclude the use of these drugs in patients with glaucoma?

Indicate which of the following are true and which are false.

1. In the eye of a normal person
- a) the intraocular pressure is about 4 mmHg
- b) the intraocular pressure is about 40 mmHg
- c) aqueous humor is **purely** an ultrafiltrate of blood
- d) aqueous humor production is partly controlled by the autonomic nervous system
- e) the intraocular pressure falls when blood flow to the eye is reduced

2. In the normal eye, muscarinic receptor activation
- a) decreases intraocular pressure
- b) dilates the pupil
- c) causes mydriasis
- d) causes accommodation for near vision
- e) causes miosis

3. In the eye of a patient with open-angle glaucoma
- a) atropine will reduce intraocular pressure
- b) a mixture of epinephrine and guanethidine will reduce intraocular pressure
- c) the condition is often congenital
- d) diagnosis is based only on increased intraocular pressure
- e) timolol maleate (a β adrenoceptor antagonist) increases the intraocular pressure

4. The pupil of a normal person
- a) dilates when phenylephrine hydrochloride is applied to the conjunctiva
- b) contracts when light is shone into the contralateral eye
- c) dilates in response to topical glucocorticosteroids
- d) constricts when the person sees someone they find attractive
- e) dilates in low light levels

5. In a normal person
- a) the ciliary muscle is predominantly under sympathetic control
- b) lidocaine is a useful local topical anesthetic for the eye
- c) a pigmented iris takes longer to dilate with atropine than a non-pigmented iris
- d) pilocarpine causes accommodation for near vision
- e) oxybuprocaine hydrochloride* dilates the pupil by blocking Na^+ channels

6. Which of the following drugs has a cycloplegic effect?
- a) atropine
- b) carbachol
- c) cyclopentolate
- d) epinephrine
- e) tropicamide

7. In open-angle glaucoma
- a) pilocarpine is given as eye drops
- b) tropicamide eye drops are useful
- c) β adrenoceptor antagonists lower intraocular pressure
- d) carbachol eye drops lower intraocular pressure
- e) YAG laser surgery is commonly used

8. In the eye of a normal person
- a) the pupils constrict after instillation of a high concentration of epinephrine
- b) stimulation of muscarinic receptors reduces the near point
- c) phenylephrine hydrochloride eye drops dilate the pupil by a direct action on β_1 adrenoceptors
- d) lidocaine can be used to produce corneal anesthesia
- e) phenylephrine hydrochloride constricts the pupil

9. Increased intraocular pressure
- a) may result from the topical application of glucocorticosteroids
- b) may be reduced by systemic treatment with acetazolamide
- c) may result from the topical application of parasympathomimetics
- d) is reduced by cyclopentolate
- e) may be reduced by miotics

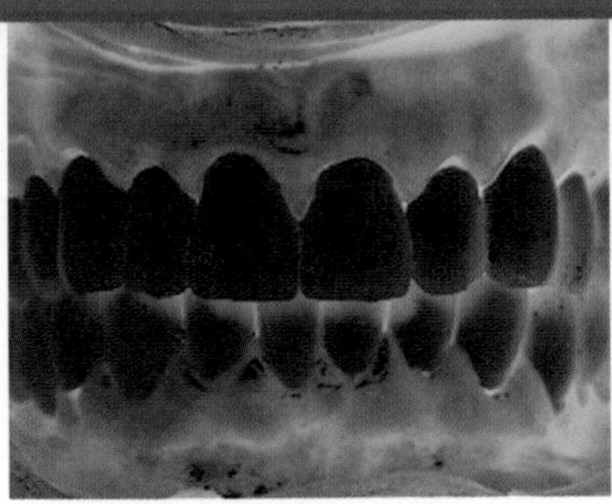

20. Drugs in Dentistry

PHYSIOLOGY OF THE ORAL CAVITY

The teeth and supporting tissues provide the initial digestive processes essential to all the body's activities. Chewing and swallowing are carried out by specialized oral tissues, which include the teeth, tongue, salivary glands, and muscles of mastication. The maxillary and mandibular dentition articulate with a specific pattern and movement to generate the forces needed for chewing. Chewing pressures and oral sensations are regulated by the trigeminal nerve in response to information provided by proprioceptive nerves in the supporting tissues of the teeth.

The salivary glands produce more than a liter of saliva daily to lubricate the oral tissues, facilitate taste, and initiate the digestive process.

TOOTH STRUCTURE AND SHAPE

Tooth structure and shape, the oral mucosa and the salivary glands are important in health and in dental disease

The tooth crown is composed of a crystalline and highly mineralized (96%) calcified tissue, the enamel. Dentin, a less-mineralized tissue, forms the bulk of the tooth structure. It is covered by enamel and protects the vital tooth pulp throughout the root length. The dental pulp contains loose connective tissue, blood vessels, and nerves. Odontoblasts, which produce the dentin, are found at the interface between the pulp tissue and dentin, with projections extending into the dentinal tubules. Finally, the root is covered with a calcified connective tissue structure, the cementum (Fig. 20.1). Carious lesions expanding into the dentin

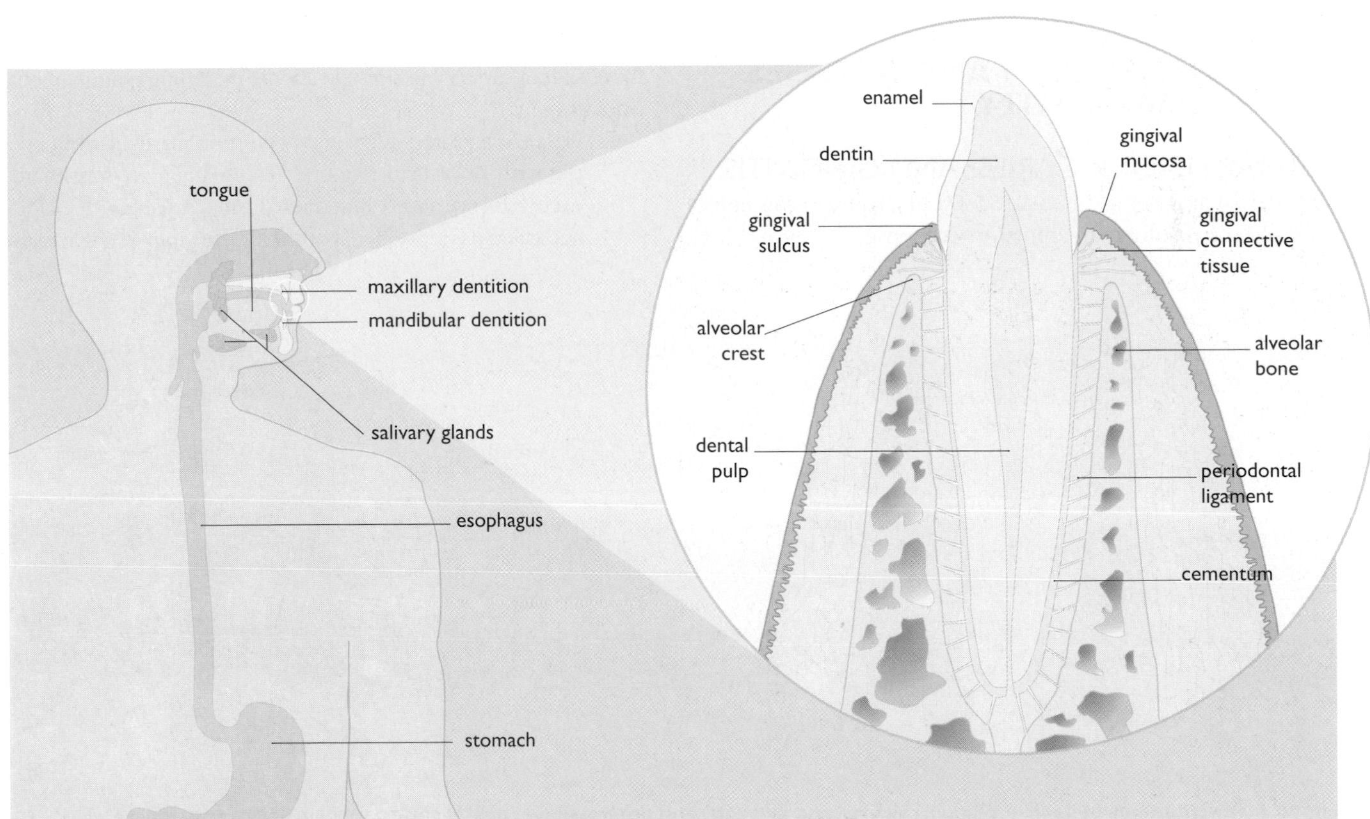

Fig. 20.1 Structure of the oral cavity. The major tissues of the oral cavity include the maxillary and mandibular dentition and supporting tissues, the tongue, and the salivary glands, all of which function together to initiate the digestion of food and nutrients.

or surgical removal of enamel during treatment exposes the dentinal tubules to external stimuli and painful sensations.

Teeth are attached to the maxillary and mandibular alveolar bone by the supporting structures of the teeth, which are termed the periodontium. Alveolar bone is unique because its primary function is to support the teeth and it gradually disappears as teeth are lost. The periodontal ligament is located between the alveolar bone and cementum and the fibers are specifically arranged to connect the teeth with alveolar bone. This arrangement allows subtle tooth movement in response to the forces of mastication.

ORAL MUCOSA

The buccal mucosa is similar to other mucosal tissues, but the gingival mucosa in proximity to the teeth and covering the periodontium is a specialized mucosa. The mucosal attachment to the tooth close to the enamel–cementum junction creates a ring of unattached gingival tissue, which forms a small space between the mucosa and tooth (i.e. the gingival sulcus or crevice). The depth of the gingival sulcus and the level of the gingival attachment are important in the treatment strategies used for periodontal disease.

SALIVARY GLANDS

Adequate salivary flow and composition are essential for maintaining healthy oral tissues. Saliva consists of water and mucin combined with minerals, enzymes, and immune components. It functions as a lubricant to protect mucosal tissues and to facilitate mastication. It is also involved in taste perception and caries prevention and is a factor determining the microbial environment of the mouth.

PATHOPHYSIOLOGY AND DISEASES OF THE ORAL CAVITY

DENTAL PLAQUE, CARIES, AND GINGIVITIS

Most dental diseases are associated with microorganisms, infection, and the resulting inflammatory response.

Dental plaque

Caries and gingivitis are common dental diseases and are related to the formation of dental plaque, which is described as a soft non-mineralized deposit consisting of microorganisms in a glycoprotein matrix that is usually found on the enamel. Plaque formation begins as a pedicle of salivary proteins adhering to the enamel surface. Oral microorganisms colonize the pedicle, forming the plaque, and can account for up to 70% of the plaque content. The varieties of dental plaque microorganisms therefore play a key role in the development of dental disease. If plaque is removed or reduced through regular dental hygiene practice, the incidence of dental caries, gingivitis, and periodontitis is significantly reduced. Plaque that has become mineralized is called dental calculus.

Dental caries

Dental caries or decay is probably the most universal and common of all reported dental diseases. Caries development is a time-dependent event involving a critical relationship between the host, plaque microorganisms, and diet. *Streptococcus mutans* species are generally regarded as the most cariogenic microorganism, but *Lactobacillus* species are also implicated in some types of carious lesions. The combination of cariogenic microorganisms with a cariogenic diet including sucrose or other carbohydrates furthers the progression of demineralization and the development of carious lesions. Factors that reduce saliva production can also contribute to the development of dental caries (Fig. 20.2). Once caries reaches the dentinal tissues, it progresses in a more diffuse pattern.

Gingivitis (inflammation of the gingiva)

Gingivitis describes the inflammatory reaction of the gingival mucosa to a variety of etiologic agents including plaque microorganisms.

- Plaque-associated gingivitis is common, particularly in people with poor oral hygiene. It is usually asymptomatic except for localized bleeding during brushing. If plaque and calculus deposits expand into the gingival crevice, the

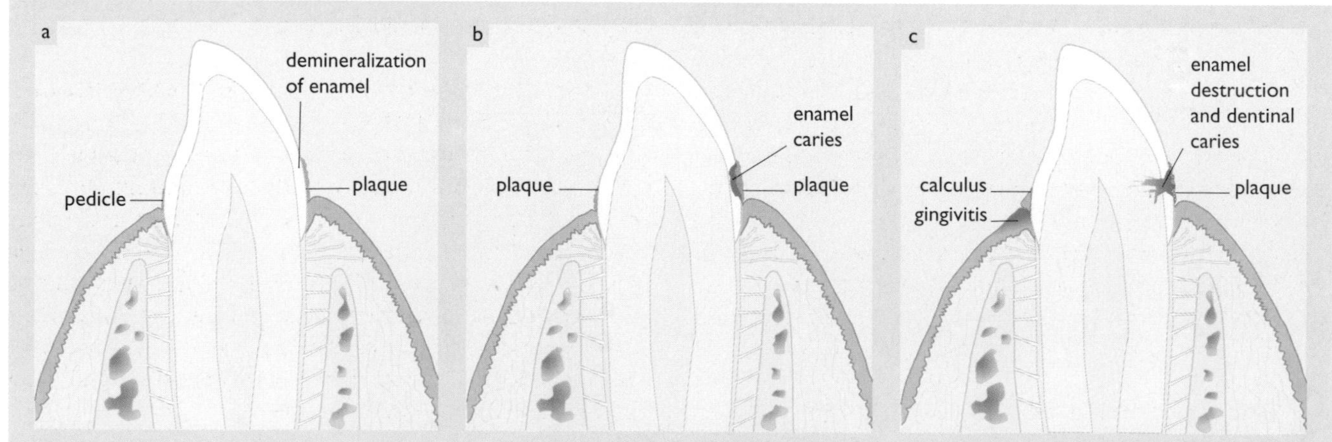

Fig. 20.2 Development of pedicle, plaque, calculus, and gingivitis and progression of dental caries. Colonization of dental plaque with cariogenic microorganisms can progress to demineralization (a), enamel caries (b), and dentinal caries (c). Plaque bacteria can induce an inflammatory gingivitis.

nature of the microorganisms changes to an anaerobe-dominated population and leads to more serious infections of the periodontium.

- Acute necrotizing ulcerative gingivitis (ANUG) is an acute painful form of gingival infection associated with fusiform and spirochete organisms, with a clinical presentation very different from that of the inflammatory gingivitis of plaque. Ulcerated and highly inflamed gingival tissues are typically observed. Fever and lymphadenopathy may also be part of the acute presentation.

Systemic factors may also play a role in gingivitis.

Management

Dental plaque, caries, and gingivitis are three distinct presentations of dental disease, but are uniquely linked as a focus for preventive dental medicine.

> **Diseases of the oral cavity**
>
> - Plaque is an important factor in dental disease
> - Caries is the most common dental disease
> - Gingivitis is the inflammatory reaction to plaque microorganisms
> - Preventive dental medicine can reduce the incidence of these diseases
> - Early dental intervention is the key to controlling dental disease

Removal of plaque and calculus (oral prophylaxis and scaling) from tooth surfaces is a major part of the overall preventive program

Over-the-counter (OTC) mouth rinses have questionable benefits in controlling plaque and calculus, but chlorhexidine is an effective topical chemotherapeutic agent with a broad spectrum of activity including plaque microorganisms and yeast. Chlorhexidine gluconate in a 0.2% or 0.12% oral rinse reduces plaque bacteria and gingivitis with twice-daily rinsing. Up to 30% of chlorhexidine is retained in the oral cavity after rinsing and is slowly released over 12 hours. Its use in oral mucosal diseases is discussed later. Dentifrices containing other antibacterial agents, including triclosan* and fluoride, are also promoted for plaque control. Calculus-control toothpastes containing pyrophosphate or zinc salts are designed to prevent calculus formation and do not affect existing calculus.

Treatment and prevention of dental caries includes plaque control and the use of systemic and/or topical fluorides

Fluorides in the water supply and in a multitude of dental products have significantly reduced the incidence of dental caries in children in developed countries, but dental caries in adults and in areas where fluoride is not available remain a major dental concern.

The mechanism of action of fluoride ions is debated but, whether systemically or topically applied, fluoride is incorporated into the crystalline apatite structure of enamel to produce a less-soluble enamel. Fluoride has also been shown to have an antibacterial affect against plaque cariogenic bacteria.

The use of supplemental systemic sodium fluoride by children must be carefully balanced against their total daily fluoride intake, including the amount in natural or artificially fluoridated water supplies. Excessive exposure to systemic fluorides is related to the development of stained or mottled enamel.

Treatment and prevention of dental caries includes:

- Removal of all carious lesions.
- Oral hygiene to reduce dental plaque.
- Dental sealants to cover pits and fissures in tooth structure.
- Cariogenic diet control.
- Systemic or topical fluorides.

ACUTE DENTAL PAIN

Pain as a general topic, and the principles of its treatment are covered in detail in Chapter 7.

Acute pain associated with dental disease is probably the most common complaint of dental patients. Any injury to the oral tissues leads to the release of chemical mediators, signs of inflammation, and tissue edema. Prostaglandins have been implicated in the genesis of dental pain because their production is associated with sensitization of trigeminal afferent nerve endings to other mediators, such as bradykinin or histamine (Fig. 20.3).

Early carious lesions are often associated with acute transient pain that is readily alleviated by dental treatment. However, untreated carious lesions continue to destroy tooth structure, allowing oral microorganisms to invade pulpal tissues. Pulpal infection often leads to the development of an acute periapical abscess and persistent pain.

Acute oral pain is a symptom of many orofacial diseases including periodontal abscesses, mucosal lesions, obstructed salivary gland ducts, and tissue trauma.

Determining the etiology of dental pain is complicated because pain can be referred from other tissues such as the sinuses, the ears, and temporomandibular joint.

Oral surgery, periodontal therapy, or other dental treatment can cause pain

The pain caused by oral surgical intervention, periodontal therapy, or other dental treatment is invariably accompanied by inflammation. Indeed, the fear of pain from dental treatment prompts many to avoid or defer treatment. Dental pain intensity can range from mild to severe depending on the individual patient, the disease presentation, and the type of dental treatment, and can be as unbearable as any other type of pain. Acute pain following dental treatment is usually most intense during the first 12–24 hours after treatment and declines over the next 2–3 days.

Management

Management of acute orofacial pain begins with its diagnosis and appropriate dental treatment.

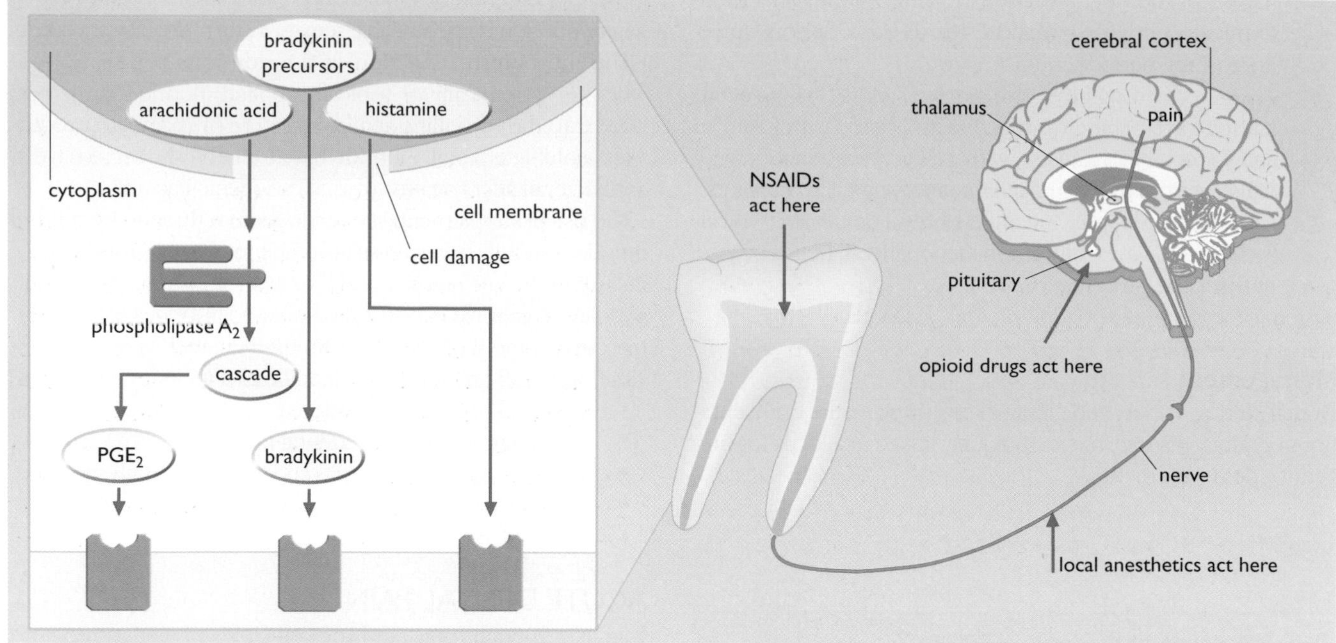

Fig. 20.3 Diagrammatic representation of the sites of action of opioids, nonsteroidal anti-inflammatory drugs (NSAIDs), and local anesthetic drugs when used for acute dental pain. Opioids act within the central nervous system to alter pain perception; aspirin and NSAIDs inhibit prostaglandin (PG) synthesis at the site of injury, and local anesthetics block transmission of the noxious stimulus.

Opioid, nonopioid, or local anesthetic drugs, either alone or in combination, are most frequently used for controlling acute orofacial pain

Opioid analgesics Acute orofacial pain of moderate intensity or greater can be effectively managed with opioid drugs. Opioids act centrally to modify pain perception by interacting with multiple opiate receptors and mimicking endogenous opioid peptides (see Chapter 7). Sedation and euphoria often accompany opioid analgesia as an added benefit in controlling the emotional component of pain. Opioids with favorable oral-to-parenteral effectiveness ratios are preferred, as is the oral route of administration. They are rarely used alone for acute dental pain and are frequently combined with aspirin or acetaminophen. Opioids used for acute orofacial pain include:

- Codeine.
- Hydrocodone.
- Oxycodone.
- Dihydrocodeine.

Codeine, hydrocodone, and dihydrocodeine probably differ very little from one another in the quality of pain relief and have comparable adverse effects (see below). Oxycodone is generally preferred for more intense pain. Increasing the opioid dose can improve the quality of pain relief, but with an increased incidence of adverse effects.

Synthetic opioids, tramadol, propoxyphene, and meperidine are also used for acute dental pain. Propoxyphene should only be used in combination with nonopioid analgesics because its analgesic efficacy is variable, while oral meperidine may not provide adequate analgesia for orofacial pain because oral administration produces variable plasma levels. A mixed agonist/antagonist such as pentazocine is infrequently used and should not be used for mild pain.

Common adverse effects of oral opioids are nausea, dizziness, and drowsiness. Sedation is variable, depending on the dose and patient response. Severe adverse effects are usually not observed in the doses used for dental analgesia. Opioid drugs should be used only during the episode of acute pain to avoid any risk of tolerance and addiction. Parenteral opioid administration is usually limited to hospital cases.

Nonopioid analgesics Aspirin and acetaminophen have been the main nonopioid analgesics used in dentistry. However, over the past 15 years, other nonsteroidal anti-inflammatory drugs (NSAIDs) have provided predictable and effective outcomes in the management of mild to moderate dental pain. Many NSAIDs (e.g. ibuprofen, fenoprofen, naproxen, diclofenac, naproxen sodium, ketoprofen, etodolac, ketorolac, meclofenamate, diflunisal) are now available as oral analgesics and differ from one another mainly in dose and duration of action.

Evaluation of NSAIDs in the oral surgery pain model (third molar extraction) has consistently shown better pain relief than with single doses of codeine, aspirin, or acetaminophen and comparable analgesia to that achieved with combinations of opioids with either aspirin or acetaminophen. Parenterally administered ketorolac has been promoted for severe postsurgical pain. As a group, the mechanism of action of NSAIDs is related to inhibiting prostaglandin synthesis in injured or diseased tissue. These drugs therefore modify initiation of the pain response close to the site of tissue injury. More recent evidence suggests a central nervous system component as part of their action.

NSAIDs should be prescribed using a by-the-clock dosing scheme to provide a sustained analgesic response, rather than used as needed.

Gastrointestinal complaints are the most commonly observed adverse effects of the nonopioid drugs, but consideration should be given to their action in inhibiting platelet aggregation (Fig. 20.4). Most of the adverse effects of NSAIDs result from nonselective inhibition of other tissue prostaglandins.

Local anesthetics Controlling pain during dental treatment using local anesthetics with vasconstrictors is paramount to dental practice. The major local anesthetics used for intraoral injection techniques are classified as amides. Ester-type local anesthetics are infrequently used, except as topical analgesics or if amides are not available. Dyclonine is an exception to this classification. Distinguishing between the chemical classes is important in those rare cases where there is a history of a local anesthetic allergy. However, evidence of a cross allergy between groups and among the amide class is lacking. Common local anesthetic drugs used for dental applications are:

- Amides (local and topical lidocaine, mepivacaine, prilocaine, etidocaine, bupivacaine).
- Esters (procaine, topical tetracaine, topical benzocaine).
- Ketones (topical dyclonine).

Local anesthetics are also discussed in Chapter 21.

The primary action of local anesthetic administration is to produce a reversible blockade of nerve conduction from a noxious stimulus site. Local anesthetic solutions must therefore be deposited close to those branches of the trigeminal nerve that innervate the area to be treated. Local anesthetics are supplied as aqueous solutions of hydrochloride salts to improve solubility and stability. Once injected, the ionized local anesthetic solution interacts with tissue buffers to allow free base formation. Adequate amounts of the free base are needed to block membrane Na^+ channels and distribute the anesthetic across the nerve cell membranes. Tissue inflammation that compromises the capacity of tissue buffers and

Drug interactions of oral analgesics

Opioids	All opioids increase the risk of CNS depression
	Meperidine is contraindicated with MAOIs or within 14 days of the last dose of an MAOI
	Propoxyphene may decrease carbamazepine clearance
	Small risk of increased sedation with cimetidine
	Increased risk of constipation, urinary retention, dry mouth with anticholinergics
Aspirin	Increased risk of bleeding with anticoagulants or other drugs that affect the clotting mechanism
	Avoid use with methotrexate unless plasma levels are monitored
	Urinary alkalinizers increase salicylate clearance
	Ethanol or NSAIDS increase risk of GI bleeding or GI adverse effects
	Large doses of aspirin may enhance the hypoglycemic effect of oral antidiabetic drugs
	Antagonism of uricosuric effect of probenecid
Acetaminophen	Concomitant high dose use with ethanol or other potentially hepatotoxic drugs
Other NSAIDs	Possibly impaired antihypertensive effects of β adrenoceptor antagonists, ACE inhibitors, and diuretics
	Can increase bleeding time with anticoagulant or other drugs that affect clotting mechanisms
	Avoid use with methotrexate unless plasma levels are monitored
	Ethanol increases risk of GI bleeding or GI adverse effects
	Antagonism of uricosuric effect of probenecid
	Suspected risk of increase in serum lithium levels

Fig. 20.4 Drug interactions of oral analgesics. (CNS, central nervous system; MAOI, monoamine oxidase inhibitor; NSAID, nonsteroidal anti-inflammatory drug; GI, gastrointestinal; ACE, angiotensin-converting enzyme)

renders the milieu acidic will substantially reduce formation of free anesthetic base and can significantly impair the achievement of adequate regional analgesia.

Considering the many administrations of local anesthetic in dental surgeries and the use of correct injection techniques, the incidence of severe adverse reactions to local anesthetic administration is extremely small. Typical reactions tend to be psychogenic responses associated with fear of the injection and include anxiety and syncope. Local reactions include trismus, injury, or infection at the site of injection. Systemic reactions depend on the amount and rate of drug absorbed and are most often associated with accidental intravascular injection or overdose. For local anesthetics, adverse central nervous system symptoms can include slurred speech, drowsiness, and muscle twitching. More severe reactions are tonic and clonic seizures, disorientation, and respiratory depression. Severe myocardial depression can occur with increasing plasma levels, but is rare.

Vasoconstrictors Some local anesthetics have a vasodilator effect on blood vessels. As local anesthetics are removed from the injection site by the vascular system, retention of the local anesthetic drug close to the target nerve tissue is important for achieving quality analgesia with a reasonable working time. The clinical working time for local anesthetic solutions without a vasoconstrictor is usually less than 10–20 minutes when used in the oral cavity. This is inadequate for most dental procedures. Small quantities of vasoconstrictors are therefore combined with local anesthetics:

- To increase the duration of action.
- To reduce the risk of systemic toxicity.
- To lessen soft tissue hemorrhage associated with oral surgical procedures.

Vasoconstrictors used in dental anesthetic solutions are epinephrine and levonordefrin, but felypressin* is also used in some countries (Fig. 20.5). Epinephrine interacts with both α and β adrenoceptors but α_1-mediated vasoconstriction dominates at the injection site.

Vasoconstrictor adverse effects are associated with intravascular injection or rapid tissue uptake of higher doses. They include tachycardia, palpitation, increased blood pressure, nervousness, and anxiety. Because the duration of the systemic action of vasoconstrictors is very short, these symptoms rapidly disappear.

There are a few contraindications to the judicious use of vasoconstrictors in dentistry. The dose of vasoconstrictor must be reduced by 50% or more in medically compromised patients who have a significant reduction in exercise or stress tolerance, or who have coronary artery disease. The key to avoiding systemic reactions to local anesthetic solutions with a vasoconstrictor is to use the smallest effective dose and careful injection after aspiration (Fig. 20.6).

Drug combinations An alternative strategy for controlling postoperative dental pain has been advocated using combinations of NSAIDs and long-acting local anesthetics. Of the latter, both etidocaine and bupivacaine provide analgesia well into the post-treatment period when the anticipated pain response is greatest. A normal dose of an NSAID is taken soon after treatment and before the return of normal sensation. This combination of drugs has been shown to reduce the intensity of pain in the immediate post-treatment period and the need for opioid medications. Pretreatment NSAIDs have also been advocated to help reduce the intensity of pain in the immediate post-treatment period.

Vasoconstrictor doses in health and in patients who have cardiovascular disease

Vasoconstrictor	Concentration used	Amount per dental cartridge (1.8 ml)	Maximum dose per dental visit
Epinephrine	1:50,000	0.036 mg	0.2 mg
	1:100,000	0.018 mg	
	1:200,000	0.009 mg	
Levonordefrin	1:20,000	0.09 mg	0.5–1 mg

Doses in health and with cardiovascular disease

The following doses allow sufficient use of local anesthesia with vasoconstrictor for quality pain control during treatment:

- For the healthy patient the dose of epinephrine is calculated at 3 μg/kg, not to exceed 0.2 μg.
- For a patient with cardiovascular disease that does not impair activities the recommended dose of epinephrine is 1.5 μg/kg not to exceed 0.1 mg.
- For a patient with cardiovascular disease that limits daily activity or reduces exercise tolerance the recommended dose of epinephrine is 0.75 μg/kg, not to exceed 0.04 mg.
- Levonordefrin doses can be similarly reduced.

Fig. 20.5 Vasoconstrictor doses in health and in patients who have cardiovascular disease

Adverse effects of analgesic drugs

- The most common adverse effects of opioids at pharmacotherapeutic doses are nausea, sedation, and dizziness
- The most common adverse effect of nonsteroidal anti-inflammatory drugs is gastrointestinal irritation
- The most common adverse effects of local anesthetics are usually psychogenic, such as syncope and anxiety

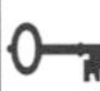 **Management of acute dental pain**

- Match choice of drug to intensity of pain
- Nonsteroidal anti-inflammatory drugs are effective for controlling dental pain
- Use combination of long-acting local anesthetics and nonsteroidal anti-inflammatory drugs
- Consider pain referred from other orofacial tissues

Limitations to vasoconstrictor use with local anesthesia
Contraindicated in:
Uncontrolled hyperthyroidism
Significant risk of adverse reactions associated with:
Uncontrolled severe hypertension
Unstable/untreated angina pectoris
Myocardial ischemia and infarction in the previous 3–6 months
Cerebrovascular accident in last 3–6 months
Uncontrolled cardiac arrhythmias
Uncontrolled congestive heart failure
General anesthesia with halogenated general anesthetics
Reduce dose due to risk of drug interactions with:
Tricyclic antidepressants
Noncardioselective β adrenoceptor antagonists

Fig. 20.6 Limitations to vasoconstrictor use with local anesthesia.

CHRONIC OROFACIAL PAIN

In contrast to acute pain, chronic orofacial pain is complicated by a myriad of patient and diagnostic issues. It may result from conditions that initiate acute pain, but many other causes must be considered because the etiology can be elusive.

The pattern of chronic orofacial pain, its persistent nature, and the patient's frustration with unsuccessful treatment modalities are associated with psychologic and behavioral developments that must be considered in all management schemes.

Chronic orofacial pain can arise from:

- Inflammation or internal derangements of the temporomandibular joint.
- Myalgia associated with the oral and facial musculature.
- Lesions in the central nervous system.

The diagnosis and management of chronic orofacial pain therefore requires a multidisciplinary approach. Examples of therapy can include selected medications, restoration of occlusal disharmony with dental appliances, surgical intervention, psychologic intervention, and physiotherapy.

Management

In chronic facial pain, drugs are used to control the pain and associated symptoms

The NSAIDs are used for the symptomatic management of pain associated with injury or inflammatory processes. The best results are usually obtained using adequate doses to control the symptoms and regular administration. Opioids should be limited to longer-acting drugs or completely avoided because of the possibility of dependence, unless the pain is due to cancer. Longer-acting NSAIDs with once- or twice-daily dosing are generally preferred.

Tricyclic antidepressants (see Chapter 7) may be used to alleviate the pain and symptoms such as depression and altered sleep patterns.

The pain of trigeminal neuralgia responds to the anticonvulsant drugs carbamazepine and phenytoin (see Chapter 7).

Centrally acting skeletal muscle relaxants are sometimes useful if there is myalgia.

Drugs used for chronic facial pain should not be considered as curative, but a positive symptom response can be useful in making a diagnosis.

ACUTE ODONTOGENIC INFECTIONS

The general principles of treatment of bacterial and viral infections are described in Chapters 23 and 24.

Dental caries, periodontal disease, acute periapical abscesses, salivary gland infections, and many other oral infections are caused by microorganisms that are part of the normal oral flora. Other oral infections are caused by microorganisms introduced into the oral cavity by trauma or other means.

Separate microenvironments within the oral cavity account for the growth of both facultative and obligate anaerobic microorganisms existing in a commensal relationship. As a result, most odontogenic bacterial infections are caused by a mix of pathogens with significant involvement of both facultative and obligate anaerobes. Aerobic streptococci and staphylococci along with fungi (yeast) are also part of the normal oral flora and are potential pathogens.

Odontogenic oral infections cause fever, malaise, swelling, pain, and pus formation

Odontogenic oral infections can present with acute symptoms of fever, malaise, swelling, and pain. Redness and pus formation may be evident, depending on the site of the infection. Pulpal infection often expands to periapical tissue, with involvement of alveolar bone if dental treatment is delayed. At this point, pain will usually prompt the patient to seek dental care, but the abscess may continue to spread from the alveolar bone until it opens onto a soft tissue surface as an intraoral fistula. With an avenue of drainage for the abscess, either through the tooth or soft tissue fistula, acute symptoms often abate and the infection assumes a chronic status. However, the infection may also spread diffusely in soft tissues with resulting cellulitis. Rarely, the infection will spread from a mandibular site, dissecting along the facial planes into the neck or, from a maxillary site, it may spread to the cavernous sinus of the brain. These latter infections can create life-threatening situations and require aggressive treatment.

Management

Acute odontogenic infections are best managed with a combination of dental intervention and antibiotic therapy.

If an abscess is pointing, surgical incision and drainage are indicated

The same effect can be created by opening into the pulp chamber of an infected tooth if soft tissue incision is not feasible.

Self-limiting infections may respond to the dental treatment without the use of antibiotic drugs.

How to manage an acute dental infection

- Recognize the cardinal signs of infection
- Consider the integrity of the patient's immune system
- Know which are the potential oral pathogens
- Match the antibiotic's spectrum to the causative pathogens
- Incise and drain any abscess if possible

For most dental infections, selection of an antibiotic drug is empirical

For most dental infections, antibiotic drug selection is based on the presenting symptoms, the location of the infection, a knowledge of the microorganisms usually associated with the type of infection, and experience (Fig. 20.7) (see below). Antibiotic drugs selected for acute odontogenic infections should have a spectrum that includes streptococcal species and anaerobic organisms. Fortunately, most microorganisms that cause common oral infections have remained sensitive to traditional antibiotic drugs. However, laboratory culturing and sensitivity tests should be performed if the infection fails to respond as expected, when sampling without contamination can be accomplished, and in osteomyelitis. As sophisticated deoxyribonucleic acid probes become available, dentists should be able to identify causative pathogens more readily to facilitate drug selection.

Penicillin V potassium remains a drug of first choice for most acute odontogenic infections

Penicillin V potassium is bactericidal and has a spectrum that includes the streptococcal and anaerobic organisms frequently encountered in acute infections. Amoxicillin is also a choice because of its bioavailability when given orally and its effectiveness against some Gram-negative organisms. Penicillin G or ampicillin is preferred for parenteral administration. Erythromycin and related macrolides are used as alternative drugs for the penicillin-allergic patient and if the infection is less severe.

Cephalosporins are seldom drugs of first choice, but are used when staphylococcal organisms are involved, for example in cases of osteomyelitis or oral trauma.

Clindamycin has a spectrum of activity that includes many anaerobic organisms associated with oral infections, while metronidazole, which has an anaerobic spectrum, is rapidly becoming a drug of choice for selected periodontal infections.

Tetracyclines are generally limited to infections associated with the periodontium, but are also used as an alternative to pencillin V in the treatment of actinomycosis.

The role of the quinolone antibiotics for common dental infections remains to be established.

Drug interactions of antibiotics used in dentistry are given in Fig. 20.8.

Antibiotic drugs used for oral infections

Penicillins	Penicillin V potassium Amoxicillin Amoxicillin with clavulanate Ampicillin
Tetracyclines	Tetracycline Doxycycline Minocycline
Cephalosporins	Cephalexin Cefaclor
Macrolides	Erythromycin Azithromycin Clarithromycin
Clindamycin	
Metronidazole	

Fig. 20.7 Antibiotic drugs used for oral infections.

Adverse effects of antibiotics

- All antibiotics can cause gastrointestinal adverse effects and diarrhea
- Allergic reactions occur more frequently with the penicillins
- Anti-infectives alter the normal flora causing a risk of opportunistic candidiasis, especially in immunosuppressed patients
- Tetracycline use in children causes permanent gray–yellow mottling of teeth

PERIODONTAL INFECTIONS

Periodontitis (infection of the periodontium) can present in several acute or chronic forms and with different etiologies. In adults it is typically chronic with symptoms limited to an erythematous-appearing gingiva that bleeds on probing or brushing. The distinguishing feature of periodontal disease is a continuing infection of the supporting tissues of the teeth, resulting in a progressive loss of gingival attachment and alveolar bone. It is the most common cause of tooth loss in adult patients.

Periodontitis often goes undetected until the patient presents with loose teeth or an acute exacerbation. People reporting bleeding gums or the presence of blood on the toothbrush should be referred for dental evaluation. In the younger age group it can present as a juvenile periodontitis.

Management

Periodontal disease is controlled by reducing the numbers of microorganisms infecting the periodontium

Controlling periodontal disease involves a variety of treatment modalities, all of which are designed to reduce the numbers of microorganisms infecting the periodontium. Earlier in this chapter, the control of plaque and gingivitis was presented as a way of reducing the numbers of supragingival microorganisms, and bacteria in plaque contribute to the inflammatory aspect of periodontal disease. However, if there is microbial invasion of the deeper tissues of the periodontium, systemic anti-infective drugs, irrigation with anti-infectives, and surgical débridement may be required to control the disease.

Systemic anti-infective drugs should include drugs that are effective against multiple anaerobic organisms. A tetracycline-containing monofilament fiber has been developed for refractory periodontal disease. The fiber is placed into the periodontal pocket around the tooth while the drug is slowly released over 10–14 days. Other release systems using either metronidazole or chlorhexidine are being evaluated. Combinations of metronidazole with amoxicillin or ciprofloxacin have been used in refractory periodontal disease with limited success.

Drug interactions of antibiotics used in dentistry

All antibiotics	Reduced effectiveness of oral contraceptives Effectiveness of bactericidal drugs may be reduced when combined with bacteriostatic antibiotics
Penicillins and cephalosporins	Probenecid inhibits renal excretion and prolongs duration of action Allopurinol increases the risk of non-allergic skin rashes in patients taking ampicillin Bioavailability of atenolol may be decreased by ampicillin
Macrolides	Concurrent use with terfenadine, astemizole, or cisapride may result in serious cardiac arrhythmias (torsades de pointes syndrome) May increase serum levels of theophylline, lithium, carbamazepine, valproic acid, cyclosporine, and digoxin Compete with clindamycin for 50S ribosomal binding site in microorganisms Increase bioavailability of triazolam enhancing the level of sedation Erythromycin may increase the effects of oral anticoagulants, therefore monitor blood clotting times
Tetracylines	Absorption impaired when given concurrently with antacids, dairy products, or iron salts Barbiturates, phenytoin, ethanol, and carbamazepine may increase hepatic metabolism of doxycycline
Clindamycin	Increases effects of nondepolarizing neuromuscular junction blockers Absorption impaired when given with kaolin or antacids Competes with erythromycin for 50S ribosomal binding sites in microorganisms
Metronidazole	Avoid concurrent use with ethanol, ethanol-containing products, and disulfiram May potentiate warfarin oral anticoagulants, so monitor blood clotting times Barbiturates can decrease its effectiveness Can increase serum lithium levels

Fig. 20.8 Drug interactions of antibiotics used in dentistry.

PROPHYLACTIC USE OF ANTI-INFECTIVE DRUGS IN DENTISTRY

Patients who have a normal immune system and do not show symptoms of acute dental infection are not routinely treated with anti-infective drugs during dental procedures. Extractions, oral and maxillofacial surgery, periodontal therapy, deep scaling, and other dental procedures are associated with an uneventful transient bacteremia that usually lasts less than 15–30 minutes. However, selected patients may develop an infection secondary to the bacteremia. The notable example is the patient with pre-existing myocardial or valvular pathology who may develop an endocarditis.

Advisory groups throughout the world have established guidelines for antibiotic prophylaxis for patients at risk. Amoxicillin, penicillin V potassium, clindamycin, or a suitable alternative drug is usually recommended for prophylactic use and given as a single high dose before the dental procedure. This is also mentioned in Chapter 8 in relation to the treatment of myocarditis.

Prophylaxis guidelines to prevent bacterial endocarditis are not intended for other 'at risk' patients

There is considerable debate about the risks and benefits and drug choice for patients with joint prostheses; however, prophylaxis should be considered for patients with a compromised immune system. Recommended guidelines cannot address every patient situation, and consultation between the physician and dentist is advised. 'At risk' patients with poor oral hygiene, extensive caries, gingivitis, or periodontitis should be placed on a dental treatment program that includes the treatment and prevention of dental disease (Fig. 20.9).

COMMON DISEASES OF THE ORAL MUCOSA

Candida infections

Candida albicans is the most common cause of an oral yeast infection. The incidence of oral candidiasis has increased in recent years, and is particularly common among people with human immunodeficiency virus (HIV), in whom virally induced immune suppression increases the risk of this infection. It presents as an opportunistic pathogen in people with a compromised immune system or when drug therapy alters the usual oral flora.

The lesions of candidiasis are seen on the buccal and palatal oral mucosa and the tongue (Fig. 20.10), and can produce an angular cheilitis. Erythematous mucosal lesions appearing on a tissue-bearing surface for a denture prosthesis are typically the result of a *Candida* infection.

Management Antifungal drugs used for the treatment of candidiasis include:

- The topical agents nystatin, clotrimazole, and chlorhexidine.
- The systemic agents fluconazole and ketoconazole.

Nystatin is the drug of choice for acute candidiasis

The drug of choice for acute candidiasis is nystatin, which can be used as a topical rinse, ointment, or lozenge. Chlorhexidine rinse is also effective. Candidiasis in denture wearers can also be treated with topical nystatin, but resolution of the infection can be difficult because the organism attaches to the denture base and is a potential source of reinoculation. Soaking the denture in nystatin or chlorhexidine or remaking the denture is usually required. Patient compliance for a topical regimen can become a problem. Systemic ketoconazole or fluconazole (Fig. 20.11) may be required for:

- The noncompliant patient.
- The treatment of chronic atrophic candidiasis.
- Candidiasis in the immunocompromised patient.

Patients 'at risk' of spreading bacterial infection and requiring antibiotic prophylaxis
Bacterial endocarditis can develop in patients with:
Prosthetic cardiac valves (bioprosthetic and homograft) A previous history of bacterial endocarditis Surgically constructed systemic–pulmonary shunts Complex congenital cyanotic cardiac malformations Rheumatic and other acquired valvular dysfunction Hypertrophic cardiomyopathy Mitral valve prolapse with regurgitation
Other types of infection may develop in patients with:
A compromised immune system
Need for prophylaxis and antibiotic choice made after consultation between the physician and dentist if the patient has:
Organ or tissue transplants Traumatic orofacial wounds Chemotherapy for cancer Vascular grafts A major joint prosthesis Renal dialysis Insulin-dependent diabetes mellitus

Fig. 20.9 Patients 'at risk' of spreading bacterial infection and requiring antibiotic prophylaxis.

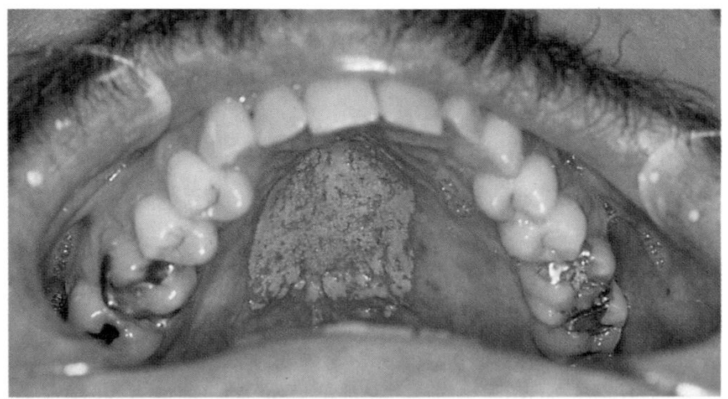

Fig. 20.10 Acute candidiasis of the palatal mucosa. The lesions produce an erythematous oral mucosa covered with white patches. (Courtesy of Dr John Wright.)

Oral viral infections

Viral infection and its treatment in general terms are dealt with in detail in Chapter 24.

Herpes viruses cause most oral viral infections

An initial herpes infection can manifest in a child as an acute herpetic gingivostomatitis or in the adult as pharyngotonsillitis. Both are associated with fever and lymphadenopathy with significant pain and ulcerative-like acute lesions. However, the most common manifestation of herpes infection is recurrent herpes labialis (cold sore, fever blisters). It appears with a prodromal onset of tingling or burning, which is usually followed by vesicle formation and rupture, pain, and finally crusting (Fig. 20.12).

Other members of the herpes virus group such as herpes zoster, Epstein–Barr virus, and, rarely, coxsackie viruses can also produce oral lesions. Hairy leukoplakia, which is observed in patients with HIV, is associated with the Epstein–Barr virus.

Drug interactions with systemic antifungal drugs
Ketoconazole
Concurrent use with terfenadine, astemizole, and cisapride not indicated due to high risk of arrhythmias (torsades de pointes)
May increase serum levels of cyclosporine
Risk of hepatotoxicity with ethanol and other hepatotoxic drugs
Decreased bioavailability when given with antacids and histamine H_2 antagonists
Fluconazole
Increases effects of warfarin oral anticoagulants, so monitor blood clotting times
Increases plasma levels of phenytoin, tacrolimus, and possibly cyclosporine

Fig. 20.11 Drug interactions with systemic antifungal drugs.

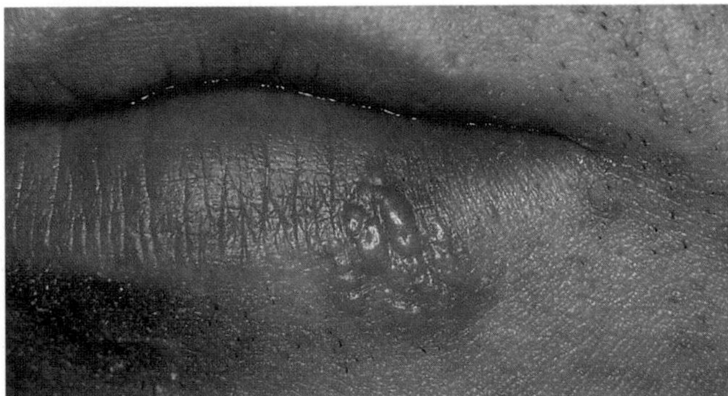

Fig. 20.12 Recurrent herpes labialis. The lesions present with multiple vesicle formation at the vermilion border of the lip extending to the skin of the face. (Courtesy of Dr John Wright.)

Management Management of initial herpetic infections is usually symptomatic and includes topical local anesthetics, systemic analgesics, and chlorhexidine rinses. Repeated episodes of recurrent herpes labialis can sometimes be controlled with systemic acyclovir. Topical acyclovir applied during the early prodromal stage may reduce the pain and duration of the lesion.

Acute aphthous ulceration

Recurrent aphthous stomatitis (canker sores) is probably one of the most prevalent oral mucosal diseases, with a general population incidence of 20%. Minor aphthous ulcers are the most common and appear as small (5 mm diameter or less) painful ulcerative lesions covered with a gray pseudomembrane (Fig. 20.13). They are seen on the nonkeratinized oral mucosa and the lateral borders of the tongue. Major aphthous ulcers occur less frequently, but are larger (over 1 cm in diameter) and extremely painful. Herpetiform ulcers occur as clusters of ulcers on the palate but are rarely observed. Their etiology remains unknown, but emotional stress, trauma, and nutritional deficiencies have been implicated. Oral ulcers are also associated with malabsorption diseases (see Chapter 14). Ulcers that persist and fail to respond to treatment require biopsy because they may be a cancer.

Ulceration of the oral mucosa

- Commonly due to oral tissue trauma
- If painful may be due to aphthous ulcers
- May be a manifestation of a systemic disease (e.g. HIV infection)
- May be a cancer if it fails to heal

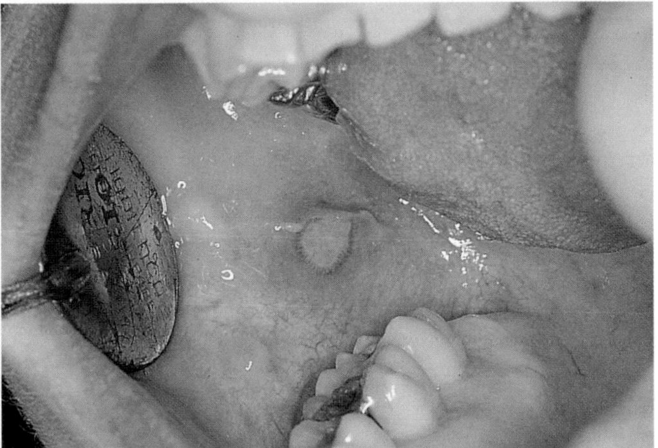

Fig. 20.13 A minor aphthous lesion on the buccal mucosa. It has a characteristic appearance with an erythematous halo surrounding the ulcer, which is covered with a gray pseudomembrane. Aphthous ulcers make it painful to eat. Minor aphthous lesions tend to heal without scarring. (Courtesy of Dr John Wright.)

Management No magical cures exist and treatment is symptomatic, usually with topical medications (Fig. 20.14). Systemic glucocorticosteroids are sometimes required for frequent and repeated episodes.

OTHER MUCOSAL LESIONS

Lichen planus and benign mucous membrane pemphigoid are chronic mucocutaneous diseases

Lichen planus and benign mucous membrane pemphigoid cause inflammation of the oral mucosa as well as other tissues. Pemphigoid is an autoimmune disease. Lichen planus has an immune component, but the etiology is less clear.

Lichen planus occurs in 0.5–1.5% of adults and is manifest as painful red ulcerative lesions (erosive or bullous) or as an asymptomatic nonerosive form on the buccal, palatal, gingival, or tongue mucosa. Nonerosive lesions include white striae (Wickham's striae) and a reticular pattern (Fig. 20.15). There may or may not be skin lesions.

Pemphigoid also causes painful red ulcerative lesions along with desquamation of the mucosal epithelium, but without the striae (Fig 20.16). Immunofluorescent staining of tissue samples is required for confirming the diagnosis.

The oral lesions of both lichen planus and pemphigoid are not always clearly defined and pemphigus, lupus erythematosus, lichenoid drug reactions, and, rarely, squamous cell carcinoma should be considered in the differential diagnosis.

Management

The acute symptoms of lichen planus are usually treated with topical anti-inflammatory glucocorticosteroids. Treatment objectives include eradicating the ulcerative lesions and controlling symptomatic exacerbations. High potency topical glucocorticosteroids (Fig. 20.17) in gel form seem to produce the most

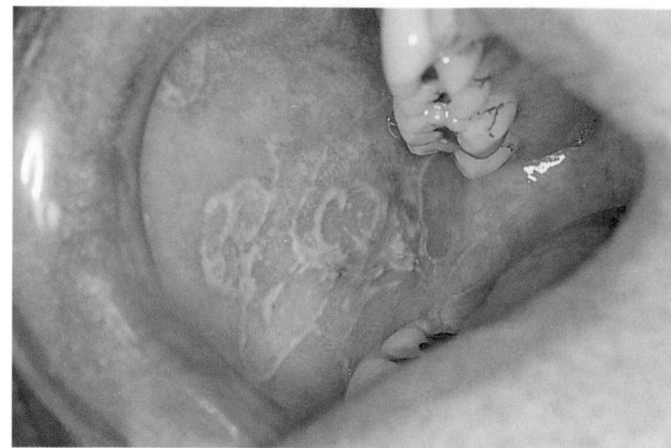

Fig. 20.15 Reticular or nonerosive lichen planus. The lesion on the buccal mucosa has a white lace-like appearance. This type of lichen planus is likely to be symptom free, unlike the ulcerative form of the disease. (Courtesy of Dr John Wright.)

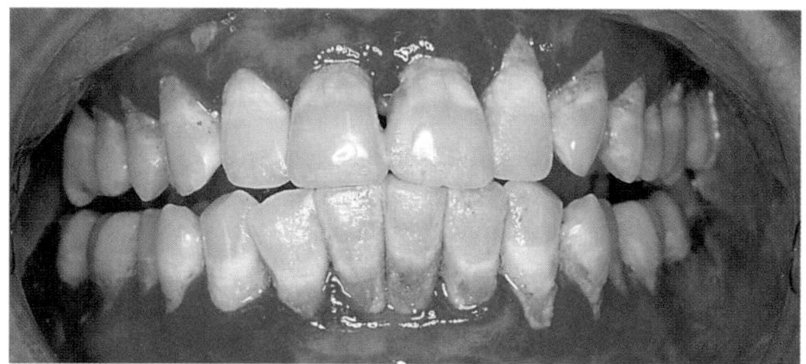

Fig. 20.16 Mucous membrane pemphigoid. This patient shows a rather diffuse presentation on the gingival mucosa with extensive desquamation of the epithelium. Antibodies attack components of the basement membrane, resulting in loss of the epithelium. This type of presentation is painful and it is difficult to maintain oral hygiene. (Courtesy of Dr John Wright.)

Topical and systemic medications for aphthous ulceration

Topical medications	
Local anesthetics	Lidocaine rinse or ointment
	Dyclonine rinse
	Diphenhydramine rinse
Anti-inflammatory glucocorticosteroids	Triamcinolone ointment
	Fluocinonide gel
Anti-infectives	Chlorhexidine rinse
	Tetracycline rinse
Systemic medications	
Anti-inflammatory glucocorticosteroids	Prednisone

Fig. 20.14 Topical and systemic medications for aphthous ulceration.

High-potency and highest-potency topical glucocorticosteroids

High-potency topical glucocorticosteroids
0.25% Desoximetasone
0.20% Fluocinolone
0.05% Fluocinonide
Highest-potency topical glucocorticosteroids
0.05% Betamethasone
0.05% Clobetasol
0.05% Halobetasol

Fig. 20.17 High-potency and highest-potency topical glucocorticosteroids.

favorable response and least risk of systemic absorption. If the lesions are not responding, higher-potency topical glucocorticosteroids (see Fig. 20.17) are used and sometimes systemic prednisone is indicated. An intralesional injection of triamcinolone is sometimes given.

Pemphigoid generally responds well to topical anti-inflammatory glucocorticosteroids. However, severe refractory pemphigoid requires more aggressive treatment with a systemic glucocorticosteroid such as prednisone or the use of an immunosuppressive drug such as azathioprine. Dapsone has occasionally been used.

The long-term use of systemic glucocorticosteroids or the use of immunosuppressive drugs should be managed by a physician as the adverse effects can be more severe and need to be carefully monitored. The use of topical glucocorticosteroids for any of these lesions may suppress the immune system and lead to the development of candidiasis, which should then be treated with nystatin or chlorhexidine oral rinses.

Topical drugs used in dentistry

- Chlorhexidine alters taste and causes easily removed staining of the teeth
- Local itching, burning, and erythema of the oral mucosa may occur with topical glucocorticosteroids
- Excessive topical local application to a large denuded surface may produce systemic toxicity

Systemic drugs used for oral mucosal diseases

- Suppression of adrenal cortical activity with systemic glucocorticosteroids
- Azathioprine can cause bone marrow depression, secondary infection, and neoplasia
- Dapsone has been associated with severe cutaneous reactions and hematologic defects

DRUG-INDUCED ORAL DISEASE

Many dental patients will be taking one or more prescribed medications, which may produce adverse effects that can manifest as painful oral mucosal reactions (stomatitis). Such adverse effects include mucositis and oral ulcerations associated with cancer chemotherapy, lichenoid drug reactions, lupus erythematosus-like reactions, pemphigus-like drug reactions, and erythema multiforme (Fig. 20.18).

Contact allergic reactions may also be observed, but occur with less frequency. Angioedema has been observed with some drugs and cinnamon-based ingredients in dentifrices. Dental materials, including metals and acrylic polymers, have also been implicated in soft tissue allergic reactions.

Phenytoin, cyclosporine, and the Ca^{2+} antagonists can cause gingival hyperplasia (Fig. 20.19), which develops in approximately 40% of patients who take phenytoin. The gingival mucosa begins to enlarge and cover the teeth. In severe cases the overgrowth will almost cover the teeth and must be surgically reduced.

Drug-induced adverse effects involving the mouth

Adverse effect	Causative drugs
Lichenoid-drug eruptions	Allopurinol, furosemide, chloroquine, chlorpropamide, gold salts, methyldopa, lithium salts, mercury, penicillamine, phenothiazines, propranolol, quinidine, spironolactone, thiazides, tetracyclines, tolbutamide
Lupus erythematosus-like eruptions	Gold salts, phenytoin, griseofulvin, isoniazid, penicillin, primidone, procainamide, thiouracil, hydralazine, streptomycin, methyldopa
Pemphigus-like drug eruptions	Penicillamine, phenobarbital, rifampin, captopril
Erythema multiforme	Antimalarials, barbiturates, carbamazepine, salicylates, chlorpropamide, sulfonamides, clindamycin, tetracyclines
Gingival hyperplasia	Phenytoin, cyclosporine, nifedipine (and other Ca^{2+} antagonists)
Xerostomia	Anorexiants, antidepressants, isotretinoin, anticholinergics, anticonvulsants, antihistamines, captopril, clonidine, prazosin, reserpine, diflunisal, piroxicam, antiparkinsonian drugs, antipsychotics, diuretics, cyclobenzaprine, opioids, albuterol

Fig. 20.18 Drug-induced adverse effects involving the mouth.

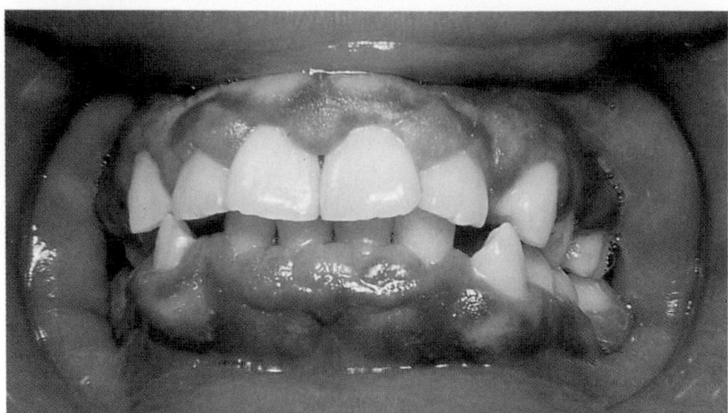

Fig. 20.19 Drug-induced gingival hyperplasia. The gingival papillae show mild hyperplasia associated with the use of phenytoin. Attention to dental hygiene and routine dental scaling to control local factors help to reduce the severity of the hyperplasia. Cyclosporine and Ca^{2+} antagonists produce a similar hyperplasia.

Drugs with anticholinergic effects frequently reduce salivary flow, leading to a drug-induced xerostomia. A dry mouth can also be due to systemic disease and must be considered in these cases.

Xerostomia

- Commonly causes a 'burning tongue'
- Carries a high risk for dental caries
- Carries a high risk for candidiasis
- May be caused by prescribed medications

Management

Management of drug-induced oral adverse effects includes:

- Identifying the suspect drug.
- Working with the physician and patient to seek an alternative drug whenever possible.

Otherwise, palliative care and efforts to improve dental hygiene and control plaque are needed. Acute inflammatory symptoms often respond to topical or systemic anti-inflammatory glucocorticosteroids. An antifungal agent such as nystatin or a chlorhexidine rinse can be used for opportunistic candidiasis. Local anesthetic rinses may be beneficial for stomatitis associated with cancer chemotherapy.

A dry mouth presents a significant challenge as there are no suitable artificial saliva substitutes, and drug-stimulated salivary flow is less than satisfactory. Oral pilocarpine may produce some benefit in patients who have a reduced salivary flow following head and neck radiation.

ANXIETY

A visit to the dentist is such an intimidating experience for many patients that they avoid dental care until the pain demands emergency attention. Dentists have long been portrayed as the harbingers of pain, so reinforcing the patient's anxiety.

Management

To overcome fear and anxiety, both behavioral and pharmacologic methods of pain and anxiety control have been developed. The use of anxiolytics and their cellular and molecular mechanisms of action are described in detail in Chapter 7.

Sedation techniques include the use of central nervous system depressants given by a variety of routes.

The drug and route of administration depend on a variety of factors

The selection of drug and route of administration depends on the degree of anxiety, the patient's medical status, the dental procedure, and the professional training of the dentist. Mild anxiety can be effectively controlled with oral doses of benzodiazepines, sedative antihistamines, or chloral hydrate. However, the quality of oral sedation is not always predictable and is inadequate for an extremely anxious patient. Nitrous oxide/oxygen sedation, which is effective for mild anxiety, has the advantage of allowing a rapid control of sedation levels. Modern gas delivery equipment is designed to limit the percentage (50%) of nitrous oxide that can be given, making this one of the safest sedation techniques.

Other techniques are required for the very anxious patient or for more complex surgical procedures. Parenteral, preferably intravenous, administration, and the use of benzodiazepines, opioids, or ultra short-acting barbiturates allow a controlled induction and dose titration to maintain and adjust the depth of sedation. The desired level of sedation is typically marked by the appearance of ptosis and slurred speech. Patients are sedated, but remain conscious so they can respond to commands and protective airway reflexes are not obtunded. The intramuscular route can be used, but drug absorption is not always predictable and sedation levels cannot be titrated.

Vital signs (blood pressure, respiration) need to be monitored at regular intervals during intravenous parenteral sedation and recovery to ensure patient safety. Adequate sedation for most dental procedures can be accomplished without producing general anesthesia. Anesthetic, anxiolytic, and sedative–hypnotic drugs used for dental sedation include:

- Inhalational drugs (nitrous oxide/oxygen).
- Opioids (meperidine, fentanyl, morphine).
- Nonbarbiturates (chloral hydrate).
- Benzodiazepines (diazepam, lorazepam, midazolam, triazolam).
- Antihistamines (promethazine, hydroxyzine).
- Barbiturates (methohexital).

Minor adverse effects associated with office conscious sedation techniques include nausea, emesis, dizziness, tremors, and dysphoria. More severe reactions such as respiratory depression, aspiration, laryngospasm, allergic drug reactions, and cardiac events can also occur. In one study, respiration depression was the most frequent severe adverse effect and occurred with a prevalence of 12/10,000 cases of intravenous conscious sedation. Careful airway management, dose titration, avoidance of unconsciousness, and patient selection are therefore fundamental to the safe and effective use of this form of sedation.

FURTHER READING

Dionne RA. New approaches to preventing and treating postoperative pain. *J Am Dent Ass* 1992; **123:** 27–34. [Paper describing the use of long-acting local anesthetics and nonsteroidal anti-inflammatory drugs in the dental pain model.]

Jastak JT, Yagiela JA, Donaldson D. *Local Anesthesia of the Oral Cavity*. Philadelphia: WB Saunders; 1995. [Excellent textbook with a comprehensive coverage of local anesthetics in dentistry.]

Millard HD, Mason DK (eds) *World Workshop on Oral Medicine*. Chicago: Year Book; 1989. [An excellent commentary by world experts on the etiology, pathophysiology, and treatment of diseases of the oral mucosa.]

Neubrun E. *Cariology*. Chicago: Quientessence; 1989. [Comprehensive textbook on caries development and prevention, and fluoride use.]

Peterson LJ. Principles of antibiotic therapy. In: Topazian RG, Goldberg MH (eds) *Oral and Maxillofacial Infections*. 3rd edn. Philadelphia: WB Saunders; 1994, pp. 160–197. [A detailed review of potential pathogenic microorganisms of the oral cavity, and antibiotic selection and use.]

Wright JM. Oral manifestations of drug reactions. In: Gage TW (ed.) Symposium on Pharmacology and Dental Therapeutics. *Dent Clin North Am* 1984; **28:** 529–543. [A well-organized and succinct review of the response of oral mucous membranes to medications.]

Make a provisional diagnosis and determine a rational pharmacologic treatment for the following hypothetical case.

A 65-year-old woman reports to the clinic with a persistent dry mouth and acute pain of 4 days' duration. She is postmenopausal and has a history of hypertension, congestive heart failure, anxiety, and anemia. Current medications include clonidine, hydrochlorothiazide, digoxin, estrogen, a potassium supplement, and alprazolam. Other symptoms include malaise, a loss of appetite, and altered taste. Her temperature is not increased and she has no lymphadenopathy. Oral examination reveals a diffusely red oral mucosa with white patches and angular cheilitis. Her tongue is inflamed and has a smooth dorsal surface lacking papillae with a white coating. The coating and white patches are easily rubbed off, but the underlying oral mucosa is red and painful.

1. Would you reassure the patient and tell her that she has a local allergic reaction that can be managed with a systemic antihistamine? Explain your answer.
2. Would you prescribe a systemic antibiotic as the patient has a generalized stomatitis, which will resolve after a few days? Explain your answer.
3. Would you prescribe a topical or systemic antiviral agent for a primary viral infection? Explain your answer.
4. Would you prescribe a topical antifungal rinse, instruct her to avoid hot spicy foods and to increase her fluid intake, and reassure her that her symptoms will quickly resolve with the use of medication? Explain your answer.
5. Suppose you prescribed a topical antifungal rinse (such as nystatin oral suspension), what is the class of drug, why is it administered topically, how long should it be continued, what is the endpoint of therapy, and what adverse effects/drug interactions can you anticipate?
6. Would you order laboratory tests and, if so, what and why?
7. How could this woman's drug therapy have contributed to her oral symptoms?

?

Indicate which is the correct answer for each question.

1. The following drug and use-pairs are correctly matched, except
- a) chlorhexidine and gingivitis
- b) fluoride and dental caries
- c) carbamazepine and trigeminal neuralgia
- d) nystatin and recurrent herpes labialis
- e) pilocarpine and radiation-induced xerostomia

2. Select the statement that is false
- a) lidocaine is an amide-type local anesthetic
- b) inflammation or infection at the site of local anesthetic administration decreases the degree of regional analgesia
- c) vasoconstrictors increase perfusion of tissues
- d) epinephrine adverse effects can include tachycardia and palpitation
- e) vasoconstrictors increase the duration of action of injected local anesthetics

3. Xerostomia is associated with all of the following classes of drugs, except
- a) cholinesterase inhibitors
- b) antidepressants
- c) antipyschotics
- d) opioids
- e) antihistamines

4. Nonsteroidal anti-inflammatory drugs
- a) mimic naturally occurring brain opioids
- b) inhibit prostaglandin synthesis
- c) block genesis of the nerve action potential
- d) interfere with the release of histamine and bradykinin
- e) cause microvasculature vasoconstriction

5. Adverse effects of antibiotic drugs can include all of the following, except
- a) hypersensitivity reactions including anaphylaxis
- b) superinfections including candidiasis
- c) antibiotic-induced diarrhea
- d) tachycardia, palpitations, and a modest elevation of blood pressure
- e) diarrhea with erythromycin

6. All of the following drug and oral adverse effect pairs are correctly matched, except
- a) fluorides and mottled enamel
- b) acyclovir and herpes labialis
- c) phenytoin and gingival hyperplasia
- d) allopurinol and lichenoid drug reaction
- e) nifedipine and gingival hyperplasia

7. The most important reason for adding vasoconstrictors to local anesthetic solutions is
- a) to increase the quality and duration of the regional analgesia
- b) to overcome the patient's anxiety and fear of dental treatment
- c) to prevent adverse drug reactions
- d) to prevent adverse drug interactions
- e) to ensure nerve conduction blockade in the presence of acute infection

8. Select the drug combination least likely to result in adverse effects
- a) metronidazole and ethanol
- b) sulfonamide and warfarin
- c) metronidazole and penicillin V
- d) erythromycin and terfenadine
- e) tetracyclines and antacids

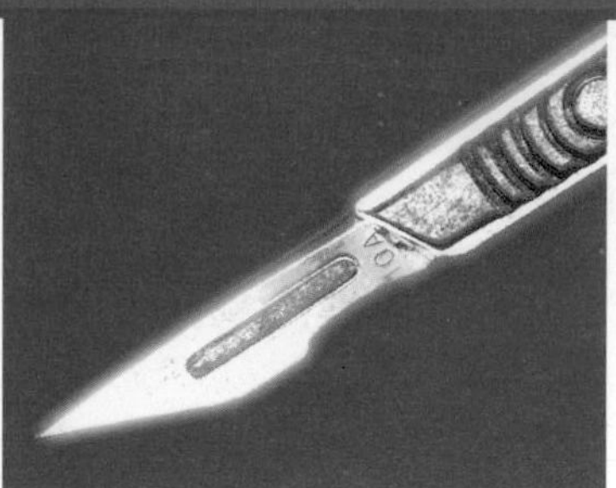

21. Drugs Used in Surgery

PATHOPHYSIOLOGY OF SURGERY AND SURGICAL DISEASE

Surgery is carried out:

- To repair, remove, or replace damaged or diseased tissues.
- To remove healthy tissue, as in organ donation for transplantation or delivery in obstetrics.

Paradoxically, surgeons achieve healing by inflicting injury. However, surgery differs from accidental trauma because the nature and extent of injury are carefully controlled and the body's responses are attenuated by anesthesia. The unconsciousness of general anesthesia is accompanied by a depression of the respiratory and cardiovascular responses to surgery. Cardiorespiratory monitoring and treatment during anesthesia parallel the basic strategies of resuscitation used to treat injured and critically ill patients.

Perioperative drugs including anesthetics are used to maintain fluid balance, treat disease, prevent sepsis, and suppress awareness and pain.

Resuscitation and anesthesia have analogous treatment strategies

Patients requiring emergency surgical and obstetric procedures present with different combinations of past and present disease. Irrespective of the type of emergency, potentially fatal conditions such as hypoxemia and hemodynamic instability can arise. Management of concurrent life-threatening conditions requires a risk–benefit approach: do the benefits of preoperative evaluation and treatment outweigh the risks of surgical delay?

LIFE SUPPORT

Prompt life support is critical in the unconscious patient and preempts surgical evaluation. An unobstructed airway is of paramount importance. The unconscious patient will not perceive airway obstruction, and hypoxemia can lead to brain damage, cardiac arrest, or death, while in patients with intracranial space-occupying lesions, hypercarbia can produce cerebral vasodilation, increased intracranial pressure, and further cerebral ischemia. Provided that there is no suspicion of spinal instability, restoring an unobstructed airway involves placing the patient on their side and pulling the mandible and therefore the tongue forward. Breathing must also be maintained to ensure oxygen delivery and carbon dioxide elimination. If the patient remains unconscious, tracheal intubation is required to protect the airway from aspiration of gastric contents.

'ABC' approach to the unconscious patient

- **Airway:** maintain patency
- **Breathing:** provide ventilation and oxygenation
- **Circulation:** give chest compressions if pulseless, obtain intravenous access, administer fluids and drugs as appropriate
- Defibrillate if necessary, consider differential diagnosis, treat reversible causes

Patients with trauma to multiple systems and those with critical illnesses typically have impaired oxygen delivery. For example:

- Chest crush injuries or pneumonia cause atelectasis and 'hypoxic hypoxia.'
- Bleeding decreases oxygen-carrying capacity and leads to 'anemic hypoxia.'
- Inadequate blood flow due to circulatory failure produces 'ischemic hypoxia.'

Carbon dioxide can also be retained in many of these situations, for example as a result of depressed ventilatory control due to head trauma or ineffective respiration due to chest trauma. Initial management of critical illness includes routine oxygen therapy and close observation of vital signs.

Oxygen therapy and mechanical ventilation

Simple oxygen devices provide a variable fraction of inspired oxygen (F_iO_2) since their low flow of oxygen is inspired along with room air.

Supplemental oxygen can be administered via nasal prongs (F_iO_2 0.24 to 0.4 with oxygen flows 1 to 6 liters/min) or vented mask (F_iO_2 0.4 to 0.6 with oxygen flows 5 to 8 liters/min). Since the development of pulse oximetry, air entrainment devices that deliver a restricted F_iO_2 are seldom used for patients with chronic carbon dioxide retention (Fig. 21.1). Oxygen toxicity of the lung (and the eye in premature neonates) may follow the use of a prolonged and high F_iO_2 (F_iO_2 1.0 for 12 hours for lung; higher sensitivity for eye).

Although the need for mechanical ventilation is often obvious in patients with severe head or chest trauma, a diagnosis of acute and progressive respiratory failure in patients with preexisting cardiorespiratory disease can be difficult. An increasing respiratory rate and increasing pCO_2 and decreasing pO_2

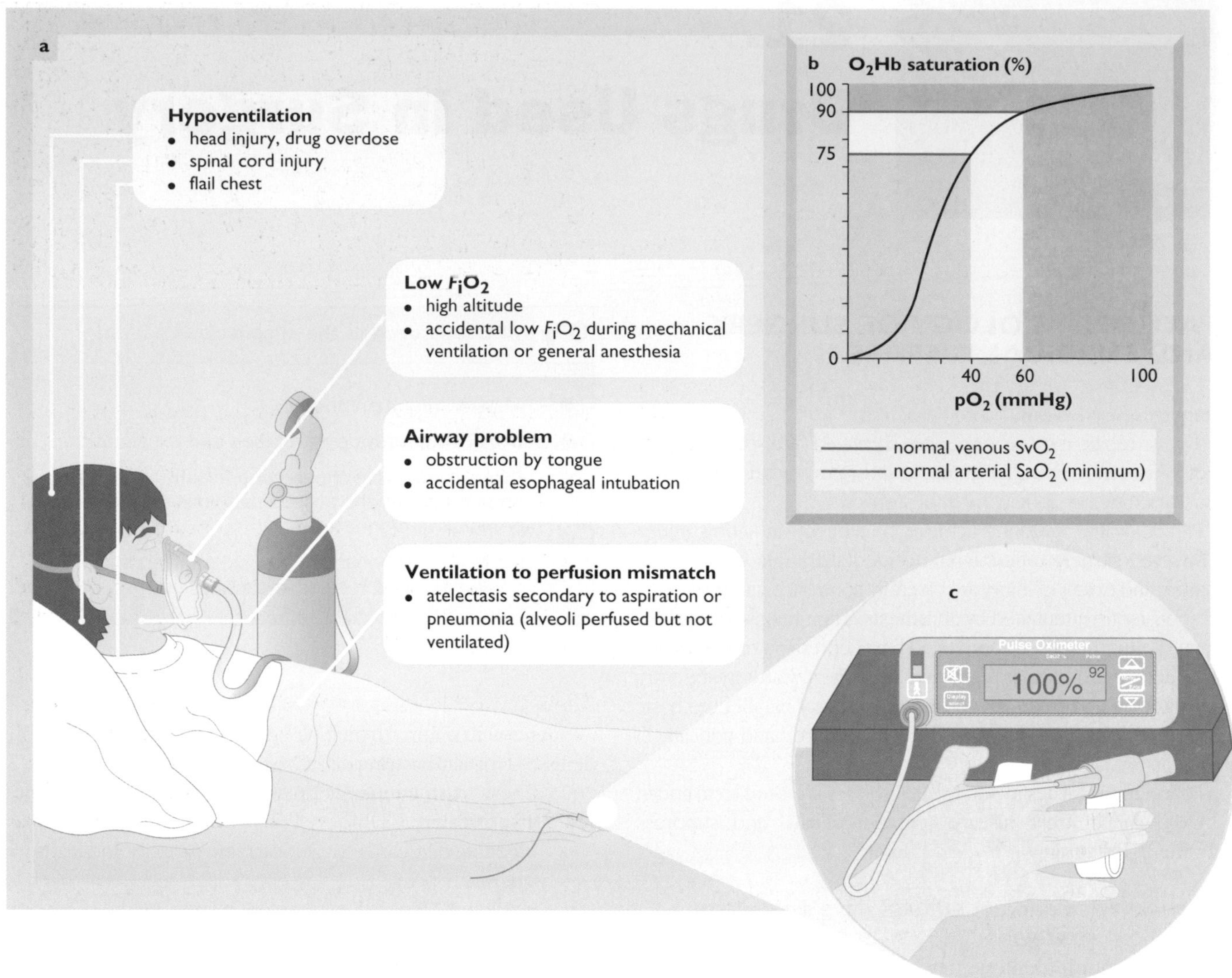

Fig. 21.1 Hypoxemia, oxygen saturation of hemoglobin, and clinical monitoring. (a) Possible causes of hypoxemia. Normal oxygenation requires sufficient inspired oxygen, a patent airway, an intact respiratory center, an innervated and stable chest wall, and ventilated and perfused alveoli. (b) Oxyhemoglobin (O_2Hb) dissociation curve and pulse oximetry. The O_2Hb dissociation curve describes the relation between the saturation of Hb with oxygen. The flat portion at the top of the sigmoid-shaped curve indicates near-maximal oxygen capacity. Saturation of Hb with oxygen is about 90% when pO_2 is 60 mmHg and about 100% when pO_2 is 100 mmHg or greater. (c) Pulse oximetry can provide a noninvasive monitor of oxygen content of arterial blood as well as pulsatile perfusion. However, pulse oximetry does not necessarily indicate circulatory adequacy. (SaO_2, percentage saturation of arterial Hb; pO_2, partial pressure of oxygen; SvO_2, percentage saturation of venous Hb)

in arterial blood may allow an early diagnosis before the development of a life-threatening emergency. Intubation and mechanical ventilation are not without risk in critically ill patients as anesthesia is often needed, with resultant cardiovascular depression and decreased organ perfusion.

MANAGEMENT OF HEMODYNAMIC INSTABILITY

Oxygen delivery depends on an intact circulation, therefore inadequate tissue perfusion must be diagnosed and treated promptly. The basic mechanisms of acute circulatory failure comprise either:

- Hypovolemia (decreased preload).
- Compromised cardiac function (decreased heart rate, very high heart rate, decreased contractility) (Fig. 21.2).

Septic shock resulting from the release of vasoactive substances is associated with hypovolemia because vasodilation and leaking capillaries decrease preload.

Management of hemodynamic instability begins with an assessment of heart rate, blood pressure, and preload. Although many causes of hypovolemia are hemorrhagic, non-hemorrhagic hypovolemia and cardiogenic circulatory failure must also be looked for since there can be multiple coexisting etiologies. For example, an elderly patient with a bowel obstruction can become hypovolemic as a result of gastrointestinal fluid accumulation and sepsis; associated circulatory failure can then lead to tachycardia and coronary hypoperfusion, which in turn can produce acute heart failure.

Healthy adults compensate for rapid losses of up to 15% of the blood volume (i.e. 15% × 70 ml/kg body weight) by increasing cardiac output. However, these sympathetic reflexes can be depressed by anesthesia, resulting in a precipitous decrease in blood pressure and tissue perfusion. It is therefore crucial to restore intravascular volume before anesthesia. Most preoperative patients will develop signs of inadequate tissue perfusion once 30% of the blood volume has been lost. Clinical markers of progressive organ dysfunction are oliguria, tachycardia, hypotension, dyspnea, metabolic acidosis, and mental changes such as agitation.

Fluid therapy and blood transfusions

The initial treatment of acute circulatory failure involves ensuring an adequate intravascular volume. Immediate surgical control is the best form of therapy for ongoing internal bleeding (e.g. ruptured ectopic pregnancy or ruptured aortic aneurysm).

> **Clinical monitoring in resuscitation and anesthesia**
>
> - Central nervous system: level of consciousness
> - **Airway** and **Breathing:** respiratory rate, pulse oximetry, expired capnometry, and arterial blood gases
> - **Circulation:** heart rate, blood pressure, electrocardiogram, urine output

Crystalloid therapy As soon as hypovolemia is diagnosed, fluid must be administered rapidly. The initial solutions should be 'crystalloids' that contain water and electrolytes at an isotonic concentration (i.e. a concentration that does not lyse or crenate red blood cells). Four times the volume of estimated blood loss must be given as crystalloid to maintain an adequate blood volume because of the rapid distribution of ions and water from the intravascular compartment to the interstitial fluid compartment (Fig. 21.3).

Colloid and blood therapy If a patient with acute circulatory failure remains hypotensive despite the rapid administration of electrolyte solution, synthetic (e.g. pentastarch) or natural colloids may be required for volume replacement. Colloid solutions provide the same oncotic pressure and intravascular

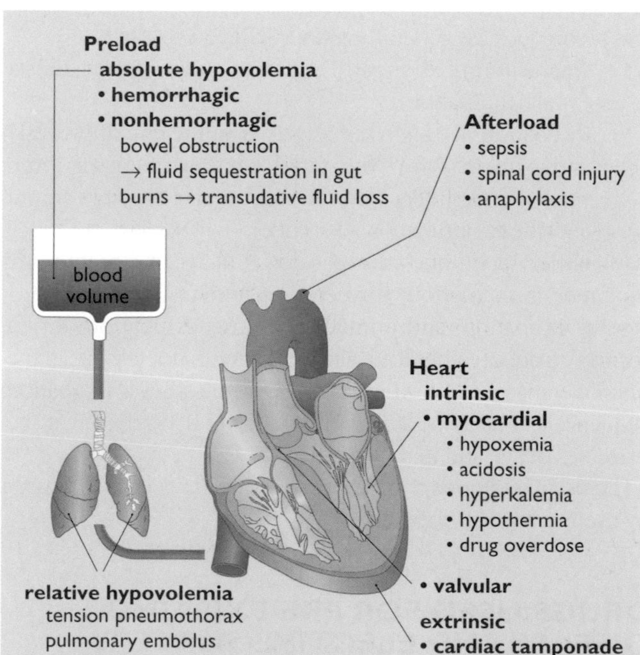

Fig. 21.2 Classification of acute circulatory failure. Clues to the correct diagnosis will be provided by the history, physical examination (CNS and pupil status; breath sounds and tracheal deviation; heart rate and flat or distended neck veins; temperature; dialysis fistulas), pulse oximetry and electrocardiography.

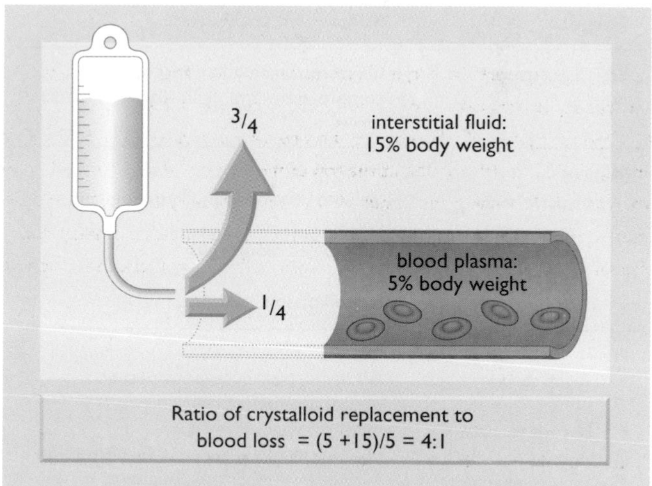

Fig. 21.3 Extracellular fluid compartments, blood loss, and crystalloid replacement. Water and electrolytes are freely diffusible between plasma and interstitial fluid through capillary pores. During bleeding, water and electrolytes are mobilized from the interstitial fluid into the circulation. Similarly, when replacing blood loss with normal saline or lactated Ringer's solution, three-quarters of the infused crystalloid will move from the circulation into the interstitial fluid. Therefore, the required crystalloid resuscitation volume is four times the blood loss.

expansion as whole blood. Ideally, blood products should not be used for simple volume expansion because of the potential immunological and infectious hazards of transfusions. Plasma and platelets should be used for coagulopathies and red blood cells to maintain arterial oxygen content (Fig. 21.4).

Monitoring fluid replacement Heart rate, blood pressure, and urine output are useful parameters of the hemodynamic efficacy of fluid replacement. Sometimes invasive methods for assessing volume status (e.g. central venous pressure and pulmonary arterial occluded pressure measurements) and cardiac output measurements are useful. The hemoglobin (Hb) concentration is an unreliable estimate of blood loss until there has been adequate fluid replacement and hemodilution. Once a steady state has been reached, however, a reduction of 1 g/dl (10 g/liter) Hb is equivalent to a one unit blood loss (500 ml whole blood, 300 ml packed red blood cells) in a 70 kg adult. Since donor blood is separated into individual components, replacement of 50% of the blood volume with crystalloid, non-plasma colloid, and packed red blood cells can dilute the clotting factors and platelets. Coagulation tests and platelet counts should therefore be monitored and plasma fraction and platelet concentrate transfusions given when needed.

Targets in the treatment of acute circulatory failure

Target	Supportive treatment
Basic life support	Oxygenation, ventilation, chest compressions and defibrillation if cardiac arrest
Preload	
Hypovolemia	Volume infusion with crystalloid and colloid
Low blood oxygen capacity	Packed red blood cells
Coagulopathy	Frozen plasma, platelets
Heart	
Bradycardia	Atropine, transcutaneous pacing, dopamine, epinephrine
Severe tachycardia	Pharmacologic slowing ± pharmacologic or electric cardioversion
Low cardiac output	Inotropes: ephedrine, dopamine, dobutamine Afterload reduction: sodium nitroprusside, nitroglycerin
Afterload	
Low brain and heart perfusion pressures	Vasopressors: phenylephrine, dopamine, epinephrine, norepinephrine

Fig. 21.4 Targets in the treatment of acute circulatory failure.

DRUG THERAPY IN ADVANCED LIFE SUPPORT

If hypotension or a low urine output persists after adequate volume expansion, drugs are given for the associated medical problems. Such drug treatment may include:

- Vasopressors for inadequate brain and myocardial perfusion pressures.
- Inotropes with or without afterload reduction for a low cardiac output.
- Antibiotics for sepsis.
- Sodium bicarbonate for acidosis.

Once the patient's circulatory status has improved, the underlying surgical cause must be identified and treated without delay.

PULMONARY ASPIRATION DURING ANESTHESIA

Anesthetics can induce regurgitation and vomiting with risk of aspiration when protective airway reflexes are obtunded. Recent food consumption therefore places patients at risk of pulmonary aspiration and death during anesthesia. However, postponing emergency surgery will not guarantee an empty stomach because pain and opioids reduce gastric motility.

Premedication to prevent pulmonary aspiration

Antacids neutralize acid, histamine H_2 receptor antagonists reduce acid production, and upper gastrointestinal motility agents promote forward emptying of the stomach. However, such premedication has limited success and is therefore not routinely used in emergency surgery (Fig. 21.5).

The best prevention of pulmonary aspiration other than using regional anesthesia involves using one of the following two airway techniques for general anesthesia:

- Tracheal intubation with sedation and local anesthesia (awake intubation).
- Intubation as soon as there is sufficient anesthesia and paralysis after the rapid administration of intravenous anesthetics and neuromuscular blockers (rapid anesthesia–intubation sequence).

With either technique, the patient is at risk of pulmonary aspiration in the period between drug administration and successful intubation, and immediately after extubation during recovery from anesthesia. Awake intubation is not feasible in the uncooperative patient, whereas the rapid anesthesia–intubation sequence can be associated with significant hypotension at the extremes of age and in the critically ill.

The risk of pulmonary aspiration is reduced in elective surgery by preoperative fasting.

DRUGS USED FOR PRE-EXISTING DISEASE AND ELECTIVE SURGERY

The patient should be as fit as possible to best withstand anesthesia and surgical injury. A thorough preoperative assessment of cardiorespiratory disease is especially important so that pre-existing disease states can be optimized prior to elective surgery.

BRONCHIAL ASTHMA, CHRONIC BRONCHITIS, AND ACUTE LARYNGOTRACHEOBRONCHITIS

Chronic obstructive pulmonary disease and a limited respiratory reserve predispose to the development of postoperative atelectasis, pneumonia, and hypoxemia, especially after upper abdominal and thoracic surgery. Reversal of bronchospasm and treatment of chronic bacterial infection using bronchodilators, antibiotics, and physiotherapy should therefore be attempted for several days preoperatively if the nature of the underlying disease permits elective surgery (see Fig. 21.5). During anesthesia, tracheal stimulation from intubation can cause life-threatening bronchoconstriction.

Patients with chronic carbon dioxide retention are susceptible to respiratory failure postoperatively since opioids and sedatives markedly decrease the ventilatory response to hypoxemia.

Acute respiratory tract infections such as viral-induced laryngotracheobronchitis should be allowed to resolve before surgery, particularly in pediatric patients. The small diameter of the airways in children means that they have an increased risk of perioperative airway obstruction from edema and laryngospasm.

HEART FAILURE, ANGINA, HYPERTENSION, ARRHYTHMIAS, AND HYPOKALEMIA

General anesthetics are myocardial depressants while epidural and spinal anesthesia are associated with vasodilation due to reduced sympathetic nervous activity. Heart failure and hypovolemia must therefore be treated preoperatively to avoid the hypotensive effect of general or spinal anesthesia. Similarly, angina, hypertension, and arrhythmias should be pharmacologically controlled, and chronic medications, with the possible exception of diuretics, should be continued on the morning of surgery (Fig. 21.6). Diuretic or adrenocorticosteroid-induced potassium depletion should be corrected over several days to minimize the perioperative risk of arrhythmias.

DIABETES MELLITUS AND ADRENAL INSUFFICIENCY

Patients with diabetes mellitus need less oral hypoglycemic drug or insulin when fasting (see Fig. 21.5) to avoid a low blood glucose, unconsciousness, and associated damage to the central nervous system (CNS). Oral diabetic drugs should therefore be withheld on the morning of surgery and sometimes, depending upon the drug's duration of action, stopped 1–2 days preoperatively (e.g. chlorpropamide). Insulin-dependent diabetic patients should have an intravenous infusion of glucose and their usual dose of insulin should be reduced on the morning of surgery. If insulin is not provided, free fatty acids are mobilized from adipose tissues and metabolized to ketones by the insulin-deficient liver, resulting in life-threatening ketoacidosis. During anesthesia, the patient's blood glucose must be measured frequently as mental status cannot be used as a monitor of hypoglycemia.

Drugs to be stopped, continued, or started preoperatively

	Drugs	Perioperative aims
Stop	Oral hypoglycemics	Avoid hypoglycemia and cerebral damage
	Monoamine oxidase inhibitors (MAOIs)	Avoid hypertensive crisis and hyperpyrexia
	Warfarin (e.g. for atrial fibrillation or prosthetic valve, convert to heparin and discontinue shortly before surgery)	Avoid excessive bleeding intraoperatively (with minimal increase in risk of cerebral embolism and stroke)
	Diuretics	Avoid hypovolemia and hypokalemia
Continue	Opioids	Avoid preoperative pain
	Anticonvulsants	Avoid seizure
	Bronchodilators	Avoid bronchoconstriction
	Antihypertensives and cardiac drugs with exception of diuretics	Avoid hypertension, angina, congestive heart failure, arrhythmia
	Adrenocorticosteroids (increase dose)	Avoid adrenal insufficiency
	Insulin (decrease dose)	Avoid ketoacidosis
Start	Histamine H_1 and H_2 receptor antagonists	Allergy prophylaxis in atopic patients
	Benzodiazepines	Provide anxiolysis and anterograde amnesia in frightened patients
	Bronchodilators (inhaled)	Avoid bronchoconstriction in stable asthmatics
	Anticholinergics	Avoid bradycardia in young children (cardiac output depends on the heart rate)
	Adrenocorticosteroids (increase dose)	Avoid adrenal insufficiency if drug history positive in past year
	Antacids, histamine H_1 receptor antagonists, gastric motility agents	Increase gastric pH and decrease gastric residual volume
	Antiemetics	Reduce risk of nausea and vomiting
	Heparin	Prevent deep vein thrombosis and pulmonary embolism
	Antibiotics	Prevent wound infection and subacute bacterial endocarditis

Fig. 21.5 Drugs to be stopped, continued, or started preoperatively.

Anesthetic interactions with pre-existing drug therapy

Body location	Drug	Anesthetic interaction
Brain	Acute alcohol intoxication Chronic alcohol abuse Clonidine	Potentiates general anesthetics Increases general anesthetic requirements Potentiates general anesthetics (but continue preoperatively to avoid intraoperative 'rebound' hypertension because of its short half-life)
Lung	Smoking Past use of bleomycin	Pulmonary injury decreases oxygen transfer and carbon monoxide decreases blood oxygen capacity High F_iO_2 can precipitate adult respiratory distress syndrome
Circulation	Diuretics β Adrenoceptor agonists, bronchodilators β Adrenoceptor antagonists Ca^{2+} antagonists Monoamine oxidase inhibitors (MAOIs) Past use of doxorubicin	Hypovolemia increases risk of hypotension and acute hypokalemia increases risk of arrhythmias during general anesthesia Potentiate arrhythmias from volatile inhaled anesthetics Potentiate myocardial depression from general anesthetics Potentiate myocardial depression from general anesthetics Sympathetic stimulants or meperidine may precipitate hypertension and hyperpyrexia Cardiomyopathy increases risk of heart failure from anesthesia
Neuromuscular junction	Aminoglycosides	Potentiate nondepolarizing neuromuscular blockers

Fig. 21.6 Anesthetic interactions with pre-existing drug therapy.

Adrenal insufficiency can occur at the time of surgical stress in patients who are taking adrenocorticosteroids or in patients who have had a past course of adrenocorticosteroids within the previous year. Parenteral replacement therapy should therefore be started on the morning of surgery and tapered as the postoperative stress resolves.

ANEMIA, BLEEDING DISORDERS, AND DEEP VEIN THROMBOSIS

Chronic anemia is usually well tolerated. For example, patients with renal failure can present with Hb concentrations as low as 6 g/dl (60 g/liter). Red blood cell transfusions should be used to treat inadequate oxygenation. Homologous transfusion is indicated when the Hb concentration is less than 6 g/dl (60 g/liter), but rarely warranted when it is greater than 10 g/dl (100 g/liter). The acceptable value, however, may be adjusted up or down depending on the patient's ability to increase cardiac output, the nature of the surgery, and the skills of the surgeon and anesthetist. Bleeding disorders and anticoagulation may need to be treated preoperatively for major surgical procedures or if epidural or spinal anesthesia is planned (see Fig. 21.5).

Postoperative deep venous thrombosis is more common in patients who are elderly or obese and in those who have malignancy or a current drug history of oral contraception. Surgical factors include hip and pelvic procedures, and prolonged immobilization during surgery or the postoperative period. Prophylactic subcutaneous heparin will decrease the incidence of deep venous thrombosis with a minimal risk of surgical bleeding (see Fig. 21.5), but should be postponed if epidural or spinal anesthesia is planned because of the risk of epidural hematoma and spinal cord compression. Warfarin is also used prophylactically, but takes longer to be effective and is not as easily reversed as heparin. Using a spinal or epidural anesthetic decreases the risk of deep vein thrombosis.

WOUND INFECTION AND BACTERIAL ENDOCARDITIS

Wound infection and postoperative sepsis are largely prevented by an aseptic surgical technique, but surgical procedures in which the respiratory, oropharyngeal, intestinal, or genitourinary cavities are entered are considered 'contaminated.' The wound infection rates in contaminated cases can, however, be reduced through the prophylactic use of antibiotics (see Fig. 21.5). In addition, patients with valvular and congenital heart disease require antibiotic coverage for contaminated surgery to prevent bacterial endocarditis.

Antibiotics are given before prosthetic implantation in clean surgery since infection would be catastrophic. For example, prophylactic antibiotics are used against skin bacteria for synthetic vascular grafts, cardiac valves, and orthopedic prostheses. In all these situations the antibiotics must be given preoperatively so that there are maximal tissue concentrations at the time of operation. The total duration of administration should be less than 72 hours.

DRUGS USED TO MODIFY THE RESPONSE TO SURGICAL INJURY

Anesthetic suppression of the physiologic response to surgery is probably beneficial, but suppression is limited to the perioperative period.

The 'stress response' to tissue injury involves local changes and stimulation of the neurologic pathways with respiratory, cardiovascular, endocrine, metabolic, and inflammatory components to increase survival from life-threatening injury. For example:

- Local tissue factors lead to vasospasm and coagulation and so reduce bleeding.
- Increases in sympathetic activity compensate for reductions in the circulating blood volume.

Following surgery, parts of the stress response can be harmful. For example:

- The accelerated clotting cascade can lead to thromboembolism.
- Increased sympathetic activity can cause angina in patients with coronary artery disease.

Other than bleeding, surgical injury is associated with significant fluid shifts during open abdominal procedures. Evaporative losses occur from the large serosal surface area of the intestines, and fluid accumulates in the intestinal interstitial compartment as the so-called 'third space loss.' These fluid losses must be replaced perioperatively with crystalloid to avoid hypovolemia and hemodynamic instability. In the initial days following surgery, however, third space losses will shift back, expand the vascular compartment, and predispose patients with heart disease to postoperative heart failure and angina.

The neurologic response to surgery is proportional to the magnitude of nociceptive stimuli and tissue injury. For example, the response to intra-abdominal surgery is greater than the response to extremity surgery. Similarly, larger quantities of anesthetic are required to suppress the response as nociceptive stimuli increase.

ANESTHESIA

Anesthesia is an insensitivity to pain involving suppression of either:

- The afferent sensory reflex (regional anesthesia).
- The central neural processing (general anesthesia).

The mechanism of general anesthetic-induced unconsciousness and suppression of motor and autonomic reflex responses to surgical stimuli is unknown. There are at least two reasons for this uncertainty: the mechanism of consciousness is undefined, and anesthetics have many actions in the CNS. The mechanism of unconsciousness appears to involve depression of synaptic transmission in the thalamus and cerebral cortex (Fig. 21.7). A drug-induced insensitivity to pain can be accomplished, however, with or without a loss of consciousness. Clinically, this means that many surgical procedures can be carried out using either general or regional anesthesia. In contrast to general anesthetics, local anesthetics block axonal conduction.

General anesthesia typically involves an intravenous induction and an inhalation maintenance, with or without opioids and neuromuscular blockers

General anesthetic drugs can be classified on the basis of their route of administration (i.e. intravenous or inhalation, Fig. 21.8):

- Intravenous anesthetics include thiopental (barbiturate), propofol (substituted isopropylphenol), midazolam (benzodiazepine), and ketamine (phencyclidine derivative).
- Inhaled general anesthetics include the inorganic gas nitrous oxide and several halogenated hydrocarbons that are liquids at room temperature. Modern examples of these volatile liquids are halothane, enflurane, isoflurane, desflurane, and sevoflurane.

Many actions of the intravenous anesthetics are mediated through specific receptor interactions, whereas the inhaled anesthetics seem to have many cellular effects.

Changing a patient's consciousness from an alert to an anesthetized state involves a transition phase, which is called induction. During this transition, airway, respiratory, and circulatory reflexes are progressively depressed in a dose-related manner by the anesthetic. Respiratory effects include a decreased ventilatory response to carbon dioxide and hypoxemia, while circulatory effects involve depression of myocardial contractility, vascular smooth muscle tone, and the autonomic nervous system.

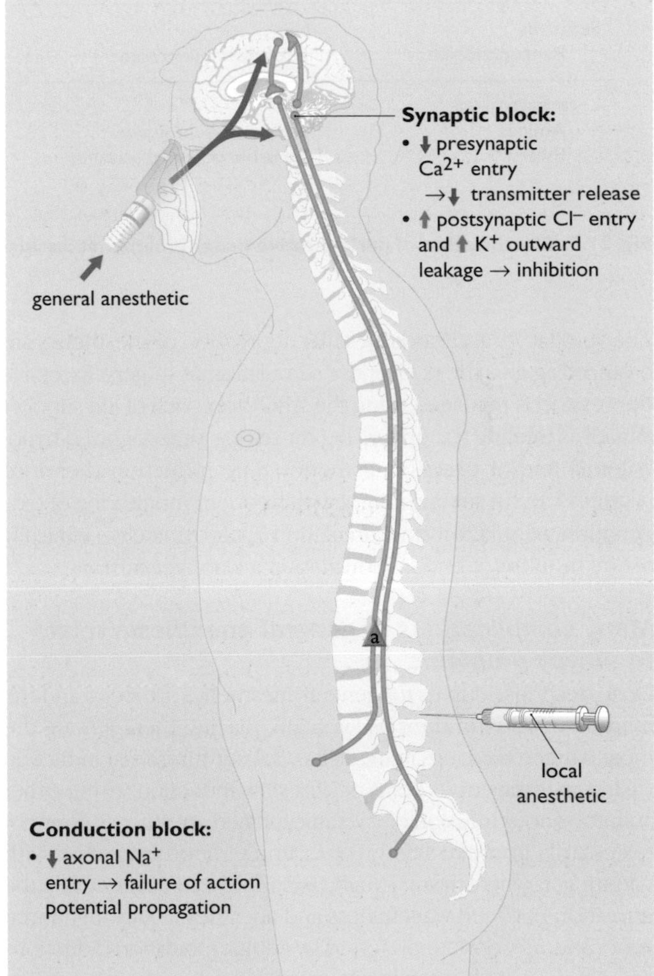

Fig. 21.7 Anesthetic suppression of the physiologic response to surgery. In regional anesthesia the afferent sensory reflex (a) is suppressed. In general anesthesia central neural processing is suppressed.

Classification of perioperative drugs

Classification	Examples	Receptor or enzyme	Most common adverse effect
Intravenous anesthetics			
Barbiturates	Thiopental, methohexital	γ Aminobutyric acid $(GABA)_A$ receptor	Respiratory/cardiovascular depression
Non-barbiturates	Propofol, etomidate		
	Ketamine	Glutamate receptor	
Inhaled anesthetics			
Volatile liquids	Halothane, enflurane, isoflurane, desflurane, sevoflurane	$GABA_A/Cl^-$ receptor channel complex, K^+ leak channels	Respiratory/cardiovascular depression
Inorganic gases	Nitrous oxide		
Neuromuscular blockers			
Depolarizing	Succinylcholine	Nicotinic acetylcholine receptor	Respiratory failure
Nondepolarizing	Pancuronium, atracurium, vecuronium, rocuronium, mivacurium		
Analgesics			
Opioids	Morphine, codeine, meperidine, fentanyl, alfentanil, sufentanil, remifentanil	Opioid receptor	Respiratory depression
Nonsteroidal anti-inflammatory drugs (NSAIDs)	Ketorolac	Cyclooxygenase	Bleeding disorders
Sedatives			
Benzodiazepines	Diazepam, midazolam	$GABA_A$ receptor	Unconsciousness
Local anesthetics			
Amides	Lidocaine, bupivacaine	Na^+ channels	Circumoral tingling, sedation, seizure
Esters	Chloroprocaine, tetracaine		

Fig. 21.8 Classification of perioperative drugs, probable mechanisms of action, and adverse effects.

The ventilatory and cardiovascular depression of anesthetics are balanced against the nociceptive stimulation of surgery. Excessive depression is managed using the 'ABC' approach of life support as well as treating the underlying cause (e.g. unrecognized hypovolemia and/or excess anesthetic). Safe induction therefore requires careful airway control with frequent monitoring of oxygenation, ventilation, and circulation. Unfortunately, a clinically useful monitor of unconsciousness does not yet exist.

Many complications of general anesthesia relate to airway problems

Dose–response curves for general anesthetics are steep and the margin of safety in their use is small, placing them among the most dangerous drugs in medicine. Substituting a fast induction (using an intravenous bolus) with a slow induction (using either an intravenous infusion or a volatile inhaled anesthetic) does not necessarily improve safety. For example, neuroexcitation with vomiting, laryngospasm, cough, and apnea can occur during the transition between wakefulness and anesthesia. Although intravenous inductions are preferred by adults, inhalation inductions are still used in children in whom intravenous access is restricted by poor patient cooperation.

An intravenous injection of thiopental is followed by rapid brain uptake and unconsciousness within 30 seconds because there is a high relative blood flow to the brain and thiopental rapidly crosses the blood–brain barrier. The concentration in brain then decreases as thiopental redistributes to other highly perfused tissues. In fact, redistribution, not metabolism, accounts for early awakening within 10 minutes from a single dose of intravenous anesthetic. Because hepatic metabolism of thiopental is slow, however, repeated administration leads to drug accumulation and slow awakening. In general, the slow metabolism of intravenous anesthetics and opioids results in postoperative drowsiness, 'hangover,' and mental impairment for at least 24 hours.

Excess anesthesia as well as inadequate suppression of the physiologic response to surgery can cause patient injury.

Inhalation agents are preferable for maintaining anesthesia

Inhalation agents do not need to be metabolized before elimination from the lung and are therefore preferred for maintaining anesthesia. This property allows a rapid decrease in the quantity of anesthetic in the brain and the heart, which in turn allows prompt treatment of anesthetic-induced cardiorespiratory depression and prompt emergence from anesthesia. In contrast to thiopental, the intravenous anesthetic propofol is rapidly metabolized and can therefore be used as both an induction and a maintenance agent.

During emergence from anesthesia neither intravenous nor inhaled anesthetics provide residual analgesia

Opioids (e.g. morphine, meperidine, fentanyl, alfentanil, sufentanil, remifentanil) are administered perioperatively to permit transition from anesthesia to a pain-free state (see Fig. 21.8). An additional benefit of opioid administration during anesthesia is a decreased need for intravenous and inhaled anesthetics and therefore less circulatory depression. Emergence can be complicated by excessive opioid administration, however, as opioids produce a dose-related respiratory depression.

The methods used to control the airway and ventilation affect anesthetic selection and dose

Manual methods for maintaining a patent airway produce painful stimuli and reflex muscle activity, which must be suppressed to reduce patient injury. When comparing the intensity of stimulation produced by airway manipulation, a face mask with an oropharyngeal airway produces least, while a laryngeal mask produces intermediate, stimulation. An endotracheal tube produces the most stimulation (Fig. 21.9).

Inhalation anesthetics

- Halothane-induced hepatotoxicity is a diagnosis of exclusion
- Fluoride-induced nephrotoxicity is a hazard with enflurane and sevoflurane
- Nitrous oxide can induce transient bone marrow depression and peripheral nerve neuropathy as a result of reduced activity of vitamin B_{12}-dependent enzymes
- Nitrous oxide may cause abortions among operating room staff and therefore waste gas scavenging systems have been introduced

Neuromuscular blocking drugs

Intubation generally involves the use of neuromuscular blockers (NMBs), since laryngeal stimulation can be associated with reflex closure of the vocal cords and hypoxemia if intubation is not successful. Neuromuscular blockade is also needed during intra-abdominal and intrathoracic procedures to prevent reflex muscle contraction and to allow surgical exposure and wound closure. Reflex muscle responses can be suppressed by high concentrations of volatile inhaled anesthetics, but this is accompanied by circulatory depression. Intubation and mechanical ventilation are needed if long-acting NMBs are used. Spontaneous ventilation can, however, be used with most intravenous and inhalation anesthetics if long-acting NMBs or high doses of opioids are not given.

NMBs prevent normal synaptic transmission at neuromuscular junctions by acting on the nicotinic cholinergic receptor (see Fig. 21.8). Two types of receptor blockade determine drug onset, duration, and adverse effects.

Depolarizing NMBs Like acetylcholine, succinylcholine binds to postjunctional nicotinic cholinergic receptors and produces depolarization with muscle fasciculations and postoperative myalgia. However, unlike acetylcholine's brief action as a result of deactivation by acetylcholinesterase, succinylcholine remains receptor bound for several minutes and the muscle does not respond to the subsequent release of acetylcholine. After a few minutes, succinylcholine is metabolized by plasma cholinesterase and the postjunctional nicotinic cholinergic membrane repolarizes. Because of its rapid onset and short duration of action, succinylcholine is used for intubation.

Airway and breathing decisions in general anesthesia

Question	Alternatives	Rationale
Airway method?	Face mask or laryngeal mask	Less invasive but less reliable. short-duration procedure not requiring intubation or mechanical ventilation
	Tracheal intubation	Requires neuromuscular blocker (NMB) and may cause trauma Maintains secure airway (e.g. head and neck surgery, surgery in the prone position) Protects lungs from aspiration (e.g. bleeding airway, recently ingested food or swallowed blood, hiatus hernia, bowel obstruction) Facilitates mechanical ventilation (e.g. anesthetic-, NMB- or opioid-induced respiratory failure)
Breathing method?	Spontaneous	Less invasive since inspiratory pressures are negative (positive in mechanical ventilation), but breathing may be inefficient. For short-duration procedure
	Mechanical	Treats respiratory failure and decreases oxygen consumption

Fig. 21.9 Airway and breathing decisions in general anesthesia.

The 'sustained' depolarization induced by succinylcholine is associated with K^+ leakage from muscle and a slight increase in serum K^+ concentration. In patients with recent burns, spinal cord injuries, and myopathies, however, succinylcholine can lead to sudden hyperkalemia and even cardiac arrest.

Nondepolarizing NMBs compete with acetylcholine for postsynaptic nicotinic receptors and so produce paralysis without initial depolarization or fasciculations. The onset time and duration are significantly longer than for succinylcholine, making these drugs more suitable for surgical relaxation. Curare, pancuronium, vecuronium and rocuronium are metabolized by the liver; atracurium and mivacurium are broken down in the plasma. However, provided that some recovery has occurred, pharmacologic reversal of paralysis is possible by administering an anticholinesterase (e.g. edrophonium, neostigmine, or pyridostigmine) to decrease the natural metabolism of acetylcholine and overcome the competitive block. The anticholinesterase is combined with a muscarinic antagonist (e.g. atropine or glycopyrrolate) to prevent cardiac arrest and bronchospasm owing to excess stimulation of muscarinic cholinergic receptors. Patients with myasthenia gravis (an autoimmune disease characterized by antibodies to the nicotinic acetylcholine receptor) are extremely sensitive to nondepolarizing NMBs.

Regional anesthesia is an alternative to general anesthesia for major surgery on the extremities or the lower abdomen

The choice between regional and general anesthesia is based on the surgical procedure, the surgeon's and anesthetist's experiences, and the patient's medical status and preference. Regional techniques can be combined with general anesthesia to reduce general anesthetic requirements and therefore their undesirable effects, and to improve postoperative analgesia. However, except for some specific surgeries (e.g. cesarean section), regional anesthesia is not necessarily safer than general anesthesia. The similar morbidity and mortality could be due to factors other than the regional anesthetic, such as excessive sedation. General anesthesia is usually required if the nerve blockade fails to allow the surgery to proceed.

Postoperative complications of anesthesia

- General anesthesia or opioids: respiratory and CNS depression, nausea and vomiting
- Epidural or spinal anesthesia: urinary retention, hypotension
- Spinal anesthesia: postural headache, hypotension
- Operative positioning: peripheral nerve injury
- Succinylcholine: muscle pain
- Opioid-induced cough suppression: pneumonia from retained secretions

General anesthetic and resuscitative drugs and equipment should be immediately available when regional anesthesia is performed. Accidental intravascular injection of local anesthetic can cause seizures and cardiovascular instability, whereas a high spinal anesthetic can produce acute respiratory failure and cardiac arrest.

The duration of local anesthesia can be increased by using epinephrine in a concentration of 1:200,000. However, vasoconstrictor-containing solutions should not be injected into a digit, an ear, the nose, or the penis because vasoconstriction can produce local ischemia. Local anesthetics and vasoconstrictors are discussed in detail in Chapter 20 (see Fig. 21.8).

Other than as a result of inadvertent intravascular injection, systemic toxicity of local anesthetics is determined by the rate of drug absorption from the injection site in relation to drug redistribution and metabolism. The extent of drug absorption depends on:

- The drug's properties.
- The dose administered.
- The presence of epinephrine.
- The vascularity of the injection site.

Pain and temperature conduction are more sensitive to blockade by local anesthetics than touch or motor control because of the size and lack of myelination of the small nerve fibers involved. If a differential blockade occurs (i.e. pain transmission is blocked, but touch is preserved), pressure will be sensed during surgery. An anxious patient will perceive any sensation as a failure of the local anesthetic.

Supplemental oxygen is needed during regional anesthesia and sedation

Sedatives and analgesics allow many patients to tolerate unpleasant procedures by relieving anxiety and pain (see Fig. 21.8). However, a patient may suddenly become unconscious owing to excessive intravenous sedation or the use of multiple drugs. In this situation, reflex pain withdrawal may be misinterpreted as wakefulness. The unconscious state can be associated with airway obstruction or respiratory depression and must be managed rapidly to avoid hypoxemic brain damage and cardiac arrest. To minimize this risk, the preprocedure preparation involves fasting and supplemental oxygen should be used routinely during the procedure. A designated person other than the operator should monitor pulse oximetry as well as the patient's wakefulness using frequent oral commands.

Benzodiazepines (e.g. diazepam or midazolam) are used to provide intravenous sedation during regional anesthesia, invasive procedures, and for critically ill patients in the intensive care unit. Benzodiazepines potentiate the action of the neuroinhibitory transmitter γ-aminobutyric acid (GABA), and memory formation is often impaired by these drugs. Anterograde amnesia can be advantageous in the short term, but disadvantageous if persistent for several hours.

Benzodiazepine-induced respiratory or cardiovascular depression are generally minimal unless these drugs are combined with opioids or other CNS depressants. Flumazenil, a $GABA_A$-antagonist, can be useful in reversing profound sedation due to benzodiazepines.

DRUGS FOR POSTOPERATIVE PAIN, NAUSEA, AND VOMITING

Pain and opioids are discussed in detail in Chapter 7 (see Fig. 21.8). The common routes of opioid administration are intravenous, intramuscular, epidural, intrathecal, and oral. Typically, the intravenous route is used in the initial postoperative phase with a 'patient-controlled analgesia' (PCA) machine to provide on-demand delivery. Opioid adverse effects include nausea and vomiting, pruritus, and respiratory depression. Opioids impair the ventilatory response to carbon dioxide and eliminate the response to hypoxemia. Although the incidence of severe respiratory depression is low, close patient observation is mandatory since this complication can be life threatening. Airway management equipment, oxygen, and naloxone, an opioid antagonist, should be readily available.

Nonsteroidal anti-inflammatory drugs (NSAIDs) and regional analgesia with local anesthetics are additional treatments for pain.

Nausea and vomiting and their drug treatment are discussed in detail in Chapter 7.

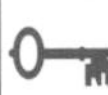

Safety measures in intravenous sedation and analgesia for invasive procedures

- Central nervous system: monitor wakefulness by designated person other than operator to ensure maintenance of consciousness
- **Airway:** preprocedure fasting to avoid aspiration during accidentally induced unconsciousness
- **Breathing:** routine use of supplemental oxygen and pulse oximetry
- **Circulation:** maintain intravenous access for emergency drug administration

Postoperative complications of surgery

- Circulation: bleeding, fluid and electrolyte imbalance, deep venous thrombosis, pulmonary embolism, pressure sores
- Wound: infection, bursting
- Gut: paralytic ileus, gastric ulceration, nutritional deficiency
- Major organ failure: brain, lungs, heart, kidneys, liver

PERIOPERATIVE DRUGS AND PHARMACOGENETICS

Important conditions to identify in the preoperative period are:

- Susceptibility to malignant hyperthermia, which is a potentially fatal disorder involving drug-induced increases in intracellular Ca^{2+} and hypermetabolism in skeletal muscle. It can be triggered by volatile anesthetics or succinylcholine. It is treated with dantrolene, which reduces Ca^{2+} release from the sarcoplasmic reticulum. The parenteral form of this emergency drug must be readily available in the operating room.
- Pseudocholinesterase deficiency, as abnormal plasma cholinesterase activity is associated with prolonged action of the depolarizing NMB succinylcholine and the nondepolarizing NMB mivacurium. This enzyme deficiency should not be life-threatening if postoperative mechanical ventilation is provided. Sedation will be required during the period of ventilation for prolonged paralysis.
- Porphyria, as acute porphyria (an inherited disease of abnormal heme precursors with gastrointestinal, neurologic, and cardiovascular clinical features) can be induced by barbiturates and possibly propofol.

FURTHER READING

Cummins RO (ed.) *Textbook of Advanced Cardiac Life Support*. Dallas: American Heart Association; 1994. [A manual of both cardiac and noncardiac resuscitation.]

Collins VJ. *Physiologic and Pharmacologic Bases of Anesthesia*. Baltimore: Williams & Wilkins; 1996. [A textbook of the basic sciences most relevant to anesthesia patient care.]

Way LW (ed.) *Current Surgical Diagnosis and Treatment 10e*. East Norwalk: Appleton & Lange; 1994. [Brief, well-written sections on fluid, infection and medical problems in surgical patients.]

Make a provisional diagnosis and determine a rational pharmacologic treatment for the following hypothetical case.

A 23-year-old female has received extensive abdominal surgery for trauma related to a motorcycle accident. Following fluid resuscitation, her general anesthetic consisted of a rapid anesthesia-intubation sequence because of the risk of aspiration of recently ingested food. Thiopental and succinylcholine were administered for induction. Oxygen, mechanical ventilation, and isoflurane were used for maintenance of anesthesia with fentanyl for analgesia and pancuronium for continued paralysis. On completion of the surgery, the anesthesiologist turns off the isoflurane and administers atropine and neostigmine intravenously to reverse the nondepolarizing neuromuscular blockade. The patient's endotracheal tube is disconnected from the ventilator and she is transferred from the operating table to the stretcher. Unexpectedly, she neither moves nor opens her eyes to command.

1. What should the immediate therapeutic approach to this unresponsive patient be?
2. Construct a differential diagnosis for 'failure to awaken and breathe' following general anesthesia.
3. How would you identify reversible causes in your differential diagnosis?

Within several minutes, the patient opens her eyes and breathes, but only on command.

4. What are the potential adverse effects of naloxone? How do these factors influence your selection of dose and rate of administration for opioid-induced respiratory depression?
5. Devise strategies to prevent complications in the immediate postanesthetic period.

Indicate which is the correct answer for each question.

1. Reducing the risk of pulmonary aspiration during surgery and anesthesia includes the following therapies, except
- a) preoperative fasting
- b) regional anesthesia
- c) laryngeal mask airway insertion
- d) rapid anesthesia-intubation sequence
- e) awake intubation

2. Which of the following statements is false?
- a) thiopental or propofol are useful in inducing general anesthesia (GA)
- b) thiopental is useful in maintaining GA
- c) nitrous oxide and isoflurane are useful in maintaining GA
- d) GA-induced ventilatory and cardiovascular depression is balanced against nociceptive surgical stimulation
- e) norphine is useful in providing postoperative analgesia

3. With regard to pharmacokinetics and short duration of clinical drug action, which of the following combinations is true?
- a) propofol: redistribution and hepatic metabolism
- b) thiopental: hepatic metabolism
- c) isoflurane: hepatic metabolism
- d) succinylcholine: renal excretion
- e) fentanyl: renal excretion

4. Neuromuscular blockers
- a) do not facilitate tracheal intubation
- b) do not facilitate intra-abdominal surgical exposure and wound closure
- c) do not prevent reflex muscle activity during surgery and light anesthesia
- d) do not prevent fractures in electro-convulsive therapy
- e) require skilled airway and breathing management

5. In the treatment of morphine-induced respiratory depression in a conscious patient on the surgical ward
- a) monitor the level of consciousness and respiratory rate
- b) administer supplemental O_2
- c) monitor oxygenation with pulse oximetry
- d) withhold sedatives
- e) all of the above

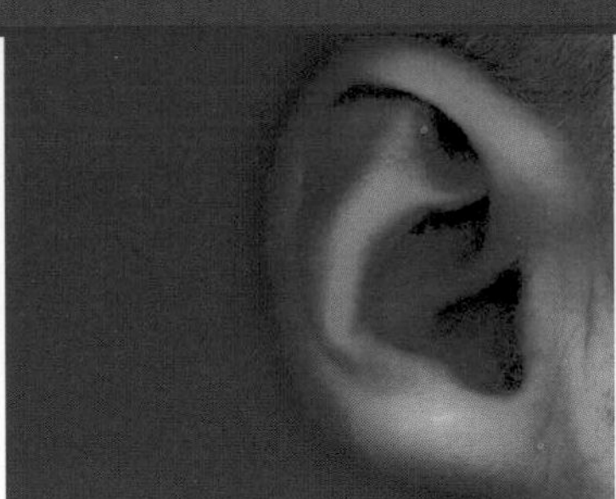

22. Drugs and the Ear

PHYSIOLOGY OF THE EAR

The ear is a sensory organ that detects sound and head position and movement

The outer ear collects sound waves and directs them to the tympanic membrane, which, with the middle ear ossicular chain, amplifies sound vibration and transforms it into fluid shifts within the inner ear (Fig. 22.1). The organ of Corti in the cochlea (Fig. 22.2) contains sensory receptor hair cells (Fig. 22.3), which are set into motion by vibration of the cochlear duct basement membrane. Hair cell motion displaces the hair cell stereocilia projecting from the cell apex. This results in cellular depolarization produced by an inward cation current (Ca^{2+}, Na^{+}) entering the apical end of the hair cell. The hair cell then releases a chemical transmitter from its basal end, leading to stimulation of the afferent bipolar neurons of the auditory nerve and their central connections. Stereocilia deflection in the opposite direction results in hair cell hyperpolarization, which inhibits basal neurotransmitter release and suppresses auditory neuron activity. Stereocilia oscillation therefore produces a train of excitatory and inhibitory impulses within the auditory nerve with the same frequency characteristics as the original sound.

Balance depends on inputs from the vestibular, visual, and proprioceptive sensory systems to the balance centers of the brain. The peripheral vestibular system (Fig. 22.4) consists of:

- The otolithic organs, the utricle, and saccule, which sense linear acceleration.
- The semicircular canals, which sense angular acceleration or rotation.

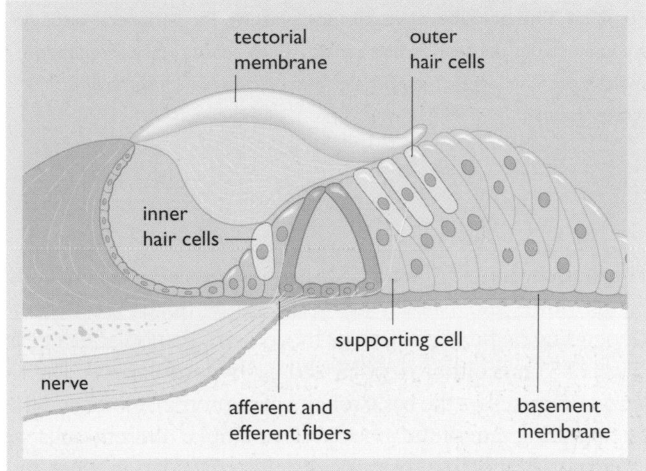

Fig. 22.2 The organ of Corti. Movement of the basement membrane results in shearing between the hair cells (fixed in their supporting cells) and the tectorial membrane.

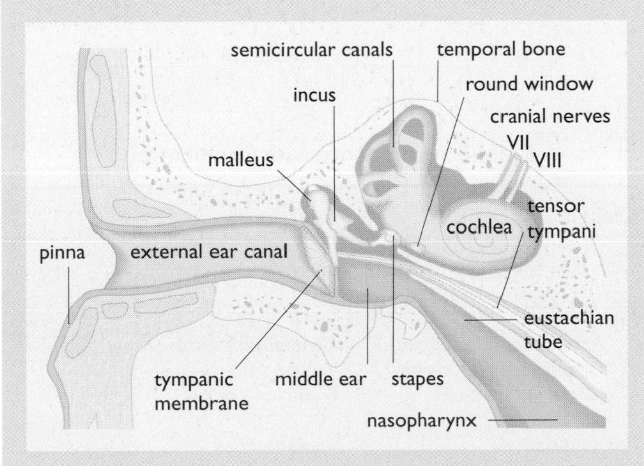

Fig. 22.1 Structure of the ear (transverse section). The ear senses sound as well as head position and motion.

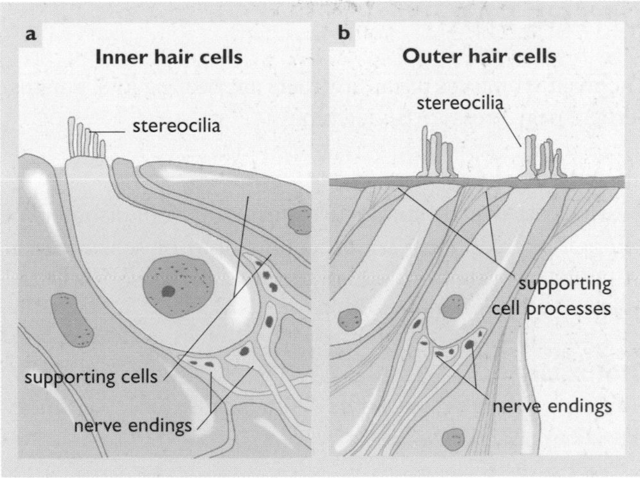

Fig. 22.3 Cochlear hair cells. There are two types of cochlear hair cells: (a) inner hair cells, which synapse with afferent nerve endings, and (b) outer hair cells, which synapse with efferent nerve endings.

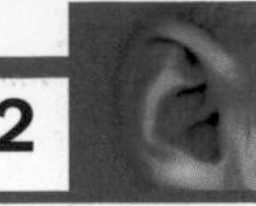

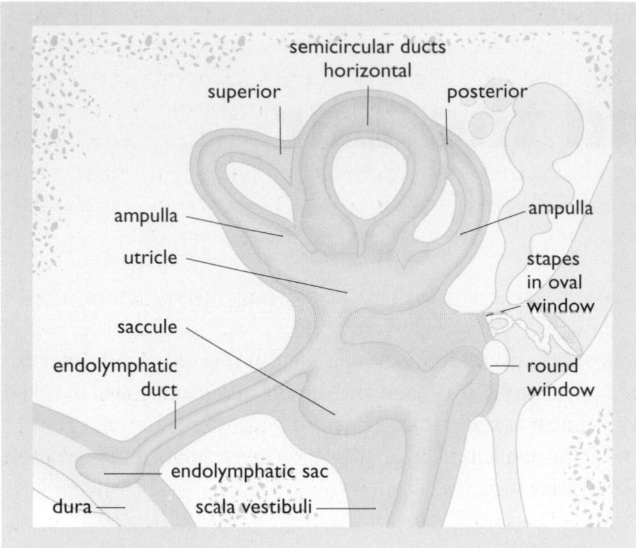

Fig. 22.4 The peripheral vestibular system. The peripheral vestibular system includes the semicircular canals (which sense rotary acceleration) and the otolithic organs, the utricle, and saccule (which sense linear acceleration).

The sensory input from these organs is critical for maintaining equilibrium and stabilizing gaze with head movement. Depending on head position or movement, vestibular hair cells (Fig. 22.5) are either depolarized or hyperpolarized. Depolarization increases the basal release of neurotransmitter and the resting firing rate of the associated vestibular afferent neuron. Hyperpolarization has the opposite effect. Head movement and position are therefore resolved into stimulatory increases or inhibitory decreases of the resting firing rate of the vestibular nerve and its central connections.

PATHOPHYSIOLOGY AND DISEASES OF THE EAR

The main symptoms of ear disorders are hearing loss, tinnitus, vertigo, pain, pressure, and itchiness.

HEARING LOSS

Hearing loss may be conductive (resulting from disorders of external or middle ear sound conduction) or sensorineural (resulting from abnormalities of the inner ear sensory cells and their central connections).

Ototoxicity

Four clinically important classes of drugs cause inner ear toxicity (Fig. 22.6).

Analgesics and antipyretics The mechanism of salicylate ototoxicity is not fully understood. However, salicylates accumulate within extracellular fluid compartments and reduce prostaglandin synthesis within the stria vascularis by inhibiting cyclooxygenase, which catalyzes the first step in prostaglandin synthesis from arachidonic acid. This causes vasoconstriction within the stria vascularis, ischemia, and inhibition of the cochlear nerve action potential.

Salicylate ototoxicity occurs at serum concentrations over 0.35 mg/ml and is reversible within 48–72 hours of salicylate withdrawal.

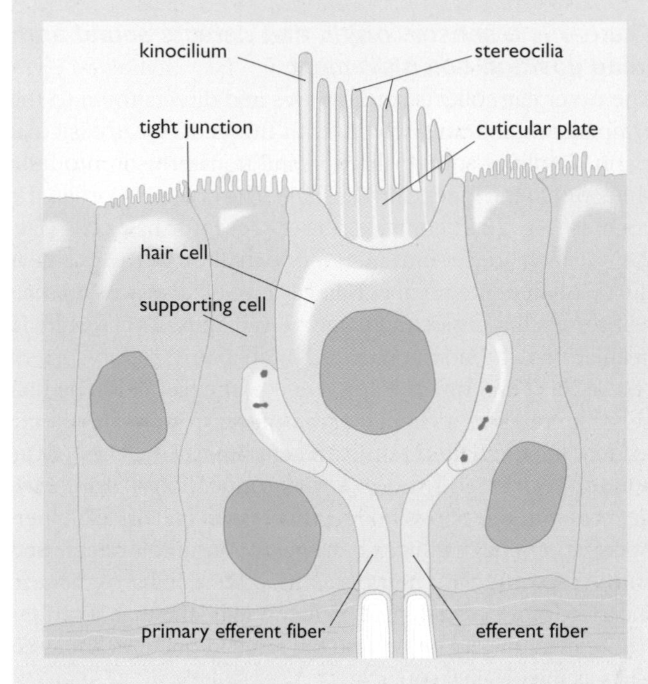

Fig. 22.5 The vestibular hair cells. In addition to having stereocilia, vestibular hair cells have a motile kinocilium. Stereocilial deflection towards the kinocilium results in hair cell depolarization, while deflection away from the kinocilium results in hair cell hyperpolarization.

Classification of ototoxic medications

Class	Examples
Analgesics and antipyretics	Salicylates, quinine
Antimicrobials	
Aminoglycoside antibiotics	Gentamicin, neomycin
Glycopeptide antibiotics	Vancomycin
Macrolide antibiotics	Erythromycin
Antineoplastics	Cisplatinum
Loop diuretics	Furosemide, ethacrynic acid

Fig. 22.6 Classification of ototoxic medications.

Antimicrobials Aminoglycoside antibiotics have adverse effects on the kidney and inner ear: streptomycin and gentamicin are more vestibulotoxic; kanamycin, tobramycin, and amikacin have more effect on cochlear hair cells. The newer aminoglycosides dibekacin* and netilmicin are less ototoxic. Aminoglycosides first bind to the outer surface of the hair cell membrane and disturb Ca^{2+} membrane channels. They then bind to phosphatidylinositol bisphosphate on the inner surface of the cell membrane. Interference with intracellular Ca^{2+} and polyamine-regulated processes causes additional membrane damage, which eventually leads to cell death. Reversible ototoxicity has been observed, but severe untreatable symptoms are common. As patients requiring aminoglycosides often have debilitating medical conditions their early complaints of 'dizziness' and tinnitus may be overlooked. Permanent disabling vestibulotoxicity is only recognized when the mobile patient complains of:

- Movement intolerance.
- Oscillopsia (difficulty in stabilizing gaze during head movement).
- Ataxia.

The best management is to identify patients with an increased risk (Fig. 22.7) and to minimize their exposure by monitoring serum drug concentrations and switching to nonototoxic antibacterials as soon as possible.

Glycopeptide antibiotics such as vancomycin are increasingly used because of the increasing resistance of bacteria to more commonly used antibiotics. Their mechanism of ototoxicity is not clear, but the pattern with outer hair cell loss preceding inner hair cell loss is similar to that seen with aminoglycosides.

High-frequency sensorineural hearing loss, 'blowing' tinnitus, and vertigo can follow large intravenous doses of erythromycin, a macrolide antibiotic, which inhibits bacterial protein synthesis by binding to the 50S ribosomal subunit. Patients with an increased risk include those with hepatic or renal failure or legionnaires' disease, and the elderly. The mechanism of this ototoxicity is unknown, but it is reversible on drug withdrawal.

Factors that increase risk of aminoglycoside ototoxicity
Impaired renal function
Prolonged course of treatment (over 10 days)
Concomitant use of other nephrotoxic or ototoxic drugs (loop diuretics, high-dose erythromycin, vancomycin)
Advanced age
Previous aminoglycoside therapy
Pre-existing sensorineural hearing loss

Fig. 22.7 Factors that increase risk of aminoglycoside ototoxicity.

Antineoplastics Cisplatin's ototoxic effect is probably due to ATPase interaction and inhibition of adenylyl cyclase resulting in labyrinthine hair cell degeneration. It is primarily cochleotoxic, causing degeneration of the outer hair cells, spiral ganglion cells, and cochlear neurons, with relative sparing of the vestibular system. The morphologic changes within the inner ear are similar to those of aminoglycoside ototoxicity. The outer hair cells of the basal turn of the cochlea are the most susceptible.

Loop diuretics (furosemide and ethacrynic acid) inhibit Cl^- reabsorption at the distal loop of Henle and promote extracellular fluid excretion. Within the inner ear they inhibit cell membrane K^+ transport within the stria vascularis and are principally cochleotoxic. Like aminoglycosides, loop diuretics have adverse effects on both the kidney and inner ear, and the toxic effects of these two medications can be synergistic.

There is an increased risk of toxicity if the drug is given too rapidly by bolus injection, or if the patient is elderly or has renal failure. Tinnitus, hearing loss, and vertigo may occur within minutes and can be reversible if the medication is withdrawn immediately.

Otosclerosis

Otosclerosis is characterized by idiopathic circumscribed endochondral otic capsule bone destruction and replacement with vascular bone and then dense lamellar bone. Characteristic sites include the anterior oval window niche, which results in stapes footplate fixation and a conductive hearing loss. Sensorineural hearing loss can result from a focus of otosclerosis adjacent to the endolymphatic space.

Epidemiologic studies indicate a lower incidence of otosclerosis in regions with high fluoride concentrations in drinking water. However, the only widely recognized indication for using fluoride is progressive sensorineural hearing loss with a high risk of otosclerosis on taking the patient's history or upon examination.

Sudden sensorineural hearing loss

Sudden sensorineural hearing loss (SSHL) is usually unilateral, progresses within hours to days, and is associated with tinnitus and, less frequently, vertigo. There are a variety of causes (Fig. 22.8). If a specific cause cannot be identified it is thought to result from a viral infection, vascular disorder, or inner ear membrane rupture.

SSHL is a medical emergency and, if specific etiologies have been excluded, many clinicians recommend a moderate course of glucocorticosteroids tapered over 10 days to 2 weeks, although they have no proven benefit. The best treatment responses occur in patients with moderate hearing losses who start glucocorticosteroids within 10 days. Treatment is not required for mild hearing loss, which routinely recovers spontaneously, and there is no proven benefit for severe hearing loss. Other agents used to treat SSHL include vasodilators, plasma expanders, and carbogen (5% CO_2, 95% O_2), but there is no convincing evidence that these are effective.

Autoimmune hearing loss

Autoimmune sensorineural hearing loss typically affects young adults, is slowly progressive over months, and is not

Conditions causing sudden sensorineural hearing loss	
Classification	**Example**
Congenital	Mondini's deformity
Acquired	
Physical factors	Barotrauma, electrical, concussion, temporal bone fracture, perilymph fistula
Chemical factors	
Metabolic	Diabetes mellitus, hyperlipidemia, hypothyroidism (Pendred's syndrome)
Ototoxic medications	Anti-inflammatory drugs, antibiotics, antineoplastics, loop diuretics
Infections and inflammation	Viral infection (measles, mumps, herpes zoster), bacterial infection (syphilis, mycoplasma, meningitis), chronic granulomatous disease (sarcoidosis)
Vascular	Vasculopathies, coagulopathies, emboli, migraine
Immunologic	Cogan's syndrome
Neoplastic	Acoustic neuroma, carcinoma
Idiopathic	Multiple sclerosis

Fig. 22.8 Conditions causing sudden sensorineural hearing loss.

accompanied by other systemic disease or hereditary defects. It appears to be due to an autoimmune reaction to a specific inner ear antigen. There is no vertigo, but more severe disease causes ataxia in dim light.

Treatment depends on the severity of the hearing loss, likelihood of autoimmune dysfunction, and the patient's general medical condition. For more severe and bilateral cases, prednisone for 2–4 weeks is the treatment of choice. A second immunosuppressive agent may be needed if:

- There is a good response and hearing recovers but the patient becomes chronically dependent on glucocorticosteroids to maintain hearing.
- There is a strong suspicion that autoimmunity is the cause. Cyclophosphamide, methotrexate, or penicillamine, can be effective, but the patient must be closely monitored for adverse effects.

TINNITUS

Tinnitus is the perception of sound in the absence of an external source. It may be:

- Objective and result from sounds generated within the body, which are audible to an observer.
- Subjective and characterized by an auditory sensation in the absence of a physical sound.

Causes include musculoskeletal and vascular sounds producing objective tinnitus, and disorders of the peripheral and central auditory systems, which usually produce subjective tinnitus. The cause may be known (e.g. noise-induced, presbycusis). Most patients also have an irreversible high-frequency sensorineural hearing loss.

Once an underlying disease has been excluded, the goal is to relieve the annoyance that tinnitus causes. If it is mild, patients may simply need information about its cause and benign nature. Masking (the use of environmental sound to 'cover over' the subjective sound), medication, and behavioral modification, may be needed for intractable tinnitus. Medications include:

- Local anesthetics (procaine, lidocaine).
- Benzodiazepines (diazepam, alprazolam, clonazepam).
- Baclofen.
- Tricyclic antidepressants (amitriptyline).
- Ca^{2+} antagonists.

The mechanism of local anesthetic control of tinnitus probably involves neuron plasma membrane Na^+ channel blockade, and the principal site is probably central at the level of the cochlear nerve and its brainstem connections. Lidocaine has dramatically suppressed tinnitus in some patients, but must be given intravenously. Tocainide is similar and can be given orally, but has intolerable adverse effects. Other 'membrane-stabilizing' agents such as carbamazepine, phenytoin, valproic acid, and amobarbital are not effective.

Benzodiazepines improve the patient's emotional response to tinnitus, but are also thought to suppress tinnitus directly. In some patients this may be due to insufficient inhibitory activity in the ascending auditory system. Benzodiazepines may act by enhancing the activity of the inhibitory neurotransmitter γ-aminobutyric acid (GABA).

Other medications used with varying success for tinnitus include Ca^{2+} antagonists and tricyclic antidepressants.

 **Anti-tinnitus drugs**

- Tocainide is the only local anesthetic that can be given orally, but can have serious adverse effects on the heart
- Benzodiazepines should be used sparingly because they can be habituating
- Tricyclic antidepressants have antimuscarinic and cardiac adverse effects (see Chapter 7)

VERTIGO

Vertigo is the hallucinatory perception of movement and can result from disorders of the peripheral or central vestibular systems. Peripherally induced vertigo is usually the more severe and associated with other aural symptoms such as hearing loss or tinnitus. It is produced by either:

- Transient fluctuations in vestibular neuron activity such as Ménière's disease and recurrent vestibulopathy.
- Constant, often permanent, hypofunction of the affected labyrinth, for example acute vestibular neuronitis, suppurative labyrinthitis, and vestibular trauma.

Centrally induced vertigo may be associated with signs of brainstem or cerebellar pathology.

Medical treatment of vertigo is aimed at stabilizing pathologic fluctuations in peripheral vestibular function and promoting central compensation if there is a permanent decrease in vestibular function.

Ménière's disease and recurrent vestibulopathy

Ménière's disease is a peripheral vestibular disorder associated with intermittent overaccumulation of endolymphatic fluid (endolymphatic hydrops). It causes episodes of severe rotary vertigo that continue for hours, hearing loss, tinnitus, and a pressure sensation in the ear. Initially these symptoms occur in 'attacks,' but eventually the condition 'burns out,' leaving the patient with a stable severe sensorineural hearing loss and a permanent, usually well-compensated, decrease in peripheral vestibular function.

Ménière's disease is managed with medication, diets to restrict Na^+ intake and prevent hydrops, and physical therapy to adapt to the loss of vestibular function. Medications include:

- Diuretics (hydrochlorothiazide, furosemide) to limit endolymphatic fluid accumulation.
- Vestibular suppressants (sedatives, antihistamines, anticholinergics, narcotics).
- Vasodilators.
- Aminoglycosides to ablate peripheral vestibular function.

Hydrochlorothiazide (with K^+ replacement) prevents recurrent vertigo in many patients, while the antihistamine meclizine moderates acute attacks, mainly through its anticholinergic effect. If an attack becomes severe, a benzodiazepine such as diazepam or lorazepam not only provides sedation but also acts directly on the medial and lateral vestibular nuclei to suppress otolithic and semicircular canal activity. More specific anticholinergic medications such as scopolamine have limited use because of their adverse effects. Some parenteral narcotics (e.g. fentanyl, droperidol) are potent vestibular suppressants and are occasionally needed for an acute incapacitating attack.

Drugs for Ménière's disease

- Hydrochlorothiazide reduces endolymph production
- Meclizine has anticholinergic effects
- Benzodiazepines are both vestibular suppressants and cerebral sedatives
- Aminoglycosides induce a stable decrease in vestibular function

Chemical ablation of vestibular function may be indicated for recurrent incapacitating vertigo not controlled by the above medications if the patient would find it easier to cope with a permanent medically induced loss of vestibular function. Streptomycin can be given parenterally for active disease in both ears, and is carefully titrated to a point of symptom control, but all peripheral vestibular function must not be ablated as this can cause incapacitating oscillopsia and ataxia. For unilateral Ménière's disease, gentamicin is injected into the middle ear, from where it is actively transported across the round window into the labyrinthine fluids. Here, it probably acts on dark cells (thought to be important in the production of endolymph) and has a toxic effect on the vestibular hair cells. Most patients adapt well after unilateral destruction of vestibular function and have no further disabling spells of vertigo.

 **Drugs used to treat Meniere's disease**

- Diuretic therapy can cause K^+ depletion, hyperglycemia, and hyperlipidemia, and exacerbate gout
- Severe permanent ataxia and oscillopsia can follow streptomycin treatment of bilateral Meniere's disease if it produces a total loss of vestibular function
- Intratympanic gentamicin treatment is associated with a 10–20% incidence of hearing loss

Recurrent vestibulopathy, also known as vestibular Ménière's disease, presents with similar recurrent vertigo, but with no auditory symptoms. The vertigo is typically more benign than that of Ménière's disease and is usually controlled with similar medication.

Vestibular neuronitis and vestibular trauma

Vestibular neuronitis results in an acute decrease in vestibular function, which may be mild and reversible or profound and permanent. It is probably caused by a virus. Vestibular trauma can have a similar range of severity, depending upon whether there has been slight concussion, total destruction of the vestibular structures, or division of the vestibular nerve.

Central adaptation must begin during the first month after onset. Patients must remain active, as forced inactivity may predispose to incomplete adaptation and permanent ataxia. Antinauseants such as dimenhydrinate may be needed for severe nausea, and the vestibular suppressants used for acute Ménière's disease can be used sparingly. No medication specifically promotes central adaptation.

FACIAL NERVE PALSY

Bell's palsy is acute unilateral facial weakness or paralysis without an identifiable cause, though herpes simplex virus type I has been implicated. Herpes zoster oticus (HZO) is acute facial paralysis with pain and varicelliform lesions, which often involve the conchal bowl. It is probably due to varicella-zoster virus infection of the geniculate ganglion and often there is eighth cranial nerve involvement, producing a profound sensorineural hearing loss and vestibular loss. Edema traps the facial nerve as it passes through the narrow fallopian canal, resulting in ischemia and neural dysfunction.

The use of glucocorticosteroids to treat acute facial paralysis is controversial. They are not indicated for incomplete facial paralysis, as this usually recovers fully without medication. If used for complete facial paralysis in Bell's palsy or HZO, they should be given within the first 10 days at a moderate dose, which is then tapered.

Acyclovir (acycloguanosine), a nucleoside analog that inhibits viral DNA replication (see Chapter 24), reduces functional deficits in immunocompromised patients with HZO, but has no proven benefit for Bell's palsy. It must be given intravenously within 72 hours of onset.

EAR INFECTIONS

Ear infections may involve the outer ear (otitis externa), middle ear (otitis media), or inner ear (labyrinthitis).

Otitis externa

Otitis externa is a bacterial or fungal infection of the soft tissue of the external ear canal. Common bacterial causes include *Pseudomonas aeruginosa, Proteus mirabilis*, staphylococci, streptococci, and various Gram-negative bacteria. *Candida* and *Aspergillus* species are the most common fungal causes. Most pathogens are inhibited by an acidic medium, and a solution of equal parts of vinegar and isopropyl alcohol prevents otitis externa. All infected debris and pus must be removed from the ear before starting any medication. Moisture should be avoided.

Treatment of otitis externa

- The external ear must be thoroughly cleaned before starting antibiotic therapy
- A combination ear drop is first-line therapy
- Severe infections may require parenteral antibiotics and narcotic analgesics

First-line medical therapy includes topical preparations combining an antibiotic and glucocorticosteroid, such as neomycin with polymyxin and hydrocortisone. Polysorbate may be included as an antifungal. Dicloxacillin, cephalexin, trimethoprim–sulfamethoxazole, or ciprofloxacin are given orally for progressive cellulitis of the external ear canal, while intravenous cefazolin, dicloxacillin, or ciprofloxacin may be needed for severe cases. A prolonged course of combination antipseudomonal therapy is required for invasive skull base osteitis, preferably aztreonam with clindamycin or a combination of ciprofloxacin with one of the following: ticarcillin, piperacillin, ceftazidime, imipenem, gentamicin, tobramycin, or amikacin (Fig. 22.9).

Otitis media

Acute purulent otitis media is a bacterial infection of the middle ear. The usual pathogens are *Streptococcus pneumoniae, Haemophilus influenzae,* and *Moraxella catarrhalis.*

Drugs used to treat otitis media

- Frequent use of antibiotics in young children can cause gastrointestinal upset and thrush
- Aminoglycoside-containing ear drops can be ototoxic in the presence of a tympanic membrane perforation and a normal middle ear mucosa
- Potentially ototoxic ear drops should be used sparingly, even in the presence of middle ear inflammation
- Repeated use of antibacterial ear drops predisposes to secondary fungal infection

First-line therapy should include amoxicillin or erythromycin plus a sulfonamide or trimethoprim–sulfamethoxazole. Second-line therapy is directed at a possible β lactamase-producing organism and may include amoxicillin–clavulanate, cefaclor, cefuroxime, cefixime, or clarithromycin (Fig. 22.10).

Treatment of otitis externa

Infection	*Pseudomonas aeruginosa, Proteus mirabilis, Staphylococcus aureus*		
	First-line: mild	**Second-line: moderate**	**Third-line: severe**
	Polymyxin/neomycin/ hydrocortisone otic solution	Dicloxacillin (po), cephalexin, ciprofloxacin	Cefazolin (iv), dicloxacillin, ciprofloxacillin

Fig. 22.9 Treatment of otitis externa. (iv, intravenous; po, oral)

Treatment of acute purulent otitis media		
Infection	*Streptococcus pneumoniœ, Hemophilus influenzae, Moraxella catarrhalis*	
First-line: po	**Second-line: po**	**Third-line: iv**
Amoxicillin, erythromycin with sulfonamide, trimethoprim–sulfamethoxazole	Amoxicillin–clavulanate, cefaclor, cefuroxime, cefixime, clarithromycin	Ampicillin/sulbactam

Fig. 22.10 Treatment of acute purulent otitis media. (iv, intravenous; po, oral)

Otitis media with an effusion is the presence of (usually sterile) fluid in the middle ear and may follow acute otitis media or occur independently. It usually clears spontaneously but, if not, a one-month course of amoxicillin or trimethoprim–sulfamethoxazole can promote fluid clearance.

Chronic otitis media is defined by the presence of a perforated tympanic membrane in the presence of middle ear infection. Bacteria that cause active infection in the presence of a perforation include *P. aeruginosa, Proteus* spp., staphylococci, Gram-negative organisms, and anaerobes (*Klebsiella* spp., *E. coli, B. fragilis*). Treatment includes ear drops with neomycin and polymyxin and an oral agent such as trimethoprim–sulfamethoxazole or cephalexin, though amoxicillin–clavulanate or ciprofloxacin with metronidazole may be required. If pseudomonas is the cause of persistent otorrhea, combining two different ear drops, one containing ciprofloxacin and the other an aminoglycoside (gentamicin, tobramycin) may be effective. Aminoglycosides can cause ototoxicity when applied to the middle ear, but this is rare in the presence of active infection.

Suppurative labyrinthitis

Bacterial infection of the spaces of the inner ear causes profound cochlear and vestibular destruction and loss of both hearing and vestibular function in the affected ear. Intralabyrinthine infection results from:

- Spread of otitis media via the round or oval windows.
- A labyrinthine fistula.
- Lateral extension of meningitis through the cochlear aqueduct and cribriform plate at the lateral end of the internal auditory canal.

If infection is due to otitis media, treatment includes surgical drainage and intravenous antibiotics (ceftriaxone for acute otitis media, nafcillin with ceftazidime plus metronidazole for chronic otitis media). If infection is due to meningitis, the appropriate intravenous antibiotic (see Chapter 23) should be given. Whether concurrent intravenous glucocorticosteroids reduce the incidence of post-meningitis hearing loss is controversial.

FURTHER READING

Alberti P, Ruben R. (eds) *Otologic Medicine and Surgery.* New York: Churchill Livingstone; 1988. [A comprehensive text with thoughtful reviews of many otologic topics.]

Fairbanks D. *Pocket Guide to Antimicrobial Therapy in Otolaryngology—Head and Neck Surgery, 7e.* Alexandria, VA: The Americal Academy of Otolaryngology—Head and Neck Surgery Foundation, Inc.; 1993. [A handy quick reference.]

Jackler R, Brackman D. (eds) *Neurotology.* St. Louis: Mosby; 1994. [A recent text with excellent basic science and thorough clinical reviews.]

Make a provisional diagnosis and determine a rational pharmacologic treatment for the following hypothetical case.

A 60-year-old man complains of left ear drainage and hearing loss. He has a long history of ear infection dating back to childhood and his ear often drains especially if he gets it wet. On examination there is purulent mucus in the ear canal and a large perforation of the eardrum. The middle ear mucosa is red and edematous. His tuning fork tests indicate a conductive hearing loss on this side.

1. Would you syringe the ear to remove the debris and tell the man to rinse it with an alcohol and vinegar solution? Explain your answer.
2. Would you prescribe an oral antibiotic alone? Explain your answer.
3. Would you prescribe a topical antibiotic? Explain your answer. Which antibiotic would you use if you did decide to prescribe one?
4. Would you take an ear swab for culture and sensitivity and while waiting for the result prescribe a topical antibiotic in combination with an oral antibiotic?
5. Two days after starting antibiotic therapy, culture and sensitivity of an ear swab reveals infection with *Pseudomonas aeruginosa* and an anaerobe. If these bacteria are not sensitive to the antibiotic therapy you have chosen, would you recall the patient to change the antibiotic, or review the patient in ten days and if the drainage persists then change the antibiotic? Explain your answer. Which antibiotic therapy would you use if you decide to change the antibiotic?

Indicate which is the correct answer for each question.

1. Each of the following medications is ototoxic, except
- a) hydrochlorothiazide
- b) tobramycin
- c) quinine
- d) cisplatin
- e) furosemide

2. A course of glucocorticosteroids is of proven benefit in the treatment of idiopathic sudden sensorineural hearing loss
- a) true
- b) false

3. Pharmacologic treatment of vertigo
- a) aims to produce transient fluctuations in vestibular neuron activity
- b) might intentionally destroy residual vestibular function
- c) can promote central adaptation following loss of peripheral vestibular function
- d) a) and c)
- e) b) and c)

4. Treatment of Bell's palsy
- a) should begin within 20 days of onset of complete facial paralysis
- b) should begin within ten days of onset of partial facial paralysis
- c) may include a combination of glucocorticosteroid and acycloguanosine
- d) b) and c)
- e) none of the above

5. Acute suppurative otitis media
- a) is often due to *Streptococcus pneumoniae* or *Staphylococcus aureus*
- b) can be caused by β lactamase producing organisms
- c) should be treated instantly with a β lactamase resistant antibiotic
- d) b) and c)

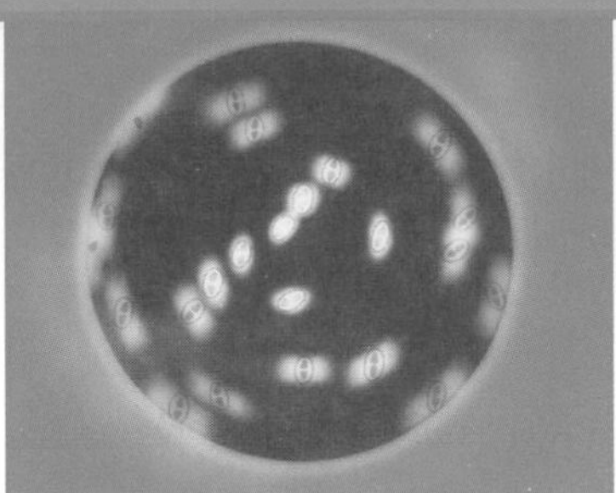

23. Bacterial Infections

Bacterial infections are exceedingly common and cause substantial morbidity and mortality. Bacterial diarrhea is a leading cause of infant mortality worldwide, and tuberculosis a very frequent cause of death due to infections.

Antibacterial drugs are among the most important therapeutic discoveries of the twentieth century and have dramatically changed the course of many illnesses, reducing mortality (e.g. of bacterial meningitis and bacterial endocarditis) and morbidity. On the other hand, antibiotics are now among the most overprescribed agents, partly because many of them have excellent safety profiles. As a result, overuse of antibiotics is a significant contributing factor to the growing international problem of antibiotic resistance by a variety of bacteria.

In practice, the term antibiotic has become synonymous with antibacterial agent

Strictly speaking, antibacterial drugs are classified as antibiotics, chemotherapeutic or synthetic agents, and semisynthetic agents, depending on whether they are:

- Byproducts of microorganisms (antibiotics).
- Entirely synthesized in the laboratory (chemotherapeutic or synthetic agents).
- A hybrid of the two (semisynthetic agents).

In practice, the term antibiotic has become synonymous with antibacterial agent, and this more liberal definition of antibiotic will be used throughout this chapter.

MECHANISM OF ACTION

The ideal antibiotic interferes with a vital function of bacteria without affecting host cells

Antibiotics are said to possess selective toxicity because they interfere with a vital function of bacteria without affecting host cells. In devising antibiotics, scientists attempt to identify functions that are specific for the bacterium as potential targets. For example, bacteria possess cell walls, whereas mammalian cells do not. Accordingly, drugs that interfere with the production of the bacterial cell wall are toxic to bacteria, but harmless to the host. Similarly, the bacterial ribosome (70S) is sufficiently different from eukaryotic ribosomes (80S) that sites on the bacterial ribosome are good targets for antibacterial drugs. Figure 23.1 shows the sites of action of the major types of antibiotics. Because of their selective toxicity, many antibiotics have a high therapeutic index (i.e. ratio of toxic dose to therapeutic dose).

Whether an antibiotic inhibits or kills bacteria depends on its concentration

The activity of a given antibiotic against a given bacterium can be readily measured in the laboratory. By exposing a standard inoculum of a bacterium to a range of concentrations of an antibiotic, the lowest concentration of the drug that inhibits bacterial growth can be determined. This is called the minimum

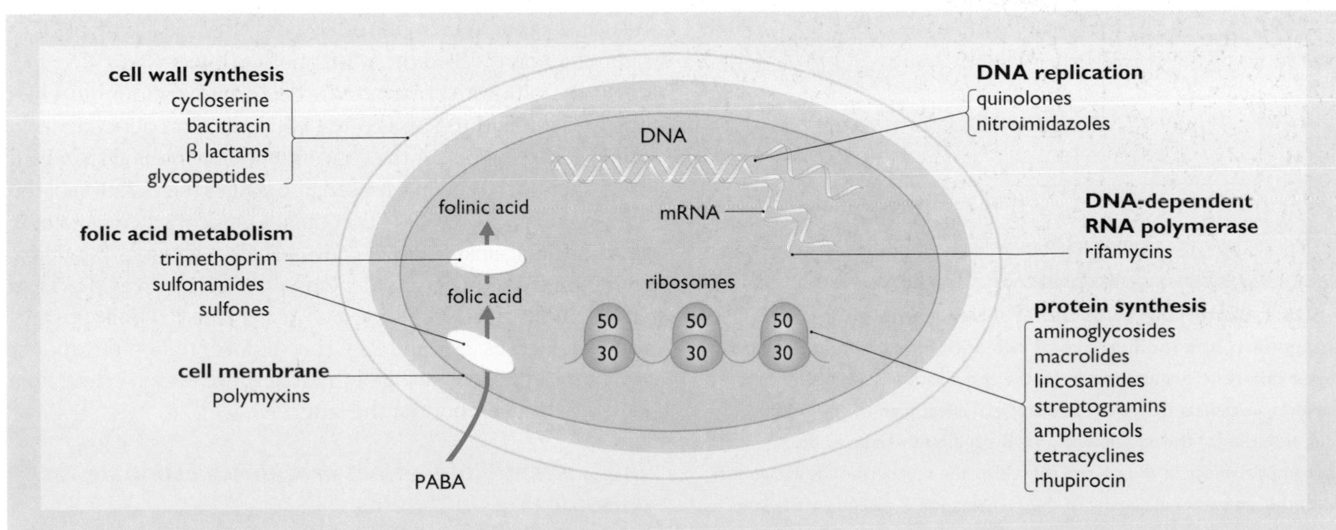

Fig. 23.1 Sites of action of different types of antibiotic agent. (PABA, *para*-aminobenzoic acid)

inhibitory concentration (MIC). As the concentration of antibiotic is increased above the MIC, a concentration is eventually reached that will actually kill the bacterium (technically a 3 $\log_{10}$-fold or 99.9% reduction in the inoculum). The lowest concentration of antibiotic required to kill the bacterium is known as the minimum bactericidal concentration (MBC). Often, the MBC is 2–8 times that of the MIC.

Antibiotics for which achievable blood concentrations regularly exceed the MBC of common pathogens are classified as bactericidal antibiotics, whereas antibiotics whose blood concentrations readily exceed the MIC but do not usually exceed the MBC are classified as bacteriostatic antibiotics. However, categorizing antibiotics as predominantly bacteriostatic or bactericidal is imperfect since there is a unique relationship between each bacterium and each antibiotic. For instance, penicillin, which is classically considered a bactericidal antibiotic, is nearly always bactericidal against streptococci, but is bacteriostatic against enterococci. Similarly, chloramphenicol, which is classically considered bacteriostatic, is bacteriostatic against most Enterobacteriaceae, but is bactericidal against most strains of *Haemophilus influenzae*.

Antibiotics may act together synergistically, antagonistically, or indifferently

Occasionally, two or more antibiotics are used together against the same pathogen. In the laboratory it is possible to categorize the relationship between two or more antibiotics against one bacterium as synergistic, antagonistic, or indifferent, depending on the effect of the drug combination on the growth of the bacterium compared with that of each drug alone (Fig. 23.2):

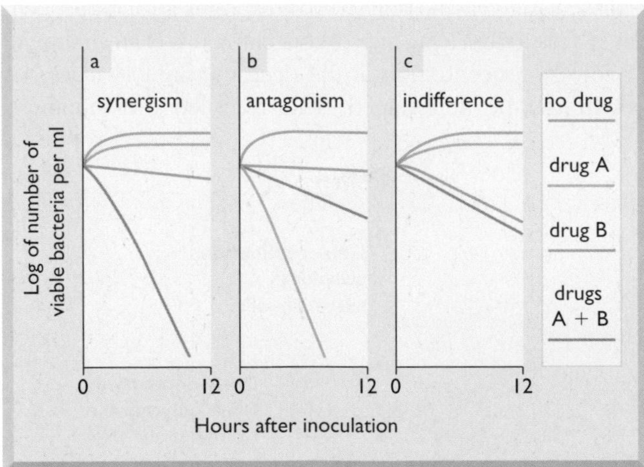

Fig. 23.2 Bacterial growth curves showing synergism, antagonism, and indifference of two antibiotics, A and B, against three different organisms. In (a) the combination is synergistic because it exerts a significantly greater antibacterial effect than the more active drug alone. In (b) the addition of drug B significantly reduces the antibacterial effect of drug A and therefore, the combination is antagonistic. In (c) the antibacterial activity of the combination is essentially the same as that of the more active drug, and the combination is therefore classified as indifferent.

- If the combination of drugs markedly increases the antibacterial effect above that of the most active drug, the combination is synergistic.
- If the combination results in less inhibition of bacterial growth than the most active agent alone, the combination is antagonistic.
- If the combination is neither synergistic nor antagonistic, it is indifferent.

In practice, most combinations are indifferent.

The clinical relevance of *in vitro* synergism and antagonism is generally unknown. However, both important synergistic and antagonistic combinations have been demonstrated clinically.

- The success rate of treating enterococcal endocarditis with a combination of penicillin plus aminoglycoside is significantly greater than that using penicillin alone, highlighting the relevance of synergy.
- The combination of penicillin and tetracycline for treating bacterial meningitis is associated with significantly higher mortality than when using penicillin alone, and is an example of antagonism *in vivo*.

Killing by bactericidal drugs can be concentration dependent or time dependent

Killing of bacteria by some bactericidal drugs (e.g. aminoglycosides and fluoroquinolones) is concentration dependent, whereas that by others (e.g. β lactams and glycopeptides) is time dependent. Concentration-dependent killing implies a greater bactericidal activity with higher concentrations of antibiotic. With time-dependent killing, there is little or no enhancement of bactericidal activity with drug concentrations above the MBC; rather, the killing depends on maintaining the concentration of antibiotic above the MBC for as much of the dosing interval as possible.

Normal bacterial replication is often delayed after an antibiotic has been stopped

When bacteria are exposed to an antibiotic at concentrations above the MIC and the antibiotic is then removed from the medium, bacterial replication often does not resume normally (as if no antibiotic were present) for a variable period of time (usually measured in hours) after removal of the antibiotic. This phenomenon is called the postantibiotic effect (PAE). The PAE does not occur with all bacterium–drug combinations but when it is present its duration is often concentration dependent. In other words, the higher the concentration of antibiotic to which the bacterium has been exposed, the longer the duration of the PAE. Aminoglycosides and fluoroquinolones consistently demonstrate a PAE against Gram-negative bacteria, whereas β lactams, with the exception of carbapenems, do not. However, β lactams do demonstrate a modest PAE against Gram-positive bacteria. Figures 23.3 and 23.4 show concentration-dependent and time-dependent killing of Gram-negative bacteria illustrating PAE in the former but not the latter.

The postantibiotic effect provides a rationale for pulse dosing antibiotics

Pulse dosing refers to the administration of relatively large doses of antibiotic to produce peak blood concentrations far higher than the MIC or MBC of the causative organism at dosing intervals longer than several serum half-lives of the drug. For example, crystalline penicillin G has a serum half-life of about 30 minutes and yet it is usually administered every 6 hours (i.e. every 12 half-lives). This dosing schedule is markedly different to that used with most other drugs (e.g. anticonvulsants), which are generally given no less frequently than every serum half-life. There are a variety of reasons why pulse dosing is effective with antibiotics.

- The therapeutic index of most antibiotics is high and it is often possible to achieve high peak serum concentrations without significant toxicity.
- Some antibiotics demonstrate concentration-dependent killing and therefore it is desirable and more efficacious to achieve high peak serum concentrations.
- It is often possible to maintain the serum antibiotic concentration above the MIC of the pathogen for the entire dosing interval, despite dosing relatively infrequently relative to the serum half-life (Fig. 23.5).
- Even if the serum antibiotic concentration does fall below the MIC for part of the dosing interval, the PAE may prevent bacterial multiplication during the brief time when the serum antibiotic concentration falls below the MIC before the next antibiotic dose (Fig. 23.6).
- Except for very immunocompromised patients, antibiotics are not the only defense against bacterial infection. The host immune system plays an active role in combatting the infection. Indeed, before the antibiotic era many people did survive bacterial infections, although their recovery was generally slower and associated with more complications than with antibiotic treatment.

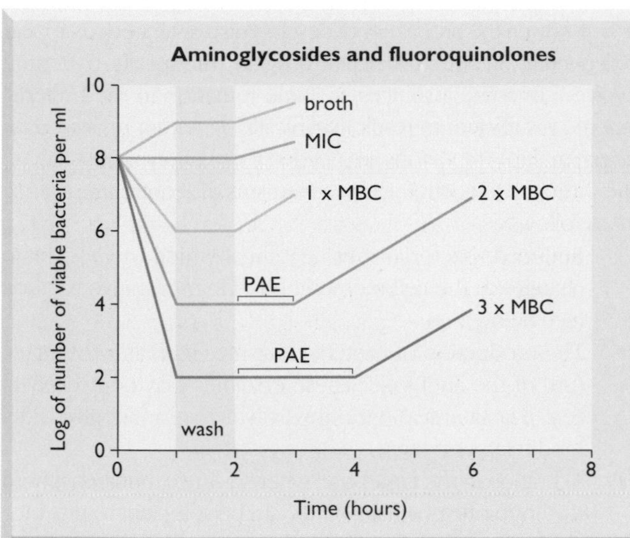

Fig. 23.3 Concentration-dependent bactericidal action and the postantibiotic effect (PAE). Time–kill study in broth containing various concentrations of an antimicrobial agent that shows concentration-dependent bactericidal action. A PAE on the residual organisms is present after washing these organisms and resuspending them in antibiotic-free broth. (MBC, minimum bactericidal concentration; MIC, minimum inhibitory concentration)

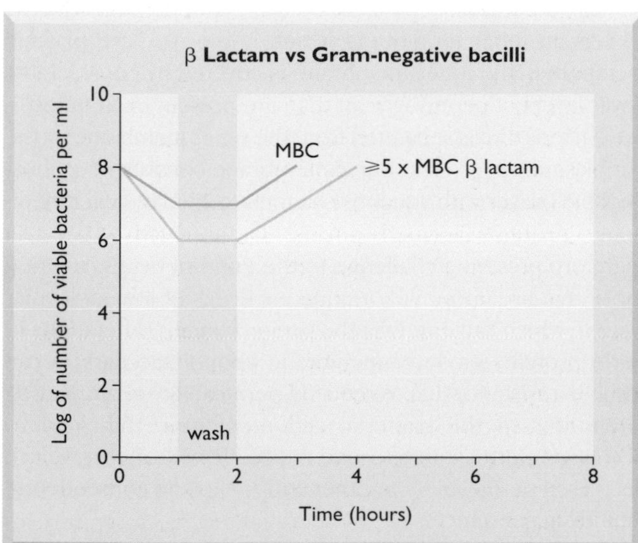

Fig. 23.4 Time-dependent bactericidal action. Time–kill study in broth containing various concentrations of a β lactam that shows time-dependent bactericidal action against a Gram-negative bacillus. There is no postantibiotic effect (PAE) on the residual organisms after washing and resuspending in antibiotic-free broth. (MBC, minimum bactericidal concentration)

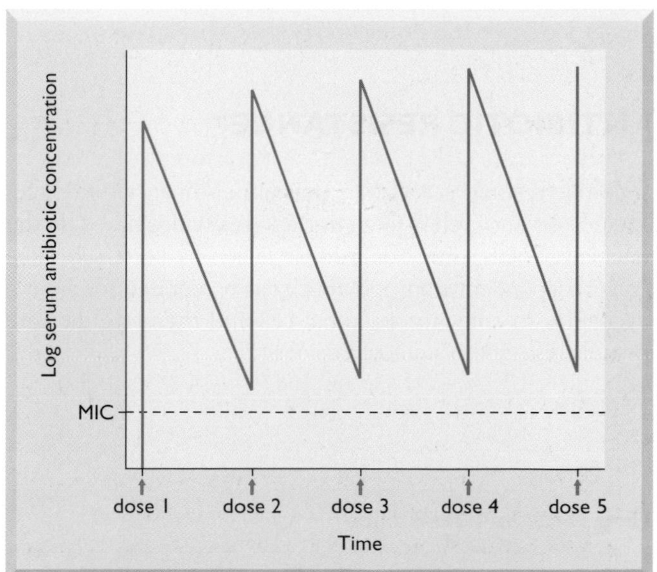

Fig. 23.5 Pulse dosing of an antibiotic. In this example, the antibiotic is very active against the pathogen and the serum antibiotic concentration remains above the minimum inhibitory concentration (MIC) at all times, despite infrequent dosing. Maintaining the serum antibiotic concentration above the MIC at all times is desirable if there is no postantibiotic effect (PAE).

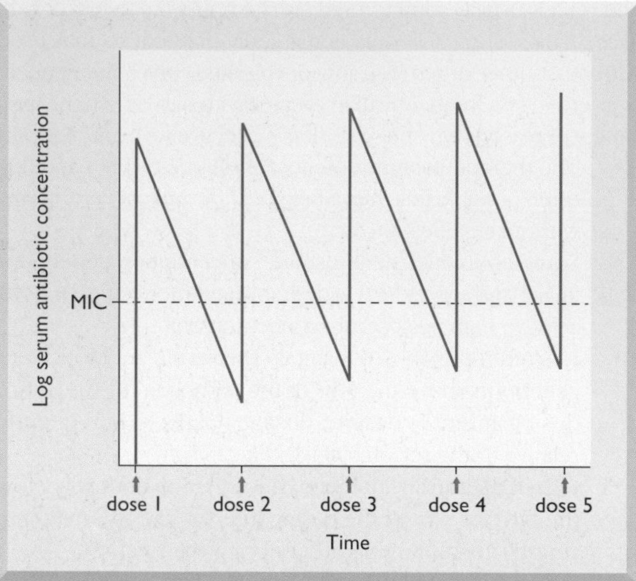

Fig. 23.6 Pulse dosing of an antibiotic. In this example, the peak serum antibiotic concentration following each dose is well above the minimum inhibitory concentration (MIC), but the serum antibiotic concentration falls below the MIC for the latter part of each dosing interval. If there is a postantibiotic effect (PAE), there is no harm in allowing the serum antibiotic concentration to fall below the MIC for a small proportion of the dosing interval.

ANTIBIOTIC SPECTRUM OF ACTIVITY

An antibiotic may have a broad or narrow spectrum of activity. Antibiotics that are active against many bacterial species are referred to as broad-spectrum antibiotics, whereas those that are active against only a few species are termed narrow-spectrum agents. However, this distinction is somewhat arbitrary.

ANTIBIOTIC RESISTANCE

Antibiotic resistance is classified as either innate or acquired. Innate resistance refers to an intrinsic resistance based on the mechanism of the drug. For example, anaerobic bacteria lack the oxygen-dependent transport mechanism required for aminoglycosides to enter the bacterial cell and therefore they are innately resistant to aminoglycosides.

> **Antibiotic resistance**
>
> - Antibiotic use is the major factor leading to antibiotic resistance
> - The three main mechanisms of antibiotic resistance are reduced bacterial permeability, enzymatic alteration of antibiotics, and altered target site

Acquired resistance refers to the acquisition of a resistance gene in a bacterium that is not innately resistant to a particular antibiotic. There is no antibiotic against which acquired resistance has not developed, at least in some bacterial species.

The major stimulus for the development of acquired antibiotic resistance is the use of the antibiotics themselves, as such use exerts selective pressure on the bacteria to develop resistance to survive. However, the probability of developing resistance does appear to depend upon both the specific drug and the specific bacterium involved. In some instances, a single mutation in the bacterial genome is sufficient to result in clinically significant resistance. In others, multiple mutations are needed for phenotypic resistance. The three main biochemical mechanisms of acquired resistance are as follows:

- Reduced bacterial permeability, which results from changes in the cell membrane of Gram-negative bacteria (see below).
- The production of bacterial enzymes that alter the structure of the antibiotic. These enzymes may be hydrolytic (e.g. β lactamases) or nonhydrolytic (e.g. aminoglycoside-modifying enzymes).
- Alteration in the target site, where a single mutation where the antibiotic normally binds can be sufficient to produce clinically significant drug resistance (e.g. methicillin-resistant staphylococci).

REDUCED BACTERIAL PERMEABILITY

There are significant differences between the structure of the cell wall and membrane of Gram-positive and Gram-negative bacteria (Fig. 23.7). Gram-positive bacteria contain many layers of peptidoglycan beneath which lies the cell membrane, and there is no appreciable barrier to the entry of antibiotics. In contrast, Gram-negative bacteria possess an outer membrane that contains copious amounts of lipopolysaccharide, as well as an inner membrane which is the true cytoplasmic membrane. The inner membrane is covered by considerably fewer layers of peptidoglycan than are present in Gram-positive bacteria and is separated from the outer membrane by the periplasmic space. The outer membrane consists of a phospholipid bilayer with aqueous channels formed by outer membrane proteins termed porins. Gram-negative bacteria therefore present a challenge to the entry of drugs, favoring those that are lipophilic or aqueous drugs of low molecular weight, which can enter via the porin channels. Alterations in porin proteins or outer membrane lipopolysaccharides can result in resistance due to reduced permeability to antibiotics. Alterations in the bacterial cell membrane that lead to decreased permeability to one antibiotic will often result in decreased permeability to other antibiotics and consequently, multidrug resistance.

SELECTING ANTIBIOTIC THERAPY

Antibiotics can be used either prophylactically or therapeutically. In either case, the same basic principles apply. Bacterial, host, and drug factors must all be considered (Figs 23.8, 23.9).

BACTERIAL FACTORS

Antibacterial therapy is effective only for bacterial infections. It is therefore important to restrict the use of antibiotics to those situations where bacterial infection is either known to be present or is highly probable. The all-too-common practice of prescribing antibiotics for infections that are probably viral is to be discouraged because it is ineffective, unnecessarily costly, generates unnecessary adverse effects, and contributes to global antibiotic resistance.

Once a bacterial infection is confirmed or is suspected, it is important to find out what the infecting organism(s) is in order to make a rational antibiotic choice. If the identity of the infecting organism(s) is not known, as is often the case when antibiotic therapy is started, it is usually possible to make a reasonable guess about the likely pathogen(s) based on statistical probabilities. For example:

- Urinary tract infection in sexually active premenopausal women is due to *Escherichia coli* in approximately 85% of cases.
- Cellulitis of an arm or leg is usually due to either *Streptococcus pyogenes* or *Staphylococcus aureus*.

To make an informed guess about the likely pathogen(s) it is important to know:

- The site of infection.
- Whether the infection is community acquired or nosocomial (hospital acquired).
- Details about the host including age, underlying illness, and/or other predisposing factors.
- The usual susceptibility trends in the local hospital or community setting (e.g. penicillin-resistant pneumococci are highly prevalent in Spain and South Africa, but much less prevalent in the US and Canada).

In selected instances, it is appropriate to start antibiotic therapy without carrying out laboratory studies to identify the pathogen (e.g. most cases of cellulitis). In other cases, particularly those where the pathogen(s) cannot be reliably predicted or in patients with severe illness, appropriate specimens should be collected before starting antibiotic therapy. The microbiology laboratory can then identify the pathogen(s) and carry out *in vitro* antibiotic susceptibility testing so that the therapy can be modified to the most appropriate regimen. Usually susceptibility results are not available until 48–72 hours after a specimen has been collected for culture.

HOST FACTORS

Many host factors need to be considered before selecting an antibiotic for a given infection.

One of the most important host factors is the site of the infection

It is essential that the antibiotic reaches the site of infection at a concentration above the MIC in all cases, and above the MBC in certain infections such as meningitis, endocarditis, and osteomyelitis, and in neutropenic patients. Only a few antibiotics

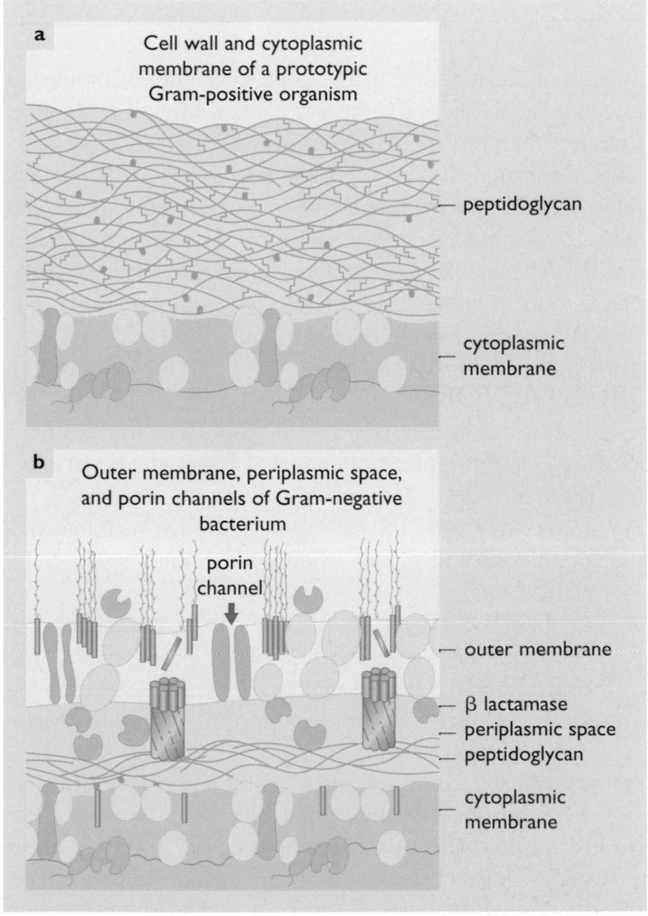

Fig. 23.7 Structure of the bacterial cell wall and membrane. (a) Gram-positive bacterium. (b) Gram-negative bacterium. Note that only Gram-negative bacteria possess an outer membrane, which provides an additional obstacle to the entry of antibacterial drugs.

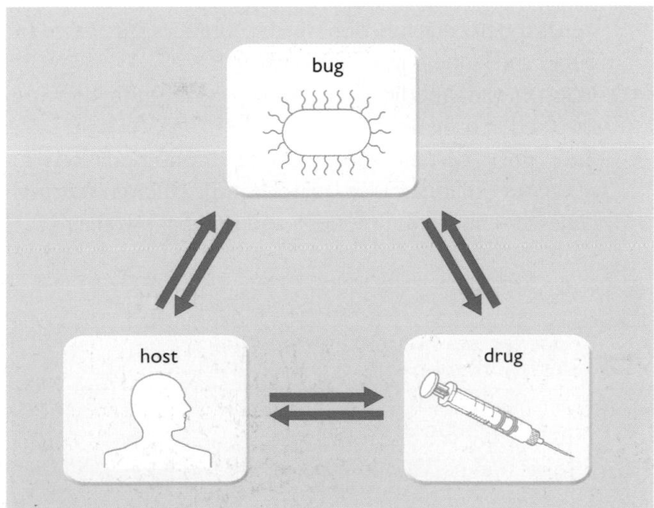

Fig. 23.8 Triangle depicting the classic bidirectional three-way interaction between a microbial pathogen ('bug'), an antimicrobial agent (drug), and the host, whose immune function is a major determinant of the outcome of an infection.

The bacterial, host, and drug factors that must be considered when selecting antibiotic therapy

Bug factors	Host factors	Drug factors
Identity of pathogen(s)†	Site of infection	Activity against pathogen(s)†
Susceptibility of pathogens†	Allergies	Ability to get to site of infection
	Renal function	Potential for drug interactions
	Hepatic function	Available routes of administration
	Neutropenia	Dosing frequency (for outpatients)
	Digestive tract function	Taste (for liquid formulations)
	Other underlying diseases	Stability at different temperatures (for liquid formulations)
	Concomitant medication	Cost
	Pregnancy	
	Desired route of administration	

† Often not known at the start of therapy.

Fig. 23.9 The bacterial, host, and drug factors that must be considered when selecting antibiotic therapy.

are able to enter the central nervous system in therapeutic concentrations to treat meningitis or a brain abscess, while urinary tract infections must be treated with drugs that are excreted by the kidney in an active form. Many antibiotics have difficulty penetrating the prostate, which is required when treating chronic bacterial prostatitis.

Other important host factors

Other important host factors include:

- Drug allergies, since certain antibiotics are relatively allergenic.
- Renal and hepatic function, since antibiotics are cleared by either the kidney or the liver.
- Concomitant medications, since some antibiotics are involved in drug interactions.
- Age, since certain antibiotics are contraindicated in neonates (sulfonamides, ceftriaxone), children (tetracyclines and fluoroquinolones), and pregnant women.

Host factors influencing the choice of an antibiotic

- Site of infection
- Renal and hepatic function
- Age
- Drug allergies
- Required route of administration

A decision must also be made about the route of administration. In general, the oral route is preferred when it is possible. Parenteral therapy is necessary if the digestive tract is nonfunctional, the patient has hypotension, therapeutic drug concentrations are required immediately (e.g. in life-threatening infections), or no oral drugs are absorbed in adequate amounts to achieve therapeutic concentrations at the site of infection. The topical route is appropriate for selected local infections (e.g. bacterial conjunctivitis).

DRUG FACTORS

Several important drug factors must be taken into account before selecting an antimicrobial agent to treat a bacterial infection. These include:

- Its activity against the pathogen(s), though such information may not be known when the treatment needs to be started.
- Its ability to reach the site of infection in a therapeutic concentration. This requires a knowledge about whether the drug should be bactericidal or bacteriostatic against the known or suspected pathogen since bactericidal activity is required for certain infections.
- Its available routes of administration and whether they are appropriate for the patient.
- Its adverse effect profile and whether this could affect underlying illnesses or result in drug interactions.
- Its dosing frequency, as acceptance of a drug in the outpatient setting is increased with dosing frequencies of two or fewer doses per day.
- When a liquid formulation is required (predominantly in young children), whether the taste is acceptable, as well as

Drug factors influencing the choice of an antibiotic

- Activity against the pathogen
- Ability to reach the site of infection
- Available routes of administration
- Adverse effect profile
- Dosing schedule
- Taste (for suspensions)
- Cost

whether it is stable at various temperatures. Some antibiotic suspensions require refrigeration to remain stable.

- Its cost, recognizing that the true cost of therapy is not merely the cost of the medication itself, but also includes the cost of administration, monitoring, and complications, including treatment failures and the cost of re-treatment.

MAJOR ANTIBIOTICS

ANTIBIOTICS THAT INHIBIT BACTERIAL CELL WALL SYNTHESIS

The bacterial cell wall is an obvious target for antibiotics. As mycoplasmas, chlamydiae and rickettsiae lack a cell wall they are innately resistant to antibiotics that inhibit bacterial cell wall synthesis. The two most important classes of antibiotics that inhibit bacterial cell wall synthesis are β lactams and glycopeptides. The topical antibiotic bacitracin and the second-line oral antituberculous agent cycloserine also inhibit this step.

β Lactams

β Lactam antibiotics possess a four-member nitrogen-containing β lactam ring and interfere with bacterial cell wall synthesis, principally by inhibiting the cross-linkage of the peptide side chains of the bacterial cell wall. β Lactams are mainly bactericidal and exhibit time-dependent killing. Most are eliminated unchanged by the kidney, so they are suitable for treating urinary tract infections.

β Lactams have a high therapeutic index, with the main adverse event being allergic reactions, most commonly a pruritic erythematous maculopapular rash. Rarely, β lactams cause anaphylaxis. They are considered safe for use in pregnancy.

There are three principal mechanisms of β lactam resistance:

- The most important is enzymatic hydrolysis of the β lactam ring by β lactamases. This mechanism occurs in staphylococci, gonococci, enterobacteriaceae, and *Bacteroides fragilis*. There are many β lactamases, which differ in their substrate specificity.
- The second most important mechanism of resistance is alteration of the target sites, called penicillin-binding proteins. Alteration in a specific penicillin-binding protein is the principal mechanism of resistance in methicillin-resistant staphylococci, as well as penicillin-resistant pneumococci.
- A third mechanism of resistance is through reduced permeability in Gram-negative cell membranes.

There are four subclasses of β lactams: penicillins, cephalosporins, carbapenems, and monobactams (Fig. 23.10).

Penicillins Penicillin was discovered by Alexander Fleming in 1928 as a byproduct of *Penicillium notatum*, from which its name originates. Penicillins consist of a β lactam ring fused to a five-member, sulfur-containing thiazolidine ring. Modification of the side chain at position six of the β lactam ring results in drugs with different antibacterial and pharmacologic properties. There are four classes of penicillins: standard penicillins, antistaphylococcal penicillins, aminopenicillins, and antipseudomonal penicillins (Fig. 23.11).

The standard penicillins are benzylpenicillin, known as penicillin G, and phenoxymethylpenicillin, known as penicillin V

Penicillin V (Fig. 23.12) is significantly more stable in the presence of acid than penicillin G and is therefore the preferred form of penicillin when oral administration is appropriate.

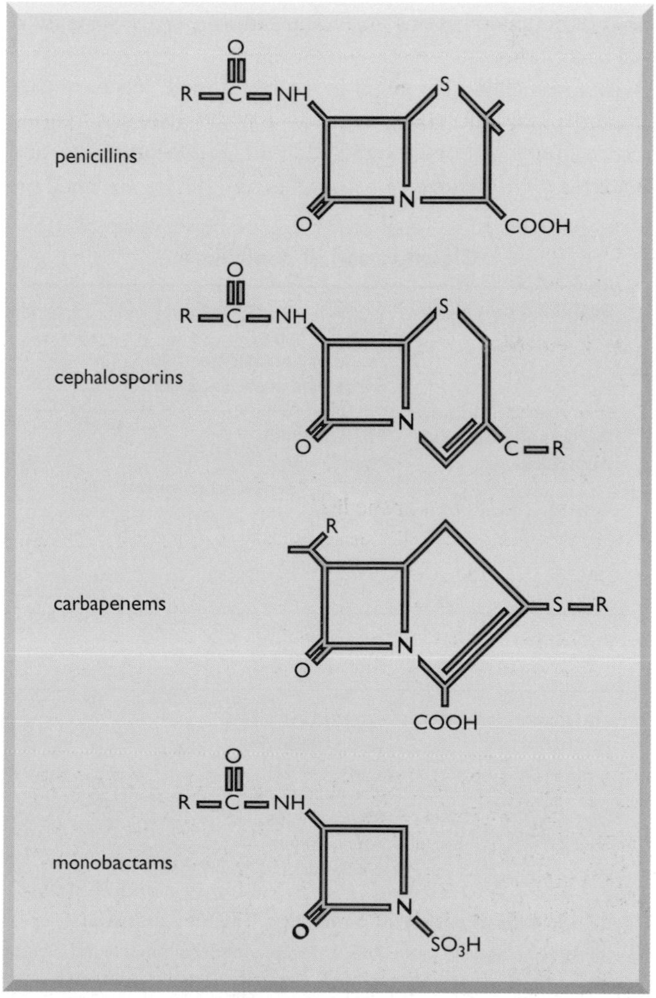

Fig. 23.10 Basic chemical structures of the four main classes of β lactam antibiotics. R denotes sites where chemical substitutions are made to create individual drugs.

Penicillin G is reserved for parenteral therapy.

In addition to crystalline penicillin G, which is used for intravenous therapy, there are two repository forms of penicillin G, which are used exclusively for intramuscular use:

- Aqueous procaine penicillin G (APPG) is a mixture of procaine and penicillin. The procaine delays the absorption of the penicillin, resulting in therapeutic blood concentrations for approximately 12 hours.
- The other repository penicillin is benzathine penicillin G, which contains penicillin G and an ammonium base. Benzathine penicillin G results in low but detectable serum concentrations of penicillin G for up to one month and is principally used in the treatment of syphilis, excluding neurosyphilis. It is also used to prevent recurrences of rheumatic fever.

Penicillin remains the drug of choice for streptococcal and meningococcal infections, syphilis, and infections due to *Pasteurella multocida*, although there is some resistance in streptococci, notably *S. pneumoniae*, and meningococci in some parts of the world.

Penicillin is useful in combination with an aminoglycoside in the treatment of infections due to enterococci and *Listeria monocytogenes*. It also remains an important drug in the treatment of dental infections, including actinomycosis, since most oral bacteria are susceptible to penicillin.

When penicillin G is given in a large dosage intravenously, cerebrospinal fluid concentrations are adequate for treating neurosyphilis and meningitis due to *S. pneumoniae* and *Neisseria meningitidis*.

Classification of penicillins

Standard penicillins	Crystalline penicillin G (iv) Penicillin V (po) Aqueous procaine penicillin G (im) Benzathine penicillin G (im)
Antistaphylococcal penicillins	Methicillin (iv) Nafcillin (iv) Isoxazolyl penicillins (iv or po) Oxacillin Cloxacillin Dicloxacillin Flucloxacillin
Aminopenicillins	Ampicillin (iv or po) Amoxicillin (po)
Antipseudomonal penicillins	Carboxypenicillins Carbenicillin (iv) Ticarcillin (iv) Ureidopenicillins Piperacillin (iv) Azlocillin (iv) Mezlocillin (iv)

Fig. 23.11 Classification of penicillins. The four classes of penicillins are standard penicillins, antistaphylococcal penicillins, aminopenicillins, and antipseudomonal penicillins. (im, intramuscular; iv, intravenous; po, oral)

Antistaphylococcal penicillins are stable to staphylococcal β lactamase

Shortly after the introduction of penicillin into clinical use, most strains of staphylococci became resistant to penicillin by producing penicillinase (β lactamase). Subsequently, several penicillins were developed that are stable to the staphylococcal β lactamase (Fig. 23.13). The first of these antistaphylococcal penicillins was methicillin, a drug that is seldom used now because it is associated with a relatively high incidence of allergic interstitial nephritis. Instead, either nafcillin or one of the isoxazolyl penicillins is preferred. The isoxazolyl penicillins are based on the parent drug oxacillin. The substitution of a chlorine atom, two chlorine atoms, and a chlorine plus a fluorine atom in place of hydrogen results in cloxacillin, dicloxacillin, and flucloxacillin, respectively.

Nafcillin and isoxazolyl penicillins are used to treat staphylococcal infections, but are not active against methicillin-resistant strains. The antimicrobial activity of the four isoxazolyl penicillins is similar, but they differ in their oral absorption, with oxacillin being considerably less well absorbed than the other three. Nafcillin, which is not an isoxazolyl penicillin, is not well absorbed orally and is reserved for parenteral use.

Aminopenicillins have enhanced activity against aerobic Gram-negative bacilli

The addition of an amino group on the penicillin side chain results in the aminopenicillins, which have enhanced activity against aerobic Gram-negative bacilli but, like standard penicillins, are not stable to staphylococcal β lactamase. Specifically, aminopenicillins are active against many strains of *E. coli*, *Proteus mirabilis*, and approximately 70% of *H. influenzae* strains. Aminopenicillins are active against some strains of

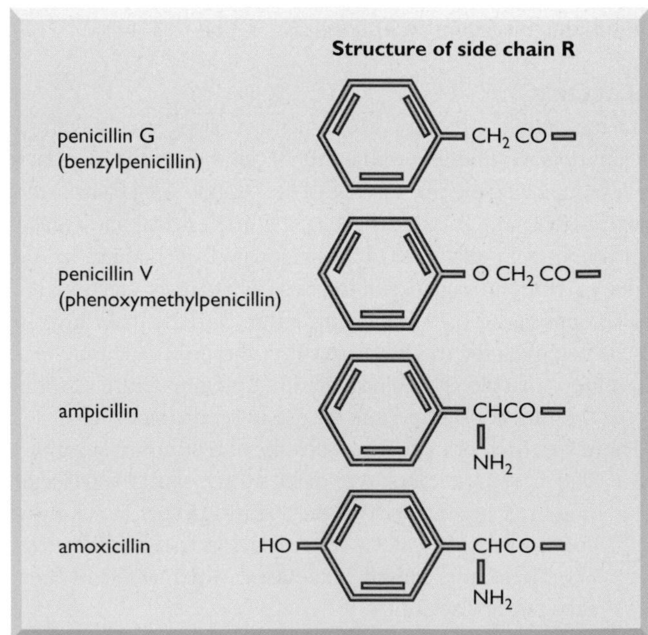

Fig. 23.12 Chemical structure of the side chain at position six of the β lactam ring of the standard penicillins and aminopenicillins.

Salmonella and *Shigella* species. They are also slightly more active than penicillin G against enterococci and *L. monocytogenes*, but both drugs are only bacteriostatic against these organisms without the addition of an aminoglycoside.

The two most important aminopenicillins are ampicillin and amoxicillin (see Fig. 23.12). Ampicillin is preferred for intravenous therapy and amoxicillin for oral therapy because of its better oral bioavailability.

Aminopenicillins are used for community-acquired respiratory tract infections because of their activity against *S. pneumoniae* and *H. influenzae*. Amoxicillin can be used to treat uncomplicated urinary tract infection, but trimethoprim–sulfamethoxazole is generally preferred, owing to its greater efficacy. Intravenous ampicillin is often used in conjunction with gentamicin in the treatment of infections due to enterococci and *L. monocytogenes*. Large intravenous doses of ampicillin result in cerebrospinal fluid concentrations that are adequate to treat meningitis due to *S. pneumoniae*, *N. meningitidis*, and susceptible strains of *H. influenzae*.

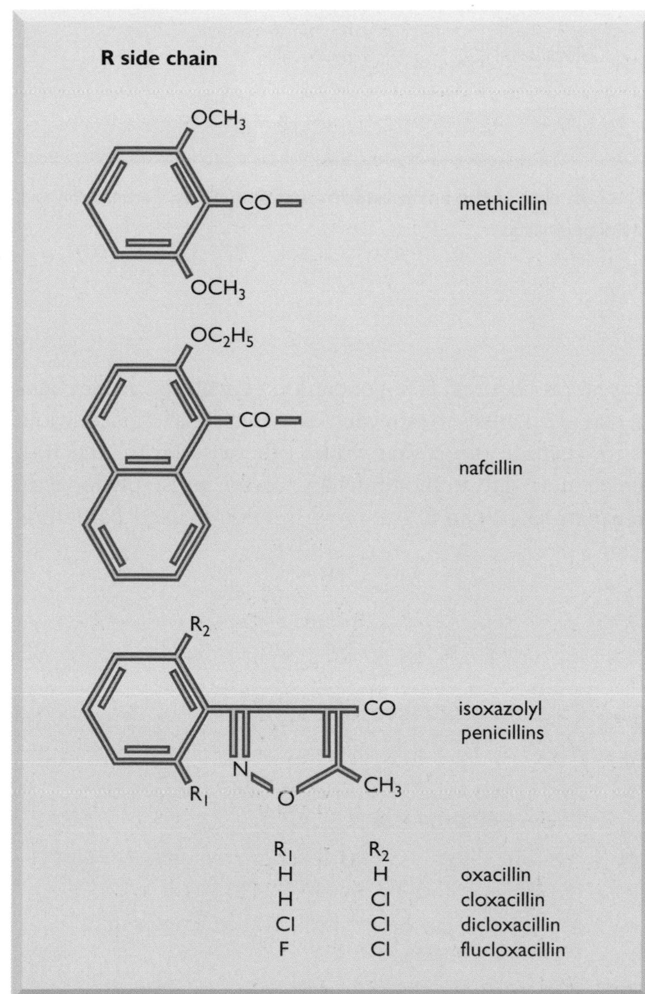

Fig. 23.13 Chemical structure of the side chain at position six of the β lactam ring of the antistaphylococcal penicillins.

Antipseudomonal penicillins are extended-spectrum aminopenicillins

The antipseudomonal penicillins are best thought of as extended-spectrum aminopenicillins, since they generally possess the same spectrum of activity as aminopenicillins plus additional activity against aerobic Gram-negative bacilli including *Pseudomonas aeruginosa*. They are not stable against staphylococcal β lactamase.

There are two subclasses of antipseudomonal penicillins, based on the chemical structure of the side chain: carboxypenicillins and ureidopenicillins (Fig. 23.14). The carboxypenicillins are carbenicillin and ticarcillin, while piperacillin, mezlocillin and azlocillin are ureidopenicillins. The ureidopenicillins have generally replaced carboxypenicillins, owing to their broader spectrum of activity and lower sodium content. Piperacillin is also active against anaerobic bacteria, including *B. fragilis*.

The antipseudomonal penicillins are used parenterally in clinical settings where infection due to *P. aeruginosa* has either been confirmed or is suspected.

Cephalosporins The first cephalosporin was discovered in 1945 by Giuseppe Brotzu from the mold *Cephalosporium acremonium*. Cephalosporins consist of a β lactam ring fused to a six-member sulfur-containing dihydrothiazine ring. Individual cephalosporins are created by side-chain substitutions at position seven of the β lactam ring and position three of the dihydrothiazine ring (see Fig. 23.10).

Cephalosporins are traditionally classified into first-, second-, and third-generation drugs based on their spectrum against aerobic Gram-negative bacilli, which increases from first to third generation (Fig. 23.15). In addition, the antistaphylococcal activity decreases from first to third generation, although there is no loss in antistreptococcal activity. Virtually all cephalosporins are stable to staphylococcal β lactamase and all have activity against aerobic Gram-negative bacilli superior to that of aminopenicillins. Unlike penicillins, cephalosporins are not active against either enterococci or *L. monocytogenes* but, like antistaphylococcal penicillins, they are not active against methicillin-resistant staphylococci.

Although cephalosporins are structurally related to penicillins, there is only approximately 10% cross-allergenicity between the two families of drugs. Accordingly, cephalosporins can often be safely used in individuals with penicillin allergy. In general, cephalosporins should be avoided in patients who have shown IgE-mediated penicillin allergy, but can usually be safely used in patients with non-IgE-mediated allergic reactions to penicillin such as a maculopapular rash.

First-generation cephalosporins are useful for skin and soft tissue infections

First-generation cephalosporins are active against streptococci, staphylococci, *E. coli*, *P. mirabilis*, and *Klebsiella pneumoniae*. They are useful in skin and soft tissue infections since these are usually due to *Streptococcus pyogenes* and/or *S. aureus*, and are commonly used as prophylaxis against infection following

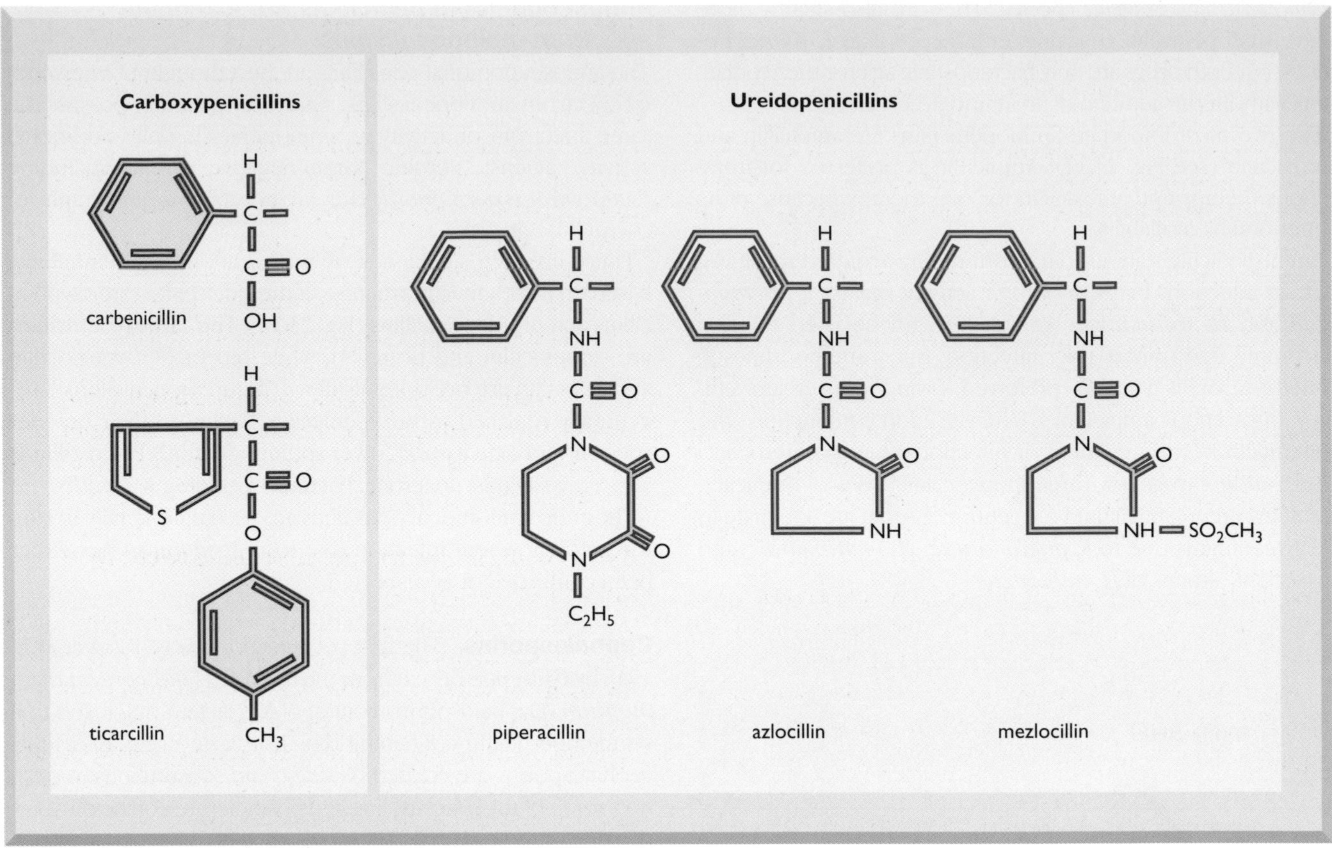

Fig. 23.14 Chemical structures of the side chains at position six of the β lactam ring of the antipseudomonal penicillins. Carbenicillin and ticarcillin are carboxypenicillins whereas piperacillin, azlocillin and mezlocillin are ureidopenicillins.

Classification of cephalosporins	
First generation	Cefadroxil (po), cefazolin, cephalexin (po), cephalothin, cephapirin, cephradine (iv/po)
Second generation with *Haemophilus influenzae* activity	Cefaclor (po), cefamandole, cefonicid, ceforanide, cefprozil (po), cefuroxime, cefuroxime axetil (po)
Second generation with *Bacteroides fragilis* activity	Cefmetazole, cefotetan, cefoxitin
Third generation	Cefotaxime, ceftriaxone, ceftizoxime, cefoperazone, moxalactam
Third generation with *Pseudomonas aeruginosa* activity	Ceftazidime, cefepime
Oral broad-spectrum	Cefixime, cefpodoxime proxetil,

Fig. 23.15 Classification of cephalosporins. This classification was based on their spectrum of activity against aerobic Gram-negative bacilli, which increases from first to third generation. The drugs are available only parenterally unless indicated otherwise. (iv, intravenous; po, oral)

surgical procedures. First-generation cephalosporins are also used as alternatives to penicillins in penicillin-allergic individuals to treat infections that would otherwise be treated with penicillin G, an aminopenicillin, or an antistaphylococcal penicillin. Cefazolin is the most frequently used parenteral agent.

First-generation cephalosporins

- Are active against streptococci and staphylococci but not enterococci
- Are active against most *Escherichia coli, Proteus mirabilis*, and *Klebsiella pneumoniae*
- Are used in the prophylaxis of wound infections following surgery
- Are useful for skin and soft tissue infections
- Are an alternative to penicillins for non-IgE-mediated penicillin allergy

There are two subtypes of second-generation cephalosporins

The two subtypes of second-generation cephalosporins are:

- Those with activity against *H. influenzae*.
- Those with activity against *B. fragilis*.

Second-generation cephalosporins with activity against *H. influenzae* are active against strains of *H. influenzae* whether or not they produce β lactamase, which inactives aminopenicillins. However, they do not achieve adequate concentrations in the cerebrospinal fluid to kill *H. influenzae* reliably, unlike third-generation cephalosporins. Otherwise, their activity is similar to that of first-generation cephalosporins. These drugs are commonly used in the empiric treatment of community-acquired respiratory tract infections in which either *S. pneumoniae* or *H. influenzae* may be a pathogen (e.g. sinusitis, otitis media, pneumonia). These drugs are also useful for the empiric treatment of a variety of infections in children in which streptococci, *S. aureus*, and *H. influenzae* may be pathogens except for meningitis.

Second-generation cephalosporins with activity against *B. fragilis* are generally used in the treatment of mixed aerobic–anaerobic infections, which are usually intra-abdominal, but are occasionally ischemic skin and soft tissue infections, such as infected lower limb cutaneous ulcers in people with diabetes mellitus.

Third-generation cephalosporins have markedly increased activity against aerobic Gram-negative bacilli

Compared with first- and second-generation cephalosporins, third-generation cephalosporins have markedly increased activity against aerobic Gram-negative bacilli, particularly Enterobacteriaceae and *H. influenzae*. They are stable to the β lactamase that can be produced by *H. influenzae* and *N. gonorrhoeae*, and to many of the β lactamases produced by Enterobacteriaceae, with the important exception of the type I chromosome-mediated inducible cephalosporinase, which may be produced by *Enterobacter cloacae*, *E. aerogenes*, *Citrobacter freundii*, *Serratia marcescens*, and *P. aeruginosa*. Therefore it is generally recommended that third-generation cephalosporins are not used as monotherapy for infections due to these pathogens, except for meningitis, where there is usually no alternative.

In general, third-generation cephalosporins have reduced activity against *S. aureus* compared with first- and second-generation cephalosporins. A few third-generation cephalosporins, particularly ceftazidime, are active against *P. aeruginosa*.

An important property of the third-generation cephalosporins is that they achieve adequate concentrations in cerebrospinal fluid to be bactericidal against Enterobacteriaceae and the three major meningeal pathogens (i.e. *S. pneumoniae*, *N. meningitidis*, and *H. influenzae*).

Third-generation cephalosporins are important drugs for treating bacterial meningitis. They are also useful for treating serious infections such as nosocomial pneumonia due to aerobic Gram-negative bacilli, particularly when aminoglycosides are contraindicated.

Oral extended-spectrum cephalosporins can be used to treat Enterobacteriaceae infections resistant to other oral β lactams

Over the last few years, a variety of oral extended-spectrum cephalosporins have become available. These drugs are sometimes called oral third-generation cephalosporins, but have considerably less activity against aerobic Gram-negative bacilli than parenteral third-generation cephalosporins. None of the oral agents is active against *P. aeruginosa* and some (cefixime, ceftibuten) are inactive against *S. aureus*. These drugs can provide an oral option for treating infections due to Enterobacteriaceae resistant to other oral β lactams.

Carbapenems Carbapenems consist of a β lactam ring fused with a five-member carbon-containing penem ring (see Fig. 23.10). The carbapenems currently available in the US are imipenem and meropenem.

Carbapenems are the most broad-spectrum antibiotics available

Carbapenems are stable to most β lactamases and active against streptococci, staphylococci, Enterobacteriaceae, *P. aeruginosa*, *Haemophilus* species and anaerobic bacteria, including *B. fragilis*. Carbapenems are active against many strains of *Enterococcus faecalis*, but not against other species of *Enterococcus*. Like cephalosporins, they are not active against *L. monocytogenes* or methicillin-resistant staphylococci.

Imipenem is broken down in the kidney by a human β lactamase called dehydropeptidase-1 to a nephrotoxic metabolite. It is therefore always co-administered with the drug cilastatin, which is a specific inhibitor of the renal β lactamase. The commercial preparation contains a fixed ratio of imipenem to cilastatin. Meropenem is not broken down by renal dehydropeptidase and does not require concomitant cilastatin. Imipenem can cause seizures in susceptible individuals, particularly those with concomitant renal insufficiency.

Carbapenems are particularly useful for treating infections due to bacteria resistant to other antibiotics. Because of their very broad spectrum of activity, they are also used to treat polymicrobial infections instead of using two or more other antibiotics.

Monobactams The name monobactam is short for monocyclic β lactam. Monobactams consist of a single ring structure, the β lactam ring, attached to a sulfonic acid group (see Fig. 23.10).

The only available monobactam is aztreonam

The only available monobactam is aztreonam, which is active only against aerobic Gram-negative bacilli including *P. aeruginosa*. Unlike other β lactams, it has no activity against Gram-positive bacteria. Aztreonam also lacks activity against anaerobes. It is available only for parenteral use.

A novel property of aztreonam is that it is essentially nonallergenic and can be used in individuals with penicillin and cephalosporin allergy.

β Lactamase inhibitors Several specific inhibitors of bacterial β lactamases have been developed for clinical use, specifically the agents clavulanate, sulbactam, and tazobactam. These drugs contain a β lactam ring (Fig. 23.16), but none has clinically useful intrinsic antibacterial activity. They act by covalently binding bacterial β lactamase, allowing β lactam drugs that would otherwise be destroyed by the β lactamase to exert their antibacterial effect. None of the β lactamase inhibitors is available for use on its own. They are only available in a fixed-dose combination with a penicillin (Fig. 23.17).

The β lactamase inhibitors inhibit most of the important bacterial β lactamases, including those produced by staphylococci, gonococci, *H. influenzae*, *B. fragilis*, and some Enterobacteriaceae. However, they do not inhibit the type I chromosome-mediated inducible cephalosporinase, which can hydrolyze all cephalosporins, including third-generation cephalosporins.

Penicillin β lactamase inhibitor combinations are useful for polymicrobial infections where the use of a single commercial product (albeit containing two drugs) may obviate the need for two or more agents. In practice, they are most frequently used in the treatment of intra-abdominal infections and infected cutaneous ulcers.

Glycopeptides

Glycopeptides are high molecular weight drugs consisting of sugars and amino acids (Fig. 23.18). Vancomycin is currently the only glycopeptide available in the US, but teicoplanin is available in parts of Europe. Vancomycin is a predominantly bactericidal antibiotic that inhibits bacterial cell wall synthesis by covalently binding to the terminal two D-alanine residues at the free carboxyl end of the pentapeptide, thereby sterically hindering the elongation of the peptidoglycan backbone (Fig. 23.19). In contrast, β lactams inhibit a later stage of cell wall synthesis by blocking the cross-linkage of pentapeptide side chains. Owing to its high molecular weight, vancomycin is unable to penetrate the cell membrane of Gram-negative bacteria and its activity is confined to Gram-positive bacteria.

Vancomycin is not absorbed from the digestive tract and is therefore used intravenously for most indications, but can be given by mouth to treat intestinal infection due to *Clostridium difficile*. When infused rapidly, vancomycin causes histamine release, resulting in an erythematous rash that is usually confined to the neck and upper trunk. This phenomenon is called the red neck syndrome and can be mistaken for allergy. It is prevented if vancomycin is infused slowly. Vancomycin is excreted unchanged by the kidney.

Because vancomycin does not contain a β lactam ring and binds to peptide side chains rather than to penicillin-binding proteins, vancomycin is unaffected by β lactamase production or penicillin-binding protein alteration. It is therefore useful in the treatment of β-lactam resistant Gram-positive infections. Acquired vancomycin resistance is uncommon, is usually confined to *E. faecium*, and due to an altered target (pentapeptide side chain).

Therapeutic indications Vancomycin is useful in the treatment of infections caused by streptococci, staphylococci, enterococci, *Corynebacterium jeikeium* and *C. difficile*. It is the drug of choice for infections caused by methicillin-resistant staphylococci and high-level penicillin-resistant pneumococci. Vancomycin is frequently used as an alternative to β lactams in patients with serious β lactam allergy as there is no crossreactivity between vancomycin and β lactams.

Vancomycin is very effective orally in the treatment of *C. difficile* enteritis, though metronidazole is usually preferred for this indication because of its markedly lower cost.

Vancomycin enters the cerebrospinal fluid in concentrations that are close to the MBC of streptococci and staphylococci, but clinical experience with vancomycin in the treatment of bacterial meningitis is limited. Vancomycin should not, therefore, be used in the treatment of meningitis unless the pathogen is resistant to third-generation cephalosporins and chloramphenicol.

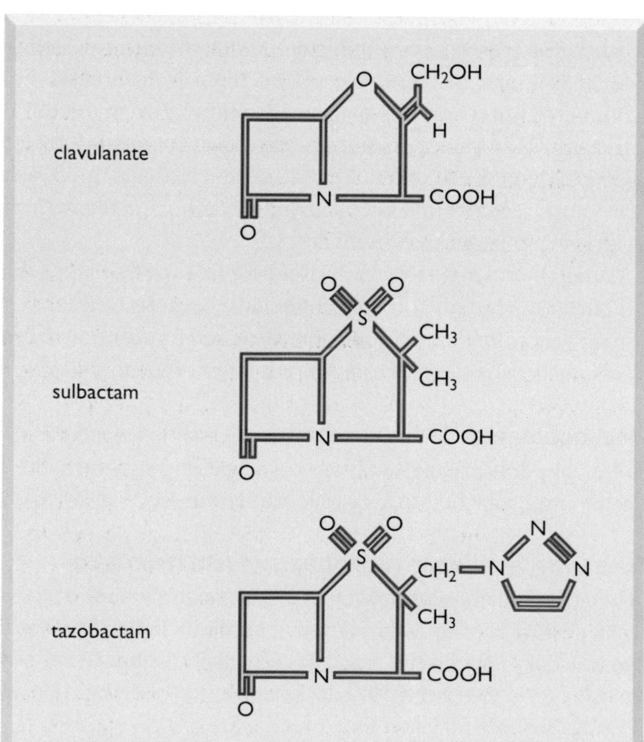

Fig. 23.16 Chemical structures of three β lactamase inhibitors: clavulanate, sulbactam, and tazobactam. Note that all three contain a β lactam ring, but none has significant antibacterial activity clinically alone. They are used in combination with aminopenicillins and antipseudomonal penicillins.

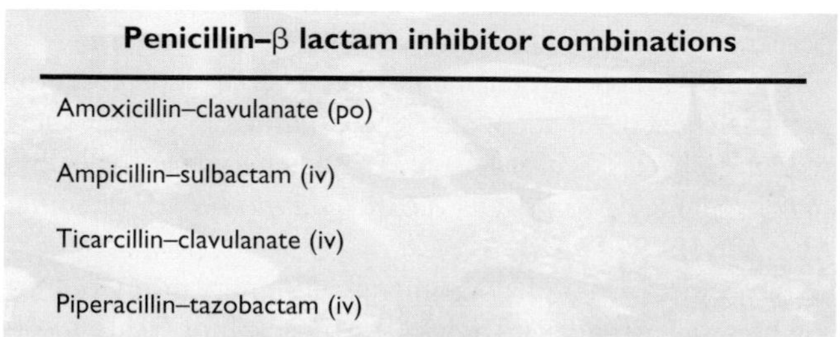

Penicillin–β lactam inhibitor combinations
Amoxicillin–clavulanate (po)
Ampicillin–sulbactam (iv)
Ticarcillin–clavulanate (iv)
Piperacillin–tazobactam (iv)

Fig. 23.17 Penicillin–β lactam inhibitor combinations. β Lactamase inhibitors are not available for use on their own, but are available in fixed-dose combinations with a penicillin. (iv, intravenous; po, oral)

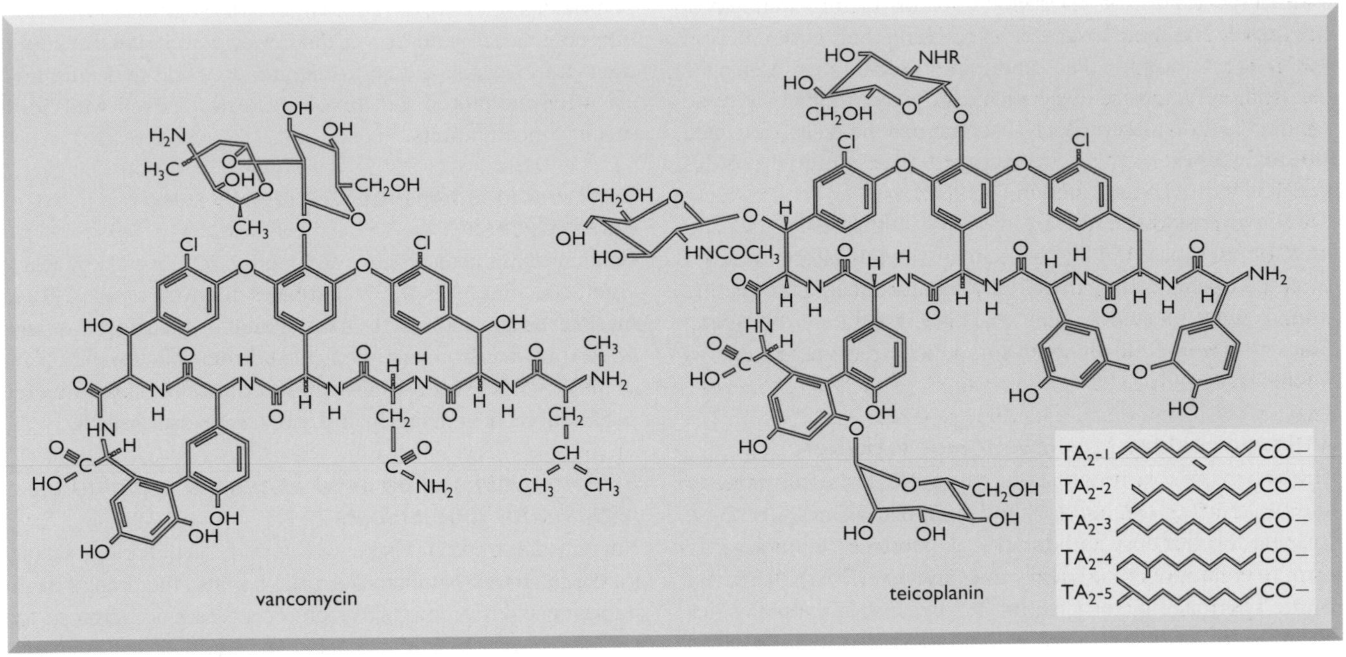

Fig. 23.18 Chemical structures of the glycopeptides vancomycin and teicoplanin. Teicoplanin comprises a mixture of five slightly different agents.

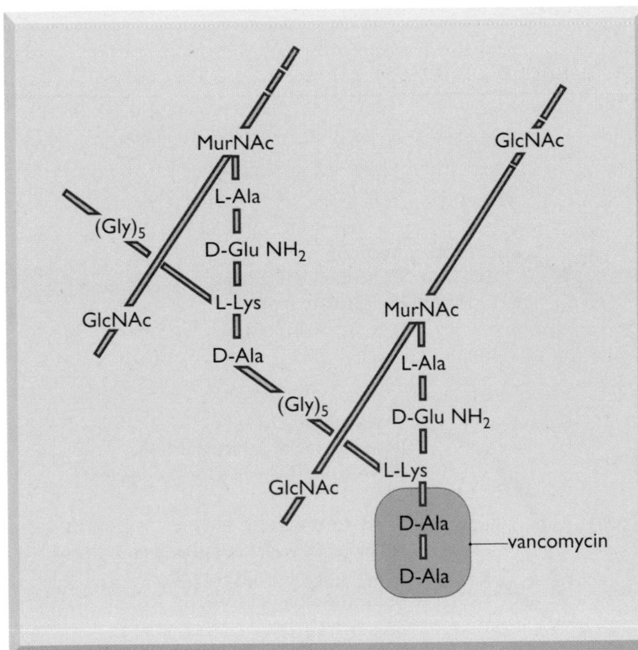

Fig. 23.19 Site of action of vancomycin on the elongating peptidoglycan polymer in bacterial cell walls.

ANTIBIOTICS THAT INHIBIT BACTERIAL CELL MEMBRANE FUNCTIONING

Polymyxin B and polymyxin E (also known as colistimethate) are octapeptides of high molecular weight that injure the plasma membranes of Gram-negative bacteria, resulting in a bactericidal effect. Because of their considerable toxicity when given systemically, their use is confined to topical therapy of infections due to aerobic Gram-negative bacilli.

ANTIBIOTICS THAT INHIBIT BACTERIAL PROTEIN SYNTHESIS

Several major classes of antibiotics act principally by inhibiting bacterial protein synthesis (Fig. 23.20). These drugs exhibit selective toxicity by inhibiting bacterial protein synthesis to a much greater extent than they inhibit host cell protein synthesis, as a result of binding to specific bacterial targets. Most of these drugs are predominantly bacteriostatic, except for the aminoglycosides, which are bactericidal.

Aminoglycosides

Aminoglycosides consist of two or more amino sugars linked by glycosidic bonds to an aminocyclitol ring. They enter bacterial cells via an oxygen-dependent transport system, which is not present in anaerobic bacteria or streptococci. Accordingly, anaerobes and streptococci are innately resistant to aminoglycosides. Once inside the bacterial cell, aminoglycosides bind irreversibly to sites on the ribosome, inhibiting protein synthesis. There is also at least one other mechanism of action that is not currently understood, which probably accounts for their bactericidal activity.

Aminoglycosides are active against aerobic Gram-negative bacilli, staphylococci, and mycobacteria. Although they are not intrinsically active against either enterococci or *L. monocytogenes*, the addition of an aminoglycoside to penicillin G, ampicillin, or vancomycin is synergistic and usually results in bactericidal activity.

The two principal mechanisms of acquired bacterial resistance to aminoglycosides are:

- Reduced bacterial permeability caused by alterations in the bacterial cell membrane.
- Production of a variety of aminoglycoside-modifying enzymes.

Aminoglycoside-modifying enzymes, which are nonhydrolytic,

add acetyl, adenyl, or phosphoryl groups to the aminoglycoside, rendering them incapable of reaching their target sites on the bacterial ribosome. Each aminoglycoside-modifying enzyme has a different substrate specificity and may modify only some aminoglycosides. Accordingly, bacteria may be resistant to one aminoglycoside and not to another. The aminoglycosides available in the US are listed in Fig. 23.21.

Aminoglycosides are not absorbed from the digestive tract and must be used parenterally to obtain a systemic effect. They are excreted unchanged by the kidney and are suitable for treating urinary tract infections. They do not enter the cerebrospinal fluid in therapeutically relevant concentrations, except in neonates.

Aminoglycosides have two major toxicities

The two major toxicities of aminoglycosides are nephrotoxicity and ototoxicity (both auditory and vestibular). The risk of these toxicities is both dose and duration dependent. Nephrotoxicity is more common, but is usually mild and reversible. Ototoxicity is often permanent (see Chapter 22). Because aminoglycosides are more toxic than most other antibiotics and must be given parenterally, their use is largely limited to serious infections due to Enterobacteriaceae and *P. aeruginosa*, and usually in the hospital setting. Aminoglycosides are also used in conjunction with penicillin, ampicillin, or vancomycin in the treatment of serious infections due to enterococci and *L. monocytogenes*. Because of their potential toxicity, serum aminoglycoside concentrations are often monitored, but toxicity can occur even with 'ideal' serum concentrations.

Gentamicin is the most frequently used aminoglycoside

Gentamicin is the most active aminoglycoside for synergy against enterococci (i.e. it is the 'workhorse' aminoglycoside). Tobramycin is usually more active than gentamicin against *P. aeruginosa*, but no more active against Enterobacteriaceae, and unlikely to be synergistic against enterococci. Ophthalmic preparations of gentamicin and tobramycin are available.

Streptomycin can be used as part of a multidrug regimen for tuberculosis

Not only can streptomycin be used as part of a multidrug regimen for the treatment of tuberculosis, but it is also the drug of choice in plague and tularemia, although recent evidence suggests that gentamicin is equally effective for these two infections. Streptomycin demonstrates synergy with penicillin, ampicillin, or vancomycin in the treatment of a few enterococcal strains for which gentamicin does not.

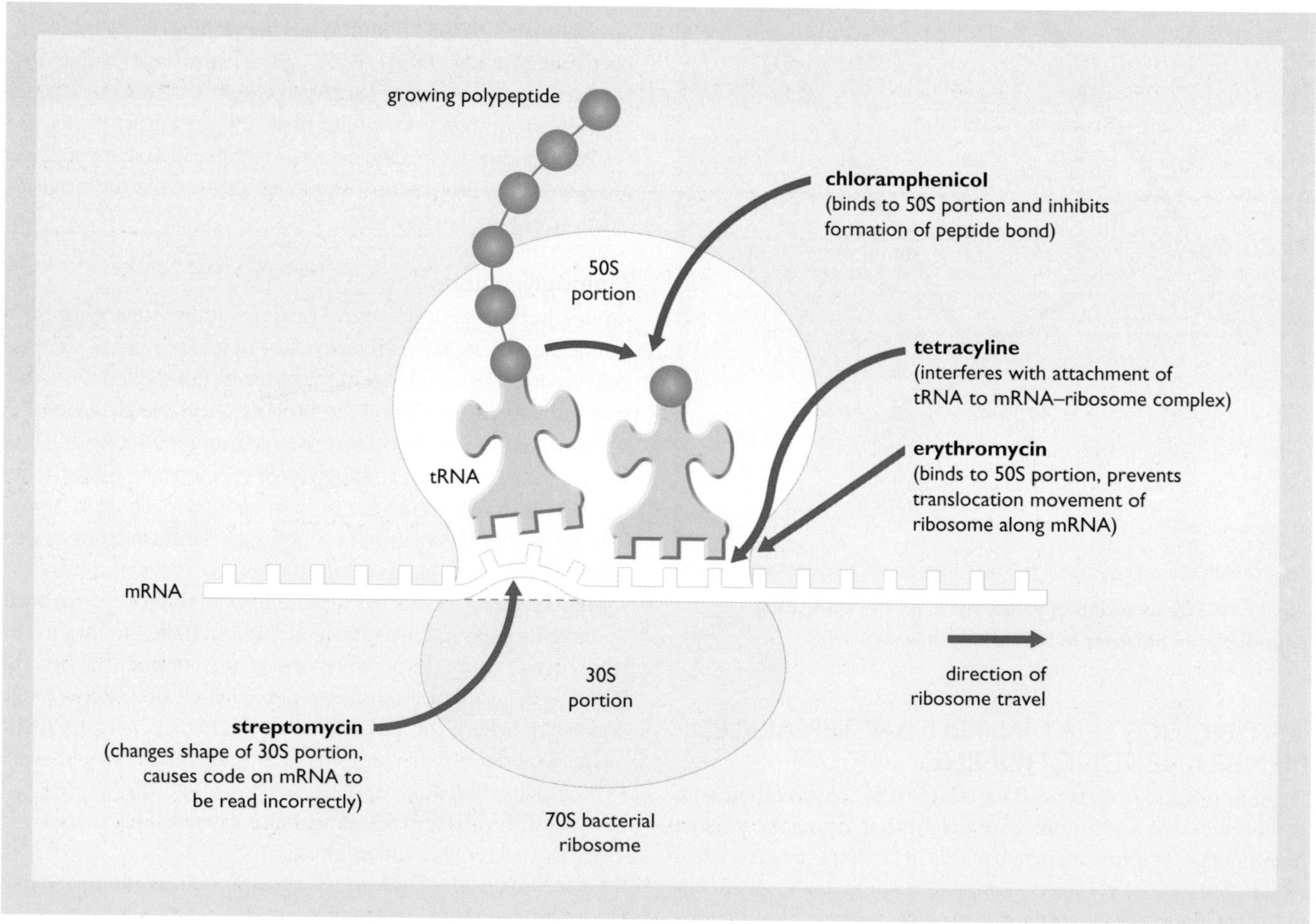

growing polypeptide
50S portion
chloramphenicol
(binds to 50S portion and inhibits formation of peptide bond)
tetracyline
(interferes with attachment of tRNA to mRNA–ribosome complex)
erythromycin
(binds to 50S portion, prevents translocation movement of ribosome along mRNA)
tRNA
mRNA
30S portion
direction of ribosome travel
streptomycin
(changes shape of 30S portion, causes code on mRNA to be read incorrectly)
70S bacterial ribosome

Fig. 23.20 Several classes of antibiotics inhibit bacterial protein synthesis.

Therapeutic indications Amikacin is the aminoglycoside least susceptible to aminoglycoside-modifying enzymes and is sometimes active against bacteria that are resistant to other aminoglycosides.

Neomycin is no longer used parenterally because of its lower efficacy and greater toxicity than other aminoglycosides. It can be used orally to reduce the intestinal load of Enterobacteriaceae (without a systemic effect) in the treatment of hepatic encephalopathy or in combination with erythromycin as a prophylactic regimen to reduce the incidence of wound infection following elective colorectal surgery.

Kanamycin is rarely used, owing to acquired resistance.

Aminoglycosides

- Are not absorbed orally
- Are active against aerobic Gram-negative bacilli
- Demonstrate concentration-dependent killing
- Cause nephrotoxicity and ototoxicity (their major adverse effects)

Paromomycin, which is related to neomycin, is used only orally to treat intestinal protozoal infections.

Macrolides, lincosamides, and streptogramins

Macrolides, lincosamides, and streptogramins (MLS drugs) are chemically unrelated but possess similar mechanisms of action, resistance, and antimicrobial activity. They reversibly bind to the 50S ribosomal subunit and so block the translocation reaction. Although classically considered as bacteriostatic antibiotics, they are bactericidal against specific isolates. The principal mechanism of acquired resistance is a specific mutation in the ribosomal ribonucleic acid (RNA) of the 50S ribosomal subunit. Resistance to one member of the MLS class does not necessarily imply resistance to others.

Macrolides are named after the macrocyclic lactone ring that forms the nucleus for these drugs (Fig. 23.22). The prototypic macrolide is erythromycin, which is available in different salts. In recent years, several newer macrolides have been introduced in the US: clarithromycin, azithromycin, and dirithromycin. Other macrolides are available in Europe and Asia. Macrolides are usually given orally, although an intravenous form of erythromycin is available, and erythromycin lotion can be used in the treatment of acne vulgaris. Macrolides are metabolized in the liver and do not penetrate the cerebrospinal fluid in therapeutically relevant concentrations.

Aminoglycosides currently available in the US, their route of administration, and their use

Agent	Routes	Comment
Streptomycin	im (iv)	For tuberculosis, plague, tularemia, severe brucellosis, some gentamicin-resistant enterococci
Neomycin	po	Used to reduce the load of Enterobacteriaceae in the bowel and to treat hepatic encephalopathy, or with erythromycin as prophylaxis in elective colorectal surgery
Paromomycin	po	For certain intestinal protozoa
Kanamycin	iv/im	Rarely used, owing to bacterial resistance
Gentamicin	iv/im	The 'workhorse' aminoglycoside; used for Enterobacteriaceae, *Pseudomonas aeruginosa*, enterococci
Netilmicin	iv/im	Similar to effect of gentamicin against Enterobacteriaceae and *P. aeruginosa*; poor synergistic activity against enterococci
Tobramycin	iv/im	Similar to effect of gentamicin against Enterobacteriaceae; more active than gentamicin against *P. aeruginosa*; poor synergistic activity against enterococci
Amikacin	iv/im	Aminoglycoside least affected by aminoglycoside-modifying enzymes; good activity against Enterobacteriaceae and *P. aeruginosa*; the most active against mycobacteria; poor synergistic activity against enterococci; the most expensive aminoglycoside

Fig. 23.21 Aminoglycosides currently available in the US, their route of administration, and their use. (im, intramuscular; iv, intravenous; po, oral)

Erythromycin is active against streptococci, staphylococci, *Bordetella pertussis*, *Corynebacterium diphtheriae*, *Campylobacter jejuni*, *Mycoplasma pneumoniae*, *Ureaplasma urealyticum*, *Legionella* species and *Chlamydia* species. Erythromycin and dirithromycin have weak activity against *H. influenzae*, but both clarithromycin and azithromycin have considerably better activity against this organism. Macrolides are not active against Enterobacteriaceae, *P. aeruginosa*, or *Mycoplasma hominis*.

Macrolides are used primarily in the treatment of respiratory tract infections. They are alternatives to penicillin for treating streptococcal pharyngitis, especially in patients who are allergic to penicillin.

Macrolides are the drugs of choice for community-acquired pneumonia as they are active against pneumococcci, *M. pneumoniae*, *C. pneumoniae* and *Legionella* species. In cases where infection may be due to *H. influenzae*, clarithromycin or azithromycin are preferred.

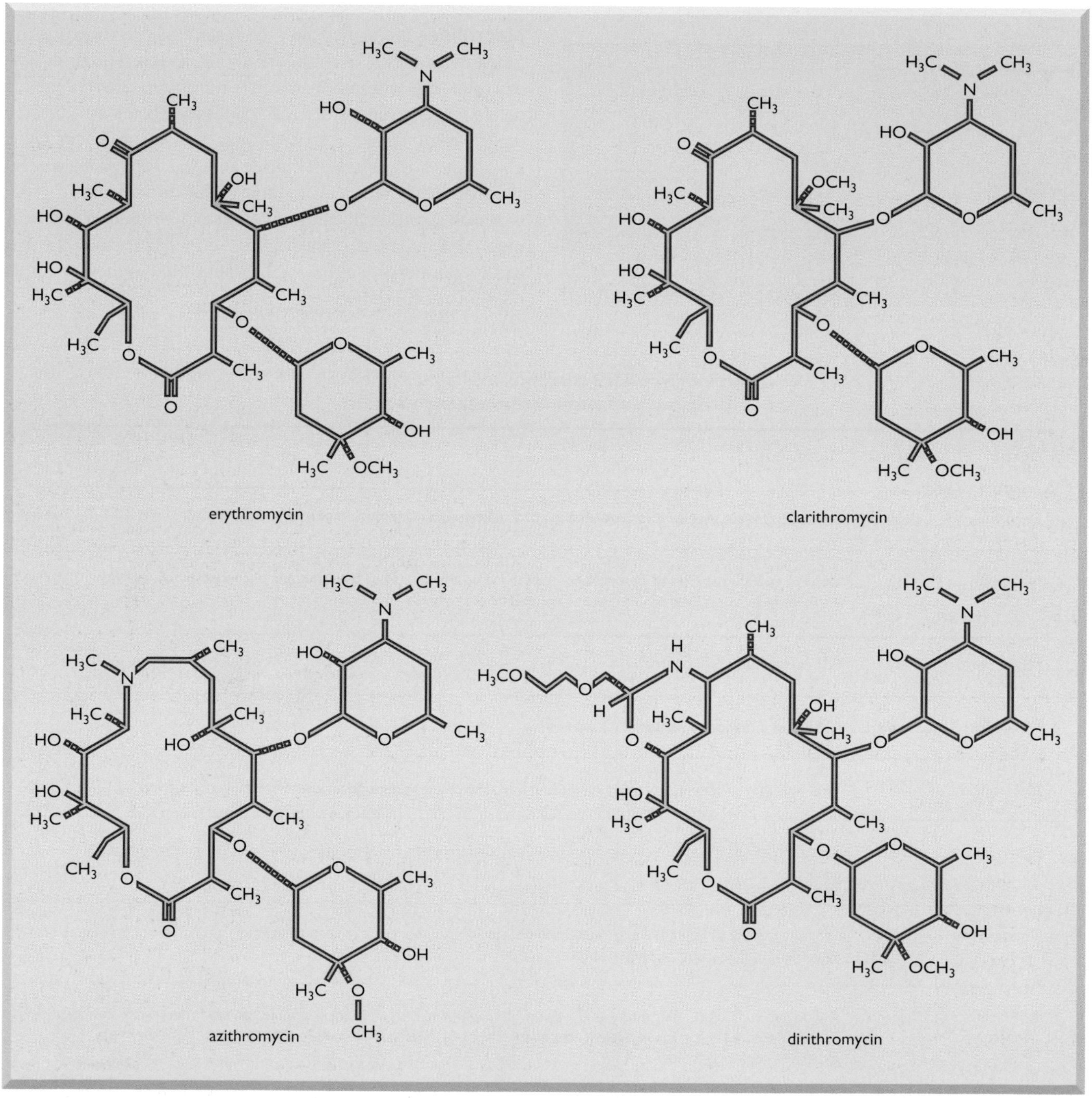

Fig. 23.22 Chemical structures of macrolides. Note the macrocyclic lactone ring, which has 14 positions except in azithromycin, where it is a 15-member nitrogen-containing ring.

Erythromycin is:

- The drug of choice for the treatment of pertussis.
- Equivalent to penicillin in eradicating the carrier state in diphtheria.
- The drug of choice for legionnaires' disease.
- Equivalent to tetracycline in the treatment of *M. pneumoniae* infections.
- The co-drug of choice for *C. jejuni* enteritis.
- The drug of choice for treating infections due to *Chlamydia trachomatis* in pregnancy, when tetracyclines are contraindicated.

Macrolides can be used as an alternative to β lactams for mild skin and soft tissue infections due to *S. pyogenes* and *S. aureus*.

Erythromycin causes gastrointestinal adverse effects

Erythromycin is probably the single most poorly tolerated oral antibiotic, owing to dyspepsia, nausea and vomiting. It interacts with motilin receptors to increase gastrointestinal motility and has been used successfully in the treatment of diabetic gastroparesis. The newer macrolides clarithromycin and azithromycin produce less severe gastrointestinal adverse effects than erythromycin, and may be suitable for individuals who have demonstrated gastrointestinal intolerance to erythromycin.

Erythromycin and clarithromycin Interact with other drugs

Erythromycin elevates serum theophylline concentrations when given concomitantly. In combination with the non-sedating histamine-H_1 antagonists astemizole or terfenadine, or the promotility drug cisapride, erythromycin and clarithromycin can lead to significant prolongation of the QT interval in the electrocardiogram. This can result in the torsades de pointes variant of ventricular tachycardia, which can be fatal.

Clarithromycin and azithromycin are more active than erythromycin against some pathogens

Clarithromycin and azithromycin, but not dirithromycin, are more active than erythromycin against *H. influenzae* and are more appropriate choices for the empiric treatment of respiratory tract infections if *H. influenzae* is a possible pathogen.

Both clarithromycin and azithromycin are active against *Mycobacterium avium* complex, an important pathogen in patients with acquired immunodeficiency syndrome (AIDS). Clarithromycin is useful in the treatment of most other nontuberculous mycobacteria. It is also very active against *Helicobacter pylori* and has been used in a multidrug regimen to treat duodenal ulcer caused by *H. pylori*.

Azithromycin is active against *C. trachomatis* and is the only drug that can cure *C. trachomatis* urethritis and cervicitis in a single dose.

Lincosamides Lincomycin and clindamycin are the two available lincosamides. Lincomycin is named after Lincoln, Nebraska where it was first isolated from the mold *Streptomycin linconensis*. The replacement of an hydroxyl group by a chlorine atom led to clindamycin (Fig. 23.23). Since clindamycin has greater activity and superior oral bioavailability, it has virtually supplanted lincomycin in clinical use.

Clindamycin is active against streptococci, staphylococci, and anaerobic bacteria, including *B. fragilis*. It is also active against *Mycoplasma hominis*, but not *M. pneumoniae* or *U. urealyticum*. It has no useful activity against enterococci or aerobic Gram-negative bacilli.

Clindamycin can be given either orally or intravenously. There is also a topical solution for the treatment of acne vulgaris and a vaginal cream for the treatment of bacterial vaginosis. Clindamycin is metabolized by the liver and does not penetrate the cerebrospinal fluid.

Clindamycin is an important antibiotic in the treatment of anaerobic infections, particularly in mixed aerobic– anaerobic infections where it is usually used in combination with other antibiotics. It can also be used as an alternative to β lactams in people who are allergic to β lactams, particularly if the oral route is appropriate.

Clindamycin is associated with a higher risk of *Clostridium difficile* enteritis than other antibiotics.

Streptogramins Although streptogramins are not currently commercially available in the US, streptogramins with activity against methicillin-resistant staphylococci and vancomycin-resistant enterococci are being developed and are expected to become available in the near future.

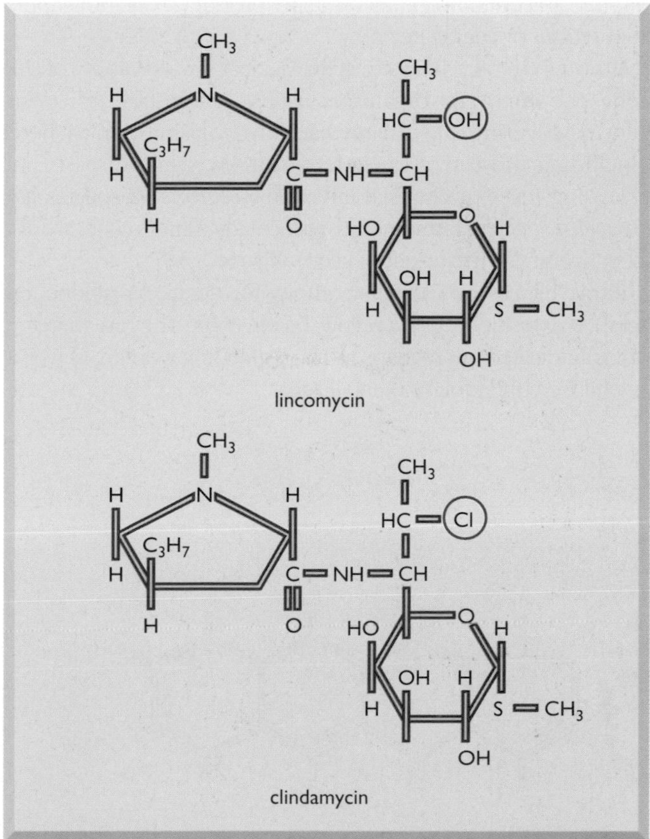

Fig. 23.23 Chemical structure of lincomycin and clindamycin. The circles denote the only difference in the compounds. Clindamycin has greater activity and oral bioavailability and is the preferred lincosamide.

Tetracyclines

Tetracyclines are moderately broad-spectrum, primarily bacteriostatic antibiotics that have a nucleus of four fused cyclic rings (Fig. 23.24), hence the name tetracyclines. Specific agents are derived from substitutions at positions five, six, and seven of the tetracycline nucleus.

As tetracyclines are concentrated intracellularly, they are useful for intracellular infections. They are excreted mainly by the kidneys and do not achieve therapeutic concentrations in cerebrospinal fluid. They are usually used orally but intravenous preparations are available, as well as a topical formulation for acne vulgaris.

Of the six tetracyclines commercially available in the US, only three are used with any frequency: tetracycline, doxycycline, and minocycline. Tetracycline is a short-acting drug that is usually administered four times daily, whereas both doxycycline and minocycline have long half-lives, allowing once- or twice-daily administration.

Tetracyclines reversibly bind to the 30S ribosomal subunit in such a manner that they block the binding of transfer RNA to the messenger RNA–ribosome complex, preventing the addition of new amino acids to the growing peptide chain (see Fig. 23.20). Acquired tetracycline resistance is usually due to changes in the transport mechanism, resulting in a lack of tetracycline accumulation within the bacterial cell.

Tetracyclines are chelated by divalent or trivalent cations. Absorption is therefore markedly decreased when these drugs are taken orally in conjunction with calcium-, magnesium-, and aluminum-containing antacids, dairy products, calcium supplementation, or sucralfate.

Although tetracyclines are active against a wide variety of bacteria, the important organisms against which they are consistently active include chlamydiae, mycoplasmas, spirochetes (including those that cause leptospirosis, Lyme disease, and relapsing fever), rickettsial infections, *Legionella* species and *Brucella* species. Tetracyclines, particularly minocycline, are also effective in the treatment of acne vulgaris.

Tetracyclines have a strong affinity for developing bone and teeth, to which they give a yellow–brown color. They are therefore contraindicated in pregnant and breastfeeding women, as well as in children under eight years of age.

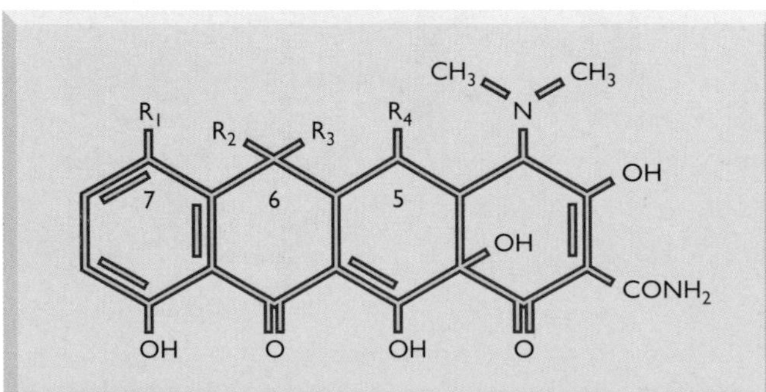

Fig. 23.24 Chemical structure of tetracyclines. Substitutions at positions five, six, and seven result in different drugs, including the three common agents tetracycline, doxycycline, and minocycline.

Amphenicols

Chloramphenicol (Fig. 23.25) is the only amphenicol available in the US. The related drug, thiamphenicol, is available in parts of Europe. Chloramphenicol is a relatively broad-spectrum, predominantly bacteriostatic antibiotic that reversibly binds to the 50S ribosomal subunit to prevent the attachment of the amino acid-containing end of transfer RNA to the peptide chain (i.e. it blocks peptidyl transferase) (see Fig. 23.20).

Acquired chloramphenicol resistance results from either:

- Reduced bacterial permeability.
- Production of the chloramphenicol-modifying enzyme, chloramphenicol acetyltransferase.

Chloramphenicol is available both orally and parenterally as well as in a topical ophthalmic preparation.

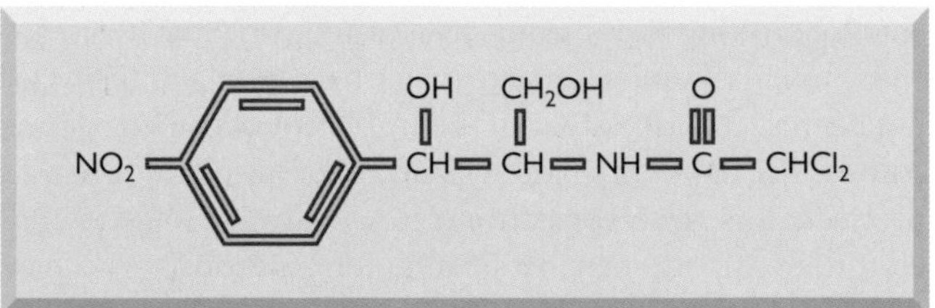

Fig. 23.25 Chemical structure of chloramphenicol.

Chloramphenicol's main adverse effect is hematologic

Chloramphenicol exerts a dose-dependent myelosuppression, which is common and reversible. Approximately 1 in 30,000 recipients develop irreversible aplastic anemia. Although this idiosyncratic reaction is rare, it is the major reason why chloramphenicol is seldom used in developed countries. Chloramphenicol is more widely used in developing countries because of its low price, broad spectrum of activity, and efficacy in enteric fever. Chloramphenicol enters the cerebrospinal fluid in therapeutically effective concentrations for the three principal meningeal pathogens (i.e. *S. pneumoniae*, *N. meningitidis* and *H. influenzae*), but not for Enterobacteriaceae. Chloramphenicol also enters brain parenchyma in concentrations sufficient to be useful in the treatment of brain abscess.

Chloramphenicol is conjugated in the liver to its inactive glucuronide. Neonates are less able to conjugate chloramphenicol; this sometimes results in high serum chloramphenicol concentrations, with resultant toxicity. Such toxicity is manifest as the gray baby syndrome, which is characterized by abdominal distension, vomiting, cyanosis, and circulatory collapse. If chloramphenicol must be used in neonates, serum concentrations need to be monitored closely.

Therapeutic indications Chloramphenicol is seldom used in developed countries, but:

- Is an acceptable alternative for the treatment of bacterial meningitis, particularly in patients with cephalosporin allergies.

- May be used in the treatment of brain abscess or enteric fever, although a variety of *Salmonella* strains around the world are resistant to chloramphenicol.
- Is an alternative to tetracycline for the treatment of Rocky Mountain spotted fever.

ANTIBIOTICS THAT INHIBIT BACTERIAL DEOXYRIBONUCLEIC ACID SYNTHESIS

Quinolones

The quinolones are synthetic antibiotics that consist of a nucleus of two fused six-membered rings (Fig. 23.26). The first drug of this class was nalidixic acid, which was of limited clinical value because of its relative inactivity and the rapid emergence of resistance. The addition of a fluorine atom at position six of the quinolone nucleus markedly enhances activity against Gram-negative bacteria and led to a new generation of drugs known as fluoroquinolones.

Quinolones inhibit bacterial deoxyribonucleic acid (DNA) gyrase, the enzyme responsible for supercoiling, nicking, and sealing bacterial DNA. Acquired resistance may develop through either decreased permeability or alterations in DNA gyrase.

Fluoroquinolones are predominantly bactericidal, exhibit concentration-dependent killing, and are renally excreted. Most have excellent oral bioavailability. They penetrate the prostate in therapeutically useful amounts. Although cerebrospinal fluid concentrations appear to be therapeutic, there is very little clinical experience in the use of quinolones for meningitis and their use is not recommended for bacterial meningitis.

Fluoroquinolones are highly active against aerobic Gram-negative bacilli including Enterobacteriaceae, *Haemophilus* species, *Moraxella catarrhalis* and, in the case of ciprofloxacin, *P. aeruginosa*. They are active against some mycobacteria, including most strains of *M. tuberculosis*, but have weak activity against streptococci and staphylococci, and no activity against anaerobes.

Like tetracyclines, fluoroquinolones are chelated by divalent and trivalent cations.

Fluoroquinolones are perhaps the best tolerated of all oral antibiotics, although more expensive than most.

Therapeutic indications Fluoroquinolones are useful in the treatment of infections due to aerobic Gram-negative bacilli that are not susceptible to less expensive agents. In many instances, they will be the only oral agents active against certain aerobic Gram-negative bacilli, particularly *P. aeruginosa*, in which case fluoroquinolones can obviate the need for parenteral therapy. Of the currently available agents, ciprofloxacin is the most active and the most commonly used. It is available in oral, parenteral, and ophthalmic formulations.

Adverse effects Some quinolones, including ciprofloxacin, increase serum concentrations of theophylline. In addition, as fluoroquinolones cause cystic lesions in the articular cartilage of growing animals, they are relatively contraindicated in children and pregnant women.

Ciprofloxacin

- Is the most commonly used fluoroquinolone
- Has excellent oral bioavailability
- Is very active against aerobic Gram-negative bacilli
- Is not active against anaerobes
- Has only limited activity against streptococci and staphylococci

4-quinolone

nalidixic acid

norfloxacin

ciprofloxacin

ofloxacin

enoxacin

lomefloxacin

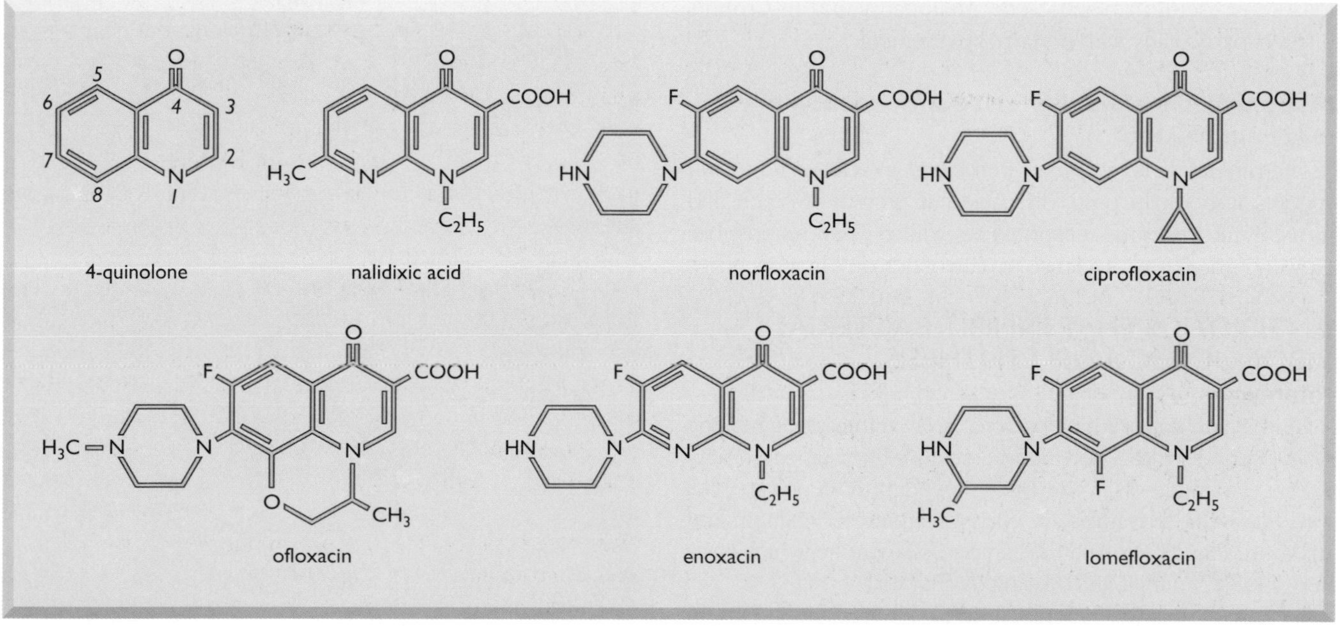

Fig. 23.26 Chemical structure of quinolone antibiotics. Note the fluorine atom at position six in the agents other than nalidixic acid. These drugs are fluoroquinolones and are much more active against aerobic Gram-negative bacilli than nalidixic acid.

Nitroimidazoles

Nitroimidazoles are well-absorbed, predominantly bactericidal agents with antimicrobial activity restricted to strict anaerobes and certain protozoa. They can enter most bacteria but only susceptible organisms produce nitroreductase, which is needed to reduce these agents to the short-lived cytotoxic intermediates that bind to DNA and inhibit its synthesis. Aerobic bacteria are innately resistant owing to their lack of nitroreductase activity. Acquired resistance can develop as a result of either:

- Decreased uptake of the drug.
- Decreased nitroreductase production.

Metronidazole is the only nitroimidazole currently licensed in the US

Both oral and intravenous preparations of metronidazole are available, with the oral form having close to 100% bioavailability. A topical formulation is available for the treatment of acne rosacea. Metronidazole achieves therapeutic concentrations in both cerebrospinal fluid and brain parenchyma

Metronidazole is active against most anaerobic bacteria, but has greatest activity against Gram-negative anaerobes including *B. fragilis*. It has no activity against aerobic bacteria. It is also very effective in the treatment of three important protozoal infections: giardiasis, amebiasis, and trichomoniasis.

Therapeutic indications Metronidazole is useful in the treatment of a variety of anaerobic infections including bacterial vaginosis, which is the most common cause of abnormal vaginal discharge. In bacterial vaginosis the bacterial flora of the vagina, which is normally dominated by *Lactobacillus* species, is replaced by an abnormal polymicrobial flora comprising predominantly anaerobes.

Metronidazole is usually considered the drug of choice for *C. difficile* enteritis.

In addition to its use against specific microorganisms, metronidazole is useful in hepatic encephalopathy and in Crohn's disease, particularly with perianal involvement.

Metronidazole should be used with caution in pregnant women

As metronidazole is mutagenic in bacteria and causes tumors in rodents, it should be used with caution in pregnant women, and its use in the first trimester should be avoided wherever possible. However, there is no evidence to date of human carcinogenicity.

ANTIBIOTICS THAT INHIBIT BACTERIAL RIBONUCLEIC ACID SYNTHESIS

Rifamycins

Rifamycin antibiotics inhibit bacterial RNA synthesis by inhibiting DNA-dependent RNA polymerase. Acquired resistance is usually due to a mutation in the DNA-dependent RNA polymerase. Two rifamycin derivatives are currently available: rifampin and rifabutin (Fig. 23.27). A third rifamycin, rifapentine, which has a very long serum half-life, is being developed.

The rifamycins are all metabolized in the liver and impart an orange color to most body fluids, especially urine.

Rifampin Rifampin was originally developed for the treatment of tuberculosis and remains a mainstay of antituberculous therapy. It is also useful in the treatment of several nontuberculous mycobacterial infections, particularly *M. leprae* (the cause of leprosy), *M. kansasii*, and *M. marinum*.

Rifampin is usually used orally, but an intravenous formulation is also available.

Rifampin must never be used alone for the treatment of mycobacterial infections, since acquired resistance will usually develop; it must be used in combination with at least one other antimycobacterial drug. Rifampin achieves concentrations in the cerebrospinal fluid adequate to treat tuberculous meningitis.

Rifampin is also active against a number of conventional bacteria, notably staphylococci, *N. meningiditis*, *H. influenzae*, and *Legionella pneumophila*. It is:

- The drug of choice for eliminating the nasal carriage state of *N. meningiditis*, *H. influenzae* type b, and *S. aureus*.
- Sometimes used as a second antistaphylococcal agent in combination with a β lactam or vancomycin in the treatment of serious staphylococcal infections, particularly endocarditis and osteomyelitis.
- Sometimes added as a second agent to erythromycin in the treatment of severe legionnaires' disease.

Rifampin may cause hepatotoxicity, a 'flu-like' syndrome, or fever (drug fever).

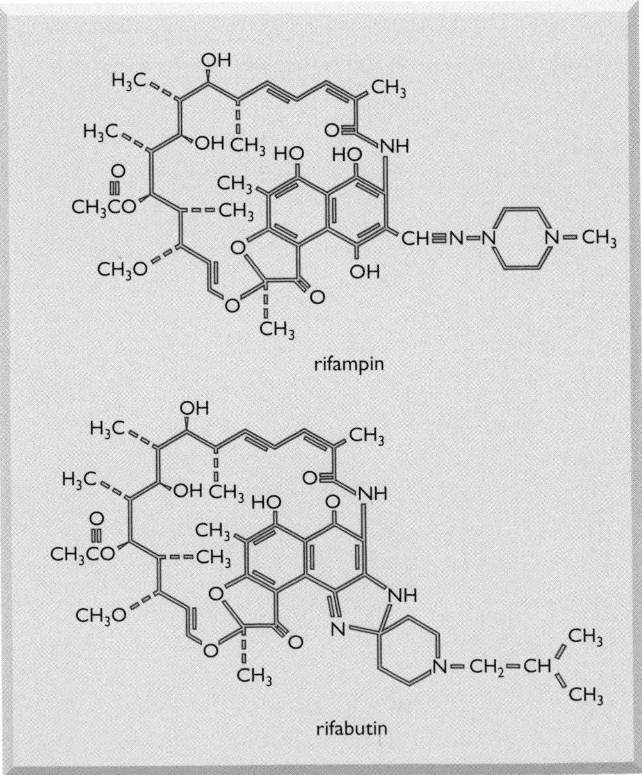

Fig. 23.27 Chemical structures of the rifamycins rifampin and rifabutin.

Rifampin is a potent inducer of hepatic microsomal enzymes

Rifampin is a potent inducer of hepatic microsomal enzymes. As a result, the metabolism of many other drugs is increased. Such drugs include glucocorticosteroids, oral contraceptives, quinidine, phenytoin, barbiturates, theophylline, clarithromycin, ketoconazole, itraconazole, cyclosporine, and warfarin.

Rifabutin Rifabutin is active against most strains of *M. tuberculosis,* including 30% of the strains that are resistant to rifampin. It is significantly more active than rifampin against *M. avium* complex and is effective as a single agent in the prevention of *M. avium* complex bacteremia in patients with AIDS. It is also useful as part of a multidrug combination in the treatment of established *M. avium* complex infection.

Although there is much more clinical experience with rifampin, rifabutin is useful in the treatment of tuberculosis as part of a multidrug regimen.

Rifabutin is available only as an oral formulation.

In comparison with rifampin, rifabutin causes less hepatic microsomal enzyme induction, so the magnitude of the drug interactions (see above) are less than those that occur with rifampin.

Rifabutin can cause a reversible uveitis, particularly when it is used in combination with clarithromycin, which is known to increase the serum concentration of both rifabutin and rifabutin's biologically active metabolite. The antifungal drug fluconazole and the human immunodeficiency virus (HIV) protease inhibitors indinavir and ritonavir also increase serum rifabutin concentrations.

PABA
sulfonamides or sulfones
DHPS
folic acid
precursors
trimethoprim (or pyrimethamine or trimetrexate)
DHFR
folinic acid
DNA
purines

Fig. 23.28 The folate biosynthetic pathway. Sulfonamides and sulfones compete with *para*-aminobenzoic acid (PABA) for dihydropteroate synthetase (DHPS). Trimethoprim and the antiprotozoal drugs pyrimethamine and trimetrexate inhibit dihydrofolate reductase (DHFR).

ANTIFOLATES

Folates are necessary cofactors in the synthesis of purines, and consequently of DNA. Although mammalian cells can use exogenous preformed folate, bacteria must synthesize their own from *para*-aminobenzoic acid (PABA). The folate synthetic pathway is outlined in Fig. 23.28. This pathway can be antagonized at two steps, by inhibition of either dihydropteroate synthetase (DHPS) or dihydrofolate reductase (DHFR).

Sulfonamides

Sulfonamides were developed in the 1930s as the first modern anti-infective drugs. These agents compete with PABA (Figs 23.28, 23.29) for DHPS, thereby inhibiting folate synthesis. Their effect is bacteriostatic. Acquired resistance can occur as a result of:

- Decreased permeability.
- Increased PABA production.
- Altered DHPS for which the drugs lack affinity.

Although many sulfonamides were once produced, the use of sulfonamides alone is no longer recommended, owing to the relatively high rates of bacterial resistance and the availability of superior antibiotics. Few laboratories routinely perform susceptibility testing of clinical isolates to sulfonamides alone. However, sulfonamides can be used alone in the treatment of infections due to *Nocardia* species, since the addition of a DHFR antagonist does not improve the activity against these organisms. Ophthalmic preparations of sulfacetamide are useful in the treatment of bacterial conjunctivitis.

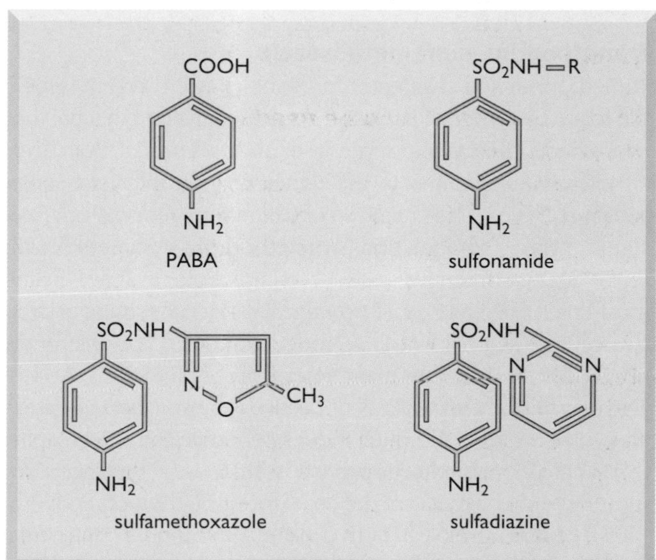

Fig. 23.29 Chemical structures of *para*-aminobenzoic acid (PABA) and sulfonamides. Note the similarity between PABA and sulfonamide drugs, which compete for the same bacterial enzyme, dihydropteroate synthetase (DHPS).

Sulfonamides are perhaps the most allergenic of antibiotics

Sulfonamide allergy is most frequently manifest as a diffuse pruritic maculopapular rash. The risk of an allergic reaction with sulfonamides is substantially greater in people infected with HIV. Rarely, sulfonamides can cause Stevens–Johnson syndrome or toxic epidermal necrolysis, both of which are life-threatening desquamating skin disorders. Of all the drugs that can cause toxic epidermal necrolysis, sulfonamides carry the highest risk.

Sulfones

Sulfones are synthetic agents related to sulfonamides and also compete with PABA for DHPS. The only commercially available sulfone is diaminodiphenyl sulfone (DDS), which is better known as dapsone.

Dapsone is active against most strains of *M. leprae*, but few conventional bacteria. It is used as part of a multidrug regimen for the treatment of leprosy. It can also be used in the prevention and treatment of *Pneumocystis carinii* pneumonia and in the treatment of some noninfectious skin diseases such as dermatitis herpetiformis.

There is only partial cross-allergenicity between sulfonamides and sulfones.

Dihydrofolate reductase inhibitors

Of the three DHFR inhibitors available to treat human infections (i.e. trimethoprim, pyrimethamine, and trimetrexate), only trimethoprim is useful for bacterial infections. Trimethoprim is a bacteriostatic agent and is active against many Enterobacteriaceae. It is excreted unchanged in the urine and, as it enters the prostate in therapeutic concentrations, it is useful in the treatment of chronic bacterial prostatitis. Trimethoprim can be used alone in the treatment of urinary tract infection and may be useful in individuals who are allergic to sulfonamides. More often, trimethoprim is used in combination with sulfamethoxazole (see below).

Trimethoprim–sulfamethoxazole

Trimethoprim and sulfamethoxazole block two different steps of the folate biosynthetic pathway. When used in combination, their antibacterial effect is often synergistic and bactericidal. Both drugs are excreted unchanged by the kidney. Because they have similar serum half-lives, their relative concentrations remain fairly constant. The combination trimethoprim–sulfamethoxazole (TMP–SMZ), sometimes called cotrimoxazole, is active against most Enterobacteriaceae, *H. influenzae*, and many strains of streptococci and staphylococci. At concentrations achievable in the urine, TMP–SMZ inhibits many enterococci. TMP–SMZ is also very active against *P. carinii*. It is not active against *P. aeruginosa* or anaerobic bacteria. Although it does penetrate the cerebrospinal fluid, there is only limited experience with its use in meningitis, and therefore other agents are preferred for this indication.

TMP–SMZ is available in both oral and intravenous formulations.

Therapeutic indications TMP–SMZ:

- Is a very important drug for the treatment of urinary tract infection, and is usually the drug of choice for urinary tract infections caused by susceptible bacteria.
- Can also be used to treat infections caused by susceptible organisms at other body sites.
- Is the drug of choice for the prevention and treatment of P. carinii pneumonia.
- May be useful for acute exacerbations of chronic bronchitis, shigellosis, and enteric fever.

MISCELLANEOUS ANTIBACTERIAL DRUGS

Nitrofurantoin

Nitrofurantoin is a synthetic nitrofuran and is used exclusively for the treatment of urinary tract infection. Its mechanism of action is unknown. It is active against most Enterobacteriaceae and enterococci, but not *P. aeruginosa*.

Nitrofurantoin is available only as an oral formulation. It is almost completely absorbed, after which approximately two-thirds are rapidly metabolized in the tissues with about one-third excreted unchanged in the urine. Blood concentrations of nitrofurantoin are very low and inadequate to treat infection, but urinary and renal concentrations are relatively high and sufficient to treat urinary tract infections. Nitrofurantoin does not enter the prostate in adequate concentration to treat chronic bacterial prostatitis. Because the activity of nitrofurantoin is reduced in an alkaline pH, it is not suitable for treating urinary tract infections due to *Proteus* species since this genus produces urease, which reduces urea to ammonium, thereby alkalinizing the urine.

Nitrofurantoin may be useful in the treatment of urinary tract infections in patients who have allergies and/or intolerance to both sulfonamides and β lactams, but trimethoprim alone and fluoroquinolones are also options for such patients. Nitrofurantoin should never be used to treat a urinary tract infection if there is any possibility of a concomitant bacteremia, because of its lack of therapeutic serum concentrations.

Adverse effects With prolonged use, nitrofurantoin can cause peripheral neuropathy and pulmonary fibrosis.

Mupirocin

Mupirocin is a unique agent, binding to bacterial isoleucyl–tRNA synthetase and preventing incorporation of isoleucine into the protein chains of the bacterial cell wall. It is available only as a topical formulation and is active against streptococci and staphylococci, with predominantly bactericidal activity. Acquired resistance is uncommon and due to altered isoleucyl-tRNA synthetase.

Mupirocin ointment is useful in the treatment of impetigo, folliculitis, secondarily infected burns, infected lacerations, and infected skin ulcers, as well as for eradicating nasal carriage of *S. aureus*.

ANTIMYCOBACTERIAL DRUGS

The rifamycins, aminoglycosides, fluoroquinolones, dapsone, and the two newer macrolides clarithromycin and azithromycin noted above, all have a role to play in the treatment of mycobacterial infections. There are three additional agents with activity restricted to mycobacterial infections that are important first-line drugs in the treatment of *M. tuberculosis* infection: isoniazid, pyrazinamide, and ethambutol (Fig. 23.30).

Isoniazid

Isoniazid (isonicotinic acid hydrazine, INH) is a critical drug in the treatment of tuberculosis. Mycobacteria differ from conventional bacteria in having a cell wall that contains large quantities of lipid. One of the most important lipid constituents of mycobacteria is mycolic acid. Isoniazid inhibits the synthesis of mycolic acid and is predominantly bactericidal against *M. tuberculosis*. It has relatively poor activity against nontuberculous mycobacteria.

Isoniazid is well absorbed orally and is metabolized in the liver by acetylation. It achieves concentrations in the cerebrospinal fluid sufficient to treat tuberculous meningitis.

Isoniazid is a cornerstone drug in the treatment of tuberculosis

In general, the treatment of active tuberculosis requires a combination of isoniazid plus rifampin, plus at least one other antimycobacterial drug until susceptibility results are available. Many experts choose to start with four antimycobacterial drugs pending susceptibility results, to minimize the risk of acquired resistance. In addition, an important principle of modern antituberculous therapy is the use of directly observed therapy whereby the ingestion of every dose of antituberculous medication is witnessed by a health care worker.

Individuals with positive tuberculin skin tests (indicative of tuberculosis infection) in whom active tuberculosis is excluded are treated with isoniazid alone (i.e. INH preventive therapy) to prevent the development of active tuberculosis.

Isoniazid causes hepatitis and peripheral neuropathy

Isoniazid causes hepatitis, the risk of which increases with age and underlying liver disease. It may also cause a peripheral neuropathy, particularly in malnourished individuals. This peripheral neuropathy can be prevented or reversed by pyridoxine administration.

Isoniazid can also cause drug fever and increases serum concentrations of phenytoin.

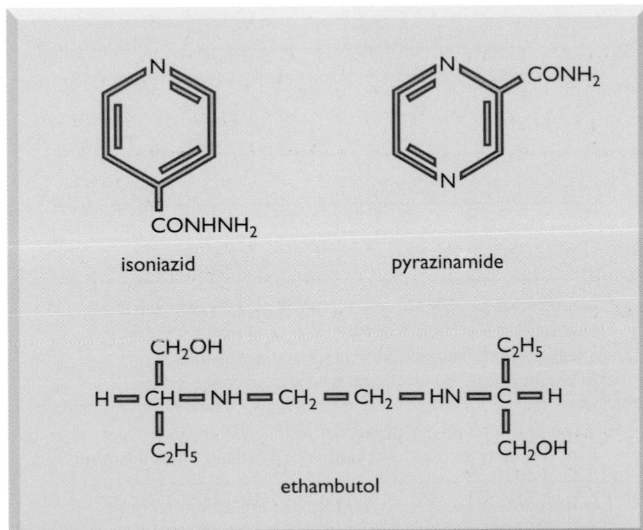

Fig. 23.30 Chemical structures of isoniazid, ethambutol, and pyrazinamide. All these agents are first-line drugs for the treatment of tuberculosis.

Pyrazinamide

Pyrazinamide (PZA) is a synthetic analog of nicotinamide with bactericidal activity against *M. tuberculosis* and is commonly used together with isoniazid and rifampin as a first-line agent. It is a prodrug that must be converted by pyrazinamidase present in *M. tuberculosis* to pyrazinoic acid, which acts against intracellular organisms. It is not useful for other mycobacterial species. PZA is available only as an oral formulation and is metabolized in the liver.

Pyrazinamide can be hepatotoxic and cause hyperuricemia

PZA can be hepatotoxic but, curiously, there is no increased hepatotoxicity of a regimen consisting of isoniazid, rifampin, and PZA compared with a regimen of isoniazid and rifampin without PZA. PZA also causes hyperuricemia, but rarely leads to acute gouty arthritis.

Ethambutol

Ethambutol is an oral drug and is bacteriostatic against *M. tuberculosis* and several other slow-growing mycobacteria. Its precise mechanism of action is not known, but it is believed to inhibit bacterial RNA synthesis. It is primarily excreted by the kidneys.

Ethambutol is never used alone, but is used in combination with other drugs in the treatment of disease due to *M. tuberculosis* and several nontuberculous mycobacterial species, particularly *M. avium* complex, *M. kansasii*, and *M. marinum*.

Ethambutol can cause retrobulbar neuritis

Ethambutol is usually very well tolerated, but a unique toxicity is retrobulbar neuritis, which is usually manifest first as red–green color blindness and later as reduced visual acuity. The risk of this adverse effect is both dose and time dependent. Baseline and serial visual acuity and color perception tests should be performed when long-term ethambutol therapy is anticipated.

Other antituberculous drugs

In cases of multidrug-resistant *M. tuberculosis* or if there are allergies, intolerance, or contraindications to the use of the main antituberculous drugs, second-line antituberculous drugs may need to be used. These include:

- Capreomycin and viomycin, which are parenteral polypeptide antibiotics.
- Ethionamide, an oral drug that is chemically related to isoniazid.
- Cycloserine, an oral drug that inhibits cell wall synthesis but causes considerable central nervous system toxicity.
- *para*-Aminosalicylic acid, an oral PABA analog that inhibits DHPS and is similar to sulfonamides and sulfones.
- Clofazimine, an oral agent, that has a role in the treatment of leprosy.

ANTIBIOTICS OF CHOICE

The principles of antibiotic selection have been outlined in the first part of this chapter. Bacterial, host, and drug factors all need to be taken into account. Two patients infected with the identical organism may require different antibiotics because of:

- Differences in the site of infection.
- Drug allergies.
- Underlying illness.
- Concomitant drug therapy.
- Age.
- Pregnancy status.

In the absence of allergies, pregnancy, underlying illness, and potential drug interactions, there are often accepted antibiotics of choice for common bacterial infections, and the appropriate antibiotic choices for selected common pathogens are presented in Fig. 23.31.

Adverse effects of antibiotics

- Nearly all can cause *Clostridium difficile* enteritis
- Aminoglycosides can cause nephrotoxicity and ototoxicity
- Chloramphenicol can cause irreversible aplastic anemia and the gray baby syndrome
- Sulfonamides can cause a skin rash, Stevens–Johnson syndrome, and toxic epidermal necrolysis
- Tetracycline can discolor the teeth if given to children under eight years of age

Drugs of choice and alternatives for selected common bacterial pathogens

Bacterium	Drug(s) of choice	Alternatives	Comments
Streptococcus species	Penicillin	First-generation cephalosporin Erythromycin Clindamycin Vancomycin	A few strains are penicillin resistant, especially some *S. pneumoniae* Erythromycin is only for mild infections Vancomycin is only for serious infections
Enterococcus species	Penicillin or ampicillin plus gentamicin	Vancomycin plus gentamicin	There are some strains for which streptomycin is synergistic but gentamicin is not Some strains are resistant to synergy with any aminoglycoside
Staphylococcus species	Antistaphylococcal penicillin	First-generation cephalosporin Vancomycin	Vancomycin is required for methicillin-resistant strains Rifampin is occasionally used to eradicate the nasal carriage state
Neisseria meningitidis	Penicillin	Chloramphenicol Third-generation cephalosporin	Rare strains are penicillin resistant
Neisseria gonorrhoeae	Cefixime	Ciprofloxacin Third-generation cephalosporin	Some strains are fluoroquinolone resistant (especially in Asia)
Bordetella pertussis	Erythromycin	TMP–SMZ	
Pasteurella multocida	Penicillin	First-generation cephalosporin	
Haemophilus influenzae	Aminopenicillin	Cefuroxime Third generation cephalosporins Chloramphenicol	Approximately 30% are aminopenicillin-resistant; therefore aminopenicillins should not be used empirically in serious infections until susceptibility results are available Rifampin is used to eradicate the nasal carriage state
Enterobacteriaceae in urine	TMP–SMZ	Ciprofloxacin Gentamicin	β Lactams are less effective than TMP–SMZ or fluoroquinolones for the treatment of urinary tract infection
Enterobacteriaceae in cerebrospinal fluid	Third-generation cephalosporin	TMP–SMZ	In neonates only, aminoglycosides are equivalent to third generation cephalosporins Experience with TMP–SMZ in meningitis is limited

Fig. 23.31 Drugs of choice and alternatives for selected common bacterial pathogens. (Continued over.)

Drugs of choice and alternatives for selected common bacterial pathogens (*continued*)

Bacterium	Drug(s) of choice	Alternatives	Comments
Enterobacteriaceae elsewhere (blood, lung, etc.)	Gentamicin or third-generation cephalosporins or ciprofloxacin	TMP–SMZ	Two-drug therapy is sometimes used in serious infection Monotherapy with a third-generation cephalosporin should be avoided if the pathogen is *Enterobacter cloacae, E. aerogenes, Serratia marcescens* or *Citrobacter freundii*
Pseudomonas aeruginosa	Antipseudomonal penicillin plus aminoglycoside	Ceftazidime Ciprofloxacin	Two-drug therapy recommended except for urinary tract infection
Bacteroides fragilis	Metronidazole or clindamycin	Imipenem Penicillin β lactamase inhibitors	*B. fragilis* is usually involved in polymicrobial infections; therefore another antibiotic active against Enterobacteriaceae is often required
Mycoplasma pneumoniae	A macrolide (e.g. erythromycin)	Tetracycline	Although tetracyclines are as effective as macrolides, the latter are recommended because of better activity against *Pneumococcus*, which can mimic this infection
Ureaplasma urealyticum	Tetracycline	Erythromycin	A few strains are tetracycline resistant
Mycoplasma hominis	Tetracycline	Clindamycin	Erythromycin is not active against *M. hominis*
Chlamydia trachomatis	Tetracycline	Azithromycin Erythromycin	Azithromycin is the only therapy effective in a single dose Erythromycin is used in pregnancy
Rickettsial species	Tetracycline	Chloramphenicol	
Listeria monocytogenes	Ampicillin plus gentamicin	Vancomycin plus gentamicin	
Legionella species	Erythromycin	Tetracycline	Rifampin is occasionally used as a second agent in severe cases
Clostridium difficile	Metronidazole	Vancomycin (oral)	
Mycobacterium tuberculosis	Isoniazid plus rifampin plus pyrazinamide plus ethambutol	Streptomycin Fluoroquinolones Ethionamide Cycloserine Viomycin Capreomycin	Directly observed therapy (DOT) is recommended Isoniazid is used alone for preventive therapy
Mycobacterium avium complex	Clarithromycin plus ethambutol ± rifabutin	Ciprofloxacin Amikacin	
Mycobacterium leprae	Dapsone plus rifampin ± clofazimine	Clarithromycin	Thalidomide is useful for erythema nodosum leprosum

Fig. 23.31 Drugs of choice and alternatives for selected common bacterial pathogens (*continued*).

FURTHER READING

Kaye D (ed.) Antibacterial therapy: *in vitro* testing, pharmacodynamics, pharmacology, new agents. *Infect Dis Clin North Am* 1995; **9(3)**: 463–810. [Essentially a small textbook on antibacterial therapy.]

Levy SB. *The Antibiotic Paradox: How Miracle Drugs are Destroying the Miracle.* New York: Plenum Publishing Corp; 1992. [A more detailed account written for the educated layperson about global antibiotic resistance.]

Levy SB. Confronting multidrug resistance. A role for each of us. *JAMA* 1993; **269**: 1840–1842. [A brief overview of the problem of global antibiotic resistance.]

Mandell GI, Bennett JE, Dolin R (eds) *Mandell, Douglas and Bennett's Principles and Practice of Infectious Diseases. 4th edn.,* New York: Churchill Livingstone; 1995. [An excellent and comprehensive textbook for the discipline of infectious diseases.]

Nell HC. The crisis in antibiotic resistance. *Science* 1992; **257**: 1064–1073. [This article gives a historic overview of the most common types of antibiotic resistance over time.]

Make a provisional diagnosis and determine a rational pharmacologic treatment for the following hypothetical case.

A four-year-old boy is brought to the emergency department of your hospital with a two-day history of fever, lethargy, headache and poor appetite. Physical examination reveals marked nuchal rigidity, a temperature of 39.7°C, but no focal neurologic deficits.

1. Would you diagnose a viral infection and advise the parents that the illness will resolve over the next few days without intervention? Explain your answer.
2. Would you prescribe antibiotic therapy without further information? Explain your answer.
3. Would you perform a complete blood count, collect blood for culture, and cerebrospinal fluid for examinations including culture? Explain your answer.
4. If this child's cerebrospinal fluid is cloudy, would you await initial laboratory results before starting antibiotics or start antibiotic therapy at once? Explain your answer.
5. If you start antibiotic therapy at once or if the cerebrospinal fluid Gram stain shows no organisms, which antibiotic would you use?
6. Would you use the same antibiotic if the child had previously had anaphylactic reaction to amoxicillin and, if not, what would be the alternative?
7. If the cerebrospinal fluid grew *Streptococcus pneumoniae* with a high level of resistance to penicillin (MIC > 2.0 mg/ml), what would be the treatment of choice?

Indicate which is the correct answer for each question.

1. Which of the following antibiotics demonstrate concentration-dependent killing of bacteria?
a) penicillin G
b) amoxicillin
c) cefotaxime
d) gentamicin
e) vancomycin

2. The treatment of choice for serious infections due to methicillin-resistant *Staphylococcus aureus* is
a) cloxacillin
b) cefazolin
c) clindamycin
d) chloramphenicol
e) vancomycin

3. The addition of clavulanate to amoxicillin results in activity against all the following β lactamase-producing organisms, except
a) *Enterobacter cloacae*
b) *Staphylococcus aureus*
c) *Haemophilus influenzae*
d) *Neisseria gonorrhoeae*
e) *Bacteroides fragilis*

4. An oral drug that is effective for the treatment of urinary tract infections due to *Pseudomonas aeruginosa* is
a) amoxicillin
b) cefixime
c) ciprofloxacin
d) gentamicin
e) ceftazidime

5. All the following statements about erythromycin are true, except
a) it produces a relatively high incidence of gastrointestinal toxicity
b) it is an alternative to penicillin for treating pneumococcal meningitis
c) in combination with terfenadine it can cause ventricular tachycardia
d) it is an alternative to penicillin for streptococcal pharyngitis
e) it is the drug of choice for legionnaires' disease

6. All the following antibiotics are active against *Bacteroides fragilis*, except
a) metronidazole
b) clindamycin
c) amoxicillin–clavulanate
d) trimethoprim–sulfamethoxazole
e) imipenem

7. Tetracyclines
a) are considered safe in pregnancy
b) are recommended in infancy
c) should be given with antacids
d) are active against *Pseudomonas aeruginosa*
e) are useful in the treatment of chlamydial infections

8. All of the following antibiotic drug combinations result in significant drug interactions, except
a) erythromycin and astemizole
b) clindamycin and phenytoin
c) ciprofloxacin and theophylline
d) rifampin and warfarin
e) tetracycline and sucralfate

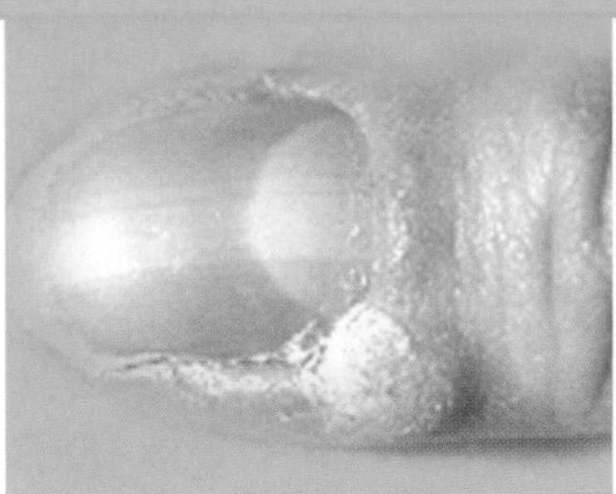

24. Viral Infections

BIOLOGY AND DRUG RESPONSIVENESS OF VIRUSES

Viral infections can involve any part of the body. Most are asymptomatic. Symptomatic infection can range from a short benign illness such as the common cold to a protracted lethal infection such as that caused by human immunodeficiency virus, type 1 (HIV-1).

Symptoms and signs are due to a variety of host responses

Host responses to viral infections range from acute inflammation (e.g. meningoencephalitis) to hypertrophy and hyperplasia (e.g. warts) and oncogenesis (e.g. human T-cell lymphotropic virus-1 leukemia).

The inflammatory response evoked by cell lysis usually terminates viral replication and leads to recovery from the infection. In contrast, an impaired host immune response can be associated with a prolonged and more severe illness. Occasionally, the normal host immune response is pathogenetic and causes disease manifestations (e.g. in dengue hemorrhagic fever). Rarely, virus replication causes little or no inflammatory reaction, but nevertheless the infection is fatal (e.g. rabies).

Viruses can be selectively inhibited by drugs

Selective inhibition of viruses by drugs depends upon either:

- Inhibition of unique steps in the viral replication pathways, such as adsorption of the virus to a cell receptor, penetration, uncoating, assembly, and release.
- Preferential inhibition of steps shared with the host cell, which include transcription and translation.

The potential therapeutic efficacy of an antiviral drug can be evaluated *in vitro*; however, *in vitro* susceptibility testing of viruses to drugs, either singly or in combination, is less predictive than similar testing for bacteriologic sensitivity to antimicrobials. Lack of standardized *in vitro* testing and insufficient knowledge of the pharmacokinetic–pharmacodynamic relationships preclude rigorous interpretations of associations between drug concentrations and their antiviral effect.

Antiviral drugs are effective against some common viral infections

Antiviral chemotherapy is effective for infections caused by:

- Herpesviruses.
- Influenza A virus.
- Respiratory syncytial virus.
- Hepatitis viruses.
- Papilloma virus.
- The arenavirus of Lassa fever.
- HIV-1.

The development of resistance often limits the usefulness of these agents. A reduction or loss of antiviral susceptibility *in vitro* may be associated with pharmacotherapeutic failure. Such antiviral resistance has been reported during therapy with all currently available antiviral drugs except ribavirin and sorivudine.

Drug-resistance in viruses is due to development of nucleotide mutations. Occasionally, such mutant strains are still susceptible to other antiviral drugs. Sometimes, the emergence of resistant strains can be minimized by using combination therapy, as demonstrated by the use of multidrug therapy for HIV-1 infection.

Successful antiviral chemotherapy depends upon host immunocompetence

Currently available antiviral drugs are virustatic only. Removal of the drug from an *in vitro* test system is invariably followed by viral replication. This contrasts with the situation in bacteriology and mycology where cell-wall active agents such as the β-lactam antibiotics (e.g. penicillins) and antifungal agents (e.g. amphotericin B), respectively, can kill all organisms in a test system and produce a clinical cure with a minimal contribution from the host's defense system. In viral infections, an intact host immune response is essential to obtain a clinical cure.

HERPESVIRUS INFECTIONS

There are seven human herpesviruses (HHV) and these cause a wide spectrum of illness (Fig. 24.1). An eighth, HHV-8, has been proposed recently as the cause of Kaposi's sarcoma and deep body cavity lymphoma in patients with HIV-1 infection.

Except for varicella (chickenpox) due to varicella zoster virus (VZV), the majority of initial infections are asymptomatic. Epstein–Barr virus (EBV), and perhaps HHV-8, are oncogenic. EBV can transform B lymphocytes *in vitro* and cause B-lymphocytoproliferative disease in immunosuppressed hosts with diminished tumor surveillance capacity. This may respond to antiviral therapy.

Some initial and recurrent infections respond to chemotherapy

Initial infections caused by herpes simplex virus type 1 (HSV-1), HSV-2, VZV, and EBV respond to antiviral therapy, but this does not prevent the development of latent infection. As a consequence, herpesviruses cannot be eradicated. Reactivation of

Commonest diseases caused by human herpesviruses

Herpesvirus	Initial	Recurrent
Herpes simplex virus, type 1	Gingivostomatitis	Orolabial herpes-'cold sores'
Herpes simplex virus, type 2	Vulvovaginitis and penile ulceration	Genital herpes
Varicella zoster virus	Chickenpox	Zoster (shingles)
Cytomegalovirus	Congenital CMV inclusion disease	Retinitis in HIV-1 infection
Epstein–Barr virus	Infectious mononucleosis	None
Human herpesvirus 6	Exanthem subitum	None
Human herpesvirus 7	?Exanthem subitum	None
Human herpesvirus 8†	Kaposi sarcoma in HIV-1 infection	None

†New proposed human herpesvirus

Fig. 24.1 Diseases caused by human herpesviruses.

latent infection causes a spectrum of disorders ranging from asymptomatic viral shedding to recurrent disease. Recurrent cold sores, genital herpes lesions, and shingles are relatively benign, but may be more severe and prolonged in hosts whose cell-mediated immunity is suppressed by drugs or disease. Reactivation-induced disease caused by herpesvirus often needs treatment with antiviral drugs.

Herpes simplex virus infections are acquired by direct contact with infectious exudate

Mucocutaneous infections (gingivostomatitis, vulvovaginitis, or anogenital infection), skin infection such as herpes gladiatorum and whitlow (around the fingernail), and keratitis (corneal infection), are the commonest manifestations. Occasionally, unilateral frontotemporal necrotizing encephalitis is the first manifestation of HSV-1 infection, probably due to virus that migrates centripetally through the cribiform plate via the ipsilateral olfactory nerve.

Neonates who develop HSV infection during vaginal delivery may acquire it from contact with the virus on the exocervix or in vulvar lesions. In two-thirds of these neonates, the infection disseminates hematogenously to cause visceral infections with a high mortality.

This wide spectrum of HSV infections has stimulated the development of topical and systemic drug treatments for HSV infections.

Varicella zoster virus infection is acquired by inhaling infectious respiratory secretions

Inhalation of infectious respiratory secretions from individuals with chickenpox leads to VZV infection evident as chickenpox or varicella. This results in a latent sensory ganglion infection, which on reactivation causes a vesicular dermatomal eruption called herpes zoster or shingles. Chickenpox and shingles can both be successfully treated with antiviral drugs.

TREATMENT

Antiherpes drugs can be classified as nucleoside analogs and nonnucleoside agents

The nucleoside analogs (Fig. 24.2), idoxuridine, trifluorothymidine and adenine-arabinoside are generally toxic and relatively ineffective by injection, but some can be used topically.

Topical drugs

Healing of herpes simplex virus keratitis is accelerated by topical antiviral agents

Idoxuridine (5-iodo-2'-deoxyuridine) applied to the cornea of patients with HSV keratitis accelerates healing of the epithelial ulcer, but its prolonged use causes epithelial dystrophy. Topical trifluorothymidine, adenine-arabinoside, and acyclovir have since been shown to be more effective and less toxic. However, only idoxuridine, adenine-arabinoside and trifluorothymidine are commercially available as topical ophthalmic formulations. Successful treatment requires frequent application of the antiviral drug solution or ointment to the eye. This is effective, but also increases the risk of adverse effects of the drug on corneal epithelial cells.

Topical idoxuridine, adenine-arabinoside and trifluorothymidine impair corneal ulcer healing to some extent during prolonged use. Additional adverse effects include conjunctivitis with pain and itching and, occasionally, allergic reactions.

Idoxuridine interferes with virus replication and cell metabolism

Idoxuridine is an iodinated thymidine analog that undergoes phosphorylation to yield the active triphosphate nucleotide. The precise role of 'viral' as opposed to 'cellular' thymidine kinases in this reaction is unclear. Idoxuridine triphosphate is incorporated as a thymidine substitute into both viral and cellular DNA, thereby interfering with virus replication and cell metabolism.

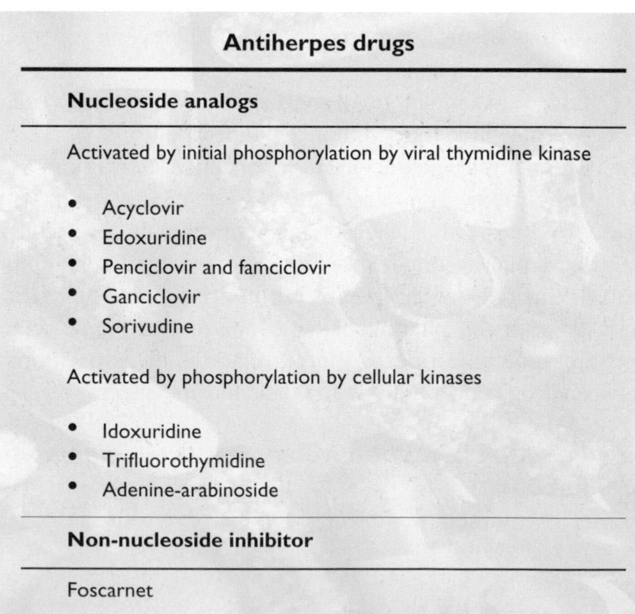

Antiherpes drugs

Nucleoside analogs

Activated by initial phosphorylation by viral thymidine kinase

- Acyclovir
- Edoxuridine
- Penciclovir and famciclovir
- Ganciclovir
- Sorivudine

Activated by phosphorylation by cellular kinases

- Idoxuridine
- Trifluorothymidine
- Adenine-arabinoside

Non-nucleoside inhibitor

Foscarnet

Fig. 24.2 Antiherpes drugs.

The effectiveness of idoxuridine applied topically to cutaneous herpesvirus infection is enhanced by dissolving it in dimethylsulfoxide (DMSO). Frequent application of idoxuridine in DMSO reduces the pain and shortens the healing time of herpes labialis and shingles. A less pronounced effect has been observed in patients with genital herpes. A solution of idoxuridine in DMSO applied to shingles lesions by brush or in gauze to keep it moist for up to three days not only hastens healing but also reduces post-herpetic neuralgia.

Adverse effects include mild local irritation, discomfort, and a garlic taste and body odor due to DMSO excretion in saliva and sweat.

Trifluorothymidine is incorporated into viral and cellular DNA to produce a faulty DNA structure

Trifluorothymidine is a fluorinated thymidine analog. It is activated by phosphorylation by cellular enzymes to its active triphosphate moiety, which inhibits HSV and CMV, including acyclovir-resistant HSV strains. It inhibits thymidylate synthetase and viral (and cellular) DNA polymerase, and is incorporated into viral and cellular DNA to produce a faulty DNA structure. Preclinical studies indicate that it is mutagenic and teratogenic.

Trifluorothymidine is available only for the topical treatment of HSV keratitis and primary keratoconjunctivitis (Fig. 24.3). It is the treatment of choice for these conditions.

Adverse effects include edema, burning, keratopathy, and occasionally allergic reactions.

Systemic drugs

Safe and effective systemic therapy for HHV infections has become possible as a result of the development of highly selective inhibitors of viral replication.

Adenine-arabinoside has been found to be significantly more effective than placebo for therapy of HSV-1 encephalitis and neonatal herpes. It is nontoxic, but needs to be infused in large volumes of solution, which can be potentially harmful in patients with encephalitis and cerebral swelling.

Acyclovir, a guanosine analog, has been shown to be a more effective treatment than adenine-arabinoside for HSV encephalitis; it is nontoxic and easier to give intravenously (Fig. 24.4). For the latter two reasons, it has replaced adenine-arabinoside for the treatment of neonates with HSV infection (Figs 24.5, 24.6).

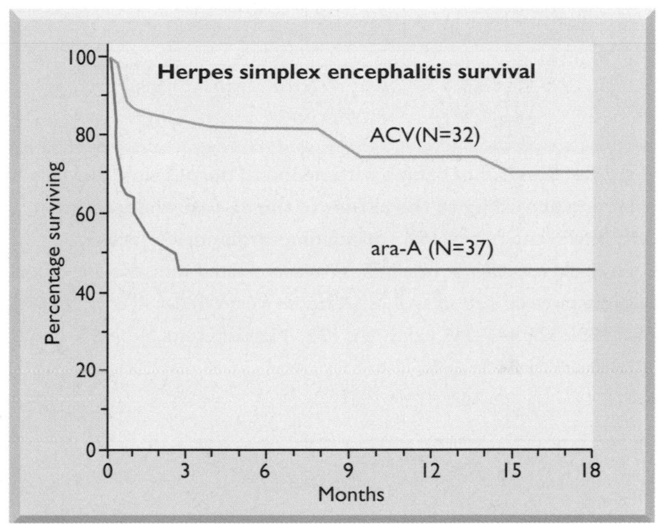

Fig. 24.4 Comparison of survival rates of patients with herpes simplex encephalitis treated with either intravenous acyclovir (ACV) or adenine-arabinoside (ara-A) for ten days. Acyclovir therapy was more effective than adenine-arabinoside (Adapted from Whitley RJ *et al.* *N Engl J Med* 1986; 314: 144–149. Copyright 1986. Massachusetts Medical Society. All rights reserved.)

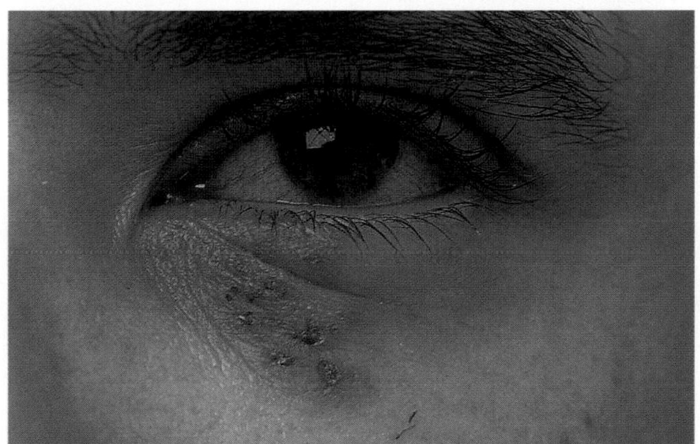

Fig. 24.3 Herpes simplex virus conjunctivitis. This resulted from spread of a contiguous infection of the cheek and lower lid. The infection responded to combined therapy with oral acyclovir and topical trifluorothymidine.

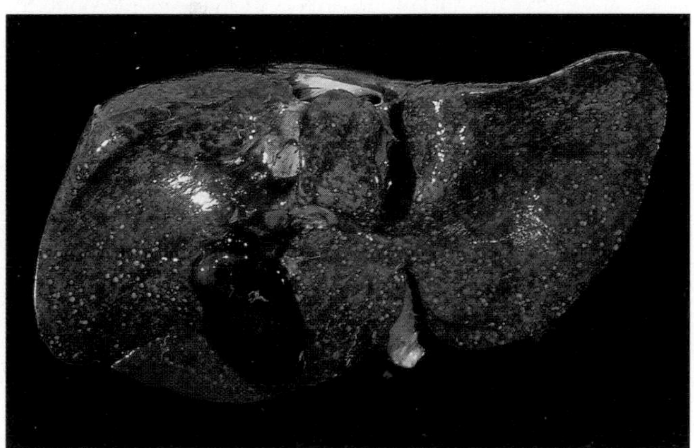

Fig. 24.5 Inferior surface of the liver of an infant who died of disseminated neonatal herpes simplex virus infection. The yellow areas are foci of hepatic necrosis caused by the virus.

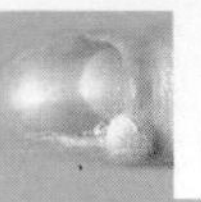

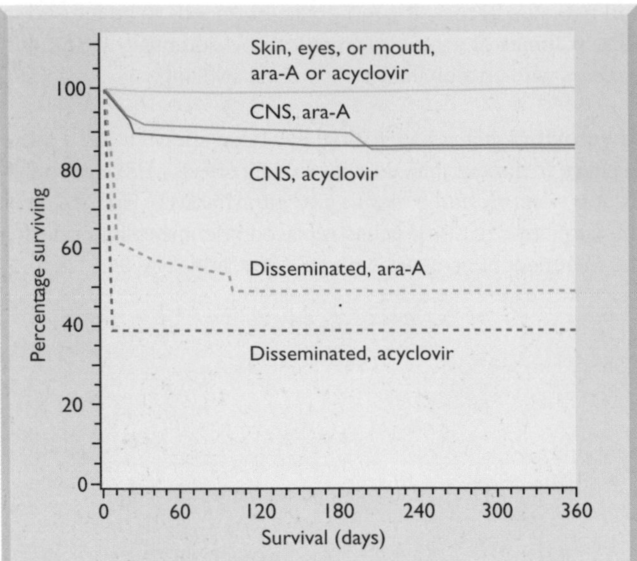

Fig. 24.6 Survival of babies with neonatal herpes simplex virus infection according to the extent of the disease and treatment with intravenous acyclovir or adenine-arabinoside (ara-A). Survival did not differ between those infants treated with acyclovir or ara-A in the three disease categories. (Adapted from Whitley RJ *et al. N Engl J Med* 1991; 324: 444–449. Copyright 1991. Massachusetts Medical Society. All rights reserved.)

Acyclovir belongs to a group of nucleoside inhibitors of herpesviruses that includes ganciclovir, edoxuridine, penciclovir, famciclovir, and sorivudine

These drugs are characterized by their selective phosphorylation by a viral thymidine kinase rather than host kinase as the first step of activation. Phosphorylation yields a triphosphate nucleotide that exerts the antiherpes effect. Acyclovir consists of guanine bound to an acyclic ribose molecule that lacks the 2' and 3' carbon molecules. Absence of the -OH group on the 3'-C molecule accounts for a large part of its antiherpes effect. *In vitro*, acyclovir is a potent inhibitor of HSV-1 and HSV-2, VZV, and EBV at concentrations that can be achieved in plasma with conventional doses.

Acyclovir selectively inhibits herpes simplex virus with a toxic:therapeutic ratio of 300–3000:1

The selectivity of acyclovir for HSV is due to three properties:

- First, it is selectively concentrated in virus-infected cells due to the catalytic action of the virus-encoded thymidine kinase enzyme (Fig. 24.7).
- Second, the active antiviral molecule, acyclovir triphosphate has a higher affinity for HSV than cellular DNA polymerase, resulting in selective competitive inhibition of the enzyme.
- Third, a complex forms between acyclovir triphosphate incorporated into the elongating DNA chain and the viral DNA polymerase that irreversibly inactivates the enzyme.

Acyclovir interferes with three steps in the herpes simplex virus DNA replicative cycle

The mechanism of action of acyclovir is interference with three steps in the HSV DNA replicative cycle:

- Acyclovir triphosphate competitively inhibits HSV DNA polymerase utilization of deoxyguanosinetriphosphate.
- Acyclovir triphosphate terminates elongation of the HSV DNA strand when incorporated as a guanosine analog substitute because absence of the 3'-OH group (see above) precludes formation of the 3'-5'-phosphodiester linkage needed to allow addition of the next nucleotide (Fig. 24.8).

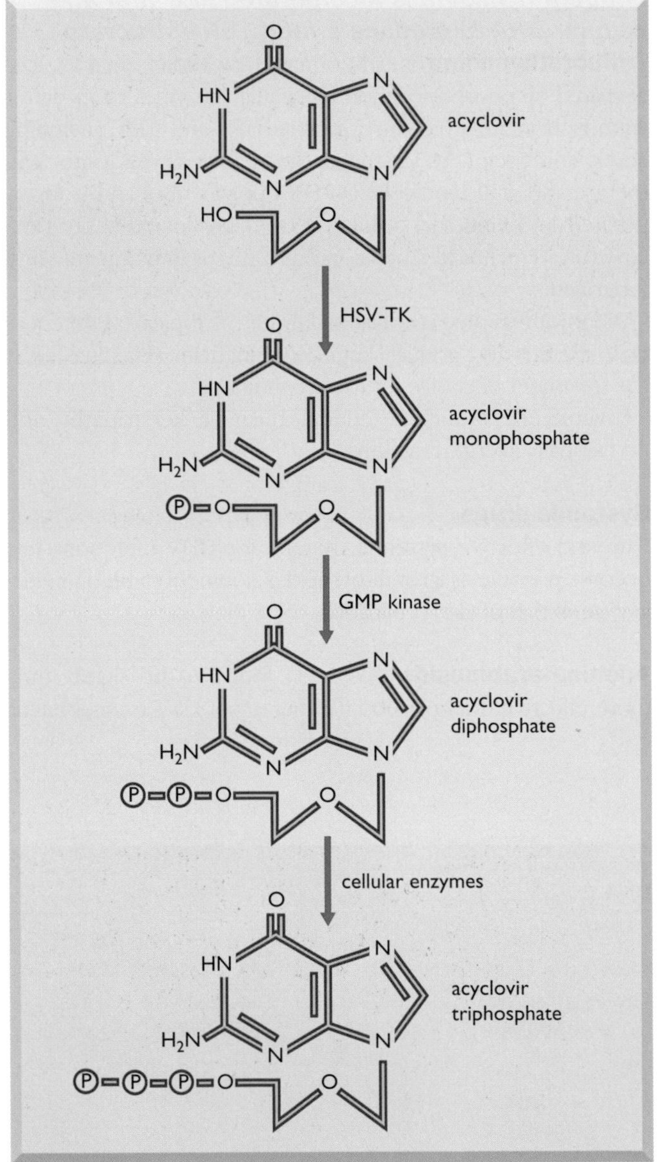

Fig. 24.7 Enzymatic conversion of acyclovir to its mono-, di-, and triphosphate forms. Herpes simplex virus thymidine kinase (HSV–TK) avidly catalyzes the formation of acyclovir monophosphate. Cellular kinases convert the monophosphate compound to the di- and triphosphate forms. Acyclovir triphosphate is the active antiviral moiety (Adapted from Elion GB. Mechanism of action and selectivity of acyclovir. *Am J Med* 1982: Acyclovir Symposium: 7–13.)

- HSV DNA polymerase is noncompetitively inhibited by forming a complex with acyclovir triphosphate on the DNA template.

Acyclovir is available in intravenous, oral, and topical, but not ophthalmic, formulations

Acyclovir is poorly absorbed from oral and topical skin formulations and is eliminated as unchanged drug by glomerular filtration and renal tubular secretion. Although dose-related adverse effects are uncommon, it is prudent to reduce intravenous doses in patients with renal disease to minimize potential adverse effects.

Pharmacologic bases for the selective inhibition of herpesvirus replication by acyclovir

- Selective concentration or trapping in infected cells due to avid phosphorylation by herpesvirus thymidine kinase
- Preferential affinity of acyclovir triphosphate for viral rather than cellular DNA polymerase
- Irreversible inactivation of viral DNA polymerase

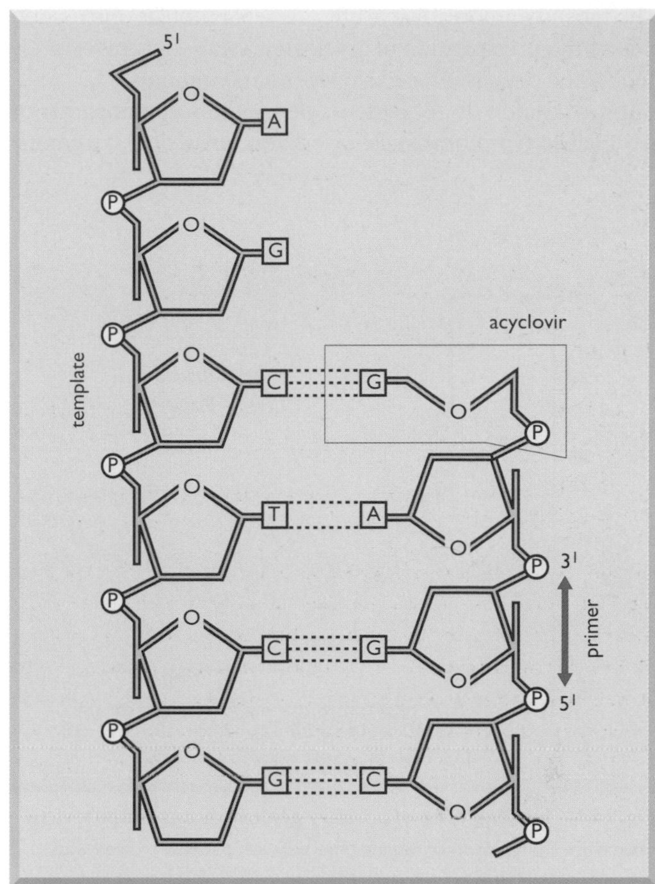

Fig. 24.8 Representation of acyclovir triphosphate termination of DNA chain elongation. Absence of the 3'-C molecule on the acyclic ribose molecule precludes formation of the 3'-5'-phosphodiester linkage needed to allow DNA chain elongation. (Adapted from Elion GB. Mechanism of action and selectivity of acyclovir. *Am J Med* 1982; Acyclovir Symposium: 7–13.)

The pharmacotherapeutic indications of acyclovir are as follows:

- Intravenous acyclovir is the drug of choice for severe HSV infection (see Figs 24.4, 24.6, 24.9–24.11).
- Oral acyclovir is effective for HSV mucocutaneous infections such as vulvovaginitis and gingivostomatitis (Fig. 24.12) and, in larger doses, for chickenpox and herpes zoster.
- Oral acyclovir accelerates the healing of herpetic whitlow, but not that of recurrent orolabial and genital HSV infections.
- Daily oral acyclovir tablets are dramatically effective in preventing recurrent genital and orolabial HSV infection (Fig. 24.13).

Acyclovir in cream and ointment formulations has different pharmacokinetic characteristics and pharmacotherapeutic effects. Acyclovir in cream penetrates the stratum corneum better than it does from the ointment; this is associated with a slightly greater therapeutic effect on cold sore healing. Oral or intravenous therapy is preferred for severe genital HSV infections because topical treatment has no effect on the systemic symptoms. Oral acyclovir produces only modest improvements in pain relief and healing compared to placebo. Overall, the role of topical acyclovir for treating herpes skin infections is limited.

The adverse effects of acyclovir are uncommon, mild, and reversible. Topical acyclovir ointment and cream may cause mild local discomfort when applied to ulcerated skin. Oral acyclovir is generally very well tolerated, but can cause nausea.

Intravenous acyclovir can cause local discomfort and phlebitis due to the alkalinity (pH 9–11) of the formulation.

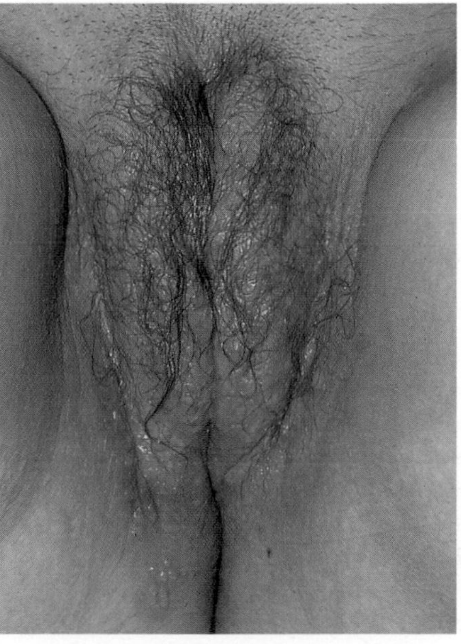

Fig. 24.9 Primary herpes simplex virus vulvovaginitis. Clusters of vesicles are visible on the labia and perineal skin.

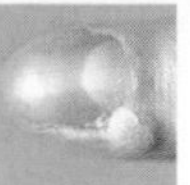

The most common adverse effect is renal tubular obstruction due to the precipitation of acyclovir crystals, but this is rarely seen if the drug is infused slowly over 60 minutes.

Approximately 1% of patients develop encephalopathic or psychiatric symptoms such as lethargy, drowsiness, tremors, confusion, hallucinations, seizures, or coma. These symptoms appear to be partly related to accumulation of acyclovir because they are most commonly seen in patients with renal failure. These symptoms also occur during therapy with adenine-arabinoside and ganciclovir.

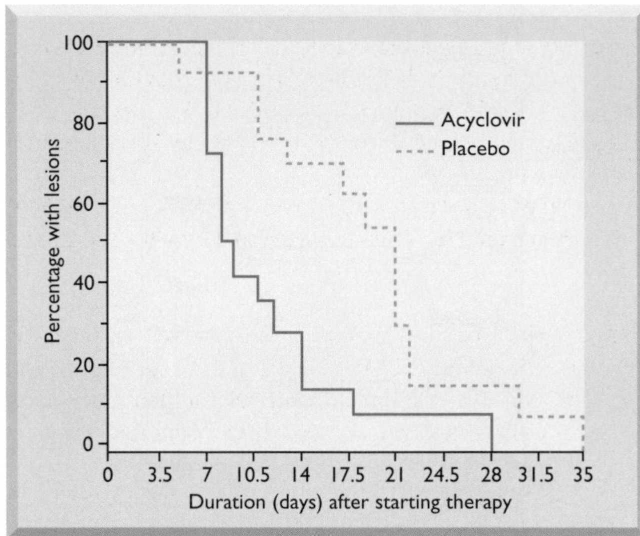

Fig. 24.10 Healing time of primary genital herpes simplex virus infection. Comparison of healing time between patients treated with intravenous acyclovir or placebo. (Adapted from Corey L *et al.* Intravenous acyclovir for the treatment of primary genital herpes. *Ann Int Med* 1983; 98: 914–921.)

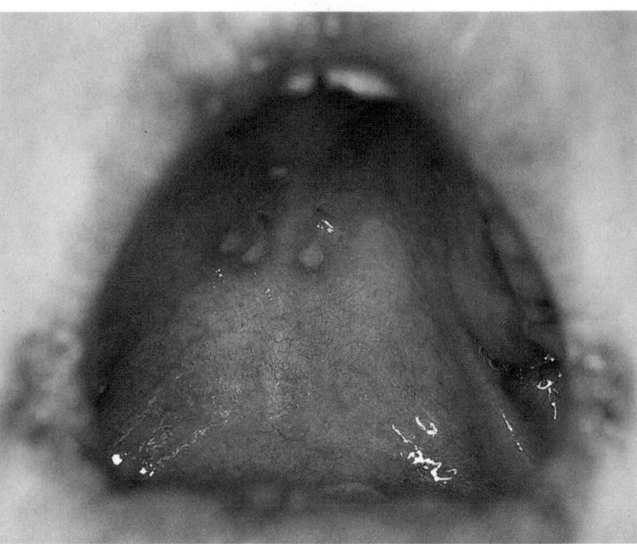

Fig. 24.12 Primary herpes simplex virus gingivostomatitis in a child. The infection responded to treatment with oral acyclovir.

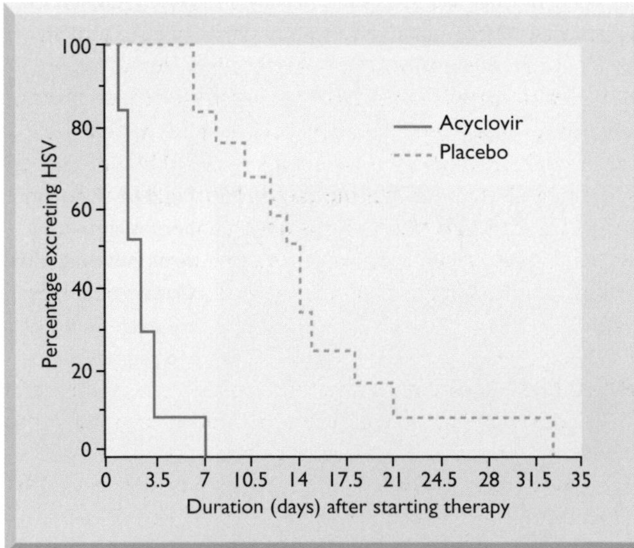

Fig. 24.11 Duration of shedding of herpes simplex virus from primary genital herpes simplex virus lesions. Comparison between patients treated with intravenous acyclovir or placebo. (Adapted from Corey L *et al.* Intravenous acyclovir for the treatment of primary genital herpes. *Ann Int Med* 1983; 98: 914–921.)

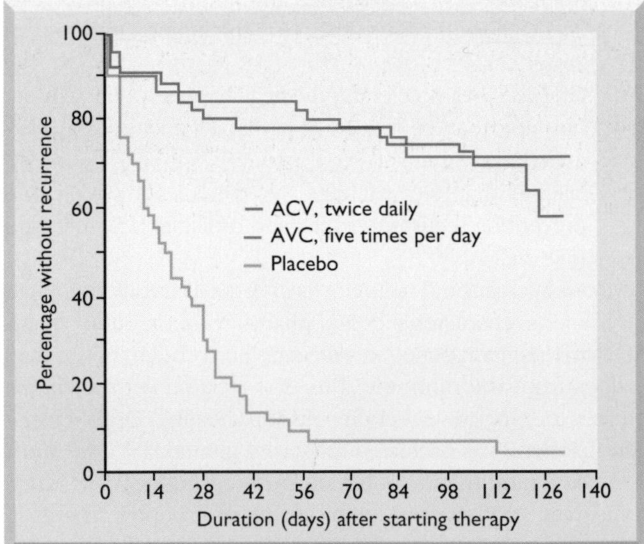

Fig. 24.13 The effect of acyclovir (ACV) and placebo ingested daily to prevent recurrence of genital herpes. The graph shows the duration before the development of recurrent genital herpes simplex virus infection in patients taking two or five acyclovir capsules or placebo daily for four months. (Adapted from Douglas JM *et al. N Engl J Med* 1984; 310: 1551–1556. Copyright 1984. Massachusetts Medical Society. All rights reserved.)

Acyclovir resistance has developed during prolonged use of acyclovir in immunocompromised patients

During prolonged use in immunocompromised patients, acyclovir-resistant HSV infections have been observed. Most acyclovir-resistant strains of HSV have lost the capacity to phosphorylate acyclovir owing to alterations in thymidine kinase. Thymidine kinase may be undetectable (thymidine kinase-negative strains). Less commonly, thymidine kinase may be detectable (thymidine kinase-positive strains), but possess an altered substrate affinity. Finally, rare mutants can have normal thymidine kinase activity, but altered DNA polymerase activity. Infection caused by thymidine kinase-negative or resistant thymidine kinase-positive strains are crossresistant to all other drugs that require thymidine kinase for activation.

Valacyclovir is a prodrug of acyclovir esterified with L-valine. Esterification increases the oral bioavailability of acyclovir fourfold. It is nearly completely converted to acyclovir by first-pass hydrolysis in the intestinal wall and liver, and so only acyclovir can be detected in the systemic circulation.

Valacyclovir appears to be as effective as acyclovir for treating HSV infections. However, its increased bioavailability probably accounts for its greater therapeutic effect compared with that of acyclovir in the treatment of shingles since VZV that causes shingles is approximately tenfold less susceptible to acyclovir than HSV.

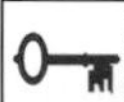

Mechanisms of action of the antiviral effect of acyclovir triphosphate

- Competitive inhibition of herpesvirus DNA polymerase
- Viral DNA chain termination
- Noncompetitive inhibition of herpesvirus DNA polymerase

Adenine-arabinoside is currently of limited therapeutic importance for herpesvirus infection. It is composed of the purine base adenine combined with a sugar, arabinose. *In vitro*, it inhibits:

- A wide range of DNA viruses including HSV, VZV, EBV, CMV, adenoviruses, vaccinia, and hepatitis B.
- A single RNA virus, Rous sarcoma virus.
- Strains of HSV and VZV resistant to acyclovir.

After intravenous administration, adenine-arabinoside is rapidly converted to arabinosyl-hypoxanthine, which is 30-fold less potent than adenine-arabinoside. Both moieties probably contribute to the antiviral effect by inhibiting DNA polymerase and causing chain termination after incorporation into DNA as an adenine substitute.

Adenine-arabinoside is an effective treatment for HSV and VZV infection but, at present, it is approved only for use:

- Parenterally to treat HSV encephalitis or neonatal HSV infection.
- Topically to treat HSV keratitis.

Although adenine-arabinoside is an effective treatment for acyclovir-resistant HSV infections, intravenous foscarnet is superior in producing more rapid lesion healing.

Edoxuridine is a nucleoside analog that preferentially inhibits HSV-2 more than HSV-1. The inhibitory concentration required *in vitro* is twofold less for HSV-2 than for HSV-1. Like acyclovir, edoxuridine is activated by viral thymidine kinase-initiated phosphorylation.

Edoxuridine is available as a 3% cream for the topical treatment of early recurrent HSV-2 genital infection during the prodromal stage.

Penciclovir is an acyclic guanosine derivative with potent activity against HSV, VZV, and EBV comparable to that of acyclovir. Like acyclovir, it is activated by intracellular phosphorylation initiated by viral thymidine kinase and has a similar mechanism of action.

Famciclovir is the diacetyl ester oral prodrug of penciclovir. Deacetylation and oxidation of famciclovir during its first-pass through the liver delivers approximately 70% of the ingested drug as penciclovir into the systemic circulation.

Penciclovir is 75% eliminated as unchanged drug into urine and 25% in feces as a deoxy metabolite with no antiviral activity. Doses need to be reduced in patients with moderate or severe renal insufficiency. Like acyclovir, penciclovir precipitates in renal tubules and causes renal obstruction when injected rapidly intravenously.

The therapeutic effect of famciclovir is similar to that of oral acyclovir tablets in initial and recurrent genital herpes infection and acute herpes zoster. Famciclovir given for ten days to patients with chronic hepatitis B virus infection reduces plasma hepatitis B virus DNA titres in 50% of patients. However, circulating hepatitis B virus DNA reappears within three weeks of stopping therapy so that the value of famciclovir in chronic hepatitis B virus infection remains uncertain.

Adverse effects of famciclovir are uncommon and mild: headache in 10%, nausea, diarrhea, and somnolence in less than 2%.

Sorivudine is a pyrimidine nucleoside analog that can inhibit VZV *in vitro* at concentrations more than 1000-fold lower than those required with acyclovir. It is only as potent as acyclovir against HSV-1. It is inactive against CMV and HSV-2, the latter being due to the lack of affinity of HSV-2 thymidine kinase for sorivudine.

Sorivudine is converted to its active triphosphate form by sequential phosphorylation, which is initially mediated by viral thymidine kinase. Sorivudine triphosphate competitively inhibits viral DNA replication, but is neither a substrate for viral DNA polymerase nor incorporated into viral DNA.

Sorivudine oral bioavailability is approximately 75%. Most of the drug is eliminated unchanged into the urine.

Studies have demonstrated the efficacy of sorivudine in healthy adults with chickenpox and HIV-1-infected adults with shingles. Sorivudine is licensed for VZV infections.

Tolerance to sorivudine is good: mild nausea, vomiting and diarrhea, and occasional elevations in hepatic enzymes are observed. Fatal myelosuppression can occur in patients treated concurrently with sorivudine and 5-fluorouracil, probably due to sorivudine inhibition of the metabolism of hepatic 5-fluorouracil, which can then accumulate to toxic levels.

Non-nucleoside analogs

Foscarnet is the only non-nucleoside antiherpes drug currently available for therapy

Foscarnet (trisodium phosphonoformate) is an inorganic pyrophosphate compound stereochemically identical to a product released from nucleotide triphosphates by the action of DNA polymerases. It inhibits:

- HSV, VZV, CMV, EBV, and HIV-1.
- Acyclovir-resistant HSV and VZV.
- Ganciclovir-resistant CMV.

The efficacy of foscarnet for treating nucleoside-resistant viruses results from its ability to inhibit herpesvirus DNA polymerase and HIV reverse transcriptase directly without the need for previous intracellular metabolism, unlike the nucleoside antiviral drugs. Foscarnet reversibly binds to the pyrophosphate binding site of these polymerases, inhibits cleavage–release of the pyrophosphate moiety from the incoming nucleotide triphosphate molecules, and prevents DNA chain elongation. Selectivity results from its 100-fold higher affinity for viral polymerases than for cellular polymerases.

Foscarnet oral bioavailability ranges from 12 to 22%. It distributes throughout the body, including the cerebrospinal fluid, and is incorporated into bone, though this is of unknown clinical importance. It is eliminated in the urine, almost exclusively as unchanged drug. Doses must therefore be reduced in patients with renal insufficiency.

Foscarnet is effective only by intravenous administration

Because of its limited oral bioavailability, foscarnet is effective only by intravenous administration. It must attain high concentrations in the tissues to inhibit virus replication and is the treatment of choice for patients with:

- Acyclovir-resistant HSV or VZV infections.
- Ganciclovir-resistant CMV disease.

Its role in chronic HIV infection is minimal as its effects on clinical endpoints and duration of pharmacotherapeutic effect remain uncertain.

Topical foscarnet is ineffective for the treatment of recurrent HSV infection of the orolabial or genital skin.

Some HSV, VZV, and CMV infections are foscarnet resistant. The resistance in CMV appears to be due to alterations in the DNA polymerase that reduce its affinity for foscarnet. CMV disease unresponsive to ganciclovir or foscarnet may respond to their combined use.

Properties of foscarnet, the only available non-nucleoside herpesvirus inhibitor drug

- **Antiviral effect does not require intracellular metabolism**
- **Directly inhibits herpesvirus DNA polymerase**
- **Particularly valuable for treating nucleoside-resistant herpes simplex virus, varicella zoster virus, and cytomegalovirus infection**
- **Requires intravenous administration**
- **Causes reversible, but serious, multiple organ toxicity**

Foscarnet infusion commonly produces adverse effects, which are reversible but serious. They involve the kidneys, calcium–phosphate homeostasis, the hematologic system, and the central nervous system:

- Nephrotoxicity due to renal tubular injury resulting in proteinuria or azotemia occurs in up to 50% of patients. Occasionally nephrogenic diabetes insipidus and acute renal failure occur.
- Hypo- and hypercalcemia and hyperphosphatemia are observed in up to 65% of patients, possibly owing to phosphate displacement from bone, Ca^{2+} chelation by foscarnet, or impaired renal tubular phosphate handling. Hypocalcemia may cause paresthesia, tetany, and seizures.
- Reversible hematologic toxicity includes anemia in 20–50% of patients, thrombocytopenia in 15–25%, and leucopenia in up to 25%. The mechanism of this hematologic toxicity is unknown.

Other adverse effects include:

- Reversible painful penile ulcers attributed to a direct irritant effect of foscarnet in urine under the foreskin.
- Thrombophlebitis due to chemical irritation during infusion.
- Gastrointestinal problems such as nausea, vomiting, and diarrhea.
- Rarely, central nervous system adverse effects such as paresthesia, confusion, ataxia, and seizures.

TREATMENT OF CYTOMEGALOVIRUS INFECTIONS

Ganciclovir

Ganciclovir, a deoxyguanosine analog, inhibits CMV and is useful for treating a variety of CMV infections. Whereas it is 10–50-fold more potent than acyclovir against CMV, it inhibits HSV and VZV *in vitro* in concentrations similar to those for acyclovir.

The antiviral effect of ganciclovir requires its conversion to the triphosphate nucleotide form, a process initiated by a kinase encoded in the UL97 gene and completed by cellular enzymes. Ganciclovir triphosphate inhibits CMV DNA replication by:

- Competitively inhibiting deoxyguanosine triphosphate incorporation by the viral DNA polymerase.
- Terminating viral DNA chain elongation following incorporation.

Ganciclovir is eliminated by renal tubular secretion and glomerular filtration. Doses must be reduced in renal insufficiency to prevent drug accumulation and toxicity.

Pharmacotherapeutic indications Ganciclovir is available in intravenous and oral forms and as a slow-release formulation for intravitreal insertion. Intravenous ganciclovir is the treatment of choice for serious CMV infections that accompany immunosuppression. Discontinuation of the therapy is, however, often followed by a relapse of the CMV disease, which can be prevented by continuous intravenous administration of the drug in a reduced dose. CMV retinitis infection may be suppressed by oral administration, but doses tenfold higher than suppressive intravenous doses are required owing to the limited oral bioavailability of the drug. CMV retinitis can also be controlled by the slow release formulation of the drug implanted intravitreally.

Resistance Ganciclovir resistance has been related to the selection of mutant strains with an altered kinase encoded by the UL97 gene or a DNA polymerase with reduced affinity for ganciclovir triphosphate.

Adverse effects Human bone marrow progenitor cells appear uniquely susceptible to ganciclovir at concentrations that inhibit CMV. As a result the commonest and most important adverse effects of intravenous ganciclovir are neutropenia (defined as <1000 neutrophils/ml) and anemia. These effects are, however, reversible on stopping the drug and are reversed, in some of those in whom ganciclovir therapy cannot be discontinued, by the administration of granulocyte–macrophage colony stimulating factor.

Central nervous system adverse effects, including confusion, seizures and hallucinations similar to those reported for acyclovir and adenine-arabinoside, have been described in 5% of patients treated with ganciclovir, while abnormal liver function tests have been observed in 2%.

RESPIRATORY TRACT INFECTIONS

Influenza A and respiratory syncytial virus respiratory tract infections are responsive to drug therapy.

INFLUENZA A

Influenza A viruses undergo continuous minor ('antigenic drift') and major ('antigenic shift') variations in the hemagglutinin and neuraminidase antigens that induce protective antibodies. As a result, populations become susceptible to new mutant strains and previously available vaccines are ineffective. Chemoprophylaxis is therefore needed if the vaccine is not available, contraindicated, or not immunogenic, while chemotherapy may be needed in the management of individuals who develop influenza.

Treatment

Currently, two drugs, amantadine (1-adamantanamine) and rimantadine (α-methyl-1-adamantanamine), are approved for influenza A chemoprophylaxis and therapy. These drugs are primary amines with a large carbon ring. Both these features are essential for their antiviral effect.

Amantadine and rimantadine prevent uncoating of the influenza virion

Uncoating of the influenza virion after it has been transported intracellularly within endosomes is essential for releasing the viral genome before it is transported into the cell nucleus where genomic replication occurs. Amantadine and rimantadine exert their antiviral effect by binding specifically to the hydrophobic domain of the M2 protein of the virus, a transmembrane polypeptide tetramer that functions as an ion channel for H^+ diffusion into the virion. Amantadine and rimantadine block the ion channel and thereby prevent acidification of the virion, which is necessary for dissociation of the influenza ribonucleoprotein from the M1 protein before its transport into the nucleus.

Amantadine also releases dopamine from central dopaminergic neurons

This effect is unrelated to its antiviral effect, but is relevant to its pharmacotherapeutic effect in Parkinson's disease and its adverse effects involving the central nervous system (see Chapter 7).

Both amantadine and rimantadine are available only as oral formulations

Amantadine and rimantadine are absorbed slowly (but well) but have different pharmacokinetic characteristics (Fig. 24.14):

- Amantadine is eliminated by glomerular filtration and renal tubular secretion and can be recovered in urine as unchanged drug after oral administration.
- Approximately 75% of ingested rimantadine is metabolized in the liver to hydroxylated metabolites, while 25% of the drug is excreted in the urine unchanged.

Amantadine doses must be reduced in patients with reduced renal function, while rimantadine doses need to be reduced in patients with severe hepatic dysfunction.

Rimantadine's apparent volume of distribution and plasma disappearance half-life are approximately twice those of amantadine. Amantadine concentration in nasal mucus approaches

Selected pharmacokinetic characteristics of amantadine and rimantadine

	Amantadine	Rimantadine
Oral bioavailability	Good	Good
Elimination	As unchanged drug in urine	Extensive hepatic hydroxylation
Effect of renal disease	Accumulation and toxicity	Minimal accumulation and toxicity
Effect of hepatic disease	None	Accumulation and toxicity

Fig. 24.14 Selected pharmacokinetic characteristics of amantadine and rimantadine.

that in the plasma, but rimantadine concentration in nasal mucus is 2.5 times greater than that in the plasma. This may be clinically relevant to the prophylactic and pharmacotherapeutic efficacy of these drugs.

Pharmacotherapeutic indications

Both amantadine and rimantadine are effective for the prophylaxis and treatment of acute influenza A infection

For treatment, amantadine and rimantadine must be started within 48 hours of the onset of symptoms. Both drugs attenuate the symptoms of acute influenza A infection and reduce the duration of virus shedding in nasal secretions. Treatment should be for five days. They are 70–95% more effective than placebo, but their efficacy in individuals who have the highest risks of developing the complications of influenza, such as patients with significant cardiorespiratory disease, has not been determined. For prophylaxis, the drugs may be ingested over prolonged periods.

Resistance

Resistance to amantadine and rimantadine is associated with point mutations in the amino acid composition of the M2 protein that result in loss of drug binding in the ion channel. Emergence of resistance associated with clinical failure has been demonstrated in 25–50% of patients within days of starting treatment with either agent. Therefore, during the course of therapy for family members, treatment-resistant infections may appear in other household members.

There are currently no alternative drugs available to treat amantadine- or rimantadine-resistant influenza A virus infection.

Adverse effects

Amantadine and rimantadine are well tolerated and have no serious renal, hepatic, or hematologic adverse effects. Chronic rimantadine use is more acceptable for the prevention of influenza than chronic amantadine use, especially by the elderly, because it has fewer central nervous system adverse effects. In college students, central nervous system adverse effects, primarily insomnia, jitteriness, and difficulty in concentrating have been reported in 13%, 6%, and 4% of amantadine, rimantadine and placebo recipients, respectively. These symptoms generally clear rapidly on discontinuing the medication. In elderly subjects, dose-related central nervous system adverse effects to amantadine are more troublesome. Seizures have been reported in individuals with a history of convulsive disorders. Reducing the doses given to the elderly, especially small women, has been only partly successful in increasing the acceptability of amantadine.

RESPIRATORY SYNCYTIAL VIRUS DISEASE

Respiratory syncytial virus (RSV) is the major cause of outbreaks of severe lower respiratory tract illness in young children

Not only is RSV the major cause of outbreaks of severe lower respiratory tract illness in young children, but it also causes outbreaks of upper respiratory tract infection in older children and adults. In 3–5% of infants and those with underlying cardiopulmonary and congenital immunodeficiency disorders, RSV infection can be fatal. While good supportive care is of the utmost importance in the management of severely ill infants, ribavirin administered as an aerosol may reduce the morbidity and mortality of these children.

Treatment

Ribavirin (1-β-D-ribofuranosyl-1,2,4-thiazole-3-carboxamide) is a broad-spectrum, well-tolerated antiviral drug with a controversial therapeutic role. It is a guanosine analog that inhibits a wide range of RNA and DNA viruses including HIV-1 *in vitro*, but its only approved indication is for the treatment of RSV disease.

Ribavirin interferes with intracellular ribonucleotide and deoxyribonucleotide pool sizes

The precise mechanism of action of ribavirin's antiviral effect is uncertain. Ribavirin is converted to its triphosphate nucleotide form by cellular kinases. Ribavirin triphosphate inhibits 5'-guanylylation of synthesized uncapped mRNA, an essential step in the processing of mRNA. Ribavirin monophosphate inhibits inosine-5-phosphate dehydrogenase, thereby interfering with guanosine triphosphate synthesis; this inhibition may partly account for the inhibition of viral nucleic acid synthesis. The triphosphate moiety inhibits influenza RNA polymerase and HIV reverse transcriptase. Ribavirin triphosphate is not incorporated into DNA and only slightly, if at all, into RNA. The selectivity of ribavirin for inhibiting viral functions by interfering with mRNA synthesis might relate to the fact that virus-infected cells are synthesizing mRNA at a much higher rate than resting uninfected cells.

Ribavirin may be given intravenously, orally, or by aerosol

Intravenous administration The pharmacokinetic characteristics of ribavirin after intravenous administration include a very large apparent volume of distribution suggesting sequestration in a non-vascular compartment. This compartment is probably the circulating red blood cell mass in which ribavirin concentration as the triphosphate exceeds the plasma concentration by 60-fold. Oral bioavailability averages 45%.

Ribavirin is primarily eliminated by metabolism and subsequent excretion into urine. Only 24% of an intravenous dose is eliminated into the urine as unchanged drug. The plasma elimination half-life approaches two weeks, and an initial loading dose may therefore be therapeutically beneficial.

Aerosol administration The efficacy and fate of ribavirin inhaled as an aerosol in patients with acute lower respiratory tract illness depends on the particle size and the mode of delivery. Optimal results require particles of 1.5 μm diameter. It is estimated that 46% of such particles are deposited in the lower respiratory tract. Ribavirin attains levels of 250–1900 μg/ml in endotracheal secretions, while plasma levels resulting from the absorption of ribavirin after aerosol administration average 2 μg /ml.

Pharmacotherapeutic indications Aerosol ribavirin is approved for the treatment of severe RSV lower respiratory tract infection in neonates and infants with underlying cardiovascular, pulmonary, or immune deficiency. Ribivarin is also effective when given intravenously or by mouth to patients with acute Lassa fever, but is not approved for this indication. It must not be combined with zidovudine for patients with HIV-1 infection (see p. 456) because the two agents are antagonistic *in vitro*.

The main adverse effect of oral and intravenous ribavirin is dose-related anemia. The anemia is mild (i.e. a 6% decrease in hematocrit) and is accompanied by reticulocytosis and hyperbilirubinemia due to extravascular hemolysis. The precise mechanism is unclear. High ribavirin triphosphate red blood cell concentrations may be relevant. The anemia usually appears after two weeks of high-dose therapy and is reversed within two weeks of stopping ribavirin.

During chronic oral therapy in patients with HIV, gastrointestinal and central nervous system adverse effects have been noted. A dry mouth, increased thirst, a metallic taste, anorexia, nausea, and flatulence have been reported, in addition to fatigue unrelated to anemia. Central nervous system symptoms include headache, insomnia, irritability, mood lability, and poor concentration, which appear to be directly related to the dose and plasma concentration. Ribavirin inhaled as aerosol can provoke cough and bronchospasm.

Intravenous ribavirin has been given mainly to patients with Lassa fever. A moderate reversible anemia (i.e. a 20% reduction in red blood cells) appears 4–7 days after the initiation of therapy and is the only identified adverse effect.

MISCELLANEOUS VIRUS INFECTIONS TREATED WITH INTERFERONS

Interferons are naturally occurring antiviral substances with a broad spectrum of activity, but limited therapeutic use

Interferons (IFNs) are naturally occurring glycoprotein cytokines that inhibit viral replication. Three major classes have been identified and characterized as have their immunomodulatory and antiproliferative effects. These latter effects of IFN and their resulting pharmacotherapeutic uses are discussed in Chapter 15.

The production of IFN in large quantities by cell culture and recombinant DNA techniques has allowed their evaluation and prescription as exogenous antiviral agents.

The three major classes of IFN are designated α, β, and γ

The IFN classes are based on the cell types from which they were initially derived:

- IFN-α from leucocytes.
- IFN-β from fibroblasts.
- IFN-γ from antigen-stimulated, sensitized lymphocytes.

There are four subtypes of IFN-α, two of IFN-β and one of IFN-γ. IFN-α and -β are secreted by almost all nucleated cells in response to a viral infection, and these two types of IFN are effective in treating a variety of chronic viral infections.

Natural secretion of IFN appears within hours of viral infection and protects neighboring cells against infection. It therefore plays a critical early role in terminating a virus infection. In addition, cells produce IFN-α and -β in response to stimulation by exogenous agents such as double-stranded RNA (dsRNA) and some polyanions. This knowledge has been used to produce IFN-α and -β in large quantities by stimulating cells in culture with agents such as inactivated Sendai virus and polyinosinic:polycytidilic acid (poly I:C), a synthetic dsRNA.

In contrast, IFN-γ secreted by sensitized lymphocytes exposed to the sensitizing antigen (viral or other) as well as some mitogens is primarily used to enhance the immune response to infection (e.g. in patients with chronic granulomatous disease).

All interferons have variable broad-spectrum antiviral effects

Only human- or subhuman-primate (e.g. ververt monkey) cell-derived interferons are active in humans. The antiviral effect is initiated by binding to specific cell surface receptors. This stimulates the synthesis of a variety of proteins, which mediate the antiviral effect.

The mechanism of the antiviral effect of IFN varies for different viruses and cells. IFNs have been shown to interfere with viral penetration, uncoating, synthesis or methylation of mRNA, translation of viral protein, viral assembly, and viral release. The major effect is to inhibit the translation of viral protein. In some systems this is due to the induction of an enzyme that catalyzes the synthesis of 2',5'-linked oligoadenylates, which in turn activates a ribonuclease that degrades viral mRNA. The detection of 2',5'- oligoadenylate in serum may be used as a marker of a biologic response to IFN.

In other virus–cell systems, IFN induces the synthesis of a protein kinase that phosphorylates and inactivates a protein (ElF_2) needed for the initiation of viral protein synthesis.

Interferons must be injected to obtain their antiviral effects

Within 1–3 hours of an intravenous injection, 2',5'-oligoadenylate can be detected in the plasma and in cells that now are resistant to virus infection. This state of resistance of the cells to virus infection, or antiviral state, wanes over 2–4 days, long after the IFN has disappeared from plasma. IFN distributes throughout the body, but it is not certain whether detection of IFN in a body fluid (e.g. cerebrospinal fluid) correlates with an antiviral state (e.g. in the central nervous system). IFN is eliminated primarily by local inactivation.

Interferons are effective treatment for a variety of viral infections

IFN-α and -β are effective treatment for:

- Chronic active hepatitis B (HBV) infection.
- Hepatitis C infection.
- Non-A non-B viral hepatitis.
- Condylomata acuminata.
- Juvenile laryngeal papillomatosis due to human papilllloma virus infection.
- Epidemic Kaposi's sarcoma, now thought to be due to HHV-8.

The IFNs are injected intralesionally into warts and intramuscularly or subcutaneously for treatment of the other infections listed. IFNs also prevent rhinovirus colds when sprayed intranasally.

The usefulness of IFNs for treating viral infections has been limited by the need for repeated injections, dose-limiting adverse effects, and a relative lack of efficacy compared with that of other antiviral drugs. The antiviral effect of IFNs may, moreover, be impaired by the development of neutralizing antibody.

ADVERSE EFFECTS

Adverse effects are associated with the injection of both natural and recombinant formulations

The adverse effects of IFNs are dose related and may diminish with continued therapy. Doses of 1–2 million units or more, consistently produce an immediate, acute influenza-like syndrome with fatigue, fever, chills, headache, anorexia, myalgia, arthralgia, nausea, vomiting, diarrhea, and diaphoresis.

Prolonged therapy, especially with large doses, can cause myelosuppression with pancytopenia, hepatitis (occasionally fatal), neurotoxicity with psychologic depression (occasionally causing attempted suicide), ataxia, tremor, seizures, sedation and coma, cardiac toxicity with arrhythmias (usually supraventricular), and neurasthenia with chronic fatigue.

Other uncommon reactions include acute hypersensitivity reactions with urticaria, angioedema, bronchospasm and anaphylaxis, rash and alopecia.

HIV-1 INFECTION

Pandemic HIV-1 infection has led to an intensive search for antiviral agents to control this disease

Several unique HIV-1 replicative steps have been identified that might be effectively targeted by antiviral drugs (Fig. 24.15). Cumulative data have shown the importance of controlling the emergence of drug resistance and using combinations of two and three different drugs for treatment. Two different classes of drugs have already been demonstrated to be effective in the treatment of HIV-1 disease:

- Nucleoside reverse transcriptase inhibitors.
- Protease inhibitors.

NUCLEOSIDE REVERSE TRANSCRIPTASE INHIBITORS

Zidovudine

Zidovudine is the prototype for a group of nucleoside human immunodeficiency virus inhibitors

Zidovudine is a thymidine analog that inhibits HIV-1, HIV-2, human T-cell leukemia/lymphoma virus-1, and other mammalian retroviruses. Other members of this group of nucleoside HIV inhibitors include dideoxyadenosine, stavudine, dideoxycytidine, and lamivudine. These agents share the following characteristics:

- They require intracellular conversion to the corresponding triphosphate nucleotide for activation.
- All interfere with HIV replication by competitively inhibiting HIV-1 reverse transcriptase and terminating DNA chain elongation after incorporation.
- All lose antiviral activity due to the development of mutations in the reverse transcriptase, although the rate of emergence of resistance and its degree vary for different drugs.

Selectivity is attributable to the greater affinity of zidovudine triphosphate for reverse transcriptase than for cellular DNA polymerases. Zidovudine inhibits HBV and EBV *in vitro*, but not HSV or VZV. The concentrations needed in patients are toxic to human myeloid and erythroid progenitor cells, which explains the common occurrence of anemia and granulocytopenia during therapy. Incorporation of zidovudine into mitochondrial DNA may explain the myopathy seen in some patients.

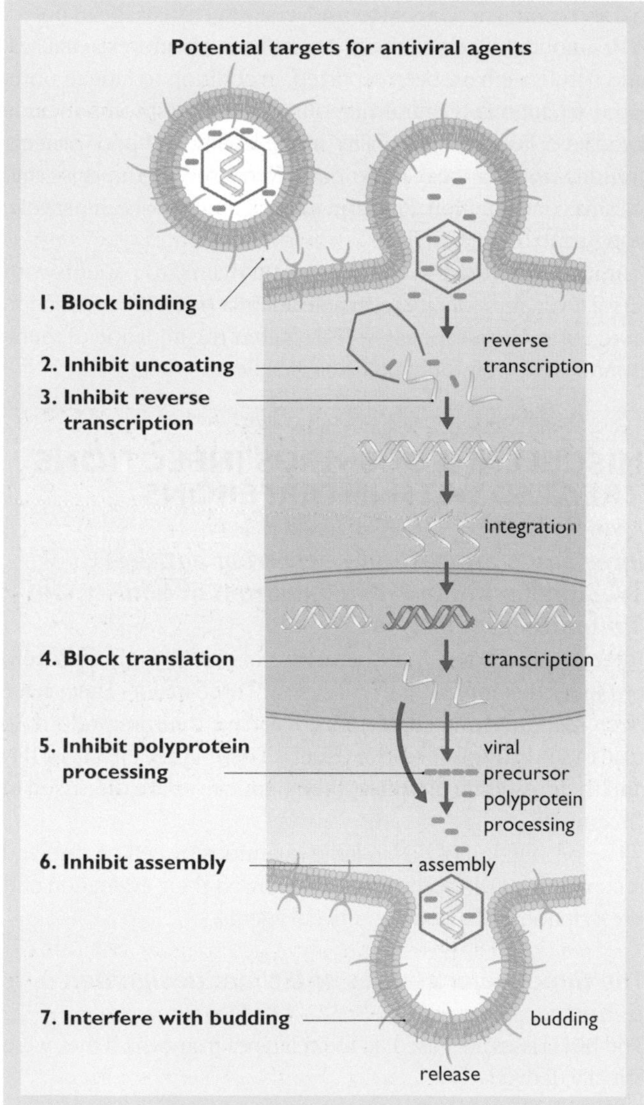

Fig. 24.15 The HIV-1 replicative cycle. This diagram illustrates the steps in the HIV-1 replicative cycle, beginning with adsorption of an HIV-1 virion to a receptor on the surface of a susceptible cell and ending with budding of a daughter virus particle. It shows potential sites for antiviral drug action including that of reverse transcriptase inhibitors (site 3) and protease inibitors (site 5).

Both oral and intravenous formulations of zidovudine are available

Oral zidovudine is 60–70% bioavailable. Elimination from the plasma is rapid, with a half-life of 1–1.5 hours, but depletion of intracellular zidovudine nucleotides is slower, making thrice-daily dosing practicable. Zidovudine undergoes first-pass hepatic metabolism with glucuronidation to yield a metabolite without HIV-inhibiting activity. Unchanged drug and the *O*-glucuronide metabolite account for 15% and 75% of the drug found in urine, respectively.

Pharmacotherapeutic indications Zidovudine prolongs the survival of patients with acquired immunodeficiency syndrome (AIDS). It was the first anti-HIV drug evaluated clinically, so placebo-treated patients were studied concurrently as controls. These initial studies established the value of zidovudine in patients with HIV-1 infection as it:

- Prevents opportunistic infections in patients with AIDS and advanced AIDS-related complex.
- Slows the progression of disease in asymptomatic or mildly symptomatic patients with 200–500 CD4 cells/ml.

Zidovudine administered orally to HIV-positive pregnant women beginning at 14–34 weeks of gestation, and given intravenously during labour and orally to the newborn, reduces the frequency of neonatal HIV infection.

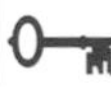

Characteristics of nucleoside reverse transcriptase inhibitors of HIV-1 replication

- Activated intracellularly by phosphorylation by cellular kinases
- Triphosphate forms competitively inhibit reverse transcriptase
- Incorporation into HIV-1 DNA causes chain termination
- Resistant strains emerge with variable facility

Zidovudine may improve the cognitive and neurologic function of patients with AIDS encephalopathy and dementia, and platelet counts in patients with HIV-associated thrombocytopenia. Zidovudine is effective for the initial treatment of:

- HIV-infected adults with less than 500 CD4 cells/ml.
- Children over three months of age.
- HIV-infected pregnant women and their newborn infants.

It is approved for combination therapy of HIV-1 with other drugs.

Resistance with clinical failure is observed in approximately 50% of patients after six months of monotherapy and in almost all patients after two years of treatment. Resistant strains of HIV-1 result from sequential point mutations in the reverse transcriptase and are not uniformly crossresistant to other nucleoside retrovirus inhibitor drugs. Zidovudine combined with didanosine or zalcitabine (see below) synergistically inhibits zidovudine-resistant virus.

Zidovudine's adverse effects are more common in patients with advanced HIV-1 disease. They are uncommon in asymptomatic or mildly symptomatic HIV-infected patients, especially those receiving the currently recommended lower daily dose of zidovudine. Macrocytic anemia and neutropenia occur 4–6 weeks after the initiation of therapy in 2% and 37% of patients with asymptomatic and advanced HIV infection treated with 600 mg/day, respectively, and in 6% and 50% of patients with asymptomatic and advanced HIV infection treated with 1200 mg/day, respectively. Thrombocytopenia has been observed in 12% of those treated with zidovudine compared with 5% of placebo-treated controls, although it increases platelet concentrations in patients with HIV-related thrombocytopenia. These effects are reversible on stopping zidovudine therapy.

Severe headache, myalgia, nausea, and insomnia also occur more frequently with zidovudine than with placebo. Other uncommon but serious adverse effects that have been observed include myopathy and myositis, hepatomegaly with steatosis and lactic acidosis, and anaphylaxis.

Newer nucleoside reverse transcriptase inhibitors

The newer nucleoside reverse transcriptase inhibitors differ from zidovudine primarily by causing a different spectrum of adverse effects

These drugs, therefore, can be used with zidovudine in combinations that have the potential to produce additive pharmacotherapeutic effects without additive adverse effects. These agents include:

- Didanosine (2',3'-dideoxyinosine).
- Zalcitabine (2,'3'-dideoxycytidine).
- Stavudine (2',3'-didehydro-2'-deoxythymidine).
- Lamivudine ({-}-2'-deoxy-3'-thiacytidine).

They are converted to active triphosphate forms by cellular kinases. All are adequately bioavailable so chronic oral therapy is practical. Elimination into urine as unchanged drug is an important route of elimination. The percentage excreted as unchanged drug in the urine varies from 45% for stavudine to 70% for lamivudine.

Pharmacotherapeutic indications Clinically, these agents have generally been prescribed in combination with zidovudine or as an alternative agent to it. Recent data on the potent immunoenhancing and antiviral effect of lamivudine with zidovudine have, however, emphasized the advantage of their use in combination. Lamivudine is unique in this group of drugs in producing sustained reductions in hepatitis B virus DNA in patients with chronic hepatitis B infection.

Resistance has limited the long-term effectiveness of these agents as monotherapy, but the kinetics and frequency of crossresistance varies for the different drugs.

Adverse effects Significant dose-limiting reversible toxicity is a feature of all these agents except lamivudine, but the basis for these adverse effects is unknown. The absence of hematologic toxicity means that these agents can be used with zidovudine. However, the propensity of several of these agents to cause peripheral neuropathy precludes their use interchangeably (e.g. stavudine should not be prescribed for a patient with a history of zalcitabine-associated neuropathy).

Main dose-limiting toxic effects of nucleoside inhibitors of HIV-1 reverse transcriptase

Drug	Main toxic effect
Zidovudine	Myelosuppression
Didanosine	Pancreatitis and peripheral neuropathy
Zalcitabine	Peripheral neuropathy
Stavudine	Peripheral neuropathy
Lamivudine	None

PROTEASE INHIBITORS

Saquinavir is the prototype of a class of potent and well-tolerated human immunodeficiency-1 drugs called protease inhibitors

This class of drugs also includes ritonavir and indinavir. They interfere with HIV replication by inhibiting post-translational processing of viral precursor polypeptides, a locus of action that differs from that of the reverse transcriptase inhibitors.

Pharmacotherapeutic indications

Administration of these protease inhibitors together with nucleoside reverse transcriptase inhibitors can theoretically increase the antiviral and immunoenhancing effects of reverse transcriptase inhibitors. Initial clinical trial results are consistent with this hypothesis:

- Ritonavir given alone yielded the highest increases in CD4 counts observed with any other anti-HIV-1 drug administered alone, and the effect was sustained for the 12 weeks of therapy.
- Saquinavir given with zidovudine to previously untreated patients with HIV-1 infection or with zalcitabine to patients previously treated with zidovudine increased CD4 levels for at least 52 weeks.
- Indinavir given together with zidovudine and lamivudine produced the most marked sustained suppression of HIV load and elevation of CD4 levels yet reported. This antiviral effect was maintained for 24 weeks.

The effect of protease inhibitors on clinical (i.e. nonlaboratory) outcomes remains to be demonstrated.

Renewed optimism for the treatment of HIV-1 infection is based on the new availability of two classes of retrovirus inhibitors with different mechanisms of action, improved adverse effect profiles, and demonstrated enhanced pharmacotherapeutic effects when used in combination.

Resistance

The propensity for these protease inhibitors to induce HIV strains resistant to other protease inhibitors is unknown, as is the effect of combination therapy on inhibiting the development of resistance.

Adverse effects

The adverse effects of combination therapy with protease inhibitors plus a nucleoside reverse transcriptase inhibitor are similar to those previously observed with the nucleoside reverse transcriptase inhibitor alone.

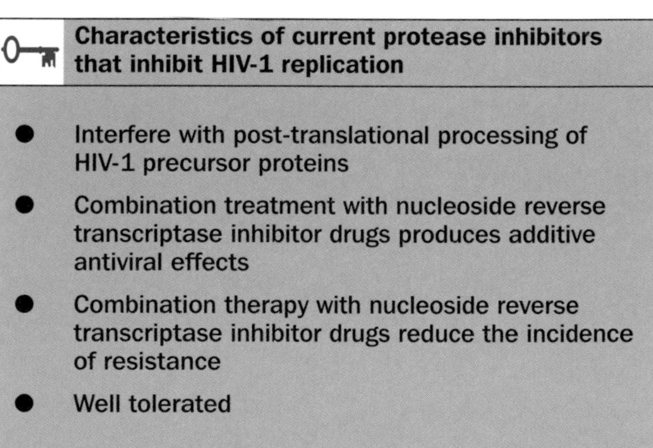
Characteristics of current protease inhibitors that inhibit HIV-1 replication

- Interfere with post-translational processing of HIV-1 precursor proteins
- Combination treatment with nucleoside reverse transcriptase inhibitor drugs produces additive antiviral effects
- Combination therapy with nucleoside reverse transcriptase inhibitor drugs reduce the incidence of resistance
- Well tolerated

FURTHER READING

Coen DM. The implications of resistance to antiviral agents for herpesvirus drug targets and drug therapy. *Antiviral Res* 1992; **12:** 245–264. [A useful review of the data concerning resistance to herpesvirus drugs and strategies for treating infection caused by such viruses.]

Gazzard BG, Moyle GJ. Individualization of HIV therapy: the clinician's perspective. *Br J Clin Pract* 1995; **49:** 145–147. [Expert opinion on how and when to treat HIV-1-infected patients with retrovirus-inhibitor drugs.]

Hayden FG. Antiviral agents. In: Mandell GL, Bennett JE, Dolin R (eds) *Principles and Practice of Infectious Diseases*. New York: Churchill Livingstone; 1995: 411–449. [Comprehensive, authoritative text on antiviral drugs for the practitioner.]

Hayden FG, Couch RB. Clinical and epidemiological importance of influenza A viruses resistant to amantadine and rimantadine. In: Hannoun C (ed.) *Options for the Control of Influenza.II*. Amsterdam: Elsevier Science Publishers; 1993: 333–342. [A useful review of our current understanding of the data and implications relating to influenza A virus resistance to drugs and the potential applications of same in respect of epidemic control.]

Moyle GT. Resistance to antiretroviral compounds: implications for the clinical management of HIV infection. *Immunol Infect* Dis 1995; **5:** 170–182. [A valuable contemporary view of an evolving area of HIV-1 pharmacotherapy.]

Whitley RT, Gnann JW Jr. Acyclovir: a decade later. *N Engl J Med* 1992; **327:** 782–789. [A comprehensive review of the mainstay of our therapeutic armamentarium for herpesvirus infections.]

Make a provisional diagnosis and determine a rational pharmacologic treatment for the following hypothetical case.

A 28-year-old man presents with multiple painful clusters of vesicles on red patches on the shaft of his penis, malaise, fever, nausea, and occasional vomiting. These symptoms began 5 days after he had sexual intercourse with a new partner. He has had a cadaveric renal transplant for two years for renal failure due to glomerulonephritis. His medications include prednisone and cyclosporine. His usual serum creatinine concentration is 200 mmol/l (normal 80–110).

On examination he is in some discomfort, his blood pressure is 145/85 mmHg, his pulse is 96 beats/min, and his temperature is 38.3°C. He appears slightly Cushingoid, and he has genital lesions as described above with tender bilateral inguinal lymphadenopathy.

1. What is the clinical diagnosis?
2. How would you confirm the diagnosis?
3. What is the natural history of this infection?
4. Which of the following drugs—acyclovir, foscarnet, valacyclovir, ganciclovir, adenine-arabinoside, sorivudine, edoxuridine, penciclovir, famciclovir—could theoretically be prescribed for the infection?
5. What is the drug of choice for this infection?
6. What is the preferred route for acyclovir administration?
7. Although prednisone and cyclosporine may be limiting the host response to this infection, it is decided to keep the cyclosporine dose as is, and to increase the dose of prednisone. Why are these recommendations appropriate?
8. Is knowledge of the patient's renal function critical to determine the size of the first dose? Explain why or why not.
9. Is knowledge of the patient's renal function critical for prescribing subsequent doses? Explain why or why not.

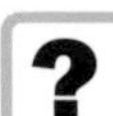

Indicate which is the correct answer for each question.

1. Properties of acyclovir include all the following, except
a) has excellent oral absorption
b) inhibits herpes simplex virus and varicella zoster virus
c) is eliminated largely unchanged in the urine
d) has modest adverse effects after oral administration
e) may cause renal tubular obstruction

2. Both amantadine and rimantadine share all the following characteristics, except
a) inhibit replication of influenza A virus
b) have good oral absorption
c) are eliminated largely unchanged in the urine
d) are effective for the prophylaxis and treatment of influenza A virus infection
e) are commonly associated with the development of resistance during therapy

3. Resistance to acyclovir in herpes simplex virus is likely to be resistant to all the following, except
a) penciclovir
b) edoxuridine
c) ganciclovir
d) valacyclovir
e) adenine-arabinoside

4. The properties of interferons include all the following, except
a) are cytokines
b) have common adverse effects resembling a flu-like illness
c) are not effective when administered orally
d) inhibit viral replication indirectly
e) cause renal failure at high doses

5. Treatment of a patient with HIV-1 infection with zidovudine alone for one year is associated with all the following, except
a) a sustained inhibition of HIV-1 replication
b) anemia as the likeliest adverse effect
c) emergence of zidovudine-resistant virus
d) a probable improved response if lamivudine is added
e) a probable improved response if saquinavir is added

6. Protease inhibitors of HIV-1, such as saquinavir, have all the following properties, except
a) inhibit HIV-1 replication by blocking uncoating of the virus during cell penetration.
b) produce an additive antiviral effect when given with zidovudine
c) may prevent emergence of zidovudine-resistant virus when given with zidovudine
d) are associated with the ready development of resistance if used alone
e) have minimal adverse effects

7. Properties of zidovudine include all the following, except
a) undergoes phosphorylation to generate the molecule that inhibits HIV-1 replication
b) has a narrow toxic therapeutic ratio for red blood cell progenitor cells
c) is well absorbed after oral administration
d) crosses the blood–brain barrier
e) does not cross the placenta

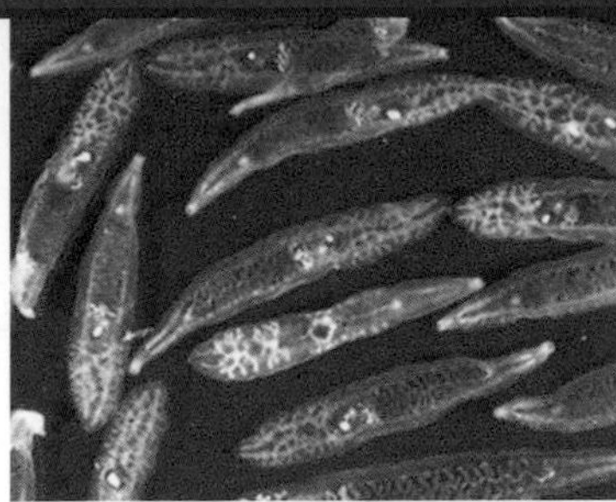

25. Parasitic Infections

Parasitism is a type of symbiosis characterized by an intimate and obligatory relationship between two organisms. The parasite is generally the smaller of the two and is usually metabolically dependent on its host. The term parasite is generally reserved for protozoa, helminths, and arthropods.

The six major tropical diseases defined by the World Health Organization

- Parasitic malaria
- Parasitic schistosomiasis
- Parasitic filariasis
- Parasitic trypanosomiasis
- Parasitic leishmaniasis
- Leprosy

The treatment of protozoan and helminthic diseases is complicated by the variable structure and metabolism of the different forms of these organisms during their life cycle

Knowledge of the biochemistry and molecular biology of protozoa and helminths has recently expanded and new compounds to treat these diseases are being developed.

PROTOZOAN DISEASES

Protozoa are small and unicellular and are among the simplest organisms of the animal kingdom

Parasitic protozoa can replicate within the host's body and are usually divided into four subphyla according to their type of locomotion:

- Sarcodina (amebae) are characterized by ameboid movements producing pseudopods (e.g. *Entamoeba histolytica*).
- Mastigophora (flagellates) are characterized by flagella producing a whip-like motion (e.g. *Giardia lamblia, Trichomonas vaginalis, Trypanosoma* spp. and *Leishmania* spp.).
- Ciliophora (ciliates) are characterized by cilia to produce movement (e.g. *Balantidium coli*).
- Sporozoa typically have no locomotor organs in the adult stage (e.g. *Plasmodium* spp., *Toxoplasma gondii, Pneumocystis carinii*).

MALARIA

Malaria is a protozoan disease that is usually transmitted by mosquitoes

Malaria is the most important parasitic disease in tropical medicine. Worldwide there are 200 million malaria cases each year and two million deaths due to malaria. It is endemic in more than 100 countries in Africa, Asia, Occania, Central and South America, and certain Caribbean islands, and approximately 60% of the world's population live in these countries.

There are four species of malaria parasites

Malaria is usually transmitted by anopheline mosquitoes and rarely by congenital transmission, transfusion of infected blood, or the use of contaminated syringes. It is caused by four species of plasmodial parasites:

- *Plasmodium falciparum*, which is widely distributed, results in the most severe infections, and is responsible for nearly all malaria-related deaths (Fig. 25.1a).
- *P. vivax*, which is also widespread and causes more benign disease than the other two species (Fig. 25.1b).
- *P. malariae* is also widespread.
- *P. ovale* is confined mainly to Africa.

The clinical features of infection depend on the species of the parasite and the immunologic status of the patient

Acute falciparum malaria is a potentially fatal disease, and non-immune travelers to malarious areas risk severe attacks. Acute malaria occurs where exposure is limited or seasonal and where the collective immunity is relatively low. In these circumstances it can occur in epidemic proportions and affect all age groups in the endemic community. Complications include cerebral malaria, hypoglycemia, pulmonary edema, acute renal failure, and massive intravascular hemolysis. Chronic repeated infection often leads to splenomegaly and progressive anemia (Fig. 25.1c). There is a particularly high risk of death among untreated pregnant women with falciparum malaria, especially where transmission is intermittent. The fetus is inevitably exposed to the effects of placental insufficiency.

Infants born to immune mothers living in holoendemic areas are unlikely to acquire malaria for several months after birth, largely owing to the passive transfer of maternal antibodies

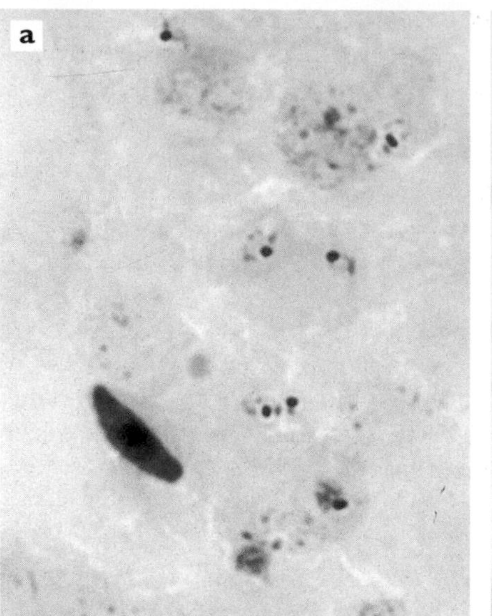

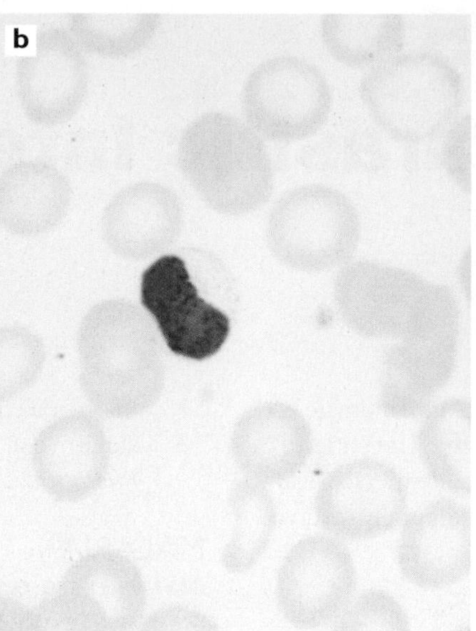

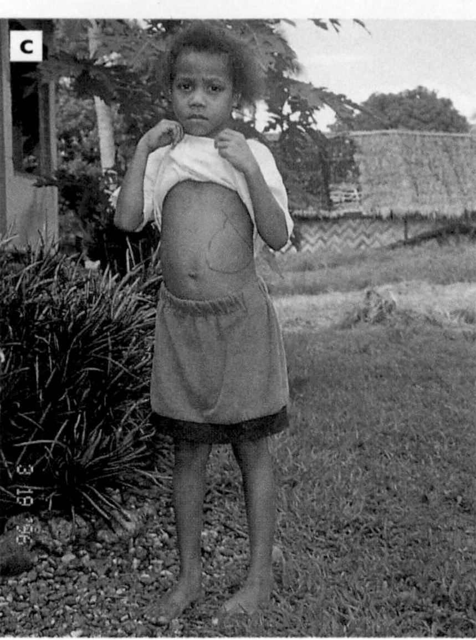

Fig. 25.1 Malaria. (a) *Plasmodium falciparum*, ring forms and a gametocyte. Giemsa stain, thick smear. (b) *P. vivax*, a mature trophozoite in an enlarged erythrocyte. Giemsa stain, thin smear. (c) A schoolgirl with anemia and splenomegaly, Vanuatu, the Southwest Pacific.

across the placenta, Thereafter, they are subject to severe and recurrent acute potentially fatal attacks during infancy and early childhood. From the age of 5 years until adulthood, the severity and frequency of these attacks decrease as immunity develops.

Clinically significant malaria is uncommon among adults (other than pregnant women and immunocompromised individuals) who have always lived in areas of high transmission.

Antimalarial drugs target different phases of the malarial life cycle

The malarial life cycle is as follows:

- Sporozoites are produced in the mosquito vectors from sexual forms of the parasite and migrate to the salivary glands (sporogony).
- Once injected into the human blood stream, the sporozoites rapidly penetrate the parenchymal cells of the liver, where they transform and grow into large tissue schizonts containing considerable numbers of merozoites (exo-red blood cell schizogony).
- The large tissue schizonts begin to rupture after 5–20 days, depending upon the species, and the released merozoites invade circulating red blood cells and rapidly multiply within the red cells.
- The host red blood cells rupture, releasing the merozoites, which then invade and destroy further red blood cells in the same way.
- Some merozoites develop into male and female gametocytes, so the infected human becomes a reservoir of infection for mosquitoes and completion of the transmission cycle is assured.

The destruction of the red blood cells and the release of the waste products of the parasites produce the episodic chills and fever that characterize the disease. Certain tissue forms of *P. vivax* and *P. ovale* persist in the liver for many months and even years (hypnozoites) and are responsible for the relapses that are characteristic of these forms of malaria. Such latent forms are not generated by *P. falciparum* or *P. malariae*. Recrudescence of these infections results from persisting blood forms in inadequately treated or untreated patients.

The four species of malaria

- *Plasmodium falciparum* causes the most severe infection; its resistance to antimalarial drugs is a major problem
- *P. vivax* causes more benign diseases, same as *P. malariae* and *P. ovale*
- *P. vivax* and *P. ovale* have relapse forms in liver
- *P. ovale* is mainly confined to Africa

The chemotherapy used to treat malaria depends on the infecting parasite, the drug's adverse effects, and the host's immunity

The effectiveness of a chemotherapeutic agent in treating malaria depends on the interactions between the malaria parasites, the antimalarial drugs, and the human host (Fig. 25.2). The choice of drug therefore depends on:

- The species of infecting parasite and its stage of development. Parasite resistance is becoming a worldwide problem. There are also differences in effectiveness between strains of the same species in different geographic areas.

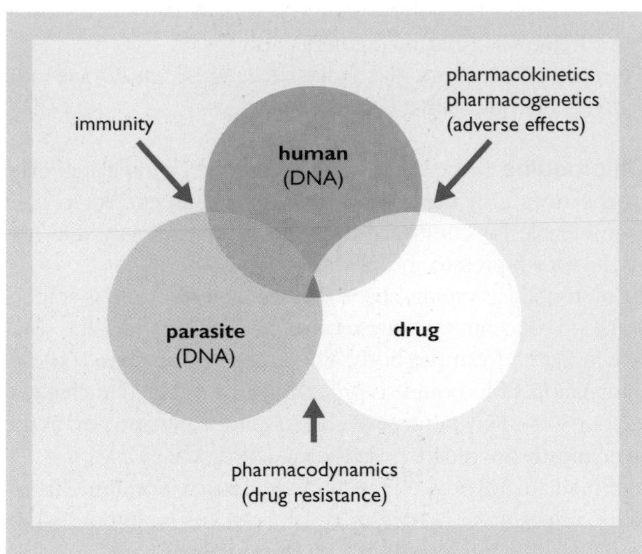

Fig. 25.2 Antimalarial drugs act at different stages of the malaria parasite's life cycle.

- The drug's adverse effects, which must be balanced against their beneficial therapeutic effects.
- The host's immunity, since people with a degree of immunity as a result of prolonged exposure to the infection can be cured or protected much more easily than those who have not and may respond to lower drug doses.

Antimalarial drugs are classified according to where they act in the malaria parasite's life cycle

Antimalarial drugs have a selective action on the different phases of the parasite's life cycle (Fig. 25.3) and may be classified as:

- Tissue schizontocides, which act on exo-red blood cell forms in the liver.
- Blood schizontocides, which attack the parasite in the red blood cell, thereby preventing or terminating the clinical attack.
- Gametocytocides, which are drugs that destroy the sexual forms of the parasite (gametocytes) in the blood to prevent transmission.
- Hypnozoitocides, which kill the dormant hypnozoites of *P. vivax* and *P. ovale* in the liver and are used as antirelapse drugs.
- Sporontocides, which interrupt the development of the sporogonic phase in mosquitoes that have fed on gametocyte carriers so that the mosquitoes cannot transmit the infection.

There are no drugs available that act against sporozoites in the blood.

Antimalarial drugs are used to protect against or cure malaria or to prevent transmission

Protective (prophylactic) use To prevent infection, antimalarial drugs are used before infection occurs or before it becomes evident, and the aim is to prevent the occurrence of the infection and any of its symptoms:

- Suppressive prophylaxis involves the use of blood schizontocides to prevent acute attacks of malaria.

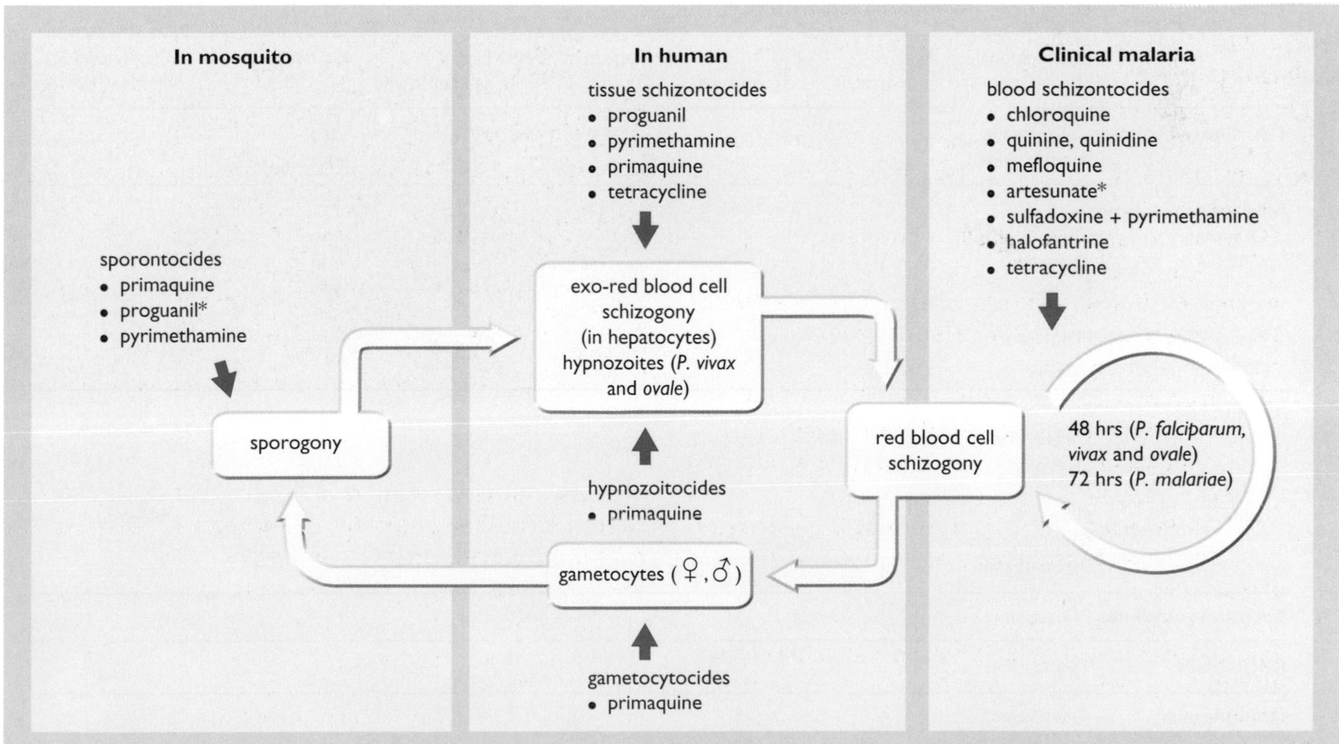

Fig. 25.3 Malaria chemotherapy. The choice of drug depends on the interactions between the malaria parasites, the antimalarial drugs, and the human host.

- Causal prophylaxis involves the use of tissue schizontocides or drugs against the sporozoite to prevent the parasite from becoming established in the liver.

Curative (therapeutic) use refers to the use of drugs to act against established infection. It consists of suppressive treatment of the acute attack, usually with blood schizontocides. Radical treatment of the dormant liver forms with hypnozoitocides is needed for relapsing malaria.

Prevention of transmission refers to eradication of infection in mosquitoes using either gametocytocides or sporontocides. This is important for controlling malaria epidemiologically.

Several chemical groups of antimalarial compounds are in general use

The actions of antimalarial drugs are summarized in Fig. 25.4.

4-Aminoquinolines

Chloroquine and amodiaquine* are active against blood schizontocides and are thought to act by:

- Being concentrated in the parasite's lysosomes where hemoglobin is being digested.
- Inhibiting the polymerization of toxic hemin into insoluble hemozoin (malaria pigment).

They are gametocytocidal against *P. vivax, P. malariae,* and *P. ovale,* but not against *P. falciparum.*

Chloroquine is the most widely prescribed antimalarial drug in the tropics. If the malaria parasite is susceptible to it, it is invaluable for curative use because it acts rapidly, and it is useful for suppressive prophylaxis.

Chloroquine is rapidly absorbed after ingestion and therapeutic blood concentrations are reached within 2–3 hours. It is slowly eliminated from the body. The kidney is the main route of elimination. Chloroquine is predominantly excreted unchanged (about 50%). Fifty percent of chloroquine is metabolized in the liver, mostly by oxidation via the cytochrome P-450 sytem.

Immediate adverse effects include nausea, vomiting, headache, uneasiness, restlessness, blurred vision, hypotension, and pruritus. It is considered to be relatively safe for use in pregnancy.

Resistant *P. falciparum* transports chloroquine out of its food vacuole more rapidly than susceptible strains. Ca^{2+} channel blockers (e.g. verapamil and nifedipine) suppress the efflux of chloroquine and, if given with chloroquine, could theoretically allow effective therapy against chloroquine-resistant strains.

Antimalarial drugs and their mechanisms of action

Class	Drug	Pharmacodynamics					
	(International generic name)	Against sporozoites	Tissue schizontocide	Hypnozoitocides	Blood schizontocide	Gametocytocide	Sporontocide
4-Aminoquinolines	Chloroquine	–	–	–	+	vmo	–
	Amodiaquine	–	–	–	+	vmo	–
Arylaminoalcohols							
Quinoline methanols	Quinine	–	–	–	+	vmo	–
	Quinidine	–	–	–	+	vmo	–
	Mefloquine	–	–	–	+	vmo	–
Phenanthrene methanol	Halofantrine	–	–	–	+	–	–
Antifolates							
Type 1	Sulfadoxine	–	–	–	+	–	–
	Dapsone	–	–	–	+	–	–
Type 2	Proguanil	–	f	–	+	–	+
	Chlorproguanil	–	f	–	+	–	+
	Pyrimethamine	–	f	–	+	–	+
8-Aminoquinolines	Primaquine	–	+	+	±	+	+
Antibiotics	Tetracycline	–	f	–	+	–	–
Quinghaosu	Artemisinin*	–	–	–	+	?	–

Fig. 25.4 Antimalarial drugs and their mechanisms of action. (–, no effect; ±, slight effect; +, marked effect ; ?, unknown effect; f, effective against *P. falciparum*; vmo, effective against *P. vivax, P. malariae,* and *P. ovale*)

Amodiaquine* is similar to chloroquine in many ways, but appears to retain some activity against chloroquine-resistant strains of *P. falciparum*. However, this advantage is usually short lived, and one of its metabolites, a quinoneimine, produces toxic hepatitis and potentially lethal agranulocytosis. Its use is now discouraged.

Arylaminoalcohols

The quinoline methanols (quinine, quinidine, and mefloquine) and the phenanthrene methanol (halofantrine) are blood schizontocides that are effective only on the blood stages of the malaria parasite engaged in digesting hemoglobin. They are used to treat acute disease because of their rapid effect on the blood stages.

Quinine and quinidine are alkaloids extracted from the bark of the *Cinchona* tree. They remain the drug of choice for the treatment of severe and complicated malaria and should always be given by rate-controlled infusion. Quinine is considered to be relatively safe in pregnancy.

Mild adverse effects are common, notably cinchonism (i.e. tinnitus, hearing loss, nausea, uneasiness, restlessness, and blurring of vision), though hypoglycemia is the most serious frequent adverse effect.

Mefloquine is structurally similar to quinine and is a long-acting blood schizontocide that is effective against all malarial species including multidrug-resistant *P. falciparum*. It can also be used for suppressive prophylaxis. It is available only in tablet form.

Adverse effects include nausea, vomiting, abdominal colic, sinus bradycardia, sinus arrhythmia, and postural hypotension. Serious but relatively rare adverse effects are acute psychosis and a transient encephalopathy with convulsions. It has been suggested that mefloquine may cause fetal abnormalities when taken during the first trimester of pregnancy.

Halofantrine is another synthetic antimalarial drug that is active against multiresistant *P. falciparum*. Its oral bioavailability is poor and variable, but can be increased if it is taken with a fatty meal. There is no parenteral preparation.

Halofantrine is usually well tolerated, with minor and reversible events such as nausea, abdominal pain, and diarrhea. However, it has been shown to prolong the electrocardiographic QTc interval at the standard recommended dose and there have been rare reports of serious ventricular arrhythmias, sometimes fatal.

Antifolates

The sulfonamides (sulfadoxine, sulfalene, and co-trimoxazole), a sulfone (dapsone), the biguanides (proguanil and chlorproguanil), and a diaminopyridine (pyrimethamine) are drugs that affect parasite folate metabolism and are divided into two groups:

- The sulfonamides and dapsone are known as type 1 antifolate drugs. They compete for the enzyme dihydropteroate synthetase, which is found only in the parasites.
- The biguanides and the diaminopyridines are known as type 2 antifolate drugs since they specifically inhibit malaria dihydrofolate reductase (Fig. 25.5).

Since both type 1 and type 2 antifolates inhibit all growing stages of the malaria parasite, these drugs are used for causal prophylaxis and treatment, and are also sporontocides as they prevent the growth of sporogonic stages in the mosquito. Mixtures of type 1 and type 2 antifolates are used in the treatment of chloroquine-resistant *P. falciparum* infections.

Sulfadoxine has a long half-life of 120–200 hours. It is less effective against *P. vivax* than against *P. falciparum*. It is synergistic in combination with pyrimethamine in a ratio of 20:1, though as the combination acts only on the late red blood stages, it seems to have a much slower action than chloroquine. This combination may cause systemic vasculitis, Stevens–Johnson syndrome, or toxic epidermal necrosis in patients who are hypersensitive to sulfonamide, and should preferably not be given in late pregnancy, during lactation, or to newborn infants because of the theoretic risk of provoking kernicterus.

Sulfalene has a half-life of 65 hours and it is often used in combination with pyrimethamine.

Dapsone has a half-life of 25 hours. It is mainly used in combination with pyrimethamine as the chemoprophylactic drug maloprim. This combination is often prescribed for travelers from the UK and Australia.

Co-trimoxazole (trimethoprim and sulfamethoxazole) is an antibacterial combination with significant antimalarial activity.

Proguanil (and the analog chlorproguanil, which has a considerably longer half-life) are prodrugs and are converted in the liver into the active triazine metabolites, cycloguanil and chlorcycloguanil. There appear to be two groups in the population, which results in conversion of the prodrug to the active metabolite by the hepatic enzyme CYP2C19 being either extensive or limited.

Proguanil has a half-life of 11–20 hours. It has a slow schizontocidal action on the red blood cell forms of malaria parasites, but is highly effective against the exo-red blood cell forms in the liver and has sporontocidal effects on *P. falciparum*.

Because of its safety, proguanil (200 mg/day) is widely prescribed in combination with chloroquine (300 mg/week) as a causal prophylactic agent. This combination can be used in pregnancy. Proguanil given alone is no longer recommended for the treatment of malaria, but recently there has been renewed interest in its use in combination with sulfones, sulfonamides, or atovaquone.

Pyrimethamine is used only in combination with sulfonamides or sulfones for treatment and prophylaxis, as resistance to it is now widespread.

8-Aminoquinolines

Primaquine is particularly active against the nongrowing stages of malaria (i.e. gametocytes and hypnozoites). It is currently the only drug available as a gametocytocide for *P. falciparum* and a hypnozoitocide (antirelapse) for *P. vivax* and *P. ovale*.

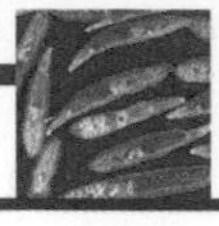

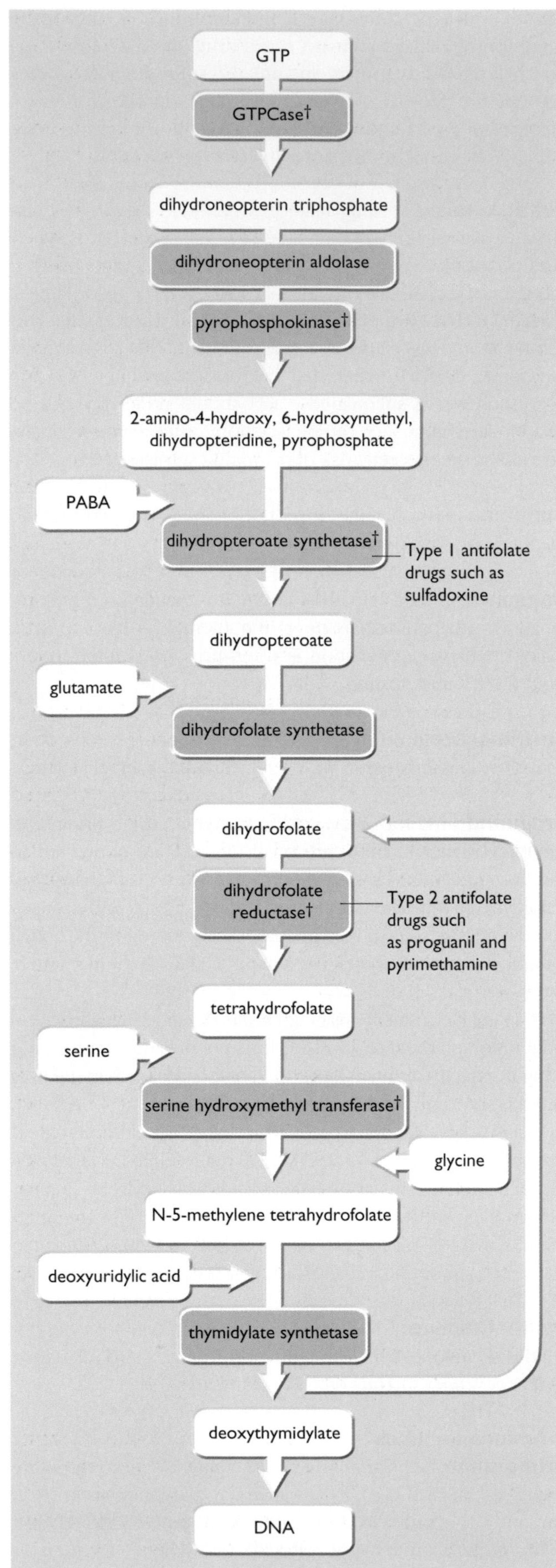

Fig. 25.5 Sites of action of antifolate drugs. Synthesis of DNA from guanosine triphosphate (GTP) by malaria parasites. The enzymes indicated with a dagger have been detected in malaria parasites, the others are presumptive. (GTPCase, GTP cyclohydrolase; PABA, *para*-aminobenzoic acid) (Adapted with permission from Warhurst DC, *Parasitology Today* 1986; 2: 58–59.)

Adverse effects include acute intravascular hemolysis in people with glucose-6-phosphate dehydrogenase (G6PD) deficiency (a hereditary deficit of this red blood cell enzyme), but severe hemolysis is unusual.

Primaquine can cross the placenta and is excreted in breast milk and should not, therefore, be used during pregnancy or lactation. A single dose of 30–45 mg base is adequate for eliminating gametocytes of *P. falciparum*, but 15 mg base is given daily for 14 days to kill the hypnozoites and achieve a radical cure of *P. vivax* and *P. ovale* malaria.

Antibiotics

These drugs (i.e. tetracycline, doxycycline, clindamycin, see Chapter 23) have a slow but marked action on the red blood cell stages of malaria. They are all inhibitors of ribosomal protein synthesis:

- Tetracycline has proved a useful addition to quinine in the treatment of multidrug-resistant *P. falciparum*.
- Doxycycline is used as a suppressive prophylactic, especially in areas where mefloquine resistance is now common, such as Thailand and Cambodia, but may have a photosensitizing effect in some individuals.

Tetracyclines should not be used in pregnant or lactating women or children under 8 years of age, because tetracyclines may produce ossification disorders of developing bones and teeth.

Clindamycin is a synthetic derivative of lincomycin and has proved effective in the treatment of uncomplicated falciparum malaria. It may also be used for the treatment in combination with quinine.

Mechanisms of action of antimalarial drugs

- 4-Aminoquinolines such as chloroquine act by concentrating in the parasite's lysosomes where hemoglobin is being digested
- Arylaminoalcohols such as quinine and mefloquine act on parasites digesting hemoglobin
- Antifolate drugs such as sulfadoxine, pyrimethamine, and proguanil affect parasite folate metabolism
- Antibiotics such as tetracycline inhibit ribosomal protein synthesis
- Primaquine is particularly active against the non-growing stages (i.e. gametocytes and hypnozoites)
- Artemisinin and its derivatives have a peroxide (trioxane) configuration that is responsible for its action

Serious adverse effects of antimalarial drugs

- Chloroquine and proguanil: mainly mild adverse effects; may be relatively safe in pregnancy
- Amodiaquine: lethal agranulocytosis
- Quinine: hypoglycemia; appropriate in pregnancy with severe malaria
- Mefloquine: acute psychosis and a transient encephalopathy with convulsions
- Halofantrine: electrocardiographic prolongation of the QT interval
- Sulfadoxine and pyrimethamine: Stevens–Johnson syndrome
- Primaquine: acute intravascular hemolysis in people with glucose-6-phosphate dehydrogenase deficiency
- Tetracycline: damaging development of bones and teeth in children under 8 years of age
- Artemisinin: relatively safe to date

New antimalarial drugs

Artemisinin (quinghaosu) is a sesquiterpene lactone extracted from the herb *Artemisia annua* (sweet wormwood), which has been used in China as an antipyretic for over 2000 years. The active component was isolated and characterized in 1971. Its peroxide (trioxane) configuration is responsible for its antimalarial activity. Clinical trials of artemisinin and its derivatives (artemether*, which is an intramuscular preparation, and artesunate*, which is available as an oral and intravenous preparation) suggest that they are rapidly acting blood schizontocides against malaria parasites including multiresistant strains of *P. falciparum,* but recrudescences are common. They have an important potential in the treatment of severe and complicated malaria, including cerebral malaria. In a recent trial in Thailand, artesunate* tablets combined with mefloquine proved more effective for the treatment of multiresistant *P. falciparum* than artesunate* or mefloquine alone. Artemisinin derivatives are now among the most promising drugs for malaria chemotherapy because of their novel molecular structure, rapidity of action, and relative safety to date.

Pyronaridine* is a mannich base that was synthesized in 1970 at the Institute for Parasitic Diseases, Shanghai. Although it is structurally similar to amodiaquine*, it may have a different mechanism of action and differing toxicity. It is effective against multiresistant *P. falciparum*, and is available as oral and injectable intramuscular and intravenous formulations.

The main adverse reactions of the oral formulation include headache, dizziness, gastrointestinal disorders, and transient electrocardiographic changes.

Benflumetol was synthesized in the 1970s by the Academy of Military Medical Sciences, Beijing. It is formulated for oral administration as a solution in linoleic acid. However, there is marked variation in its pharmacokinetic parameters, indicating poor bioavailability. It is now being given orally in China with artemether* for the treatment of *P. falciparum* infections and preclinical studies show that this combination is synergistic.

Hydroxynaphthoquinones (atovaquone) The antimalarial potential of the naphthoquinones was recognized in the mid-1940s. The most interesting compound in this group is now atovaquone, which clears resistant *P. falciparum* parasites. Early human studies showed a high incidence of recrudescence, but combination with proguanil may prevent this.

Parasite resistance to antimalarial drugs

P. falciparum was noted to be resistant to chloroquine in 1959 in Thailand and in Colombia in 1960, and the rapid worldwide spread of chloroquine-resistant falciparum malaria has posed serious problems. The problem of chloroquine resistance has been further complicated by the increasing prevalence of parasite resistance to the combination of sulfadoxine–pyrimethamine and quinine. There are also mefloquine-resistant strains of *P. falciparum* in South-East Asia and some African countries. However, despite the extensive spread of chloroquine-resistant strains of *P. falciparum* and the recent emergence of chloroquine-resistant *P. vivax* in Papua New Guinea, chloroquine is still the most widely used antimalarial drug in the world, but there is a need for alternative antimalarials.

The resistance of the parasites to antimalarials ranges from a minimal loss of effect, detected only by delayed recrudescence, to a high level of resistance, at which the drug has no suppressive effect. In 1967 the WHO proposed a grading system based on the response of *P. falciparum* parasites to normally recommended doses of chloroquine (Fig. 25.6). This grading is also used for other blood schizontocides and other species of human malaria.

AFRICAN TRYPANOSOMIASIS (SLEEPING SICKNESS)

African trypanosomiasis is a protozoan disease transmitted by tsetse flies

Two subspecies of *Trypanosoma brucei* (*T. brucei gambiense* and *T. brucei rhodesiense*) cause African trypanosomiasis, which is a serious health risk to at least 50 million people in sub-Saharan Africa. The early acute disease is a systemic illness characterized by hemolymphatic involvement with intermittent fever, skin rashes, edema, and anemia. Later, there is invasion of the central nervous system (CNS) with meningoencephalitis leading to apathy, lethargy, and somnolence. Untreated patients ultimately die from malnutrition, intercurrent infection, or deepening coma.

African trypanosomiasis is treated with suramin, pentamidine isetionate, melarsoprol, or eflornithine

If there are no CNS changes, suramin or pentamidine isetionate are the drugs of choice during the early stage of infection, while melarsoprol was until recently the only substance that could be used to treat patients with CNS involvement. Recent studies, however, have shown that eflornithine may be preferable for *T. gambiense* CNS disease.

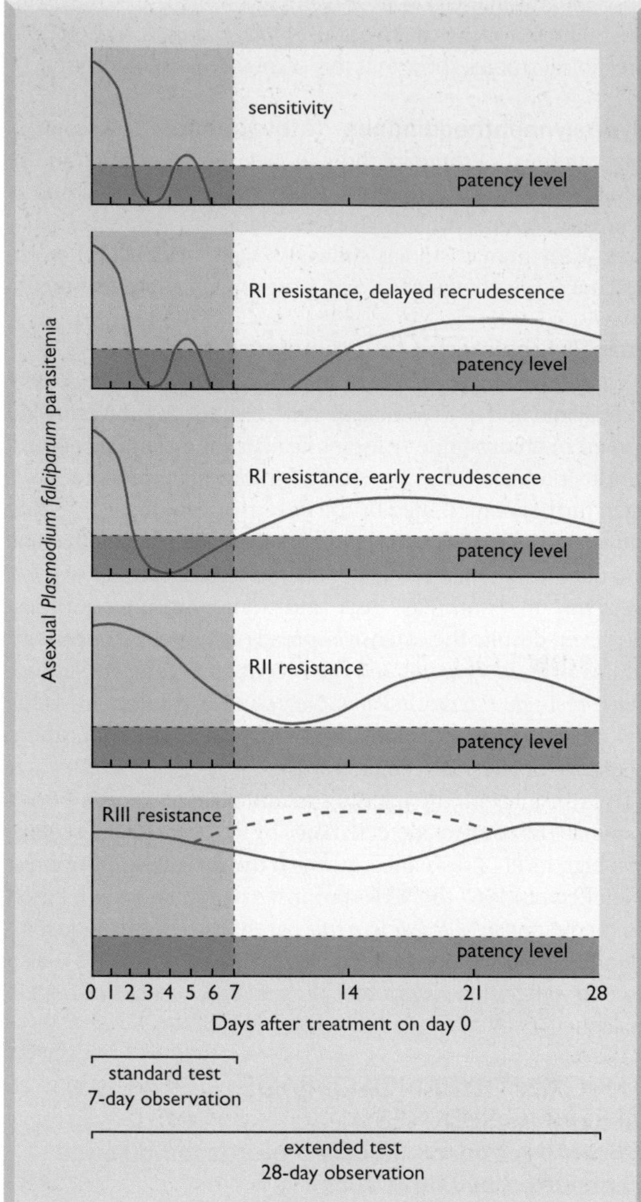

Fig. 25.6 The response of malaria parasites to chloroquine. The diagram shows degrees of response ranging from sensitivity to the highest resistance (RIII). (Adapted with permission from *WHO Technical Report Series No. 529*, by WHO Scientific Group, 1973.)

Suramin After intravenous administration, suramin binds to plasma proteins and persists at low concentrations for as long as 3 months. It does not penetrate into the CNS and is therefore restricted to the treatment of early acute disease. The mechanism of its action is uncertain, but inhibition of many enzymes is probably important because it is a polyanion that readily complexes with proteins.

Suramin causes a variety of adverse effects. Direct adverse effects that call for immediate withdrawal of treatment include rare cases of potentially fatal collapse during the first injection, heavy albuminuria, stomal ulceration, exfoliative dermatitis, severe diarrhea, prolonged high fever, and prostration. Less serious symptoms include anorexia, malaise, polyuria, urticaria, paresthesia, and hyperesthesia.

Suramin is also active against adult *Onchocerca volvulus*.

Pentamidine isetionate is a diamidine compound and is administered intravenously. It is highly tissue bound, excreted slowly, and does not penetrate into the CNS. Some interactions, such as selective adherence to the DNA of trypanosomal kinetoplasts and inhibition of ribosomal RNA polymerase, may be important to its mechanism of action.

Adverse effects include tachycardia, nausea, rash, hypotension, hypoglycemia or insulin-dependent diabetes mellitus due to direct pancreatic damage, and reversible renal failure.

Pentamidine isetionate may also be used to treat *Pneumocystis carinii* pneumonia.

Melarsoprol is a trivalent arsenical compound and is administered intravenously to treat CNS trypanosomiasis. Arsenicals react with sulfhydryl groups and therefore bind to proteins. It may inactivate pyruvate kinase, a critical enzyme in the metabolism of trypanosomes. It is largely metabolized to nontoxic pentavalent compounds and is excreted in the urine and feces within a few days.

The most serious adverse effect of melarsoprol is encephalopathy, which is fatal in about 6% of patients. Other severe adverse effects include myocardial damage, renal failure, hepatotoxicity, and hemolysis in people with G6PD deficiency. Less serious adverse effects include hyperthermia, urticarial rashes, headache, diarrhea, and vomiting.

Eflornithine (DL-*d*-difluoromethylornithine) is a relatively new agent for the treatment of African trypanosomiasis in patients with CNS involvement. Polyamine synthesis in *T. brucei* and *Leishmania* species, as in mammalian cells, is initiated by ornithine decarboxylase (ODCase). Eflornithine inhibits this enzyme. Its therapeutic use is based on the evanescence of human ODCase (which has a half-life of less than 1 hour) compared with that of trypanosomal ODCase (which has a half-life of more than 6 hours). Human cells are capable of regenerating ODCase after eflornithine is eliminated. Eflornithine hydrochloride can be given either intravenously or orally, and 80% is excreted unchanged in the urine. The ratio of cerebrospinal fluid to serum concentrations ranges from 0.09 to 0.45.

Adverse effects of eflornithine hydrochloride are usually mild and reversible. They include anemia, thrombocytopenia, vomiting, diarrhea, and a transient loss of hearing. It is a safer drug than suramin, pentamidine isetionate, or melarsoprol.

AMERICAN TRYPANOSOMIASIS (CHAGAS' DISEASE)

American trypanosomiasis is a protozoan disease transmitted by triatomine bugs, blood transfusion, organ transplantation, and congenital infection

American trypanosomiasis is caused by *T. cruzi* and affects approximately 16–18 million people and a variety of animals in Central and South America. Many people with the infection have no clinical manifestations. The infection starts with an acute parasitemic phase lasting a few weeks and continues with a chronic lifelong phase. *T. cruzi* multiplies in the amastigote phase in body tissues, particularly the heart muscles. Life-threatening manifestations in the acute phase include myocarditis and meningoencephalitis. Chronic sequelae include myocardial damage and intestinal tract involvement.

American trypanosomiasis is treated with nifurtimox or benznidazole

Both nifurtimox and benznidazole are useful drugs in the treatment of acute American trypanosomiasis. The value of therapy in the chronic phase is not clear.

Nifurtimox reduces the duration of symptoms in the acute phase of American trypanosomiasis and decreases the associated mortality due to myocarditis and meningoencephalitis. It is well absorbed after oral administration and extensively metabolized; little is excreted in the urine. Metabolic reduction of the nitro group yields a nitro anion radical. In the presence of oxygen, the nitro compound is regenerated with the production of superoxide, which is toxic to the parasite and host.

Adverse effects of nifurtimox are frequent, dose related, and reversible. They include nausea, vomiting, gastric pain, anorexia, vertigo, myalgia, convulsions, and polyneuritis.

Benznidazole is another nitroimidazole derivative used in the treatment of acute American trypanosomiasis. Its efficacy and toxicity are similar to those of nifurtimox, but its mechanism of action is unclear.

LEISHMANIASIS

Leishmaniasis is a group of protozoan infections of the viscera, skin, and mucous membranes transmitted by sandflies

Leishmaniasis is caused by protozoa of the *Leishmania* species. It is estimated that approximately 12 million people are infected worldwide.

Leishmaniasis is treated with pentavalent antimonial compounds

Leishmaniasis is usually responsive to pentavalent antimonial compounds. Patients who have relapsed and become unresponsive to antimonials alone have been successfully treated with antimonials combined with allopurinol, pentamidine, or amphotericin B.

Pentavalent antimony

Meglumine antimoniate or sodium stibogluconate are two forms of antimony used to treat leishmaniasis. Their efficacy varies according to the leishmanial species, the geographic area, and the nutritional status and immunocompetence of the host.

The pentavalent antimonials are relatively well tolerated. Dose-related electrocardiographic changes are T-wave inversion and prolonged QT intervals. Nausea, anorexia, malaise, and lethargy are uncommon, except when high doses (more than 20 mg sodium stibogluconate/kg/day) are administered.

Serious adverse effects of drugs for trypanosomiasis and leishmaniasis

- **Suramin: fatal collapse, heavy albuminuria, stomal ulceration, exfoliative dermatitis, severe diarrhea, prolonged fever, prostration**
- **Pentamidine: hypotension, hypoglycemia, insulin-dependent diabetes mellitus, reversible renal failure**
- **Melarsoprol: encephalopathy, myocardial damage, renal failure, hepatotoxicity, hemolysis in people with glucose-6-phosphate dehydrogenase deficiency**
- **Eflornithine: usually mild and reversible adverse effects**
- **Nifurtimox: myalgia, convulsions, and polyneuritis**
- **Pentavalent antimony: relatively well tolerated**

HELMINTHIC DISEASES

The helminths are large multicellular organisms with complex tissues and organs

Helminth is derived from the Greek word *helmins* and means worm. The three groups of helminths that parasitize humans are:

- Nematoda (roundworms).
- Trematoda (flukes).
- Cestoda (tapeworms).

NEMATODE (ROUNDWORM) INFECTIONS

Ascariasis

Ascariasis is caused by an intestinal nematode and is acquired by ingesting contaminated vegetables and drinking-water

Ascariasis is caused by *Ascaris lumbricoides* and is the most prevalent helminthic infection in the world. It is acquired by ingesting mature eggs contaminated vegetables and drinking-water. The adult worm usually lives in the small intestine, but can migrate to the main bile duct, gall bladder, and pancreatic duct, or can penetrate the small intestinal wall, resulting in erratic infection. The clinical manifestations include a dull upper abdominal pain, loss of appetite, nausea, vomiting, and abdominal distension.

Ascariasis is treated with pyrantel pamoate or piperazine*

Pyrantel pamoate is a broad-spectrum anthelmintic and is the drug of choice for treating ascariasis. It is also used to treat *A. lumbricoides, Enterobius vermicularis,* and hookworm infections. It is a depolarizing neuromuscular-blocking agent and inhibits cholinesterase, causing a spastic paralysis and slow contracture of these worms, respectively. Pyrantel pamoate is poorly absorbed from the gastrointestinal tract and the majority of the drug is excreted in the feces.

Adverse effects of pyrantel pamoate are usually rare when it is used in normal doses. Pyrantel pamoate is usually given as a single dose of 5–10 mg/kg.

Piperazine* is highly effective against *A. lumbricoides* and *E. vermicularis* infections. It blocks the neuromuscular junction and causes a flaccid paralysis in *A. lumbricoides*. Piperazine is rapidly absorbed after oral administration.

Adverse effects of piperazine are occasional dizziness and an urticarial reaction. It is contraindicated in people with known hypersensitivity, epilepsy, or a renal or hepatic disorder. Piperazine is given as a single dose of 30–80 mg/kg or as divided doses amounting to 50–80 mg/kg in total.

Pyrantel pamoate and piperazine have antagonistic effects and should not be used together.

Hookworm infection

Hookworm disease is also one of the most common helminthic infections. It is caused by *Ancylostoma duodenale* (Old World hookworm) or *Necator americanus* (New World hookworm). *A. duodenale* occurs predominantly in temperate zones such as the Mediterranean Basin, the Middle East, northern India, China, and Japan, while *N. americanus* occurs in the tropical and subtropical areas of Africa, Asia, and the Americas. The adult worms live in the human intestine as bloodsuckers. The life cycles of both are similar, but the penetration sites by infective larvae (filariform) are different. Old World hookworm larvae penetrate the oral mucosa, whereas New World hookworm larvae penetrate the skin. The major symptoms of infection are related to iron deficiency anemia and a loss of plasma protein.

Hookworm infection is treated with pyrantel pamoate

Pyrantel pamoate is reported to be more effective against *A. duodenale* than against *N. americanus* and the anthelmintic action of this drug is discussed above. A single dose will decrease the number of worms harbored, but complete cure may require several courses of treatment.

Enterobiasis (oxyuriasis, pinworm infection)

Enterobiasis is a worldwide infection caused by *E. vermicularis* and is the most common helminthic infection in the developed countries of the northern hemisphere, especially among schoolchildren. The parasite rarely causes serious complications. The major clinical symptom is pruritus ani.

Enterobiasis is normally treated with pyrantel pamoate.

Strongyloidiasis

Strongyloidiasis (*Strongyloides stercoralis* infection) has a worldwide distribution, particularly in tropical and subtropical areas. The infective form (filariform larvae) can penetrate through intact skin and cause an itchy erythema at the point of penetration. These larvae are carried in the blood to the lung and the sputum contaminated with these larvae is swallowed. The larvae then enter the small intestine, penetrate the mucosa, and mature into adult worms. The fertilized female discharges partially embryonated eggs. Larvae are excreted in the stools and some may penetrate the mucous membrane of the lower bowel and the anal skin (autoinfection).

The host immune mechanism and the parasite reproductive mechanism remain in balance so that neither is seriously affected. If this balance is disrupted, massive numbers of larvae can penetrate into all parts of the body (hyperinfection).

Strongyloidiasis is treated with albendazole or thiabendazole, but these should not be given to pregnant women

Albendazole Is a benzimidazole derivative that is highly effective in treating strongyloidiasis and is considered to be the drug of choice. It is thought to exert its anthelmintic effect by blocking glucose uptake in susceptible helminths, and studies have shown that it has vermicidal, ovicidal, and larvicidal activity. Less than 5% is absorbed after oral administration. A 3-day course of 400 mg once daily is normally prescribed.

Albendazole is well tolerated by both adults and children over 2 years of age, though gastrointestinal discomfort and headache have been reported. It has, however, shown a teratogenic and embryotoxic potential experimentally and should not therefore be given to pregnant women.

Thiabendazole is a benzimidazole derivative that inhibits the helminth-specific mitochondrial fumarate reductase system of various helminths. It is rapidly absorbed from the gastrointestinal tract and treatment with two divided doses of 50 mg/kg/day for 3 days is very effective against strongyloidiasis. It should be taken for at least 5 days to treat hyperinfection of strongyloidiasis.

Thiabendazole is associated with a high incidence of acute adverse effects such as vertigo and gastrointestinal discomfort (e.g. nausea, a loss of appetite, and vomiting). It also has a teratogenic and embryotoxic potential experimentally and should not be given to pregnant women. Ivermectin can be used as an alternative drug.

Infection with nematode larva

Visceral larva migrans (toxocariasis), angiostrongyliasis, and trichinosis are examples of infection with nematode larvae:

- Visceral larva migrans is a syndrome caused by the migration of the larvae of *Toxocara canis* in the viscera. Most patients are infected with only a small number of larvae and are usually asymptomatic. The infection is frequently associated with eosinophilia.
- Trichinosis is much more common in Europe and America than in Africa and Asia and is caused by *Trichinella spiralis*. The initial phase of the infection can cause transient gastrointestinal complaints such as nausea, diarrhea, vomiting, and abdominal pain. The phase of muscle invasion by the larvae typically causes the triad of myalgia, palpebral edema, and eosinophilia.
- Angiostrongyliasis is caused by *Angiostrongylus cantonensis*. Approximately 2000 cases have now been reported in the Asian Pacific area. The major clinical manifestations of cerebral angiostrongyliasis are eosinophilic meningitis with peripheral eosinophilia.

These infections are all treated with thiabendazole for at least 1–2 weeks.

Filariasis (Bancroftian filariasis, Brugian filariasis, loiasis)

Bancroftian filariasis and Brugian filariasis are caused by *Wuchereria bancrofti* and *Brugia malayi*, respectively, and have different geographic distributions:

- Bancroftian filariasis occurs in tropical areas (e.g. Central Africa, South America, India, southern China).
- Brugian filariasis is restricted to Indonesia, the Malay peninsula, Vietnam, southern China, central India, and Sri Lanka.

Both Bancroftian and Brugian filariasis are referred to as lymphatic filariasis since the organisms are found in the lymphatic system and are diagnosed mainly by detecting microfilariae in the peripheral blood.

- Loiasis is caused by the African eye worm (*Loa loa*). It is endemic only to the rain forest areas of central and west Africa. The major clinical features (fugitive swelling or carabar swelling) result from the continuous migration of the adult worm into subcutaneous tissues.

Diethylcarbamazine is used to suppress and cure infections with W. bancrofti, B. malayi *and* Loa loa

Diethylcarbamazine kills both the microfilariae and the adult worms of Bancroftian and Brugian filariasis and loiasis. A total cumulative dosage of 72 mg/kg is needed to eliminate *W. bancrofti* infections, but a lower dosage is recommended for treating *B. malayi*.

Adverse effects of diethylcarbamazine are anorexia, nausea, headache, and vomiting, They are not severe and usually disappear within a few days despite continued therapy.

Onchocerciasis

Onchocerca volvulus is the parasite that causes river blindness and is common in all parts of West and Central Africa, particularly along the rivers of the savanna in south Sahara.

Ivermectin has replaced diethylcarbamazine as the drug of choice to treat onchocerciasis.

Ivermectin immobilizes *Onchocerca volvulus* by producing a tonic paralysis of the peripheral muscle system (Fig. 25.7). It is given as a single oral dose of 0.15–0.20 mg/kg every 6–12 months.

Adverse effects are generally not reported with ivermectin, although a mild ocular irritation, transient nonspecific electrocardiographic changes, and somnolence have been reported. An immediate inflammatory reaction resulting from the death of microfilariae (Mazzotti reaction) can be severe.

Trichuriasis and capillariasis

Trichuriasis (whipworm disease) is distributed worldwide, but is most prevalent in tropical and subtropical areas. It is caused by *Trichuris trichiura*. The eggs are usually stained with bile and are barrel shaped, and transparent bipolar mucoid plugs are characteristic and diagnostic features. Patients with mild infection are usually asymptomatic, but may have gastrointestinal symptoms such as abdominal pain, diarrhea, nausea, anorexia, anemia, rectal prolapse, weakness, and cachexia.

Intestinal capillariasis is caused by *Capillaria philippinensis* and is reported in the Philippines, Thailand, Japan, and Iran. Symptoms include watery stools, malaise, anorexia, nausea, and vomiting.

Both trichuriasis and capillariasis can be treated by albendazole (as described above) or by mebendazole.

Mebendazole is a benzimidazole derivative that inhibits glucose transport. Its site of action is cytoplasmic microtubules and intestinal cells of nematodes, where it binds to the colchicine receptor on tubulin dimers (Fig. 25.8). The small amounts absorbed after oral ingestion are extensively metabolized within the liver to inactive moieties.

TREMATODE INFECTIONS

Schistosomiasis (bilharziasis)

Schistosomiasis is caused mainly by *Schistosoma japonicum, S. mansoni,* and *S. haematobium,* the type depending on the geographic location:

- *S. japonica* infection is endemic to China, the Philippines, Thailand, Laos, and the Indonesian island of Celebes.
- The endemic area of *S. mansoni* infection includes the Middle East, Africa, and South America.
- The endemic area of *S. haematobium* infection includes Africa and the Middle East.

Infected snails are the intermediate hosts for fresh water transmission.

S. japonica and *S. mansoni* primarily involve the liver, spleen and gastrointestinal tract, whereas *S. haematobium* affects the genitourinary tract.

Schistosomiasis is treated with praziquantel.

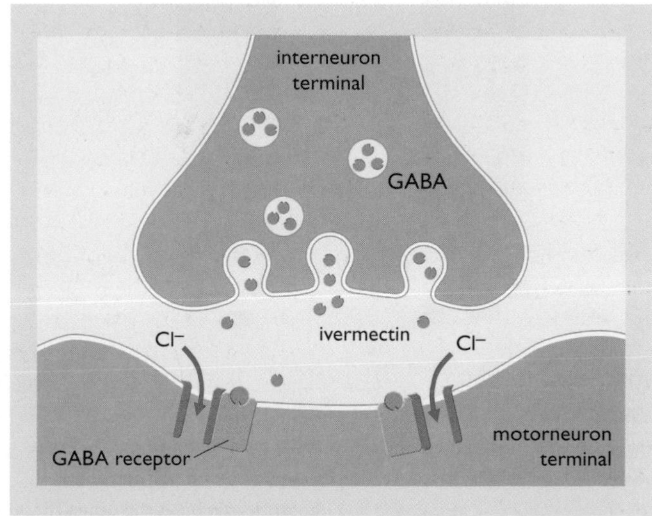

Fig. 25.7 Interaction between the nematode synapse and ivermectin. Potentiation of γ-aminobutyric acid (GABA) results in an influx of Cl^- and motor neuron hyperpolarization. Ivermectin also potentiates GABA release, which may explain its anthelmintic mechanism of action in causing worm paralysis.

Praziquantel is highly active against a broad spectrum of trematodes, including all species of schistosomes pathogenic to humans. At the lowest effective concentrations it increases muscular activity, and this is followed by contraction and spastic paralysis. At slightly higher but still therapeutic concentrations, it causes vacuolization and vesiculation of the tegument of susceptible parasites (Fig. 25.9). It is given at a daily dose of 50 mg/kg divided into three portions after meals for 2 days only.

Praziquantel is well tolerated and safe when given in one to three doses during the same day for single or mixed infections with all species of *Schistosoma*. Adverse effects include abdominal discomfort, nausea, headache, and dizziness, and may occur shortly after administration. It is preferable to delay treatment of pregnant women until after delivery, though praziquantel has not been reported to be mutagenic, teratogenic, or embryotoxic.

Clonorchiasis and opisthorchiasis

Clonorchiasis is caused by *Clonorchis sinensis* and is endemic to China, Taiwan, Hong Kong, Japan, and Korea. Opisthorchiasis is caused by *Opisthorchis viverrini,* which is distributed in Thailand, Laos, and Kampuchea, and *O. felineus* in Russia and Central and Eastern Europe. Most infections are asymptomatic in the acute stage, but may sometimes cause acute signs and symptoms including chills, fever, epigastralgia, hepatosplenomegaly, and eosinophilia. In the chronic stage, patients often have nonspecific gastrointestinal symptoms, including nausea, vomiting, a loss of appetite, and abdominal pain. The most frequent complication is recurrent cholangitis. These diseases are also a common cause of pancreatitis.

Clonorchiasis and opisthorchiasis are treated with praziquantel, 50–75 mg/kg, divided into three portions after meals for 2 days.

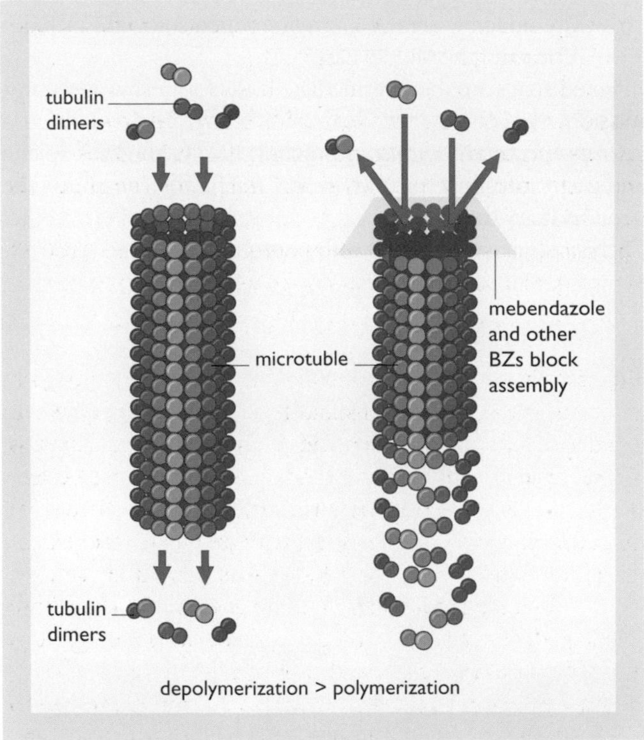

Fig. 25.8 Mechanism of action of mebendazole and other benzimidazoles (BZs). Microtubules are polar, with polymerization continually occurring at one end and depolymerization at the other. These drugs bind with high affinity to a site on the tubulin dimer, so preventing polymerization. Depolymerization leads to complete breakdown of the microtubule. (Adapted with permission from Brody, Larner, Minneman and Neu, *Human Pharmacology Molecular to Clinical*, Mosby-Year Book Inc.; 1994.)

Paragonimiasis

Paragonimiasis is caused by a lung fluke of a variety of *Paragonimus* species, most commonly *P. westermani*. However, many other pathogenic species have been reported:

- In Asia, *P. skrjabini, P. hueitungenesis, P. heterotrema, P. philippinensis,* and *P. miyazakii*.
- In Latin America, *P. kellicotti, P. mexicanus, P. ecuadoriensis,* and *P. calilensis*.
- In Africa, *P. africanus* and *P. uterobilateralis*.

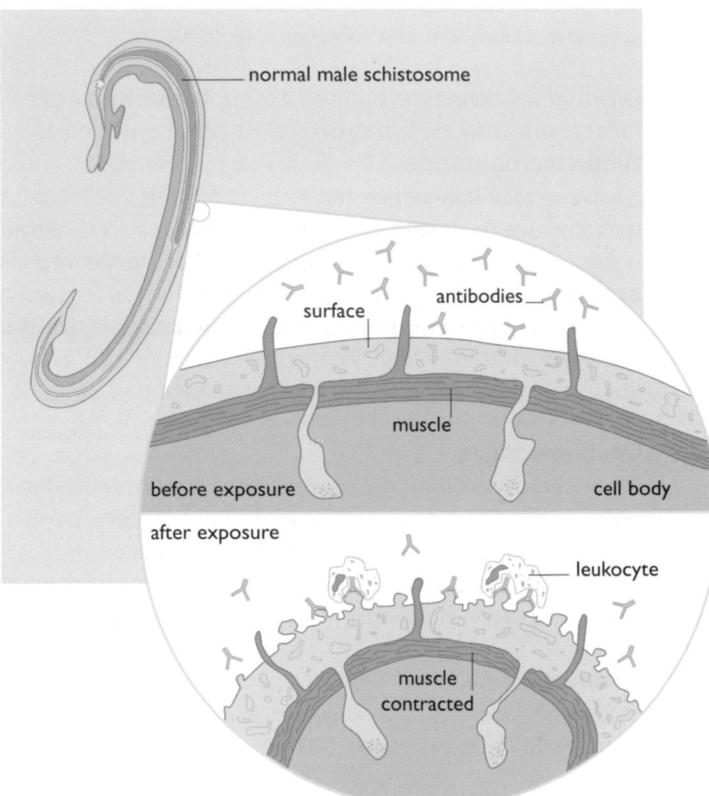

Fig. 25.9 Mechanism of action of praziquantel. (a) Before exposure the schistosome is unaffected by the numerous antibodies directed towards its surface. (b) Exposure to praziquantel increases membrane permeability to certain monovalent and divalent cations, particularly Ca^{2+}, inducing an influx of Ca^{2+} into the schistosome tegument within 1–2 seconds. The resultant change in permeability of the schistosome surface towards external ions causes small holes and balloon-like structures to form, making the schistosome vulnerable to antibody-mediated adherence of host leukocytes, killing the schistosome. (Adapted with permission from Brody, Larner, Minneman and Neu, *Human Pharmacology Molecular to Clinical*, Mosby-Year Book Inc.; 1994.)

Paragonimiasis is contracted by ingesting infected uncooked crustaceans, which are the second intermediate host of Paragonimus. In Japan, flesh meat of wild boars (the paratenic host of *P. westermani*) is a source of infection.

The major clinical manifestations of paragonimiasis are pulmonary signs and symptoms (e.g. pleural pain, dyspnea, bloody sputum, cough). Complications include pleural effusion, pneumothorax, pulmonary abscess, and empyema. Eosinophilia is common. Chest radiographs may show diffuse infiltration and nodular or ring shadows. Ectopic migration of the parasites has been reported in practically all internal organs. The most important complication is cerebral paragonimiasis. It is most frequently encountered in children in Japan and Korea.

Paragonomiasis is treated with praziquantel as a daily dose of 50–75 mg/kg, divided into three portions for 3 days, or bithionol.

Bithionol is used in a dosage of 50 mg/kg divided into two or three portions after meals on alternate days for a total of 10–15 doses. Its mechanism of action is inhibition of the respiratory actions of the parasite's mitochondria.

Adverse effects of bithionol are common and are generally mild and transient, but these symptoms are occasionally severe (e.g. anorexia, diarrhea, nausea, vomiting, dizziness, headache, and abdominal cramps).

Fascioliasis

Fascioliasis is caused by *Fasciola hepatica, F. gigantica* and *F.* sp. (Japanese large liver fluke). It occurs worldwide, is common in cows, goats, and horses, and is endemic in Europe, South and Central America, Africa, and Asia. *F. gigantica* has been reported mainly in Africa. These worms incidentally infect the biliary system of humans, and freshwater plants such as watercress, lettuce, and alfalfa, and cow's liver have been reported as sources of infection. These worms are harbored in intrahepatic bile ducts and patients with fascioliasis usually have hepatomegaly, fever, and eosinophilia.

Fascioliasis is treated with bithionol at a dose of 50 mg/kg divided into three portions after meals on alternate days for a total of 10–15 doses or praziquantel at a dose of 75 mg/kg divided into three portions for 7 days.

Fasciolopsiasis

Fasciolopsiasis is caused by *Fasciolopsis buski* and the endemic areas of this disease are eastern China, Taiwan, Thailand, Vietnam, Laos, India, and Indonesia. People become infected by eating contaminated aquatic plants, and the parasite then lodges in the duodenum and jejunum. Most infections are asymptomatic, but clinical signs and symptoms such as fever, eosinophilia, generalized edema, intestinal obstruction and malnutrition can occur in severe infection.

Fasciolopsiasis is treated with praziquantel at a dose of 50–75 mg/kg divided into three portions for 3 days.

Heterophyiasis

Heterophyiasis is caused by the members of the family Heterophyidae (e.g. *Heterophyes heterophyes* and *Metagonimus yokogawai*). *H. heterophyes* is found mainly in Egypt, the Mediterranean basin, and Japan, while *M. yokogawai* is most common in the Far East and is contracted by eating raw fish. These two parasitic infections are asymptomatic, though severe infection may produce gastrointestinal signs and symptoms (e.g. colic, abdominal tenderness, and diarrhea).

Heterophyiasis is treated with praziquantel at a dose of 50 mg/kg divided into three portions for 1–2 days.

CESTODE INFECTIONS

Large intestinal tapeworms (except *Taenia solium*)

Taeniasis is caused by adult *Taenia saginata*, which is known as the beef tapeworm, and humans are the definitive hosts. The adult worms are 5–8 m long and are made up of 1000–2000 proglottides. *T. saginata* is distributed worldwide. The adult worm is harbored in the small intestine of the host, and the gravid proglottides are expelled. Taeniasis is common in Ethiopia and in Mexico, and relatively common in South America and East and West Africa. It rarely produces severe clinical features, but must be distinguished from taeniasis caused by *T. solium*.

Diphyllobothriasis is caused by the adult *Diphyllobothrium latum,* which is known as the fish tapeworm. The infection is seen in most parts of the world (e.g. in many European countries, the Near East, Siberia, Japan, and North America). People can become infected by eating poorly cooked fillets of salmon, trout, and pike, which are intermediate hosts. The adult worm is the longest tapeworm that infects man, measuring 4–10 m in length. Most patients are asymptomatic, but in Finland some patients with this disease are anemic owing to a lack of vitamin B_{12}.

These large tapeworm infections can be treated with praziquantel, niclosamide, or Gastrografin

Praziquantel The day before the treatment, the patient is given a barium enema to reduce the quantity of feces in the intestinal lumen. Praziquantel is given as a single dose of 10 mg/kg. Magnesium sulfate is taken as a rapid-acting laxative to expel the tapeworm 2–3 hours after the praziquantel.

Niclosamide has an anthelmintic action, stimulating oxygen uptake at low concentrations and blocking glucose uptake at higher concentrations. When the parasite dies, the scolex is released from the intestinal wall and the segments are digested. Niclosamide is a safe drug because very little is absorbed from the gastrointestinal tract. On the day of treatment, the patient is fasted until treatment. The adult dose is 2 g as a single dose. Children weighing more than 34 kg are given 1.5 g, while those weighing 10–34 kg are given 1 g, and those under 10 kg, 0.6 g. The tablets should be chewed thoroughly before swallowing and washed down with a little water. Post-treatment purges to expel the worm are not necessary because the scolex and proglottides may be digested by the effect of this drug.

Adverse effects of niclosamide are not severe, though mild gastrointestinal disturbances can occur.

Gastrografin is a water-soluble contrast material for the gastrointestinal tract that has recently been shown to have an anthelmintic effect on intestinal tapeworm (*Taenia saginata, Diphyllobothrium latum, Diplogonoporium grandis*). Its mechanism of action has not been reported. Enemas and laxatives are used to decrease the volume of feces in the intestine the day before Gastrografin treatment. Gastrografin (300 ml) is injected through a duodenal tube inserted through the mouth until the tip reaches the duodenal flexure. Under fluoroscopic monitoring, the tapeworms are evident as radiolucent shadows descending in the intestine treated with Gastrografin. When the parasites reach the rectum, the patient is encouraged to defecate.

Taenia solium and *Cysticercus cellulosae*

Taeniasis is also caused by *T. solium* (pork tapeworm). The adult lives in the human intestine, like *T. saginata* and *D. latum*. Adult *T. solium* possesses 800–900 proglottides and measures approximately 2–3 m in length. Taeniasis caused by *T. solium* has a worldwide distribution. Cysticercosis is caused by the larvae of *T. solium* (*Cysticercus cellulosae*), which live subcutaneously in the orbit and brain. Most cases result from ingestion of food and water contaminated with the eggs of *T. solium*. Taeniasis and cysticercosis occur in Latin America, Eastern Europe, India, Pakistan, Indonesia, China, and Korea. The clinical manifestations of cerebral cysticercosis depend on the location of the cyst.

Drugs used to treat taeniasis and cysticercosis include Gastrografin, praziquantel, niclosamide, and albendazole

Gastrografin is the drug of choice for taeniasis because it does not cause any damage to the worm and therefore dangerous live eggs of *T. solium* are not released into the intestinal lumen. The anthelmintic action and dose for therapeutic use of Gastrografin are as described above for *Diphyllobothrium latum* above.

Cysticercosis must be treated after the treatment with Gastrografin. Praziquantel and niclosamide are also useful. Praziquantel is administered in a daily dose of 50–95 mg/kg divided into three portions for 7 days. After a further 7 days, it is given again at the same dose. Prednisolone (15 mg daily divided into three portions) should be given throughout the treatment period to prevent or reduce allergic reactions that may result from the destruction of the cysticerci.

Albendazole is a benzimidazole carbamate that blocks glucose uptake by the larval and adult stages of susceptible parasites, depleting their glycogen stores and decreasing the formation of ATP. It is a good choice for treating cysticercosis and hydatid disease and is the preferred treatment of neurocysticercosis because it is more effective than praziquantel. Albendazole is absorbed from the gastrointestinal tract and is rapidly and extensively metabolized in the liver. It is recommended that it is taken on an empty stomach when it is used against intestinal parasites, but with a fatty meal when used against tissue parasites. Two 7-day courses of 10–15 mg/kg/day divided into three portions are separated by treatment-free periods of 7 days. Prednisolone should be given throughout the treatment period to reduce allergic reactions.

Adverse effects of albendazole include transient gastrointestinal discomfort and headache.

Echinococcosis (hydatid disease)

Echinococcosis is caused by the larval forms of the tapeworms Echinococcus granulosus *and* E. multilocularis *and is acquired by ingesting the eggs*

E. granulosus is found worldwide and echinococcosis (cystic hydatid disease) is seen in East Africa, the Mediterranean littoral, South America, the Middle East, Australia, India, and Russia. *E. multilocularis* is the second most common species. Echinococcosis from *E. multilocularis* (alveolar hydatid disease) occurs in Canada, central Europe, Siberia, Alaska, and northern Japan. The adult worms of *E. granulosus* and *E. multilocularis* measure 2–7 mm and 1.2–4.5 mm in length, respectively. The scolex of these worms possesses four suckers and a rostellum with two rows of hooklets.

The adult worms live in the small intestine of a final host (e.g. dog, fox, wolf). Humans are the intermediate hosts and ingest the eggs excreted by an infected final host. The clinical manifestations depend on the size of the cyst (*E. granulosus*) and the degree of infiltration (*E. multilocularis*) in the liver, lung, and other organs. Echinococcosis from *E. multilocularis* resembles carcinoma in its ability to metastasize and is frequently fatal.

Surgery is still the treatment of choice for operable cases of echinococcosis. Chemotherapy with albendazole can be effective, given as four 30-day courses of 10–15 mg/kg/day divided into three portions separated by treatment-free periods of 15 days.

Hymenolepiasis

Hymenolepiasis is caused by *Hymenolepis nana* (the dwarf tapeworm) and *H. diminuta*. *H. nana* is the smallest tapeworm that infects humans, measuring 1–4 cm, and commonly infects children in tropical and subtropical regions. The infection is acquired by ingesting eggs in food and water. Autoinfection and rapid reproduction increase the worm population in malnourished or immunocompromised children, who experience gastrointestinal manifestations including nausea, vomiting, diarrhea, and abdominal pain.

H. diminuta is a common parasite of rats and mice that occasionally infects humans. The adult worm measures 20–60 cm in length. Its life cycle requires an intermediate host (fleas) and final host (rats and mice). People acquire the infection by accidentally ingesting infected fleas.

Treatment is with praziquantel administered as a single dose of 10–25 mg/kg. Niclosamide can be used alternatively:

- On 7 consecutive days for *H. nana* infections, using 2 g on the first day and 1 g on the remaining 6 days.
- As for large intestinal tapeworms, for *H. diminuta* infections (i.e. a single dose of 2 g).

OTHER PROTOZOAN DISEASES

AMEBIASIS

Amebiasis is caused by *Entamoeba histolytica,* which is a protozoan parasite and is worldwide in distribution. It is usually transmitted from person to person through cyst-contaminated food and drink or hands, and may also be transmitted by sexual contact. There are two groups of parasite that cannot be distinguished morphologically—a pathogenic parasite (*E. histolytica)* and a non-pathogenic parasite (*E. dispar)*. The clinical features of intestinal amebiasis due to *E. histolytica* infection range from mild diarrhea to fatal dysentery. The stools are usually soft, have a foul smell, and are often mucopurulent and bloody (i.e. look like strawberry jelly).

Amebic liver abscess is most frequently seen in extraintestinal amebiasis. Clinical manifestations commonly include right hypochondrial or epigastric pain, fever, chills, anorexia, and weight loss. Liver aspiration is a useful diagnostic and therapeutic procedure. The aspirated pus, which looks like anchovy paste or chocolate milk, is mixed with blood and necrotic liver tissue. Pleuropulmonary amebiasis, amebic brain abscesses, and amebic skin ulcers are sometimes seen.

Drugs used to treat amebiasis are metronidazole, tinidazole, or dehydroemetine. Metronidazole and tinidazole are contraindicated in people with known hypersensitivity or chronic alcohol dependence, and in early pregnancy. If dehydroemetine is used, the heart rate and blood pressure should be carefully monitored and treatment should be stopped immediately if tachycardia, severe hypotension, or electrocardiographic changes develop.

Metronidazole (see Chapter 23) is a nitroimidazole derivative with antiprotozoan activity. It also has antibacterial activity against all anaerobic cocci and both anaerobic Gram-negative bacilli and anaerobic spore-forming Gram-positive bacilli. Its mechanism of action is inhibition of DNA synthesis and degradation of existing DNA, and therefore it is potentially teratogenic.

Adverse effects of metronidazole are usually mild, but headache and gastrointestinal symptoms are common. More serious reactions are stomatitis, leukopenia, peripheral neuritis, and ataxia. When taken with alcohol it can cause abdominal pain, vomiting, flushing, and headache.

Metronidazole is given at a daily dose of 30 mg/kg divided into three portions, from 5–10 days.

Tinidazole is also a nitroimidazole derivative that has recently been developed as an antiprotozoan drug. Its mechanism of action is the same as that of metronidazole, but its adverse effects are less severe.

Tinidazole is given at a daily dose of 2 g, divided into two portions from 6–days.

Dehydroemetine Emetine is an alkaloid extracted from ipecac. Dehydroemetine is a derivative of (and is less toxic than) emetine. Following intramuscular injection it is widely distributed in body tissues. Dehydroemetine has been one of the most widely used drugs in the treatment of severe invasive intestinal amebiasis, amebic liver abscess, and other extraintestinal types of amebiasis.

Adverse effects primarily involve:

- The neuromuscular system, producing weakness (e.g. dyspnea and muscular pain).
- The gastrointestinal tract.
- The heart and cardiovascular system, producing hypotension, precordial pain, tachycardia, and dysrhythmias (e.g. flattening and inversion of the T wave and prolongation of the QT interval).

Dehydroemetine should not, therefore, be used unless the nitroimidazoles are ineffective or contraindicated. Injections should always be given intramuscularly.

GIARDIASIS

Giardiasis is an infection caused by the flagellated protozoon *Giardia lamblia*. It is transmitted through cyst-contaminated water or food and occurs worldwide, particularly where sanitation is poor. The infection is usually asymptomatic, but moderate to heavy infection usually causes anorexia, nausea, malaise, abdominal muscle cramps, vomiting, abdominal distension, and diarrhea. The clinical signs and symptoms of chronic infection are those of a malabsorption syndrome, with weight loss, steatorrheic stool, and debility.

Giardiasis is treated with either metronidazole or tinidazole.

Four major signs of congenital toxoplasmosis

- Retinochoroiditis
- Hydrocephalus
- Intracranial calcification
- Psychomotor disorders

TOXOPLASMOSIS

Toxoplasmosis is a protozoan infection caused by *Toxoplasma gondii.* It occurs worldwide, but is particularly common in warm humid areas. The sexual reproduction of *T. gondii* takes place in the intestinal epithelium of the cat, which is its final host. Toxoplasmosis is transmitted to humans in several ways, for example through:

- The feces of infected cats (transmitted via oocysts).
- Ingestion of infected raw meat, usually pork (transmitted via cysts).
- Transplacental transmission, to cause congenital toxoplasmosis.

The most common clinical manifestation is cervical lymphadenopathy, but other clinical features are fever, malaise, lymphadenopathy, atypical lymphocytosis, and myalgia. The infection has serious implications in immunocompromised hosts. Congenital infections are generally severe and can result in a fatal syndrome characterized by hydrocephalus, hepatosplenomegaly, icterus, mental retardation, and chorioretinitis.

Toxoplasmosis is treated with pyrimethamine, which is normally used in combination with sulfadiazine

Pyrimethamine and sulfadiazine are inhibitors of folate metabolism that kill the tachyzoites but do not eradicate encysted organisms. A combination of pyrimethamine and sulfadiazine is particularly effective because both drugs penetrate the cerebrospinal fluid in therapeutically active concentrations. Pyrimethamine alone has been used to treat toxoplasmic encephalitis in patients who are hypersensitive to sulfadiazine. In adults, the daily dosage is 2–4 g of sulfadiazine, along with 50 mg of pyrimethamine. The dose of pyrimethamine should be halved after 3 days and treatment should continue for 30 days. Since pyrimethamine is an inhibitor of folic acid, leukocyte counts should be checked at least twice a week.

Adverse effects of pyrimethamine are anorexia, abdominal cramps, vomiting, ataxia, tremor, and seizures. It can induce thrombocytopenia, granulocytopenia, and a megaloblastic anemia due to folic acid deficiency at the high dosage needed to treat toxoplasmosis. Adverse effects of sulfadiazine are nausea, vomiting, diarrhea, headache, and occasionally hypersensitivity reactions (e.g. Stevens–Johnson syndrome). Both pyrimethamine and sulfadiazine are contraindicated in people with known hypersensitivity or severe hepatic or renal dysfunction and in the first 3 months of pregnancy.

TRICHOMONIASIS

Trichomoniasis is a flagellate protozoan disease caused by *Trichomonas vaginalis*. It is sexually transmitted and is the commonest protozoan infection in the world. *Trichomonas* species have only a trophozoite stage, which multiplies by longitudinal binary fission and is transmitted from host to host. The infection can be asymptomatic in men, but usually causes vaginitis, cystitis, and cervicitis in women.

Drug treatment of trichomoniasis is with metronidazole or tinidazole.

PNEUMOCYSTOSIS

Pneumocystosis is caused by *Pneumocystis carinii,* which has been classified as both a protozoan parasite and a fungus. *P. carinii* is a common cause of opportunistic infection in patients who are immunocompromised, prostrated, and malnourished. *P. carinii* pneumonia is the most frequent immediate cause of death in patients with AIDS. The typical clinical manifestations are severe respiratory symptoms (e.g. dyspnea, tachypnea, cough, and cyanosis).

Drug treatment of pneumocystosis is trimethoprim–sulfamethoxazole or pentamidine isetionate

Trimethoprim–sulfamethoxazole Most cases of *P. carinii* pneumonia respond to trimethoprim–sulfamethoxazole given in a high daily dosage. These two drugs have a similar antiprotozoan spectrum and independently inhibit different steps in the enzymic synthesis of tetrahydrofolic acid.

Adverse effects of trimethoprim–sulfamethoxazole are common and include nausea, vomiting, glossitis, and skin rashes. Hypersensitivity reactions can be severe (e.g. Stevens–Johnson syndrome), while agranulocytosis, aplastic anemia, and thrombocytopenic purpura may also occur. Trimethoprim–sulfamethoxazole is contraindicated in people with known hypersensitivity and severe renal dysfunction.

Pentamidine isetionate is a diamidine compound with antiprotozoan activity and appears to be an effective treatment for *P. carinii* infection. The recommended dose is 4 mg/kg/day for 14 days, either by slow intravenous infusion over at least 60 minutes or by intramuscular injection.

Adverse effects of pentamidine isetionate include nephrotoxicity, which is common and usually completely reversible. Other common adverse effects are hypotension, hypoglycemia, and syncope, which occur after rapid intravenous infusion. Pentamidine isethionate is contraindicated in people with known hypersensitivity and severe renal dysfunction.

FURTHER READING

Karbwang J, Harinasuta T. *Chemotherapy of Malaria in Southeast Asia*. Bangkok: Mahidol University; 1992. [A useful publication for explaining the clinical pharmacology of antimalarials.]

Marr JJ. Antiprotozoal and antihelminthic chemotherapy. In: Hoeprich PD, Jordan MC, Ronald AR (eds) *Infectious Diseases 5e,* pp. 289–298. Philadelphia: J.B. Lippincott Company; 1994. [An explanation of the chemotherapy of trypanosomiasis and leishmaniasis.]

Warrell DA. Treatment and prevention of malaria. In: Gilles HM, Warrell DA (eds) *Bruce-Chwatt's Essential Malariology 3e,* pp. 164–195. London: Edward Arnold; 1993. [This book discusses the general principles of malaria chemotherapy.]

World Health Organization. *Practical Chemotherapy of Malaria, Report of a WHO Scientific Group, Technical Report Series no. 805.* Geneva: WHO; 1990. [This report provides the latest scientific advice on specific medical and public health problems related to malaria chemotherapy.]

World Health Organization. *WHO Model Prescribing Information: Drugs Used in Parasitic Diseases.* Geneva: WHO; 1990. [This publication provides practical and clinical information on essential drugs in the treatment of parasitic infections.]

Make a provisional diagnosis and determine a rational pharmacologic treatment for the following hypothetical case.

A 49-year-old man complained of intermittent pain in his epigastrium and abdominal right upper quadrant. The pain had been present for 4 weeks. He was admitted to hospital because the right upper quadrant pain had become more severe. He had not travelled outside of Japan and had lived most of his life in Mie prefecture, a rural location. An abdominal echogram demonstrated an actively mobile worm in the gall bladder. A stool exam revealed eggs with thick mamillated shells.

1. What is the probable diagnosis?
2. What is the Latin name of the worm and to which group of helminths does it belong?
3. How might this condition have been contracted?
4. What anthelmintics would you choose to treat this condition?
5. How do these anthelmintics exert their effects?

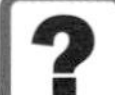

Indicate which is the correct answer for each question.

1. Which one of the following statements about metronidazole is incorrect?
   a) it is extremely useful in the treatment of trichomoniasis and amebiasis
   b) it has disulfiram-like effects (producing nausea and vomiting), when alcohol is consumed while the drug is still within the body
   c) because of its possible mutagenic effects, its use is contraindicated in the first trimester of pregnancy unless absolutely necessary (e.g. severe life-threatening infection)
   d) it is poorly absorbed from the gastrointestinal tract, and therefore has to be given parenterally
   e) its mechanism of action appears to involve disruption of the structure of DNA in susceptible organisms, resulting in strand breakage and the loss of DNA's helical structure

2. Which one of the following statements about chloroquine is correct?
   a) it is active against exo-red blood cell forms of malaria
   b) it is used to prevent initial malarial infection as well as subsequent relapse
   c) prolonged high-dosage therapy may cause corneal and retinal changes and optic atrophy
   d) its principal sites of action are Ca^{2+} channels within the cell membranes of malarial organisms, leading to increased Ca^{2+} permeability and cell death
   e) it is commonly used in the treatment of filarial worm and roundworm infections

3. Which one of the following drugs is the drug of choice for treating late African trypanosomiasis with central nervous system involvement?
   a) pentamidine
   b) melarsoprol
   c) nifurtimox
   d) suramin
   e) praziquantel

4. Which of the following drugs is combined with pyrimethamine to produce an antimalarial action by sequential blockade of folic acid biosynthesis in sensitive *Plasmodium* strains?
   a) chloroquine
   b) primaquine
   c) mefloquine
   d) sulfadoxine
   e) quinacrine

5. The mechanism of action of praziquantel against schistosomes is believed to be
   a) alteration of Ca^{2+} handling by the schistosome
   b) alteration of Na^{+} handling by the schistosome
   c) alteration of glucose handling by the schistosome
   d) alteration of ATPases in the schistosome
   e) activation of lytic enzymes in the schistosome

6. Which one of the following statements about cerebral malaria is incorrect?
   a) intravenous quinine can be useful.
   b) derivatives of *Artemisia* can be useful
   c) children are a major group affected by it
   d) children are less likely to die from it than adults
   e) *Plasmodium falciparum* is the major cause

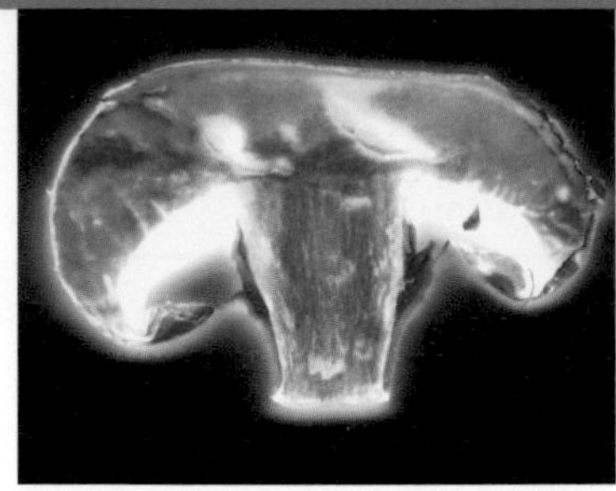

26. Fungal Infections

BIOLOGY OF FUNGI

Fungi differ from higher plants in their structure, reproduction, and nutrition. They lack chlorophyll, leaves, true stems, and roots, reproduce by spores, and live as saprophytes or parasites. The method of sexual reproduction of most pathogenic fungi is unknown (i.e. they are Fungi Imperfecti). Fungi that infect skin (dermatophytes) are classified according to their predominant ecologic site (Fig. 26.1).

Relatively few species of fungi are pathogenic and pathogenicity results from:

- Mycotoxin production.
- Allergenicity.
- Tissue invasion.

Zoophilic species tend to cause highly inflammatory skin reactions, while anthropophilic species produce mild chronic lesions. The reactions are site dependent and altered by the host's immune status. Opportunistic pathogens are important causes of disease in immunosuppressed patients.

Classification of fungi according to site of origin

Origin	Name
Soil	Geophilic
Animals	Zoophilic
Human skin	Anthropophilic

Fig. 26.1 Classification of fungi according to site of origin.

MANAGEMENT OF FUNGAL INFECTIONS

Most fungi are not affected by antibacterial drugs. There are few specific antifungal agents and the use of many of these is restricted by their relative toxicity.

The diagnosis of systemic fungal infection must be established before starting treatment because many systemic antifungal treatments have significant adverse effects

Certain fungi causing skin lesions, including *Microsporum* (e.g. *M. canis, M. audouinii, M. distortum*), produce brilliant green fluorescence under Wood's ultraviolet light, while *Trichophyton schoenleinii* causes a paler green fluorescence of infected hair (Fig. 26.2). Wood's light can also be used to diagnose pityriasis versicolor as the scales usually fluoresce yellow.

Superficial skin mycoses can be diagnosed by microscopy and culture of skin scrapings, plucked (not cut) hairs, or nail clippings, while systemic mycoses can be diagnosed by microscopy and culture of pus, exudate, tissue biopsy, feces, urine, sputum, spinal fluid, or blood. If possible, specimens should be inoculated directly onto the media.

Serologic tests are mainly available only in specialist laboratories, but help establish the diagnosis of many mycoses (Fig. 26.3).

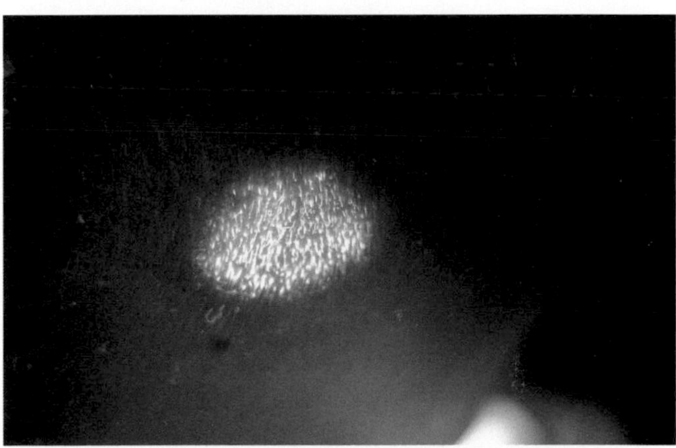

Fig. 26.2 Tinea capitis. Note the characteristic fluorescence under Wood's light. (Courtesy of Dr Richard Staughton.)

Availability and usefulness of serologic tests in diagnosing fungal infections

Serologic test useful	Serologic test useful for deep-seated infection	Serologic test useful, but not widely available
Histoplasmosis	Candidiasis	Sporotrichosis
Coccidioidomycosis	Cryptococcosis	Mycetoma
Blastomycosis		Nocardiosis
Aspergillosis (sometimes)		Chromomycosis
		Zygomycosis

Fig. 26.3 Availability and usefulness of serologic tests for diagnosing fungal infections.

Skin tests are useful diagnostically only if a patient has recently visited an endemic area for the first time, but may be of value for sporotrichosis and *Aspergillus* hypersensitivity. Positive tests have no diagnostic value in ringworm and candidal infections and are of limited significance in histoplasmosis and coccidioidomycosis.

GENERAL MEASURES FOR INFECTED PATIENTS

Spread of infection must be minimized (e.g. children should stay away from school until treatment is established [*M. canis*] or until there is no fluorescence and the hair has regrown [anthropophilic species]), and topical treatment should be used. Schoolchildren should be screened with Wood's ultraviolet light and scalp massage techniques for early diagnosis and treatment.

Advice regarding a likely source of infection can be given if the species of fungus is known (e.g. treatment of infected pets or prophylactic antifungal dusting powder after swimming).

Preventive measures should be taken for patients at high risk (e.g. frequent oral toilet, adequate denture care, and careful attention to drying and ventilation of intertriginous areas in the seriously ill can help prevent candidiasis).

SPECIFIC ANTIFUNGAL TREATMENT

The three main classes of antifungal medicines are the polyene macrolides, the antifungal azoles, and the allylamines (Fig. 26.4).

Polyene macrolide antibiotics

Amphotericin B is an antifungal antibiotic produced by *Streptomyces nodosus*. It binds to ergosterol in the fungal cell membrane (Fig. 26.5), with the formation of 'amphotericin pores' (Fig. 26.6), resulting in a loss of macromolecules and ions from the fungus and irreversible damage. Binding to

Antifungal medicines and their routes of administration

Drug class	Drug name	Routes of administration
Polyene macrolides	Amphotericin B	T, I, P
	Nystatin	T (O for GI tract only)
	Natamycin	T
	Candicidin	T
Azoles		
Imidazoles	Clotrimazole	T
	Miconazole	T, I
	Ketoconazole	T, O
	Isoconazole*	T
	Tioconazole	T
	Econazole	T
	Sulconazole	T
	Terconazole	T
	Oxiconazole	T
	Butoconazole	T
Triazoles	Fluconazole	O
	Itraconazole	O
Allylamines	Naftifine	T
	Terbinafine	T, O
Other	Griseofulvin	O
	Amolorfine	T
	Flucytosine	O

Fig. 26.4 Antifungal medicines and their routes of administration. (GI, gastrointestinal; I, intravenous; O, oral; P, parenteral; T, topical)

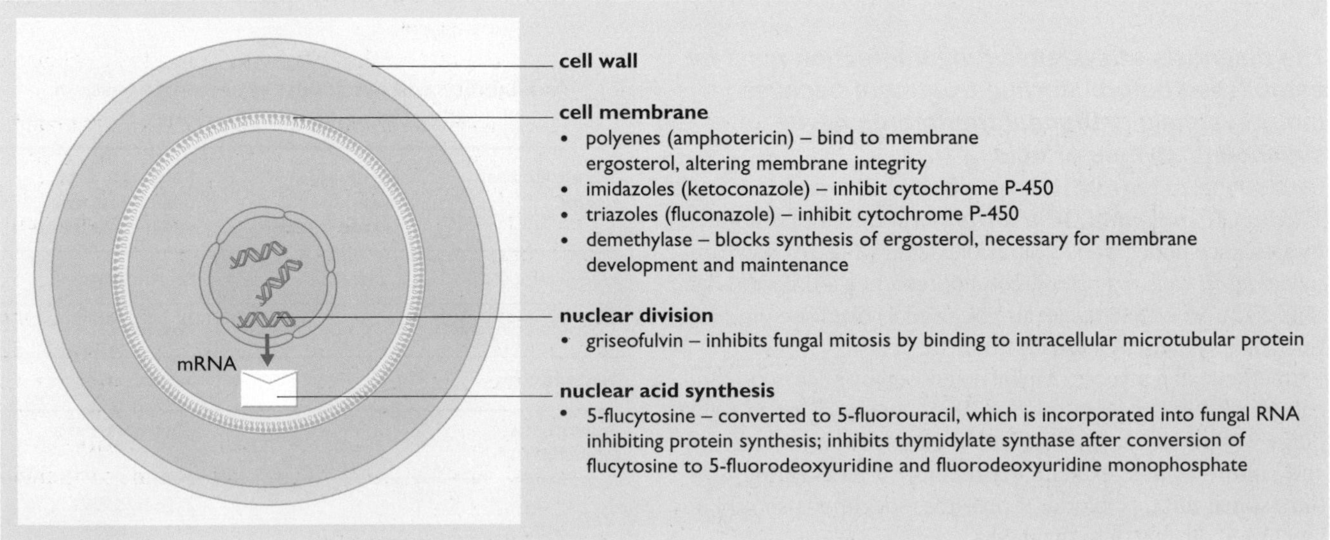

Fig. 26.5 Sites of action of antifungal drugs. (Adapted with permission from *Human Pharmacology: Molecular to Clinical* by Brody, Larner, Minneman, and Neu, Mosby-Year Book Inc., 1994.)

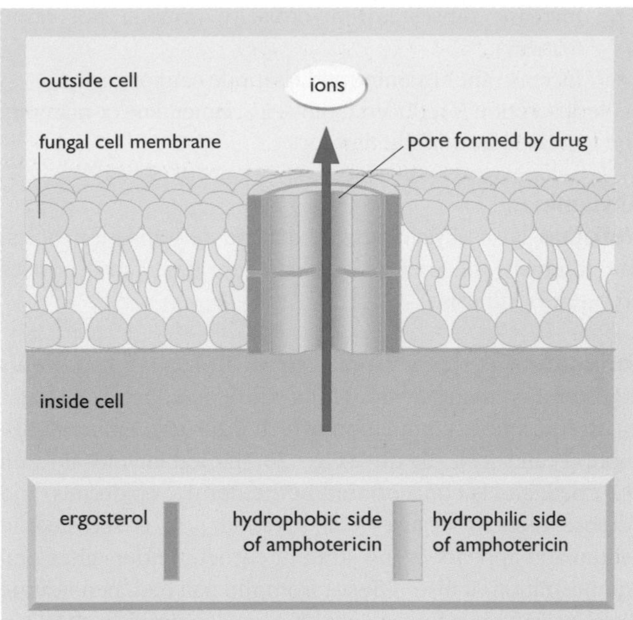

Fig. 26.6 Mechanism of action of polyene antifungal agents. Binding to ergosterol damages the membrane with leakage of ions and irreversible fungal cell damage. (Adapted with permission from *Human Pharmacology: Molecular to Clinical* by Brody, Larner, Minneman, and Neu, Mosby-Year Book Inc., 1994.)

cholesterol (e.g. on red blood cell membranes) may account for some of amphotericin's adverse effects.

Amphotericin is poorly absorbed from the gastrointestinal (GI) tract and is therefore effective orally only for GI fungal infections, is 90% protein bound, and is excreted in the urine over several days. Only 2–3% of the blood level is achieved in the cerebrospinal fluid (CSF) after intravenous injection, so intrathecal (or intracisternal) injection is necessary for fungal meningitis.

Topical amphotericin is used to treat mucosal candidiasis. Intravenous amphotericin for the treatment of systemic fungal infections (see Fig. 26.9) must be given cautiously. An initial test dose is administered, with careful monitoring, and then a slow infusion, with gradual incremental increases in dose, is delivered until there is a therapeutic response. Daily treatment often has to be continued for 6–12 weeks. Longer-term treatment on alternate days (this is sufficient once a steady state is achieved) is often needed to maintain blood levels.

Amphotericin resistance can develop if the fungus alters the amount of ergosterol on its membrane or modifies its structure so that the drug binds less avidly.

Adverse effects following intravenous infusion of amphotericin

- Fever
- Chills
- Hypotension
- Vomiting
- Dyspnea
- Headaches
- Thrombophlebitis at the site of injection
- Renal toxicity is invariable, but treatment can be continued to a creatinine concentration of 200 μmol/liter

Nystatin is a polyene macrolide with a similar mechanism of action to amphotericin. It is stable when dry, but quickly disintegrates on contact with water or plasma. It is not absorbed from skin, mucous membranes, or the GI tract, and orally administered nystatin is excreted in the feces. It is too toxic for parenteral administration. Its clinical use is limited to topical applications for the skin and mucous membranes (buccal and vaginal), and oral administration to suppress *Candida* in the lumen of the gut in infants and those with impaired immunity. Resistance to nystatin does not develop *in vivo*, but some *Candida* species are not susceptible.

Natamycin is a polyene antifungal agent used as a 5% ophthalmic suspension.

Candicidin is a polyene antibiotic used topically for vaginal candidiasis.

Antifungal azoles

Imidazoles and triazoles:

- Inhibit fungal lipid (especially ergosterol) synthesis in cell membranes.
- Interfere with fungal oxidative enzymes (primarily the 14α-demethylase microsomal P-450-dependent enzyme) resulting in accumulation of 14α-methyl sterols, which may disrupt the packing of acyl chains of phospholipids, inhibiting growth and interfering with membrane-bound enzyme systems.

Triazoles have greater selectivity against fungi than imidazoles, and cause less endocrine disturbance.

These agents are available for topical use, but clotrimazole is too toxic to use systemically. Intravenous miconazole can be used for disseminated mycoses, but is limited by its adverse effects (vomiting, hyponatremia, hyperlipidemia, thrombophlebitis, hematologic disturbances).

Ketoconazole was the first orally active azole antifungal agent. It is less toxic and less effective than amphotericin. It is well absorbed (but see interactions below), although CSF concentrations are low; it is largely protein bound, and is metabolized by the liver. Ketoconazole is indicated for:

- *Candida* (1–2 weeks; 4–10 months for mucocutaneous candidiasis).
- Dermatophytes (3–8 weeks).
- Systemic infections, particularly disseminated blastomycosis, but not fungal meningitis.

Adverse effects of ketoconazole

- Nausea
- Vomiting
- Photophobia
- Skin rashes
- Hepatotoxicity
- Mild elevation of hepatic enzymes (5–10%)
- Symptomatic hepatitis is rare, but progressive fatal hepatotoxicity reported with high doses so liver function tests required at regular intervals
- Gynecomastia and reduced libido
- Menstrual irregularities (10% of women)
- Hypertension and fluid retention
- High dose ketoconazole should be avoided in patients with tuberculosis, histoplasmosis, paracoccidioidomycosis, and AIDS

Fluconazole (a bistriazole) is more readily absorbed from the GI tract than ketoconazole and penetrates the blood–brain barrier producing CSF concentrations 50–80% of those in the blood. It is excreted by the kidneys unchanged and its half-life is considerably prolonged in renal insufficiency. It can be used for systemic infections including cryptococcal meningitis, although relapse is common and maintenance treatment is often required. Adverse effects include vomiting, diarrhea and rashes (including Stevens–Johnson syndrome). Thrombocytopenia and transient abnormalities of hepatic function are also described, but there seem to be no endocrine effects. Animal studies suggest that it is teratogenic.

Itraconazole is a synthetic dioxolane triazole. Absorption from the GI tract is incomplete, but increases when it is taken with food. It is 99% protein-bound and is concentrated in tissues such as lung, liver, and bone, but has limited CSF penetration. It is excreted by the liver and has one active metabolite with a half-life of 20–40 hours, which is also excreted by the liver. In neutropenic pateints, a loading dose should be given for the first four days and a maintenance dose of 400 mg is often required to achieve adequate serum levels. Itraconazole is well tolerated, though nausea, vomiting, headaches, abdominal pain, and transient increases in hepatic enzymes have been reported.

Resistance to the azole drugs is rare, but resistant *Candida* strains have been recovered from patients with chronic mucocutaneous candidiasis and AIDS.

Important drug interactions Azole drugs:

- Increase the phenytoin, oral hypoglycemic, anticoagulant and cyclosporine concentrations (by inhibition of P-450).
- Increase simvastatin myotoxicity (muscle not bone marrow).
- Increase antihistamine and cisapride cardiotoxicity.

Azole absorption is reduced by antacids, cimetidine or rifampin, and increased by thiazide diuretics.

Allylamines

Naftifine is an allylamine naphthalene derivative for topical use. It inhibits the enzyme squalene epoxidase and decreases ergosterol synthesis.

Terbinafine is the first orally active allylamine. It prevents ergosterol synthesis by inhibiting squalene epoxidase, resulting in squalene accumulation, which leads to membrane disruption and cell death (Fig. 26.7). Terbinafine is well absorbed, and is concentrated in the dermis, epidermis, and adipose tissue (because it is lipophilic). It is secreted in sebum and appears in the stratum corneum hours after oral administration. It also diffuses from the nail bed, penetrating distal nails within four weeks. It is metabolized in the liver and the inactive metabolites are excreted in the urine. It is effective mainly against dermatophytes. Early trials show impressive clinical and mycologic cure and relapse rates (Fig. 26.8). Terbinafine is well tolerated. Nausea, abdominal pain, and allergic skin reactions can occur, but are often mild. Loss of taste has been reported. Terbinafine concentrations are increased by cimetidine and reduced by co-administration with rifampin.

Other antifungal agents

Griseofulvin was the first, orally active, antifungal agent isolated from *Penicillium griseofulvum*. Its mechanism of action is not established, but it probably interferes with microtubule function or nucleic acid synthesis and polymerization. It inhibits dermatophyte growth, but has no effect on the fungi producing deep mycoses or on *Candida* species. Absorption varies according to the preparation, but microparticle preparations are better absorbed, peaking 1–3 hours after ingestion. Serum concentrations drop after 30 hours. It is concentrated in active metabolizing cells near the hyphal tip and passes rapidly into fully keratinized cells, reaching the outermost cells in eight hours, but is not thought to bind firmly to keratin. As sweat transports griseofulvin in the stratum corneum, excessive sweating can cause rapid clearance. Griseofulvin is metabolized in the liver to 6-demethyl griseofulvin, which is then excreted via the kidneys and perhaps bile.

Griseofulvin is the treatment of choice for childhood dermatophyte infections, but the treatment schedules are prolonged because the drug is fungistatic rather than fungicidal. Long-term relapse rates are high (40–70% for toenails).

Adverse effects are uncommon, but a hypersensitivity reaction with fever, skin rash, leukopenia and a serum sickness-like illness is well recognized. Headaches are common, and irritability and nightmares can be a problem, but usually improve on continuing the drug. If not, the dose can be reduced to 125 mg daily for a few days and then gradually increased, giving most of the treatment at night. Griseofulvin can cause light sensitivity eruptions and petechial rashes, and has also been associated with urticarial rashes, which settle despite continuing treatment. Hepatotoxicity, peripheral neuritis, bone marrow suppression, proteinuria and estrogen-like effects in children have been described, and griseofulvin is teratogenic.

Griseofulvin resistance can develop during treatment.

Griseofulvin interacts with other drugs including:

- Warfarin, increasing warfarin metabolism and reducing the anticoagulant effect.
- Phenobarbital, with simultaneous treatment reducing the blood concentration of griseofulvin after oral administration.

Griseofulvin exacerbates porphyria, and reportedly precipitates or exacerbates systemic lupus erythematosus.

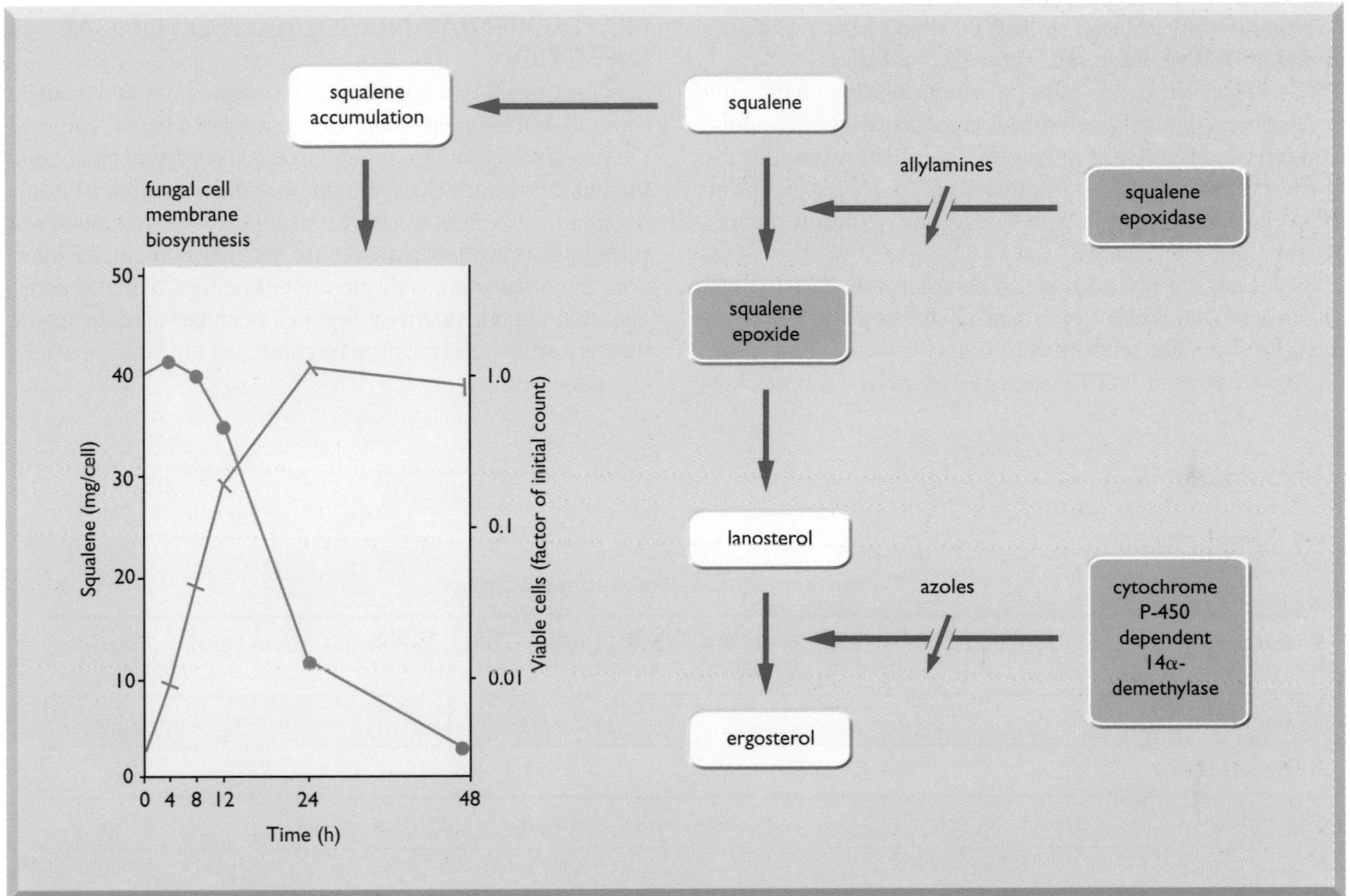

Fig. 26.7 Terbinafine inhibits squalene epoxidase, resulting in the accumulation of squalene inside the fungal cell. This accumulation of squalene (red line) correlates with cell death (blue line). (Adapted with permission from Ryder NS, *Clin Exp Dermatol*, 1989, 14, 98–100.)

Effectiveness of terbinafine

Infection	Dosage	Clinical cure (%)	Mycologic cure (%)	Relapse rate (%)
Tinea unguium	250 mg 12 wks		81–88	
Tinea pedis	250 mg 2 wks	87	78	Low 6/52 later
Tinea corporis/cruris	250–500 mg	85	92	
Onychomycosis (hands)	250–500 mg	85	95	80% cure at 3–12 month follow-up
Onychomycosis (toes)	250–500 mg	80	80	
Candidiasis	500 mg 4 wks	70	80	

Fig. 26.8 Effectiveness of terbinafine.

Amolorfine is a recently introduced antifungal available as a nail lacquer that is fungicidal for dermatophytes and has some activity against molds.

Flucytosine is active orally and interferes with nucleic acid syntheisis by inhibiting thymidylate synthetase. It is active only in cells able to transport it into the cell via a cytosine permease and convert flucytosine to 5-fluorouracil. This is then metabolized by uridine monophosphate pyrophosphorylase and can be incorporated into RNA or metabolized to 5-fluorodeoxyuridylic acid, a potent thymidylate synthetase inhibitor. DNA synthesis is disrupted as a result.

The clinical usefulness of flucytosine is limited by the rapid development of resistance, which is partly delayed by co-administration of amphotericin B. Proposed mechanisms include loss of the permease for cytosine transport or decreased uridine monophosphate pyrophosphorylase or cytosine deaminase activity.

Flucytosine is well absorbed and penetrates the CSF (60–80% serum levels). It is excreted largely unchanged in the urine, so the dose should be reduced in renal impairment.

Adverse effects include hepatotoxicity (enzyme abnormalities occur in about 5% of patients, but are usually reversible), enterocolitis, hair loss, and bone marrow suppression. Blood counts should be monitored weekly. Uracil reduces bone marrow suppression without reducing antifungal efficacy. The plasma concentration should be monitored.

Treatment indications of antifungal agents

A summary of the effectiveness of antifungal agents is shown in Fig. 26.9.

NEUTROPENIA AND SUSPECTED FUNGAL INFECTION

Antifungal treatments must be started in any neutropenic patient with a fever resistant to antibiotics before knowing the nature of the fungal infection. Amphotericin B is the drug of choice and the full therapeutic dose should be achieved within 24 hours because treatment of established candidiasis or aspergillosis in such patients is often unsuccessful. Furthermore, fungal infections often reactivate with subsequent periods of neutropenia. Empirical amphotericin treatment before antileukemic treatment may be justified, and needs to be continued until the neutrophil count recovers.

Treatment indication of antifungal agents

Infection	Amphotericin B	Ketoconazole	Fluconazole	Itraconazole	Terbinafine	Griseofulvin	Flucytosine
Dermatophytes		x		x	x	x	
Pityrosporum		x		x			
Candidiasis	xC	x	x	x	x		x
Aspergillus	x	x		x			x
Blastomycosis	x	x		x			
Coccidioidomycosis	x	x		x			
Cryptococcosis	xC	x	x				x
Histoplasmosis	x	x		x			
Paracoccidioidomycosis	x	x		x			x
Chromoblastomycosis							
Sporotrichosis	x			x			
Mucormycosis	x						x
Toluropsis							
Pseudoallescheriasis		x					
Zygomycosis		x					

Fig. 26.9 Treatment indication of antifungal agents. (C, amphotericin B used in combination with flucytosine)

Prophylaxis

Fluconazole can be used prophylactically against candidiasis in neutropenic patients, but ketoconazole is not recommended for transplant recipients because it interferes with cyclosporine concentrations. Itraconazole seems to afford some protection against aspergillosis and candidiasis, but absorption is a problem. It is recommended in units without high-efficiency particulate air filters, and should be used in preference to fluconazole for patients who remain neutropenic for more than 3 weeks.

NONSPECIFIC TREATMENT OF FUNGAL INFECTIONS

A variety of topical preparations are available for skin infections and can be effective if used regularly.

Compound benzoic acid ointment (Whitfield's ointment) is effective, but less acceptable cosmetically, than some newer preparations. It must be diluted by 50% for use in the scrotum and groin (in emulsifying ointment). Antiseptic paints such as Castellani's paint, undecenoate fatty acids and their salts, benzoyl peroxide, salicylic acid, ciclopirox olamine, iodochloroxolamine, triacetin, haloprogins and tolnaftate are alternatives for dermatophyte infections. Contact dermatitis is a rare adverse effect with all these treatments, and irritant dermatitis can pose problems, especially in patients with raw skin and fissures.

Selenium sulfide 2.5% in a detergent base is widely used for pityriasis versicolor. It stains clothing and can be irritant, but is considerably cheaper than topical azoles. Alternatively 20% sodium hyposulfite solution and 50:50 propylene glycol in water can be used long term to prevent relapses

Saturated potassium iodide solution given orally remains the treatment of choice for lymphocutaneous sporotrichosis.

FURTHER READING

Bickers DR. Antifungal therapy: potential interactions with other classes of drugs. *J Am Acad Dermatol* 1994; **31**: S87–90. [A useful review of the clinically relevant interactions of commonly used antifungal drugs with other drug classes.]

Bjorkholm M. Chemoprophylaxis of fungal infections in neutropenic patients. *Ann Oncol* 1994; **5**: 571–574. [A review of the prevention of fungal infections in neutropenic patients.]

Filler SG, Edwards SG. When and how to treat serious candidal infections: concepts and controversies. *Curr Clin Top Infect Dis* 1995; **15**: 1–8. [A review of the treatment of candidal infections.]

Finlay AY. Global overview of Lamisil. *Br J Dermatol* 1994; **43**: 1–3. [An extensive review of the clinical trial data with Terbinafine.]

Make a provisional diagnosis and determine a rational pharmacologic treatment for the following hypothetical case.

A 7-year-old school girl was taken to her family practitioner by her mother who was concerned about her daughter's hair loss and itchy scalp. The child's scalp was inflamed, with hair loss and scaling. Many of her school friends had reported similar symptoms over the previous few months.

1. How would you confirm whether the infection was a fungal infection?
2. What general measures would you recommend to the child's mother?
3. What drug would be most useful to treat this child?

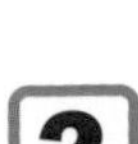

Indicate whether the following answers are true or false.

1. The following statements are correct
- a) fungi reproduce by spore formation
- b) zoophilic fungi are likely to produce less inflammation than anthropophilic species
- c) most fungi that are pathogenic to man are Fungi Imperfecti
- d) microscopy and culture of skin or tissue is the most important investigation of fungal disease
- e) Wood's light examination can help in the diagnosis and management of fungal infection

2. The following mechanisms of action are correct
- a) amidazoles and triazoles inhibit the synthesis of fungal lipids, especially ergosterol
- b) terbinafine prevents the synthesis of ergosterol by inhibiting the action of squalene epoxidase
- c) amphotericin B acts by binding to ergosterol in cell membranes
- d) amidazoles and triazoles interfere with fungal oxidative enzymes
- e) griseofulvin is thought to act by interfering with microtubule function or with nucleic acid synthesis and polymerization

3. The following statements about the metabolism of antifungal agents are correct
- a) amphotericin B and itraconazole are largely protein bound in the blood
- b) the azole antifungal agents are orally active and penetrate the blood–brain barrier
- c) doses of fluconazole need to be modified in renal failure
- d) terbinafine is concentrated in skin, nails, and fat
- e) blood flucytosine concentration should be monitored

4. Oral candidiasis
- a) is more common in people with diabetes mellitus
- b) is a common complication of inhaled anti-asthma medication
- c) is treated with amphotericin B
- d) treatment in patients with dentures includes treatment of the dentures as well as the mouth
- e) suggests immunosuppression or chronic mucocutaneous candidiasis if the patient fails to respond to topical treatment

5. In cryptococcal meningitis
- a) combination treatment with amphotericin B and flucytosine is the treatment of choice in non-AIDS patients
- b) combination therapy delays the development of resistant organisms
- c) in patients with AIDS requires long-term therapy to prevent relapse
- d) fluconazole can be used to induce clinical remission
- e) oral itraconazole and fluconazole suppress recurrences after induction of remission

6. The following statements about adverse effects are correct
- a) headaches can be experienced with amphotericin B, griseofulvin, and itraconazole
- b) thrombophlebitis can be a problem with intravenous amphotericin B and miconazole
- c) amphotericin B is nephrotoxic
- d) hepatotoxicity is the major adverse effect of ketoconazole
- e) fluconazole and itraconazole interfere less with androgen steroid synthesis than ketoconazole

7. The following statements are correct
- a) in pityriasis versicolor shampoo preparations (e.g. ketoconzole shampoo) are a useful first line treatment
- b) tinea pedis infection at swimming pools can be reduced by the use of tolnaftate powder
- c) topical treatment of scalp ringworm limits spread, but systemic treatment is needed to eradicate the infection
- d) cure rates and relapse rates of nail infections are better with terbinafine than with griseofulvin
- e) ketoconazole can be used instead of amphotericin B for histoplasmosis and paracoccidiomycosis of the lung

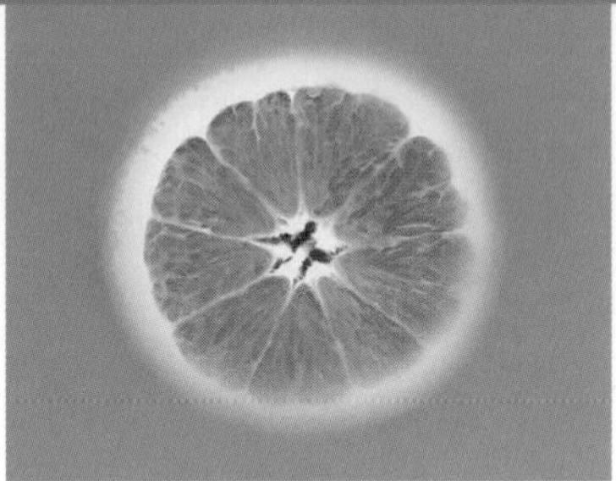

27. Vitamins

Vitamins are defined as structurally unrelated organic compounds that must be provided in small quantities in the diet. Although diet is the principal source, there are other sources: for example, vitamin D is synthesized in skin exposed to ultraviolet light and vitamin K is synthesized by intestinal flora.

Vitamins differ from:

- Minerals, which are also nutrients required in small quantities, because minerals are inorganic substances.
- Essential amino acids, which are also organic nutrients, because essential amino acids are needed in large quantities.

The discovery of vitamins has important historical roots. The recognition of deficiency states, seen only rarely today, often led to the isolation of the individual vitamins.

Rickets, beriberi, and scurvy are all examples of deficiency diseases which ultimately led to the discovery of vitamins D, B, and C, respectively. Historical background is often a useful beginning for a clear understanding of the individual vitamins.

CLASSIFICATION

Vitamins are a heterogeneous group of compounds with very different structures, sources, daily requirements, and modes of action. There are two major types based on solubility: water-soluble vitamins (e.g. vitamin B complex, vitamin C) and fat-soluble vitamins (e.g. vitamins A, D, E, and K) (Fig. 27.1). Subclassification of vitamins takes into account features other than solubility, for example storage capacity in the body, mode of action, and potential toxicity.

The body's storage capacity for different vitamins varies

The body's storage capacity is high for fat-soluble vitamins and lower for water-soluble vitamins. An exception to this rule is the body's storage capacity for the water-soluble vitamin B_{12}, which is normally sufficient for about 3–6 years.

Some vitamins are more toxic than others

Toxicity due to either long-term accumulation in the body or a short-term administration of a high dose is more likely with fat-soluble vitamins (e.g. vitamins A and D).

Classification of vitamins

Water-soluble vitamins	Fat-soluble vitamins
Vitamin C	Vitamin A
B complex vitamins Vitamin B_1 (thiamine) Vitamin B_2 (riboflavin) Vitamin B_3 (nicotinic acid) Vitamin B_6 (pyridoxine) Vitamin B_{12} (cobalamin) Pantothenic acid Biotin Folic acid	Vitamin D Vitamin E Vitamin K

Fig. 27.1 Classification of vitamins. The two major groups based on solubility are water-soluble and fat-soluble vitamins.

Diseases caused by vitamin deficiency

- Beriberi (vitamin B_1)
- Hemorrhage (vitamin K)
- Megaloblastic anemia (vitamin B_{12}, folic acid)
- Night blindness (vitamin A)
- Osteomalacia (vitamin D)
- Pellagra (vitamin B_3)
- Rickets (vitamin D)
- Scurvy (vitamin C)

VITAMINS AS THERAPY

Vitamins maintain growth and normal body functions

There are large variations in the daily requirements of the different vitamins. An inadequate supply is associated with specific deficiency diseases. Some people, such as pregnant women, alcoholics, and strict vegans have an increased risk of developing vitamin deficiency.

People at risk of vitamin deficiency

- Pregnant women
- Infants
- The elderly
- People with chronic disease
- People who take drugs, such as oral contraceptives, or anticonvulsants, on a regular basis
- Alcoholics
- Strict vegans
- Undernourished populations

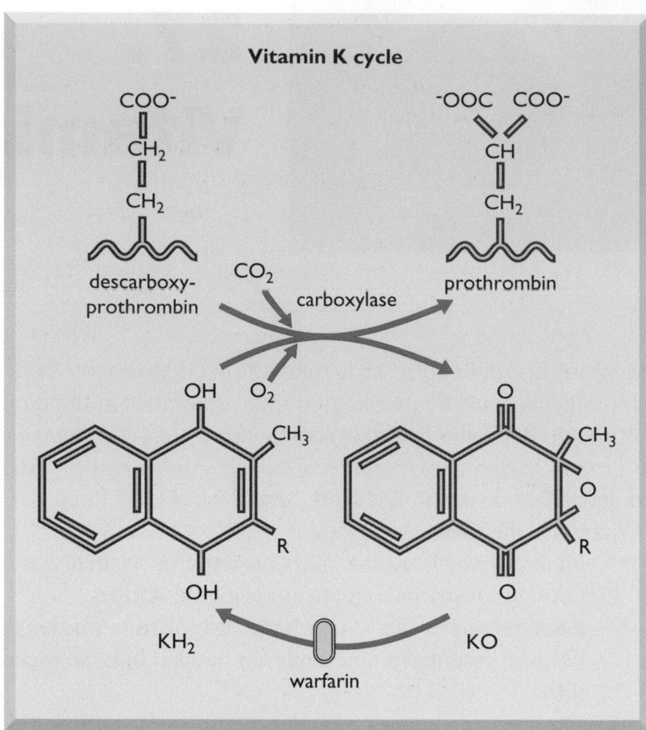

Fig. 27.2 The vitamin K cycle. Vitamin K acts as a coenzyme in the conversion of descarboxyprothrombin to prothrombin catalyzed by carboxylase. During the carboxylation process, vitamin K is converted to its inactive oxide and then metabolized back to its active form. The reductive metabolism of the inactive vitamin K epoxide back to its active hydroquinone form is warfarin sensitive. Warfarin and related drugs block the γ-carboxylation and this results in molecules that are biologically inactive for coagulation.

HOW VITAMINS WORK

Vitamins exert their effects in three main ways: as coenzymes, as antioxidants, or as hormones.

Most water-soluble vitamins act as coenzymes for specific enzymes

Many enzymes are inactive without the presence of small amounts of substances called cofactors. These cofactors can be trace metals or organic molecules, and organic molecules that function as cofactors are called coenzymes. Coenzymes take part in the reaction being catalyzed. During the process they are transformed into an intermediate form and are subsequently generated back to their active form (Fig. 27.2). Most water-soluble vitamins act as coenzymes for specific enzymes.

Some vitamins act as antioxidants, others as hormones

Vitamin C and vitamin E function as antioxidants, while the two fat-soluble vitamins, vitamin A and vitamin D, act as hormones. Specific binding sites have been identified for vitamin A and vitamin D for exerting their hormonal activity.

RECOMMENDED DIETARY ALLOWANCES AND DAILY INTAKE

Recommended dietary allowances (RDAs) of vitamins (as well as minerals and other nutrients) have been established in most countries. RDAs are aimed at maintaining maximal stores of the vitamins without causing toxicity and are intended to meet the requirements of normal persons with respect to age and sex. The recommended daily intake has been based on a daily intake of 2000 kcal (Fig. 27.3). In the US, RDAs are published periodically by the Food and Nutrition Board, National Academy of Sciences, and National Research Council.

Daily vitamin requirements

Vitamin A	5000 IU
Vitamin B_1	1.5 mg
Vitamin B_2	1.7 mg
Vitamin B_3	20 mg
Vitamin B_6	2 mg
Vitamin B_{12}	0.003 mg
Vitamin C	60 mg
Vitamin D	400 IU
Vitamin E	30 IU
Vitamin K	0.08 mg
Pantothenic acid	10 mg
Biotin	0.3 mg
Folic acid	0.4 mg

(Daily values based on 2000 kcal daily intake)

Fig. 27.3 Daily vitamin requirements.

INTERACTION OF VITAMINS WITH DRUGS AND FOODS

There are several examples of common food interactions. For example, ingestion of large doses of vitamin C-containing fruits interferes with the absorption of vitamin B_{12}. Likewise, certain fish and blueberries may contain thiaminase, which inactivates vitamin B_1.

Drug–vitamin interactions are discussed in the appropriate sections for the individual vitamins. In general, long-term ingestion of unabsorbed lipids such as mineral oil (used as a laxative) may dramatically decrease the absorption of the fat-soluble vitamins and may lead to the related vitamin-deficiency disease. Other drug–vitamin interactions include:

- Estrogen-containing oral contraceptives and vitamins B_1, B_2, and folic acid.
- Antibiotics and sulfonamides with vitamin B_3 (tetracyclines), vitamin B_{12} (neomycin), vitamin C (tetracyclines), vitamin K (sulfonamides), and folic acid (sulfonamides).
- Anticonvulsants and vitamin D, vitamin K, and folic acid.

VITAMINS AS DIETARY SUPPLEMENTS

Dietary supplements may contain over-the-counter drugs, plant extracts, and vitamins. At present, they are not covered by Food and Drug Administration regulations and are often marketed without accurate content and composition labeling and without instructions for safe use. These substances may have adverse effects and interact with drugs and foods.

Vitamin pills are mostly consumed by children, the elderly, and exercising adults, and about 40% of the adult population in the US and Canada supplement their diet with vitamins daily.

The usefulness of vitamin pills for purposes other than correcting deficiency symptoms has not been established. An intake of fat-soluble vitamins at doses exceeding the RDA has a potential risk of producing hypervitaminosis. Ingestion of megadoses of vitamin C carries a risk of causing kidney stones, while immediate adverse effects, such as increased clotting tendency, may arise from vitamin K ingestion by patients taking a stable dose of warfarin.

WATER-SOLUBLE VITAMINS

VITAMIN B_1 (THIAMINE)

Source

Vitamin B_1 is found in dried yeast, whole grains, whole brown rice, and wheat germ.

Functions

Thiamine, in the form of thiamine diphosphate, acts as a coenzyme in carbohydrate metabolism in reactions involving decarboxylation of α-ketoacids, such as pyruvate and α-ketoglutarate. Thiamine also acts as a coenzyme for the transketolase reactions of the hexose monophosphate shunt for using pentose.

Deficiency

The deficiency state of vitamin B_1 is beriberi (Fig. 27.4). This deficiency disease became more common with increasing consumption of polished rice prepared from brown rice by husking off the outer germ layer, which contains most of the vitamin B_1 activity. In the 1880s, dietary supplements of meat and grains were used to cure beriberi in sailors in the Japanese Navy. There are two forms of beriberi: dry and wet beriberi.

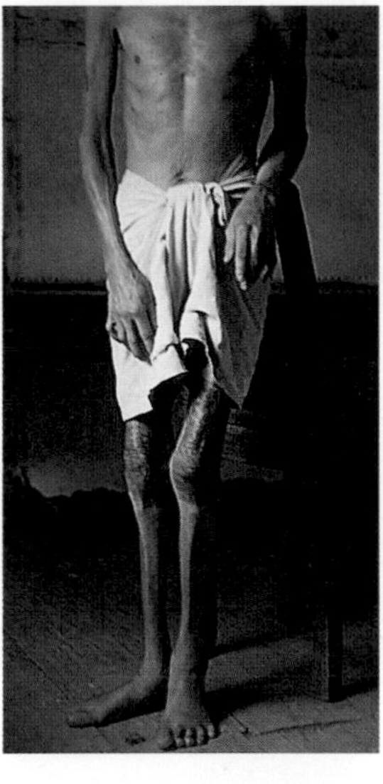

Fig. 27.4 Beriberi showing peripheral neuropathy. Some patients develop wrist drop and marked wasting of the lower extremities. (Courtesy of Dr A. Bryceson.)

- Dry beriberi relates to nervous system deficiency resulting in a degenerative neuropathy characterized by general neuritis, paralysis, and atrophy of the muscles (see Fig. 27.4).
- Wet beriberi describes involvement of the cardiovascular system resulting in edema partly due to myocardial insufficiency, palpitations, tachycardia, and an abnormal electrocardiogram.

Apart from insufficient intake, vitamin B_1 deficiency may result from heavy alcohol consumption, when it may cause Wernicke's encephalopathy and Korsakoff's psychosis.

Infantile beriberi may result from a low content of thiamine in the breast milk of thiamine-deficient women.

Pharmacotherapeutic use

The main use of thiamine is to treat or prevent thiamine deficiency, especially in alcoholics. It may be infused intravenously in an emergency situation (e.g. in acute Wernicke's encephalopathy).

VITAMIN B_2 (RIBOFLAVIN)

Source

Vitamin B_2 is found in yeast, organ meat such as liver, dairy products, and green leafy vegetables.

Functions

Riboflavin, in the form of flavin mononucleotide (FMN) or flavin adenine dinucleotide (FAD), acts as a coenzyme for various respiratory flavoproteins.

Deficiency

The symptoms of deficiency include cheilosis (inflamed lips), stomatitis, corneal vascularization, amblyopia, and sebaceous dermatosis.

Phenothiazines, tricyclic antidepressants, and quinine (an antimalarial) inhibit flavokinase, which converts riboflavin to FMN, and may therefore increase requirements for riboflavin.

Pharmacotherapeutic use

Vitamin B_2 is given in a dose of 5–20 mg/day to treat deficiency.

VITAMIN B_3 (NICOTINIC ACID)

Source

Vitamin B_3 is found in meat, fish, legumes, and whole grains. Tryptophan may serve as a source for nicotinic acid (niacin) since it can be converted to nicotinic acid with an efficiency of 60:1 (i.e. 60 tryptophan molecules to form one nicotinic acid molecule).

Functions

Nicotinic acid is converted in the body into two physiologically active forms: nicotinamide adenine dinucleotide (NAD) and nicotinamide dinucleotide phosphate (NADP). The main function of vitamin B_3 is in oxidation–reduction reactions using NAD or NADP. It is an essential coenzyme for many dehydrogenases in the Krebs cycle, for anaerobic carbohydrate metabolism, and for lipid and protein metabolism.

Deficiency

Pellagra, the deficiency disease of vitamin B_3, was first described in 1735 by Casal as the *mal de la rosa* disease (i.e. sickness of the rose) because of the roughness and color of the skin. The term pellagra is translated from Latin as rough (agra) skin (pelle). The etiology of pellagra as a deficiency disease, rather than an infection, was established in the early 1910s when pellagra patients were successfully cured by diet supplementation.

The primary symptoms of pellagra are dermatitis, diarrhea, and dementia (the three Ds). Pellagra is occasionally observed in populations who use corn, which has a low tryptophan content, as a major protein source.

Pharmacotherapeutic use

Nicotinic acid is effective for treating pellagra. It is also pharmacologically useful in the treatment of certain plasma lipid disorders (see Chapter 12).

Toxicity

Nicotinic acid may produce unpleasant flushing and vasodilation when treating hyperlipidemia with pharmacologic doses. Severe hepatotoxicity has been associated with the use of long-acting formulations.

VITAMIN B_6 (PYRIDOXINE)

Source

Vitamin B_6 is found in meat, fish, legumes, dried yeast, and whole grains.

Functions

Vitamin B_6 is the coenzyme for a variety of essential reactions in the metabolism of certain amino and fatty acids. Impaired formation of γ-aminobutyric acid due to impaired glutamate decarboxylase is believed to cause the tendency to convulsions seen in vitamin B_6 deficiency.

Deficiency

Deficiency of vitamin B_6 may result from dietary insufficiency. It may also occur in patients being treated with penicillamine, oral contraceptives, and isoniazid. Isoniazid combines with pyridoxal to form pyridoxal hydrazone, which has no coenzyme activity. Signs of deficiency include seborrhea-like skin lesions, anemia, neuropathy, and convulsions in infancy.

Pharmacotherapeutic use

Although vitamin B_6 is essential, clinical syndromes of isolated deficiency are rare. It may be given as an addition to the therapy of patients with other vitamin B complex deficiencies.

Toxicity

Long-term ingestion of excessive dosages of vitamin B_6 can cause peripheral neuritis.

VITAMIN B_{12}

Source

Muscle meats, liver, and dairy products are the exclusive source of vitamin B_{12}. The dietary source of vitamin B_{12}, in these animal products, is derived microbially from normal gut flora.

Structure

The basic structure of vitamin B_{12} is complex. Hodgkin was awarded the Nobel prize for elucidating this structure (Fig. 27.5). It consists of a corrin nucleus (a porphyrin-like ring structure with four reduced pyrrole rings linked to a central cobalt atom), 5,6-dimethylbenzimidazolyl nucleotide, and variable R groups. Different substitutions covalently bound to the cobalt atom, result in different cobalamins (see Fig. 27.5). The active forms of vitamin B_{12} are 5-deoxyadenosylcobalamin and methylcobalamin.

Absorption

Dietary vitamin B_{12} is absorbed in the distal ileum by a receptor-mediated process. A prerequisite to vitamin B_{12} absorption is its combination with an intrinsic factor secreted into the lumen of the stomach by the parietal cells of the gastric mucosa. Once absorbed, vitamin B_{12} is transported to the various cells of the body, bound to a plasma glycoprotein, transcobalamin II. Excess vitamin B_{12} is stored in the liver, and only trace amounts are normally lost in the urine and stools. There are sufficient stores in the liver to provide about 3–6 years' supply of the daily requirement of about 2–3 μg.

Functions

Vitamin B_{12} is vital for cell growth and mitosis. It is essential for the conversion of methylmalonyl coenzyme A (CoA) to succinyl CoA and for folate regeneration. Accumulation of methylmalonyl CoA in vitamin B_{12} deficiency with the resulting synthesis of abnormal fatty acids and their incorporation into cell membranes may account for the neurologic manifestations of vitamin B_{12} deficiency.

The role of vitamin B_{12} in folate regeneration is the biochemical link between vitamin B_{12} and folic acid metabolism. This explains the functional deficiency of folic acid metabolites in vitamin B_{12} deficiency. In vitamin B_{12} deficiency there is an accumulation of 5-methyltetrahydrofolate due to impaired regeneration of folic acid and this results in impaired DNA synthesis and megaloblastic anemia.

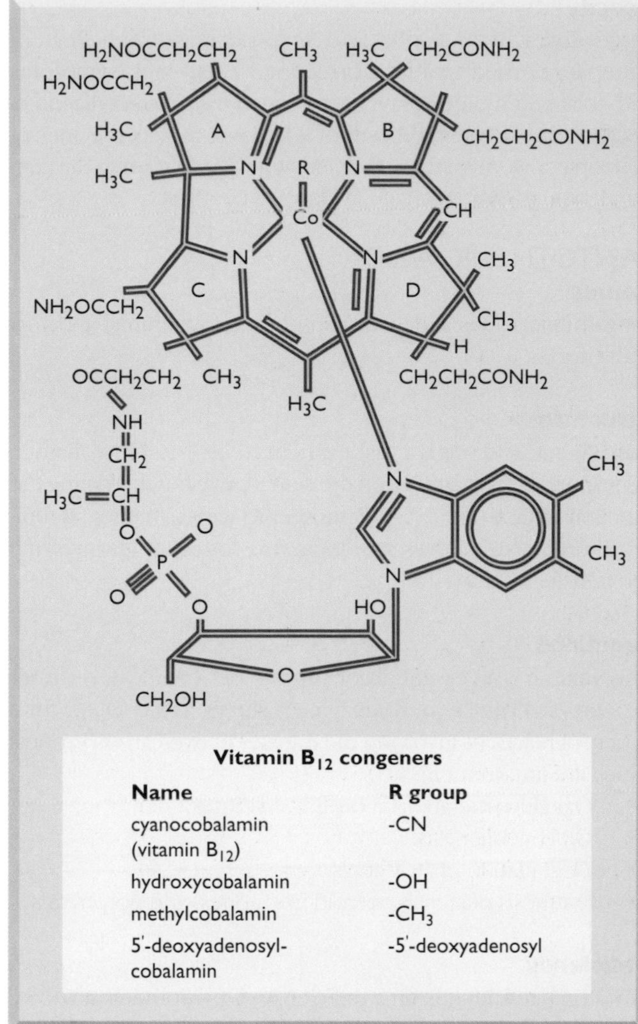

Vitamin B_{12} congeners

Name	R group
cyanocobalamin (vitamin B_{12})	-CN
hydroxycobalamin	-OH
methylcobalamin	$-CH_3$
5'-deoxyadenosyl-cobalamin	-5'-deoxyadenosyl

Fig. 27.5 Chemical structure of vitamin B_{12} and cobalamins. The basic structure of vitamin B_{12} consists of a corrin nucleus (a porphyrin-like ring structure with four reduced pyrrole rings linked to a central cobalt atom), 5,6-dimethylbenzimidazolyl nucleotide and variable R groups. Different substitutions covalently bound to the cobalt atom result in different cobalamins.

Deficiency

Ever since the 1820s the disease pernicious anemia (deficiency of vitamin B_{12}) was associated with digestive or absorptive problems in the gastrointestinal tract. Vitamin B_{12} deficiency results mainly from impaired absorption due to one of the following:

- A deficiency of intrinsic factor.
- Defects in absorption of the vitamin B_{12}–intrinsic factor complex.

The most common causes of vitamin B_{12} deficiency are pernicious anemia (due to defective secretion of intrinsic factor following destruction of secretory cells in the stomach as a result of autoimmune disease), partial or total gastrectomy, malabsorption syndrome, inflammatory bowel disease, gastrointestinal resection, fish tapeworm infection, and a strict vegan diet.

Common causes of vitamin B_{12} deficiency

- Pernicious anemia
- Partial or total gastrectomy or gastrointestinal resection
- Malabsorption syndrome
- Inflammatory bowel disease
- Fish tapeworm infection
- A strict vegan diet

Deficiency impairs DNA synthesis, cell division, and function, and so the effect is most apparent in tissues where cells are rapidly dividing (e.g. bone marrow, gastrointestinal epithelium). Megaloblastic anemia is the main hematologic finding. Other clinical features are sterility, organic brain syndromes (hallucinations, emotional lability, and dementia), spinal cord degeneration, and peripheral neuropathies.

Pharmacotherapeutic use

Treatment of vitamin B_{12} deficiency involves replacing vitamin B_{12} by injection and treating the cause, if possible.

FOLIC ACID

Source

Folic acid is found in organ meat, liver, dried yeast, and fresh green leafy vegetables.

Functions

Folic acid (pteroylglutamic acid) is composed of a pteridine ring, *p*-aminobenzoic acid, and glutamic acid. Once absorbed, it is reduced to tetrahydrofolic acid (THF), which acts as an acceptor of one-carbon units. The role of vitamin B_{12} in folate regeneration is shown in Fig. 27.6. Folate cofactors are essential for the one-carbon transfer reactions necessary for DNA synthesis. Folic acid is a coenzyme for the:

- Conversion of homocysteine to methionine.
- Conversion of serine to glycine.
- Synthesis of thymidylate (a rate-limiting step in DNA synthesis).
- Metabolism of histidine.
- Synthesis of purines.

Deficiency

In 1919, Osler showed that anemia associated with pregnancy differed from that caused by vitamin B_{12} deficiency. During the 1940s, folic acid was purified and synthesized and found to be responsible for megaloblastic anemia.

Folate deficiency is mainly expressed as megaloblastic anemia, and is often seen in alcoholics and in people with extensive small bowel disease. The daily requirement in normal adults is approx-

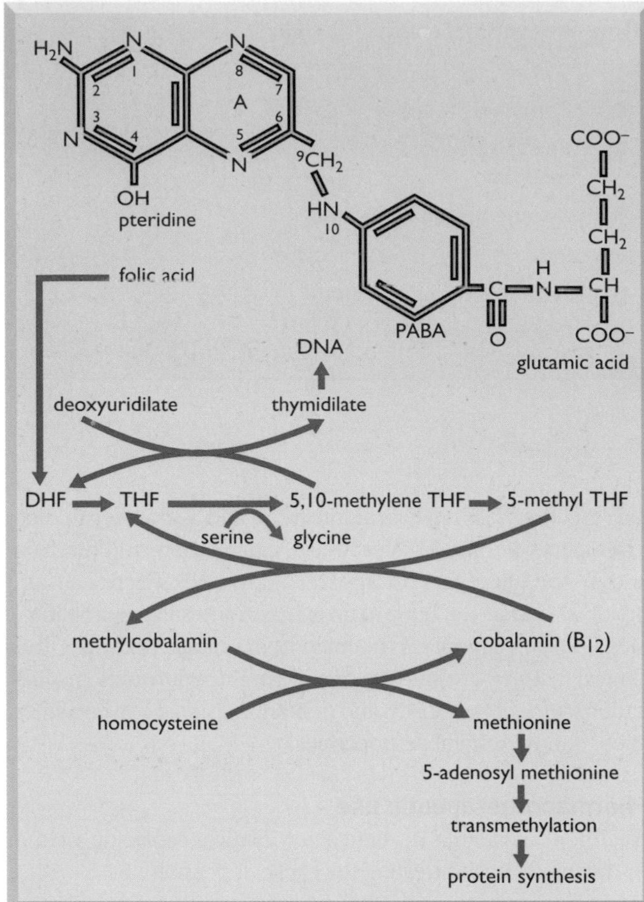

Fig. 27.6 Structure and regeneration of folic acid by vitamin B_{12}. Folic acid is reduced first to dihydrofolic acid (DHF) and subsequently to tetrahydrofolic acid (THF) by folate reductase. In the process serine is converted to glycine, THF accepts one carbon unit to form 5,10-methylene THF. The latter can either be converted to 5-methyl THF or donate the methylene group to deoxyuridilate and revert to DHF. Kinetically, the formation of 5-methyl THF is more favorable. The transfer of the methylene group from 5,10-methylene THF to deoxyuridilate is an essential step for DNA synthesis. 5-Methyl THF must be transformed to THF to maintain the required supply of 5,10-methylene THF. This is carried out by donating the methyl group to vitamin B_{12} to form methylcobalamin. This in turn donates the methyl group to homocysteine, forming methionine. Methionine is then transformed to 5-adenosylmethionine which is important for protein synthesis. 5-Methyl THF accumulates in vitamin B_{12} deficiency.

imately 50–100 μg. Pregnant or nursing women require 200–400 μg or more daily.

Pharmacotherapeutic use

The usual oral dose is 1 mg/day for deficiency states. In addition, prenatal supplements of folic acid may help prevent neural tube defects when given three months before conception and during the first trimester.

Toxicity

Large doses of oral folic acid may decrease the effect of antiepileptic medications. Correcting hematologic symptoms with folic acid should always be preceded by a correct diagnosis because, although large doses of folate will correct the anemia of people with vitamin B_{12} deficiency, it will not correct the central nervous system damage, which will continue.

PANTOTHENIC ACID

Source

Pantothenic acid is widely distributed in both animal and vegetable foods.

Structure

Pantothenic acid was the last nutrient to be listed as a vitamin. Lipmann and Kaplan received the Nobel prize for elucidating the function of CoA (Fig. 27.7). Pantothenic acid is an integral moiety in CoA, which serves as a coenzyme for reactions involving the transfer of acetyl groups.

Functions

This vitamin is an essential constituent of CoA and acyl carrier protein (see Fig. 27.7). Coenzyme A serves as a cofactor for a variety of reactions involving the transfer of two-carbon groups, which are important in:

- Oxidative metabolism of carbohydrates.
- Gluconeogenesis.
- Degradation of fatty acids.
- Synthesis of sterols, steroid hormones, and porphyrins.

Deficiency

Symptoms resulting from a deficiency of pantothenic acid are uncommon because it is so plentiful in foods, but may develop in people with liver disease or who drink excessive alcohol. They include paresthesia of the limbs, muscle weakness, and 'burning feet' syndrome.

BIOTIN

Source

Biotin is found in yeast, egg yolk, meat, and dairy products. Intestinal microflora are an additional source.

Functions

Biotin acts as a coenzyme in reactions involving carbon dioxide fixation, β-decarboxylation, and deamination.

Deficiency

Biotin defiency is rare, but may occur during long-term total parenteral nutrition (TPN). Symptoms include anorexia, nausea, vomiting, general lassitude, and a dry dermatitis.

Pharmacotherapeutic use

Large doses (5–10 mg/day) are usually given for deficiency.

VITAMIN C

Source

Vitamin C is found in citrus fruits, tomatoes, potatoes, cabbage, and green peppers.

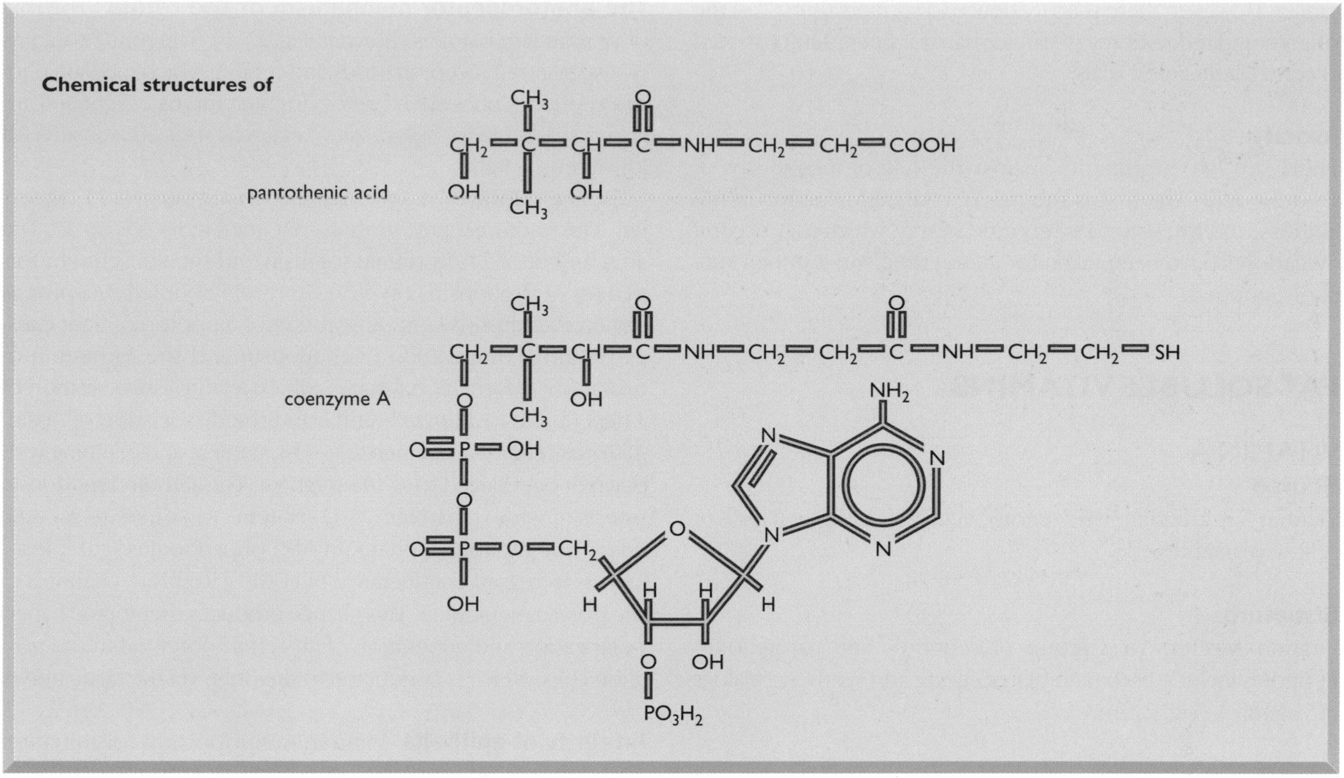

Chemical structures of

pantothenic acid

coenzyme A

Fig. 27.7 Structural correlation between pantothenic acid and coenzyme A.

Structure

There are two active forms of vitamin C: L-ascorbic acid or dehydroascorbic acid. Ascorbic acid is easily oxidized to dehydroascorbic acid.

Absorption

Vitamin C is readily absorbed in the ileum by a Na^+-dependent carrier-mediated mechanism. It is stored in all tissues, with the highest concentrations in the adrenal and pituitary glands. In all tissues, ascorbic acid is reversibly converted to dehydroascorbic acid. The main metabolite is excreted by the kidneys as an oxalate salt. Massive doses of vitamin C may cause kidney stones and diarrhea.

Functions

Vitamin C acts as a reducing agent. It is required for:

- Collagen formation; without it, protocollagen does not cross-link properly, resulting in impaired wound healing.
- Synthesis of biogenic amines, norepinephrine, and epinephrine.
- Synthesis of carnitine, the carrier protein that facilitates the transport of fatty acids into mitochondria for β-oxidation.

Deficiency

Vitamin C deficiency is called scurvy and results from either increased requirements or a low intake. Scurvy (Fig. 27.8) became prevalent in the 1500s when long sea voyages became common. As a result, oranges and lemons were prescribed for long sailing voyages, and subsequently in the 1740s, citrus fruits, which contain citric acid, were used to prevent scurvy. Scurvy is characterized by hemorrhages, loose teeth, gingivitis (see Fig. 27.8), and swollen joints.

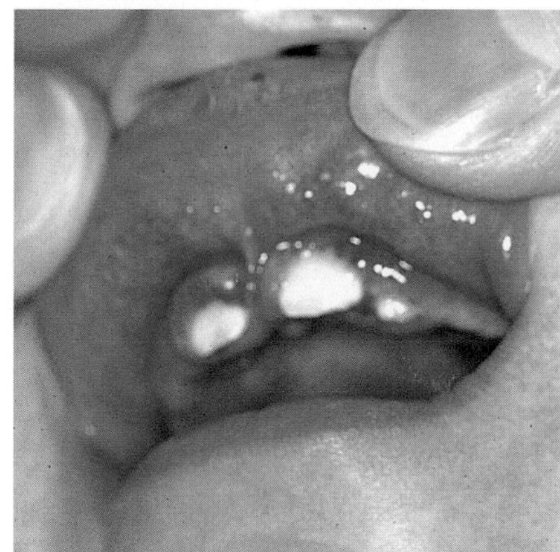

Fig. 27.8 Scurvy. Vitamin C deficiency is rare. Features of scurvy include severe gingivitis and loosening of the teeth. (Courtesy of Professor R. Waterlow.)

Pharmacotherapeutic use

Doses of 100–1000 mg/day orally have been used to treat ascorbic acid deficiency disease. Large doses have been proposed as being useful for general well-being and in the treatment of cancer. However, there is no evidence to support this use of the vitamin; indeed, efficacy in cancer has not been demonstrated in controlled clinical trials.

Toxicity

There are two arguments against the use of megadoses of ascorbic acid. The first is the risk of oxalate formation in the kidneys, and the second is rebound scurvy, which may occur if megadoses have been taken for a long time and are then suddenly stopped.

FAT-SOLUBLE VITAMINS

VITAMIN A

Source

Vitamin A is found in fish liver oils, egg yolk, and green leafy or yellow vegetables.

Structure

Vitamin A refers to a group of retinoids and carotenoids. Retinoids include both naturally occuring and synthetic analogs of vitamin A (Fig. 27.9).

Clinically available retinoids

Chemical name	Alternative name	Clinical use
Retinol		Vitamin A deficiency
Retinoic acid (all-*trans*)	Tretinoin	Acne (topical treatment)
Retinoic acid (13-*cis*)	Isotretinoin	Acne (systemic treatment)
Etretinate		Psoriasis

Fig. 27.9 Clinically available retinoids.

Absorption

Retinoid esters are hydrolyzed in the intestinal lumen and absorbed by a carrier-mediated mechanism. The absorbed retinyl esters are taken up by the liver, hydrolyzed, and transported in the circulation bound to retinol-binding protein. This complex is taken up by various organs, especially the intestine, liver, and eye, where it binds to specific sites on the cell membrane. At certain sites, such as the retina, retinol is converted to 11-*cis* retinal and incorporated into rhodopsin (see below).

Functions

Vitamin A plays a role in:

- The photoreceptor mechanism of the retina.
- The integrity of epithelia.
- Lysosome stability.

The photoreceptor mechanism of the retina The role of vitamin A in vision is shown in Fig. 27.10. The retina contains two specialized receptors (rods and cones), which mediate photoreception. Cones are receptors for high-intensity light and are also responsible for color vision, whereas rods are sensitive to low-intensity light.

The active form of vitamin A in the visual system is 11-*cis* retinal. The photoreceptor protein contained in rods is opsin. The attachment of 11-*cis* retinal to opsin and the subsequent formation of rhodopsin, a typical G protein-coupled receptor, is required to absorb light. Absorption of a photon of light causes photodecomposition of rhodopsin and the formation of unstable conformational states, which lead to isomerization of 11-*cis* retinal to all-*trans* retinal and the dissociation of opsin. All-*trans* retinal can isomerize to 11-*cis* retinal and combine with opsin or be reduced to all-*trans* retinol. The activated rhodopsin interacts with transducin, a G protein, to stimulate a cyclic guanosine monophosphate (cGMP) phosphodiesterase, leading to decreased conductance of cGMP-gated Na^+ channels in the plasma membrane. This change produces membrane hyperpolarization and generation of an action potential in the ganglion cells, which is conducted to the brain via the optic nerve.

Integrity of epithelia Vitamin A is important for initiating and controlling epithelial differentiation in mucosal and keratinized tissues.

Role in carcinogenesis Vitamin A prevents or reverses the transformation of pre-malignant cells into malignant cells *in vitro*, but the clinical significance of this observation is not yet clear.

Deficiency

The link between night blindness and vitamin A deficiency became clear only relatively recently. During the 1900s and 1920s it was shown that a fat-soluble material in egg yolk and cod liver oil was essential to promote growth and cure night bindness. However, it was not until the 1930s that the structures of β retinol and related compounds were elucidated. On the other hand, vitamin A toxicity was observed in arctic explorers who consumed large amounts of polar bear livers.

Symptoms of vitamin A deficiency include xerophthalmia (dry and lusterless cornea and areas covering the eye, Fig. 27.11), keratomalacia (dryness and ulceration of the cornea, Fig. 27.12), Bitot's spot, and night blindness. The health and integrity of the skin is also decreased in vitamin A deficiency.

Deficiency can result from a low intake or from fat malabsorption due to a variety of diseases. Alcohol consumption may decrease the vitamin A stores in the liver.

Pharmacotherapeutic use

Retinoic acid (tretinoin, all-*trans* retinoic acid) is the acid form of vitamin A. It is an effective topical treatment for acne vulgaris (see Fig. 27.9). A topical application of retinoic acid usually irritates the skin, producing dryness and erythema. These adverse effects are common during the first few weeks of therapy, and usually diminish with continued therapy.

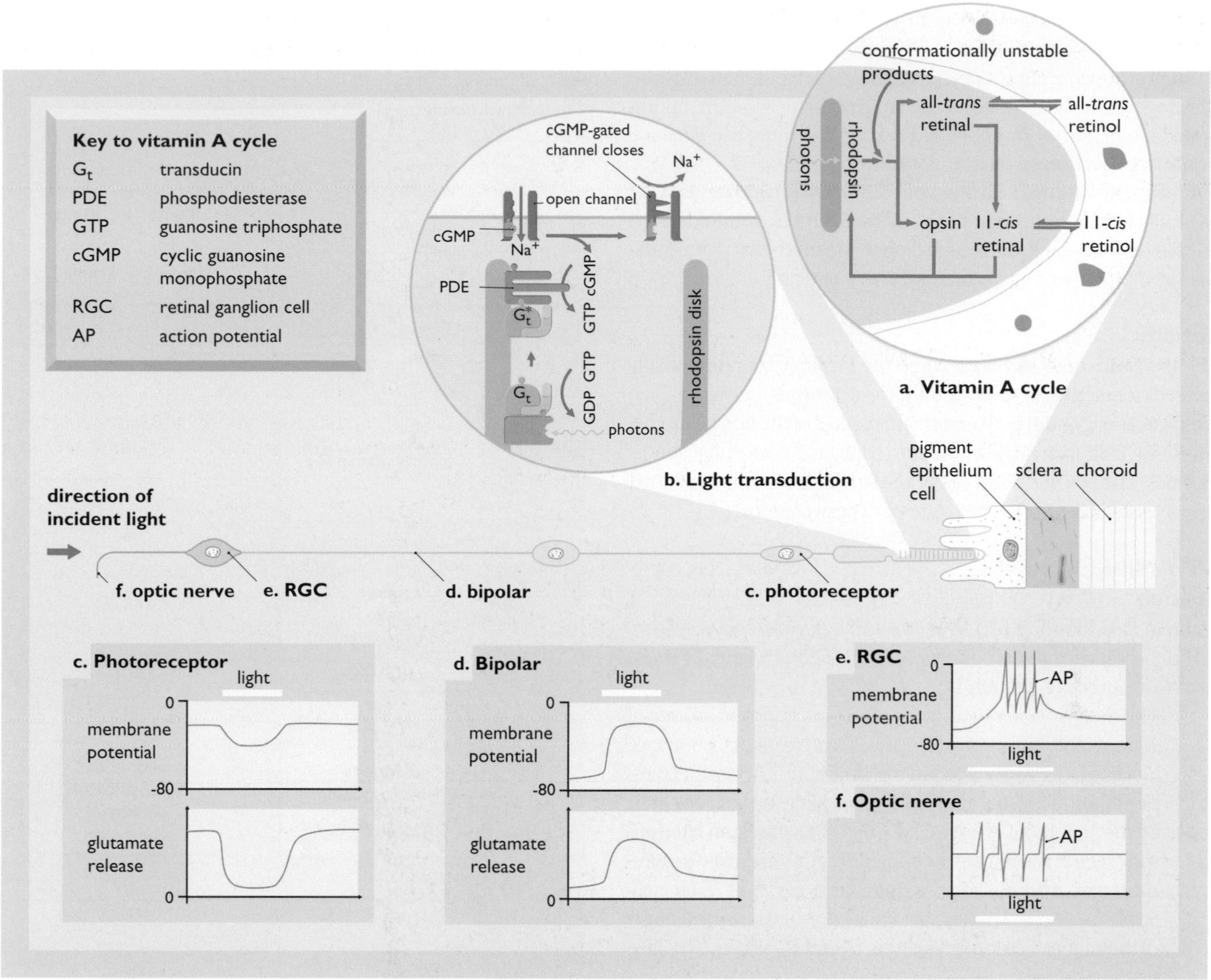

Key to vitamin A cycle

G_t	transducin
PDE	phosphodiesterase
GTP	guanosine triphosphate
cGMP	cyclic guanosine monophosphate
RGC	retinal ganglion cell
AP	action potential

Fig. 27.10 Role of vitamin A in vision. The attachment of 11-*cis* retinal to opsin to form rhodopsin is required for the absorption of light (a). Absorption of a photon of light results in a photodecomposition of rhodopsin and formation of unstable conformational states, leading to isomerization of 11-*cis* retinal to all-*trans* retinal and the dissociation of opsin. All-*trans* retinal can isomerize to 11-*cis* retinal and combine with rhodopsin or be reduced to all-*trans* retinol. The activated rhodopsin interacts with transducin, a G protein, to stimulate a cGMP phosphodiesterase, leading to a decreased conductance of cGMP-gated Na^+ channels in the plasma membrane (b). This change produces membrane hyperpolarization and generation of an action potential in the retinal ganglion cells, which is conducted to the brain via the optic nerve (c–f).

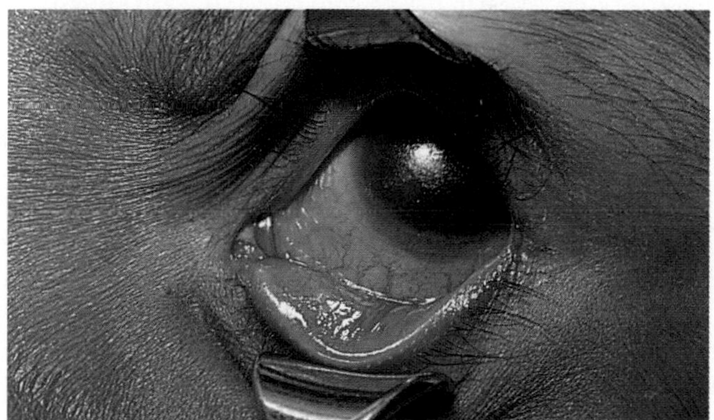

Fig. 27.11 Xerophthalmia. Vitamin A deficiency is a common cause of blindness in pre-school children in the tropics. The dryness of the cornea and conjunctiva gives the eye a dull hazy appearance. (Courtesy of Professor W. Peters.)

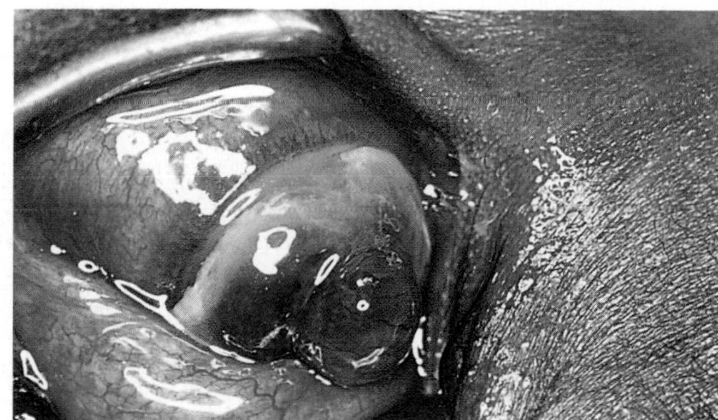

Fig. 27.12 Keratomalacia. This is a softening or coagulative necrosis of the cornea that occurs in chronic severe vitamin A deficiency. (Courtesy of Professor J. Waterlow.)

A synthetic analog of vitamin A, 13-*cis* retinoic acid (isotretinoin), is effective orally and used for severe cystic acne. Common adverse effects resemble those of hypervitaminosis A. Teratogenicity is a major risk in pregnant women taking isotretinoin, and women of childbearing age must use effective contraception before starting retinoids.

Another synthetic derivative of vitamin A, etretinate, is used topically for the treatment of psoriasis. Synthetic retinoids used in skin diseases have enhanced activity on epithelial differentiation combined with decreased systemic toxicity.

Toxicity

Hypervitaminosis A develops when the intake of retinoids greatly exceeds requirements. Symptoms include pruritus, dermatitis, skin desquamation, disturbed hair growth, fissures of the lips, headache, anorexia, fatigue, irritability, hemorrhage, and congenital abnormalities. The adverse effects of systemic acne treatment described above essentially represent a state of hypervitaminosis A.

VITAMIN D

Source

Vitamin D is found in fish liver oils and egg yolk, and is synthesized in skin exposed to ultraviolet (UV) light. Essentially there are two sources of vitamin D:

- The diet provides vitamin D_3 (cholecalciferol) from animal sources and vitamin D_2 (ergocalciferol) from plant sources.
- Vitamin D_3 is synthesized in the skin from 7-dehydrocholesterol (produced in the wall of the intestine from cholesterol) by the action of UV light. Exposure of the face and hands to sunlight for 15 minutes is enough to supply the daily requirement of vitamin D. Dietary requirements of vitamin D are negligible for people who live in sunny areas or who spend much of their times outdoors. Vitamins D_2 and D_3 are equally effective as vitamins.

Structure and metabolic activation

Vitamin D is a family of sterol derivatives. It is a prehormone, which is converted in the body into a number of biologically active metabolites (Fig. 27.13). Vitamin D_3 is first converted to 25-hydroxyvitamin D_3 (25[OH]D_3, calcifediol) in the liver, and this is further converted in the kidneys to 1,25-dihydroxyvitamin D_3 (1,25[OH]$_2D_3$, calcitriol). A further metabolite with activity is 24,25-dihydroxyvitamin D_3 (24,25[OH]$_2D_3$); however, its physiologic role is less well understood.

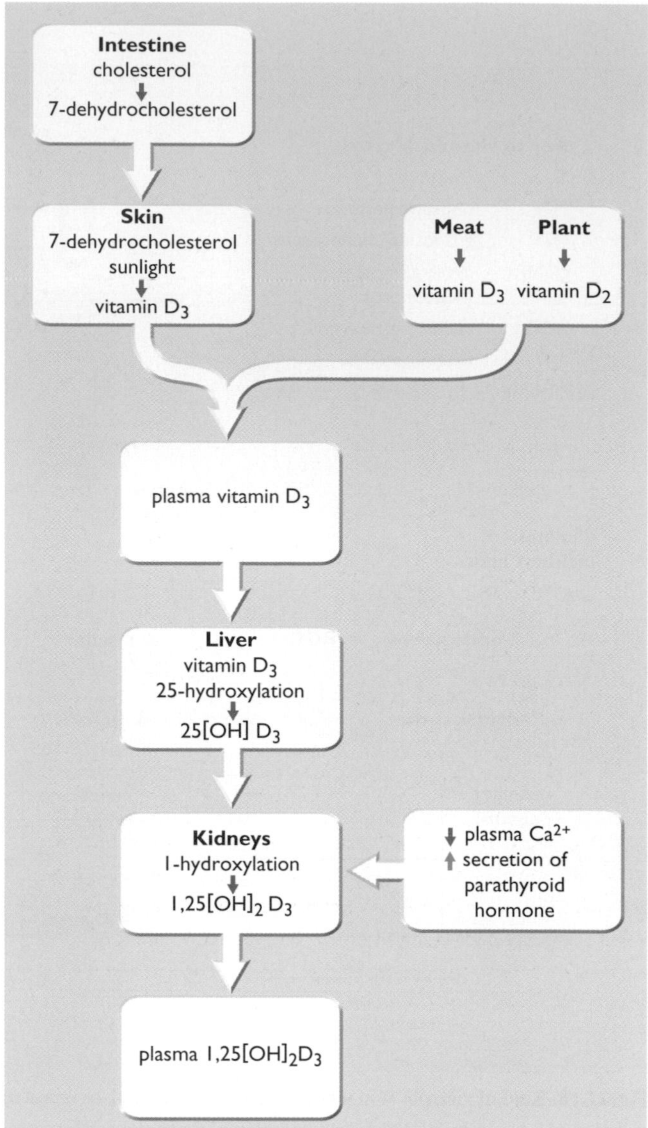

Fig. 27.13 Activation of vitamin D. Vitamin D (dietary and that synthesized in the skin) is converted in the body into a number of biologically active metabolites. Vitamin D_3 is first converted to 25-hydroxyvitamin D_3 (25[OH]D_3) in the liver, and this is further converted in the kidneys to 1,25-dihydroxyvitamin D_3 (1,25[OH]$_2D_3$).

Absorption

As with other fat-soluble vitamins, vitamin D is only optimally absorbed by the intestine when there is fat in the diet. After absorption, vitamin D_3 is transported in chylomicrons to the liver and stored with a carrier protein, vitamin D-binding protein. Vitamin D and its metabolites circulate in plasma bound to this protein. Excess vitamin D is stored in adipose tissue.

There are two major steps in the metabolism of vitamin D.

- The first process is 25-hydroxylation, which occurs in the liver.
- The second process is 1-hydroxylation in the kidney, which is stimulated by parathyroid hormone (PTH). A decreased ionized Ca^{2+} concentration in the plasma stimulates PTH secretion from the parathyroids (Fig. 27.14).

Biliary excretion is the major pathway of elimination and 24-hydroxylation in the kidney is a preliminary step.

Functions

1,25[OH]$_2D_3$ acts as a hormone and plays an important role in Ca^{2+} homeostasis. Together with PTH, it maintains plasma levels of Ca^{2+} by:

- Promoting intestinal absorption of Ca^{2+}.
- Increasing Ca^{2+} mobilization from bone.
- Decreasing Ca^{2+} excretion from the kidney (by enhancing renal reabsorption).

Physiologic concentrations of calcitonin have a negligible role in

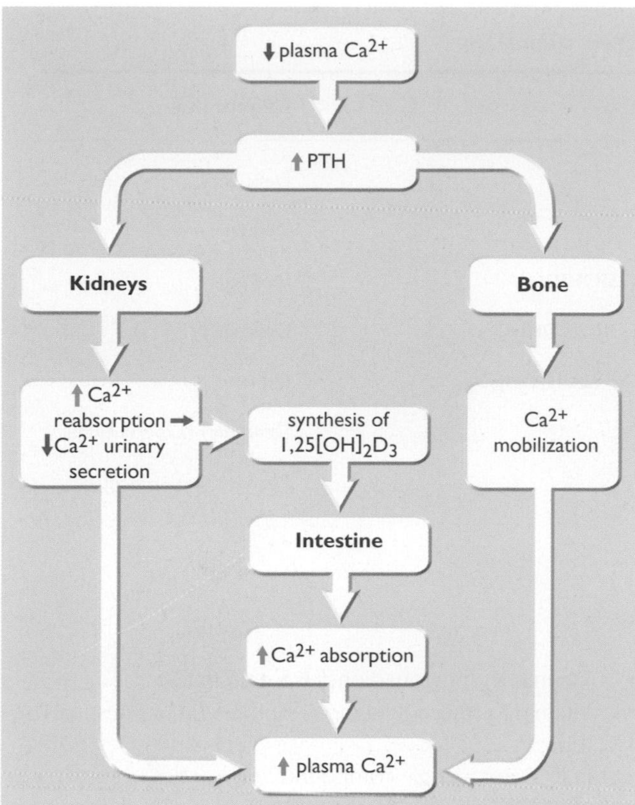

Fig. 27.14 Regulation of Ca^{2+} plasma concentration by vitamin D and parathyroid hormone (PTH). Vitamin D and PTH regulate plasma Ca^{2+} concentrations by acting on three main target tissues: intestine, kidney, and bone. A decrease in plasma Ca^{2+} concentration triggers increased secretion of PTH, which acts on the kidneys and bones. PTH in the kidneys promotes the synthesis of 1,25-dihydroxyvitamin D_3 (1,25[OH]$_2$D$_3$), which in turn increases gastrointestinal absorption of Ca^{2+}. Consequently, decreased plasma Ca^{2+} concentration leads to enhanced Ca^{2+} mobilization from bone, increased reabsorption in the kidneys, and facilitated absorption in the gut.

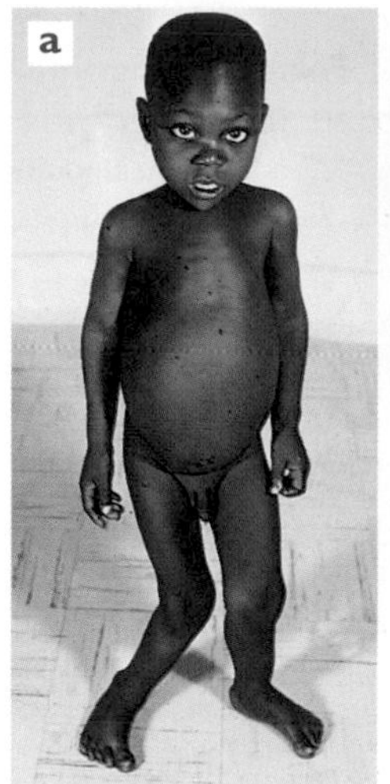

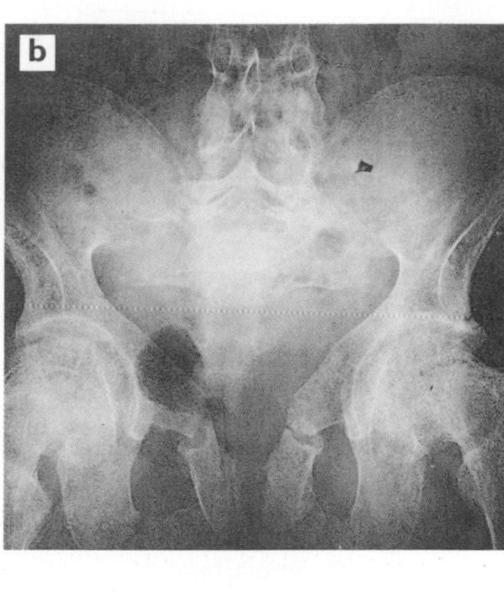

Fig. 27.15 Vitamin D deficiency. (a) Rickets causing gross deformity of the legs and pigeon chest in this boy. (Courtesy of Professor R. Hendrickse.) (b) Osteomalacia. The increased demands of pregnancy may result in gross deformity of the pelvis. (Courtesy of Dr G.D. Scarrow.)

Ca^{2+} homeostasis in humans.

The reciprocal relations between 1,25[OH]$_2$D$_3$ and PTH are shown in Fig. 27.14. These processes maintain plasma Ca^{2+} concentration at approximately 10.0 mg/dl (2.5 mmol/liter).

Other functions of 1,25[OH]$_2$D$_3$ include:

- Enhanced bone formation by promoting osteoclast maturation and indirectly stimulating osteoclast activity.
- Cell differentiation.
- Inhibition of the growth of some carcinomas, especially breast cancer and malignant melanoma.

Deficiency

In the 1810s it was discovered that cod liver oil would cure rickets, the classical deficiency disease of vitamin D (Fig. 27.15a). The adult form of rickets is osteomalacia (Fig. 27.15b). Demineralization of bones results from the release of calcium into the plasma, which is triggered by PTH. People with a high risk of vitamin D deficiency include infants in whom dietary deficiency may be worsened by a lack of sunlight exposure, the elderly, and patients with renal failure in whom a deficiency of 1,25[OH]$_2$D$_3$ results from a lack of synthesis in the kidneys. Hypoparathyroidism and estrogen administration can decrease PTH levels and have similar effects. Fat malabsorption and alcohol consumption may also result in deficiency. The general signs of hypocalcemia are increased excitability including paresthesia, tetany, and increased neuromuscular excitability, laryngospasm, and convulsions.

Causes of vitamin D deficiency

- Lack of sunlight exposure (infants)
- Renal failure (elderly)
- Hypoparathyroidism
- Estrogens, phenytoin, or phenobarbital
- Fat malabsorption
- High alcohol consumption

Pharmacotherapeutic use

Plasma levels of Ca^{2+} provide the definition for hyper and hypocalcemic states. The pharmacotherapeutic uses of vitamin D (Fig. 27.16) are:

- To treat rickets (nutritional and metabolic), osteomalacia, and hypoparathyroidism. Metabolic rickets is usually treated with agents that do not require renal 1-hydroxylation to become activated (e.g. calcitriol).
- To treat psoriasis when derivatives with no vitamin D activity (e.g. calcipotriol) may be used.

Toxicity

Hypercalcemia may be caused by excess vitamin D. Prolonged hypercalcemia produces initially reversible, but subsequently irreversible,

Name	Chemical name	Clinical use
Cholecalciferol	Vitamin D_3 (D_3)	Deficiency
Ergocalciferol	Vitamin D_2 (D_2)	Deficiency
Calcifediol	25-hydroxyvitamin D_3 (25[OH]D_3)	Deficiency
Calcitriol	1,25-dihydroxyvitamin D_3 (1,25[OH]$_2D_3$)	Deficiency
Secalcifediol	24,25-dihydroxyvitamin D_3 (24,25[OH]$_2D_3$)	None
Dihydrotachysterol		Deficiency (experimental)
Calcipotriol		Psoriasis (experimental)

Fig. 27.16 Forms of vitamin D and their clinical use.

renal damage and calcification of soft tissue, including that of the cardiovascular system. Hypervitaminosis may be accompanied by growth retardation in children, fetal defects, reduced parathyroid function, and aortic stenosis.

VITAMIN E

Source

Vitamin E is found in vegetable oils, wheat germ, leafy vegetables, egg yolk, margarines, and legumes.

Structure

α-Tocopherol is the most active of eight naturally occurring tocopherols with vitamin E activity. β-Tocopherol (wheat) and γ-tocopherol (corn and soya bean oils, margarines) are at least half as potent as the α form, whereas δ-tocopherol (sunflower oil) has almost no biologic activity.

Function

Vitamin E acts as an antioxidant, but this effect is of uncertain significance.

Deficiency

Premature infants are at risk of vitamin E deficiency because there is poor transplacental transport.

Pharmacotherapeutic use

The only indication for vitamin E therapy is hemolytic anemia of the newborn.

VITAMIN K

Source

Vitamin K is found in leafy vegetables, vegetable oils, and liver, and is synthesized by intestinal flora.

Structure

Vitamin K is a quinone derivative and there are two natural forms:

- Vitamin K_1 (phytonadione) is found in food.
- Vitamin K_2 (menaquinone) is synthesized by intestinal bacteria.

Vitamin K_2 is not a single compound, but a series of substances with varying lengths of side chain (n=1–13); menaquinone-4 is the most biologically active form. Vitamin K_3 is a synthetic water-soluble derivative.

Functions

Vitamin K is essential for the formation of prothrombin and factors VII, IX, and X, which are glycoproteins with a number of γ-carboxyglutamic acid residues clustered at the N-terminal end of the peptide chain. Vitamin K is needed as a cofactor for this post-translational modification. During the carboxylation process, vitamin K is converted to its inactive oxide and then metabolized back to its active form (see Fig. 27.2). The reductive metabolism of the inactive vitamin K epoxide is warfarin sensitive. Warfarin and related drugs block the γ-carboxylation and this results in molecules that are biologically inactive for coagulation. Broad-spectrum antibiotics that alter gut bacterial flora decrease vitamin K production and can increase the effects of warfarin anticoagulation.

Deficiency

In 1935, Dam found that a factor was required to cure coagulation defects and this was named vitamin K ('koagulation factor').

Vitamin K deficiency causes hemorrhage due to prothrombin deficiency leading to a prolonged prothrombin time. Drug therapy with anticonvulsants (hydantoins) and antibiotics (neomycin) may result in a vitamin K deficiency. Newborns, especially those that are premature, are at risk of deficiency because of the low amount of vitamin K in breast milk and low intestinal synthesis. Fat malabsorption or dietary consumption of unabsorbed lipids such as mineral oil can also cause vitamin K deficiency.

Hepatic insufficiency precipitates the consequences of vitamin K deficiency as a result of the already compromised liver synthesis of coagulation factors.

Causes of vitamin K deficiency

- Anticonvulsants (hydantoins) and antibiotics (neomycin)
- Low intestinal synthesis (infants)
- Fat malabsorption
- Dietary consumption of unabsorbed lipids
- Hepatic insufficiency

Pharmacotherapeutic use

The major clinical use of vitamin K is to treat and/or prevent vitamin K deficiency especially in newborns. It can be given parenterally to antagonize the effects of warfarin rapidly, but reversal of the anticoagulant effects is delayed owing to the time required to replenish the decreased plasma concentrations of vitamin K-dependent clotting factors.

Toxicity

Kernicterus, which is an abnormal accumulation of bilirubin in the central nervous system, may be caused by excess vitamin K.

TRACE ELEMENTS

Some elements, including certain metals, are essential for life. The most obvious example of such a metal is iron, without which, oxygen-carrying molecules and certain enzymes are unable to function. Iron is discussed in detail in Chapter 9. Other important elements such as potassium, sodium, magnesium, and iodine are discussed throughout the book.

Some elements serve analogous functions to those of iron in terms of acting as essential cofactors for enzymes. These elements include the metals copper, zinc, selenium, manganese, molybdenum, and cobalt, as well as the element fluoride.

DEFICIENCIES OF TRACE ELEMENTS

Copper deficiency has hematologic effects

Copper deficiency is very rare since the trace amounts required by the body occur in most foods. However, it can occur in Menkes' syndrome or following intestinal bypass surgery or can be induced by an excessive intake of zinc. In copper deficiency, enzymes such as cytochrome oxidase are less active than normal, resulting in hematologic consequences such as leukopenia and mild anemia. Minute quantities (1–2 mg) of cupric sulfate added to the diet will resolve the deficiency.

Zinc deficiency affects nucleic acid metabolism

Zinc is important for nucleic acid metabolism and a lack of zinc is unusual because it is a common component of many foods. Genetic factors or inadequate parenteral nutrition can, however, cause deficiency. This results in a distinctive rash and a variety of unrelated conditions including hypogonadism, impaired wound healing, altered immune function, and depressed mental function. Oral zinc rapidly alleviates these symptoms.

Selenium is a component of glutathione peroxidase

Selenium is an important component of glutathione peroxidase. Only microgram quantities (10–75 μg depending upon age) are required. This quantity is usually ingested in a normal diet, and so selenium deficiency is rare.

Whether reduced activity of glutathione peroxidase is associated with the myopathies (particularly cardiac) caused by selenium deficiency is unknown.

Manganese deficiency can retard growth

Manganese plays an important role in mucopolysaccharide metabolism and deficiency can retard growth.

Molybdenum deficiency produces symptoms of gout

Molybdenum deficiency produces symptoms of gout due to its role in purine metabolism. In gout, urate crystals settle into the joints, and produce swelling of the joints accompanied with fevers.

Fluoride deficiency leads to faulty tooth enamel and abnormal bone structure

Addition of fluoride to drinking water deficient in fluoride and to dental products, such as toothpaste, appears to reduce the incidence of caries in a population dramatically. This is a direct effect of fluoride's role in the development of tooth enamel. Fluoride deficiency not only results in the production of faulty tooth enamel, but also causes abnormal bone structure. Where fluoride is not added to drinking water, the ingestion of fluoride tablets can be of value.

FURTHER READING

Deluca HF (ed.) *The Fat-Soluble Vitamins*. New York: Plenum Press; 1978. [Biochemical and clinical aspects of fat-soluble vitamins.]

Guyton A (ed.) *Textbook of Medical Physiology*. Philadelphia: WB Saunders Company; 1991. [An excellent textbook on medical physiology.]

Rolfes SR, Debruyne IK, Whitney EN (eds) *Life Span Nutrition, Conception Through Life.* St Paul: West Publishing Company; 1990. [Detailed and comprehensive information on the role of vitamins in nutrition.]

Sherwood L (ed.) *Human Physiology*. St. Paul: West Publishing Company; 1993. [A well-written and highly illustrated textbook on human physiology.]

Make a provisional diagnosis and determine a rational pharmacologic treatment for the following hypothetical case.

A 27-year-old woman is considering having another child. Her previous pregnancy ended in miscarriage because the fetus had a neural tube defect. She wants to know whether the defect is genetic and whether her next baby will have the same problem. On examination the patient looks healthy, but pale, and when asked about her eating habits she discloses she is a vegetarian.

1. Should you advise her to seek genetic advice and, if so, why?
2. Should you reassure her that there is nothing to worry about and that her next pregnancy will be fine and, if so, why?
3. As the patient is a vegetarian, should you prescribe a multivitamin preparation and reassure the patient about her next pregnancy and, if so, why?
4. Does the patient have a high risk of vitamin B_{12} deficiency and, if so, what would should you do and why?
5. In view of this patient's desire to become pregnant, which drugs would you recommend and for how long would you recommend them?

Indicate which is the correct answer for each question.

1. Which of the following coagulation factors depends on vitamin K for synthesis by the liver?
a) prothrombin (factor II)
b) factor VIII
c) factor XII
d) factor V

2. All of the following are correct, except
a) large doses of vitamin C increase the incidence of oxalate stones in kidneys
b) absorption of vitamin B_{12} requires the presence of intrinsic factor
c) deficiency of folic acid causes megaloblastic anemia
d) the active form of vitamin A in the vision cycle is 11-*cis* retinal
e) osteomalacia is an expression of hypervitaminosis D in adults

3. All of the following are correct, except
a) fat-soluble vitamins require the presence of fat in the diet for proper absorption
b) body stores of vitamin B_{12} are sufficient for 3–6 months
c) storage capacity in the body is higher for fat-soluble vitamins and less for water-soluble vitamins
d) activation of vitamin D_3 occurs in the liver and kidneys
e) Wernicke's encephalopathy is associated with thiamine deficiency

4. Which one of the following vitamin D forms is synthesized by the kidneys?
a) calcitriol
b) calciferol
c) calcipotriol
d) cholecalciferol
e) ergocalciferol

5. All the following vitamins are correctly matched with the condition for which they are used pharmacotherapeutically, except
a) vitamin B_3 and pellagra
b) folic acid and peripheral neuropathy
c) vitamin C and scurvy
d) vitamin E and hemolytic anemia
e) vitamin A and acne

6. All the following terms are associated with vitamin A, except
a) retinoids
b) acne
c) rhodopsin
d) keratomalacia
e) osteomalacia

7. All the following terms are associated with vitamin D, except
a) parathyroid hormone
b) osteoclasts
c) kernicterus
d) Ca^{2+} homeostasis
e) ultraviolet light

8. All the following terms are associated with vitamin B_{12}, except
a) megaloblastic anemia
b) intrinsic factor
c) folic acid regeneration
d) hemolysis
e) transcobalamin II

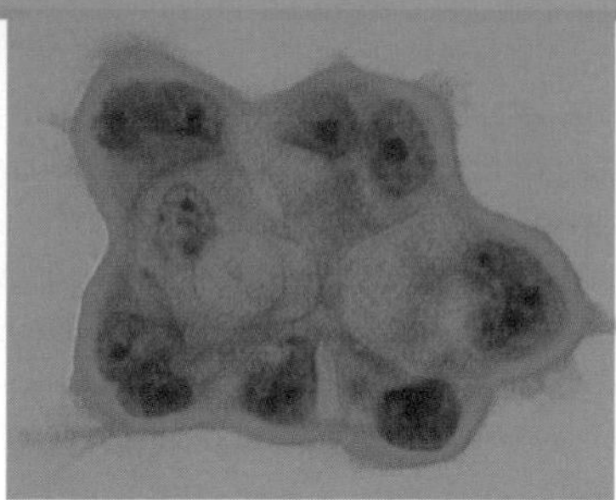

28. Neoplasms

TUMORIGENESIS

Tumors are neoplastic growths ('new growths') of cells. Benign tumors do not spread or metastasize from their original site. Malignant tumors, which are also known as cancers, spread or metastasize by:

- Direct extension into surrounding tissues.
- Via the lymphatic system.
- Via the blood (hematogenously).

Cancer is an increasing mass of abnormal cells derived from a single normal cell as a result of clonal expansion that invades surrounding normal tissues and spreads throughout the body via the lymphatic system or the blood. The growth of a cancer is known as carcinogenesis or tumorigenesis and is a multistep process (Fig. 28.1).

Genetic mutations contribute to approximately 50% of all human cancers

Although many specific and identifiable events must occur to cause cancer, there is also a stochastic (random) element.

Oncogenes are DNA sequences that code for the key proteins involved in tumorigenesis. They were first isolated from viruses that caused cancers in laboratory animals and are over expressed in cancer cells. Oncogenes can code for growth factors and mitogenic factors and therefore cancer cells can stimulate their own proliferation (Fig. 28.2).

Functional growth factor receptors can be expressed constitutively on the surface of cancer cells, but other growth factors may be needed to initiate expression and activation of some receptors.

Proliferative pathways are normally linked to antiproliferative pathways, leading to feedback control of proliferation. Some

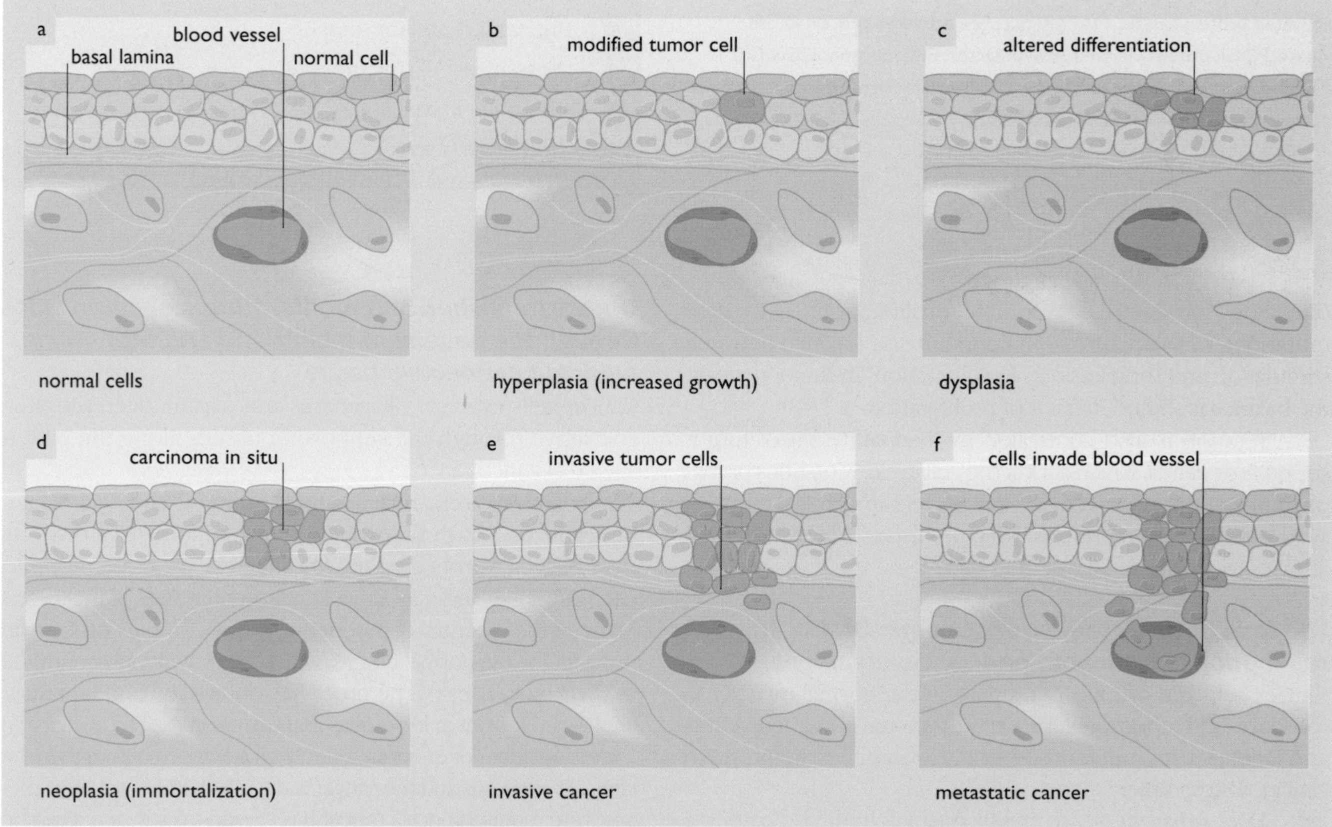

Fig. 28.1 Hypothetical progression from normal to malignant cells.

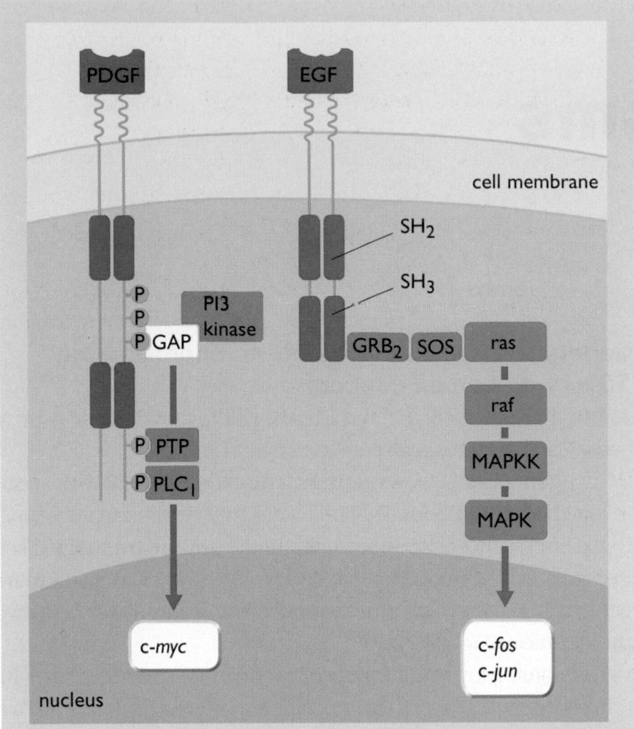

Fig. 28.2 Two schemes showing how extracellular growth factors stimulate cancer cell proliferation. Overexpression of any of these cellular homologues of oncogenes or a mutation that produces constitutive activation may contribute to enhanced growth. (EGF, epidermal growth factor; PI3, phosphoinisitol-3-kinase; GAP, GTP-ase activating protein; GRB_2, G (protein) related protein B_2; MAPK, mitogen-activated protein kinase; MAPKK, mitogen-activated protein kinase kinase; PDGF, platelet-derived growth factor; PLC, phospholipase C; PTP,phosphotyrosine phosphatase; ras, raf, cellular signal transducers; c-*fos*, c-*jun*, c-*myc*, inducers of DNA synthesis)

oncogene products can inhibit proliferation. Oncogene mutations or overexpression can shift the balance between stimulation and suppression of proliferation. In tumorigenesis, the balance is shifted in favor of proliferation.

Proliferation is also controlled by a separate set of tumor suppressor genes, which act via the cell cycle. Mutations or loss of tumor suppressor genes, such as *p53* in the Li–Fraumeni syndrome or *rb* in retinoblastoma, predisposes individuals and families to an increased risk of cancer.

The loss of the integrity of genomic DNA replication is critical to cancer development

Cancer cells can propagate only when the normal capacity to recognize and repair mutations in the genome is lost. Individuals and families with mutations in DNA repair genes are prone to cancer, for example:

- DNA repair genes to repair mismatched base pairs are mutated in hereditary nonpolyposis colon cancer.
- DNA repair to helicases are absent or defective in xeroderma pigmentosum, a genetic disease characterized by defective repair of ultraviolet radiation damage.

p53 may have a crucial role in the cellular response to DNA damage or mutation. Normally, *p53* arrests cells before DNA replication to allow repair to take place and also initiates apoptosis (programmed death of obsolete or damaged cells). Loss of normal *p53* function allows flawed DNA to replicate and the survival of flawed cells.

Cancer cells are immortalized cells

Every cell in the body, except for the germ cells of the gonads, is programmed for a finite number of cell divisions before senescence. This cellular program is the telomere. Telomeres are at the ends of the chromosome and must pair and align at mitosis. They are produced and maintained by an enzyme, telomerase, in germ cells and embryonic cells. This enzyme loses its function during normal development. A portion of the telomere is therefore lost with each cell division and such telomeric loss serves as a cellular clock. Cancer cells re-express telomerase, which allows them to proliferate endlessly. Loss of the normal cell cycle controls imposed by *rb* and *p53* facilitate the re-emergence of telomerase expression. As many as 95% of cancer cells express telomerase, making it a potential target for therapeutic intervention.

Characteristics of cancer

- Increased proliferation
- Loss of regulatory proteins
- Genomic instability
- Immortalization

Once established and proliferating, cancer invades through the basement membrane and into adjacent connective tissue

Cancer cells express collagenases and plasminogen activators and move through the supporting tissues along the path of least resistance.

Angiogenesis is essential to supply nutrients and is stimulated by fibroblast growth factor and vascular endothelial growth factor. Collagen, vitronectin, and fibronectin expression promotes cell scaffolding and may aid in attachment at sites of metastasis. Many of the essential components of this complex process are provided by the normal tissues, which can unwittingly contribute to their own demise. The processes of invasion and metastasis are less important in leukemias and lymphomas (blood cancers).

Invasion and metastasis are often well advanced before there are clinical symptoms and the cancer is detected. Pharmacologic therapies are required once a cancer has spread overtly or microscopically beyond its site of origin and has become a systemic disease.

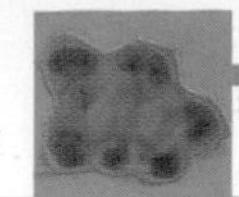

Expert histologic diagnosis is an essential component of cancer chemotherapy

The histologic diagnosis of some tumors is essential to establish whether the objective of therapy is palliation or cure, for example:

- If a non-Hodgkin's lymphoma (NHL) has a low-grade favorable histologic subtype it is incurable, but its growth is relatively indolent. Treatment of any symptoms is therefore conservative, with one chemotherapeutic agent rather than aggressive multiagent chemotherapy with its attendant risks of morbidity and mortality.
- If a NHL has an intermediate- or high-grade histologic subtype it has a rapidly fatal natural course, but is often cured by multiagent chemotherapy, while single agent or less intensive regimens have no effect.
- Extensive, even metastatic, small-cell lung cancer can be cured with multiagent chemotherapy, but nonsmall-cell lung cancer at the same stage is incurable.
- Histologic typing in acute leukemia to show whether it is lymphoblastic or nonlymphoblastic determines the choice of chemotherapeutic agents and the outcome.

Staging is the accurate determination of the extent of tumor spread by local invasion and lymphatic and hematogenous metastases

There is a precise staging system for each histologic type of cancer based upon its unique clinical and anatomic characteristics, and the use of biochemical, cytologic, and molecular biologic determinants is increasing accuracy. Accurate staging serves two purposes:

- It allows precise comparisons between patients and patient groups for a more accurate evaluation of the effectiveness of treatment.
- It is a guide for deciding which treatment to use for an individual patient.

Patients with an early stage of cancer and a favorable prognosis may require less intensive treatment (e.g. less extensive surgery and/or avoidance of chemotherapy). This reduces short-term morbidity and long-term adverse effects, which have become apparent as the treatment of cancer has become increasingly effective and more patients, especially children, survive. Such unanticipated long-term consequences include infertility, growth retardation, and second malignancies.

PRINCIPLES OF CELL PROLIFERATION AND CHEMOTHERAPY

A knowledge of the basic processes of cellular proliferation is essential to understand the mechanisms of action of anticancer drugs. Cells in a tissue are in one of the following three stages:

- Actively dividing (cycling).
- Differentiating (dying).
- Dormant (can actively divide if cellular environmental conditions allow).

Four distinct cell cycle phases are recognized: the S, G_1, G_2, and M phases (Fig. 28.3). The activity of replicative enzymes such as thymidine kinase, DNA polymerase, dihydrofolate reductase, ribonucleotide reductase, RNA polymerase II and topoisomerases I and II is increased during the S phase. Control of a G_2/M checkpoint to allow DNA repair or completion of replicative DNA synthesis is a crucial element in cell cycle control. The G_1 phase may be virtually absent, as in embryonic cells, or so prolonged that it produces dormancy (G_0).

Techniques for measuring cell cycles include the use of tritiated thymidine (^{3}H-TdR)-uptake pulse labeling to determine the fraction of cells actually synthesizing DNA. The S phase can also be measured by using a cell sorter to identify chromosome number (i.e. 2n, 4n). These measurements are used clinically in the staging of breast cancer.

Cancer cell populations do not grow in a linear manner with time

The growth of a tumor population is best described by Gompertzian kinetics (Fig. 28.4).

Growth retardation and cell loss correlates with cytologic and spatial factors. Proximity to blood vessels and access to oxygen are important determinants of cell viability and growth and have a significant therapeutic impact on:

- Radiation therapy, where oxygen is an essential intermediate.
- Chemotherapy, where many drugs target growing cycling cells.

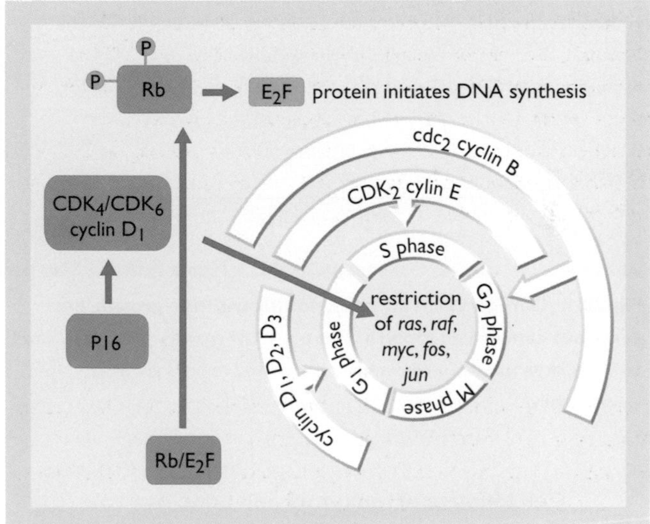

Fig. 28.3 The cell cycle and some of the important regulatory proteins. The S phase refers to the active synthesis of DNA and lasts approximately 12–18 hours. The G_2 phase lasts 1–8 hours and the DNA complement is 4n (twice the normal number of chromosomes). Mitosis (M) lasts about 1–2 hours. The duration of the G_1 phase is variable, and the late G_1 phase is associated with an increase in DNA synthesis enzymes. The complex regulation of the restriction point for the start of S phase involves cyclins and CDKs (cyclin-dependent kinases), which continue to regulate the CDKs through the entire cell cycle. (cdc_2, cell division cycle protein 2, an essential controlling gene for cell cycle progression; *ras, raf, myc, fos, jun,* cellular homologs of viral oncogenes involved in cellular proliferation; Rb, retinoblastoma protein; E_2F, a transcription factor)

The dose-limiting toxicity of anticancer drugs on normal tissue is often directly related to the rate of its cell growth

Normal tissues can be divided into different types on the basis of their cell proliferation kinetics:

- Rapidly proliferating tissues (labeling index [LI] > 5%) include the bone marrow, gut mucosa, reproductive organs, and hair follicles.
- Slowly proliferating tissues (LI < 1%) include the trachea, bronchial epithelium, liver, kidney, and endocrine organs.
- Nonproliferating tissues in adults include skeletal muscle, heart, bone, and nerve tissue.

The bone marrow is commonly the organ most sensitive to the antiproliferative effects of cancer chemotherapy.

Different tumors have different labeling indexes and doubling times

A comparison of the growth kinetics of normal bone marrow granulocytes and leukemic cells (Fig. 28.5) shows that the rate of cell proliferation in leukemia is less than in normal bone marrow. However, the cell population in leukemia expands because cell proliferation exceeds cell maturation and death. Solid tumors typically have a much lower fraction of actively growing cells. The LI is 1–5% in slow-growing adenocarcinomas, but up to 30% in Burkitt's lymphoma, testicular carcinoma, Ewing's sarcoma, NHL, and subclinical breast cancer.

Doubling times are 30–70 days in Hodgkin's disease, osteosarcoma, and fibrosarcoma, while slow-growing adult carcinomas with doubling times longer than 70 days include lung cancer, colon and gastrointestinal cancers, and advanced breast cancer. The slower rate of growth results from the presence of many nonproliferating cells and a high rate of cell death.

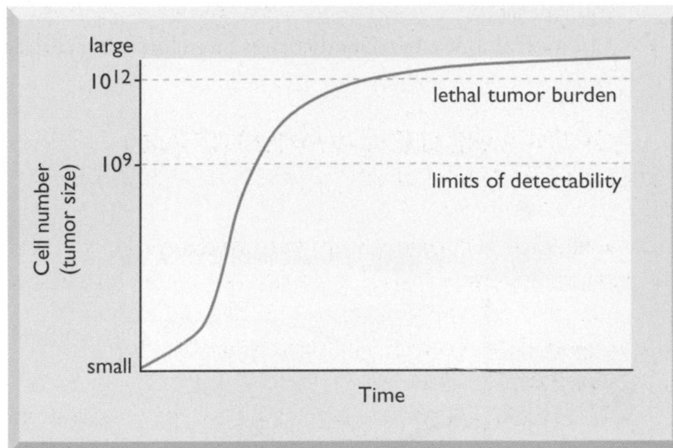

Fig. 28.4 Gompertzian kinetics, not logarithmic growth, best describes cancer cell growth. There is a low growth rate in very small and very large tumors, while intermediate-sized tumors grow exponentially.

Cell kinetics of leukemia and bone marrow

Cell type	Labeling index (%)	Cell cycle time (h)
Acute leukemia	3–12	48–72
Chronic myelogenous leukemia	6–25	48–72
Chronic lymphocytic leukemia	0–1	48–72
Normal myeloblasts	32–75	16–24
Normal myelocytes	18–25	16–24

Fig. 28.5 Cell kinetics of leukemia and bone marrow.

Several fundamental principles of clinical cancer therapy are determined by cell proliferation kinetics

The log kill hypothesis postulates that drugs kill a constant fraction of tumor cells (related to the log number of cells) and not a constant number of cells (Fig. 28.6). A proportion of cells in a cancer can survive a course of treatment by chance without being specifically drug resistant. Therefore, each drug or combination of drugs has a certain cytotoxic capacity. As a result, combination therapy is more likely to provide a cure than single drug therapy.

The log kill varies with cell growth rate and so there is a progressive decrease in log kill in the late stages of tumor growth when cells stop cycling. Early recurrences of slow-growing tumors occur because the log kill is small. Late recurrences of rapidly growing tumors may occur despite effective treatment if too few courses of treatment are given. This is referred to as the period of risk.

Some cancer therapies kill cells at specific phases of the cell cycle

Certain classes of intervention (i.e. antineoplastic drugs and radiotherapy) show phase-specific lethality.

In cancer chemotherapy there are several characteristic curves of dose versus cell survival (Fig. 28.7). In exponential curves, the proportion of surviving cells is exponentially related to the dose of the intervention. As the dose increases, the cell kill increases.

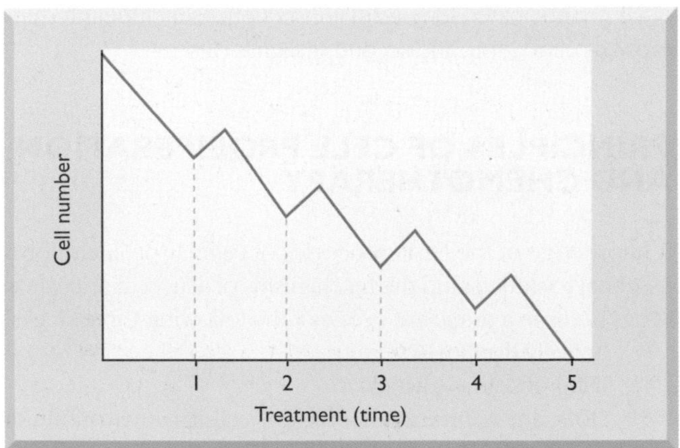

Fig. 28.6 Log kill hypothesis. A drug or drug combination can kill a constant fraction of cancer cells. Certain cells survive each treatment by chance alone and are sensitive to subsequent treatments.

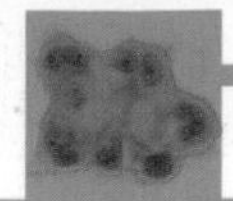

Such interventions are not cycle or stage specific (i.e. they kill cells anywhere in the cell cycle, even resting cells) and include:

- 5-Fluorouracil, cisplatin, glucocorticosteroids, nitrogen mustard, and melphalan.
- Radiotherapy.

Cyclophosphamide and other alkylating agents are active in all cells, but have increased activity in cells at the G_1/S boundary.

Phase-specific survival curves show a plateau with no increase in kill at higher doses. Further kill can be obtained, however, by increasing the exposure time, but not the dose. Drugs producing this type of curve are:

- The antimetabolic cytotoxic drugs such as cytarabine, thioguanine, and hydroxyurea, which are active only in the S phase.
- Methotrexate, doxorubicin, epipodophyllotoxins, and vinca alkaloids, which have maximum lethal toxicity during the S phase.
- Bleomycin, which has maximum activity in the G_2 and M phases.

Cytotoxic drugs block the cell cycle

All cytotoxic cancer drugs can interfere with progression of cells through the cell cycle, leading to synchronization and slowing of rapidly proliferating cells. This results in decreased sensitivity to S phase drugs.

Cytotoxicity is proportional to the total drug exposure

The pharmacokinetics of cancer chemotherapeutic agents can be complex, and cytotoxicity is proportional to the total drug exposure (area under the curve [AUC]), and not the peak plasma concentration of drug (Fig. 28.8). The drug has first to penetrate into individual cancer cells and then to interact with its molecular target. As this interaction is often reversible, at least initially, a cytotoxic concentration must be maintained at this time. In addition, the number of individual interactions between a drug and target molecules needed to kill a single cell can be enormous. It is estimated that one million molecules of cisplatin must bind to the DNA of a single cell to kill it.

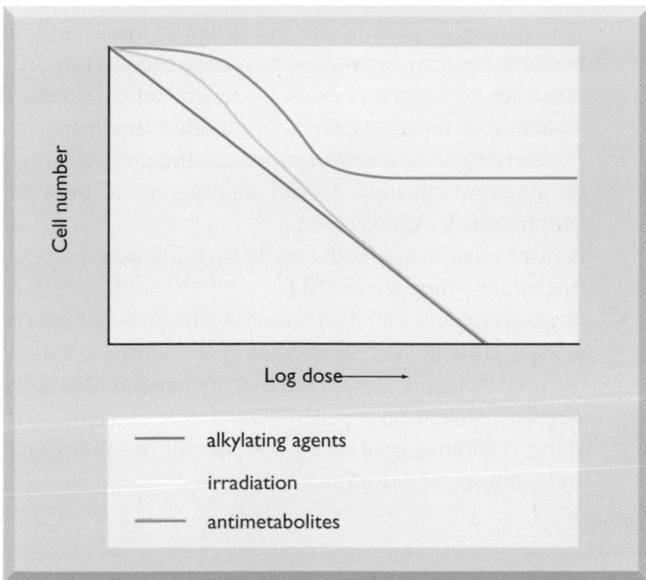

Fig. 28.7 Cycle-specific drug lethality. For noncycle-dependent agents like irradiation or alkylating agents, increasing dose produces increasing cell kill. For cycle-specific agents, like antimetabolites, which kill only actively growing cells, increasing doses have a plateau effect as cell growth slows with chemotherapy. Prolonging the duration of exposure will increase the cell kill.

Principles of cytotoxic cancer therapy

- **Drugs kill a constant fraction, not a constant number, of cells**
- **Cells may have discrete periods of vulnerability to cytotoxic drugs**
- **Cytotoxic drugs slow the progression of cells through the cell cycle**
- **Cytotoxic drugs are not selectively toxic toward cancer cells**
- **Cytotoxicity is proportional to total drug exposure**

PRINCIPLES OF COMBINATION CHEMOTHERAPY

Combinations of anticancer drugs were introduced because it was found that single agents did not produce significant remissions or cures except for choriocarcinoma.

Drugs used for combination therapy should:

- Be effective when used alone.
- Preferably produce a high fraction of a 'complete response' (defined as a 100% kill of cells in a tumor) rather than a partial response (e.g. less than a 50% kill).
- Have different biochemical mechanisms of action to attack a tumor containing a heterogeneous population of cells.

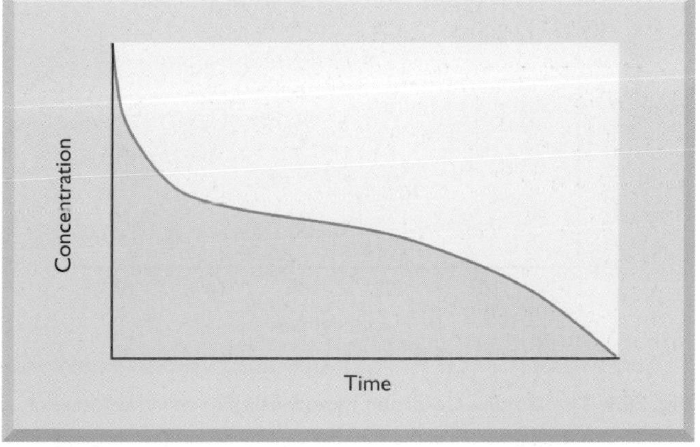

Fig. 28.8 Cytotoxicity is due to the total drug exposure or area under the curve (shaded).

- Not have similar adverse effects, otherwise the dosage will need to be reduced, resulting in a loss of the added benefit of the combination.

Tumors are heterogeneous in a variety of ways, including drug sensitivity, as a result of their unstable genetic makeup. Most drug resistance is innate for the tumor type. It may become clinically apparent when sensitive clones in the tumor are killed and the resistant clones propagate and become dominant. Curability is proportional to the tumor cell number and, in accordance with the Goldie–Coldman hypothesis, there is a greater probability of (drug-resistant) mutations in a larger population of cells (Fig. 28.9).

Principles of combination chemotherapy

- Drugs used have individual anticancer actions, nonoverlapping toxicity, and different mechanisms of action
- Optimal dose and schedule regimens used
- Shortest possible dosing interval

Benefits of combination therapy over single interventions

- Increases maximum cell kill and decreases toxicity
- Kills cells in tumors with heterogeneous cell populations
- Reduces the chance of development of resistant clones

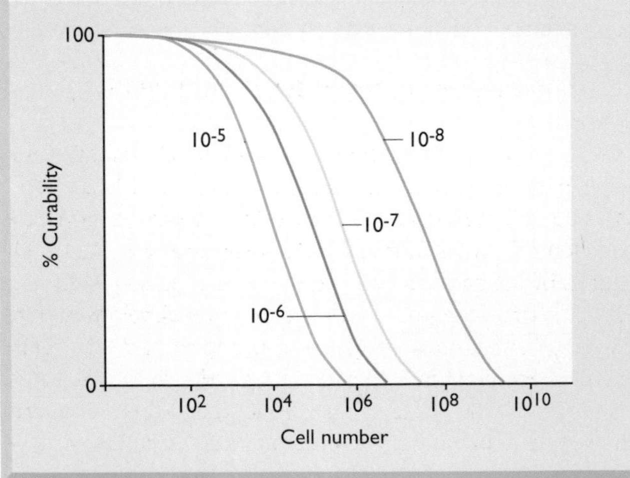

Fig. 28.9 The Goldie–Coldman hypothesis. For an intrinsic rate of mutation to drug resistance, the chances of drug failure (incurability) increase with size of the tumor (10^{-5} to 10^{-8} indicate mutation rate per cell division, i.e. 10^{-5} is one mutation per 100,000 divisions).

LATE COMPLICATIONS OF CANCER CHEMOTHERAPY

GONADAL DYSFUNCTION

The cancer therapies most likely to produce gonadal dysfunction are alkylating agents (and irradiation), and this is dose related.

About 80% of males with Hodgkin's disease treated with MOPP (mustine*, vincristine [Oncovin], procarbazine, and prednisolone) become oligo- or azoospermic, and about 50% recover within 4 years. Procarbazine is the principal cause.

In females, amenorrhea, vaginal atrophy, and endometrial hypoplasia are dose and age related. Irreversible changes and menopause due to ovarian failure are more likely with increasing age. Alkylating agents (and irradiation) are the most common causes.

Gonadal dysfunction is less severe and more reversible in prepubertal children, but boys at puberty appear to be more susceptible than any other patient group.

CARCINOGENESIS

Cancer can be caused by carcinogenic chemicals and some therapeutic drugs. One common factor in their mechanism of action is interaction with DNA.

Testing for environmental and occupational carcinogens involves examining the capacity of an agent to produce mutations in bacteria (Ames test) or to produce sister chromatid exchanges (translocations of genomic sequences from one chromosome to its identical, diploid counterpart) in cultured mammalian cells. Clinical proof of carcinogenesis is difficult to establish.

Drugs have high, low, or unknown risks of producing malignancies, and anticancer drugs are the drugs most commonly associated with drug-induced cancer (Fig. 28.10).

- The alkylating agents are particularly implicated in hematopoietic malignancies, and those used in low daily doses for prolonged periods are most likely to produce leukemia, characteristically 3–7 years after treatment.
- Ovarian cancer treated with any chemotherapy is followed by an approximately 27-fold increase in acute nonlymphocytic leukemia (ANLL).
- Breast cancer treated with melphalan is followed by an up to sevenfold increase in ANLL.
- Myeloma treated with melphalan is followed by an approximately 214-fold increase in ANLL at 50 months (17.4% of the total incidence), but there is no increase in ANLL after 20 years of follow-up in patients with breast cancer treated with a combination of cyclophosphamide, methotrexate, and 5-fluorouracil (CMF).

Late complications of cancer therapy

- Leukemogenesis/myelodysplasia
- Testicular and ovarian failure
- Secondary cancers

An increased incidence of early leukemias (ANLL less than 2 years after treatment) with a different chromosomal translocation at 11q23 has been noted in patients treated with drugs acting on topoisomerase II, such as etoposide and doxorubicin.

RESISTANCE TO CHEMOTHERAPY

If a cancer is incurable, some fraction of the cancer cells must be resistant to treatment. Resistance that is clinically apparent at the time of initial treatment because the majority of cells in the tumor are resistant is called *de novo* resistance. If the treatment initially kills nonresistant cells in the tumor, resistance is said to be acquired.

De novo resistance can be *de novo* genetic (i.e. the cells are initially inherently resistant) or can arise because drugs are unable to reach the target cells because of permeability barriers such as the blood–brain barrier (i.e. the cancer cells reside in pharmacologic 'sanctuaries').

De novo *genetic resistance is a property of an individual cell and is transferable to its progeny*

One widely studied form of genetic resistance produces abnormal transport mechanisms, resulting in either decreased cellular uptake or increased cellular efflux at the cell membrane level. The substrates for such transporters are primarily natural products like plant alkaloids and include anthracyclines, epipodophyllotoxins, vinca alkaloids, and paclitaxel. Multiple drug resistance arises from a single mutation or amplification of the *mdr 1* gene. The *mdr* gene is a member of the functionally diverse ABC transmembrane superfamily of transport proteins and ion channels, including the membrane resistance protein (MRP) and cystic fibrosis genes.

Many drugs are retained in cells after alteration or activation, for example after the kinase addition of phosphate groups to nucleosides (cytarabine) or polyglutamation of methotrexate. Absent or diminished levels of these enzymes decrease the cellular retention of these drugs and may confer *de novo* resistance.

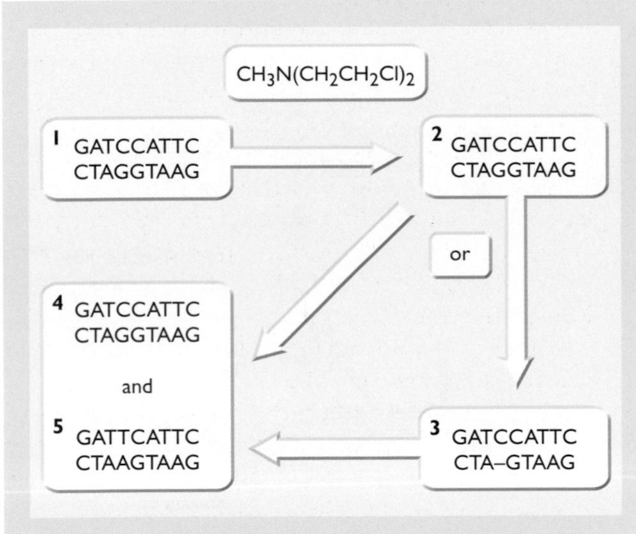

Fig. 28.10 Carcinogenesis or leukemogenesis occur because drugs, especially the alkylating agents, cause permanent genetic mutations. This is exemplified by the G to A transition shown. (1) Correct base pair sequence (hypothetical). (2) Alkyl adduct binds to guanine (white). (3) Spontaneous loss of the adducted guanine (depurination), producing a strand break. (4) Repair/removal of the alkyl adduct and return to correct base pair sequence. (5) G to A transition producing a mutation. A mutation in a proto-oncogene or tumor suppressor gene would confer a proliferation to that cell and its clonal progeny.

Pharmacologic sanctuaries include the inaccessible compartments of the blood–brain barrier and the testes

Pharmacologic sanctuaries can occur in solid tumors because their blood supply and diffusion (and therefore drug delivery) are limited by the palisading effect (cells piling up in successive rows) that occurs in tumors. Inappropriate H^+ concentrations (pH) can also confer resistance, as extracellular acidosis in a tumor will ionize some drugs (e.g. doxorubicin) and decrease their cross-membrane movement into cells.

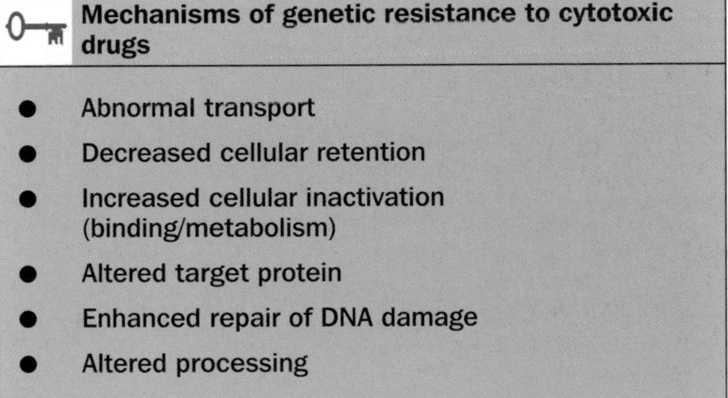

Mechanisms of genetic resistance to cytotoxic drugs

- Abnormal transport
- Decreased cellular retention
- Increased cellular inactivation (binding/metabolism)
- Altered target protein
- Enhanced repair of DNA damage
- Altered processing

Acquired resistance never develops in non-cancerous cells

Acquired resistance is an imprecise term. It fails to distinguish between the unmasking of innate genetic resistance in the initial heterogeneous tumor that becomes evident only as sensitive cells are killed off, and acquired genetic resistance that is actually induced by the chemotherapy itself, or emerges spontaneously during treatment. Acquired resistance never develops in non-cancerous cells and is therefore a property of the unstable mutable genome of transformed cancer cells. In clinical terms, acquired resistance means that the therapeutic ratio (the ratio between the minimum therapeutic and toxic doses) is not constant.

Multiple acquired drug resistance is expressed as a dominant phenotype. Drug resistance can be conferred to cells by gene transfer. The amount of p-glycoprotein of 170 kD (p-Gp 170) found on the surface of multiple drug resistance cells correlates with the degree of resistance. The expression of this protein may be increased by oncogenes like *ras* or mutant *p53*.

Membrane resistance protein is a 190,000 kD ATP binding plasma membrane protein that can confer acquired multidrug resistance similar to the p-Gp 170 mdr protein. Decreased uptake due to deletion or altered kinetics of a transport mechanism, as in methotrexate and melphalan resistance, has been described in experimental tissue culture.

Increased intracellular metabolism produces acquired resistance (Fig. 28.11). Enzymes inactivate many drugs by chemical processes such as oxidation, deamination, and reduction, and their enhanced activity may inactivate drugs. For example, aldehyde dehydrogenase oxidizes cyclophosphamide to inactive metabolites and cytidine deaminase inactivates cytarabine.

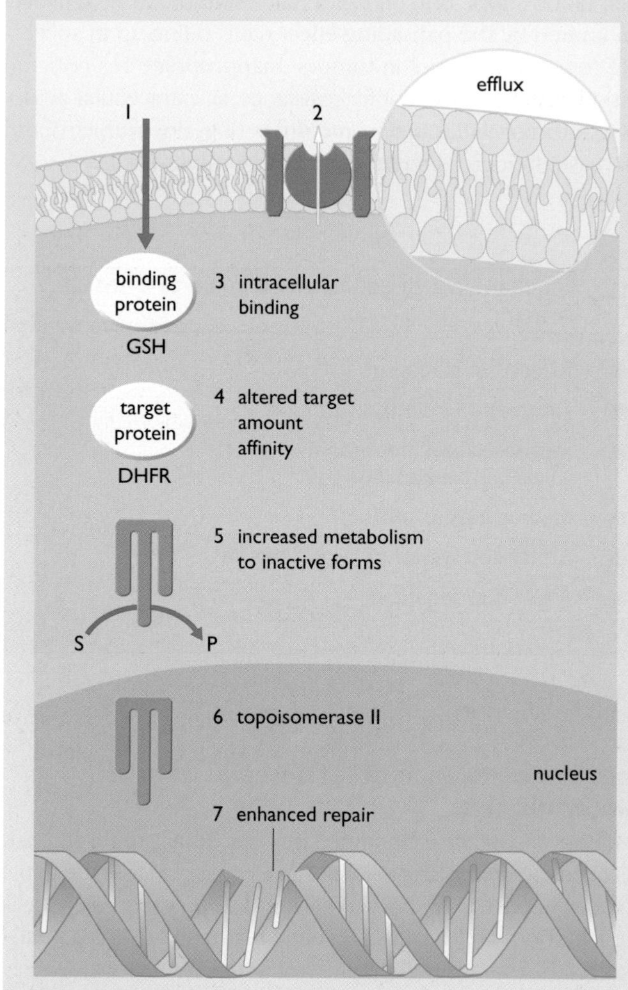

Fig. 28.11 Diagram showing several possible mechanisms of drug resistance. The classical biochemical view. Resistance can occur because of: (1) decreased uptake; (2) rapid efflux via membrane transport proteins; (3) increased intracellular binding to glutathione (GSH); (4) an altered target protein, either an increased amount or decreased binding affinity; (5) inactivation by intracellular detoxifying enzymes; (6) altered topoisomerase II, either a decreased amount or reduced affinity for a drug; and (7) enhanced repair of DNA damage. (DHFR, dihydrofolate reductase)

Altered intracellular concentrations of target protein may result in acquired resistance (see Fig. 28.11):

- An increased concentration of target protein by gene amplification, such as dihydrofolate reductase amplification in methotrexate-resistant cells, may exceed the capacity for drug uptake and binding.
- Decreased topoisomerase concentrations reduce DNA damage and alter cytotoxicity caused by drugs that use topoisomerase I and II as the essential intermediate in producing DNA damage and lethality.
- Compartmentalization of target proteins away from the site of cytotoxic interaction can also produce resistance.

Altered target proteins are frequently encountered in highly resistant tumor cell lines. Mutations in the amino acid sequence of target proteins may change the active site and decrease or abolish drug binding, as in topoisomerase I (camptothecins) and II (etoposide), dihydrofolate reductase (methotrexate), and thymidylate synthetase (5-fluorouracil).

Mutation to a doubly resistant phenotype is stepwise. If there are two effective therapies, resistance may be prevented or delayed by alternating the treatments.

ANTINEOPLASTIC CHEMOTHERAPY AGENTS

ALKYLATING AGENTS

Mechanism of action

All alkylating agents (Fig. 28.12) produce covalent bonding of alkyl (saturated carbon atoms) group(s) to cellular molecules and have

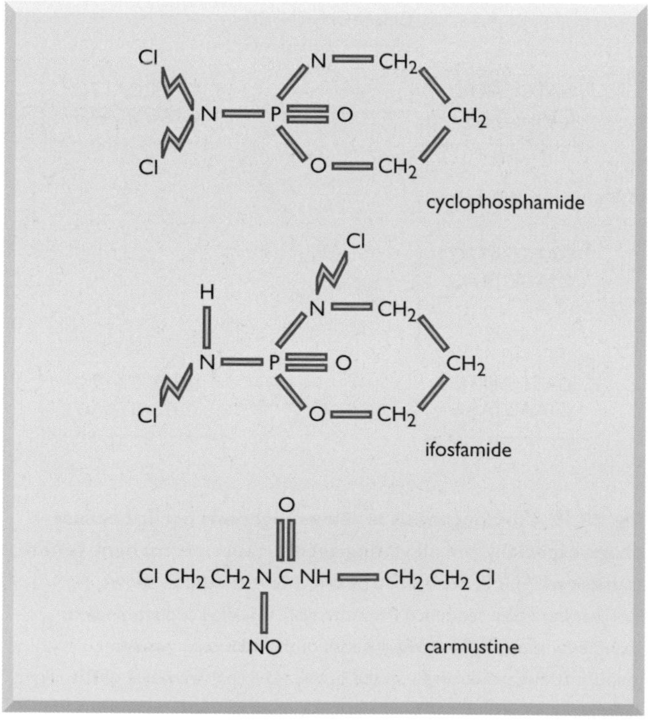

cyclophosphamide

ifosfamide

carmustine

Fig. 28.12 Chemical structures of alkylating agents. Amost all clinically useful alkylating agents spontaneously eliminate a Cl^- and have two active alkylating moieties.

reactive electrophilic intermediates, which bind to nucleophiles such as DNA (Fig. 28.13). People with genetic defects in DNA repair, such as ataxia–telangectasia, Fanconi's anemia, Bloom's syndrome, and xeroderma pigmentosa are highly sensitive to DNA-damaging agents.

Mechlorethamine, melphalan, cyclophosphamide, chlorambucil, and ifosfamide are in widespread clinical use (see Fig. 28.12). Aziridines, such as thiotepa, epoxides (dibromodulcital), and alkyl alkane sulfonates such as busulfan are less frequently used. The nitrosoureas such as carmustine, lomustine, and semustine* are highly lipophilic and easily cross the blood–brain barrier and can therefore be used to treat brain tumors. Streptozocin is a monofunctional alkylating agent with no bone marrow toxicity, but it destroys the β cells of the pancreas, causing diabetes mellitus.

Cellular uptake of alkylating agents is by active transport into cells via physiologic transporters (for nitrogen mustards) or passively for nitrosoureas. For example mechlorethamine uses the choline transporter, melphalan the L-glutamine transporter, and cisplatin the methionine transporter.

The molecular mechanism of action of alkylating agents is alkylation with nucleophilic substitution of DNA

The molecular and cellular pharmacology of the alkylating agents is well understood. The molecular mechanism of action is alkylation with nucleophilic substitution (SN_1 or SN_2) of DNA, preferentially the ^{7}*N*-guanine, ^{6}*O*-guanine, and ^{3}*N*-cytosine (see Figs 28.13, 28.14). Drug decomposition occurs spontaneously at physiologic pH and chloroethyl-diazonium or carbonium ions alkylate DNA or protein. Alkylating agents are therefore really prodrugs. Isocyanate moieties produced by spontaneous decomposition carbamoylate DNA polymerase and protein.

Sites of alkylation are widespread and include proteins (enzymes, cell membranes) and nucleotides, accounting for adverse as well as therapeutic effects. All O and N atoms of purines and pyrimidines are preferred substrates, such as ^{6}O-guanine, ^{7}N-guanine, ^{3}N-cytosine, ^{3}N-thymidine, and ^{1}N-adenine.

Bifunctional alkylating agents produce more DNA damage than monofunctional agents. Formation of interstrand cross-links (ISCs) correlates best with cytotoxicity. Some evidence suggests that these ISCs may preferentially alkylate transcriptionally active genomic regions. ISCs prevent DNA replication and RNA transcription. Monofunctional adducts produce single-strand DNA breaks as a result of depurination by endonucleases or spontaneously. Tautomerization of adducted bases produces mismatched base pairing, which is a major cause of mutations and possible carcinogenesis/leukemogenesis in normal cells.

Resistance

Alkylating agent resistance is often multifactorial:

- Membrane transport may be decreased (e.g. for melphalan, cisplatin).
- The drug may be bound by glutathione (GSH) via GSH-S-transferase or metallothioneins in the cytoplasm and inactivated.
- The drug may be metabolized to inactive species (e.g. by enzymes such as aldehyde dehydrogenase I, or the chloroethyl groups of the active binding residues of cyclophosphamide or melphalan may be hydroxylated).

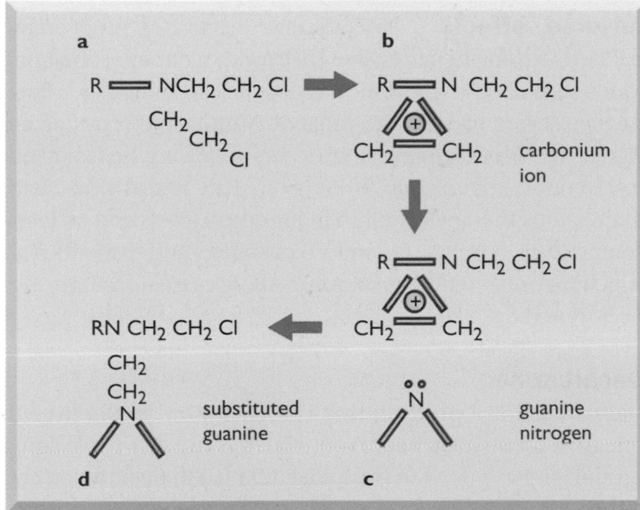

Fig. 28.13 Formation of a reactive carbonium ion (b) from an alkylating agent such as nitrogen mustard (a), and intermediate SN_1 nucleophilic attack of a guanine nitrogen (c,d). The resulting adduct can cause the base to hydrolyze and produce an apurinic site, cause a change in base pair formation by tautomerization with a resulting mutation, or a second adduct can bond to another base and make a covalent cross-link. This reaction requires SN_1 and depends only on the concentration of drug.

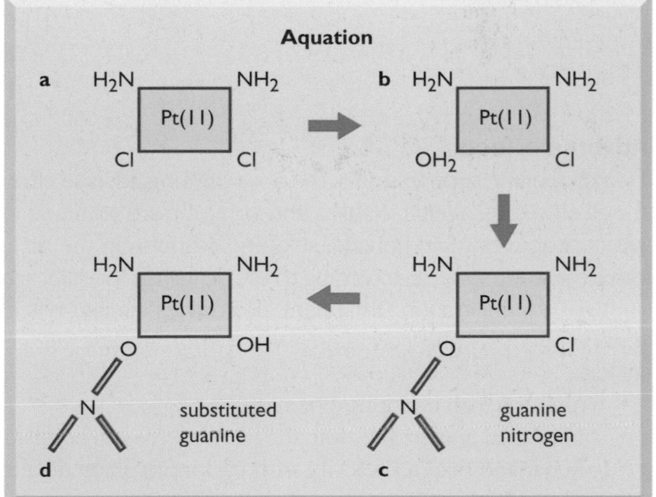

Fig. 28.14 An SN_2 reaction of cisplatin on a guanine nucleotide after aquation. Cisplatin (a) loses a Cl^- and bonds to water (b), this OH_2 group then bonds to an electron rich nitrogen molecule and displaces the OH_2 group to form a covalent bond (c). Since cisplatin is bifunctional, cross-links may be formed and, since the reaction rate depends on both the concentration of cisplatin and a neutrophile (d), it is an SN_2 kinetic reaction. (Pt (II), platinum)

Pharmacokinetics

The alkylating agents, exept for cyclophosphamide, have very short half-lives in plasma. Nitrogen mustard has a half-life of 10 minutes. Melphalan gives variable blood levels when taken orally owing to poor absorption, and a half-life of 1.8 hours when given intravenously. Chlorambucil is well absorbed orally with a half-life of 1.5–3 hours. Cyclophosphamide peak levels are dose dependent (500 nM with 60 mg/kg). The parent drug, which is well absorbed orally (97%), has a half-life of 3–10 hours whereas the half-life for its alkylating activity is 8 hours. Of all the metabolites, hydroxycyclophosphamide exhibits the highest therapeutic index. Repeated oral doses of phenobarbital or cyclophosphamide itself may increase total drug exposure and increase both activation and inactivation. Ifosphamide has a longer half-life which increases at higher doses (4–5 g/m^2) than cyclophosphamide which is 15 hours. Stearic hindrance to the hydroxylation of the chloroethyl side chains is clinically important. Nitrosureas have peak levels of 5 μM with a distribution phase of 5 minutes and a serum half-life of 70 minutes.

Characteristics of alkylating agents

- Directly damage DNA
- Have a broad spectrum of antitumor activity and immunosuppression
- Active against proliferating and nonproliferating cells
- Cause dose-limiting myelosuppression
- Are genotoxic and associated with an increased risk of leukemogenesis

Adverse effects

Hematopoietic suppression is the dose-limiting adverse effect for all alkylating agents. Nausea and vomiting are common as are teratogenesis and gonadal atrophy, although in the latter cases these are variable according to the drug, its schedule, and route of administration. Treatment also carries a major risk of leukemogenesis and carcinogenesis. Other adverse effects include:

- Alopecia with cyclophosphamide.
- Interstitial pneumonitis with the nitrosoureas and busulfan.
- Renal and bladder toxicity with cyclophosphamide and ifosfamide.

Cyclophosphamide

Cyclophosphamide is a prodrug that requires oxidation to active 4-hydroxycyclophosphamide in the liver via the hepatic microsomal cytochrome P-450 system. This is followed by the spontaneous reversible formation of aldophosphamide in the blood, and then an elimination reaction to yield phosphoramide mustard, the active alkylating form of the drug intracellularly and in the blood. Induction of cytochrome P-450 enzymes by cyclophosphamide itself, or other drugs such as phenobarbital or cimetidine, results in increased levels of active cyclophosphamide. Of all the metabolites of cyclophosphamide, 4-hydroxycyclophosphamide has the highest therapeutic index.

The alkylating agents, except for cyclophosphamide, have very short half-lives in plasma.

NONCLASSICAL ALKYLATING AGENTS

Procarbazine

Mechanism of action Procarbazine is not itself cytotoxic or mutagenic, but is activated in the liver to an azo intermediate, which is converted to alkylating azoxy compounds. The molecular mechanism of action is DNA alkylation. However, DNA methylation, free radical-mediated damage, and inhibition of DNA and protein synthesis may be additional molecular mechanisms of action. The primary cellular mechanism of action is chromatid breakage and translocation, and the tissue mechanism of action is termination of cell cycle progression due to the secondary cellular action, which is inhibition of the G_1/S phase transition.

Pharmacokinetics Procarbazine and its metabolites are cleared from plasma within 2 hours. Phenytoin and phenobarbital increase both the clearance and antitumor effect of procarbazine by accelerating production of its cytotoxic metabolites.

Resistance develops rapidly to procarbazine and may be due to nucleic acid synthesis to replace adducted bases, which is more rapid during active DNA synthesis.

Adverse effects Procarbazine inactivates monoamine oxidase, causing hypertensive crises with tyramine-containing foods (e.g. cheese, red wine). It also has an 'Antabuse' effect, causing severe nausea with ethanol. Nausea and vomiting are significant. Myelosuppression occurs following oral, but not intravenous, administration. Neurotoxicity is also worse with intravenous therapy owing to higher peak levels and includes somnolence, confusion, mood changes, and paresthesias, which may respond to pyridoxine. Allergic reactions have also been noted.

Dacarbazine

Dacarbazine is a prodrug that is metabolized in the liver to release a methyldiazonium ion, which is the active alkylating product. It has poor cerebrospinal fluid (CSF) penetration and is therefore of no use for central nervous system (CNS) cancers. Its major adverse effects are severe nausea and vomiting.

Hexamethamelamine

Hexamethamelamine is a prodrug that is activated in the liver. Its major adverse effects are nausea and vomiting, and myelosuppression occurs in 50% of all patients. Neurotoxicity 1–3 months after treatment includes mood changes and paresthesias.

PLATINUM COMPOUNDS

In 1968, it was observed that electric currents through platinum electrodes caused filamentous growth in bacteria, which is a sign of inhibited DNA synthesis.

Cisplatin

Clinical trials of cisplatin in the early 1970s went on to revolutionize the treatment of genitourinary tumors.

Cisplatin (dichloro-diamino-*cis* platinum II) requires the replacement of Cl^- with water (aquation) for activation. Activation is slow (2.5 hours) and only the *cis* enantiomer is cytotoxic.

Mechanism of action Cisplatin binds to guanine in DNA and RNA, and the interaction is stabilized by hydrogen bonding. The molecular mechanism of action is unwinding and shortening of the DNA helix. Although ISCs occur (10% of all adducts), the cellular mechanism of action, cell inactivation, appears to be principally due to the formation of intrastrand links (75–80%). A relationship exists between the number of cross-links, ability to repair cross-links, and cytotoxicity.

Resistance to cisplatin may involve protein repair and/or topoisomerase II binding.

Pharmacokinetics Cisplatin is inactivated in blood and intracellularly by covalent interaction with the sulfhydryl groups in glutathione and metallothioneins. Protein binding to tissue, blood cells, and plasma proteins also inactivates cisplatin. Cisplatin is filtered by glomeruli and actively secreted in the proximal convoluted tubules. Approximately 25% of a dose is excreted within 24 hours, 90% in the urine.

Adverse effects The major adverse effect of cisplatin is renal toxicity with renal tubular damage and necrosis, similar to that seen with heavy metals. Protective procedures to avoid this involves hydration and diuresis. Myelosuppression, usually thrombocytopenia, is less common. If there is adequate renal protection, peripheral neuropathy is dose limiting, if not, then renal toxicity is dose limiting. Ototoxicity with hearing loss, allergic reactions, severe nausea, and vomiting are common.

Carboplatin

Carboplatin is an analog of cisplatin with the same mechanism of cytotoxicity. It was developed to be less nephrotoxic and less likely to cause vomiting.

ANTIMETABOLITES

Methotrexate

Mechanism of action The molecular mechanism of action of methotrexate (Fig. 28.15) is inhibition of the enzyme dihydrofolate reductase. It has been in use since 1948 when it was first demonstrated that folate antagonists could induce complete (but transient) remissions of childhood acute leukemia.

Folates are one-carbon cofactors in purine and pyrimidine biosynthesis and include:

- Pteridine.
- *para*-Aminobenzoic acid.
- Glutamate complexes.

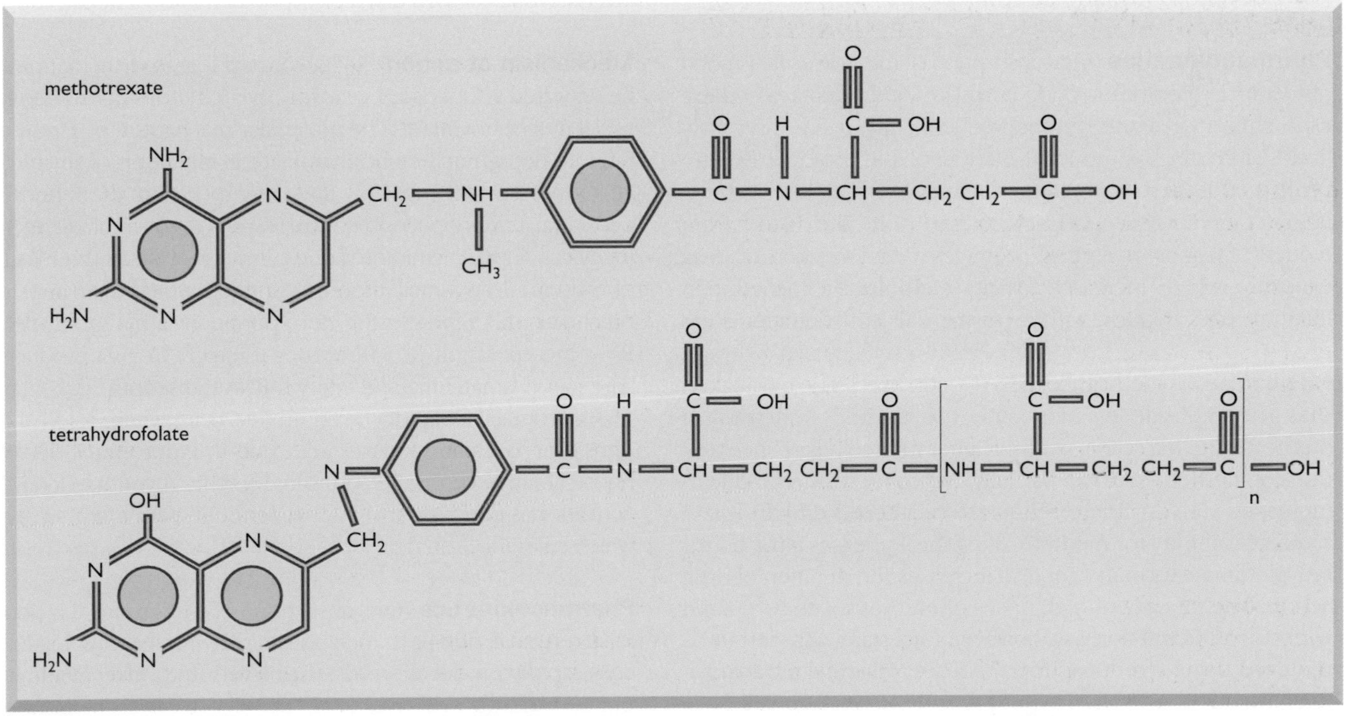

Fig. 28.15 Chemical structure of methotrexate and tetrahydrofolate. Methotrexate is an analog of tetrahydrofolate and binds to dihydrofolate reductase. The NH_2 group at position 4 converts methotrexate from a substrate to a tight binding inhibitor of dihyrofolate reductase.

Polyglutamates are more efficient cofactors because they are retained longer in the cells. The tetrahydro (reduced) folates are the active forms and the essential role of dihydrofolate reductase is to maintain a supply of reduced folate cofactors. Dihydrofolate and formyl dihydrofolate, which accumulate after inhibition of dihydrofolate reductase, directly inhibit folate-dependent enzymes.

Methotrexate is actively transported via a ^{5}N-methyl tetrahydrofolic acid (reduced folate) system through the cell membrane into the cytoplasm, where it binds and inactivates dihydrofolate. Free methotrexate competes with increased concentrations of dihydrofolate (from decreased thymidylate synthase activity) to inhibit dihydrofolate reductase. The cellular mechanism of action is a reduction in the availability of thymidylate synthase. Methotrexate also has effects on purine synthesis, where 10-formyl dihydrofolate is a necessary cofactor in two steps of *de novo* purine synthesis. The required intracellular concentration of methotrexate for inhibiting pyrimidine synthesis is 1×10^{-8}M, while that for inhibiting purine synthesis is 1×10^{-7}M.

In general, cytotoxicity is directly proportional to the duration of exposure, although increased drug concentrations may overcome resistance and increase cytotoxicity

Resistance Multiple mechanisms have been described for methotrexate resistance. These include:

- Decreased membrane transport.
- Decreased affinity of dihydrofolate reductase for methotrexate.
- Increased concentration of dihydrofolate reductase.
- Decreased polyglutamation due to decreased folate polyglutamyl synthase.
- Decreased thymidylate synthesis.

Pharmacokinetics Oral absorption of methotrexate is good but variable. Poor absorption correlates with increased relapses in childhood acute lymphocytic leukemia. It has three half-lives (5 minutes, 2–3 hours, 8–10 hours), and the latter two are prolonged if there is impaired renal function or fluid accumulation. Re-emergence of methotrexate into the blood from pleural effusions or ascites, produces a prolongation of drug exposure which increases toxicity Methotrexate penetration into the CNS is poor, with a plasma:CSF concentration ratio of 31:1.

High doses of methotrexate have been used. The rationale is that the high doses overcome the limited transport of methotrexate into cancer cells. Higher intracellular concentrations of methotrexate can partially overcome resistance due to increased dihydrofolate reductase or altered dihydrofolate reductase affinity for methotrexate. This increases intracellular polyglutamate formation and so increases the duration of drug action. The efficacy of high doses of methotrexate compared with conventional doses is, however, uncertain, and 'rescue' is required using a reduced folate source, 5-formyl tetrahydrofolic acid (leucovorin). Thymidine and blockade of cell cycle progression with l-asparaginase have also been tried to allow the use of high doses of methotrexate.

Adverse effects Myelosuppression and mucositis are the major adverse effects of methotrexate. CNS damage is most severe when methotrexate is given intrathecally with irradiation and may manifest as one of the following:

- Chemical arachnoiditis, which is characterized by headache, fever, and nuchal rigidity and is the most common and most acute adverse effect. It may be due to additives in the diluent (benzoic acid in sterile water).
- Subacute CNS toxicity, which occurs 2–3 weeks after administration and is characterized by motor paralysis, cranial nerve palsy, seizures, and coma.
- Chronic demyelinating encephalitis, which produces dementia and spasticity with cortical thinning, enlarged cerebral ventricles, and cerebral calcifications.

The latter two adverse effects may be worsened by radiotherapy. Cirrhosis and portal vein fibrosis result from prolonged oral use. Chemical hepatitis is reversed by choline administration.

Trimetrexate

Trimetrexate is a methotrexate analog that enters cells by diffusion. It is therefore active against reduced folate transport-resistant mutants and polyglutamation-deficient mutants that are resistant to methotrexate. It is also used to treat *Pneumocystis carinii* pneumonia.

10-EDAM (10-ethyl-10-deaza aminopterin)

This drug has a wider spectrum of activity and more selective uptake and retention (due to an increased rate of polyglutamation) in tumor cells relative to normal tissues than methotrexate.

Fluorinated pyrimidines (5-fluorouracil)

5-Fluorouracil (Fig. 28.16) was developed in 1957 on the basis of an observed increased uracil incorporation into rat hepatomas.

Mechanism of action 5-Fluorouracil is a prodrug that must be activated (ribosylated, phosphorylated) to 5-fluoro-deoxyuracil monophosphate. The molecular mechanism of action of 5-fluoro-deoxyuracil monophosphate is inhibition of thymidylate synthase (Fig. 28.17). RNA incorporation of 5 fluoro-deoxyuracil monophosphate corresponds to cytotoxicity in many cell lines. Thymidine alone cannot reverse all the effects of 5-fluoro-deoxyuracil monophosphate, which also impairs precursor rRNA processing and polyadenylation of nuclear RNA. Incorporation of 5-fluorouracil into DNA also produces base pair mismatching and faulty mRNA transcripts.

5-Fluorouracil is rapidly taken up into cells, where a series of phosphorylases and kinases act upon it. Fluorouracil deoxyribose is activated in one additional step by thymidine kinase. Activation is complex and interdependent, with many sites at which resistance can develop.

Pharmacokinetics Oral absorption of 5-fluorouracil is poor as a result of first-pass metabolism. An intravenous loading dose rapidly produces steady-state levels. Intra-arterial administration allows selective drug delivery to liver metastases where a first-pass metabolism by the tumor reduces systemic drug levels, and adverse effects.

Fig. 28.16 Chemical structures of cytarabine, deoxycytidine, uracil, thymidine, and 5-fluorouracil. Like methotrexate, cytarabine and 5-fluorouracil are analogs of nucleotides which are taken up and actuated by normal cellular processes. However, because of a unique feature, they become inhibitors of DNA synthesis rather than building blocks of DNA. There are many potential sites of resistance because of the complex biochemistry.

Combination chemotherapy 5-Fluorouracil has been used in combination with many drugs in the treatment of solid tumors.

Methotrexate increases 5-fluorouracil triphosphate formation and increases cytotoxicity. Thymidine inhibits 5-fluorouracil degradation and thereby increases its half-life. Infusions of thymidine triphosphate, a feedback inhibitor of ribonucleotide reductase, increases 5-fluorouracil triphosphate incorporation into RNA. Inhibitors of *de novo* purine synthesis such as pyrazofurin, *L*-phosphonoacetyl-l-alanine, and allopurinol increase 5-fluorouracil triphosphate production.

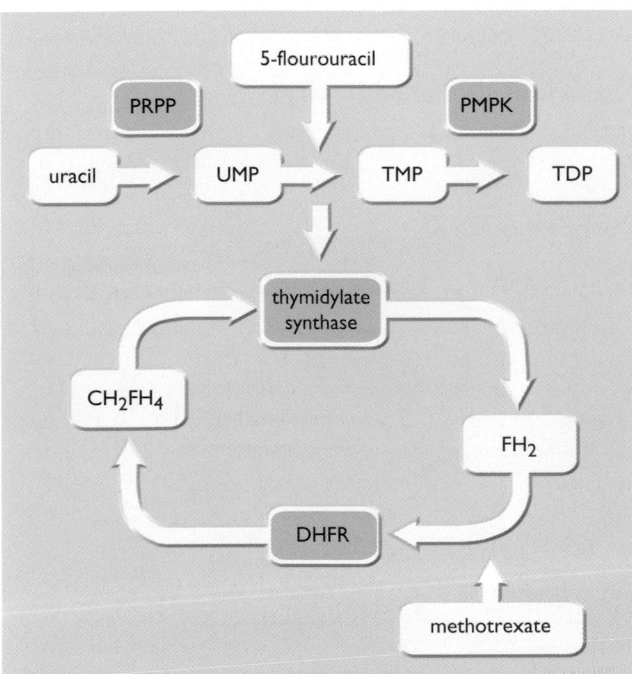

Fig. 28.17 The thymidine pathway showing the inhibition of thymidylate synthase by 5-fluorouracil. Methotrexate and 5-fluorouracil both act to decrease the synthesis of thymidine (DHFR, dihydrofolate reductase; CH_2FH_4, methylene tetahydrofolate, the donor of a methyl group to uracil; FH_2, dihydrofolate; PMPK, pyrimidine monophosphate kinase; PRPP, phosphoribosyl pyrophosphatase; TDP, thymidine diphosphate; TMP, thymidine monophosphate; UMP, uracil monophosphate)

Leucovorin increases the inhibition of thymidylate synthase, which requires reduced folate cofactors to form a tight ternary complex with 5-fluorouracil. Leucovorin increases the cytotoxicity in 5-fluorouracil-insensitive tumors by stabilizing the ternary complex, slowing the reversibility of the reaction, and increasing deoxythymidine monophosphate (dTMP). Leucovorin doubles the effectiveness of 5-fluorouracil in the treatment of colon and breast cancers. 5-Fluorouracil significantly prolongs survival when used in the treatment of locally advanced rectal and pancreatic cancers.

Adverse effects Reversible myelosuppression, mucositis, and diarrhea are the major adverse effects of 5-fluorouracil. Prolonged intravenous infusions ($\geq$ 21 days) cause palmar erythema and desquamation. People with dihydropyrimidine dehydrogenase deficiency, with an enzyme activity less than 5% of normal, have an increased risk of a severe and even fatal reaction to 5-fluorouracil.

Purine antimetabolites

Purine antimetabolites were discovered in the 1940s and 1950s and have been in clinical use for over 40 years.

Characteristics of antimetabolites

- Mimic essential cellular 'metabolites'
- Usually effective against actively proliferating cells
- Have common toxicities of myelosuppression and mucositis
- Are teratogenic, but not usually leukemogenic

Mechanism of action The general cellular mechanism of action is a reduction in purine levels in tumor cells. This is achieved in a variety of ways:

- The ribonucleotide 6-mercaptopurine (Fig. 28.18) inhibits *de novo* purine biosynthesis. Its molecular mechanism of action is inhibition of glutamine 5-phosphoribosylpyrophosphate aminotransferase, the first step in purine synthesis, by negative feedback through mimicking a purine nucleoside (see Fig. 28.19). 6-Mercaptopurine also inhibits the interconversion of inosinate to adenylate, and inosinate to xanthylate, the precursor to guanylate.
- Azathioprine, a widely used immunosuppressant, is a prodrug of 6-mercaptopurine.
- 6-Thioguanine (Fig. 28.18), when converted to the active form thioGMP, inhibits glutamine 5-phosphoribosyl-pyrophosphate aminotransferase and inosinic acid dehydrogenase.

Adverse effects include myelosuppression, mucositis, teratogenesis, and reversible cholestatic jaundice.

Thiopurine *S*-methyltransferase catalyzes the *S*-methylation of thiopurines such as 6-mercaptopurine and 6-thioguanine. Synthesis of this enzyme is genetically polymorphic and 1 in 300 people have an autosomal recessive deficiency. In these people, usual doses cause severe hematopoietic toxicity due to the accumulation of thiopurines.

As 6-mercaptopurine is metabolized via xanthine oxidase, allopurinol can interfere with its metabolism, resulting in toxicity.

Selective adenine deaminase inhibitors

New purine analogs have been designed to inhibit adenine deaminase inhibition selectively as their molecular mechanism of action. Their cellular mechanism of action is a decrease in *de novo* purine synthesis. These agents have proved beneficial in previously refractory diseases.

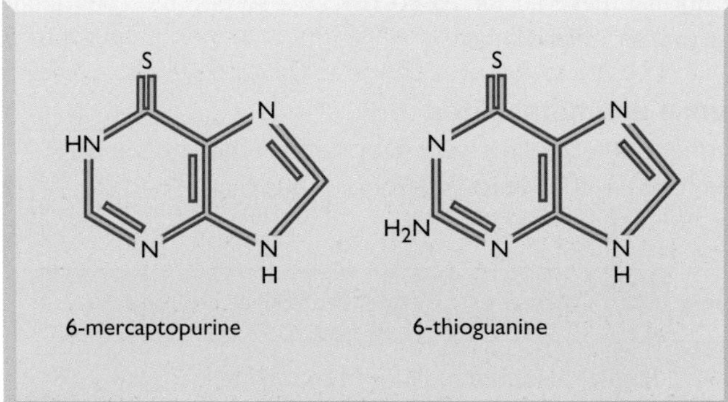

Fig. 28.18 Chemical structures of 6-mercaptopurine and 6-thioguanine. Thiopurines are triphosphorylated and act as feedback inhibitors of *de novo* purine synthesis; they are also potent immunosuppressant drugs.

Deoxycoformicin (pentostatin) causes dose-related adverse effects of profound immunosuppression due to T cell cytolysis, somnolence, and coma. Approximately 30–40% of patients have decreased renal function after receiving the drug.

Fludarabine is a prodrug that is converted to its triphosphate form. Its cellular mechanism of action is inhibition of DNA polymerase and ribonucleotide reductase. Its adverse actions are predominantly restricted to severe reversible myelosuppression and an extreme suppression of cell-mediated immunity.

2-Chlorodeoxyadenosine (2-CDA) is a purine analog and prodrug that is metabolized to the active product 2-CDA triphosphate (2-CDA-TP), which accumulates intracellularly. Its cellular mechanism of action is inhibition of purine synthesis. 2-CDA-TP is preferentially retained in leukemic cells (chronic lymphocytic leukemia, hairy cell leukemia, and ANLL) and its main adverse effect is severe neutropenia.

Cytarabine

Cytarabine (cytosine arabinoside, also known as ara-C) is a nucleoside analog of cytosine. It is a prodrug that requires phosphorylation to produce the active monophosphate product, ara-CMP and subsequently the triphosphate (ara-CTP). The molecular mechanism of action of ara-CMP is ultimately via ara-CTP competition with cytosine triphosphate for DNA polymerases. The resultant cellular mechanism of action is incorporation of ara-CTP into DNA. This produces cytotoxicity. The secondary cellular mechanism of action is premature chain termination.

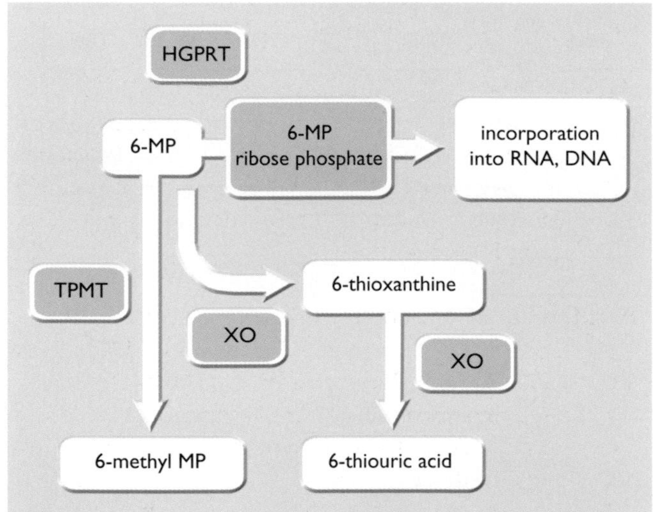

Fig. 28.19 The purine nucleoside pathway. 6-Mercaptopurine (6-MP) is activated to the triphosphate to be incorporated into DNA and RNA or to produce negative feedback on *de novo* purine synthesis. Metabolism is via xanthine oxidase (XO) to thiouric acid (allopurinol can interfere with this reaction and produce excessive toxicity), and via methylation and desulfuration to 6-methylpurine. One in 300 people lack thiopurine methyltransferase (TMPT) and can have excessive toxicity to the usual clinical dose.(HGPRT, hypoxanthine guanine phosphoribosyltransferase)

Resistance to cytarabine correlates with the formation and retention of ara-CMP. Genetic resistance occurs because cytarabine cytotoxicity is cell cycle and S phase specific.

Pharmacokinetics Cytarabine is deaminated in the intestines so it cannot be given orally. It is actively transported across cell membranes and rapidly phosphorylated in a stepwise fashion by deoxycytidine kinases to the active triphosphate. Deamination by cytidine deaminase inactivates the drug. The major plasma half-life is 2 hours.

Adverse effects of cytarabine include myelosuppression, which is dose limiting, severe, and reversible. Cholestatic jaundice and mucositis are less common. Cerebellar dysfunction due to a loss of cerebellar Purkinje cells occurs in up to 30% of patients treated with a high-dose regimen > 3 g/M^2 for six or more twice daily doses. This occurs more fequently in elderly patients with renal insufficiency and the syndrome is usually irreversible.

Combination chemotherapy Synergism, due to decreased DNA repair, has been reported with cyclophosphamide, cisplatin, carmustine, and thiopurines.

5-Azacytidine

Structurally and functionally, 5-azacytadine is an analog of cytosine. It is chemically unstable and after phosphorylation to a triphosphate is incorporated into RNA and DNA (its molecular mechanism of action) where it cleaves spontaneously. This cleavage product prevents cytosine methylation. Hypomethylation of cytosine occurs preferentially in actively transcribed regions of DNA. Unlike cytarabine, it is phosphorylated by uridine–cytidine kinase. It is inactivated by cytidine deaminase.

Hydroxyurea

Hydroxyurea was first synthesized over 100 years ago. Its use is limited to chronic myelogenous leukemia, myeloproliferative diseases, hypereosinophilic syndrome, and intracerebral leukostasis in acute leukemia. It may be mildly synergistic with radiotherapy in cervical cancer.

Mechanism of action The molecular mechanism of action of hydroxyurea is inhibition of ribonucleotide reductase (Fig. 28.20). As a result, its cellular mechanism of action is inhibition of S phase cells and synchronization of cells at the G_1/S interface. The effects of hyrdroxyurea are reversed by deoxyribonucleotides.

Hydroxyurea rapidly enters the CSF and ascitic fluid and is therefore effective for CNS cancer.

Adverse effects Leukopenia is a common adverse effect. Hydroxyurea is very short acting and rapidly reversible. A lichen planus-like skin change has been noted.

Gemcitibine* (2´-2´,difluorodeoxycytidine)

Gemcitibine* is a cytidine analog developed to treat solid tumors. It is similar to cytarabine in that it is a prodrug, is deaminated, and activated by cytidine dexoyribose kinase. Its cellular mechanism of action is inhibition of DNA synthesis. It is less effective as a DNA chain terminator than cytarabine, but is much less easily removed from DNA once incorporated. The triphosphate form of gemcitibine* is retained intracellularly much longer than cytarabine and its feedback inhibition of cytidine deaminase prevents removal of the activated species. Gemcitibine* is active throughout the cell cycle and active against resting/noncycling cells (unlike cytarabine, which is S phase selective).

TUBULIN-BINDING AGENTS

Vinca alkaloids

Vincristine, vinblastine, vindesine*, and vinorelbine are all alkaloids derived from the periwinkle plant (*Vinca rosea*).

Mechanism of action The cellular mechanism of action of vinca alkaloids is the prevention of microtubule assembly, causing cells to arrest in the late G_2 phase by preventing formation of mitotic filaments for nuclear and cell division. They achieve this by the molecular mechanism of action of binding to and inactivating tubulin. Their basic structure is a complex alkaloid of vindoline and catharanthine, which differ by only one or two substituents, but have widely varying spectra of activity and toxicity (Fig. 28.21).

Vinca alkaloids enter cells by nonsaturable energy-independent membrane transport and then bind to tubulin. This inhibits microtubule assembly. Tubulin polymerizes to form microtubules and is important in mitosis, transport, and cell structure (Fig. 28.22). Very low concentrations induce a metaphase arrest. Although the alkaloids act throughout the cell cycle, they are especially effective in the late S phase or G_2/M. The cytotoxic dose is low and is selective for transformed lymphocytes.

Experimental work suggests that prolonged exposure to vincristine is necessary to achieve maximal cytotoxicity and so continuous infusions are now being evaluated in lymphomas.

Resistance to vinca alkaloids involves mutations in tubulin-binding sites.

Adverse effects Sensory and motor peripheral neuropathies are characteristic adverse effects of all vinca alkaloids. Autonomic

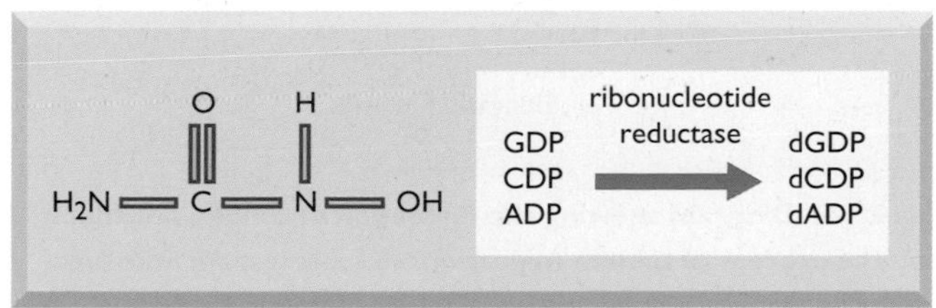

Fig. 28.20 Hydroxyurea and its target of inhibition, ribonucleotide reductase. By decreasing the pool of deoxyribonucleotides, hydroxyurea can stop or slow DNA synthesis and cellular proliferation.

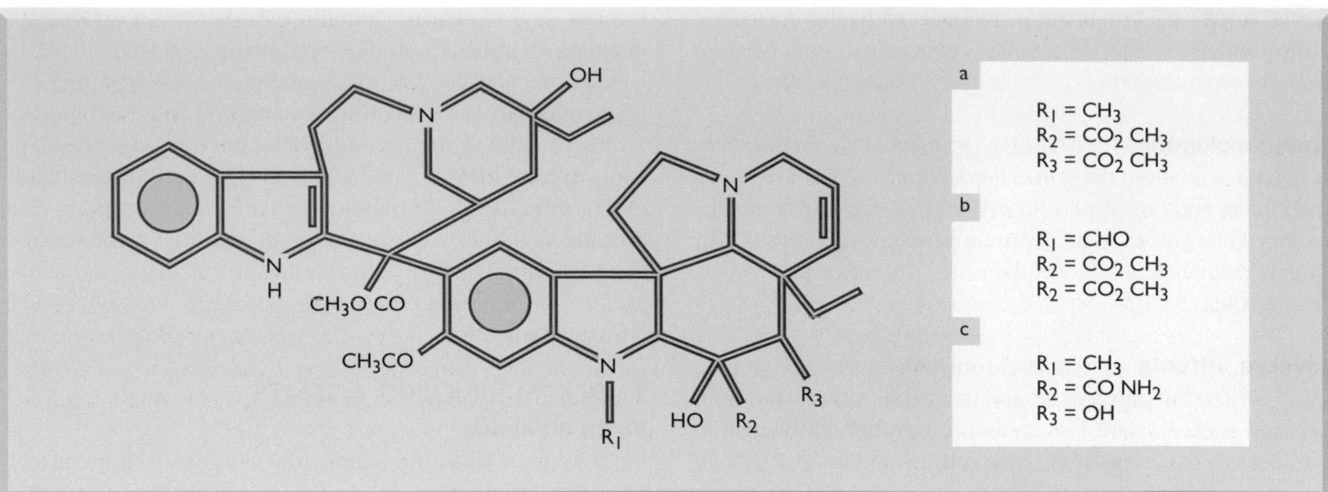

Fig. 28.21 Chemical structures of the vinca alkaloids. The vindaline backbone is unchanged between the various agents of this class, but small substitutions on the catharantine group markedly shift the toxicity profile but have less effect on therapeutic activity. (a) Vinblastine, (b) vincristine, and (c) vindesine. The CH_3 instead of CHO at R_1 produces myelosuppression, which is not seen with vincristine.

neuropathy after a high single dose and hepatic failure have been reported. Toxicity is cumulative and its severity is dose related. The spectrum of neurotoxicity and additional toxicities varies between the alkaloids:

- Vincristine is the most neurotoxic, followed by vindesine* and then vinblastine, with vinorelbine being the least neurotoxic.
- Vinblastine is the most myelotoxic, followed by vindesine* and then vinorelbine. Vincristine is not myelosuppressive.
- All cause mild alopecia, but this is more more severe with vinblastine and vindesine* than for vincristine and vinorelbine.
- All induce the syndrome of nephrogenic inappropriate antidiuretic hormone secretion.
- All cause equally severe local extravasation injury.

L-Asparaginase decreases hepatic metabolism and increases toxicity, so vinca alkaloids should be given 12–24 hours before L-asparaginase.

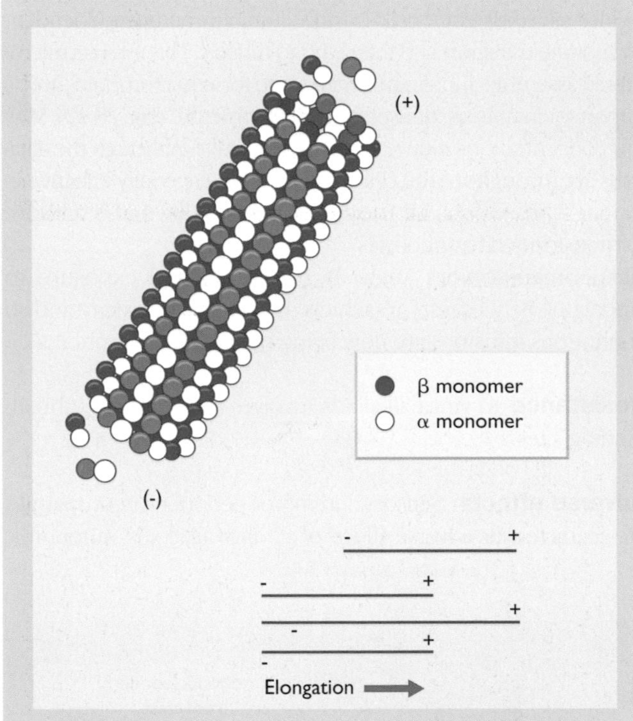

Fig. 28.22 Diagram showing the formation of tubulin polymers and the process of tubulin migration. The polymers are made up of α and β monomers and the process of tubulin migration involves elongation at a (+) end and shortening at a (–) end. Vinca alkaloids decrease the association rate at the (+) end and prevent polymerization of α and β dimers. Toxanes stabilize multimers and prevent dissociation at the (–) end, resulting in increased polymerization. Either effect on the dynamic equilibrium is cytotoxic.

Paclitaxel

Paclitaxel (Fig. 28.23) is a complex diterpine taxane originally isolated from the bark of the Western yew. It is insoluble in water and therefore is emulsified in cremophor, an emulsifier that can induce a severe anaphylactic reaction.

Taxanes enhance all aspects of tubulin polymerization, a cellular mechanism of action that is the opposite effect to that of vinca alkaloids, but they are also cytotoxic, emphasizing the dynamic importance of tubulin polymerization as a target for cytotoxic drugs. Taxanes stabilize tubulin polymers and do not prevent polymerization.

A low concentration of paclitaxel increases both the microtubule number and the formation of bundles, changes cell shape, and produces mitotic arrest in actively dividing cells. Altering the microtubule ↔ tubulin equilibrium by irreversible polymerization of tubules is the major mechanism for the antineoplastic actions of the taxanes.

Taxanes act as a substrate for multidrug resistance-mediated cellular efflux. At appropriate concentrations cremophor itself can inhibit the p-Gp/mdr efflux pump. Alterations in tubulin itself may reduce or even prevent taxane binding or, *in vitro*, produce a mutant tubulin that requires a taxane for normal polymerization kinetics.

Adverse effects Anaphylactic reactions due to cremophor are frequent and can be controlled by pretreatment with a glucocorticosteroid and antihistamine. Major adverse effects of paclitaxel are neutropenia and neuropathy, particularly with 24-hour infusion.

Interactions have been reported with several antineoplastic agents. These have occurred only with the prolonged (24-hour) infusion. More severe neutropenia is produced when cisplatin is used before paclitaxel than when paclitaxel is used before cisplatin, because paclitaxel clearance is reduced by cisplatin. For the same reason there is an increased incidence and severity of mucositis when doxorubicin is used before paclitaxel than when paclitaxel is used before doxorubicin.

TOPOISOMERASE-ACTIVE DRUGS

Topoisomerases I and II are nuclear enzymes that cleave one (Top I) or two (Top II) strands of DNA to allow DNA strand passage to unwind DNA and relieve torsional stress and to decatenate intertwined segments of DNA (Top II). Top I and/or Top II are necessary for DNA replication and RNA transcription. Top II is necessary for the completion of mitosis. Top II plays a crucial role in the tertiary structure of chromatin. Two isoforms have been isolated. The predominant isoform, Top IIa is tightly cell cycle regulated (increased in S phase and increased further in M phase). Top IIa and especially Top I can be elevated in neoplastic cells independently of increased proliferation.

Topoisomerases form a covalent bond with DNA through a tyrosine transester linkage. Drugs stabilize this transient intermediate, preventing religation of the DNA strands. The exact molecular mechanism of cytotoxicity is uncertain, since enzyme inhibition is fully reversible. Possible cellular mechanisms include:

- Inappropriate recombination of topoisomerase-bound DNA strands (sister chromatid exchange[SCE]).
- Apoptosis due to unreplicated DNA or unrepaired DNA strand breaks, and/or decreases in mitotic promotion factor (MPF), which is a complex of two proteins, a cyclin and cdc_2 (p34), a phosphokinase, which phosphorylates other proteins to regulate the passage into mitosis.

Etoposide and teniposide

Structurally, etoposide and teniposide are semisynthetic epipodophyllotoxins, which are derivatives of podophyllotoxin, a tubulin-binding extract of the mandrake plant (*Mandragora officinarum*) (Fig. 28.24). All are poorly soluble in water and are emulsified in Tween and polyethylene glycol.

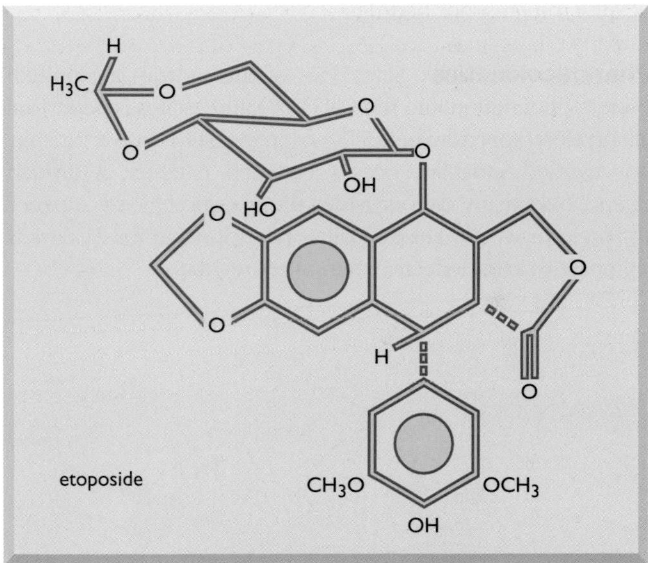

Fig. 28.24 Chemical structure of etoposide, an epipodophyllotoxin that acts on topoisomerase II. The podophyllotoxin backbone is a product of the mandrake root and herbalists have used it for centuries as an emetogenic agent.

Fig. 28.23 The chemical structure of paclitaxel. The 8-membered taxane ring required 35 years to synthesize. The molecule is insoluble in water.

Mechanism of action The molecular mechanism of action of epipodophyllotoxins is the ability to stabilize transiently a 'cleavable complex' of Top II and DNA, which is reversible after drug withdrawal (Fig. 28.25). Top II is a necessary intermediary since the drugs do not interact directly with DNA. Although the cellular mechanism of cytotoxicity is unclear, there is a linear relationship between drug concentration, double-strand DNA breaks, and cytotoxicity.

Resistance Mechanisms of resistance include increased levels of p-Gp 170 and *mdr* gene amplification/overexpression with enhanced efflux, an enhanced capacity to repair DNA strand breaks, decreased topoisomerase II levels (with a collateral increase in Top I), and altered (mutant) topoisomerase II enzymes capable of religating the separated DNA strands despite the presence of drug.

Pharmacokinetics Since 95% of these drugs are protein bound, penetration into the CNS (5%) and ascites is poor. Oral absorption (approximately 50%) of an ingested dose is variable, but marked variability occurs between patients. A divided course over many days provides therapeutic efficacy superior to single or weekly doses. Daily oral etoposide for 21 days is significantly more effective than other regimens.

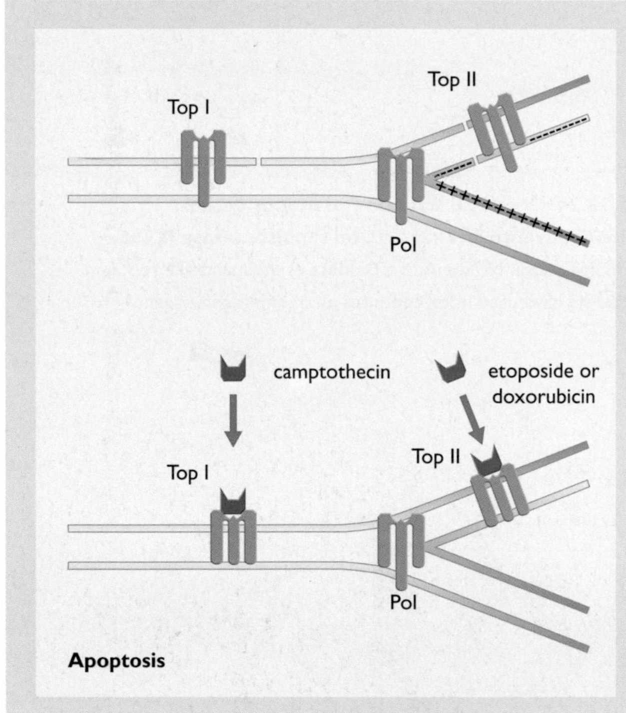

Fig. 28.25 Diagram showing sites of action of camptothecin and etoposide or doxorubicin. They stabilize the normally transient covalent cleavage in replicating DNA produced by topoisomerase I (Top I) and/or topoisomerase II (Top II), which produces a double-strand DNA break by collision with the DNA replication apparatus of DNA polymerase a (leading strand 5′→3′) and polymerase d (lagging strand 3′→5′) (Pol).

Adverse effects include myelosuppression, especially neutropenia, which is dose limiting, and oral mucositis. Toxicity depends on the regimen.

Camptothecin and derivatives

Mechanism of action Camptothecin (Fig. 28.26) is a plant alkaloid derived from a Chinese tree, *Camptotheca accuminata*. It was first introduced in clinical trials in the 1970s, but it was then abandoned because it lacked clinical efficacy and caused severe hemorrhagic cystitis. Interest was renewed 15 years later with the discovery that the molecular target of camptothecin is Top I, which is highly expressed in neoplastic tissues. All Top I inhibitors have an intact lactone E ring. Hydrolysis of the lactone to produce a carboxylate inactivates the drug. Multiple analogs, as well as camptothecin itself, are now in clinical trials. As S-phase-specific agents (cellular mechanism of action), camptothecins have to be present in the cell over a prolonged period.

Common properties of the camptothecins include:

- Activity in a wide variety of epithelial cancers.
- A high degree of binding to serum albumin (> 80%).
- Severe reversible myelosuppression.
- Marked interpatient variability in pharmacokinetics.
- Significant schedule dependency (activation is greater with a divided dose schedule).

Camptothecins have a wide spectrum of activity in solid tumors, including nonsmall-cell lung cancer (NSCLC), small-cell lung cancer (SCLC), and colon, cervical, and ovarian cancers. They are also effective against leukemias and lymphomas.

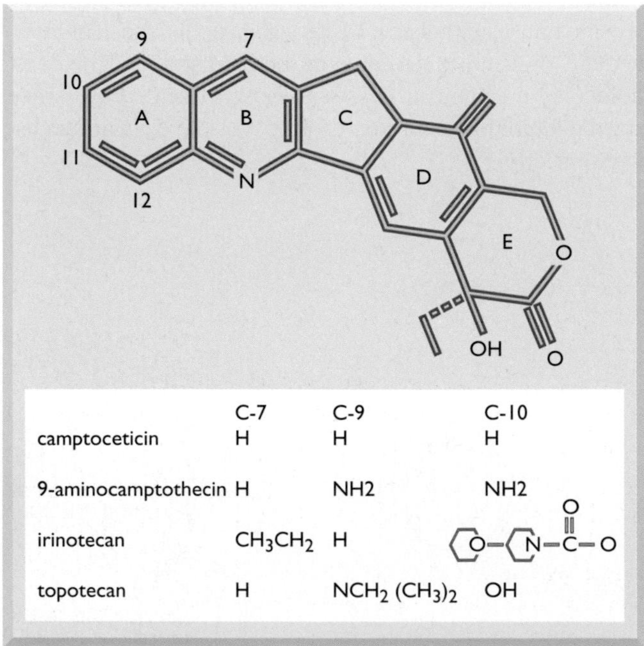

	C-7	C-9	C-10
camptoceticin	H	H	H
9-aminocamptothecin	H	NH2	NH2
irinotecan	CH_3CH_2	H	(piperidino-piperidine)–N–C(=O)–O
topotecan	H	$NCH_2\ (CH_3)_2$	OH

Fig. 28.26 Chemical structures of the camptothecins, which act on topoisomerase I. The lactone E ring must be intact for topoisomerase I interation. Substitutions at C-7, -9 and -10 increase water solubility. The C-10 substitution of irinotecan is hydrolyzed to OH. This metabolite, called SN-38, is 200 times more active than the parent drug.

Resistance Mechanisms of resistance include:

- Decreased Top I levels.
- An altered/mutant topoisomerase that cannot bind the drug or one that can religate in the presence of camptothecin.
- Enhanced membrane efflux via p-Gp 170 for water soluble analogs such as topotecan* (see Fig. 28.26), which is a semisynthetic water-soluble camptothecin analog.

Irinotecan* (CPT-11) (see Fig. 28.26) is a prodrug and is cleaved by ubiquitous carboxylesterases to a metabolite which is a significantly more effective Top I inhibitor. Irinotecan* causes a particularly severe diarrhea, which is responsive to octreotide and preventable with high-dose loperamide. Less frequently it causes severe myelosuppression, which is not related to serum drug levels, but is associated with weekly dosing schedules.

9-Aminocamptothecin (see Fig. 28.26) is a poorly soluble analog of camptothecin with pronounced actions against experimental colon cancer, thereby providing an impetus for the development of analogs. Because it is poorly soluble it is given as a colloidal suspension, and the optimal dosing schedule is a continuous infusion for 72 hours every 3 weeks. Adverse effects include neutropenia, mild nausea, and alopecia.

ANTITUMOR ANTIBIOTICS

Dactinomycin

Dactinomycin (actinomycin D) has significant anticancer actions against solid tumors in children, such as Wilms' tumor, Ewing's tumor, neuroblastoma, rhabdomyosarcoma, and choriocarcinoma.

Mechanism of action Structurally, dactinomycin is two symmetric polypeptide chains attached to a phenoxazone ring. The molecular mechanism of action is intercalation of the phenoxazone ring perpendicular to the long axis of DNA while the peptide chains lie in the minor groove. The resulting cellular mechanism of action is inhibition of RNA and protein synthesis by prevention of chain elongation.

Dactinomycin enters cells by passive diffusion. Drug resistance is due to increased expression of *p-Gp/mdr*.

Adverse effects of dactinomycin include nausea, vomiting, mucosal ulceration, dose-limiting myelosuppression, and dermatologic manifestations. Dactinomycin is a severe vesicant and a radiation sensitizer, and can produce severe radiation 'recall injury.'

Mitomycin C

Mitomycin C has widespread but limited clinical usefulness in the treatment of a broad range of solid tumors, including those of the gastrointestinal tract, breast, lung, head, neck, and bladder, and gynecologic tumors. It is synergistic with 5-fluorouracil and with radiotherapy. Experimentally, initial trials with mitomycin C were disappointing because of severe cumulative bone marrow, pulmonary, and renal toxicity. However, it can be used in combination with other agents using an intermittent schedule.

Mechanism of action The mechanism of action of mitomycin C depends on bioreductive alkylation under anaerobic, reducing conditions as it needs to be reduced at quinone sites to form unstable intermediates, which react monofunctionally at the guanine 2N position. It is therefore a prodrug. About 10% of adducts can form ISCs. Free radical formation under aerobic conditions (a second basis for prodrug activity) may lead to single-strand DNA breaks, or these may result from unsuccessful alkylation repair.

Resistance The mechanisms of resistance to mitomycin include:

- Decreased bioactivation.
- Increased DNA repair.
- Increased *p-Gp/mdr* gene product expression.

Pharmacokinetics Mitomycin C is used intravenously since oral absorption is erratic. Impaired liver or renal function does not change its pharmacokinetics.

Anthracyclines and anthracenediones

Doxorubicin and daunorubicin (Fig. 28.27) have a wide spectrum of usefulness in cancer chemotherapy which is second only to the usefulness of alkylating agents. Doxorubicin is effective against:

- Non-Hodgkin's lymphoma.
- Hodgkin's disease.
- Acute leukemias.
- Carcinomas of the breast, lung, stomach, and thyroid.
- Sarcomas.

Doxorubicin is used to treat solid tumors, and in leukemia, where it causes less mucositis. Doxorubicin is a prodrug. The active metabolite idarubicin is effective against leukemia and is itself used therapeutically because it can be given orally.

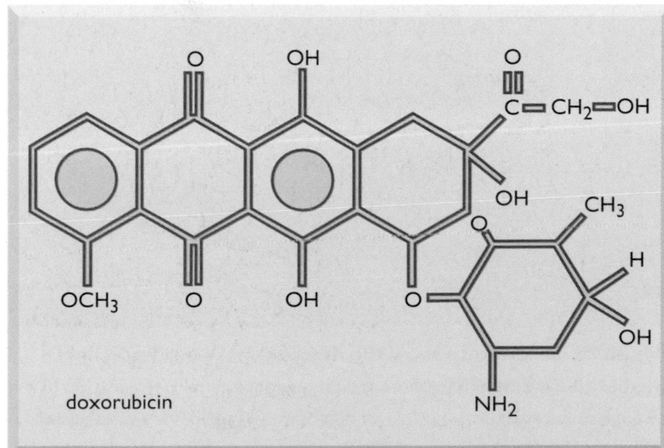

Fig. 28.27 Chemical structure of the anthracyclines. The flat planar chromophore in the center intercalates DNA at specific base pair sequences. This allows interaction with topoisomerase II.

Anthracyclines have a unique cumulative cardiotoxicity (Fig. 28.28), which may be blocked by the iron chelator, desrazoxane. Epirubicin* is less cardiotoxic than other anthracyclines and is widely used in Europe. It is particularly effective in breast cancer. Anthracycline cytotoxicity does not depend on the dosing regimen.

Mechanism of action Anthracyclines and anthracenediones intercalate with DNA and bind avidly to nuclear chromatin, forming a ternary complex of drug intercalated into DNA and Top II to produce strand cleavage. This is their molecular mechanism of action. The Top II-mediated mechanism is probably the most important.

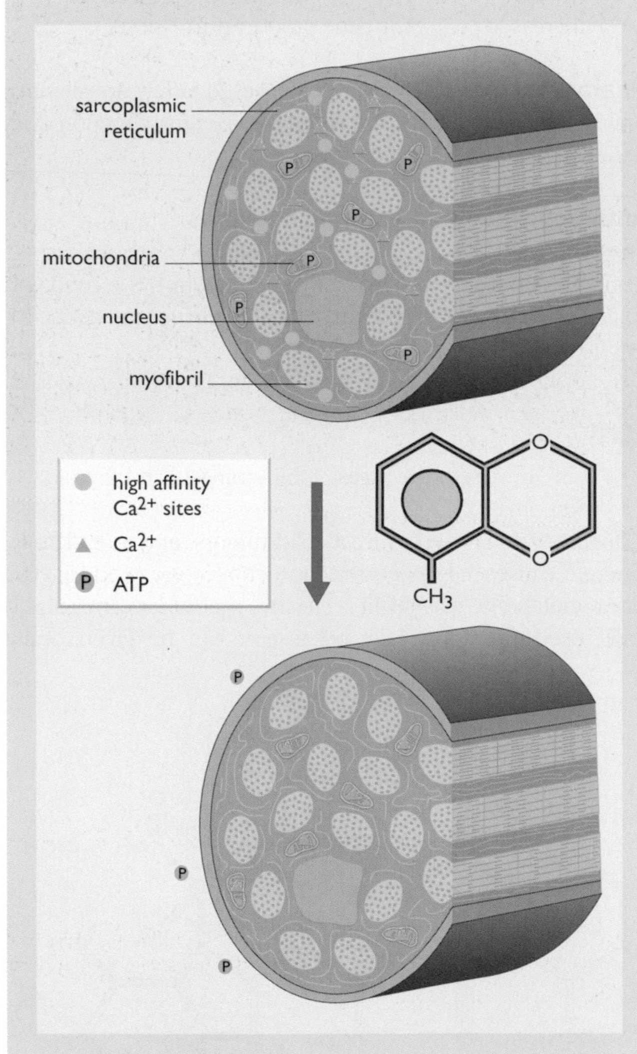

Fig. 28.28 Diagram to show the mechanism of anthracycline-mediated cardiotoxicity. Free radical quinones cause peroxidation of the sarcoplasmic reticulum with loss of high-affinity Ca^{2+} binding sites and the release of Ca^{2+} into the cytoplasm. Excess intracellular Ca^{2+} is toxic, resulting in the disruption of actin and myosin and uptake of Ca^{2+} into the mitochondria to displace ATP (P), resulting in a loss of contractility, death of cells and, later, thinning of the heart wall.

Free radical formation via electron reduction is a second cytotoxic mechanism. All anthracyclines are quinones capable of producing free radicals, which damage membranes, proteins, and lipids. Glutathione and catalase can detoxify the free radical quinones, and lack of catalase in cardiac tissue is the basis for anthracycline cardiotoxicity. Complexes of iron and anthracycline bind tightly to cell membranes to cause spontaneous membrane destruction. Recently, activation of a ceramide synthetase pathway that produces apoptotic cell death has been described. The relevance of this to the beneficial effects of these drugs in cancer treatment is not certain.

Resistance Mechanisms of resistance to anthracyclines include:

- *p-Gp 170/mdr* gene glycoprotein-mediated drug efflux.
- Altered Top II concentrations.
- A mutant topoisomerase II.
- Increased glutathione concentration.
- Increased glutathione peroxidase activity (this enzyme detoxifies free radicals).
- Decreased glucose-6-phosphate dehydrogenase concentration.

Pharmacokinetics Anthracyclines and anthracenediones diffuse passively into cells in an un-ionized form. The compounds become charged and are prevented from diffusing into cells if there is extracellular acidification, which is common with solid tumors.

Doxorubicin is a potent radiation sensitizer. Heparin binds the daunosamine sugar and increases clearance. Doxorubicin decreases paclitaxel clearance.

Adverse effects of anthracyclines include myelosuppression, mucositis, and stomatitis (especially with doxorubicin and with a continuous infusion rather than bolus doses. Cardiac toxicity, a particular and potentially lethal problem, causes heart failure. Factors increasing the risk of heart failure include pre-existing heart disease, hypertension, and cardiac radiation therapy. Cardiac toxicity is a function of peak dose concentration, and continuous infusions or weekly dosing decrease the risk. Desrazoxane, an iron chelator, decreases cardiotoxicity.

Idarubicin

Idarubicin is effective against acute leukemia and breast cancer. It has the same mechanism of action and resistance as doxorubicin, and its oral bioavailability is 30%. Its effectiveness depends on its metabolism to an active metabolite, 13-epirubicinol. Idarubicin is less cardiotoxic than doxorubicin.

Mitoxantrone

Mitoxantrone is an anthracenedione that is less cardiotoxic than anthracyclines. Its molecular mechanism of action is interaction with Top II and DNA, resulting in its cellular mechanism of action of producing breaks in DNA strands. Mitoxantrone does not produce free radical generation. The mechanisms of resistance to mitoxantrone are the same as for doxorubicin.

Adverse effects of mitoxantrone include extravasation injuries, alopecia, and nausea, and dose-limiting myelosuppression. Overall, the adverse effect profile is much more favorable than that for anthracyclines, especially with respect to cardiotoxicity. However, cardiotoxicity is seen in patients who have previously been treated with doxorubicin. Cardiotoxicity is less frequent, but just as severe, than with anthracyclines.

Bleomycins

The bleomycins are a family of complex glycopeptides isolated from a *Streptomyces* which avidly chelate metals. Bleomycin A_2 is the main bleomycin used clinically. Bleomycin is used to treat Hodgkin's disease, NHL, and testicular, cervical, head, and neck cancers. It is an essential drug in the chemotherapy of germ cell cancers when its omission from the regimen results in a significant decrease in cure rate.

Mechanism of action All active bleomycin compounds bind reduced iron (Fe^{2+}), so their molecular mechanism of action is not directed towards tissue. Their cellular mechanism of action is to produce single- and double-strand DNA breaks. Such breaks are reflected as DNA chromosomal gaps, deletions, and fragments. These result from a secondary molecular mechanism of action in which free radical formation from Fe^{2+}–bleomycin–oxygen forms an intercalated complex between DNA strands. Intercalation of drug into DNA is the initial step, before Fe^{2+} is oxidized, and oxygen is reduced to the radicals $\cdot O_{2-}$ or $\cdot OH$. DNA cleavage occurs after the intercalated bleomycin complex is assembled and DNA strand breaking absolutely requires oxygen.

Pharmacokinetics Bleomycins are large cationic molecules and penetrate cell membranes poorly via a bleomycin-binding membrane protein. Internalized bleomycins are either translocated to the nucleus or hydrolyzed by bleomycin hydrolase, a cysteine protease present in normal and malignant cells, but found in decreased concentrations in lung and skin.

Specific cytotoxic drug interactions

- Procarbazine inhibits monoamine oxidase
- Allopurinol inhibits 6-mercaptopurine metabolism
- Barbiturates and cimetidine increase activation of cyclophosphamide
- Cisplatin and doxorubicin enhance paclitaxel toxicity when given before paclitaxel
- Asparaginase inhibits the metabolism of vinca alkaloids

General principles of cancer chemotherapy administration

- Allow for full recovery of myelosuppression before resuming dosing, though this may not apply for aggressive leukemias and lymphomas
- Avoid concomitant administration of platelet-inhibiting drugs
- Avoiding drug interactions involving cytochrome P-450 metabolism
- The dose of certain drugs needs adjustment if there is hepatic and renal impairment
- There is no evidence that hematopoietic cytokines given to ameliorate myelosuppression improve outcome, but they markedly increase costs

Adverse effects Bleomycin toxicity is confined to the lungs and skin. Pulmonary toxicity is the major problem and is manifest as a subacute or chronic interstitial pneumonitis and, at a later stage, fibrosis.

FURTHER READING

Chabner BA, Longo DL. *Cancer Chemotherapy and Biotherapy 2e*. Philadelphia: Lippincott–Raven; 1996. [This is the most comprehensive and current textbook on cancer pharmacology.]

DeVita VT Jr, Hellman S, Rosenberg SA. *Cancer: Principles and Practice of Oncology 4e*. Philadelphia: JB Lippincott; 1993. [Excellent review of the principles of cancer pharmacology and major chemotherapeutic agents. The remainder of the book is an excellent guide to clinical cancer medicine,]

Darnell J, Lodish H, Baltimore D. *Molecular Cell Biology 3e*. New York: W.H. Freeman and Co., Scientific American Books; 1995. [Superbly illustrated, expertly written text on molecular biology. The best in the field.]

Perry, MD. *The Chemotherapy Source Book*. Baltimore: Williams and Wilkins; 1992. [Very good review of cancer pharmacology with guides to the treatment of various malignant diseases.]

Skeel RT. *Handbook of Cancer Chemotherapy*. Boston: Little, Brown; 1991. [Very good short pocket size text with excellent practical information.]

Make a provisional diagnosis and determine a rational pharmacologic treatment for the following hypothetical case.

A 55-year-old woman was diagnosed 3 years ago with a stage II (T_2 N_1, Mo) breast cancer. She received 4 months of adjuvant chemotherapy with cyclophosphamide and doxorubicin. She presents now with right upper gradient pain, weight loss, fevers, and jaundice. A computed tomography scan of the abdomen reveals portal hepatitis, prepancreatic, precaval, and para-aortic adenopathy.

1. Is it essential to establish a tissue diagnosis?
2. What is a differential diagnosis?
3. Why would a complete blood count be indicated?
4. Needle biopsy shows non-Hodgkin's lymphoma. What is the preferred treatment?
5. Is there anything in the patient's history which raises concerns about additional chemotherapy?

Indicate which is the correct answer for each question.

1. All of the following drugs are correctly matched with a major adverse effect, except
   a) prednisone: bone marrow suppression
   b) cyclophosphamide: hemorrhagic cystitis
   c) vincristine: neurologic toxicity
   d) doxorubicin: cardiomyopathy
   e) 5-fluorouracil: bone marrow suppression

2. All of the following drugs are correctly matched with their mechanism of action, except
   a) 5-fluorouracil: antimetabolite
   b) lomustine: alkylating agent
   c) dactinomycin: antimetabolite
   d) vincristine: antimitotic agent
   e) 6-mercaptopurine: antimetabolite

3. All of the following statements regarding doxorubicin are correct, except
   a) it has a narrow spectrum of antitumor activity
   b) it is a natural product
   c) it acts on topoisomerase II
   d) it can generate free radicals
   e) it can cause cardiotoxicity

4. Which one of the following statements concerning the adverse effects of anticancer drugs is false?
   a) many anticancer drugs initially cause nausea and vomiting as a result of their direct gastrointestinal toxicity
   b) many anticancer drugs are potential carcinogens
   c) anticancer drugs can cause amenorrhea or impair spermatogenesis
   d) patients undergoing chemotherapy who develop leukopenia are susceptible to opportunistic infections
   e) hyperuricemia can occur when anticancer drugs produce a high tumor cell kill

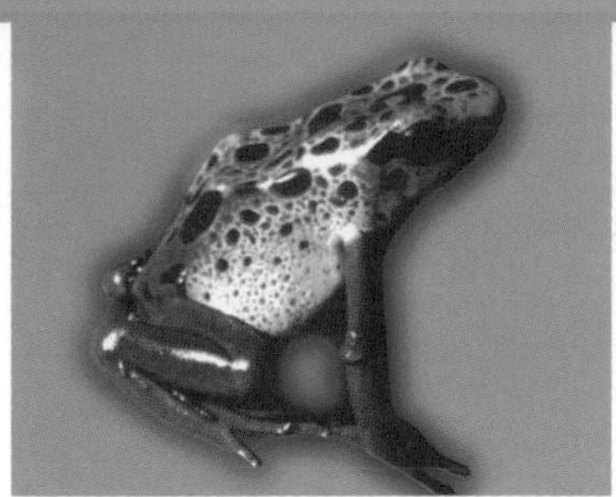

29. Toxins and Poisons

Every natural or synthetic chemical can cause injury if the dose is high enough.

Clear definitions for venoms, toxins, and poisons are not available since every chemical can cause injury if the dose is high enough (Fig. 29.1). Whether the chemical is a venom, a toxin, or a poison depends mainly on its source, not its actions:

- Venoms are substances injected by one species into another.
- A poison is a chemical that can injure or impair body functions.
- Toxins were originally described as being produced by microorganisms, but the word is also used more broadly (e.g. the ω conotoxins from coneshells). However, an antitoxin refers to an antibody to a toxin produced by bacteria.

Venoms and toxins are usually proteins or polypeptides, particularly those produced by vertebrates. Invertebrates and plants produce a wide diversity of toxins and poisons. Many are alkaloids.

Generally, acute toxicity results from brief exposure, chronic toxicity from months or years of exposure

Exposure to venom involves direct contact, whereas ingestion is the most common route of exposure to a toxin and is an important route for poisons. Chemicals in the air, water, and food (e.g. pesticides, heavy metals, chlorinated hydrocarbons) lead to chronic low-level exposure, and inhalation exposure is a common route in the workplace. The skin is an effective barrier to most water-soluble poisons, but not necessarily to fat-soluble substances.

Chemicals hazardous to man

- Venoms from animals
- Toxins from animals and plants
- Poisons from natural and man-made sources

Toxins and poisons can have direct and indirect mechanisms of action

Many toxins and poisons act on target organs, possibly as the result of the particular physiologic and biochemical functions of these organs (Fig. 29.2). The kidneys are particularly vulnerable although metallothioneins, a unique protein class, protect the kidney, and other organs, by avidly binding some poisons (e.g. cadmium).

Whether damage is reversible or irreversible often depends upon the repair and regenerative abilities of the target tissue. Liver damage is often reversible, because the liver can regenerate. However, central nervous system (CNS) damage is usually irreversible because neurons do not regenerate. In addition, the axon has limited metabolic functions and relies on the transport, often over long distances, of materials from the cell body. Furthermore, there is a normal, age-related, loss of neurons and exposure to neuropoisons may reduce the age at which neurologic and behavioral deficits appear.

Potency of various poisons in terms of acute lethality

Lethal potency in terms of average lethal dose in mg/kg body weight	Toxins, venoms and poisons
1,000,000	Water
10,000	Ethanol, other alcohols, general anesthetics
1,000	Iron salts, vitamins
100	Barbiturates, general anesthetics
10	Morphine, some snake venoms
1	Nicotine and many plant poisons
0.1	Curare, sea snake venoms, jellyfish toxins
0.01	Tetrodotoxin
0.001	Ciguatoxin, palytoxin
<0.0001	Botulinum toxins

Fig. 29.1 Potency of various poisons in terms of acute lethality.

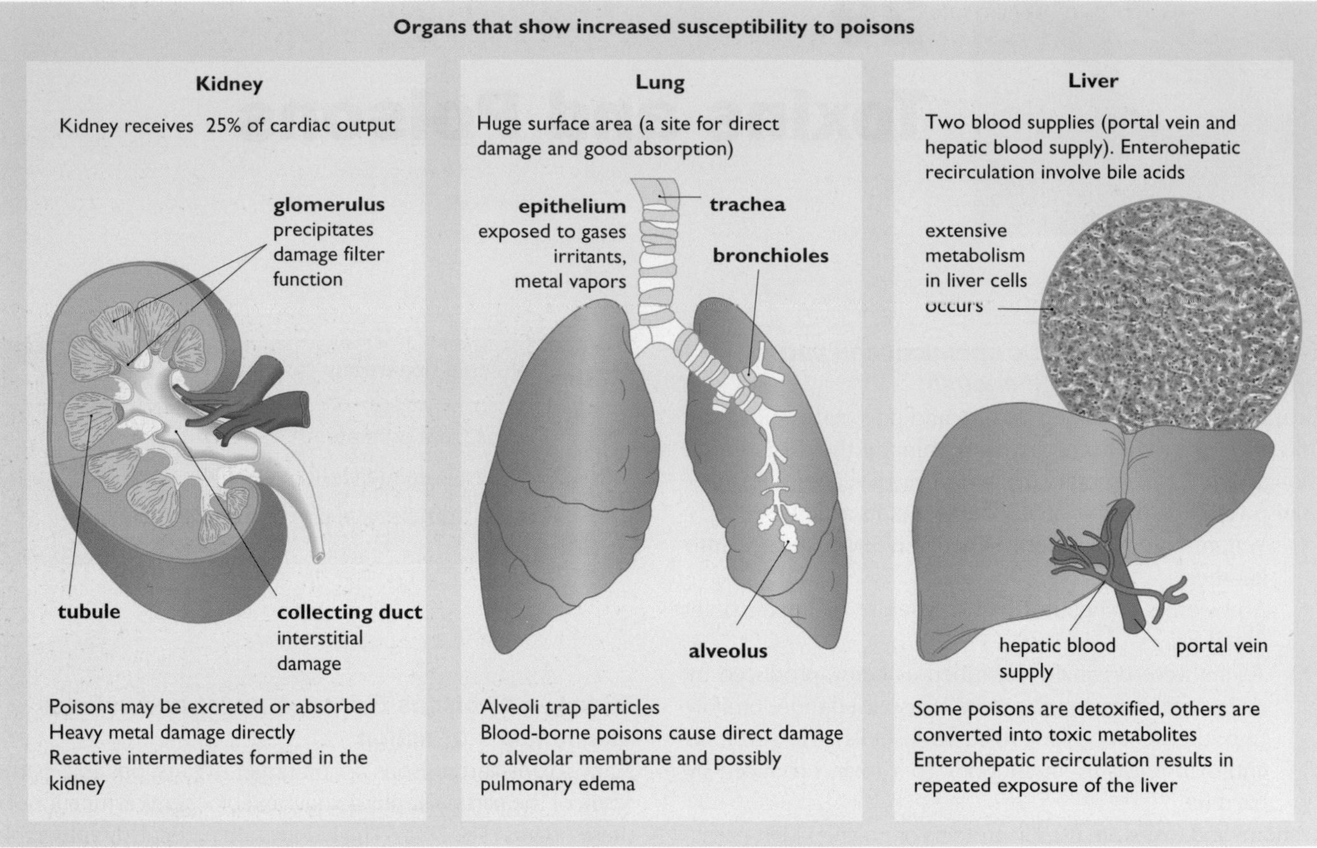

Fig. 29.2 Physiologic mechanisms that particularly expose the kidney, lung, and liver to poisons.

Poisons can act indirectly: allergic reactions are immunologically mediated adverse reactions to repeated exposure and sensitization. Poisons can also act directly on the immune system and cause immunosuppression. The activation and recruitment of phagocytic cells to sites of chemically induced injury plays a role in the progression of tissue injury.

Idiosyncratic reactions to chemicals further complicate the effects of poisons.

Approximately eight million people in the US suffer acute poisoning each year

The hazard due to exposure to toxins is regulated by government committees and agencies. A no-observed-adverse-effect level (NOAEL) of exposure to a hazard can be determined in laboratory animals and 1/100th of this amount is considered acceptable for humans (this is derived by dividing the NOAEL by 1/10 for individual differences and 1/10 for species differences). This factoring can be related to the fact that the Environmental Protection Agency (US) considers a risk of one death per million individuals exposed as the maximum acceptable exposure. As a comparison, in the US 20,000 people die each year from the effects of illicit drugs. In addition, acute toxicity due to drug or poison ingestion accounts for at least 10% of hospital admissions.

Standard medical procedures and specific therapy are needed to manage envenomation and poisoning

The obvious first step is to remove the source of exposure (Fig. 29.3). This is followed by limiting absorption or speeding excretion of the venom or poison, for example by:

- Restricting movement of venom from the envenomation site.
- Removing poisons from the stomach or skin.
- Acidification or alkalinization of the urine.
- Ingestion of water.

Treatment of poisoning

- Remove the source of poison
- Minimize absorption of the poison
- Supportive therapy
- Specific therapy, if available

The third step is the use of specific antidotes, antivenins, or antitoxins. Other steps can include hemodialysis to remove toxins by filtration, and hemoperfusion to remove toxins by circulating blood through an activated charcoal filter.

Principles for treatment of poisoning

- Remove source of poison or victim from source (e.g. rescue)
- Remove and limit absorption of poison (e.g. fresh air, wash, emesis, limit contact)
- Supportive therapy (e.g. ventilation, external cardiac massage, saline/oxygen, drugs)
- Specific therapies
  - Antivenins for animal venoms
  - Antitoxins for bacterial toxins
  - Chelators for heavy metals
  - Gases (e.g. oxygen for carbon monoxide)
- Other drug therapies
  - Ethanol for methanol
  - Digoxin antibodies for digoxin
  - Pyridoxine for isoniazid
  - Nitrite and thiosulfate for cyanide
  - *N*-acetylcysteine for acetaminophen
- Specific antagonists
  - Atropine and oximes for organophosphate anticholinesterases
  - Flumazenil for benzodiazepines
  - Opioid antagonists (naloxone) for opiates
  - Anticholinesterases for neuromuscular blockers

Fig. 29.3 Principles for treatment of poisoning.

VENOMS, TOXINS, AND POISONS FROM NATURAL SOURCES

VENOMS FROM ANIMALS

Venoms occur in all animal phyla (Figs 29.4, 29.5), usually as proteins or polypeptides with a variety of structures and actions. Specialized venom glands and injection apparatus are required to inject the venom.

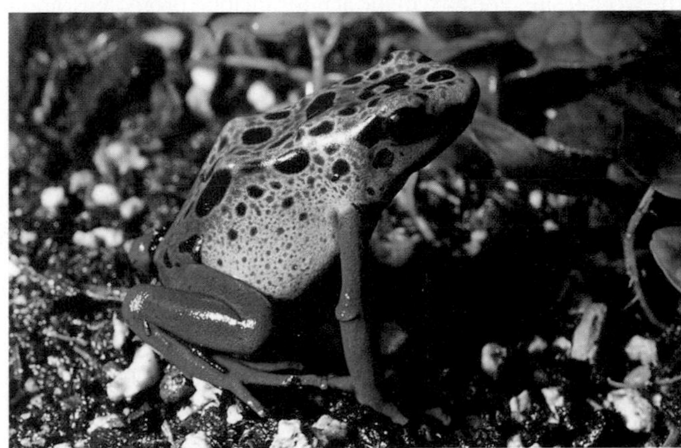

Fig. 29.4 A typical poisonous frog. Extracts from the skin of similar poisonous frogs (*Dendrobates* sp.) are painted on the tips of arrows and darts in Central and South America. Many vertebrates are capable of injecting venoms or contain poisons. (Photograph by Ron Kertesz, with permission of Vancouver Aquarium.)

The sources and mechanisms of action of various animal venoms and toxins

Toxin	Source	Mechanisms of action
Small molecules		
Tetrodotoxin	Puffer fish, octopus, salmander	Na^+ channel blocker
Saxitoxin	Shellfish contaminated with dinoflagellates	Na^+ channel blocker
Ciguatoxin	Large tropical fish contaminated with dinoflagellates	Actions on Na^+ channel
Cardiac glycosides	Toad skin	ATPase inhibitor
Batrachotoxin	Frog skin	Na^+ channel activator
Domoic acid	Shellfish (mussels)	CNS toxin
Palytoxin	Sea anemone	Ionophore
Proteins and polypeptides		
α Bungarotoxin	Elapid snakes (kraits)	Nicotinic receptor blocker
β Bungarotoxin	Elapid snakes (kraits)	Presynaptic cholinergic nerves
α Conotoxin	Coneshells	
μ Conotoxin	Coneshells	Skeletal muscle Na^+ channel blocker
ω Conotoxin	Coneshells	N-type Ca^{2+} antagonist
Cardiotoxin	Elapid snakes	Direct acting cardiotoxin
Phospholipases	Many snakes	Cell membrane destruction
Bacterial toxins		
Botulinum toxin	*Clostridium botulinum*	Synaptin in nerve endings
Cholera toxin	*Cholera vibrio*	Activation of G_s protein
Pertussis toxin	*Bordetella pertussis*	Inactivates G_o/G_s protein
Endotoxin	Gram-negative bacteria	Cell membranes
Tetanus toxin	*Clostridium tetani*	Cell membrane inophore
Staphylococcal toxin	*Staphylococcus* sp.	Enterotoxin

Fig. 29.5 The sources and mechanisms of action of various animal venoms and toxins.

Fatal allergies can develop to the venoms of bees, hornets, and wasps, but the direct effects of such stings are mainly local skin reactions and are rarely fatal.

Snake venoms

Some snake venoms are enzymes, and these account for some of the systemic toxicity and much of the local toxicity of a crotalid snake (rattlesnakes and pit vipers) bite. Crotalid venoms can affect blood coagulation and hemostasis and cause tissue necrosis at the wound site. The enzymatic actions include proteolysis, lipolysis, and phospholipase activity, resulting in cell disruption and lysis.

Nonenzyme snake venoms can have specific actions. Many elapid snakes (e.g. cobra, krait) venoms contain neuromuscular-blocking polypeptides. Some of these block nicotinic cholinoceptors with such selectivity that one such polypeptide (α bungarotoxin) was first used to identify and label nicotinic receptors. β Bungarotoxin selectively blocks the release of acetylcholine at the neuromuscular junction.

The lethality of snake venoms varies

The most dangerous snakes are probably the tropical sea snakes, which, despite small fangs, are able to inject lethal amounts of nicotinic cholinoceptor-blocking polypeptides. In addition, the venom contains phospholipases, which break down muscle membranes and cause subsequent myoglobinuria.

Antivenins exist for most snake and some other venoms. Treatment with antivenins and local procedures to limit the escape of venom from the wound site can be very effective.

Snake venoms have led to pharmacologic developments

A bradykinin-potentiating factor isolated from Brazilian snake venoms led to the development of captopril, the first clinically useful angiotensin converting enzyme inhibitor (see Chapter 8). Ancrod* is a fibrinolytic factor from Malaysian pit vipers that breaks down fibrinogen into fragments of fibrin and so produces afibrinogenemia.

Other venoms

Other well-studied venoms include those from scorpions. These can be lethal for children. They target a variety of cellular macromolecules, including K^+ channels.

Many marine animals contain venoms, including vertebrates such as fishes (e.g. stingrays), and these can inflict severe pain and injury, but are not usually lethal. Tetrodotoxin is a venom in puffer fish, which are eaten, after very careful preparation, as a delicacy (known as fugu) in Japan. Nonvertebrate species also possess dangerous venoms.

- The venoms in jellyfish and corals are contained within nematocysts (Fig. 29.7) and are injected in limited quantities unless large areas of the skin are involved. Some of the box jellyfish found in tropical Australian waters can cause fatal stings in children.
- Some species of octopus inject tetrodotoxin, a selective blocker of Na^+ channels, into their prey and this is sometimes lethal in children.
- The venoms of various tropical species of coneshells (shellfish) show molecular target selectivity. Depending upon the species (Fig. 29.6), they are either predators of fish, worms, or other coneshells. Each prey-specific species of coneshell has its own specialized conotoxins (i.e. venoms) targeted to specific molecular sites, including ion channels and receptors.

TOXINS AND POISONS FROM ANIMALS

Vertebrates contain few substances that are poisonous to other species. However, invertebrates (e.g. fungi and bacteria) often contain toxins. Bacterial toxins are produced by many species and probably serve purposes other than killing hosts. Fungi also use chemicals to deter competitors and predators. Many poisons are produced by fungi and have adverse effects on many species, especially bacteria. The sources of most antibiotics are fungi.

Bacterial toxins vary in chemical nature and actions

Botulinum toxin, an orally absorbed protein from *Clostridium*, is responsible for botulism. It is one of a group of bacterial endotoxins that includes tetanus and diphtheria toxins, and it is so potent that a single molecule can disable a single nerve ending. The mechanism appears to involve inactivation of a synaptin responsible for the exocytosis of acetylcholine.

Cholera toxin causes the massive diarrhea seen with cholera. The molecular mechanism involves ADP ribosylation of the adenylyl cyclase stimulatory G_s protein, causing irreversible inactivation

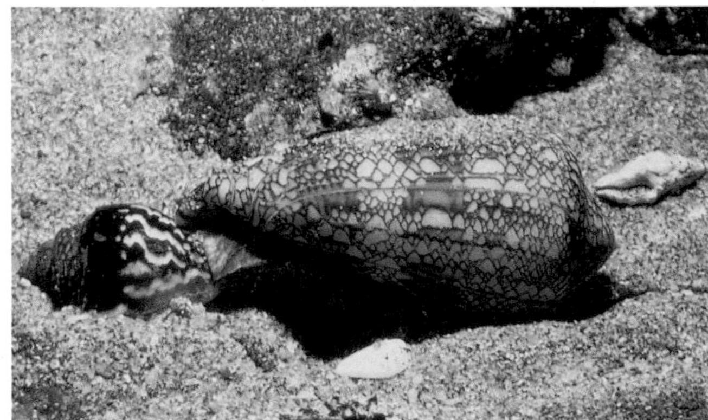

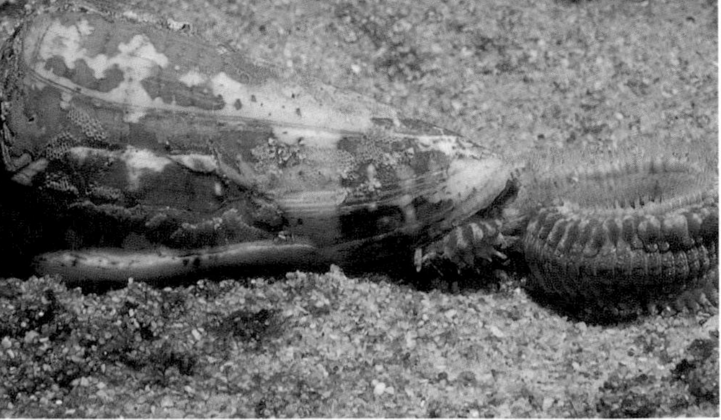

Fig. 29.6 Different coneshells have evolved venoms that are relatively specific for their prey species. Conotoxins are often highly selective for certain ion channels. (Photographs by Alex Kerstitch.)

of GTPase and therefore permanent activation of G_S protein (see Chapter 3). As a result cAMP accumulates and there is salt and water hypersecretion from gut epithelium. In contrast, pertussis toxin inactivates G_i/G_O proteins.

Exotoxins released from bacteria and endotoxins released following bacterial breakdown are often responsible for the adverse effects of bacterial infection.

POISONS FROM PLANTS

Plants use chemicals for defense, and as a result produce many poisons, and even venoms, to deter or kill predators (Fig. 29.8).

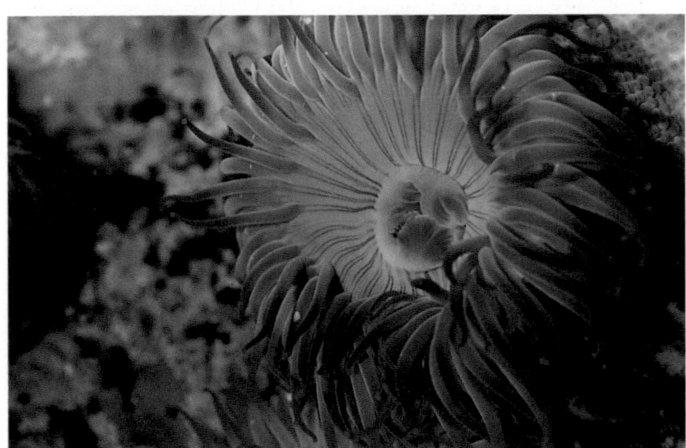

Fig. 29.7 Many marine invertebrates contain venoms and poisons. Venoms in corals, anemones, and jellyfish are contained within special cellular organelles known as nematocysts. Nematocysts also contain a stinging thread that can penetrate the skin. Many of these invertebrates are very attractive and children are particularly liable to be stung. (Photograph by Ron Kertesz, with permission of Vancouver Aquarium.)

Plant chemicals are usually small organic molecules. The diversity, availability, and ease of ingestion of plant poisons led to the discovery of the first drugs. Many drugs are still extracted from plants, or are chemical derivatives of their extracts (e.g. atropine, tubocurarine, digoxin, reserpine, morphine, caffeine, nicotine, taxol, aspirin, quinidine, quinine, vincristine).

Plant poisons are particularly dangerous to domestic animals and children. Information about the nature of the common plant poisons and their treatment is readily obtained from Poison Control Centers. Herbal concoctions can contain plant poisons.

INDUSTRIAL POISONS

Industrial poisons are either intentional products of industry or byproducts of industrial processes (e.g. air pollution). Environmental poisons are those that reach the environment and they can cause acute or chronic poisoning or be

Industrial poisoning

- The major industrial poisons are metals (elemental, salt, and organic forms), air pollutants and gases, aromatic and aliphatic hydrocarbons (liquid and vapor), insecticides, pesticides, and herbicides
- All produce both acute and chronic toxicity
- Mutagenesis and carcinogenesis are particular problems

The sources and mechanisms of action of various plant and fungal poisons

Poison	Source	Mechanism of action
Some plant poisons		
Atropine, scopolamine	Solanaceae (jimson weed, deadly nightshade)	Muscarinic receptor antagonists
Cardiac glycosides	Digitalis, strophanthus, oleander, convallaria	ATPase inhibitors
Aconitine	Hellebores	Cardiac Na^+ channel activator
Capsaicin	*Capsicum* sp. (peppers)	Substance P depleter
Ricin	Castor bean	Protoplasmic poison
Myristicin	Nutmeg and mace	Hallucinogenic
Emetine	*Ipecacuana* sp.	Stimulates vomiting center
Pennyroyal oil	*Mentha* sp.	Hepatotoxic and oxytoxic
Safrole	Sassafras tree	Animal carcinogen
Pyrrolizidines	Heliotropium, comfrey (herbal tea)	Hepatotoxic
Some fungal toxins		
Muscarine	Clitocybe, *Amanita* sp., *Inocybe* sp.	Muscarinic agonist
Phallotoxins, amatoxins	*Amanita* sp. (death cap, destroying angel)	Hepatotoxic
Coprine	*Coprinus* sp.	Blocks aldehyde dehydrogenase
Ibotenic acid	*Amanita* sp.	Hallucinogenic
Psilocybin	*Psilocybe* sp.	Hallucinogenic
Aflatoxins	*Aspergillus* sp.	Hepatocarcinogenic
Ergot alkaloids	*Claviceps* sp.	Multiple actions
Orelline	*Corinarius* sp.	Nephrotoxic

Fig. 29.8 The sources and mechanisms of action of various plant and fungal poisons.

carcinogenic. The concentrations of such substances in the environment are not usually high enough to constitute an acute toxic hazard, but the low concentrations are sufficient to produce chronic poisoning.

METALS

Heavy metals such as mercury, cadmium, and lead are toxic, the toxicity arising from both the salts and the elemental metal, particularly vapors and dusts. The mechanism of toxicity often involves their combination with specific groups on essential macromolecules (Fig. 29.9). Heavy metals such as arsenic tend to react to with the oxygen/sulfur groups on essential macromolecules such as enzymes to form metal complexes (coordination compounds).

Mercury

Mercury is used extensively in industry and is a common cause of accidental poisoning. Paints, mercury thermometers, and laboratories are a less common source. Toxic quantities of mercury vapor can be absorbed by the lungs, while inorganic and organic mercurial salts are responsible for the poisoning following oral ingestion. Methylmercury-contaminated food led to hundreds of deaths in Iraq, while its accumulation in sea food poisoned the residents of Minamata Bay in Japan.

Oral elemental Hg^{2+} is poorly absorbed, but mercury vapor is well absorbed. Acute poisoning affects the respiratory tract, producing cough, dyspnea, and interstitial pneumonitis. Acute ingestion of inorganic mercury causes corrosive damage to the gastrointestinal tract and renal damage. Symptoms of chronic poisoning are more insidious and neurologic (visual disturbances, ataxia, paresthesias, and neurasthenias). The diagnosis is based upon the symptoms and a history of exposure, and is usually associated with mercury concentrations higher than 40 μg/liter in blood and 5 μg/liter in urine (Fig. 29.10).

Mercury absorption depends upon its chemical type, with inorganic salts absorbed as Hg^{2+} (approximately 10% of the ingested dose). Organic mercurials are well absorbed from the gastrointestinal tract and distributed fairly uniformly. Mercury readily forms covalent bonds with sulfur (as -S- bonds or -SH groups) and this bonding is ultimately responsible for poisoning. Mercury also binds to phosphoryl, carboxyl, amide, and amine groups and thereby disturbs the functioning of enzymes, receptors, and other important cellular macromolecules.

Specific treatment of mercury poisoning includes the use of chelators (see p. 530) such as intramuscular dimercaprol for those with severe intoxication, and oral penicillamine for less severe exposure. Oral succimer may be useful as a replacement for penicillamine. Dimercaprol is contraindicated for organic mercurial poisoning since it can elevate mercury concentrations in the brain. The enterohepatic recirculation of mercury allows

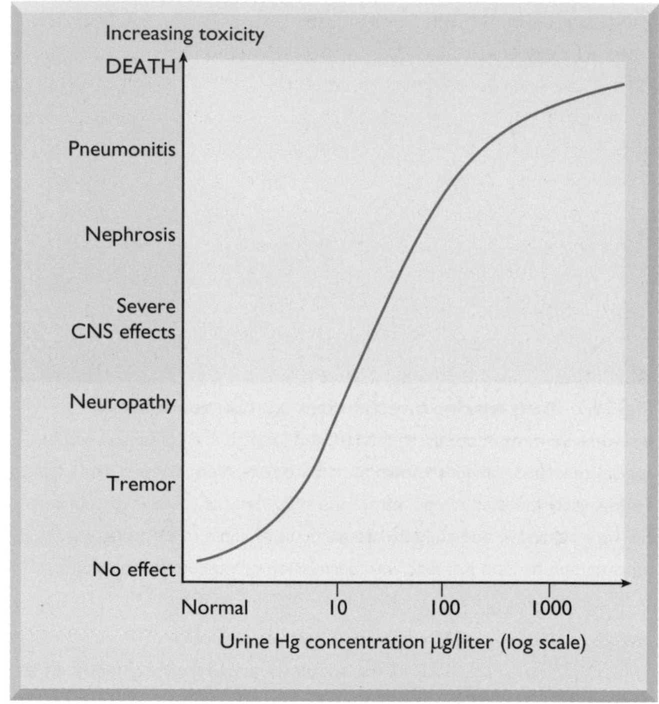

Fig. 29.10 Relationship between urine mercury concentration and symptoms of mercury poisoning.

Mechanisms of action of heavy metal toxicity

Metal	Site and mechanism of molecular actions	Tissue and organ target
Mercury	Direct toxicity Sulfhydryl binding and disruption of important macromolecules (enzymes, pumps, receptors) Also binds phosphoryl, amino, and other groups	Corrosive damage to lungs and gastrointestinal tract CNS, lung, and renal damage
Lead	Sulfhydryl group binding Impaired heme synthesis	CNS and peripheral nervous system, cardiovascular, blood, kidney and skin
Cadmium	Binds to macromolecules and disrupts function	Lung and renal damage
Arsenic	Sulfhydryl groups and oxidative metabolism uncoupling	Peripheral nervous system, CNS, gastrointestinal tract, liver, and cardiovascular system

Fig. 29.9 Mechanisms of action of heavy metal toxicity.

for the use of nonabsorbed polythiol resins, which irreversibly bind mercury so that it is lost in the feces. L-Cysteine, infused intra-arterially, forms a dialyzable complex with methylmercury.

Lead

Lead has been used for centuries in water pipes and glazes. In some countries organic lead compounds are added to gasoline to prevent premature ignition (antiknock). Older paints contain lead at up to 40% of their dry weight. Occupational exposure used to be common and still is in some countries. Chronic lead poisoning, particularly in urban regions, has led to government restrictions on lead use, especially in paint and gasoline (Fig. 29.11).

Acute lead poisoning is less common than chronic poisoning and is a result of ingestion or exposure to lead vapor. Symptoms include nausea, vomiting, a metallic taste, and severe abdominal pain. There can also be acute severe CNS symptoms, a hemolytic crisis, kidney damage, and shock. Chronic poisoning (plumbism) causes gastrointestinal, neuromuscular, renal, and CNS symptoms, as well as symptoms related to other body systems. Neuromuscular and CNS symptoms usually follow severe poisoning; gastrointestinal symptoms follow less severe poisoning (Fig. 29.12). CNS symptoms are more common in children and include disturbed motor control, restlessness, and irritability, and sometimes a progressive deterioration of mental function which may occur as a result of low-level environmental exposure and be difficult to diagnose.

Lead is absorbed from the gastrointestinal and respiratory tracts. Gastrointestinal absorption is greater in children. Lead is distributed throughout the body, and deposited in the bones, teeth, and hair.

Chelation therapy (guided by the blood concentrations of heavy metal) is useful with, in order of priority:

- $CaNa_2$ ethylenediaminetetraacetic acid (EDTA) (im or iv).
- Dimercaprol (im).
- D-Penicillamine (orally).
- Succimer.

Cadmium

Cadmium poisoning is as common as mercury and lead poisoning, owing partly to its widespread industrial use in plastics,

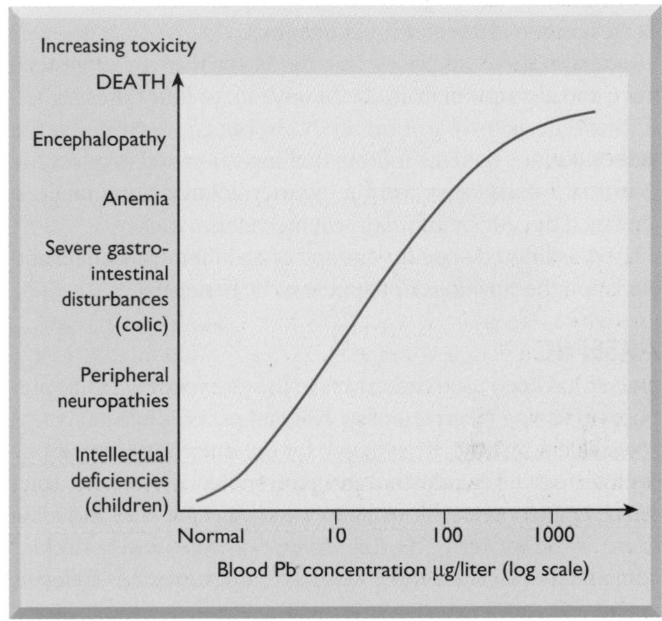

Fig. 29.12 Relationship between blood lead concentration and symptoms of lead poisoning.

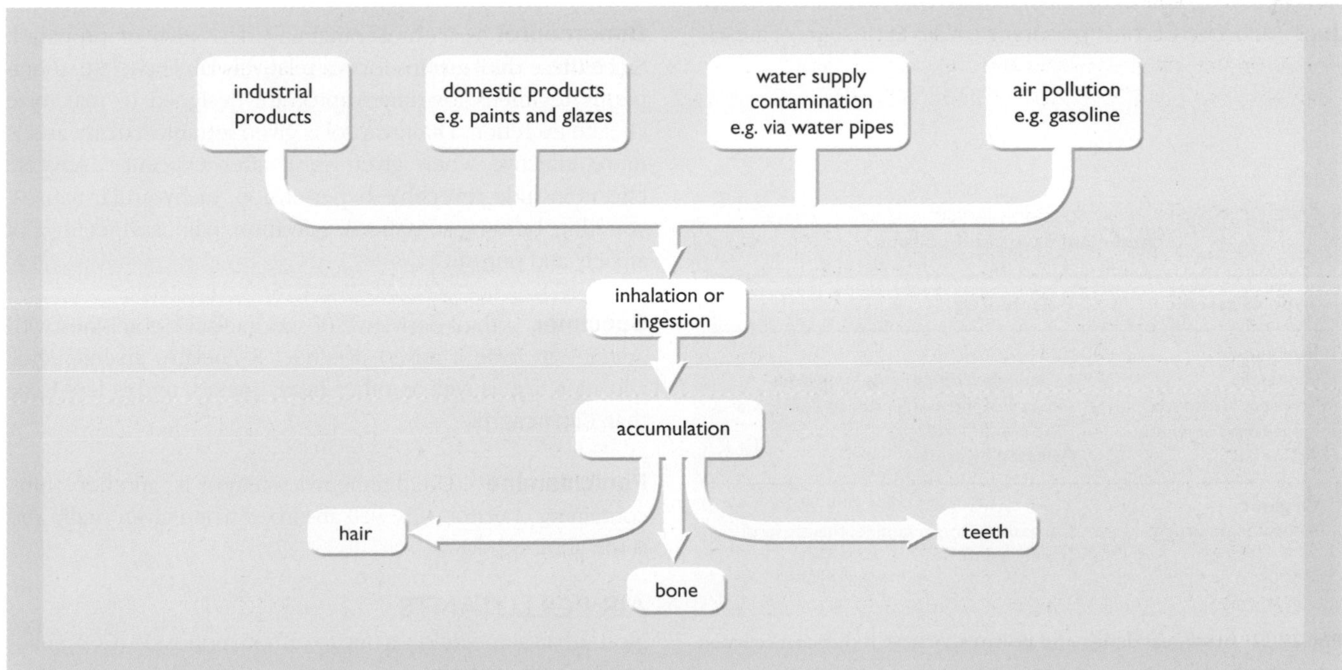

Fig. 29.11 Sources and body distribution of lead.

paints, and batteries. Cadmium accumulates in food, particularly shellfish, animal livers and kidneys, and food grains. Exposure through food is most important, but industrial workers can be exposed to cadmium vapors in the air.

Acute poisoning is generally due to airborne exposure and is associated with initial lung irritation followed by pneumonitis, chest pains, residual emphysema, and possibly fatal pulmonary edema. Oral ingestion causes vomiting, diarrhea, and abdominal cramps. The results of chronic poisoning depend upon the mode of exposure: the lung is a major target with air exposure, and the kidney and lungs following ingestion. Cadmium probably causes osteomalacia and carcinogenesis.

Cadmium (Cd^{2+}) is poorly absorbed from the gastrointestinal tract, and absorption from the lungs is up to four times higher. It distributes slowly around the body, but concentrates in the kidney. Kidney damage follows oral ingestion and involves the proximal tubules first and the glomeruli later. Lung tissue is damaged directly by an unknown mechanism.

There is limited specific therapy of cadmium poisoning and chelation therapy does not appear to be beneficial.

ARSENIC

Arsenic has been used extensively in the past for therapeutic purposes including treatment of syphilis and parasitic infections, and some arsenical drugs are still used for the latter. Most arsenic poisoning arises from industrial and environmental exposure. High concentrations of arsenic occur in some water supplies, including those of the western US, while some pesticides and herbicides contain arsenic (Fig. 29.13). Arsenicals are sometimes added to animal food stock to promote growth, and as murderous poisons.

Acute arsenical poisoning is now rare because its availability is strictly regulated. Symptoms develop over 12 hours and include severe gastric pain, projectile vomiting, and severe diarrhea. Renal collapse, anuria, and shock can lead to death. Neuropathies and encephalopathies are common if death does not occur. Chronic poisoning causes early signs of muscle weakness and myalgias, hyperpigmentation, and hyperkeratosis. Other symptoms include sweating, stomatitis, lacrimation, excessive salivation, coryza, dermatitis, and alopecia.

Arsenic absorption depends on the form ingested. It is stored mainly in heart, lung, liver, and kidney, but concentrates in the keratin of the hair and nails, as well as bones and teeth. Biochemically, arsenic uncouples oxidative metabolism by substituting for phosphates. It causes capillary leakage and myocardial damage as well as epithelial sloughing in the gastrointestinal tract and bloody feces. The renal capillaries and renal tubules are severely damaged, while cerebral vessel damage is responsible for some neuropathies. Central necrosis and cirrhosis can occur in the liver.

Arsenicals are also carcinogenic and teratogenic. They induce squamous and basal cell skin carcinomas, and possibly lung and liver cancers.

Specific treatment for arsenic poisoning includes chelation therapy with intramuscular dimercaprol, followed by oral penicillamine or succimer.

Arsenical drugs and poisons

Type of arsenic	Poison/drug
Inorganic	
Elemental	Insecticides, rat poisons, fungicides
Trivalent arsenite	(source of most arsenical poisoning via
Pentavalent arsenate	food contamination)
Arsine gas	Released by acids
Organic	
Antiparasitic drugs	Carbasone, tryparsamine, melasosprol (rarely used)

Fig. 29.13 Arsenical drugs and poisons. Arsenic is the most common cause of acute heavy metal poisoning, and is the second most common source (after lead) of chronic heavy metal poisoning.

CHELATORS

Chelators are molecules that can hold metals in inactive forms suitable for mobilization and excretion. Those used medically include EDTA, diethylenetriaminepenta-acetic acid (DTPA), dimercaprol, succimer (Fig. 29.14), penicillamine, and deferoxamine.

EDTA is usually given as the calcium disodium salt, but these ions are easily displaced by heavier toxic metals and by manganese, zinc, and iron. Administration is intravenous or intramuscular, but the latter route is painful. Treatment schedules must be followed carefully since rapid infusion can cause transient hypocalcemia. However, since the body has a huge excess of calcium ions over EDTA ions, calcium concentrations quickly return to normal.

Dimercaprol is a thiol-containing derivative of propanol. Since these thiol groups form a relatively labile chelate, therapeutic regimens for dimercaprol are designed to maximize chelate excretion. Dimercaprol is given intramuscularly and is more effective when given early after exposure. Adverse effects include reversible hypertension, tachycardia, nausea, vomiting, burning sensations, salivation, pain, and feelings of anxiety and unrest.

Succimer, a thiol derivative of succinic acid, combines with cysteine to form a mixed disulfide. It chelates arsenic, lead, and mercury, as well as other heavy metals, and is less toxic than dimercaprol.

Penicillamine (D-β,β-dimethylcysteine) is another thiol-containing chelator. It is well absorbed when given orally and is metabolized slowly.

AIR POLLUTANTS

Most urban air pollution is due to carbon monoxide (CO), sulfur oxides, hydrocarbons, and nitrogen oxides. These come from burning coal products and gasoline. Photochemical pollution (smog) contains hydrocarbons, oxides of nitrogen, and photochemical oxidants. Airborne particles account for 10% of all air pollution (Fig. 29.15).

Airborne particles

Airborne particles larger than 5 μm in diameter are usually deposited in the upper airways, whereas those 1–5 μm in size reach the terminal airways or alveoli. A mucus blanket propelled by cilia (the mucociliary escalator) carries larger insoluble particles upwards to the pharynx, from where they can be swallowed. Silica particles larger than 1 mm reach the alveoli where they are either removed, phagocytized, or absorbed into lymphatics. Pneumoconiosis is caused by inhalation of small dust particles, which are phagocytized and then form fibrotic silicotic nodules throughout the lungs. Symptomatic pneumoconiosis usually takes years to develop and increases the susceptibility of the lungs to infection. Asbestos (fibrous hydrated silicates) was widely used in industry, but bronchial cancer occurs 20–30 years after initial exposure to asbestos. Concomitant smoking increases the cancer rate (see p. 537). Mesoepithelioma in the pleura or peritoneum is a rapidly fatal malignancy that appears to be related to exposure to chrysolite asbestos fiber and occurs 25–40 years after initial exposure.

Carbon monoxide

Carbon monoxide is a colorless, odorless, tasteless, nonirritating gas formed by incomplete combustion of carbon compounds. It is a major cause of accidental and suicidal deaths. When fire occurs in an enclosed space, most victims die from acute CO poisoning, rather than from burns. CO binds to hemoglobin (Hb) to form carboxyhemoglobin (COHb), which cannot bind oxygen. The high affinity of CO for hemoglobin (220 times that of oxygen) means that even low concentrations of CO are dangerous because of their ability to impair oxygen delivery. The reduction in the oxygen-carrying capacity of blood is proportional to the amount of COHb, and the effects of poisoning are due to hypoxia. In addition to decreasing the oxygen-carrying capacity of blood ('functional anemia'), CO also impairs the capacity of Hb to deliver oxygen to the tissues. This is due to shifting the oxygen dissociation curve to the left (Fig. 29.16). Moderate concentrations have little effect on vital functions (blood pressure, heart rate) at rest

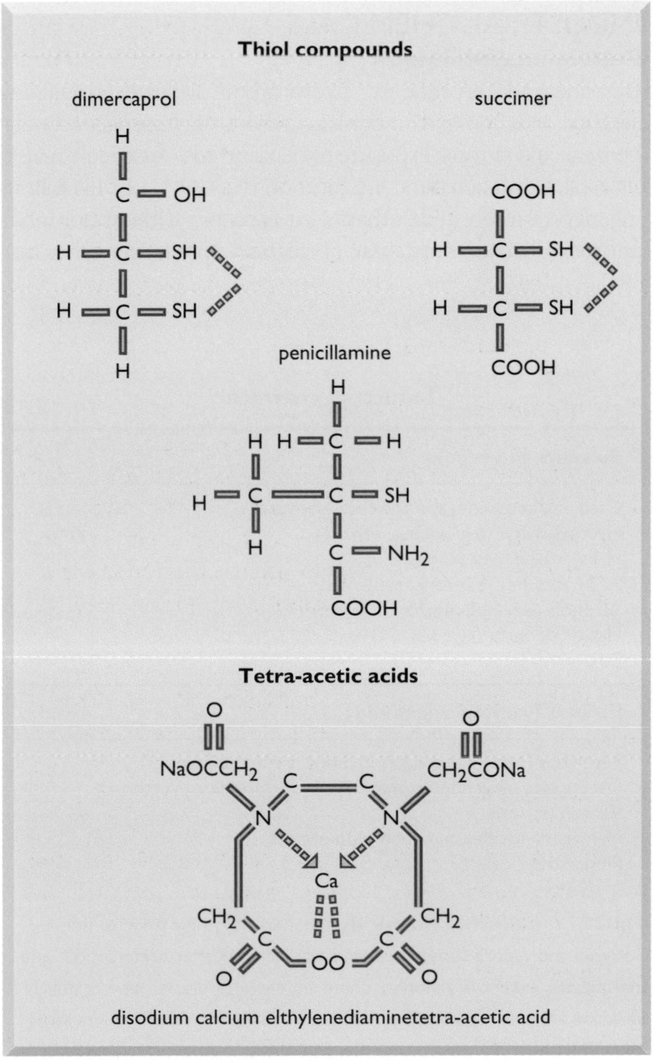

Thiol compounds

dimercaprol

succimer

penicillamine

Tetra-acetic acids

disodium calcium elthylenediaminetetra-acetic acid

Fig. 29.14 Chelator molecules.

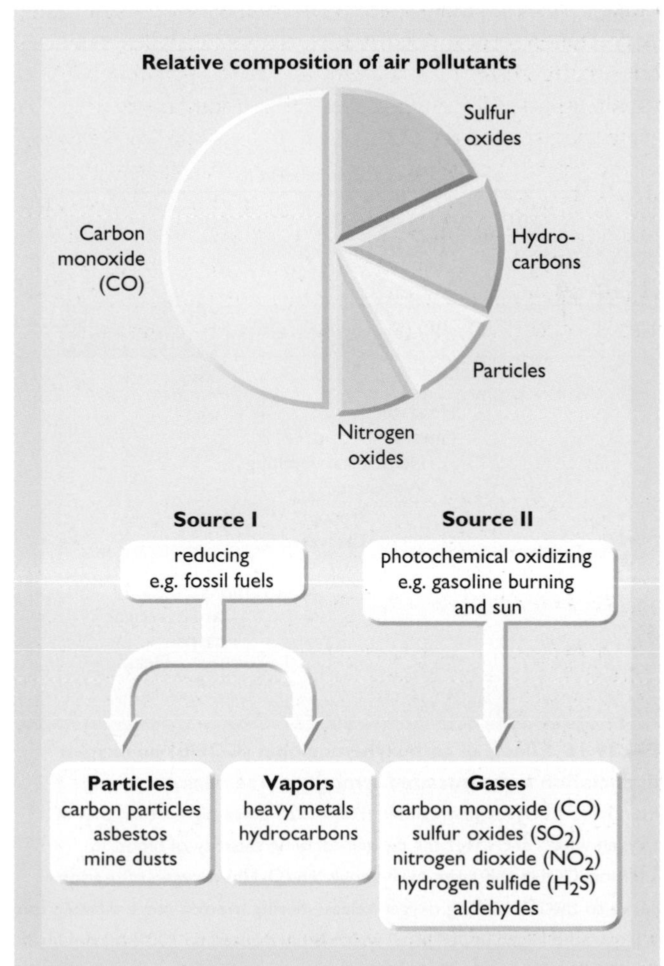

Fig. 29.15 Air pollutants.

in healthy subjects owing to the considerable reserve in oxygen-carrying capacity of blood and to the reserve in the cardiovascular system.

COHb fully dissociates and CO is excreted easily by the lungs. Treatment of CO poisoning therefore involves immediate transfer to fresh air, with artificial respiration if required. Rapid administration of 100% oxygen is often the only therapy required. The cardiovascular system, particularly the heart, is susceptible to low concentrations of CO, since the heart normally extracts a large fraction of oxygen delivered to it. Experimental and clinical studies suggest that long-term exposure to CO facilitates the development of arteriosclerosis. The fetus is especially susceptible to CO and the persistent low levels of COHb produced by smoking during pregnancy may adversely affect fetal development.

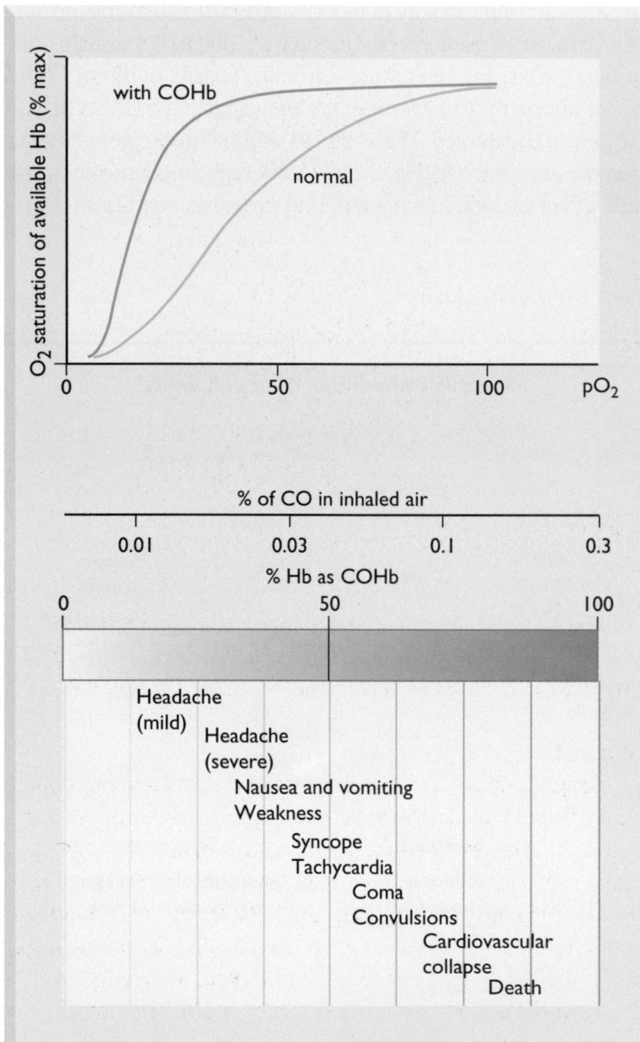

Fig. 29.16 Effects of carboxyhemoglobin (COHb) on oxygen dissociation and associated symptoms. The affinity of carbon monoxide (CO) for hemoglobin (Hb) is 220 times higher than that of oxygen which decreases the oxygen-carrying capacity of blood. In addition, COHb shifts the oxyhemoglobin (O_2Hb)–oxygen saturation curve to the left, making oxygen release during hypoxia more difficult. This is illustrated in the upper panel which is normalized to 100% maximum. If the data were expressed as absolute oxygen content, the values in the presence of COHb would be decreased compared with normal.

Other air pollutants

Other air pollutants include sulfur oxides, nitrogen oxides, and aldehydes:

- Inhaled sulfur dioxide causes a parasympathetic-dependent bronchoconstriction in normal people, but this may be very severe in asthmatics, who are sensitive to concentrations as low as 0.25 parts per million.
- Nitrogen dioxide is a lung irritant capable of causing pulmonary edema. It is a particular risk to farmers because it is released from silage and may cause pulmonary damage ('silo-filler's lung').
- Aldehydes are formed by sunlight acting on the products of incomplete combustion, or are released from aldehyde-containing resins. Formaldehyde irritates respiratory mucous membranes and can provoke skin reactions.
- Acrolein is more irritating than formaldehyde and is the major reason for the irritating quality of cigarette smoke and photochemical smog.

INDUSTRIAL CHEMICALS

Petroleum distillates

Gasoline and kerosene are hydrocarbon distillates containing aliphatic, aromatic, and other hydrocarbons. Most gasolines contain benzene and chronic exposure to benzene can cause leukemia.

Gasoline and kerosene intoxication (Figs 29.17, 29.18) following ingestion resemble ethanol intoxication, while vapor inhalation can cause ventricular fibrillation. Inhalation can cause

Industrial chemicals
Solvents and vapors
Gasoline, kerosene, and their derivatives Hydrocarbons (e.g. butane, ethane) Halogenated hydrocarbons Aromatics (e.g. benzene, toluene) Alcohols (ethanol, methanol, propanol) Higher alcohols (glycols) Ethers
Poisons (varying selectivity)
Pesticides (many synthetic and a few natural compounds) Insecticides (organophosphates, organochlorines, pyrethrins) Vermin poisons Many rodenticides and general fumigants Herbicides

Fig. 29.17 Industrial chemicals. Most are varyingly toxic to humans. Solvents and vapors sometimes have similar CNS effects. Herbicides and insecticides, except organophosphate anticholinesterases, have relatively selective actions, but vermin poisons are usually not selective. Industrial chemicals generally cause acute toxicity. There are many solvents and vapors whose chemical nature makes them ideal fuels and solvents.

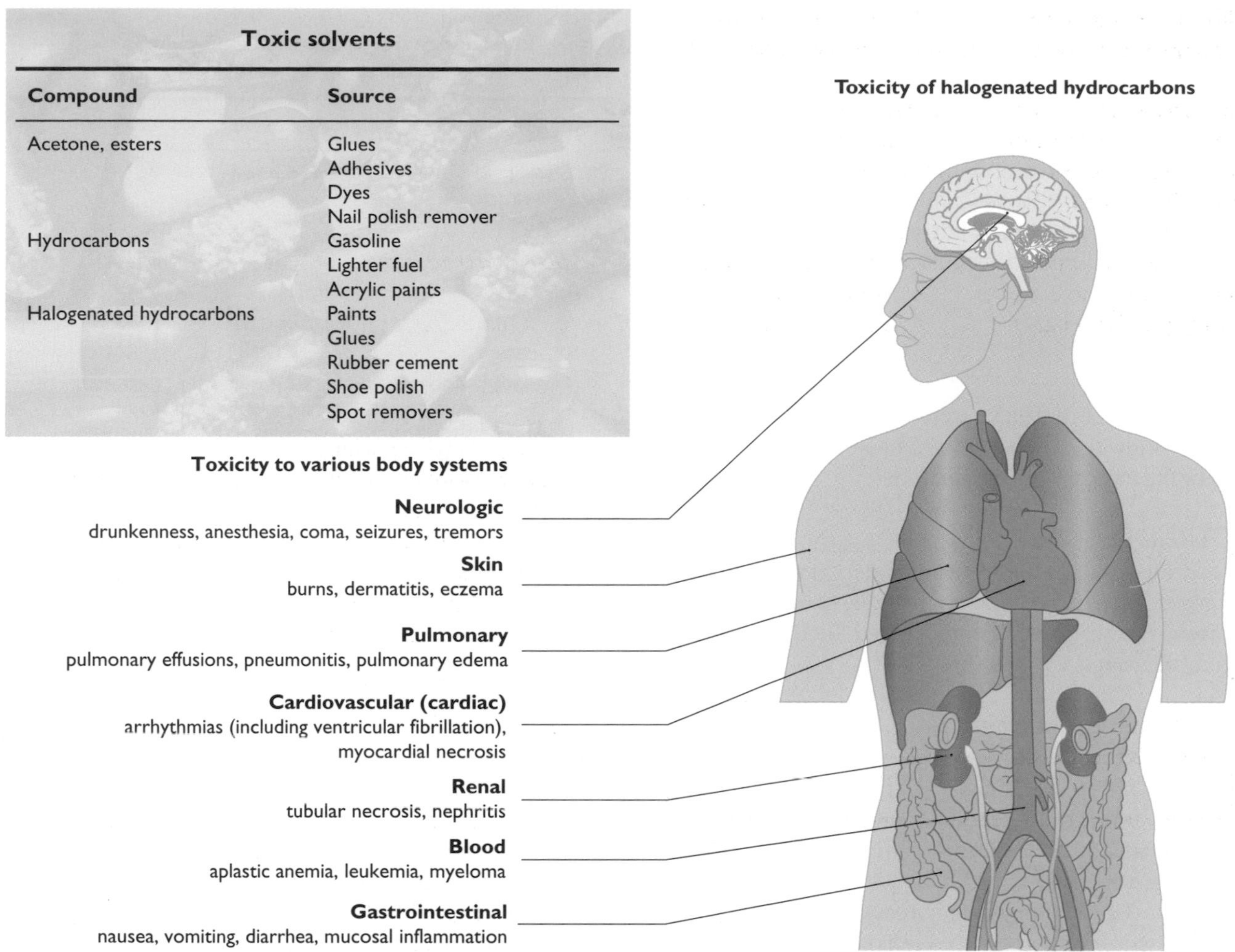

Toxic solvents

Compound	Source
Acetone, esters	Glues Adhesives Dyes Nail polish remover
Hydrocarbons	Gasoline Lighter fuel Acrylic paints
Halogenated hydrocarbons	Paints Glues Rubber cement Shoe polish Spot removers

Fig. 29.18 Toxic solvents and toxicity of halogenated hydrocarbons on various body systems.

chemical pneumonitis complicated by bacterial pneumonia and pulmonary edema. Death due to hemorrhagic pulmonary edema may occur within 24 hours. Management is symptomatic and supportive.

Contaminated drinking water can result in long-term gasoline exposure. Higher molecular weight compounds in gasoline, like most organic solvents, depress the CNS and cause dizziness and incoordination. Neuropathy is an important toxic effect of *n*-hexane.

Halogenated hydrocarbons

Halogenated hydrocarbons are widely used as industrial solvents. Several small halogenated hydrocarbons occur in drinking water as a result of chlorination. Other halogenated hydrocarbons can contaminate water supplies. Since there are correlations (casual or causal) between water chlorination and cancer of the colon, rectum, and bladder, there is concern about the exposure of large populations to chlorinated drinking water.

Transient exposure to carbon tetrachloride vapor causes ocular and nasal irritation, nausea, vomiting, dizziness, and headache. Death may result from ventricular fibrillation or respiratory depression. Serious and delayed toxic effects include liver and kidney damage.

Hepatotoxicity is common with halogenated hydrocarbons in general, but not with the more complex halogenated hydrocarbons used as inhalational anesthetics (see Chapter 21).

Alcohols

Methanol (wood alcohol) is a common industrial solvent and is added to contaminate ethanol so as to avoid taxes on drinkable ethanol. The absorption, distribution, and metabolism of methanol and ethanol are similar, and their metabolism is by zero-order kinetics (see Chapter 5). Methanol inebriates less than ethanol, and produces headache, vertigo, vomiting, upper abdominal pain, and hyperventilation. Retinal damage may be severe and lead to blindness (see Chapter 10). The other major problem is metabolic acidosis.

Ethanol has a 100-fold greater affinity for alcohol dehydrogenase than methanol. A specific treatment for methanol poisoning is therefore to maintain blood ethanol concentrations at 100 mg/100 ml to prevent the formation of methanol's toxic metabolites, formaldehyde and formic acid (causes acidosis). Dialysis may be required to decrease methanol concentrations so as to avoid blindness.

Other alcohols (isopropanol, ethylene and diethylene glycol, and propylene alcohol) are also toxic.

Aromatic hydrocarbons

Benzene is an excellent solvent but highly toxic and carcinogenic. Toxic effects following limited exposure to benzene include blurred vision, tremors, disturbed respiration, cardiac arrhythmias, paralysis, and unconsciousness. Chronic intoxication can cause aplastic anemia and even leukemia.

Toluene is a CNS depressant and low concentrations produce fatigue, weakness, and confusion, but it probably does not cause aplastic anemia or leukemia. 'Glue sniffers' inhale toluene vapors from glue.

PESTICIDES

Over 0.5 billion kg of pesticides are used in the US every year, 2.0 billion worldwide. Herbicides are most commonly used, followed by the insecticides and fungicides.

INSECTICIDES

The insecticide residues that contaminate food result in low-level exposures for the general population. Acute poisoning results from eating heavily contaminated foods or during agricultural spraying.

Organochlorine insecticides

Chlorinated ethane derivatives Dichlorodiphenyltrichloroethane (DDT) is lipid soluble and only slowly eliminated from the body. It has a wide margin of safety and there are no reports of human deaths. Methoxychlor (Fig. 29.19), a replacement for DDT, stimulates the CNS by antagonizing γ aminobutyric acid (GABA) ionotropic receptors resulting in decreased Cl^- currents and reduced inhibition. Methoxychlor and similar compounds can induce convulsions before other less serious signs of toxicity.

Cyclodienes Chlorinated cyclodienes, unlike DDT, are readily absorbed from intact skin. Aldrin and dieldrin have the greatest carcinogenic potential among the insecticides and are banned in the US, while chlordane and heptachlor are banned for use on crops.

Hydrocarbons The γ isomer of benzene hexachloride (BHC) is lindane, which causes tremors, ataxia, convulsions, and prostration. Both lindane and BHC have been implicated as a cause of aplastic anemia. Toxaphene induces tumors in mice. Other chlorinated hydrocarbon insecticides concentrate several thousandfold in the food chain.

Organophosphate insecticides Organophosphate insecticides (irreversible cholinesterases) are alternatives to organochlorine insecticides. One of them, parathion, is the most frequent cause of fatal poisoning. Cholinesterase inhibition results in massive acetylcholine accumulation and excessive muscarinic receptor stimulation results in excessive parasympathetic activity (hypersecretion, diarrhea, sweating), confusion, agitation, and coma. The specific treatment is the muscarinic receptor antagonist atropine (see Chapter 21).

a

The four major types of organochlorines and their analogs

Compound	Analogs
DDT	Methoxychlor
Benzene chloride	Lindane
Cyclodienes	Aldrin
	Chlordane
	Dieldrin
Toxaphenes	Toxaphene

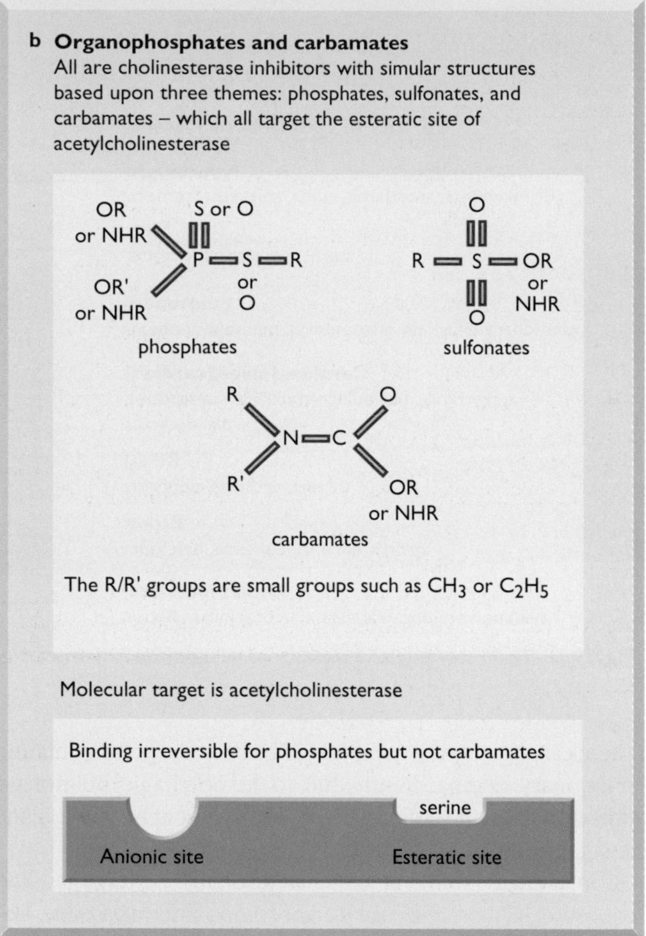

c

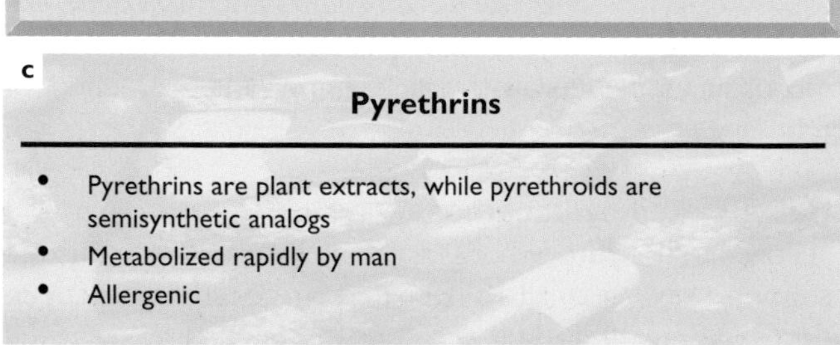

Fig. 29.19 Poisonous insecticides, pesticides, and herbicides. (a) The four major types of organochlorines and their analogs all contain a heavily chlorinated hydrocarbon backbone of MW 300–550, but have varied toxicity. They are lipid soluble and act on the CNS. They are also hepatic enzyme inducers. (b) Organophosphates and carbamates. All are cholinesterase inhibitors with similar structures based upon phosphates, sulfonates, and carbamates, and target the esteratic site of acetylcholinesterase. Over 35 different organophosphates and 20 carbamates are available. (c) Pyrethrins.

Botanic insecticides

Botanic insecticides such as pyrethrin are increasingly used. The crude extract, pyrethrum, is obtained from flowers and is considered safe in terms of direct toxicity, but can cause contact dermatitis and respiratory allergy. In the past nicotine has been used as an insecticide, but it is extremely toxic and absorbed through the skin

Rotenone, another natural product, rarely causes human poisoning and is used to treat head lice, scabies, and other ectoparasites. Local effects include conjunctivitis, dermatitis, and rhinitis. Other insecticides are used as ectoparasiticides (e.g. lindane is used as a miticide for scabies, and malathion for nits, see Chapter 18).

GENERAL PESTICIDES

The fumigants used to control insects, rodents, and soil nematodes include hydrogen cyanide (HCN), acrylonitrile, carbon disulfide, carbon tetrachloride, ethylene dibromide, ethylene oxide, and methyl bromide, all of which are very poisonous to humans.

HCN is a rapidly acting poison and kills within minutes of exposure. It is released during fires involving nitrogen-containing plastics. HCN has a high affinity for ferric iron, particularly in mitochondrial cytochrome oxidase where it inhibits cellular respiration. HCN victims die quickly or recover fully, but chronic neurologic sequelae can occur. Treatment has to be rapid. It involves giving nitrites to form methemoglobin, which has a great affinity for HCN, followed by thiosulfate to form the nontoxic thiocyanate.

Rodenticide toxicity varies. For example, the anticoagulant warfarin is relatively safe since toxicity depends on repeated ingestion, but sodium fluoroacetate and fluoroacetamide, which are among the most potent rodenticides, are very poisonous.

Strychnine*, a poisonous alkaloid, is still used as a pesticide and is a source of accidental poisoning. It increases neuronal excitability which may lead to severe seizures by selectively blocking inhibition (mediated by glycine).

Other rodenticides include white or yellow elemental phosphorus spread onto bait. Zinc phosphide reacts with water and acid in the stomach to produce the extremely poisonous phosphine. Thallium sulfate, which is hazardous and not selective for rodents, is now strictly regulated in many countries.

HERBICIDES

Most herbicides have low toxicity, but some have caused human fatalities. Dioxin (plus byproducts, CDD and TCDD) occurs in herbicides, but is a byproduct of manufacturing (e.g. paper making). Several epidemiologic studies of people exposed to high concentrations of dioxin suggest low toxicity, but other studies suggest that TCDD might be carcinogenic and teratogenic.

Several substituted dinitrophenols are used to kill weeds, and human poisoning with dinitro-orthocresol (DNOC) has occurred. The short-term toxicity of dinitrophenols is due to uncoupling of oxidative phosphorylation, and death or recovery occurs within 24–48 hours.

Paraquat is responsible for many accidental or suicidal poisonings. It damages the lungs, liver, and kidneys. The serious nature of its delayed pulmonary toxicity makes prompt treatment mandatory.

Many other herbicides have relatively low acute toxicities.

FUNGICIDES

Fungicides are a heterogeneous group of chemical compounds, but few have been extensively investigated for toxicity. Dithiocarbamates have some teratogenic and/or carcinogenic potential.

CARCINOGENESIS AND MUTAGENESIS

Chemicals known to cause cancer in humans after prolonged exposure include vinyl chloride, benzene, and naphthylamine. Cigarette smoke contains cancer-causing chemicals, and chronic consumption of ethanol increases the risk of esophageal and liver cancer. Charcoal broiling contaminates food with carcinogenic polycyclic aromatic hydrocarbons (those found in coal tars). Some foods contain carcinogens and these probably partly account for regional differences in cancer incidence.

Multiple steps are involved in chemical carcinogenesis. The nature of exposure to carcinogens is important (i.e. duration, dose, and frequency). Chemical induction of cancer involves initiation, promotion, and progression. Initiation (by initiating agents) is the conversion of normal cells into neoplastic cells via actions on DNA. However, additional events convert transformed cells to malignant cells. In animals, promoter chemicals increase the incidence of cancers or decrease the latency to tumor growth, although they do not act on DNA, or produce mutations.

A mutation is an alteration in DNA sequence that may change the cellular phenotype. Spontaneous mutagenesis occurs by mostly unknown mechanisms, but this natural rate can be increased 10–1000-fold by mutagens. Mutations are more likely to cause cancer in cells with deficient DNA repair enzymes or in which division is so rapid that DNA repair is incomplete. Many cancers are thought to begin as a routine mutation or are a hereditary trait.

Chemical carcinogens are either genotoxic or epigenetic

Genotoxic carcinogens (Fig. 29.20) react covalently with DNA to produce genetic mutations. Mutagenic potential can be detected by tests such as the Ames test for bacterial mutagenicity. Genotoxic carcinogens can be further subclassified on the basis

Carcinogens, cocarcinogens, and promoters

Genotoxic agents (mutagenic)	Chemical alkylating agents Ionizing and ultraviolet (skin) radiation Nickel, cadmium Hydrocarbons (polycyclics) and polyamines (arylamines, nitrosamines)
Epigenetic agents	Hormones such as estrogens Promoters such as phorbol esters Trauma Alcohol ingestion

Fig. 29.20 Carcinogens, cocarcinogens, and promoters.

of whether they require biotransformation before they become active. Most genotoxic agents are procarcinogens or activation-dependent genotoxic agents. Nitrosamines are typical procarcinogens.

An epigenetic agent enhances the effects of genotoxic carcinogens. It may act by:

- Increasing effector concentrations of genotoxin.
- Enhancing metabolic activation of a genotoxin.
- Decreasing detoxification of a genotoxin.
- Inhibiting DNA repair.
- Increasing proliferation of DNA-damaged cells.

Tumor promoters enhance carcinogenic activity when given after a genotoxin. Phorbol esters are tumor-promoting agents that act by binding to protein kinase C. TCDD (dioxin) is also a potent tumor promoter.

Immunosuppressive drugs are epigenetic agents that suppress the immune system and thereby 'allow' carcinogenesis.

Asbestos is an epigenetic carcinogen

Asbestos fibers are centers of mitotic activity and these add to smoking as a carcinogenic mechanism. Smokers have a 10-fold greater risk of developing lung cancer than nonsmokers and asbestos increases this risk to 50-fold.

Mechanisms of action of chemical mutagens and carcinogens

- **Genotoxins cause genetic damage, which many lead to cancer**
- **Epigenetic compounds amplify the cancer-forming actions of genotoxins**
- **Promoters (chemical, physical, and biologic) amplify the adverse effects of mutagens and carcinogens**

FURTHER READING

Amdur MO, Doull J, Klassen CD, et al. (eds) *Casarett & Doull's Toxicology: The Basic Science of Poisons, 4e*. New York: Pergamon Press; 1991. [A standard toxicological reference book.]

Gosselin RE, Smith RP, Hodge HC (eds) *Clinical Toxicology of Commercial Products 5e*. Baltimore: Williams and Wilkins; 1984. [Source of information on toxic commercial products.]

Hay A. How to identify a carcinogen. *Nature* 1988; **332**: 782–783. [Procedures for identifying potential carcinogens.]

Sullivan JB, Krieger GR (eds) *Hazardous Materials Toxicology*. Baltimore: Williams and Wilkins; 1992. [Source for material on toxicological hazards in the environment.]

Tu AT (ed.) *Handbook of Natural Toxins, Volumes 1–5*. New York and Basle: Marcel Dekker Inc; 1988. [An extensive source of information on toxins and venoms.]

Make a provisional diagnosis and determine a rational pharmacologic treatment for the following hypothetical case.

While on holiday in Indonesia a friend has spent the day swimming over coral reefs. The surrounding land is agricultural, and streams from fields and villages flow into the sea. Your friend leaves the sea complaining of coral cuts and has a variety of skin abrasions, cuts, and skin lesions on his lower legs. He has a shower and a snack of local hot foods and drinks. Shortly afterwards he says he feels weak and appears to have ptosis. He grows increasingly weak, but his pulse remains strong and he has no other symptoms.

1. What would you do first?
2. What supportive measures should be taken?
3. Is the probable cause of your friend's problems an octopus bite, envenomation by a snake or coneshell, botulism from contaminated food, organophosphate insecticide from run-off or food contamination, or general food poisoning?
4. What specific therapy is available?

?

Indicate which is the correct answer for each question.

1. 2,3,7,8-Tetrachlorodibenzodioxin (TCDD) is not
   a) a carcinogen in some experimental animals
   b) a teratogen in some experimental animals
   c) a toxic hazard
   d) more potent than botulinum toxin as a lethal agent in man
   e) a byproduct of manufacturing

2. Lead poisoning is not associated with
   a) severe abdominal pain
   b) disturbances of mood
   c) peripheral neuropathy
   d) red blood cell abnormalities
   e) abnormal patterns of bone growth

3. A 26-year-old male presents as an emergency in a semi-conscious state. He is arousable, but unable to answer questions. Investigations reveal a severe metabolic acidosis. He has most probably ingested
   a) carbon tetrachloride
   b) ethanol
   c) methanol
   d) cyanide
   e) benzene

4. Which of the following statements is false?
   a) parathion is an organophosphate insectide used in agriculture and horticulture
   b) pyrethrins (chrysanthemic acids) are obtained by extraction from flowering plants
   c) dioxin is a toxic byproduct of chlorine bleaching of wood pulp
   d) dichlorodiphenyltrichloroethane (DDT) is an organophosphate insectide used in agriculture and horticulture
   e) carbon monoxide is a common air pollutant

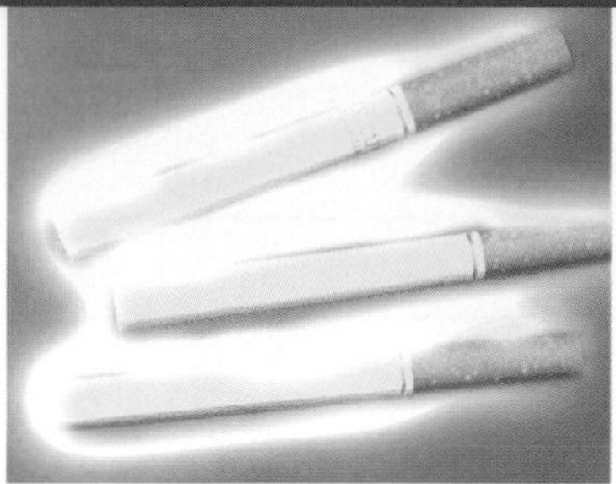

30. Drug Dependence and Drugs of Abuse

Drug dependence can be defined as 'repeated, compulsive use of a drug in order to receive its chemical rewarding effects or to avoid the punishing effects of drug withdrawal.' 'Compulsive' implies a lack of control, i.e. the behavior cannot be stopped even if the drug taker desires this.

There are many other definitions of drug dependence, but all recognize that the rewarding and punishing effects of drugs are central to the concept. These two characteristics can also be used to classify different types of dependence:

- Taking a drug primarily to receive its rewarding effects is described as psychological dependence.
- Taking a drug to avoid withdrawal is described as physiological dependence—its diagnosis is based on whether signs of drug tolerance and withdrawal are present in an individual.

Unfortunately, these are just concepts and any individual who is dependent on a drug will usually be taking it for both these reasons, to a greater or lesser extent. Similarly, no drug produces one form of dependence alone, though some are likely to produce one type more commonly than the other (see Fig. 30.8). There are many other terms used to describe behavior associated with drug taking. The most common is drug abuse. Based on the DSM IV (Diagnostic and Statistical Manual for Mental Disorders) criteria for substance abuse, drug abuse is defined as 'drug use which does not meet the criteria for dependence, but which continues in the face of harmful medical or social consequences for the drug taker.'

Furthermore, there is still confusion between drug dependence and addiction. The term 'addiction' is not used in this chapter, but it can be defined as 'an extreme form of dependence in which the need to obtain the drug has become the dominant force in an individual's life.'

All drugs that produce dependence produce rewards within the brain

All drugs that produce dependence have chemical effects within the brain that provide pleasurable sensations or rewards (Fig. 30.1). There are many such rewards, including the anti-fatigue effect of caffeine, the relaxation caused by alcohol, and even passing a stool after using a laxative! However, by far the most rewarding chemical effect is the feeling of pure pleasure produced by drugs such as cocaine and amphetamines. This is thought to result from a potentiation of dopamine transmission in the limbic forebrain, specifically in the nucleus accumbens (see Fig. 30.3). All pleasurable stimuli may eventually act through this dopaminergic pathway, and many drugs which provide other kinds of reward also indirectly increase dopaminergic transmission in the nucleus accumbens.

In addition, there are nerve pathways that use opioid peptides, which may directly mediate pleasure, but it is widely thought that these also indirectly affect the dopaminergic nerves in the nucleus accumbens.

It has been suggested that genetic differences in the dopamine receptors in the nucleus accumbens may underlie genetic differences in the rewarding effects that drugs have in different people, and consequently influence susceptibility to drug dependence.

Rewards lead to repeated behavior as a result of operant conditioning

In animals, operant conditioning is usually studied by rewarding a specific behavior (pressing a lever, for example) with something the animal needs (most commonly a food pellet). Very soon the animal 'learns' to press the lever to receive its reward. In psychological jargon, the food acts as a positive reinforcement for the behavior.

The effects of drug rewards can be studied in exactly the same way (e.g. animals will rapidly learn to press a lever to obtain an intravenous injection of heroin or cocaine, Fig. 30.2). Interestingly, they will also learn to press a lever to obtain an electrical stimulation in the nucleus accumbens or related brain areas (Fig. 30.3). This is called intracranial self-stimulation (ICSS).

Because these drug rewards (and ICSS) will induce specific behaviors to receive them, they are all capable of being positive reinforcements, and this defines how likely they are to cause psychological dependence. The 'addictive potential' of new drugs in animals can therefore be assessed, and a measure of this can be obtained by seeing how much 'work' an animal will do to get the drug. For example, rats trained to press the lever for cocaine will press the lever up to 1000 times before receiving the injection of drug, sometimes ignoring all other behavior (including eating and drinking) in order to continue pressing the lever for cocaine. On this basis, cocaine is very likely to be self-administered for its rewarding properties by humans, as is indeed the case.

Another aspect of operant conditioning that is very relevant to drug rewards is how quickly the reward follows the behavior. If a rat receives a food pellet immediately after pressing a lever it learns the appropriate behavior much more quickly than if the food follows 10 minutes later. Much the same is true of drugs: when they rapidly produce rewards, they reinforce the behavior of taking them more positively than when their rewards are delayed. This can even apply to different ways of taking the same drug. For example, nasal snorting of the hydrochloride salt of cocaine will produce a reward in the brain within a few minutes,

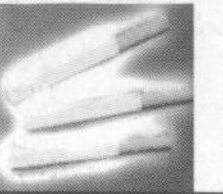

Rewards and mechanisms of drugs of dependence

Drug class	Drug	Reward	Mechanism of action	Transmitter
Stimulant	Cocaine	Euphoria, arousal	Inhibition of catecholamine reuptake	Dopamine, norepinephrine
	Amphetamines ('ecstasy')	Euphoria, arousal, perceptual disturbance	Monoamine release and inhibition of reuptake	Dopamine, norepinephrine, serotonin
	Nicotine	Euphoria, concentration, relaxation	NicAChR activation causing NT release, NicAChR desensitization	Dopamine, norepinephrine, acetylcholine
	Caffeine	Anti-fatigue, concentration	Adenosine receptor antagonism enhancing NT release	Norepinephrine
Depressants	Alcohol	Euphoria, relaxation, amnesia	Increased DA release, potentiation at $GABA_A$ Rs, inhibition at NMDA Rs	Dopamine, GABA, glutamate
	Benzodiazepines	Anxiolysis	Potentiation at $GABA_A$ Rs	GABA
	Barbiturates	Sedation	Potentiation at $GABA_A$ Rs	GABA
Dissociative anesthetic	Phencyclidine, ketamine	Relaxation, amnesia perceptual disturbance,	Channel block at NMDA Rs	Glutamate
Analgesic	Morphine, heroin, methadone	Euphoria, relaxation, analgesia	Agonists at opioid receptors	Endorphins
Cannabinoids	Cannabis, tetrahydrocannabinol	Euphoria, relaxation, perceptual disturbances	Agonist for specific G protein-linked receptors	Anandamide?
Hallucinogens	Lysergic acid diethylamide, mescaline	Perceptual disturbances	Agonist (and antagonist) at specific serotonin receptors, effects on catecholamines?	Serotonin, dopamine

Fig. 30.1 Rewards and mechanisms of drugs of dependence. (DA, dopamine; GABA, γ-aminobutyric acid; $GABA_A$ R, $GABA_A$ receptor; NicAChR, nicotinic acetylcholine receptor; NMDA R, *N*-methyl D-aspartate receptor; NT, neurotransmitter)

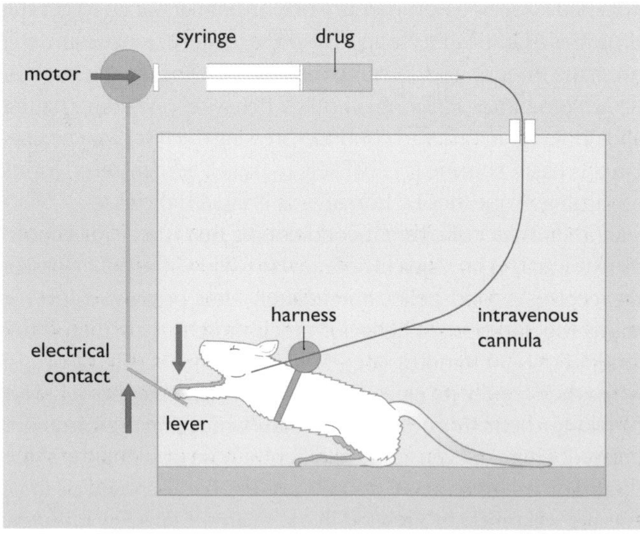

Fig. 30.2 Apparatus for self-injection of drugs by laboratory animals. The diagram shows a rat pressing a lever to receive an intravenous injection of the drug contained in the syringe above the cage. Rats and other laboratory animals in this situation will readily self-inject most of the drugs that humans regard as pleasurable, though exceptions include hallucinogens such as lysergic acid diethylamide. Because there is good agreement between the animal and human data, tests like this can be used to assess the likely 'abuse potential' for new pharmacotherapeutic agents.

but inhaling the fumes from heated 'crack' cocaine produces the reward in seconds. Crack cocaine is therefore more positively reinforcing, and the introduction of crack is one of the reasons why there is now a cocaine epidemic in the US.

In general, drugs that are smoked or taken intravenously produce rapid effects and are likely to lead to psychological

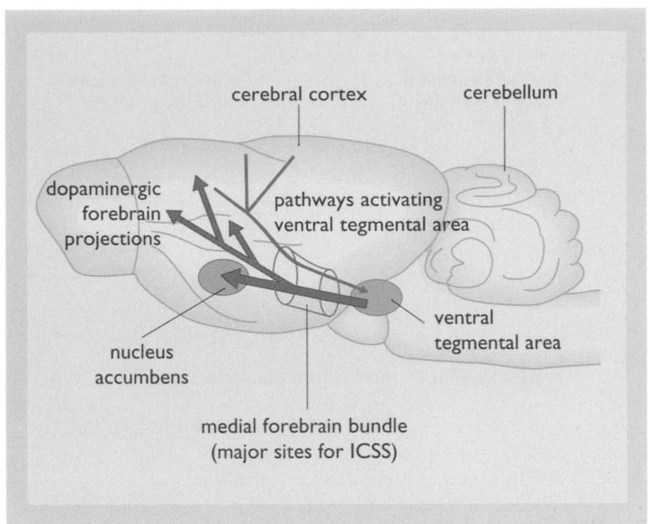

Fig. 30.3 'Reward' pathways in the brain. The diagram shows the major dopaminergic pathway thought to mediate reward in the mammalian brain (in red). This pathway is a part of the mesolimbic dopaminergic projections running from the ventral tegmental area (in green). The nerves thought to play the most important part in the rewarding effects of drugs terminate in the nucleus accumbens (in blue), which is part of the limbic system of the forebrain. Electrodes placed in these areas will support intracranial self-stimulation (ICSS) by animals, but other areas of the brain will also do this. Many are close to the medial forebrain bundle, which carries axons running to and from the ventral tegmental area.

dependence, whereas drugs taken orally are slower acting and are less likely to cause psychological dependence (see Fig. 30.8). However, many other factors are involved, including Pavlovian or classic conditioning.

In classic conditioning, conditioned stimuli induce a response

Pavlov's dogs were trained to salivate (the response) when a bell was rung (the conditioned stimulus) by repeated presentation of the bell with food. The same principles can be applied to operant conditioning because, when a reward closely follows a behavior (as in operant conditioning), and this is repeated many times, associations build up between the behavior and the reward. These associations gradually make the behavior itself take on the characteristics of a reward. Those who repeatedly smoke cigarettes for the nicotine reward eventually find that they feel more comfortable with a cigarette in their mouth (i.e. the cigarette-smoking behavior has become rewarding for its own sake).

This is very similar to the development of a 'habit,' in which a behavior that was originally performed for a purpose is carried out automatically without considering whether it is appropriate. In fact, when there is an association between the drug reward and the behavior of taking it, the drug is said to be 'habit-forming' for a behavior.

There is very little difference between a habit that is very difficult to stop (a compulsive behavior) and psychological dependence on a drug. In this situation, the behavior of taking the drug contributes to the positive reinforcement for continuing the behavior and becomes an end in itself. The associations are increased, so increasing the risk of becoming psychologically dependent, if drug taking becomes a ritual and the drug is always taken in exactly the same way.

Additionally, everything associated with the behavior (e.g. the environment, the company, the time of day) can also become conditioned stimuli associated with the drug reward. Together, all these factors are called the 'setting' for the drug-taking behavior (Fig. 30.4).

THE PROGRESSIVE NATURE OF DEPENDENCE

The first type of dependence is usually psychological dependence

The reason for starting to use a drug repeatedly is almost always because it provides a reward of some kind (including a pharmacotherapeutic reward such as relief from pain or anxiety). As a result, the first type of dependence to occur is usually a psychological dependence (i.e. repeatedly taking a drug because of the desire for its rewarding effects). Early in a drug-taking career, drug rewards, particularly from stimulant drugs, may actually seem to become greater with repeated drug use. This is referred to as 'sensitization.' This drags the user further into psychological dependence.

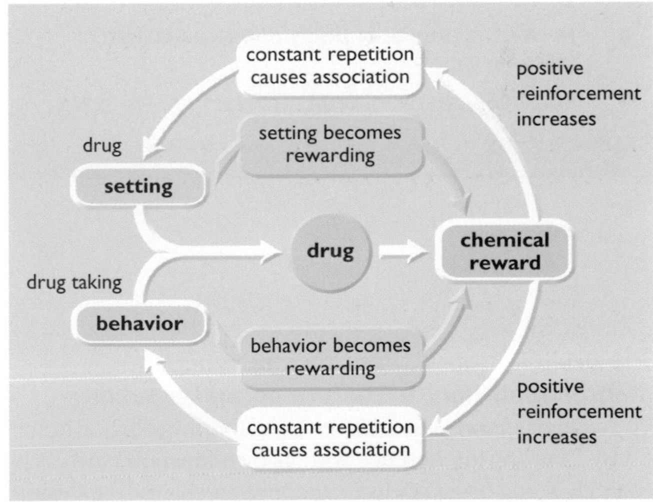

Fig. 30.4 Classic conditioning and drug rewards; the vicious circle leading to dependence. Drugs that induce pleasure do so by producing some kind of chemical reward in the brain. When the behavior of drug taking is repeated frequently, this rewarding effect becomes associated with the behavior that precedes it and the drug 'setting' in which it occurs. Gradually, this repeated association makes the drug-taking behavior and the setting become conditioned stimuli, capable of inducing the reward themselves. Now both the familiar setting and the behavior contribute to the reward, increasing the positive reinforcement for drug taking and increasing the strength of the drug habit.

Physiological dependence commonly begins after psychological dependence

On continued use of the drug, a subtle change commonly occurs in the drug-taker's motives: he or she will begin to feel unwell or unhappy as the drug is 'wearing off', and avoidance of these feelings becomes an additional reason to take the drug. Like rewarded behavior, this behavior can also be studied by operant conditioning methods (e.g. rats will readily learn to press a lever to stop something unpleasant happening to them). However, as the reinforcement for the behavior is unpleasant or negative it is called a 'negative reinforcement.' Similarly, the consequences of a drug leaving the brain are negative reinforcements for drug-taking behavior. As soon as this becomes a major motive for taking the drug, the dependence has shifted toward physiological rather than psychological dependence. This progression will then continue, because the effects of drug removal from the brain become more and more severe. At the same time, the drug rewards can become progressively less (Fig. 30.5). These changes in the relative importance of positive and negative reinforcements are related, and occur partly because the brain adapts to overcome the effects of drugs that are taken repeatedly.

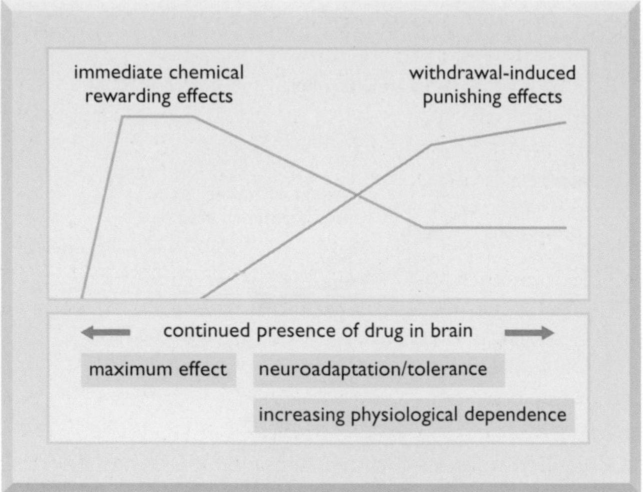

Fig. 30.5 Temporal changes in the rewards of drugs and the punishing effects of drug withdrawal during repeated administration. When a drug is taken frequently for several days there is usually a change in its effects. Initially, the first few experiences with the drug are similar (they may even increase, producing 'sensitization') and this is shown by the blue line marked 'immediate chemical rewarding effects.' At this time, punishing effects associated with a falling concentration of drug in the brain (red line) are usually minor or may be completely absent. However, as the drug is taken repeatedly, tolerance begins to develop to the rewarding effects of the drug (so the blue line gradually falls) and at the same time the punishing effects of removal of drug from the brain begin to increase (red line). The rate and extent of these two changes depend on a variety of factors including the drug, how frequently it is taken, and the route by which it is taken, but the principles are common to most drugs of dependence. They mean that someone who repeatedly takes a drug is likely to experience a gradual change in motive for taking the drug, from a compulsive desire for the positive rewarding effects of the drug (psychological dependence) to avoidance of the negative, punishing effects of drug withdrawal (physiological dependence).

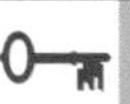
Motives for drug dependence

- Rewarding effects of drugs due to activation of dopamine systems in the limbic forebrain
- Rewarding effects of drugs due to activation of opioid systems
- Punishing effects of drug removal from the brain

The brain initiates adaptive mechanisms (neuroadaptation) to restore normal function

The central nervous system is designed for physiological homeostasis, and any interference with its own function (such as by centrally acting drugs) induces adaptive mechanisms to restore normal function. These occur at all levels of organization within the brain, but most is known about those that occur in individual nerves. This 'neuroadaptation' is sometimes simple, for example exposure to an agonist drug will often cause nerves to reduce, or 'downregulate,' the number of receptor proteins for that drug. This means that the drug has fewer receptor proteins in the brain on which it can act, and so its effects on brain function are reduced. This is one way in which chronic drug administration can lead to tolerance, in which the acute effects of the drug (e.g. a drug reward) become progressively less.

Neuroadaptation can cause physiological dependence

If a drug is rapidly removed after its long-term use, the brain is 'taken by surprise' and there is a finite period in which the adaptation (the receptor downregulation in this example) is still present, but without the reason for its existence (the agonist drug). During this time the natural agonist in the brain (e.g. a neurotransmitter) will be acting on a reduced number of receptor proteins without any help from the agonist drug. As a result, the function of the 'adapted' nerves will be altered and their activity will 'overbalance' in the opposite direction from the change that the drug caused originally. If the drug produced an acute reward of some kind, then exposure of the adaptation will produce an effect that is unpleasant or punishing.

The whole concept is a bit like a see-saw (Fig. 30.6), in which the drug perturbs the system in one direction. This is overcome by an adaptation that opposes the effect of the drug (producing tolerance), but when the drug is removed the adaptation causes the system to overbalance in the opposite direction, producing the signs and symptoms of withdrawal.

The early symptoms of withdrawal are usually considered to be the negative reinforcements that maintain drug-taking behavior in physiological dependence. Once this kind of adaptation has occurred, the consequences of preventing someone from taking their drug can be severe. The unpleasant effects of withdrawal can progress beyond the early symptoms to include specific psychological and physical signs that together make up the drug withdrawal syndrome. This differs markedly between the different classes of drugs of dependence (see Fig. 30.8).

Neuroadaptation that produces tolerance do not always produce physiological dependence

In the scheme discussed above, the same neuroadaptation that produces tolerance is also responsible for the physiological dependence because it causes the punishing effects of withdrawal. However, this is not always the case. For example, suppose nerves reacted to the presence of an agonist drug by changing their receptor proteins in a way that reduced the affinity of the drug for its receptor. Clearly, this could reduce the effects of the drug and produce tolerance, but it need not have any effect on the affinity of the natural agonist for the receptor. Removing the drug might therefore not have any functional consequences for the transmitter–receptor system. There are many adaptations like this that could lead to tolerance, but not withdrawal signs, and this is seen in the clinical situation: some people appear to be tolerant to a drug, but show no signs of withdrawal when they stop taking it. The converse can also be true.

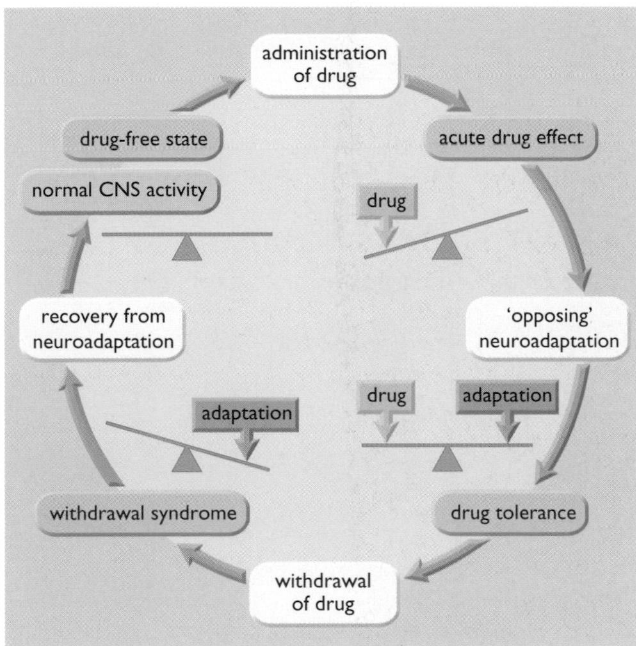

Fig. 30.6 Tolerance and withdrawal as consequences of neuroadaptation (the see-saw analogy). The cycle of drug taking begins at the upper left-hand side of the figure with central nervous system (CNS) activity in balance (the drug-free state). The first experience with the drug causes a chemical effect in the brain (the chemical reward), which unbalances the brain's chemistry in some way (the acute drug effect). If drug taking is repeated frequently, the brain begins to initiate adaptations in its chemistry to oppose the chemical effects of the drug. Now, CNS activity returns to normal despite the presence of the drug (the see-saw is balanced again), causing drug tolerance. However, if the drug is now removed rapidly (withdrawal) there is nothing to balance the chemical adaptation in the brain, and CNS activity overbalances in the opposite direction. This disturbance of brain function then causes the drug withdrawal syndrome, which will last until the brain can recover its normal function by removing the chemical adaptation.

A drug can produce withdrawal signs without much evidence of tolerance

Consider how nerves might adapt to an antagonist drug. As an antagonist will reduce the input to nerves from the natural agonist, the physiological adaptive response is to increase (upregulate) the numbers of receptor proteins shared by the antagonist and agonist. However, this does not have much effect on the response caused by the antagonist: it just increases the number of binding sites for the antagonist and agonist to compete for, and is therefore a poor explanation for tolerance. However, when the antagonist is removed from the brain, the natural agonist can act unopposed on the increased numbers of receptors, thereby causing functional changes during drug withdrawal. It is therefore possible to have withdrawal signs from a drug without much tolerance, and vice versa, but usually both occur (Fig. 30.7).

EFFECTS OF DRUG WITHDRAWAL

The explanations for the effects seen on drug withdrawal, discussed above, have some important implications for drug dependence. The signs and symptoms of a true withdrawal syndrome are usually the exact opposite to the acute effects of the drug, so stimulant drugs cause depression and lassitude on withdrawal, whereas anxiolytic drugs cause severe anxiety. Additionally, depressant drugs, including anxiolytics, alcohol, and opiates, have acute depressant effects on motor systems as well as altering feelings and emotions. As a result, neuroadaptation to depressants results in withdrawal syndromes that include overactive motor systems, leading to physical signs such as tremors and even seizures (Fig. 30.8).

Effects on the autonomic nervous system are also common during drug withdrawal, but it is not always possible to decide whether they represent neuroadaptation or are a nonspecific response to the stress of withdrawal.

Another important implication of the role of neuroadaptation in withdrawal relates to the time with which the drug leaves the brain. If this is rapid, there is less time for the brain to remove the adaptation and the consequences of withdrawal are likely to be severe. This is important when considering treatment strategies for drug dependence, because the severity of withdrawal can be limited by allowing the drug or a substitute to leave the brain very slowly.

The rate at which neuroadaptations occur may be an important factor in genetic differences in susceptibility to drug dependence. Additionally, rapidly occurring adaptations may become

Features of physiological drug dependence

- A tendency to take the drug to avoid the punishing effects of its removal
- Neuroadaptation leading to reduced effects of the drug on the brain
- Neuroadaptation leading to a syndrome of withdrawal when the drug is removed from the brain
- A withdrawal syndrome that includes signs and symptoms opposite to those induced by the drug acutely

conditioned to stimuli associated with drug taking in much the same way as for drug rewards.

CONDITIONED STIMULI FOR THE DRUG REWARD AND NEUROADAPTATION

As explained above, when drugs are taken repeatedly the drug-taking behavior and its setting can become conditioned stimuli for the drug reward. However, as the drug continues to be taken repeatedly, rapid adaptations to its effects in the brain are induced each time it is taken, and these, too, can become associated with the drug-taking behavior and setting.

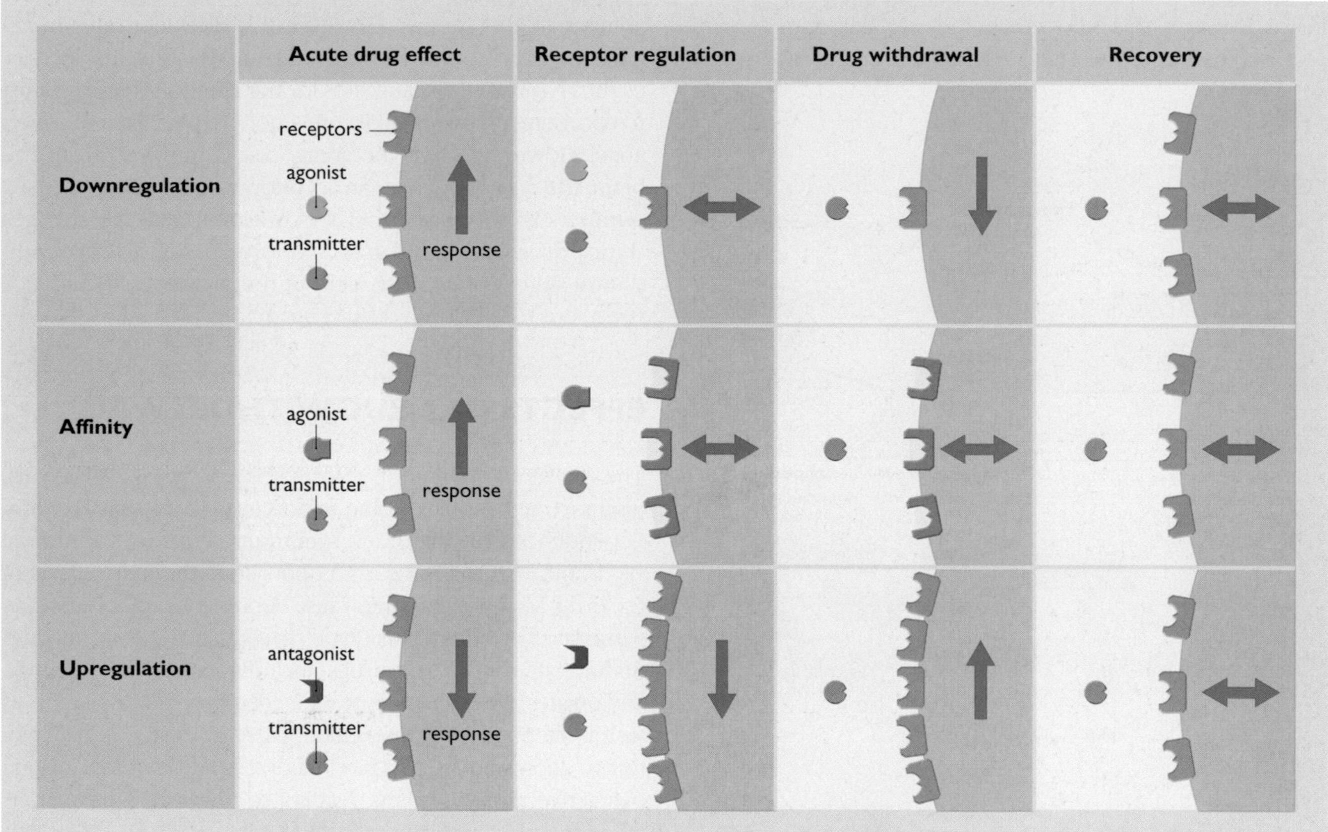

Fig. 30.7 Consequences of different types of receptor regulation for drug tolerance and withdrawal. The simplest type of receptor regulation is shown in the top panel. The acute effect of an agonist drug is to augment the receptor response (blue arrow) for the natural agonist (the transmitter) at these receptors. If this action persists (i.e. the agonist drug is taken repeatedly), the affected nerves downregulate these receptors, returning the receptor response to normal levels (horizontal arrow). Receptor regulation is therefore an effective mechanism for drug tolerance. However, when the drug is rapidly removed the transmitter is left alone with fewer receptors on which to exert its effect. The response will be reduced, providing a mechanism for functional changes associated with drug withdrawal. These may persist until the receptor population can return to the original drug-free state. A variation on this response to an agonist drug is shown in the middle panel. Here, nerves respond to the continued presence of the drug by altering their receptor population so that affinity for the drug, but not for the natural agonist, is reduced (a deeper binding pocket in the red receptors in the diagram). This effectively restores the normal response (i.e. produces tolerance), but causes no functional change on withdrawal. In the lower panel a common response to an antagonist drug is shown. Because the nerve receives a lower input (reduced receptor response) from the natural transmitter, it increases the synthesis (upregulates) the receptor proteins for this transmitter. However, this also provides the antagonist drug with more binding sites to exert its effect, and so is a relatively ineffective adaptation (i.e. it contributes little to drug tolerance). However, once the antagonist is removed, the natural transmitter has an increased number of receptors on which to exert its effect and this causes a functional increase in the receptor response associated with drug withdrawal. Receptor regulation can therefore explain either tolerance or withdrawal, or both tolerance and withdrawal, depending on the conditions.

Drug-taking behavior and its setting can elicit the reward and the adaptation to it

Consider someone who has repeatedly used alcohol in the same bar every night for years. As the environment has strong associations with the chemical reward (relaxation and euphoria), this chemical reward is anticipated as soon as this person enters the bar; as a result he feels better even before he has had a drink. However, the environment also acts as a cue to initiate the adaptive mechanisms that will oppose the effects of the alcohol as soon as it arrives in his brain. This gives his brain an advantage over the alcohol and means that the effects of the alcohol will be reduced specifically in the setting in which it is usually taken, referred to as 'environment-dependent tolerance' (Fig. 30.9).

However, what happens if the alcohol does not arrive in his

Types of tolerance, dependence, and withdrawal produced by drugs of dependence

Drug class	Drug	Reward and psychological dependence	Physiological dependence (tolerance)	Withdrawal syndrome
Stimulants	Cocaine	Strong, rapid, particularly intravenous or crack	Weak	Mainly psychological signs, severe depression, dysphoria, sleep disturbances, appetite
	Amphetamine	Strong, less rapid unless intravenous	Weak	As for cocaine
	Nicotine	Weak, rapid when smoked	Weak	Mainly psychological signs, irritability, anxiety, depression, appetite
	Caffeine	Weak, slow	Weak	Mainly psychological signs, irritability, depression, tiredness, headache
Depressants	Alcohol	Moderate, slow	Moderate	Severe; anxiety, depression, dysphoria, sleep disturbance, tremors, shakes and seizures, confusion, hallucinations
	Benzodiazepines	Weak, slow	Moderate	Moderate and variable; severe anxiety, dysphoria, sleep disturbances, feelings of unreality, tremors, seizures, hallucinations
	Barbiturates	Weak, slow	Marked	Severe; anxiety, dysphoria, sleep disturbances, tremors, seizures
Dissociative anesthetics	Phencyclidine, ketamine	Moderate	Weak?	Anxiety, dysphoria?
Analgesics	Morphine, heroin	Strong, rapid when intravenous or when smoked	Very strong	Moderate to severe; anxiety, dysphoria, sleep disturbances, muscle cramps, diarrhea, tremors and shakes
	Methadone	Less strong	Strong	Less severe (slow elimination)
Cannabinoids	Cannabis, tetrahydrocannabinol	Moderate, rapid when smoked	Moderate?	Weak; anxiety, dysphoria, sleep disturbances
Hallucinogens	Lysergic acid diethylamide, mescaline	Weak?	Weak?	Rare: unusual for use to be frequent enough to induce physiological dependence

Fig. 30.8 Types of tolerance, dependence, and withdrawal produced by drugs of dependence.

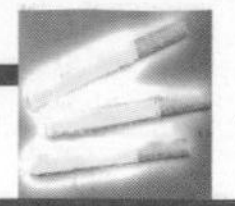

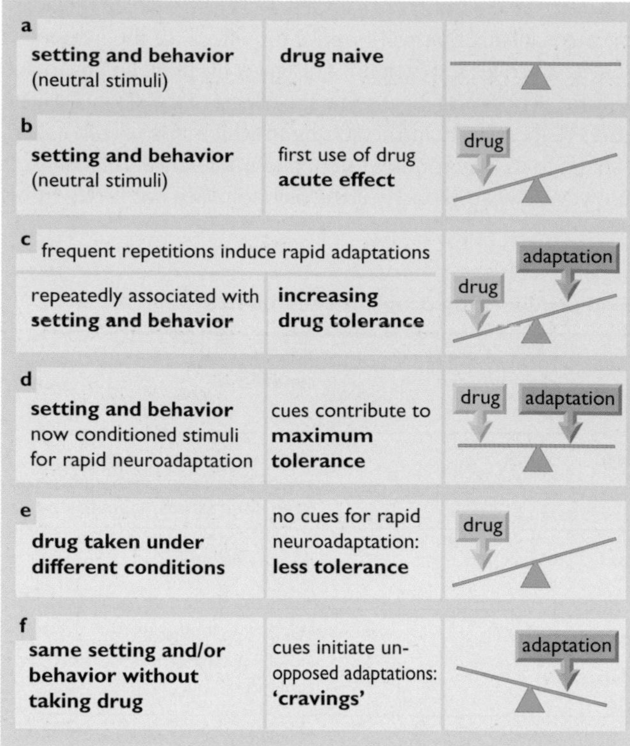

Fig. 30. 9 Contribution of conditioning to tolerance and craving: the see-saw analogy. In the drug-naive state (a), the behavior and setting that will become associated with drug taking are neutral stimuli (i.e. they produce no chemical or emotional effect on the brain). This persists during the first experiences with the drug (b), but with frequent repetitions of the drug-taking behavior in the same setting, these stimuli become associated with the drug reward (as in Fig. 30.3). However, as drug taking persists, rapid neuroadaptations are induced by each appearance of the drug in the brain and contribute to tolerance (c). Now these adaptations are repeatedly paired with the drug-taking behavior and setting, and so these become conditioned stimuli capable of initiating the neuroadaptation. Under these conditions, the behavior and setting can act as cues to initiate the adaptation even before the drug appears in the brain. At this stage they therefore contribute to the maximum tolerance attainable (d). This has two important implications. First, it means that a drug taken in an unfamiliar way and in an unfamiliar setting may produce a greater effect (an overdose) because tolerance is reduced (e). Second, it means that exposure to these cues without taking the drug (e.g. when someone is trying to quit drug taking) can initiate unopposed chemical adaptation in the brain (f), which might elicit feelings very similar to 'craving' for the drug.

brain because he has decided to quit drinking? The environment of the bar has induced adaptation to oppose the alcohol, but there is no alcohol to balance it. As a result, there will be a functional imbalance in the opposite direction from the acute effects of alcohol. This is very similar to the explanation of drug withdrawal, and the consequences can also be similar. In this case the individual may become very anxious and his hands start shaking, and these two early signs of alcohol withdrawal may overcome the resolve not to drink alcohol.

The drug setting and the drug-taking behavior have therefore become cues that act as conditioned stimuli for both the drug reward and the adaptation to it. They produce complex feelings, which are a mixture of the anticipation of the drug reward and sensations similar to withdrawal. These are very similar to the positive and negative reinforcements for drug-taking discussed above, but here they occur without having taken the drug.

The drug setting and drug-taking behavior can help produce the basis for craving

Just like the drug effects, the drug setting and drug-taking behavior can act as strong reinforcements for drug taking, and probably contribute to the phenomenon of craving, in which an irresistible desire to take a drug can resurface after months or even years of abstinence. It is essential to understand the mechanisms for craving because it often seems to be an important factor in causing a 'relapse' back to drug taking.

TREATING DRUG DEPENDENCE

There is a paradox in treating drug dependence because dependence in itself is not a problem; for example, it is accepted that up to half the population are dependent on caffeine. However, many drugs that cause dependence are:

- Harmful both acutely and chronically, so their use is associated with widespread morbidity (Fig. 30.10).
- Expensive, particularly those that are illegal, so dependence imposes a heavy financial burden, resulting in poverty and crime.

These factors make the treatment of dependence an important therapeutic goal, but success requires a dramatic and sustained change in the behavior of the dependent individual and this is difficult to achieve. Before attempting treatment, the reason why someone is taking the drug must be known. To an extent, this can be simplified into whether the individual is psychologically or physiologically dependent on the drug.

Psychological dependence is treated by interfering with the processes that have made drug taking a habit

When someone is psychologically dependent on a drug, the behavior is almost as important to them as the drug. It is the associations between the behavior (and its setting) and the drug reward that maintain drug taking, so that if these can be broken the habit can probably also be broken. This should be simple: if the dependent individual is allowed to continue his or her drug-taking behavior while gradually removing the drug, the association between the two should gradually weaken. In operant conditioning this process is called 'extinction' of behavior. An example would be a cigarette smoker trying to give up smoking by smoking cigarettes that are progressively weaker (in nicotine). This way the continued behavior of smoking becomes less and less associated with the nicotine reward and it should be easier to stop the behavior altogether when this association is lost. In practice, smokers often inhale more deeply or more frequently when they switch to low-nicotine cigarettes, titrating

Harmful effects of drugs of dependence

Drug	Acute toxicity	Chronic toxicity CNS pathology	Other pathology
Cocaine, amphetamines	Cardiac dysrhythmias, hypertension, stroke	Paranoid psychosis	Vasoconstriction and tissue anoxia at sites of injection, snorting or inhalation. Damage to fetal brain *in utero*
Ecstasy	Hyperthermia, exhaustion, dehydration	Neurodegeneration of serotoninergic nerves?	
Nicotine	Nausea, vomiting	Stroke (CVS effects), neurodegenerative diseases less common	CVS (nicotine and carbon monoxide): arteriosclerosis, hypertension, coronary heart disease
			Cancer (tar and nicotine): e.g. lung, bladder
			Respiratory (tar and nicotine): bronchitis, emphysema, asthma (passive)
			Fetus (nicotine): growth retardation (placenta?)
Caffeine	Anxiety, insomnia, gastric irritation, palpitations	'Caffeinism' (repeated acute toxicity)	Hypertension, cardiac dysrhythmia
Alcohol	Ataxia, nystagmus, coma, respiratory depression, death	Neurodegeneration (potentiated by vitamin B deficiency): e.g. dementia, cerebellar ataxia. Psychiatric illness: depression common	Neuromuscular: myopathy and peripheral neuropathy
			CVS: hypertension, cardiomyopathy, dysrhythmias (coronary thrombosis, arteriosclerosis, and thrombotic stroke less common)
			GIT: e.g. hepatitis and cirrhosis of liver, pancreatitis
			Cancer: e.g. liver, stomach
			Fetal alcohol syndrome: damage *in utero*, retarded postnatal development
Benzodiazepines	Hypotension, confusion (especially in the elderly)	Minor	Minor (fetal damage?)
Barbiturates	Confusion, sedation, coma, respiratory depression, death	Minor	Minor (fetal damage and respiratory depression in neonate?)
Dissociative anesthetics	Confusion, violent behavior, hyperthemia, paranoia, hallucinations	Flashbacks? paranoid psychosis?	Minor (fetal damage and respiratory depression in neonate?)
Heroin, morphine, methadone	Confusion, respiratory depression	Minor	Minor (respiratory depression in neonate)
Cannabis, tetrahydrocannabinols	Confusion, hallucinations	Flashbacks? psychosis? memory loss?	Lung cancer, immunosuppression, reduced testosterone secretion, (fetal developmental abnormalities?)
Hallucinogens	Confusion, terror	Flashbacks, psychosis?	Minor (fetal damage?)

Fig. 30.10 Harmful effects of drugs of dependence. (CNS, central nervous system; CVS, cardiovascular system; GIT, gastrointestinal system)

their drug reward to the same level as before. Nevertheless, this approach to breaking psychological dependence can often be successful, though it rarely forms part of a therapeutic strategy because it is assumed that people who require clinical treatment are also physiologically dependent on the drug in question.

Physiological dependence is treated by breaking the association between withdrawal phenomena and retaking the drug

In physiological dependence, drug taking is maintained by the negatively reinforcing properties of the drug (i.e. withdrawal phenomena). The objective in treatment is to break the association between these effects and the behavior of retaking the drug. The usual approach is to prevent the withdrawal phenomena by administering the same drug (or a substitute) in a different way (i.e. involving different behavior). This weakens the association between the original behavior and relief of withdrawal, and then by slowly tapering the dose of drug the patient can theoretically get to a drug-free state without developing a severe withdrawal syndrome. This whole process is called detoxification and is a very important part of treatment in all situations where withdrawal can be severe (Figs 30.10, 30.11). There are several examples of this approach:

- The treatment of cigarette smokers with a nicotine patch is a common example.
- The other common way of producing detoxification is to use a substitute drug that can prevent the withdrawal syndrome from the drug of dependence (this ability of the substitute drug is often called cross-dependence).

TREATING CIGARETTE SMOKERS WITH A NICOTINE PATCH

Here, nicotine is administered in a different way (i.e. transdermally versus smoking) so there is no association between the smoking behavior and either the positive or negative reinforcing effects of nicotine. Gradually the strength of the nicotine patch is reduced, allowing nicotine to leave the system slowly and smoothly over 2 or 3 weeks. This is another advantage of the patch as the pharmacokinetics of nicotine elimination mean that this would be very difficult during cigarette smoking. Additionally, transdermal administration of pure nicotine is much less harmful than smoking tobacco. This technique is associated with the following features, all of which are common to successful methods for detoxification (Fig. 30.11):

- Reduced association between behavior and reinforcements.
- Slower elimination.
- Reduced toxicity.

Using a substitute drug to prevent the withdrawal syndrome

Methadone is a heroin substitute

The best example of producing detoxification by using a substitute drug is the use of methadone in people who have been using heroin intravenously. Methadone, just like heroin, is an opiate receptor agonist, and so it can prevent the consequences of heroin removal. Its big advantage over heroin is that it is administered orally rather than intravenously. Not only is this a different drug-taking behavior, but it is also less dangerous than intravenous injection because it does not have the attendant risks of bloodborne diseases such as human immunodeficiency virus (HIV) infection. Additionally, methadone is less positively reinforcing, partly owing to the slow pharmacokinetics of oral administration. Also, in order to wean a patient off the drug, it can be allowed to leave the body much more slowly than heroin, again owing to the pharmacokinetics of oral administration. All these factors should make methadone substitution an ideal way to convert someone from using heroin to a drug-free condition. In practice, many people who are switched to methadone stay on this drug for years because they become physiologically

Treatments used for detoxification in drug dependence

Drug	Detoxification	Comments
Cocaine, amphetamine	Antidepressant drug (e.g. imipramine and desipramine)	Not really detoxification. Symptomatic treatment of withdrawal depression and reduction of withdrawal-induced craving?
Nicotine	Nicotine preparation with slower elimination (e.g. dermal patch, gum)	Much lower toxicity than smoking, but some cardiovascular toxicity, nightmares, skin rashes
Alcohol	Sedative/hypnotic (e.g. diazepam, chlormethiazole*)	Toxicity strongly potentiated by alcohol relapse, possibility of inducing iatrogenic dependence
Benzodiazepines	Substitute longer-acting benzodiazepine	Not all patients can cope with tapering dose of substitute drug; acceptance of dependence may be less traumatic
Heroin, morphine	Substitute a different opioid agonist (e.g. methadone, buprenorphine)	Many patients will not accept tapering of substitute drug, resulting in 'methadone maintenance' therapy. Oral route makes the substitute safer than intravenous injection

Fig. 30.11 Treatments used for detoxification in drug dependence.

dependent on methadone rather than heroin. They then stay this way because even slow withdrawal is unpleasant. Nevertheless, this treatment is much less dangerous than self-injecting heroin and in many ways methadone dependence is a successful outcome.

Benzodiazepines can substitute for alcohol

As for the substitution of methadone dependence for heroin dependence, the substitution of benzodiazepine dependence for alcohol dependence as a result of detoxification (see Fig. 30.11) is also an advance because it reduces morbidity. However, this kind of substitution (of one form of dependence for another) is not the true therapeutic aim.

ANTIDEPRESSANTS AND DRUG WITHDRAWAL

Depression is a major characteristic of withdrawal from cocaine and amphetamines, and imipramine (and similar drugs) are sometimes used at this time. This might be classified as a symptomatic treatment of withdrawal, but the close similarities between the mechanisms of these stimulants and antidepressant drugs (i.e. inhibition of catecholamine reuptake) suggests a stronger connection to substitution.

Drug dependence should probably be regarded as a chronic relapsing condition

Despite the availability of a variety of different treatments, most attempts to modify dependence therapeutically end in a relapse (see below). In fact, drug dependence should probably be regarded, in a similar way to asthma or diabetes mellitus, as a chronic relapsing condition. On this basis it would be easier to accept the idea that complete abstinence is not always an option and that any treatment outcome associated with reduced morbidity should be considered a success.

TREATMENTS TO PREVENT RELAPSE

Detoxifying a patient so that he or she is drug free is relatively easy but, even with continuing treatment, at least half will relapse into drug taking within a few months. Mark Twain summed it up nicely when he said (of smoking) 'Quitting is easy, I've done it several times.' There are several reasons why relapse occurs so frequently. First, recovering patients are very aware of the drug rewards that they have given up; their lives often feel empty and meaningless without them. If they cannot find other rewards in their lives (e.g. in personal relationships, religion, work) the pressure to return to taking drugs can be too much. This pressure is greatly increased by exposure to the drug-related cues that cause craving, such as returning to an environment in which drugs were taken, seeing friends taking drugs, and being offered drugs.

NONPHARMACOLOGIC APPROACHES

There are several nonpharmacologic approaches to counter the pressures to return to drug taking, for example:

- Emphasizing other life rewards.
- Removal from the environment and social group associated with drug taking.
- Cue exposure with psychological support.

Many of these are provided by lay support groups, e.g. Alcoholics Anonymous. All are at least as effective as any pharmacologic intervention, but some drugs are also useful, though the evidence is not always convincing.

PHARMACOLOGIC APPROACHES

Some drugs prevent the rewarding effects of the misused drug

The simplest pharmacologic approach to drug abuse is to give the patient an antagonist of some sort that will prevent the effects of the drug that is being abused (Fig. 30.12), for example:

- Naltrexone to prevent the rewarding effects of heroin.
- Dopamine antagonists may prevent the effects of cocaine (this is under investigation).

In fact, the same drugs (antagonists at opiate and dopamine receptors) can probably be used to reduce the rewarding effects of all the drugs of dependence, since they all act through the same pleasure pathways. The intention is that the patient receiving the antagonist knows that there is no point in relapsing into drug taking because it will not provide the usual reward.

In the jargon of operant conditioning, the antagonist is described as a 'negative discriminative stimulus'; while it is present, the behavior (of drug taking) will not be rewarded. Therapeutically this is an unusual concept because the antagonist has little pharmacologic effect in the absence of the agonist, yet maintaining this absence is the object of the treatment! In fact, any effect the antagonist does have alone is often a problem. All these drugs interfere with the natural systems in the brain that mediate pleasure, and someone taking them may experience anhedonia (the inability to feel pleasure). This makes patient compliance a problem and the approach is useful clinically only in patients who are highly motivated. The approach can be improved (theoretically at least) by using a partial agonist instead of an antagonist (e.g. buprenorphine instead of naltrexone). Because such a drug has some rewarding effects itself, compliance is improved, but the drug is effective therapeutically because it can still reduce the high caused by stronger agonists like heroin.

Some drugs convert the original drug reward into punishment

Another way to provide a negative discriminative stimulus for drug taking is to convert the original drug reward into punishment. The only true example is the use of the drug disulfiram in treating detoxified alcoholics. This drug prevents the breakdown of acetaldehyde (the primary metabolite of alcohol). As a result, when someone taking disulfiram drinks alcohol, he or she experiences the effects of an accumulation of acetaldehyde in the blood. This causes nausea, headache, and flushing of the face and neck, and is very unpleasant. If the treatment is successful this interaction never occurs because the patient does not drink alcohol while receiving disulfiram. However, if their resolve slackens, all they have to do is stop taking disulfiram and they are able to enjoy alcohol once again.

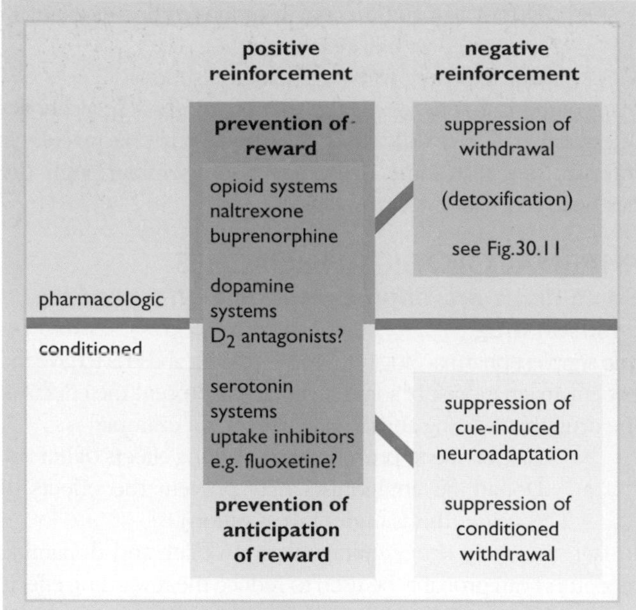

Fig. 30.12 Potential pharmacologic treatments for preventing relapse. The forces that lead to drug taking are depicted as either positive or negative reinforcements and arising either from direct pharmacologic effects of drugs of dependence (upper blue panels) or from conditioning that develops over the period of repetitive drug use (lower yellow panels). At present almost all therapeutic intervention is based on the pharmacologic effects of the drugs. This is usually capable of achieving detoxification (right blue panel), but often does not prevent relapse. Treatments that are effective against the pharmacologic positive rewarding effects of drugs (green panel) may also reduce some of the conditioned positive reinforcements for drug taking, and this may help explain why drugs like naltrexone are effective against relapse. However, for some drugs under some conditions, conditioned negative reinforcement induced by cues previously associated either with withdrawal or with drug taking (right yellow panel) may be most important in relapse, and this is a very important area for pharmacologic and psychological research.

Pharmacologic treatment of dependence

- Detoxification by removing the drug from the system very slowly so that a serious withdrawal syndrome is less likely to be precipitated, or
- Substituting a safer drug that can prevent withdrawal and then removing this slowly
- Preventing relapse into drug taking by administering an antagonist or partial agonist
- Attempts to reduce craving (combined with psychosocial treatment)

Some drugs may affect the positive and negative aspects of craving

Finally, there are some treatments that may genuinely affect the positive and negative aspects of craving. The anticipation of drug rewards (positive aspects) may well use the same neurotransmitter systems as natural pleasures, and therefore be reduced by drugs like naltrexone and dopamine antagonists. If so, these drugs may be effective against craving but will suffer from the same disadvantages of compliance, discussed above.

The pharmacology of the negative aspects of craving may be similar to that of withdrawal, but has not yet been studied in any depth. However, it seems a good avenue for investigation. Acamprosate is a drug now approved for use in recovering alcoholics in Europe that may work in this way, but until more is understood about the mechanism of craving it will be difficult to prove this or to develop new therapies.

FURTHER READING

Bertschy G. Methadone maintenance treatment: an update. *Eur Arch Psychiatry Clin Neurosci* 1995; **245**: 114–124. [The clinical use of methadone in the treatment of heroin abuse.]

Hyman SE, Nestler EJ. Initiation and adaptation: a paradigm for understanding psychotropic drug action. *Am J Psychiatry* 1996; **153**: 151–162. [A review for those interested in complex mechanisms of neuroadaptation and their role in drug dependence.]

Littleton J, Little H. Current concepts of ethanol dependence. *Addict* 1994; **89**: 1397–412. [A review on alcohol dependence, this is also in the same issue as many other relevant reviews on drug dependence.]

Mendelson JH, Mellow NK. Management of cocaine abuse and dependence. *N Engl J Med* 1996; **334**: 965–972. [This review describes some of the current issues that are important for treatment of cocaine dependence – it is also relevant to some other stimulant drugs.]

Stolerman IP, Jarvis MJ. The scientific case that nicotine is addictive. *Psychopharmacol (Berlin)* 1995; **117**: 2–10, 14–20. [This review examines the current issues surrounding nicotine use and whether or not it is addictive.]

Woods JH, Winger G. Current benzodiazepine issues. *Psychopharmacol (Berlin)* 1995; **118**: 107–115. [An account of the controversy over the incidence of dependence on benzodiazepines.]

Make a provisional diagnosis and determine a rational pharmacologic treatment for the following hypothetical case.

A 24-year-old man is admitted to the emergency room with an overdose of morphine; he is unconscious with pin-point pupils and impaired respiration. He has been an illicit user of morphine intravenously for the past 2 years, since starting work in a hospital. Over the past 6 months, his performance at work has deteriorated considerably.

1. What are the major pharmacologic issues in the urgent care of this patient (see Chapter 7 for additional information)?
2. How might the acute detoxification of this patient be managed?
3. What approaches might be taken in the long-term management of this patient?

Indicate whether the following answers are true or false.

1. The diagnostic criteria for physiological dependence include
a) tolerance
b) alterations in blood pressure
c) intravenous drug use
d) a distinct withdrawal syndrome
e) harmful medical consequences

2. Identify the correct statements about the major neuronal pathway thought to mediate drug-induced euphoria
a) cell bodies in the substantia nigra
b) terminals in the nucleus accumbens
c) serotoninergic
d) dopaminergic
e) cell bodies in the hypothalamus

3. The method of tobacco administration that provides the most rapid access of nicotine to the brain is
a) chewing/sublingual
b) dermal patch
c) snuffing/intranasal
d) smoking
e) rectal

4. The mechanism of action of cocaine involves
a) inhibition of adenosine receptors
b) release of acetylcholine
c) inhibition of monoamine transporters
d) potentiation of dopamine in the nucleus accumbens
e) enhanced nerve conduction by action on Na^+ channels

5. Recognized common sequelae of cocaine or amphetamine use include
a) hypotension
b) cerebrovascular accident ('stroke')
c) paranoid psychosis
d) cardiac dysrhythmias
e) lethargy

6. Diseases that are more common in people who abuse alcohol include
a) hypertension
b) dementia
c) arteriosclerosis
d) coronary thrombosis
e) cardiomyopathy

7. Heroin withdrawal
a) can be suppressed with naloxone
b) is commonly treated with methadone substitution
c) is usually fatal if untreated
d) can sometimes be precipitated by cues associated with drug taking
e) lasts for 2–3 hours

8. Effective neuroadaptations to the presence of an antagonist drug at receptors for transmitter X include
a) a reduction in reuptake of neurotransmitter X
b) downregulation of receptors shared by the drug and transmitter X
c) an increase in release of transmitter X
d) an increase in coupling between receptors for transmitter X and intracellular signaling
e) increased breakdown of transmitter X

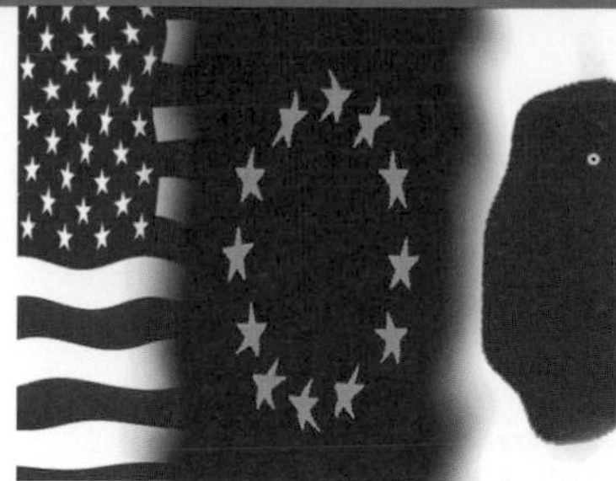

31. Regulation of Drug Use

Drug regulation seeks to ensure efficacy, safety, and chemical purity

Almost all drugs are sold for profit by pharmaceutical companies. Various methods have been developed to test whether a particular drug is effective, and most governments regulate the testing and eventual approval for sale. Drug regulations have several goals:

- To protect the public because there is a conflict of interest between the need of a pharmaceutical company to make a profit and the need of patients for a medication that is likely to benefit them.
- To apply standards of proof of efficacy and safety so that practitioners can be assured that a drug has been tested adequately.

Although it is ultimately the prescriber's responsibility to know what data support a drug's use in a particular setting and what the risks of such use are, an underlying assumption of regulation is that the prescriber needs assistance.

Drug testing progresses from animals to humans. Regulatory bodies:

- Set the policy that defines what animal data are sufficient before human studies can start.
- Enforce rules of manufacturing and purity so that the stated contents and amounts of a particular medication are accurate.
- To varying extents, limit what claims can be made about drugs in advertising.

STAGES IN DRUG DEVELOPMENT

Several stages can be defined from the discovery of a new drug to the demonstration of its clinical efficacy and adequate safety.

Animal studies set the scene for clinical trials

The presence of *in vitro* and *in vivo* pharmacologic effects forms the rationale for considering that a drug is likely to have some therapeutic benefit. Such data are needed before investigating a new drug in humans because there is always some risk to patients undergoing drug trials.

Animal experiments, often referred to as preclinical drug development, seek data from animal models of the human disease or syndrome that is the therapeutic target in humans. The success of such models to predict the outcome in humans varies widely, depending on how closely the pathophysiology in the model mimics the pathophysiology in people. For example, models of pneumonia caused by *Staphylococcus aureus* are quite predictive. The infecting organism is the same in the model and in humans, and the animal's immunologic defenses against the bacteria and pulmonary pathology are very similar to those in humans. In contrast, animal models of rheumatoid arthritis only indirectly mimic the disease in man and are less predictive. Usually, the ability to develop models in animals is related to a basic understanding of the pathophysiology of a particular disorder. In the above examples, the immediate cause of the pneumonia is known whereas in rheumatoid arthritis the immediate precipitating cause is not known.

Animals also serve other purposes in drug development. They can be used to investigate the relationship between drug dose and plasma concentration to beneficial and toxic effects. This can guide initial dosing in humans so that the first doses tested in people are not picked randomly. Animals are usually given doses that produce a much greater total exposure to the drug than that expected in people to exaggerate effects. Certain undesirable effects in people can then be anticipated during human testing. Sometimes the doses required for efficacy in the animal model produce severe adverse effects and preclude human studies. Animals are also used to screen for carcinogenic and teratogenic effects.

Human testing of drugs progresses through a series of clinical trials

Clinical trials begin after enough data have been generated to justify testing a new drug in humans. The three phases of drug development have been denoted as Phase I, Phase II, and Phase III.

Phase I denotes the first studies in humans, which are carried out under very close supervision and are usually single blind (Fig. 31.1) to find the lowest dose that cannot be tolerated because of unacceptable toxicity. Further testing is carried out with doses less than this dose. Traditionally, these studies have been carried out in healthy subjects, but healthy subjects are increasingly being replaced by the type of patients for whom the drug would eventually be used.

Phase II begins after the tolerated dose range has been defined. These studies are carried out in patients for whom the new drug is deemed to have potential benefit. The major purpose is to gather evidence that the drug has the effects suggested by the preclinical trials. Sometimes the endpoint of Phase II clinical trials is the actual goal of therapy; at other times a surrogate endpoint is used. Other purposes of Phase II trials are to define the pharmacokinetics of a drug and to relate plasma concentrations to effects. The influence of hepatic and renal disease on the elimination of the drug from the body is also investigated, and

Clinical trial terminology

Term	Definition
Control	The established therapy (or a placebo if there is no established therapy) against which the efficacy of a new agent can be compared
Randomized	Patients entering the trial have an equal probability of receiving the test or control agent so that factors that could affect the outcome, other than the therapy being tested, are equally distributed in the experimental and control groups
Double blind	Neither the health professionals nor the patient know whether the patient is receiving the experimental or control agent, to avoid any bias about which therapy might be better
Single blind	The health professionals know which treatment a patient is receiving but the patient does not know
Open label	The opposite of double blind. Both health professionals and patients know whether the drug is the experimental or the control agent and the dose that the patient is receiving
Parallel trial	At least two regimens are tested simultaneously, but patients are assigned only one therapy
Crossover trial	Patients receive each therapy in sequence and therefore serve as their own controls. For example, if therapy A is being tested against therapy B, some patients receive A before B and some receive B before A, so that the effect of the drug therapy and not of the order in which each therapy is given, can be tested
Endpoint	This is measured to assess a drug's effect (e.g. blood pressure is the endpoint for testing an antihypertensive agent, while pain relief is the endpoint for testing an analgesic)
Surrogate endpoint	An outcome of therapy that predicts the real goal of therapy without being that goal (e.g. reduction in tumor size as a surrogate for survival)

Fig. 31.1 Clinical trial terminology.

pharmacokinetic and pharmacologic interactions of the new drug with other drugs are explored. Phase II studies may be single or double blind and may be parallel or crossover in design, with patients being allocated randomly to treatment groups.

Phase III consists of the definitive clinical trials that establish efficacy and safety of the new drug. Whenever possible, the trials are double blind, randomized, and controlled. They are almost always parallel in design. Statistical considerations must be made in planning the design and size of all clinical trials, but especially Phase III trials, so that valid conclusions can be made when the trial is completed.

DRUG REGULATION

Drug regulation and approval proceeds by several steps

Although practices vary from continent to continent, drug regulation everywhere aims to ensure that marketed drugs are safe and effective. However, safe and effective are relative terms and require interpretation. Toxicity is tolerated for drugs that have beneficial effects in otherwise fatal diseases for which there are few if any cures, such as AIDS or many cancers. However, the safety requirements for an analgesic for mild to moderate pain will be quite different: only minimal and nonmedically serious adverse effects would be allowed.

In the US, the Food and Drug Administration approves drugs

In the US a pharmaceutical company submits preclinical data to the Food and Drug Administration (FDA) in a document called an Investigational New Drug (IND). The FDA then gives or withholds permission to initiate clinical trials in humans. As clinical trials proceed, the pharmaceutical company keeps the FDA informed of progress and any toxicities. When Phase III is completed, the company submits all preclinical and clinical data to the FDA in a New Drug Application (NDA). The FDA reviews the data and decides whether the data provide adequate documentation of safety and efficacy to support the use of the drug for a particular disease. The FDA will then approve the drug. If the data are not adequate, the FDA will ask for additional clinical trials. Part of the approval process consists of writing a 'label.'

The FDA also approves the manufacturing process and standards. Once an NDA is approved, the company may sell the drug.

In Europe, drug approval is obtained by centralized or decentralized processes aimed at producing more uniform practices across all member states

In Europe the regulation process is rapidly changing. Until recently, each country in Europe reviewed data and approved drugs separately, and requirements for approval differed from country to country Separate applications for approval were made to each country. With the development of the European Union, new procedures have recently replaced this country by country approval process. The result is that the prerequisites for approval have become uniform. The requirements to initiate trials in humans still differ from country to country. In general they are less restrictive than in the US. If a qualified clinical investigator deems that enough evidence has accumulated to justify testing in humans, the investigator is allowed to do so after summarizing the rationale for it. Regulatory authorities are notified that such testing is taking place, but they are less active than the FDA in actually approving such testing.

Information provided by the drug 'label' required for FDA approval in the US

- Data that support the approval
- Pharmacologic actions of the drug
- Indication (approved use) of the drug
- A description of adverse effects
- Instructions on dosing

Once clinical drug development has been completed, a pharmaceutical company can proceed by either a centralized or decentralized process, which ultimately result in more uniform practices across all member states. The process chosen by a pharmaceutical company depends on a combination of scientific, commercial, and political considerations.

THE CENTRALIZED PROCEDURE

Applications under the centralized procedure are submitted to the European Medicines Evaluation Agency (EMEA), which is responsible for administering the regulatory procedures and sending the application to the Committee on Proprietary Medicinal Products (CPMP). The CPMP, composed of representatives of all member states, then appoints a Rapporteur. The Rapporteur is identified with a particular country and the staff of that country's drug regulatory agency are responsible for the initial review. When the review is complete the Rapporteur prepares a report of the data, provides an opinion on approvability, and presents the report to the CPMP. The CPMP may then request further information and pose questions that the sponsoring company must answer. The CPMP then formulates its opinion and a decision is made on whether or not to approve the product. Approval by this centralized process entitles the pharmaceutical sponsor to sell the product throughout all the member states. The equivalent of the 'label' is the Summary of Product Characteristics, which is uniform in all member states.

THE DECENTRALIZED PROCEDURE

In the decentralized approach an application is made to one country, the so-called Reference Member State. The regulatory authority of that state reviews the data and makes a unilateral decision about whether to approve or not to approve the application. If the Reference Member State approves the application, a report is sent to each other member state; these have 90 days to accept the report and therefore approve the application, or object to the report, in which case the objections are sent to the CPMP for arbitration. The CPMP's decision is ultimately binding on all member states. Again, a uniform Summary of Product Characteristics is composed for all states.

In Japan, the approval process is carried out under the authority of the Ministry of Health and Welfare and the Central Pharmaceutical Affairs Council

Initiating clinical trials in Japan requires the approval of the Ministry of Health and Welfare (MHW). An application for approval is sent to the MHW after data have been assembled from clinical trials. The MHW acts as an administrative body and sends the data to the Central Pharmaceutical Affairs Council (CPAC) for review. The CPAC consists of experts in various disciplines such as medicine and pharmaceutical science, and recommends a course of action to the MHW, which implements the approval.

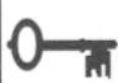

Drug development is a lengthy process

- The time taken from submitting an application for approval to receiving a decision can take from 6 months to many years, though 1–2 years is typical
- The process of drug development, from drug discovery to approval, typically takes from 6 to more than 10 years

FURTHER READING

Gogerty JH. Preclinical research evaluation. In: Guarino RA (ed) *New Drug Approval Processes*. New York: Marcel Dekker; 1987, pp. 25–54. [A thoughtful discussion of issues in preclinical research as it bears on clinical drug development.]

Japan Pharmaceutical Reference, 3e. Japan Medical Products International; 1993, pp. 14–34. [A description in detail of the requirements for approval for drugs in Japan.]

Mamelok RD. Drug discovery and development. In: *Clinical Pharmacology*, 3e. New York: McGraw-Hill; 1992, pp. 911–921. [A more detailed discussion of issues in demonstrating a drug's safety and efficacy.]

Indicate which is the correct answer for each question.

1. Regulatory agencies for drugs attempt to accomplish all of the following except?
 a) an evaluation of data on whether a drug is efficacious
 b) an evaluation of data on whether a drug's toxicity is acceptable
 c) an evaluation of preclinical data to decide if testing a new drug in people may proceed
 d) an evaluation of whether individual health care professionals are acting skilfully when administering drugs to patients

2. Controlled, randomized, double-blind clinical trials
 a) are biased because patients can choose a treatment to take
 b) do not compare a new drug either to a placebo or to an established agent
 c) are very important in Phase III of drug development
 d) are useful because health professional can draw a conclusions about a drug's efficacy while such trials are being conducted since they know which therapy the experimental patients are getting

3. A parallel trial differs from a crossover trial in that
 a) in a parallel trial, patients get all therapies and in a crossover trial patients choose which therapy to take
 b) a parallel trial is always controlled and a crossover trial is never controlled
 c) a crossover trial uses a surrogate endpoint, whereas a parallel trial uses a more definitive endpoint
 d) in a parallel trial, a patient receives only one regimen, whereas in a crossover trial, each patient receives several regimens

4. Which choice is true?
 a) the FDA has jurisdiction to approve drugs all over the world if the drug is manufactured by an American company
 b) the FDA can give advice to companies on when to initiate trials in people but can not prevent a company from doing so
 c) in Europe, both the centralized and decentralized procedure for approval more uniform among participating countries
 d) the FDA, the Committee on Proprietary Medicinal Products and the Japanese Central Pharmaceutical Affairs Council must agree before a drug is approved

5. In Japan
 a) the Ministry of Health and Welfare reviews data primarily for its scientific content
 b) the Central Pharmaceutical Affairs Council is primarily an administrative body without scientific qualifications
 c) the Central Pharmaceutical Affairs Council evaluates data and recommends a course of action to the Ministry of Health and Welfare
 d) drugs are approved by the CPMP

6. Which of the following is false?
 a) an endpoint is an indication of a drug's effect
 b) a surrogate endpoint is not the real goal of therapy but is predictive of the real goal of therapy
 c) 'open label' describes a clinical trial where both the health professional and patient know what agent the patient is getting
 d) an endpoint tells a health professional when a clinical trial is completed

Answers

7. Drugs and the Nervous System

1. This man obviously has a major mental illness and is at risk of deterioration. Admission to hospital for observation is probably the most appropriate course of management. It provides the patient with a place of safety, where the risk of harm to himself and others is minimized, and allows the healthcare team an opportunity to assess the patient more fully and gain more information about his illness. Treatment may also be started as soon as a diagnosis is made.
2. The two most likely diagnoses are acute schizophrenia (additional features required to make this diagnosis are more abnormal thought phenomena, mood incongruent delusions, and negative schizophrenic symptoms) and a major depressive disorder (any biologic symptoms of depression, a previous history of depression, and good premorbid adjustment).
3. Acute schizophrenia: any class of antipsychotic may be used. If sedation is required either a sedative neuroleptic, such as chlorpromazine, may be administered or a combination of a nonsedative antipsychotic, such as risperidone, and a short-acting benzodiazepine, such as lorazepam. There is an increasing tendency to use atypical antipsychotics, such as risperidone, sertindole, or olanzepine, as first-line treatments because they cause fewer adverse effects and therefore enhance patient compliance. Clozapine may not be used as first line. Therapy should be continued for 2–6 weeks at a therapeutic dose. If the initial medication is ineffective you may switch to another class of antipsychotic and review the diagnosis, particularly looking for an affective (mood) component. Effective therapy after a first episode should be continued for at least 6 months to 1 year. Careful monitored withdrawal may then follow. Subsequent episodes require much longer periods of maintenance but there is yet to be a clear consensus over the length of this. The adverse effects are listed in the text and are class dependent. In general. all typical neuroleptics carry a high risk of extrapyramidal adverse effects, akathisia, and tardive dyskinesias.

   Major depressive disorder: any class of antidepressant may be used to treat major depressive disorder in this patient. As he is having difficulty sleeping, a sedative tricyclic such as amitriptylline may be used. If tolerance to adverse effects is an issue, an SSRI would probably be used. This would also be the class if the patient was suicidal. The drug should be used for at least 2 weeks and usually for up to 6 weeks to determine if it is effective. If the patient does not respond to the first line of therapy, then either an antidepressant of a diferent class can be used or lithium can be added to 'augment' the continuing dose of antidepressant. The effective medication would usually be continued for 6–12 months before a gradual decrease and cessation would be monitored. The adverse efeects would depend on the class of drug used and the reader is referred to the relevant text.

8. Drugs and the Cardiovascular System

1. Yes.
2. Serum creatinine and electrolytes, electrocardiogram, chest radiograph
3. Prompt lowering of blood pressure and relative ease in titrating an appropriate safe dose. Intravenous nitroprusside is commonly used in the emergency treatment of hypertension.
4. It is important to avoid lowering blood pressure too much in patients with severe long-standing hypertension to avoid decreasing cerebral blood flow. While somewhat arbitrary, an immediate goal of around 180/110 mmHg might be appropriate in this case.
5. The first goal would be to start oral drug therapy to wean the patient from the intravenous nitroprusside. The most important long-term goal should be to educate the patient about the critical need for regular medication.

9. Drugs and Blood

1. No. Alcohol is a direct marrow suppressant and alcoholics whose caloric intake is mainly alcohol may suffer from nutritional deficiencies such as folate. It is always a good policy to encourage moderation in intake of alcoholic beverages. This patient is probably suffering from anemia and has neurologic symptoms consistent with vitamin B_{12} deficiency. It would not be appropriate to send him home without further laboratory tests to determine his complete blood count, folate and vitamin B_{12} levels.
2. No. Encouraging patient to have a better life style with a balanced diet is always good clinical practice. However, vitamin B_{12} deficiency is commonly due to pernicious anemia and lack of intrinsic factor. Dietary B_{12} or common preparations of vitamin supplements will not contain adequate vitamin B_{12} levels to treat vitamin B_{12} deficiency due to pernicious anemia.
3. No. Although the patient's symptoms suggest B_{12} deficiency, it would be inappropriate to start patient on therapy without a definitive diagnosis unless the patient is critically ill. In addition, it would be inappropriate to commit the patient to life-long treatment for pernicious anemia without an appropriate workup to confirm the disgnosis. Furthermore, by treating the patient with folate and B_{12} concurrently, the clinician will lose the benefit of confirming the diagnosis when the appropriate therapy leads to clinical improvement.
4. Yes. The patient's symptoms suggest vitamin B_{12} deficiency. The complete blood count will assess the severity of anemia and the blood smear may reveal macrocytosis and polysegmented neutrophils, which would be very helpful in confirming the diagnosis. Folate levels are indicated since alcoholic patients often have nutritional deficiencies including folate that may contribute to this patient's symptoms.
5. The patient's macrocytic anemia further supports the initial clinical suspicion that he may be vitamin B_{12} deficient. The patient's alcoholism is probably not the only or the most immediate clinical issue.
6. No. Initial vitamin B_{12} supplementation should be through the parental route although long term treatment with large doses (1 mg) of oral B_{12} has been shown to be successful despite lack of intrinsic factor needed for receptor-mediated absorption.
7. No. The patient may also be folate deficient and folate replacement may correct his anemia despite vitamin B_{12} deficiency. However, if his B_{12} deficiency remains untreated, his neurological symptoms may progress leading to irreversible damage.
8. No. Iron-deficient patients usually present with normocytic or microcytic anemia.

10. Drugs and the Renal System

1. Take a mid-stream specimen of urine for microbiologic examination (culture and sensitivity).
2. Yes.
3. Amoxicillin or nitrofurantoin, depending on microbiologic results, for 3–5 days.
4. Proteinuria resolves and a clear second mid-stream urine specimen, taken 5–7 days after cessation of treatment.
5. Common adverse effects of amoxicillin are diarrhea, nausea, and rashes. Candidiasis is also likely in pregnancy. For nitrofurantoin, adverse effects include anorexia, diarrhea, nausea, and vomiting.

11. Drugs and the Respiratory System

1. This approach assumes an inconsequential infection and that the asthma can be ignored. It avoids drug complications, but does nothing to prevent the occurrence of possibly dangerous infections or troubling symptoms.
2. In the absence of information an antibiotic could be chosen on the basis of the probable nature of the infection (organism and prognosis), probable sensitivity to the antibiotic, and risk:benefit ratios for different antibiotics. When the identity of the organism causing the infection is not known, a best guess is based on clinical judgement. When the organism and its sensitivity are known, the choice is based upon the expected adverse effects and their frequency and importance. Since antibacterial efficacy should be high, the risk:benefit ratio depends on the adverse effects.
3. The choice of bronchodilator is based on the factors considered on pp. 233–236. The choice is between β adrenoceptor agonists for symptomatic relief, glucocorticosteroids to moderate the underlying immune processes (inflammation, release of autacoids) responsible for the asthmatic response, and aminophylline, which moderates the immune process and has some bronchodilator actions. β Adrenoceptor agonists provide good symptomatic relief, but have little effect on underlying pathology and aerosols can be difficult to administer in children. The major adverse effects include tremor and tachycardia, and tachyphylaxis can occur.
4. This is a careful, but expensive, approach. The blood tests would indicate the status of the immune system with respect to infection and/or allergy, while the culture and sensitivity test would indicate whether a pathogenic bacterium is present and its sensitivity to antibiotics. Such information provides a scientific basis for planning a therapeutic strategy.

5. It is now agreed that asthma is basically an inflammatory condition and that anti-inflammatory drugs should be used early in addition to a bronchodilator. In children chromolyn is very safe and low-dose oral aminophylline reduces the inflammatory response with fewer possible adverse effects of tremor and excitement. Glucocorticosteroid given as an aerosol lacks the adverse effects seen with systemic administration.
6. The most likely diagnosis is a self-limiting viral infection, which, as a result of an allergic or other liability to asthma, has led to symptomatic bronchoconstriction. A viral infection is not treated with antibiotics, but acute symptomatic relief of the asthma can be obtained with an aerosol β adrenoceptor agonist. Since allergic asthma has an inflammatory component with hypersensitivity to bronchoconstrictor agents, topical glucocorticosteroids or oral aminophylline are more appropriate to reduce the inflammation and hypersensitivity. Aerosol glucocorticosteroids have few adverse effects, while aminophylline therapy can be titrated to known effective blood concentrations. The duration of treatment would depend upon the nature of the asthma in this patient. Most guidelines for the therapy of asthma suggest reducing medication to the lowest possible level once the patient is symptom free.

12. Drugs and the Endocrine and Metabolic Systems

1. The patient shows clinical signs of glucocorticosteroid deficiency (nausea and weight loss) and mineralocorticosteroid deficiency (volume depletion, hyperkalemia) suggestive of adrenal failure (Addison's disease). Measurement of cortisol and aldosterone concentrations, as well as their regulatory hormones ACTH and plasma renin activity would confirm this diagnosis. A careful evaluation would exclude infection or neoplasm of the adrenals. The usual cause is autoimmune.
2. A synthetic glucocorticosteroid (e.g. hydrocortisone 10 mg po at 7 a.m., 5 mg po at 3 p.m.), and a synthetic mineralocorticosteroid (e.g. fludrocortisone 0.1 mg po daily)
3. Patients should be aware of the symptoms of glucocorticosteroid deficiency (i.e. unexplained anorexia, nausea and fatigue) and should wear an identifying bracelet. Since an endogenous adrenal response is absent, glucocorticosteroids must be increased temporarily if the patient has a significant febrile illnesses or gastroenteritis or undergoes surgery. The dose of synthetic mineralocorticosteroid does not usually need adjusting.
4. Adverse effects of glucocorticosteroid therapy are osteoporosis, accelerated arteriosclerosis, glucose intolerance, obesity, myopathy, cataracts, avascular necrosis of bone, growth retardation, and infections. Adverse effects of mineralocorticosteroid therapy are hypertension and hypokalemia.

13. Drugs and the Reproductive System

1. Ultrasound of the ovary to see if it is enlarged and has multipollinar cysts. Measure plasma concentrations of LH and FSH to see if the ratio of LH:FSH is high. Measure plasma testosterone concentrations to see if they are abnormal.
2. Diagnosis will probably be polycystin ovarian syndrome (PCOS). Treatment will depend on whether the infertility is to be cured, or for hirsutism. For fertility, clomphene, if this fails gonadotropin prepartations (FSH followed by LH), or pulsatile administration of GnRH analogs. These treatments should induce ovulation. For hirsutism, an antiandrogen such as cyproterone acetate either alone, or in combination with the combined oral contraceptive. The former will antagonize the action of the testosterone, the latter will suppress ovarian function and so prevent androgen synthesis.
3. Since erection involves psychogenic, neuronal, and vascular elements, these aspects may all need to be examined. However, careful questioning and investigation for nocturnal erections give useful clues as to further investigations. Intracavernosal injections will establish whether erection is possible.
4. All aspects of failure of erection can be treated with drugs, but with varying efficacy. Thus, if erectile failure has psychogenic origins, appropriate psychotherapy may be helpful, with perhaps a trial of yohimbine. Intracavernosal injections or intrauretheral administation will show the patient that erection is possible and can be used for long-term management if the condition requires.

14. Drugs and the Gastrointestinal System

1. The classes of drug that will alleviate the symptoms of peptic ulcer, but not bring about a cure, are H_2 antihistamines, proton pump inhibitors, sucralfate, and antacids.
2. In view of the cost, the drug prescribed was probably a proton pump inhibitor (e.g. omeprazole).
3. A relapse is liable to occur since omeprazole does not eradicate the underlying cause, which is infection with *Helicobacter pylori*.
4. The treatment would probably comprise one or more antibiotics with or without an H_2 antihistamine or proton pump inhibitor. However, the optimum treatment for *H. pylori* infection has yet to be determined.
5. Eradication of *H. pylori* will cure a peptic ulcer, and there will be no relapse provided that there is no reinfection.

15. Drugs and the Immune System

1. Antinuclear antibody, anti-DNA antibody, and serum complement. The most suspected disease from her history is systemic lupus erythematosus because the young female had facial erythema, decreased white blood cell count, and massive proteinuria. Thus, these three serological tests are necessary to make a definitive diagnosis for, and determine the disease activity of, SLE.
2. Chest radiograph, renal function tests, and renal biospy.
3. Glucocorticosteroid (methylprednisolone) 'pulse' therapy and then high-dose prednisolone. For several weeks until clinical and serological remissions. With low-dose prednisolone, for several years. Infection, psychosis, ischemic necrosis of bone, osteoporosis, diabetes mellitus, hyperlipidemia, cataract, and glaucoma.

16. Drugs and the Bladder

1. Appropriate choices are trimethoprim or quinolones.
2. Since other bcateria than *E.coli* may be the cause of infection, the results of the culture may or may not modify the treatment. A change of therapy is only motivated if the causative organism is insensitive to the given antibiotic (trimethoprim or quinolones).
3. Recommended treatment time is 10 days.
4. Most probably a combination of a weak detrusor and an increased outflow resistance associated with the infection (increased dynamic component of the outflow obstruction) contributes to the retention.
5. By blocking Ca^{2+} inflow necessary for contraction of the detrusor muscle, diltiazem will weaken detrusor strength.
6. Any drug that weakens detrusor contraction (most commonly drugs with antimuscarinic adverse effects, e.g. tricyclic antidepressants, antihistamines) or increases outflow resistance (eg ephedrine, phenylpropanolamine).
7. An α_1 adrenoceptor antagonist may decrease outflow resistance and improve bladder emptying.

17. Drugs and the Musculoskeletal System

1. The aspirin dose can now be decreased to avoid tinnitus, but as she has not responded clinically, consider discontinuing aspirin and trying other NSAIDs, such as diclofenac or naproxen.
2. Low-dose prednisone is usually very effective in reducing the pain and morning stiffness associated with rheumatoid arthritis. Doses of prednisone at 5 mg po daily (or less) are relatively well tolerated with minimal short- and long-term adverse effects. With clinical improvement, the daily dose can be tapered or an alternate day regimen can be initiated to minimize the potential concern of glucocorticosteroid-induced osteoporosis.
3. A 20-week trial of intramuscular gold salts without clinical response requires re-evaluation of the disease-modifying agents. Considerations would be to discontinue the gold injections and start another second agent, such as methotrexate or sulfasalazine. If it was left and there were partial clinical improvement, continue the gold injections and add a second disease-modifying agent, such as antimalarials, methotrexate, or sulfasalazine.
4. Methotrexate liver toxicity is dose and time dependent. The long-term concern is the development of cirrhosis and subsequent liver failure. Liver enzymes and serum albumin should be monitored monthly. If there are persistent abnormalities then the dose can be held or reduced and the abnormalities followed. If there is concern of underlying liver disease, or the abnormalities do not resolve, the risks of proceeding to a liver biopsy can be discussed with the patient. The patient will ultimately need to decide whether to continue with methotrexate after being fully informed by the physician.

18. Drugs and the Skin

1. The likely diagnosis is atopic dermatitis.
2. It is important that children with eczema are bathed daily because they have more bacteria, particularly *Staphylococcus aureus,* on their skin than children with normal skin, and there is now evidence that the staphylococcus might act as a superantigen to fuel the eczema. However, children with eczema should avoid detergents and therefore should not use soaps and bubble bath and should not have their hair washed in the bath. Aqueous cream or some of the commercially available emollients can be used as soap substitutes. As eczematous skin has an impaired barrier to transepidermal water loss, further losses must be minimized by adding an emollient to the bath water and applying an emollient all over the body after bathing.

3. In addition to emollients, topical glucocorticosteroids (mild or moderate only in the case of a 2-year-old) need to be applied in the short term to control the allergic inflammation in the skin. The risk of adverse effects resulting from the use of glucocorticosteroids of the appropriate strength for the child's age short term is less than the risk of damage to the skin from constant scratching and secondary infection with potential systemic spread.
4. Sedative oral antihistamines have been shown to be beneficial in the treatment of eczema, probably because they help to break the itch–scratch–itch cycle. Cetirizine and ketotifen may have additional antiallergic properties.

19. Drugs and the Eye

1. Reduced production and increased drainage of aqueous humor.
2. Nonselective β adrenoceptor antagonists are the first-line therapy.
3. Levobunolol hydrochloride, carteolol hydrochloride, and timolol maleate reduce the rate of aqueous humor production by blocking β adrenoceptors on the ciliary body, thereby decreasing the effects of circulating epinephrine.
4. Asthma, obstructive airways disease, bradycardia, heart block, and heart failure.

20. Drugs in Dentistry

1. This is not the correct approach. Although acute allergic reactions can be manifested in the mouth there should be other typical signs of an allergic reaction or a history of allergy. Antihistamines are not indicated because they would add to the drying effect and worsen the presenting symptoms.
2. This is not the correct approach. Generalized stomatitis is rarely, if ever, a symptom of a bacterial oral infection. Acute necrotizing ulcerative gingivitis can produce generalized pain and discomfort, but the oral examination should reveal significant gingival infection with necrotic tissue and not white patches. The patient should have an elevated body temperature and possibly lymphadenopathy. Antibiotic use without appropriate symptoms is inappropriate and could worsen the existing disease.
3. This is not the correct approach. Oral viral infections are associated with vesicle formation and rupture with an acute onset of pain. There should also be a fever, pain and lymphadenopathy. The symptoms do not support a diagnosis of a viral infection. Using an antiviral drug would not be effective or alleviate the painful symptoms.
4. This approach is partially correct as the presenting symptoms do appear to resemble those of acute pseudomembranous candidiasis. However, candidiasis is an opportunistic infection in the oral cavity and underlying factors can be contributory. Correcting underlying factors as far as possible is important in preventing reinfection. Advising the patient to avoid spicy or other types of foods that are irritating an already painful oral mucosa will make the patient more comfortable during the acute phase of the disease. The sore mouth may be preventing the patient from eating properly or drinking sufficient fluids. Nutritional and fluid support are always important in acute infections.
5. Nystatin is an antifungal and is not systemically absorbed. It is effective when used topically providing the patient is compliant. The drug therapy should be continued for 14 days initially. The preferable endpoint of therapy is when the cultures are negative for *Candida* or empirically, after 14 days if there are no symptoms and signs. Because nystatin is not absorbed systemically adverse effects are usually limited to minor gastrointestinal complaints if they occur. Allergy to this drug is very rare. Drug interactions are not reported with this drug, probably because of its lack of systemic absorption. It is therefore a first choice in patients who are already taking multiple drug therapy.
6. The identification of *Candida* species with hyphae in an oral culture are diagnostic for candidiasis. Sensitivity testing is not necessary unless the infection does not respond to the intial drug. The history does not suggest an immunocompromised patient. With a vague history of anemia, it is important to request laboratory tests that could assist in the overall evaluation. Laboratory data that could rule out anemia include ferritin, iron, folic acid, and vitamin B_{12} levels. A red blood cell count along with a microscopic inspection could help confirm or deny the presence of anemia. The smooth tongue with an absence of papillae is also seen in patients with anemia. Anemia is a contributory factor to opportunistic candidiasis.
7. This patient is taking several drugs that are associated with xerostomia: in particular, the antihypertensive drugs clonidine and hydrochlorothiazide. Alprazolam is also associated with a dry mouth. This combination of drugs and the age of the patient are sufficient to reduce saliva production. Saliva contains immunoglobulins and provides protective lubrication for oral tissues. When this is impaired, tissue aging and possible anemia present opportunistic circumstances for an oral yeast infection.

21. Drugs Used in Surgery

1. The immediate goal is to ensure that brain oxygenation is taking place. The 'ABCD' mnemonic is used to organize evaluations and therapy during any critical event in anesthesia and resuscitation. In this case study, the position of the tracheal tube should be verified using auscultation and expired capnometry while oxygen is administered through bag-valve ventilation. Then, the adequacy of breathing and circulation including intravenous access should all be urgently confirmed.
2. Assuming that the ABC evaluation did not provide any concerns other than failure to awaken and breathe, your differential diagnosis should include the following: excessive anesthesia; excessive opioid administration; hypocapnia; neuromuscular blockade; hypoglycemia; and cerebral ischemic event.
3. Reversible causes in the differential diagnosis are evaluated as follows: expired inhaled anesthetic monitoring for excessive inhaled anesthetic; expired capnometry for hypocapnia; peripheral nerve stimulation for neuromuscular blockade; and blood glucometer testing for hypoglycemia.
4. Antagonism of opioid-induced respiratory depression with intravenous naloxone can be accompanied by antagonism of analgesia, sympathetic stimulation (i.e. tachycardia, hypertension, arrhythmias, pulmonary edema) and stimulation of nausea and vomiting. Since the onset of action is 1–2 minutes, intravenous naloxone should be titrated in a conscious patient to avoid the above adverse effects. Naloxone has a short duration of action (30–45 minutes) compared to most opioid agonists, so the need for additional doses of naloxone requires careful monitoring.
5. Tracheal extubation should be delayed until the patient has the cognitive and physical ability to clear her airway; this will reduce the risk of aspiration and laryngospasm. She should be in the lateral position; this will reduce the risk of upper airway obstruction from the tongue falling back and aspiration should vomiting occur. She should receive supplemental oxygen; this will reduce the risk of hypoxemia from respiratory depression and obstructed ventilation. Pulse oximetry should be used for the early detection of hypoxemia.

22. Drugs and the Ear

1. No. The moisture of irrigation could make the infection worse. The ear should be kept dry.
2. No. An oral antibiotic, if given, is best used in combination with a topical antibiotic.
3. Perhaps. In mild infections, a topical antibiotic (neomycin plus polymyxin drops) alone can be effective.
4. Yes. Taking a culture initially can help to identify the etiologic agent, which may help direct further therapy of first-line treatment not effective.
5. It would be best to review the patient in 10 days because although the cultured bacteria may not be sensitive to your choice of first-line antibiotic, the infection may settle and not need further medication. Ciprofloxacin with gentamicin or tobramycin drops given with oral ciprofloxacin would be reasonable second-line treatment if the drainage persists.

23. Bacterial Infections

1. No. The presence of nuchal rigidity strongly suggests a diagnosis of meningitis and a bacterial etiology must be pursued since bacterial meningitis is usually fatal if not treated.
2. No. It is important to collect blood and spinal fluid prior to the institution of antibacterial therapy to determine the bacterial etiology and antibiotic susceptibility of the pathogen.
3. Yes. These tests confirm the diagnosis and guide therapy.
4. No. Cloudy cerebrospinal fluid (CSF) is due to a very high number of white blood cells, which occurs almost exclusively in bacterial meningitis. As bacteria multiply in the CSF approximately every 60 minutes, it is important to institute therapy as soon as the diagnosis of bacterial meningitis is probable.
5. A third-generation cephalosporin, usually cefotaxime or ceftriaxone.
6. No. Chloramphenicol is the alternative.
7. Vancomycin.

24. Viral Infections

1. Genital herpes in an immunocompromised host.
2. Culture vesicles for herpes simplex virus, and send acute (now) and convalescent (in 2–3 weeks) serum samples to demonstrate seroconversion.
3. Slow resolution over 3 weeks.
4. All except sorivudine.
5. Acyclovir.
6. Intravenous
7. Reducing the dose of cyclosporine may increase the risk of renal homograft rejection. Prednisone is increased to avoid the relative adrenocortical insufficiency that will occur during the stress of this severe infection.
8. No, knowledge of the patient's renal function is not critical for determining the size of the first dose. This is because only the apparent volume of distribution is critical in determining the drug concentration achieved with the first dose, and it is not expected to be markedly abnormal in a patient with mild–moderate renal insufficiency.
9. Yes, knowledge of the patient's renal function is critical for prescribing subsequent doses because acyclovir causes dose-related central nervous system toxicity and is eliminated by renal excretion.

25. Parasitic Infections

1. Ascariasis.
2. *Ascaris lumbricoides*, belonging to the Nematoda (roundworms).
3. By the ingestion of either mature eggs, contaminated vegetables or water.
4. Pyrantel pamoate and piperazine.
5. Pyrantel pamoate is a depolarizing neuromuscular blocking agent which inhibits cholinesterase causing slow contracture and spastic paralysis of the worm, while piperazine blocks the neuromuscular junction causing flaccid paralysis.

26. Fungal infections

1. Scrapings of scale and plucked hairs should be sent to the laboratory for microscopy and culture.
2. The crusts should be removed and regular shampooing is recommended. The child must be kept away from school until the treatment has become established (i.e. about 1 week). If the infection is zoophilic, the child can then return to school as human-to-human transmission is limited. If the infection is arthrophilic, however, she must remain off school until repeat scrapings are negative, and the school needs to institute a screening program.
3. Griseofulvin is the drug of choice because of her age.

27. Vitamins

1. Being vegetarian, the patient has a very high risk of vitamin B_{12} deficiency. There is no need for genetic advice.
2. By no means. The patient should become aware of belonging to a high risk group.
3. A multivitamin preparation may not be sufficient.
4. The patient does have a high risk of vitamin B_{12} deficiency with resulting folate deficiency.
5. Megaloblastic anemia due to vitamin B_{12} deficiency should be treated with vitamin B_{12}. To prevent neural tube defects, folic acid should be prescribed at least 3 months before pregnancy as well as during the first trimester.

28. Neoplasms

1. Yes. Treatment and prognosis is very different for different cancers.
2. Recurrent breast cancer, non-Hodgkin's lymphoma, and pancreatic cancer.
3. Although this presentation would be unusual, a similarly acute nonlymphocytic leukemia is a possibility.
4. Combination chemotherapy. The recommended treatment is CHOP (cyclophosphamide, doxorubicin, vincristine, and prednisone).
5. Yes. Previous treatment with doxorubicin. Unless provisions are made to use a cardioprotective agent or to prolong the administration of doxorubicin by infusion, there is a lifetime maximum of 450 mg/m^2 before the risk of cardiotoxicity begins to rise.

29. Toxins and Poisons

1. First, the source of poisoning should be removed and absorption minimized. Vomiting carries a high risk of aspiration due to the impaired neuromuscular reflexes. The lesions on the legs might include envenomation sites and wrapping them tightly with bandages will limit lymphatic drainage and venom absorption.
2. Respiratory failure may develop owing to severe muscle weakness and can be fatal. It is imperative that your friend is taken to the nearest hospital in case mechanical ventilation is required.
3. The absence of symptoms other than general weakness and ptosis indicates a specific neuromuscular defect. Botulism or tetrodotoxin envenomation (from an octopus) are unlikely because of their rarity and the absence of signs of parasympathetic blockade. Food poisoning and organophosphate poisoning induce an entirely different set of symptoms. Sometimes wounds from sea snake bites and coneshell stings are very small and the victim is unaware of having been bitten or stung. The probable cause of the symptoms is sea snake envenomation and the victim did not notice the bite.
4. There are antivenins for sea snake and coneshell venoms, but their availability is limited and may have to come from Australia. Specific treatments are available for the other possible causes of the victim's condition but are not relevant to this case if it is sea snake envenomation.

   Sea snake envenomation makes artificial ventilation mandatory until no longer needed. There is a risk of skeletal muscle lysis due to phospholipase activity in the venom, and myoglobinuria can damage the kidneys. The highest level of medical care is needed.

30. Drug Dependence and Drugs of Abuse

1. The major immediate threat to this patient's life is respiratory failure with carbon dioxide retention due to suppression of the respiratory center by morphine. There are two therapeutic approaches depending on the depth of respiratory suppression. A narcotic antagonist such as naloxone may quickly reverse respiratory suppression if a sufficiently large dose is given. If the response is not prompt enough or the patient's respiratory suppression is immediately life-threatening, respiratory tract intubation and ventilator support may be required (see Chapter 7).
2. Several drugs are potentially useful in managing acute morphine withdrawal, for example, clonidine ameliorates some of the unpleasant symptoms associated with withdrawal. Alternatively, therapy can be started with a substitute drug such as methadone.
3. The major issue in the long-term care of this patient is to prevent relapse. Maintenance therapy with methadone may be useful. In addition, non-pharmacologic approaches such as psychologic support and a change of environment and social group may be critical to long-term therapeutic success.

Answers

2. Drug Names and Classification Systems

1. a
2. d
3. b

3. General Principle of Drug Action

1. b
2. d
3. b
4. a
5. b
6. c
7. d
8. d

4. Quantification of Drug Action

1. d
2. d
3. b
4. d
5. d
6. a
7. c

5. Factors Influencing the Actions of Drugs

1. d
2. c
3. c
4. e
5. b
6. d
7. c
8. a

6. Drug Safety and Pharmacovigilance

1. a) F, b) T, c) F, d) F, e) F
2. a) T, b) T, c) T, d) F
3. a) T, b) F, c) F, d) F
4. a) F, b) T, c) T, d) F, e) T
5. a) T, b) F, c) T, d) T

7. Drugs and the Nervous System

1. a) T, b) F, c) T, d) F, e) T
2. a) F, b) T, c) F, d) T, e) T
3. a) T, b) T, c) F, d) T, e) F
4. a) T, b) F, c) T, d) F, e) T
5. a) T, b) T, c) F, d) F, e) F
6. a) F, b) T, c) F, d) F, e) T
7. a) T, b) F, c) T, d) F, e) T
8. a) T, b) F, c) T, d) F, e) T

8. Drugs and the Cardiovascular System

1. c
2. b
3. b
4. a
5. d
6. e
7. c
8. a

9. Drugs and Blood

1. d
2. c
3. a
4. d
5. c

10. Drugs and the Renal System

1. a) T, b) T, c) T, d) T, e) T
2. a) F, b) F, c) T, d) T, e) F
3. a) T, b) T, c) F, d) F, e) T
4. a) F, b) F, c) T, d) T, e) F
5. a) F, b) T, c) T, d) F, e) T
6. a) F, b) F, c) T, d) T
7. a) F, b) T, c) T, d) F
8. a) T, b) T, c) T, d) F, e) F

11. Drugs and the Respiratory System

1. c
2. a
3. a
4. a
5. e
6. c
7. d
8. c

12. Drugs and the Endocrine and Metabolic Systems

1. d
2. a
3. b
4. c
5. b
6. b
7. d
8. c

13. Drugs and the Reproductive System

1. a
2. d
3. d
4. c
5. b
6. b
7. c
8. b
9. d

14. Drugs and the Gastrointestinal System

1. d
2. b
3. d
4. c
5. c
6. c
7. d
8. d

15. Drugs and the Immune System

1. a) T, b) T, c) F, d) T, e) T
2. a) F, b) F, c) F, d) F, e) T
3. a) F, b) T, c) F, d) T, e) F
4. a) F, b) T, c) T, d) T, e) F
5. a) T, b) T, c) T, d) F
6. a) F, b) T, c) T, d) F
7. a) F, b) F, c) T, d) F, e) F
8. a) F, b) T, c) T, d) F, e) F

16. Drugs and the Bladder
1. e
2. c
3. c
4. e
5. c

17. Drugs and the Musculoskeletal System
1. b
2. d
3. d
4. d
5. a
6. d

18. Drugs and the Skin
1. a) T, b) T, c) T, d) T, e) F
2. a) T, b) T, c) T, d) F, e) T
3. a) T, b) T, c) F, d) F, e) T
4. a) T, b) T, c) T, d) T, e) F
5. a) T, b) T, c) T, d) T, e) T

19. Drugs and the Eye
1. a) F, b) F, c) F, d) T, e) T
2. a) T, b) F, c) F, d) T, e) T
3. a) F, b) T, c) T, d) F, e) F
4. a) T, b) T, c) F, d) F, e) T
5. a) F, b) T, c) T, d) T, e) F
6. a) T, b) F, c) T, d) F, e) T
7. a) T, b) F, c) T, d) T, e) F
8. a) F, b) T, c) F, d) T, e) F
9. a) T, b) T, c) F, d) F, e) T

20. Drugs in Dentistry
1. d
2. c
3. a
4. b
5. d
6. b
7. a
8. c

21. Drugs Used in Surgery
1. c
2. b
3. a
4. e
5. e

22. Drugs and the Ear
1. a
2. b
3. b
4. e
5. b

23. Bacterial Infections
1. d
2. e
3. a
4. c
5. b
6. d
7. e
8. b

24. Viral Infections
1. a
2. c
3. e
4. e
5. a
6. a
7. e

25. Parsitic Infections
1. d
2. c
3. b
4. d
5. a
6. d

26. Fungal Infections
1. a) T, b) F, c) T, d) T, e) F
2. a) T, b) T, c) T, d) T, e) T
3. a) T, b) F, c) T, d) T, e) T
4. a) T, b) T, c) T, d) T, e) T
5. a) T, b) T, c) T, d) T, e) T
6. a) T, b) T, c) T, d) T, e) T
7. a) T, b) T, c) T, d) T, e) T

27. Vitamins
1. a
2. e
3. b
4. a
5. b
6. e
7. c
8. d

28. Neoplasms
1.
2.
3.
4.
5.
6.

29. Toxins and Poisons
1. d
2. e
3. c
4. d

30. Drug Dependence and Drugs of Abuse
1. a) T, b) F, c) F, d) T, e)F
2. a) F, b) T, c) F, d) T, e) F
3. a) F, b) F, c) F, d) T, e) F
4. a) F, b) F, c) T, d) T, e) F
5. a) F, b) T, c) T, d) T, e) T
6. a) T, b) T, c) F, d) F, e) T
7. a) F, b) T, c) F, d) T, e) F
8. a) T b) F, c) T, d) T, e) F

31. Regulation of Drug Use
1. d
2. c
3. d
4. c
5. c
6. d

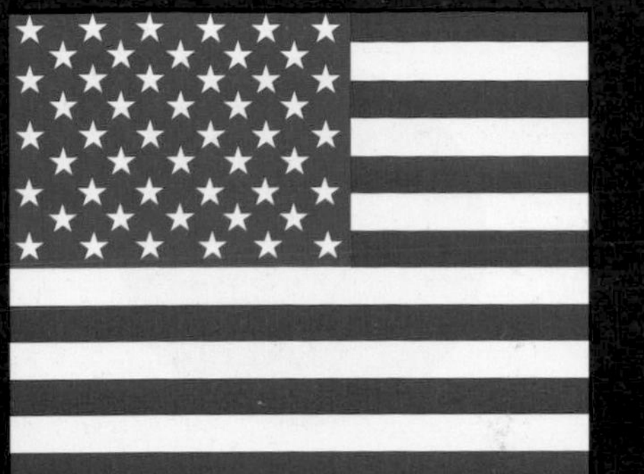

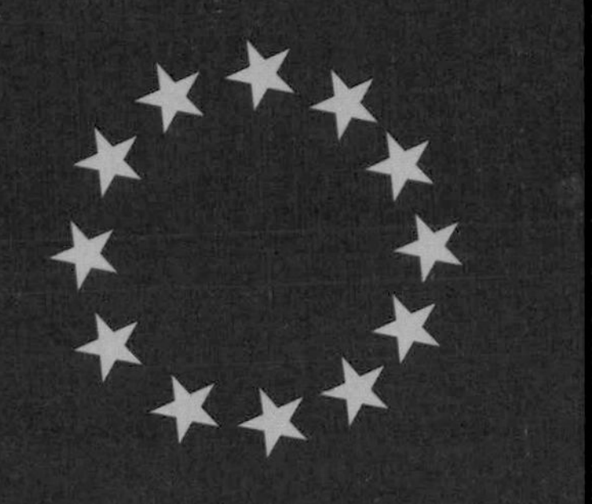

This drug index indicates the approved drug name in each of three key regions: the USA, European Union, and Japan. When a drug has not been approved in a particular region, the entry is blank.

acarbose	acarbose	acarbose
acebutolol	acebutolol	acebutolol
acetaminophen	paracetamol	acetaminophen
acetazolamide	acetazolamide	acetazolamide
acetohexamide		acetohexamide
acetylcysteine	acetylcysteine	acetylcysteine
acyclovir	acyclovir	aciclovir
adenosine	adenosine	adenosine
		alacepril
albendazole	albendazole	albendazole
albuterol	salbutamol	salbutamol
alclometasone dipropionate	alclometasone dipropionate	alclometasone dipropionate
alcohol	alcohol	alcohol
	alendronate sodium	alendronate sodium
alfentanil	alfentanil	
	alginates	sodium alginate
		alinidine
allopurinol	allopurinol	allopurinol
alprazolam	alprazolam	alprazolam
alprostadil	alprostadil	alprostadil
alteplase	alteplase	alteplase
	aluminium acetate	
amantadine	amantadine	amantadine
ambenonium		ambenonium
	amethocaine hydrochloride	
amikacin	amikacin	amikacin
amiloride	amiloride	
aminobenzoic acid	aminobenzoic acid	anthranilic acid
aminoglutethimide	aminoglutethimide	
aminoglycosides	aminoglycosides	aminoglycosides
aminopenicillins		
aminophylline	aminophylline	aminophylline
	4-aminopyridine	
amiodarone	amiodarone	amiodarone
amitriptyline	amitriptyline	amitriptyline
amlodipine	amlodipine	amlodipine
amobarbital	amylobarbitone	amobarbital
	amodiaquine	
	amorolfine	amorolfine
amoxapine	amoxapine	amoxapine
amoxicillin	amoxycillin	amoxicillin
amoxicillin-clavulanate		amoxicillin-clavulanate potassium
amphetamines	amphetamines	
amphotericin B	amphotericin B	amphotericin B
ampicillin	ampicillin	ampicillin
amrinone		amrinone
	amsacrine	
amyl nitrite		amyl nitrite

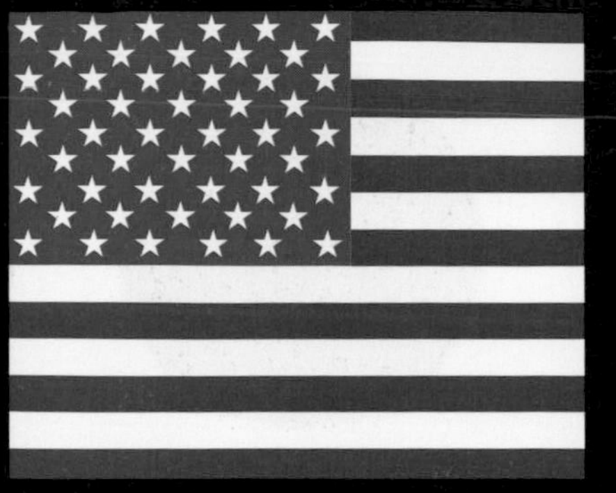	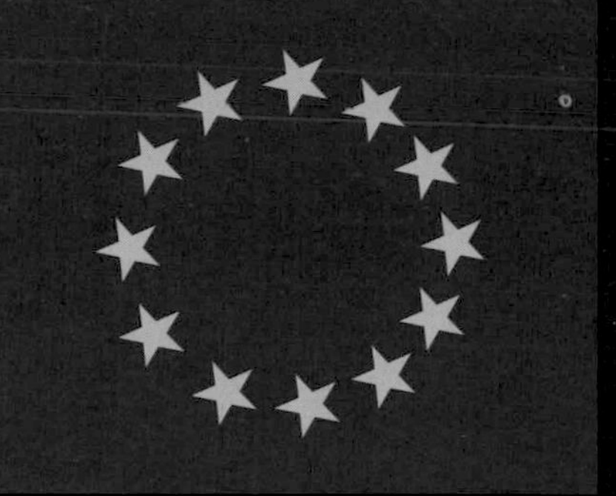	
	ancrod	
anistreplase	anistreplase	anistreplase
antazoline	antazoline	
	anthracyclines	
anthralin		
apomorphine	apomorphine	
apraclonidine	apraclonidine	
	artemether	
	artesunate	
asparaginase	asparaginase	asparaginase
aspirin	aspirin	aspirin
astemizole	astemizole	astemizole
atenolol	atenolol	atenolol
atovaquone	atovaquone	
atracurium	atracurium	
atropine	atropine	atropine
auranofin	auranofin	auranofin
aurothioglucose		
azatadine		
azathioprine	azathioprine	azathioprine
	azelaic acid	
azithromycin	azithromycin	azithromycin
aztreonam	aztreonam	aztreonam
bacitracin	bacitracin	bacitracin
baclofen	baclofen	baclofen
	bambuterol	
beclometasone dipropionate	beclomethasone dipropionate	beclomethasone dipropionate
benazepril		benazepril
bendroflumethiazide	bendrofluazide	
	benserazide	benserazide hydrochloride-levodopa
benzalkonium chloride	benzalkonium chloride	benzalkonium chloride
	benzamycin	
benznidazole		
benzocaine	benzocaine	benzocaine
benzodiazepines	benzodiazepines	benzodiazepines
benzoic acid ointment	benzoic acid ointment	
benzonatate		
benzoyl peroxide	benzoyl peroxide	
benzphetamine		
benztropine	benztropine	
	benzyl benzoate	
bepridil		bepridil
betamethasone	betamethasone	betamethasone
betamethasone valerate	betamethasone valerate	betamethasone valerate
betaxolol	betaxolol	betaxolol
bethanechol	bethanechol	bethanechol
	bethanidine	bethanidine sulfate
		bevantolol
bezafibrate	bezafibrate	bezafibrate
bicuculline	bicuculline	
biperiden	biperiden	biperiden
bisacodyl	bisacodyl	bisacodyl
bismuth		
	bismuth chelate	
bisoprolol	bisoprolol	bisoprolol
bithinol		

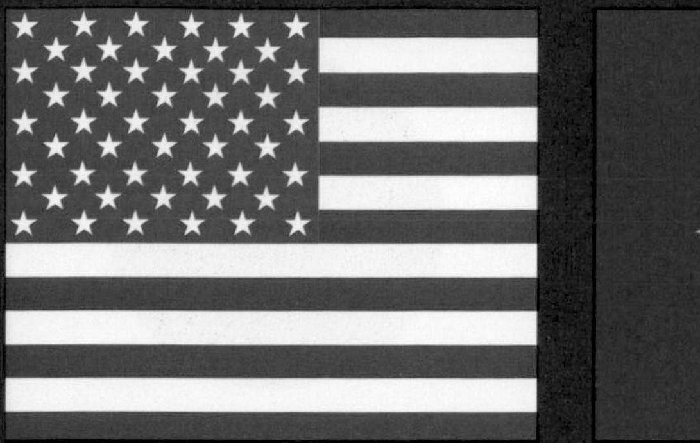
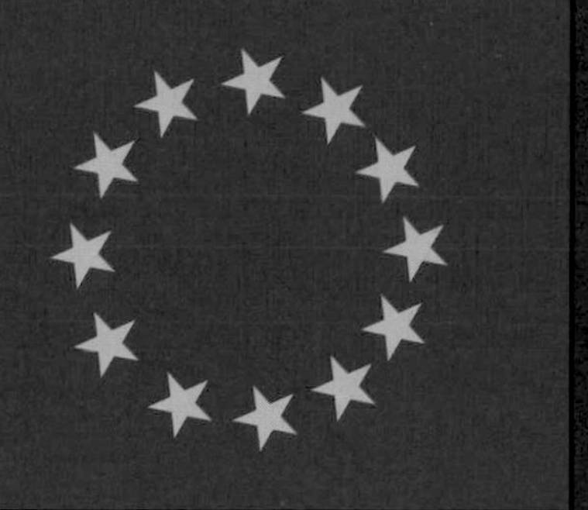

bitolterol		bitolterol mesilate
bleomycin	bleomycin	bleomycin
botulinum	botulinum	
bretylium	bretylium	
bromocriptine	bromocriptine	bromocriptine
brompheniramine	brompheniramine	
	buclizine	
budesonide	budesonide	budesonide
bumetanide	bumetanide	bumetanide
	α-bungarotoxin	
bupivacaine	bupivacaine	bupivacain
buprenorphine	buprenorphine	buprenorphine
bupropion		
buserelin	buserelin	buserelin
buspirone	buspirone	buspirone
busulfan	busulphan	busulphan
butoconazole		
butorphanol		butorphanol
caffeine	caffeine	caffeine
	calamine	calamine
calcipotriene	calcipotriol	calcipotriol
calcitonin	calcitonin	calcitonin
calcium gluconate	calcium gluconate	calcium gluconate
cannabis	cannabis	
	canrenoate	canrenoate potassium
capreomycin	capreomycin	capreomycin sulfate
	capsaicin	
captopril	captopril	captopril
carbachol	carbachol	carbachol
carbamazepine	carbamazepine	carbamazepine
carbapenem	carbapenem	carbapenem
	carbaryl	
carbenicillin	carbenicillin	carbenicillin
carbidopa	carbidopa	carbidopa
	carbomer	
carboplatin	carboplatin	carboplatin
carboprost	carboprost	
carmustine	carmustine	
carteolol	carteolol	carteolol
cefaclor	cefaclor	cefaclor
cefadroxil	cefadroxil	cefadroxil
cefamandole	cephamandole	cephamandole
cefazolin	cephazolin	cefazolin
cefixime	cefixime	cefixime
cefonicid		
cefoperazone		cefoperazone
ceforanide		
cefotaxime	cefotaxime	cefotaxime
cefotetan		cefotetan
cefoxitin	cefoxitin	cefoxitin
cefpodoxime	cefpodoxime	cefpodoxime
cefprozil		cefprozil
ceftazidime	ceftazidime	ceftazidime
ceftibuten	ceftibuten	ceftibuten
ceftizoxime	ceftizoxime	ceftizoxime
ceftriaxone	ceftriaxone	ceftriaxone

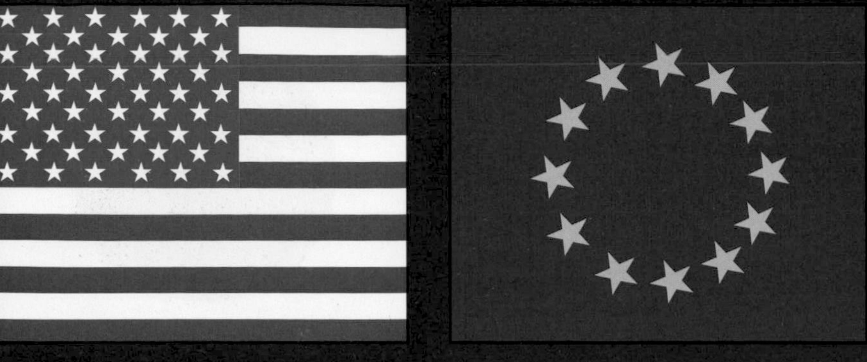

cefuroxime sodium		cefuroxime sodium
cefuroxime axetil	cefuroxime axetil	cefuroxime axetil
celiprolol	celiprolol	celiprolol
cephalexin	cephalexin	cefalexin
cephalosporins	cephalosporins	cephalosporins
cephalothin		cefalotin
cephapirin		cefapirin
cephradine	cephradine	cefradine
cetirizine	cetirizine	cetirizine
	cetrimide	cetrimide
chenodiol		
chloral hydrate	chloral hydrate	chloral hydrate
chlorambucil	chlorambucil	
chloramphenicol	chloramphenicol	chloramphenicol
chlordiazepoxide	chlordiazepoxide	chlordiazepoxide
chlorhexidine	chlorhexidine	chlorhexidine
	chlormethiazole	
chloroprocaine		
chloroquine	chloroquine	
chlorothiazide	chlorothiazide	
chlorotrianisene		
chlorpheniramine	chlorpheniramine	chlorpheniramine
chlorpromazine	chlorpromazine	chlorpromazine
chlorpropamide	chlorpropamide	chlorpropamide
chlorprothixene		chlorprothixene
chlortetracycline	chlortetracycline	
chlorthalidone	chlorthalidone	chlortalidone
cholestyramine	cholestyramine	colestyramine
ciclopirox olamine		ciclopirox olamine
cilastatin	cilastatin	cilastatin sodium imipenem
cilazapril	cilazapril	cilazapril
cimetidine	cimetidine	cimetidine
	cinnarizine	cinnarizine
cinoxacin	cinoxacin	cinoxacin
	ciprofibrate	
ciprofloxacin	ciprofloxacin	ciprofloxacin
cisapride	cisapride	cisapride
cisplatin	cisplatin	cisplatin
		citalopram
clarithromycin	clarithromycin	clarithromycin
clavulanate	clavulanic acid	clavulanate
clemastine	clemastine	clemastine
		clenbuterol
clidinium bromide		
clindamycin	clindamycin	clindamycin
clioquinol	clioquinol	
	clobazam	clobazam
clobetasol propionate	clobetasol propionate	clobetasol propionate
	clobetasone butyrate	clobetasone butyrate
clofazimine	clofazimine	
clofibrate	clofibrate	clofibrate
clomiphene	clomiphene	clomiphene
clomipramine	clomipramine	clomipramine
clonazepam	clonazepam	clonazepam
clonidine	clonidine	clonidine
clorazepate	clorazepate	clorazepate

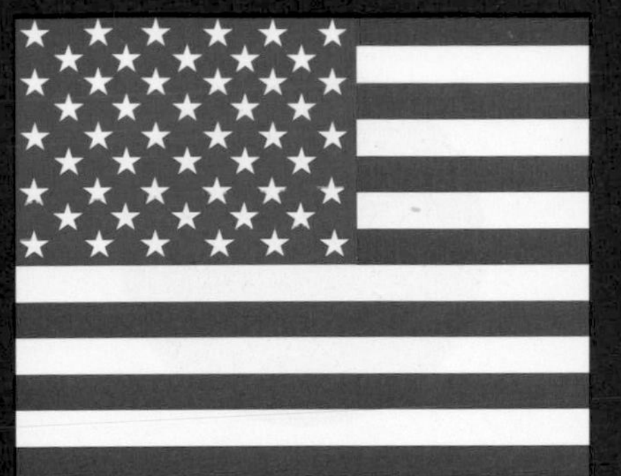
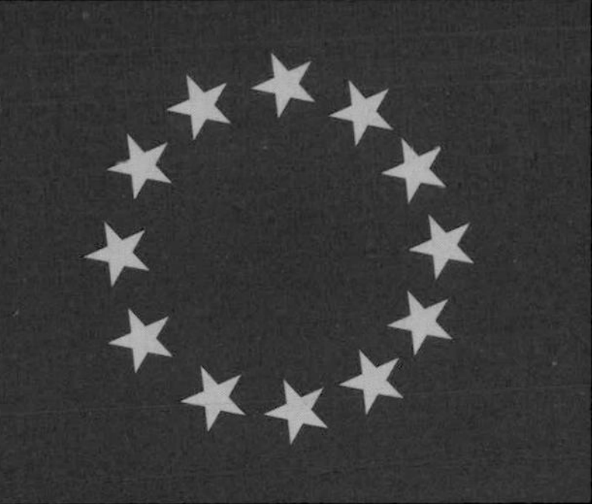

clotrimazole	clotrimazole	clotrimazole
cloxacillin	cloxacillin	cloxacillin
clozapine	clozapine	
coal tar	coal tar	
cocaine	cocaine	cocaine
codeine	codeine	codein
	co-dergocrine mesylate	
colchicine	colchicine	colchicine
colestipol	colestipol	
colistimethate		
colistin	colistin	colistin
	co-phenotrope	
corticotropin	corticotrophin	
cortisone	cortisone	cortisone
	co-trimoxazole	
	cromokalim	
cromolyn sodium	sodium cromoglycate	cromoglicate sodium
crystal violet	crystal violet	
curare	curare	tubocurarine chloride
cyclandelate		cyclandelate
cyclizine	cyclizine	
cyclobenzaprine		cyclobenzaprine
cyclopentolate	cyclopentolate	cyclopentolate
cyclophosphamide	cyclophosphamide	cyclophosphamide
	cycloserine	cycloserine
cyclosporine	cyclosporin	cyclosporin
cyproheptadine	cyproheptadine	cyproheptadine
	cyproterone	cyproterone
	cyproterone acetate	cyproterone acetate
L-cysteine	L-cysteine	L-cysteine
cytarabine	cytarabine	cytarabine
dacarbazine	dacarbazine	dacarbazine
dactinomycin	dactinomycin	dactinomycin
danazol	danazol	danazol
danthron	danthron	
dantrolene	dantrolene	dantrolene
dapsone	dapsone	
daunorubicin	daunorubicin	daunorubicin
	debrisoquine	
deferoxamine	desferrioxamine	desferoxamine
dehydroemctine	dehydroemetine	
		delapril
demecarium bromide	demecarium bromide	
demeclocycline	demeclocycline	demeclocycline
desflurane	desflurane	
desipramine	desipramine	desipramine
desmopressin	desmopressin	desmopressin
desogestrel	desogestrel	
desoximetasone	desoxymethasone	
dexamethasone`	dexamethasone	dexamethasone
	dextranomer preparations	
dextroamphetamine	dexamphetamine	
dextromethorphan	dextromethorphan	dextromethorphan hydrobromide
	dianette	
diazepam	diazepam	diazepam
diazoxide	diazoxide	

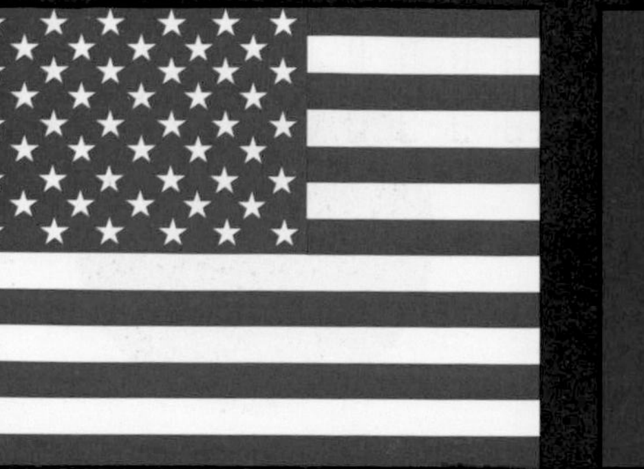 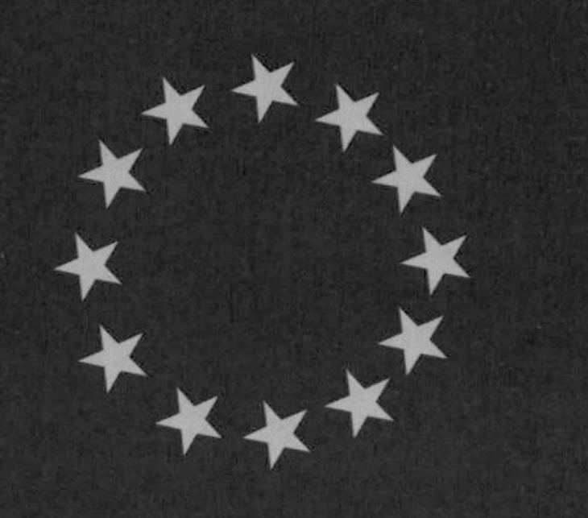 

		dibekacin
dichlorphenamide	dichlorphenamide	dichlorphenamide
diclofenac	diclofenac	diclofenac
dicloxacillin		dicloxacillin
dicumarol		
dicyclomine	dicyclomine	dicyclomine
didanosine	didanosine	didanosine
		dideoxyinosine
		dideoxycytidine
dienestrol	dienoestrol	
diethylcarbamazine	diethylcarbamazine	diethylcarbamazine
diethylpropion		
diethylstilbestrol	stilboestrol	diethylstilbestrol
	diflucortolone valerate	diflucortolone valerate
diflunisal	diflunisal	diflunisal
digitoxin	digitoxin	digitoxin
digoxin	digoxin	digoxin
	dihydrocodeine	dihydrocodeine phosphate
diltiazem	diltiazem	diltiazem
dimenhydrinate	dimenhydrinate	dimenhydrinate
dimercaprol	dimercaprol	dimercaprol
dinoprostone	dinoprostone	dinoprostone
	dioctyl sodium sulphosuccinate	dioctyl sodium sulphosuccinate
dioxin		
diphenhydramine	diphenhydramine	diphenhydramine
	diphenoxylate	
dipivefrin hydrochloride	dipivefrine	dipivefrine hydrochloride
dipyridamole	dipyridamole	dipyridamole
disopyramide	disopyramide	disopyramide
disulfiram	disulfiram	disulfiram
	dithranol	
	dizocilpine	
dobutamine	dobutamine	dobutamine
docusate sodium	docusate sodium	
	domperidone	domperidone
dopamine	dopamine	dopamine
doxacurium		
doxapram	doxapram	doxapram hydrochloride
doxazosin	doxazosin	doxazosin
doxepin	doxepin	
doxorubicin	doxorubicin	doxorubicin
doxycycline	doxycycline	doxycycline hydrochloride
droperidol	droperidol	droperidol
dyclonine		
echothiophate	ecothiophate	ecothiophate
econazole	econazole	econazole
edrophonium	edrophonium	edrophonium chloride
EDTA	EDTA	disodium edetate
eflornithene	eflornithene	
emetine	emetine	
enalapril	enalapril	enalapril
endorphilns	endorphins	
enflurane	enflurane	enflurane
enoxacin		enoxacin
enoxaparin	enoxaparin	enoxaparin
	enoximone	enoximone

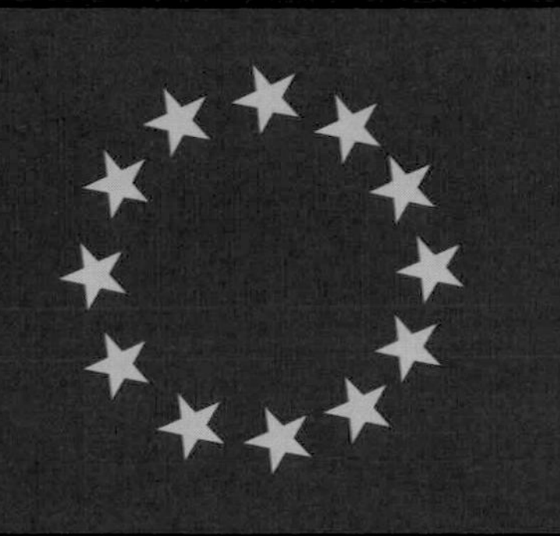

ephedrine	ephedrine	ephedrine
epinephrine	adrenaline	epinephrine
	epirubicin	epirubicin
epoprostenol	epoprostenol	
equilin		
ergocalciferol	ergocalciferol	ergocalciferol
ergonovine		
ergotamine	ergotamine	ergotamine
erythromycin	erythromycin	erythromycin
erythropoietin	erythropoietin	erythropoietin
esmolol	esmolol	
estradiol	oestradiol	estradiol
estradiol valerate	oestradiol valerate	estradiol valerate
estriol	oestriol	estriol
estrone	oestrone	estrone
ethacrynic acid	ethacrynic acid	etacrynic acid
ethambutol	ethambutol	ethambutol
	ethamsylate	ethamsylate
ethanol	ethanol	ethanol
ethchlorvynol		
ethinyl estradiol	ethinyloestradiol	ethinylestradiol
ethionamide	ethionamide	ethionamide
ethosuximide	ethosuximide	ethosuximide
ethotoin		cthotoin
etidocaine		
etidronate	etidronate	etidronate
etodolac	etodolac	etodolac
etomidate	etomidate	
etoposide	etoposide	etoposide
	etorphine	
etretinate	etretinate	etretinate
Factor concentrates	Factor concentrates	Factor concentrates
famciclovir	famciclovir	famciclovir
famotidine	famotidine	famotidine
felodipine	felodipine	felodipine
	felypressin	felypressin propitocaine hydrochloride
fenfluramine	fenfluramine	
fenofibrate	fenofibrate	fenofibrate
fenoprofen	fenoprofen	fenoprofen
	fenoterol	fenoterol
fentanyl	fentanyl	fentanyl
finasteride	finasteride	finasteride
flecainide	flecainide	flecainide
	flucloxacillin	flucloxacillin sodium
fluconazole	fluconazole	fluconazole
flucytosine	flucytosine	flucytosine
fludarabine	fudarabine	
fludrocortisone	fludrocortisone	fludrocortisone
flumazenil	flumazenil	flumazenil
flunisolide	flunisolide	flunisolide
fluocinolone acetonide	fluocinolone acetonide	fluocinolone acetonide
fluocinonide	fluocinonide	fluocinonide
	fluocortolone	
fluorescein sodium	fluorescein	fluorescein sodium
fluoride	fluoride	fluoride
	fluoroquinolones	

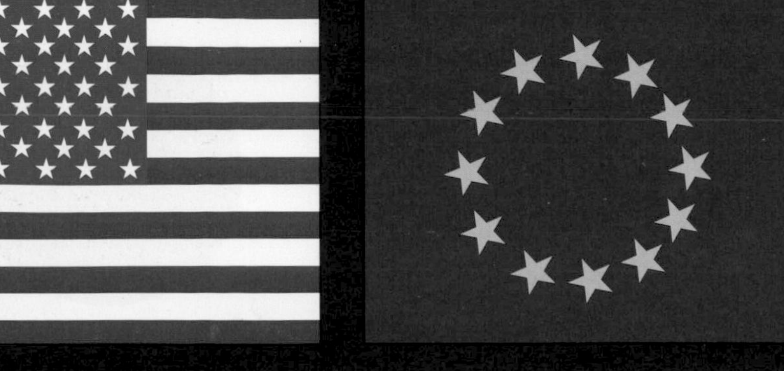

fluorouracil	fluorouracil	fluorouracil
fluoxetine	fluoxetine	
	flupenthixol	
fluphenazine	fluphenazine	fluphenazine
	flurandrenolone	
flurazepam	flurazepam	flurazepam
fluoxymesterone		fluoxymesterone
flurbiprofen	flurbiprofen	flurbiprofen
	fluorometholone	fluorometholone
flutamide	flutamide	flutamide
fluticasone propionate	fluticasone propionate	fluticasone propionate
fluvoxamine	fluvoxamine	fluvoxamine
folic acid	folic acid	folic acid
foscarnet	foscarnet	
fosinopril	fosinopril	fosinopril
	framycetin	
furosemide	frusemide	furosemide
fusidic acid	fusidic acid	fusidate sodium
GABA	GABA	GABA
gabapentin	gabapentin	
gallamine	gallamine	
	gamolenic acid	
ganciclovir	ganciclovir	ganciclovir
		gemcitabine
gemfibrozil	gemfibrozil	gemfibrozil
gentamicin	gentamicin	gentamicin
gestodene	gestodene	
	gestrinone	
glipizide	glipizide	
glutethimide		
glyburide	glibenclamide	glibenclamide
	glyceryl trinitrate	
glycine	glycine	
glycopyrrolate		
GCSF	GCSF	
GMCSF	GMCSF	
gold salts	gold salts	
gonadorelin	gonadorelin	gonadorelin acetate
goserelin	goserelin	goserelin
gramicidin	gramicidin	gramicidin
granisetron	granisetron	granisetron
griseofulvin	griseofulvin	griseofulvin
guanabenz		guanabenz acetate
guanadrel		
guanethidine	guanethidine	guanethidine
guanfacine		guanfacine
halazepam		
halcinonide	halcinonide	halcinonide
halobetasol		halobetasol
halofantrine	halofantrine	halofantrine
haloperidol	haloperidol	haloperidol
haloprogin		haloprogin
halothane	halothane	halothane
hemicholinium	hemicholinium	
heparin	heparin	heparin
heroin	diamorphine	

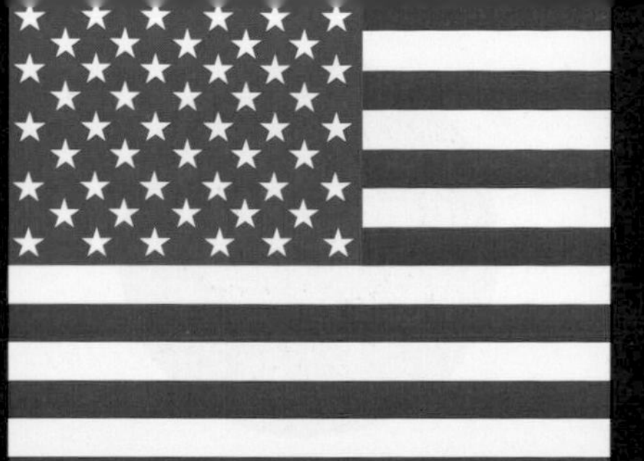

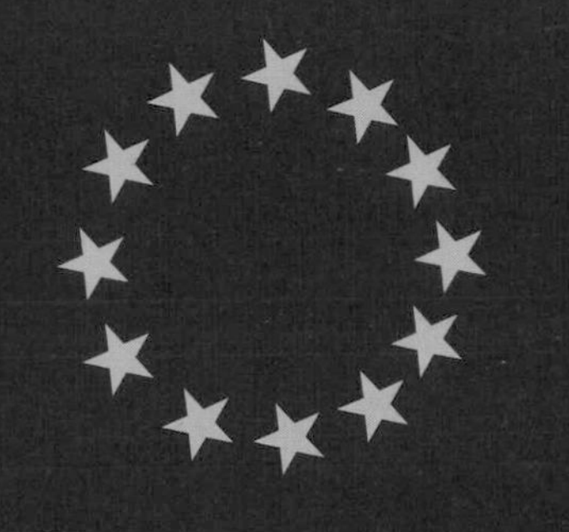

USA	EU	Japan
		hirudin
hexachlorophene	hexachlorophane	
histamine	histamine	histamine
histrelin		
homatropine	homatropine	homatropine hydrobromide
hyaluronidase	hyaluronidase	hyaluronidase
hydralazine	hydralazine	hydralazine
hydrochlorothiazide	hydrochlorothiazide	hydrochlorothiazide
hydrocodone		
hydrocortisone	hydrocortisone	hydrocortisone
hydrocortisone acetate	hydrocortisone acetate	hydrocortisone acetate
hydrocortisone butyrate	hydrocortisone butyrate	hydrocortisone butyrate
hydrogen peroxide	hydrogen peroxide	
hydromorphone	dimorphone	
hydroxychloroquine	hydroxychloroquine	
	hydroxyethylcellulose	
	5-hydroxytryptophan	
hydroxyurea	hydroxyurea	
hydroxyzine	hydroxyzine	hydroxyzine
	hypromellose	
ibuprofen	ibuprofen	ibuprofen
		ibutilide
	ichthammol	ichthammol
idarubicin	idarubicin	idarubicin
idoxuridine	idoxuridine	idoxuridine
ifosfamide	ifosfamide	ifosfamide
imipenen	imipenem	imipenem
imipramine	imipramine	imipramine
immunoglobulins	immunoglobulins	immunoglobulins
impromidine	impromidine	
indapamide	indapamide	indapamide
indinavir		
indomethacin	indomethacin	indomethacin
insulin	insulin	insulin
interferons	interferons	interferons
interleukin-2	interleukin-2	interleukin-2
iodoquinol		
	ipecacuanha	
ipratropium bromide	ipratropium bromide	ipratropium bromide
		irinotecan
iron	iron	iron
iron sulfate	iron sulphate	
isocarboxazid	isocarboxazid	
	isoconazole	isoconazole nitrate
isoetharine		
isoflurane	isoflurane	isoflurane
isoniazid	isoniazid	isoniazid
isoproterenol	isoprenaline	isoproterenol
isosorbide	isosorbide	isosorbide
isotretinoin	isotretinoin	
	ispaghula	
isradipine	isradipine	
itraconazole	itraconazole	itraconazole
ivermectin	ivermectin	
kanamycin	kanamycin	kanamycin
kaolin	kaolin	

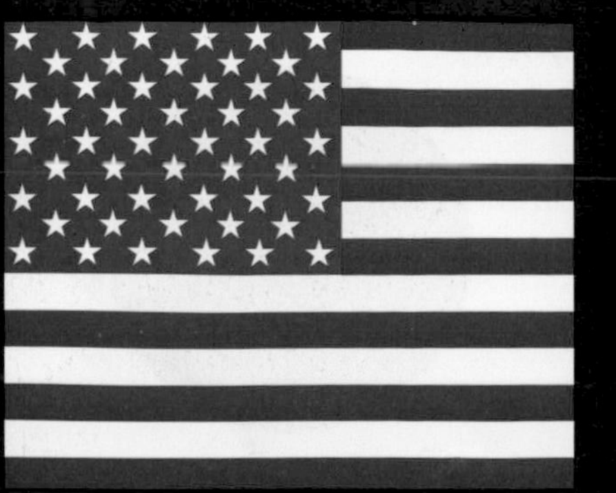

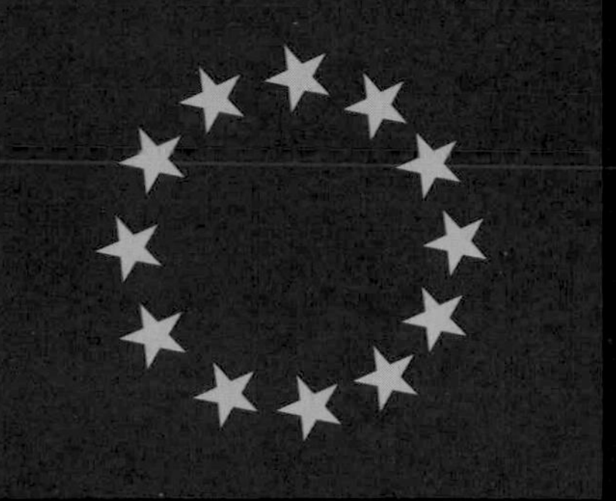

ketamine	ketamine	ketamine
ketanserin	ketanserin	ketanserin
ketoconazole	ketoconazole	ketoconazole
ketoprofen	ketoprofen	ketoprofen
ketorolac	ketorolac	ketorolac
ketotifen	ketotifen	ketotifen
labetalol	labetalol	labetalol
lactulose	lactulose	lactulose
lamotrigine	lamotrigine	lamotrigine
lansoprazole	lansoprazole	lansoprazole
leucovorin	leucovorin	leucovorin
leuprolide		leuprolide
	leuprorelin	leuproreline
levobunolol hydrochloride	levobunolol hydrochloride	levobunolol hydrochloride
levodopa	levodopa	levodopa
levonordefrin		
levonorgestrel	levonorgestrel	
levorphanol		
lidocaine	lignocaine	lidocaine
lincomycin		lincomycin hydrochloride
	lincosamides	
lindane	lindane	
	liquid paraffin	liquid paraffin
lisinopril	lisinopril	lisinopril
lithium	lithium	lithium
lithium carbonate	lithium carbonate	lithium carbonate
lomefloxacin		lomefloxacin
lomustine	lomustine	
loperamide	loperamide	loperamide
loracarbef		loracarbef
loratadine	loratadine	loratadine
lorazepam	lorazepam	lorazepam
losartan	losartan	losartan
lovastatin		
loxapine	loxapine	
	lysergide	dihidroergotoxinemesilate
	lysuride	
	macrogols	macrogols
mafenide		
malathion	malathion	
mannitol	mannitol	D-mannitol
maprotiline	maprotiline	maprotiline
mazindol		mazindol
mebendazole	mebendazole	mebendazole
mecamylamine		
mechlorethamine		
meclizine	meclozine	meclizine
meclocycline		
meclofenamate		meclofenamate hydrochloride
medroxyprogesterone	medroxyprogesterone	medroxyprogesterone
mefenamic acid	mefenamic acid	mefenamic acid
mefloquine	mefloquine	
megestrol	megestrol	
meglumine antimoniate	meglumine antimonate	meglumine amidotrizoate
melarsoprol		
melatonin	melatonin	

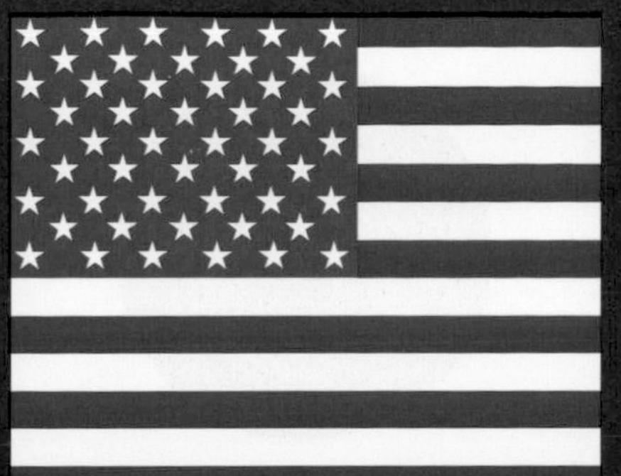
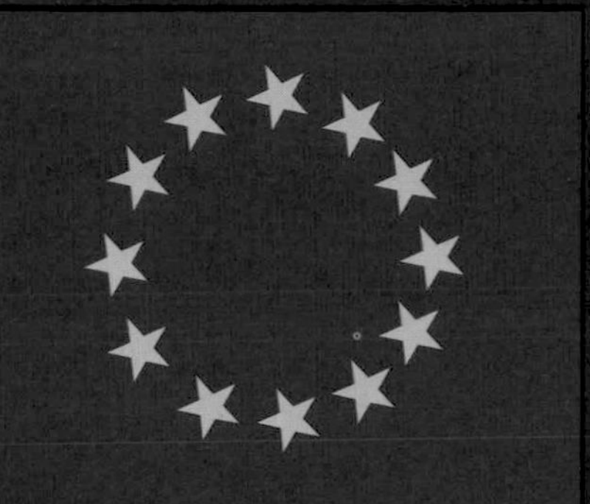

		meloxicam
melphalan	melphalan	melphalan
menotropin	menotrophin	
	menthol	l-menthol
	mepacrine	
meperidine	pethidine	pethidine
mephentermine		
mephenytoin		
mepivacaine		mepivacaine hydrochloride
meprobamate	meprobamate	
	mepyramine	
mercaptopurine	mercaptopurine	mercaptopurine
	mercilon	
meropenem	meropenem	meropenem
	mesalazine	mesalazin
mescaline	mescaline	
mesna	mesna	mesna
mesoridazine		
mestranol	mestranol	mestranol
metaproterenol		
metformin	metformin	metformin
methacholine	methacholine	
methadone	methadone	
methamphetamine		methamphetamine hydrochloride
methanol	methanol	
methantheline		
methazolamide		methazolamide
methenamine	hexamine	hexamine
methicillin	methicillin	methicillin
methimazole		
methohexital	methohexitone	
methotrexate	methotrexate	methotrexate
methoxamine	methoxamine	methoxamine
methoxyflurane		
methscopolamine	methyl hyoscine	
methylcellulose	methylcellulose	methylcellulose
methyldopa	methyldopa	methyldopa
methylphenidate	methylphenidate	
methylprednisolone	methylprednisolone	methylprednisolone
methyltestosterone		methyltestosterone
metipranolol	metipranolol	
metoclopramide	metoclopramide	metoclopramide
metolazone	metolazone	metolazone
metoprolol	metoprolol	metoprolol
	metriphonate	
	metrodin	
metronidazole	metronidazole	metronidazole
metyrapone	metyrapone	metyrapone
mexiletine	mexiletine	mexiletine
mezlocillin		mezlocillin
miconazole	miconazole	miconazole
midazolam	midazolam	midazolam
mifepristone	mifepristone	mifepristone
milrinone	milrinone	milrinone
minocycline	minocycline	minocycline
minoxidil	minoxidil	

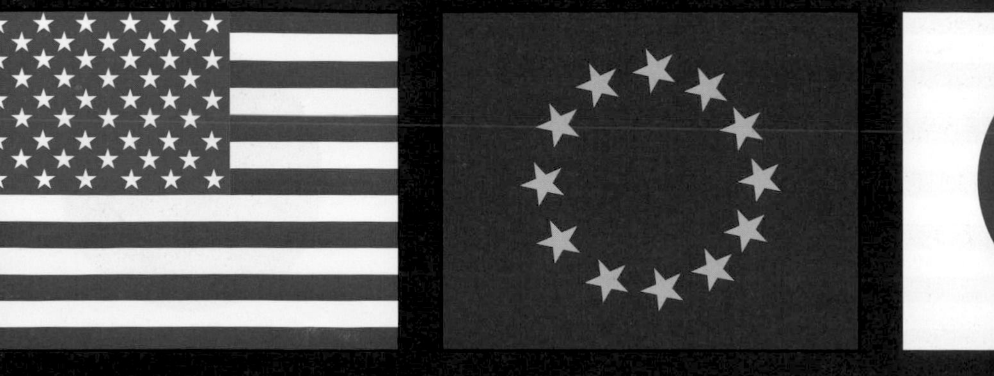

misoprostol	misoprostol	misoprostol
mitomycin	mitomycin	mitomycin C
mitotane	mitotane	mitotane
mitoxantrone	mitozantrone	mitoxantrone
mivacurium	mivacurium	
	moclobemide	moclobemide
moexipril	moexipril	
molindone		
mometasone furoate	mometasone furoate	mometasone furoate
moricizine		moricizine
morphine	morphine	morphine
moxalactam		
mupirocin	mupirocin	mupirocin
	mustine	
nabumetone	nabumetone	nabumetone
nadolol	nadolol	nadolol
nafarelin	nafarelin	nafarelin
nafcillin		
naftifine		
nalbuphine	nalbuphine	
nalidixic acid	nalidixic acid	nalidixic acid
naloxone	naloxone	naloxone
naltrexone	naltrexone	
nandrolone	nandrolone	nandrolone
naproxen	naproxen	naproxen
naproxen sodium		
natamycin		
nedocromil sodium	nedocromil sodium	nedocromil
nefazodone		nefazodone
neomycin	neomycin	trodiomycin
neostigmine	neostigmine	neostigmine
netilmicin	netilmicin	netilmicin
niacin		nicotinic acid
nicardipine	nicardipine	nicardipine
niclosamide	niclosamide	
	nicotinamide	nicotinamide
nicotine	nicotine	nicotine
nifedipine	nifedipine	nifedipine
nifurtimox		
nimodipine	nimodipine	nimodipine
nitrazepam	nitrazepam	nitrazepam
nitrofurans		
nitrofurantoin	nitrofurantoin	
nitrofurazone		
nitrogen mustard	nitrogen mustard	
nitroglycerin	nitroglycerine	nitroglycerin
nitrosoureas	nitrosoureas	
nitrous oxide	nitrous oxide	nitrous oxide
nizatidine	nizatidine	nizatidine
norepinephrine	noradrenaline	norepinephrine
norethindrone	norethisterone	norethisterone
norethynodrel		
norfloxacin	norfloxacin	norfloxacin
norgestimate	norgestimate	
norgestrel	levonorgestrel	norgestrel
nortriptyline	nortriptyline	nortriptyline

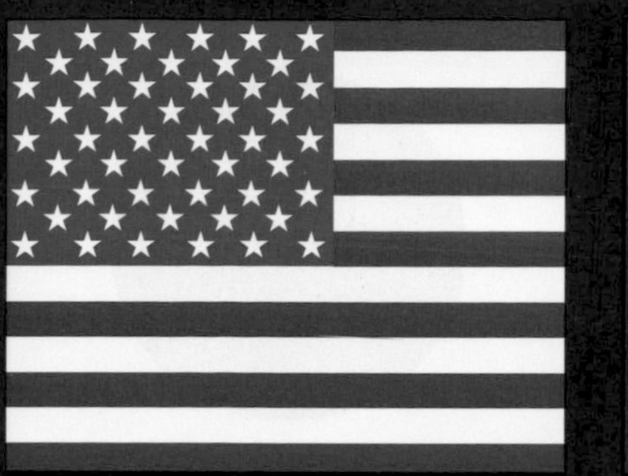	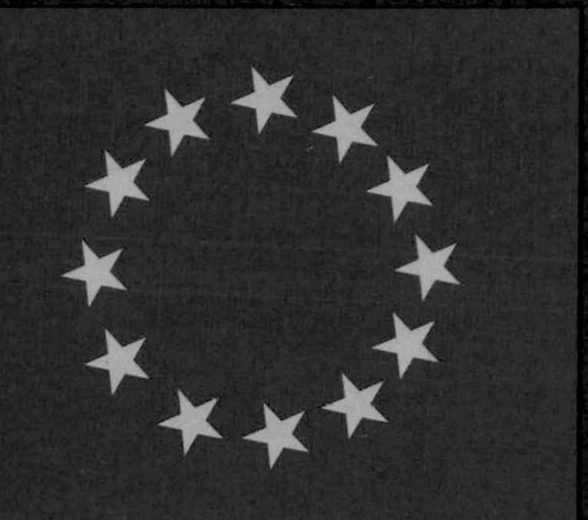	
nystatin	nystatin	nystatin
octreotide	octreotide	octreotide
ofloxacin	ofloxacin	ofloxacin
		olanzapine
olsalazine	olsalazine	olsalazine
omeprazole	omeprazole	omeprazole
	omnopon	
ondansetron	ondansetron	ondansetron
opium	opium	opium
orphenadrine	orphenadrine	
	oubain	
oxacillin		oxacillin
oxamniquine	oxamniquine	
oxandrolone		
oxazepam	oxazepam	oxazepam
oxiconazole		oxiconazole
	oxitropium	oxitropium
	oxitropium bromide	oxitropium bromide
	oxybuprocaine	oxybuprocaine hydrochloride
oxybutynin	oxybutinin	oxybutinin
oxycodone	oxycodone	oxycodone
oxygen	oxygen	oxygen
oxymetholone	oxymetholone	oxymetholone
oxymorphone		
oxytetracycline	oxytetracycline	oxytetracycline
oxytocin	oxytocin	oxytocin
paclitaxel	paclitaxel	
pamidronate disodium	disodium pamidronate	pamidronate disodium
pancuronium	pancuronium	pancuronium
papaverine	papaverine	papaverine
	paraffin	paraffin
paraldehyde	paraldehyde	
paraquat	paraquat	paraquat
parathion	parathion	
parathyroid hormone	parathyroid hormone	parathyroid hormone
paromomycin	paromomycin	paromomycin
paroxetine	paroxetine	paroxetine
pectin		
pemoline	pemoline	pemoline
penbutolol		penbutolol
		penciclovil
penicillamine	penicillamine	penicillamine
penicillin G	benzylpenicillin	benzylpenicillin
penicillin V		
pentaerythritol tetranitrate	pentaerythritol tetranitrate	
pentamidine	pentamidine	pentamidine
pentazocine	pentazocine	pentazocine
pentobarbital	pentobarbitone	pentobarbital sodium
pentostatin	pentostatin	pentostatin
pergolide	pergolide	pergolide
perindopril	perindopril	perindopril
permethrin	permethrin	
perphenazine	perphenazine	perphenazine
phenacemide		
phencyclidine	phecyclidine	
phendimetrazine		

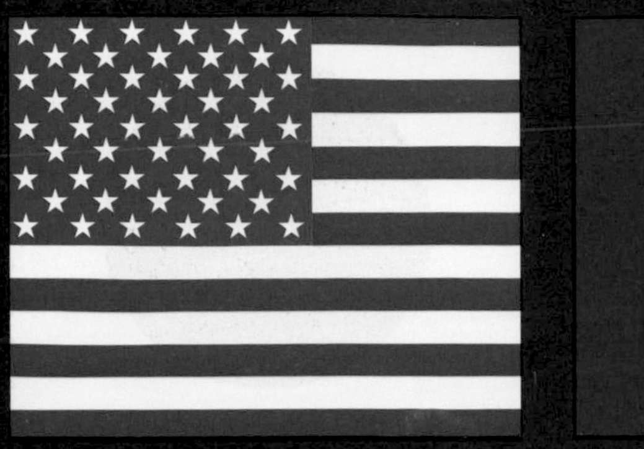
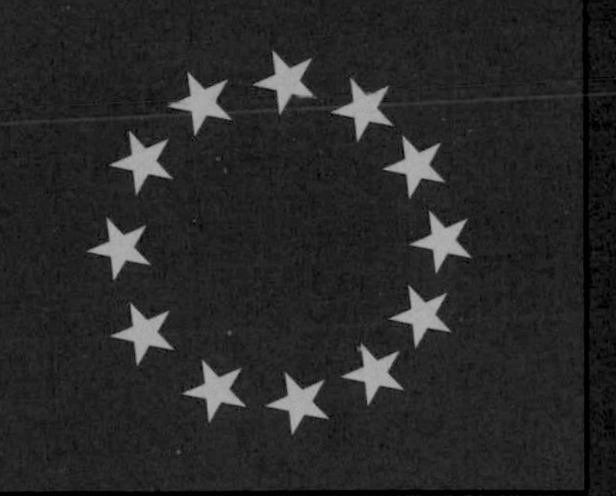

phenelzine	phenelzine	
phenobarbital	phenobarbitone	phenobarbital
	phenothrin	
phenoxybenzamine	phenoxybenzamine	
	phenoxymethylpenicillin	
phentermine	phentermine	
phentolamine	phentolamine	phentolamine
phenylbutazone	phenylbutazone	
phenylephrine	phenylephrine	phenylephrine
phenylpropanolamine	phenylpropanolamine	
phenytoin	phenytoin	phenytoin
physostigmine	physostigmine	
picrotoxin	picrotoxin	
pilocarpine	pilocarpine	pilocarpine
pimozide	pimozide	pimozide
pindolol	pindolol	pindolol
pipecuronium		pipecuronium
piperacillin	piperacillin	piperacillin
	piperazine	
pirenzepine	pirenzepine	pirenzepine
piroxicam	piroxicam	piroxicam
	pivampicillin	
plicamycin	plicamycin	
podophyllum resin	podophyllin	
	polyethylene glycol	
polymyxin B	polymyxin B	polymyxin B
		practerol
potassium iodide		potassium iodide
	potassium permanganate	potassium permanganate
povidone-iodine	povidone-iodine	povidone-iodine
	polyvinyl alcohol	
pralidoxime	pralidoxime	pralidoxime
pravastatin	pravastatin	pravastatin
prazepam		prazepam
praziquantel	praziquantel	praziquantel
prazosin	prazosin	prazosin
prednisolone	prednisolone	prednisolone
prednisone	prednisone	
prilocaine	prilocaine	
primaquine	primaquine	
primidone	primidone	primidone
probenecid	probenecid	probenecid
probucol	probucol	probucol
procainamide	procainamide	procainamide
procaine	procaine	procaine
procarbazine	procarbazine	procarbazine
prochlorperazine	prochlorperazine	prochlorperazine
procyclidine	procyclidine	
progesterone	progesterone	progesterone
	proguanil	
prolactin	prolactin	
promethazine	promethazine	promethazine
	prontosil	
propafenone	propafenone	propafenone
	propamidine isethionate	
propantheline	propantheline	propantheline

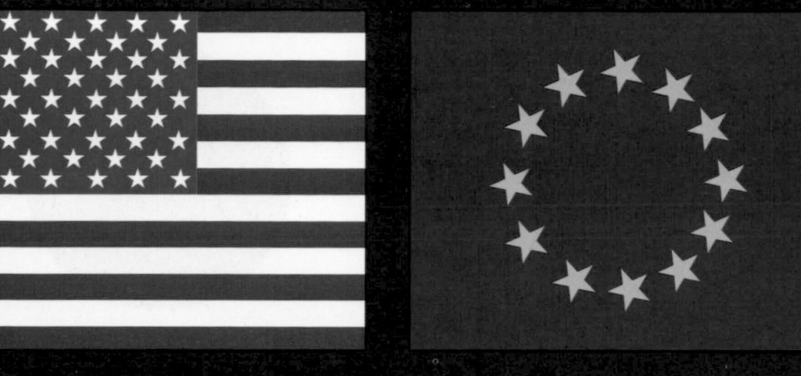

propofol	propofol	propofol
propoxyphene		
propranolol	propranolol	propranolol
propylene glycol		propylene glycol
propylthiouracil	propylthiouracil	propylthiouracil
prostacyclin	prostacyclin	prostacyclin
prostaglandins	prostaglandins	prostaglandins
protriptyline	protriptyline	
	proxymetacaine	
pseudoephedrine	pseudoephedrine	
	psoralens	
pyrantel pamoate	pyrantel pamoate	
pyrazinamide	pyrazinamide	pyrazinamide
pyridostigmine	pyridostigmine	pyridostigmine
pyridoxine	pyridoxine	pyridoxine
pyrimethamine	pyrimethamine	pyrimethamine
	pyronaridine	
quazepam		quazepam
quinacrine	mepacrine	
quinapril	quinapril	quinapril
quinghaosu	artemisinin	
quinidine	quinidine	quinidine
quinine	quinine	quinine
		raloxifene
ramipril	ramipril	ramipril
ranitidine	ranitidine	ranitidine
reserpine	reserpine	reserpine
resorcinol	resorcinol	
ribavirin	tribavirin	
rifabutin	rifabutin	
rifampin	rifampicin	rifampicin
rimantadine		
		risedronate
risperidone	risperidone	risperidone
ritodrine	ritodrine	ritodrine
rocuronium	rocuronium	
rolipram	rolipram	rolipram
	salicylate	
salicylic acid	salicylic acid	salicylic acid
salmeterol	salmeterol	salmeterol
salsalate	salsalate	sasapyrine
saquinavir		
scopolamine	hyoscine	scopolamine
secobarbital	quinalbarbitone	secobarbital
selegiline	selegiline	selegiline
selenium sulfide	selenium sulphide	
	semustine	
senna	senna	senna
serotonin	serotonin	
		sertindole
sertraline	sertraline	sertralin
sevoflurane	sevoflurane	sevoflurane
silver nitrate		silver nitrate
simethicone		
simvastatin	simvastatin	simvastatin
sodium	sodium	

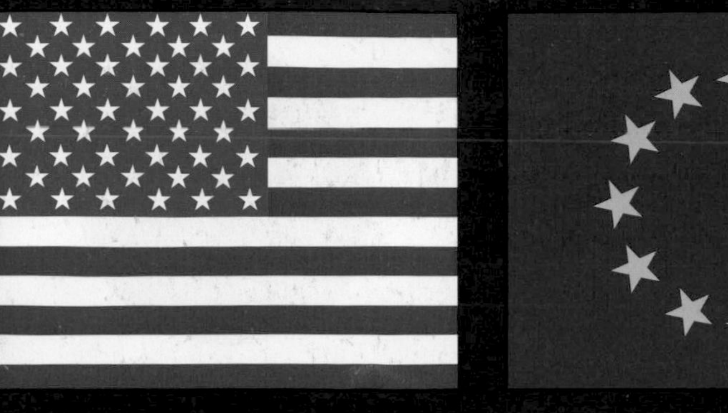

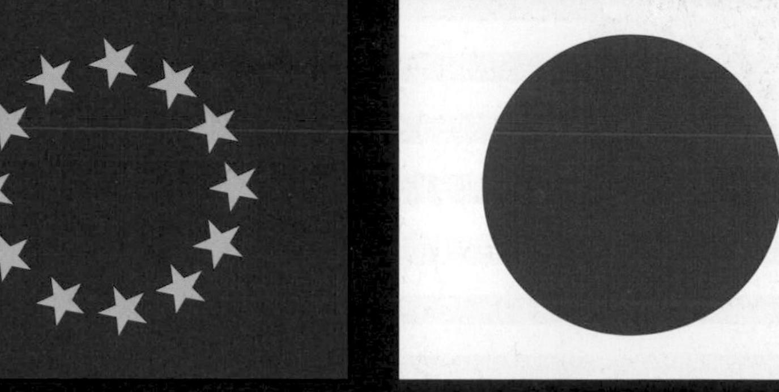

sodium bicarbonate	sodium bicarbonate	sodium bicarbonate
	sodium clodronate	clodronate disodium
sodium fluoride	sodium fluoride	sodium fluoride
	sodium fusidate	sodium fusidate
sodium nitroprusside	nitroprusside	
	sodium picosulfate	sodium picosulfate
sodium stibogluconate	sodium stibogluconate	
sodium tetradecyl sulfate	sodium tetradecyl sulphate	
		sorivudine
sotalol	sotalol	sotalol
spectinomycin	spectinomycin	spectinomycin
spirapril		spirapril
spironolactone	spironolactone	spironolactone
stanozolol	stanozolol	stanozolol
stavudine		
streptokinase	streptokinase	streptokinase
	streptokinase-streptodornase	streptokinase-streptodornase
streptomycin	streptomycin	streptomycin
streptozocin	streptozotocin	
	sterculia	
	strychnine	
succimer		
succinylcholine	suxamethonium	suxamethonium
sucralfate	sucralfate	sucralfate
sufentanil	sufentanyl	
sulbactam		sulbactam
sulconazole	sulconazole	sulconazole
sulfacetamide	sulphacetamide	
sulfadiazine	sulphadiazine	sulfadiazine
sulfadoxine	sulfadoxine	sulfadoxine
sulfamethizole	sulphamethizole	sulfamethizole
sulfamethoxazole	sulphamethoxazole	sulfamethoxazole
	sulphametopyrazine	
	sulphapyridine	
sulfasalazine	sulphasalazine	safazosulfapyridine
sulfinpyrazone	sulphinpyrazone	sulfinpyrazone
sulfisoxazole	sulphisoxazole	sulfisoxazole
sulindac	sulindac	sulindac
sulfur	sulphur	sulfur
	sulpiride	sulpiride
sumatriptan	sumatriptan	sumatriptan
suramin	suramin	
	suxamethonium	suxamethonium chloride
		tacalcitol
tacrine	tacrine	
tacrolimus	tacrolimus	tacrolimus
tamoxifen	tamoxifen	tamoxifen
taxol	taxol	taxol
tazobactam	tazobactam	tazobactam
teicoplanin	teicoplanin	teicoplanin
temazepam	temazepam	temazepam
teniposide		
terazosin	terazosin	terazosin
terbinafine	terbinafine	terbinafine
terbutaline	terbutaline	terbutaline
terconazole		

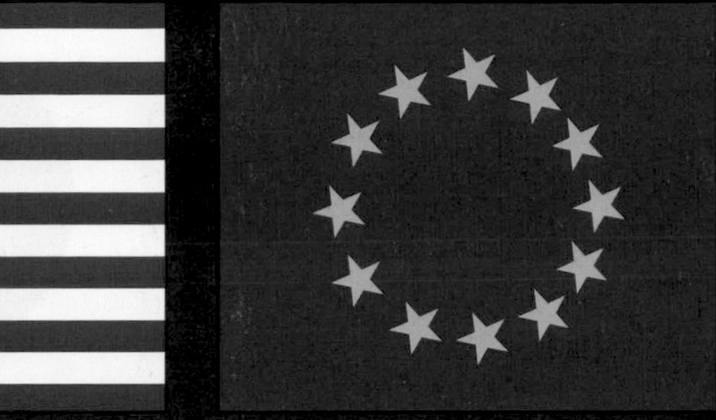

terfenadine	terfenadine	terfenadine
testolactone		
testosterone	testosterone	testosterone
	tetrabenazine	
tetracaine		tetracaine
tetracycline	tetracycline	tetracycline
tetraethylammonium	tetraethylammonium	
tetrahydrocannabinol	tetrahydrocannabinol	
	tetrodotoxin	
thalidomide	thalidomide	
theophylline	theophylline	theophylline
thiabendazole	thiabendazole	
	thiamphenicol	
thiazide	thiazide	
thioguanine	thioguanine	6-thioguanin
thiopental	thiopentone	thiopental
thioridazine	thioridazine	thioridazine
thiotepa	thiotepa	thiotepa
thiothixene		
thrombin	thrombin	thrombin
ticarcillin	ticarcillin	ticarcillin
ticlopidine		ticlopidine
		tiludronate
timolol	timolol	timolol
tinidazole	tinidazole	tinidazole
tioconazole	tioconazole	tioconazole
tissue plasminogen activator	tissue plasminogen activator	tissue plasminogen activator
	titanium dioxide	
tobramycin	tobramycin	tobramycin
tocainide	tocainide	tocainide
tolazamide	tolazamide	tolazamide
tolazoline		tolazoline
tolbutamide	tolbutamide	tolbutamide
tolmetin	tolmetin	tolmetin
tolnaftate		tolnaftate
		topotecan
torsemide		
tramadol	tramadol	
	trandolapril	trandolapril
tranexamic acid	tranexamic acid	tranexamic acid
tranylcypromine	tranylcypromine	
trazodone	trazodone	trazodone
tretinoin	tretinoin	tretinoin
triamcinolone	triamcinolone	triamcinolone
triamcinolone acetonide	triamcinolone acetonide	triamcinolone acetonide
triamcinolone diacetate		triamcinolone diacetate
triamcinolone hexacetonide	triamcinolone hexacetonide	
triamterene	triamterene	triamterene
triazolam		triazolam
trichloroacetic acid	trichloroacetic acid	
	triclosan	
trifluoperazine	trifluoperazine	trifluoperazine malate
trifluorothymidine		
triflupromazine		
trifluridine		
trihexyphenidyl	benzhexol	

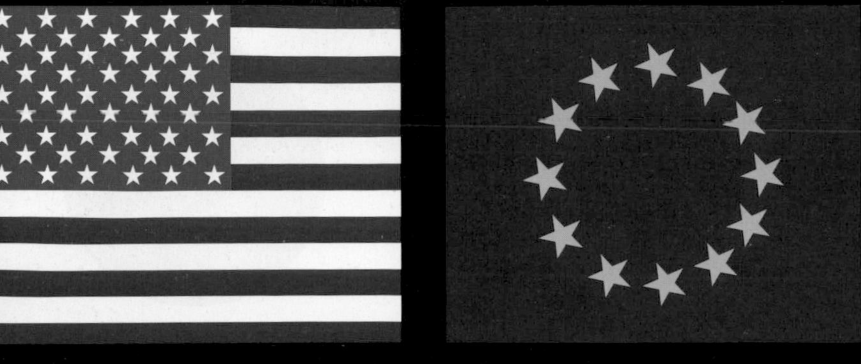

trimeprazine	trimeprazine	
trimethaphan	trimetaphan	trimetaphan
trimethoprim	trimethoprim	trimethoprim
trimetrexate		trimetrexate
tripelennamine		
triprolidine	triprolidine	triprolidine
		troglitazone
tropicamide	tropicamide	tropicamide
	tropisetron	tropisetron
tubocurarine	tubocurarine	tubocurarine
tyramine	tyramine	
urea	urea	urea
urofollitropin	urofollitrophin	
urokinase	urokinase	urokinase
ursodiol		
	valaciclovir	valaciclovir
valproate	valproate	valproate
vancomycin	vancomycin	vancomycin
vasopressin	vasopressin	vasopressin
vecuronium	vecuronium	vecuronium
		velnacrine
venlafaxine	venlafaxine	
verapamil	verapamil	verapamil
	vesamicol	
		vesnarinone
vidarabine		vidarabine
	vigabatrin	vigabatrin
vinblastine	vinblastine	vinblastine
vincristine	vincristine	vincristine
	vindesine	vindesine
vinorelbine		vinorelbine
vinpocetine	vinpocetine	vinpocetine
vitamin B_{12}	vitamin B_{12}	cyanocobalamin
vitamin D	vitamin D	vitamin D
vitamin K	vitamin K	Vitamin K
warfarin	warfarin	warfarin
yohimbine		
zalcitabine	zalcitabine	zalcitabine
zaprinast	zaprinast	zaprinast
zidovudine	zidovudine	zidovudine
zileuton	zileutin	
zinc sulfate	zinc sulphate	zinc sulfate
		ziprasidone
		zofenopril
zolpidem	zolpidem	zolpidem
	zopiclone	zopiclone
	zuclopenthixol	

Index

- Entries in **bold** refer to drugs. Entries underlined refer to diseases, disorders and infections.
- Drugs are listed by the American spellings, unless there is no American equivalent.
- Not all drugs included in the drug index are included in the subject index, only those where significant information is available.
- Readers are advised to refer to specific drugs after consulting the main drug group entries – generalized cross-references have not been inserted, and are assumed.

Index